Acquiring Medical Language

Steven L. Jones, PhD
Houston Baptist University

Andrew Cavanagh, MD
Texas A&M College of Medicine

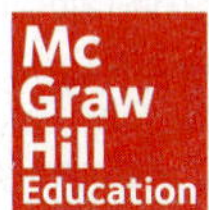

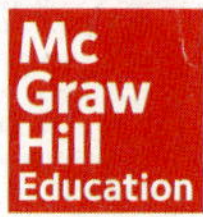

ACQUIRING MEDICAL LANGUAGE

Published by McGraw-Hill Education, 2 Penn Plaza, New York, NY 10121.

Some ancillaries, including electronic and print components, may not be available to customers outside the United States.

This book is printed on acid-free paper.

1 2 3 4 5 6 7 8 9 0 RMN/RMN 1 0 9 8 7 6 5

ISBN 978-0-07-340231-4
MHID 0-07-340231-1

Senior Vice President, Products & Markets: *Kurt L. Strand*
Vice President, General Manager, Products & Markets: *Marty Lange*
Vice President, Content Design & Delivery: *Kimberly Meriwether David*
Managing Director: *Chad Grall*
Brand Manager: *William Mulford*
Director, Product Development: *Rose Koos*
Product Developer: *Jessica Dimitrijevic*
Executive Marketing Manager: *Harper Christopher*
Digital Product Analyst: *Katherine Ward*
Director, Content Design & Delivery: *Linda Avenarius*
Program Manager: *Angela Fitzpatrick*
Content Project Managers: *Pat Frederickson, Sherry Kane, Marianne Musni*
Buyer: *Susan K. Culbertson*
Design: *Lisa King/Srdj Savanovic*
Content Licensing Specialists: *Lori Hancock*
Cover Image: *© mathisworks/Getty Images*
Compositor: *Laserwords Private Limited*
Printer: *R. R. Donnelley*

All credits appearing on page or at the end of the book are considered to be an extension of the copyright page.

Library of Congress Cataloging-in-Publication Data

Jones, Steven L., 1975-, author.
Acquiring medical language/Steven L. Jones, Andrew Cavanagh.
p.; cm.
Includes index.
ISBN 978-0-07-340231-4 (alk. paper)–ISBN 0-07-340231-1 (alk. paper)
I. Cavanagh, Andrew, author. II. Title.
[DNLM: 1. Medicine. 2. Terminology as Topic. W 15]
R123
610.1'4-dc23

2014031508

www.mhhe.com

brief contents

Table of Contents

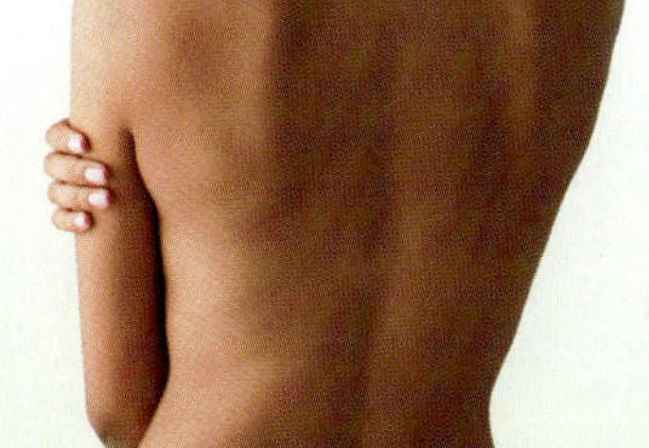

CHAPTER 4 The Musculoskeletal System–Orthopedics 179

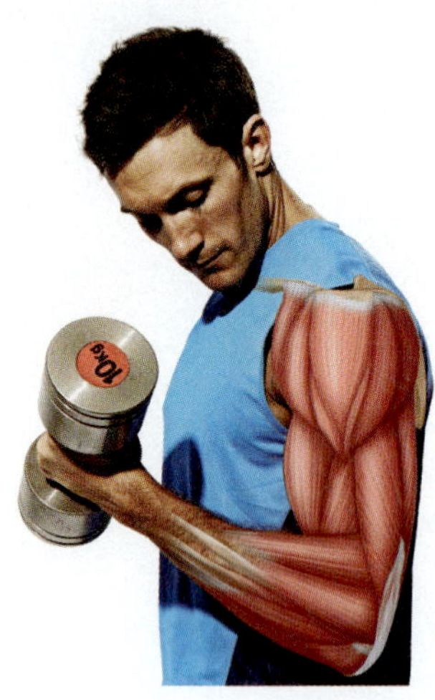

CHAPTER 5 The Nervous System–Neurology and Psychiatry 243

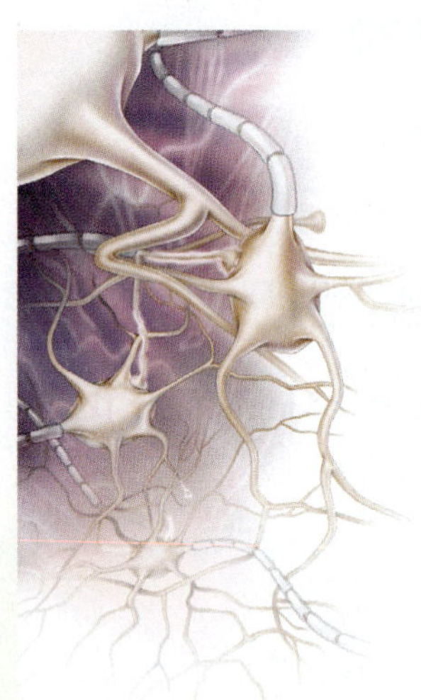

CHAPTER 6 The Sensory System–Ophthalmology and Otolaryngology 310

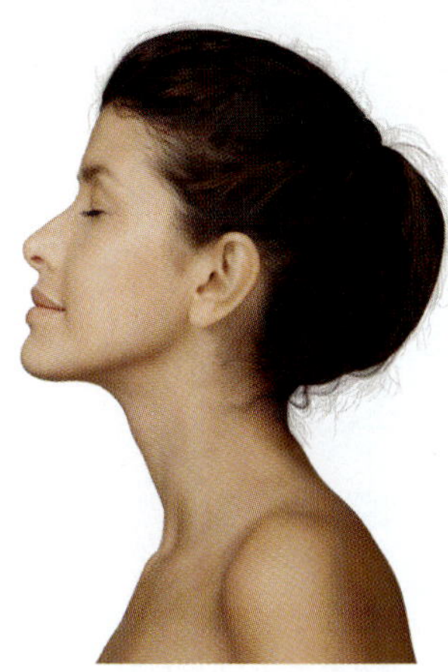

CHAPTER 7 The Endocrine System–Endocrinology 382

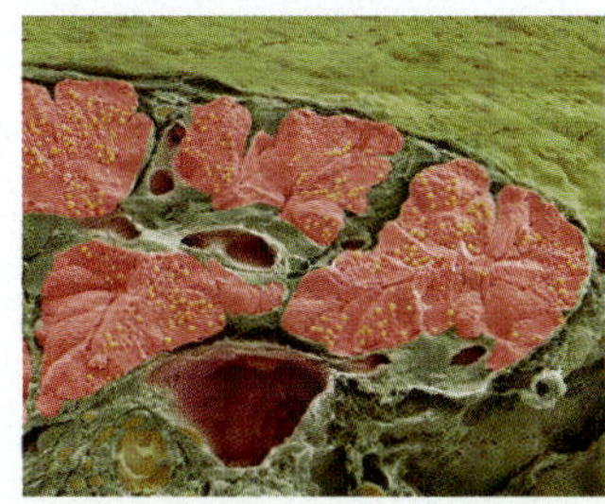

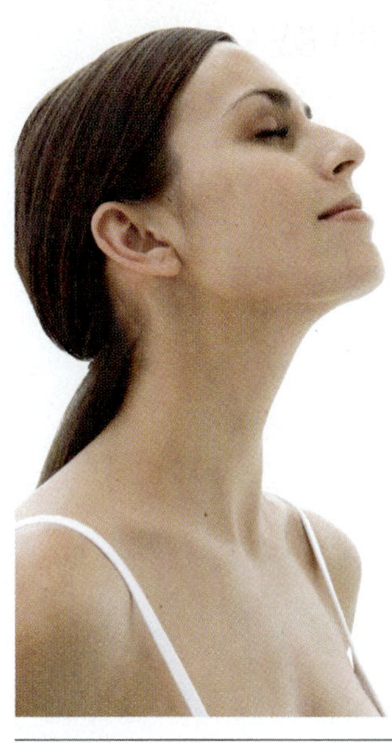

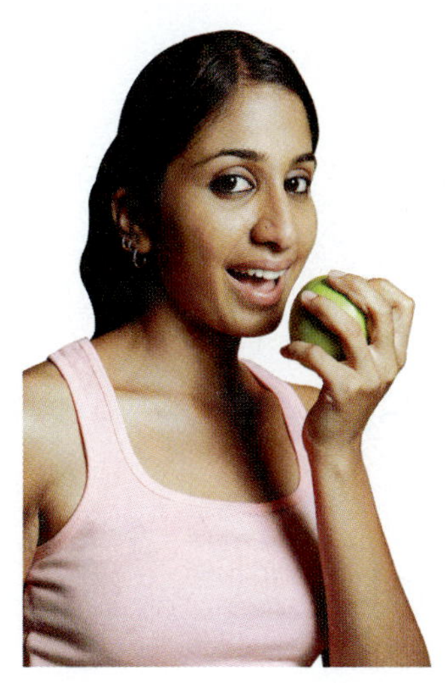

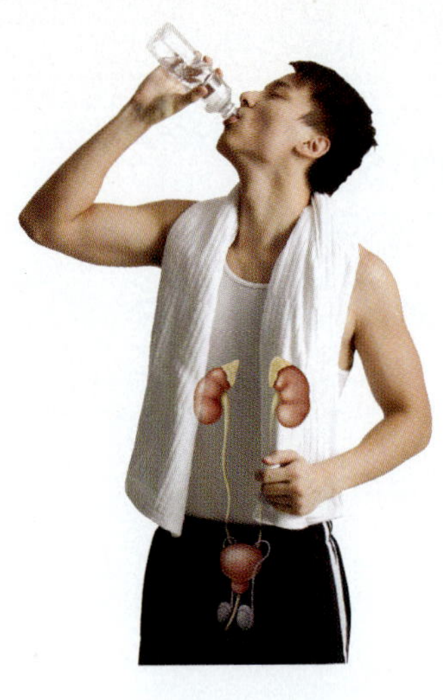

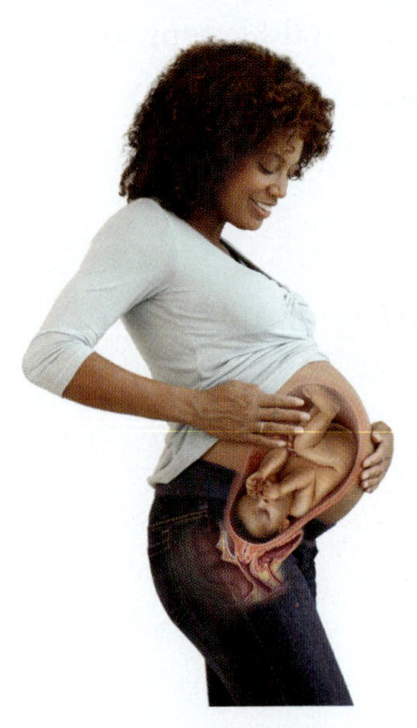

To our wives:

Tamber Jones

and

Ashley Cavanagh.

Your devotion, support, encouragement,
and assistance made this book possible.

about the authors

Steven L. Jones, PhD

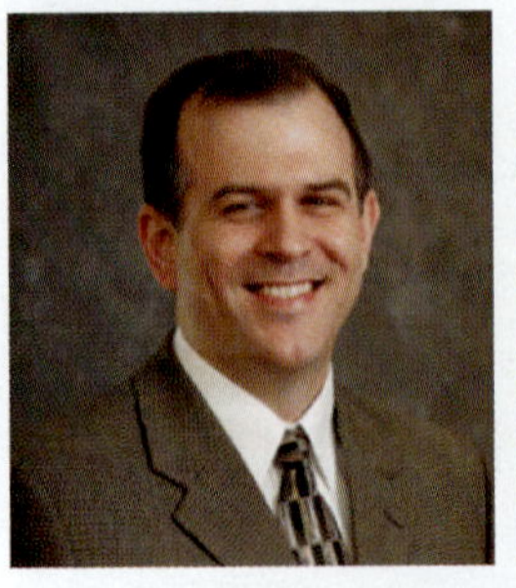

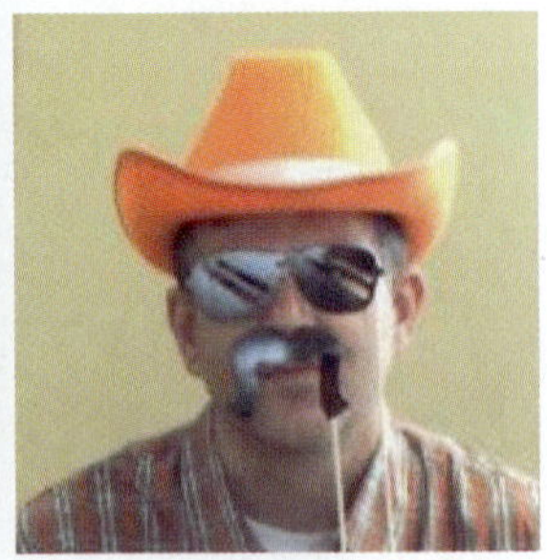

Steve holds a BA in Greek and Latin from Baylor University, an MA in Greek, Latin, and classical studies from Bryn Mawr College, and a PhD in classics from the University of Texas at Austin. Steve has held previous faculty appointments at Trinity University, the University of Texas at Austin, and Baylor University. Currently he is assistant professor of classics at Houston Baptist University in Houston, where he also serves as chair of the Department of Classics and Biblical Languages and as director of the Master of Arts in Biblical Languages Program. He teaches courses on Latin, Greek, Classical Civilization, Early Christianity, and the Classical Roots of Medical Language.

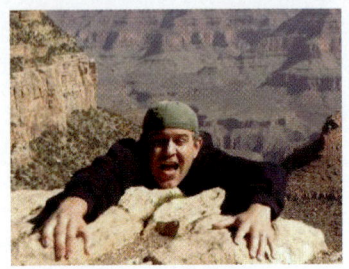

When not breaking down medical words, Steve enjoys spending time with his wife and four daughters, watching baseball, drinking ice-cold Dr Pepper, and showing off his parallel-parking skills.

Andrew Cavanagh, MD

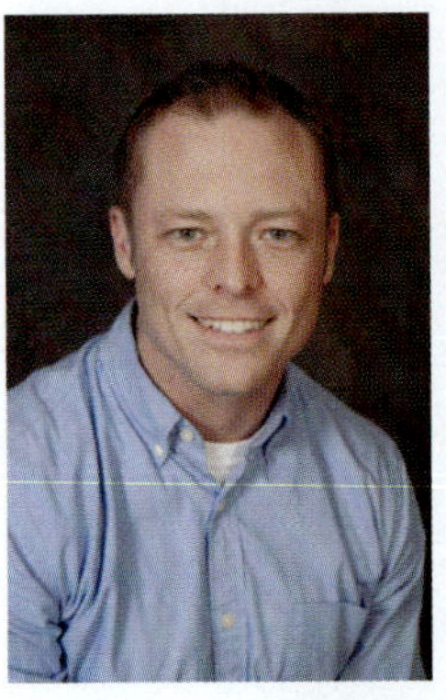

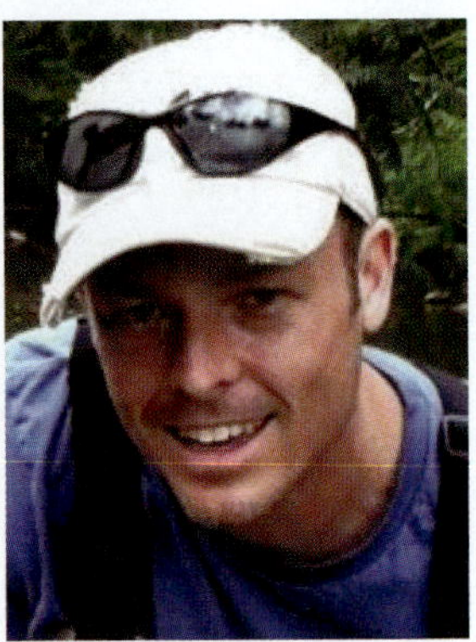

Andy holds a BS in genetics from Texas A&M University and an MD from Texas A&M College of Medicine. After completing his residency at Palmetto Health Children's Hospital, he joined the pediatric practice of the Austin Regional Clinic in Austin. In addition to being board certified in pediatrics, Andy has served as the pediatric specialty chief for Dell Children's Medical Center and on the board of Dell Children's Medical Center Executive Committee. He is currently clinical assistant professor of pediatrics at the Texas A&M College of Medicine.

When not comforting sick children at work or wrestling with his own two kids at home, Andy enjoys mountain biking, travel, Bible study, and trying to make his wife laugh.

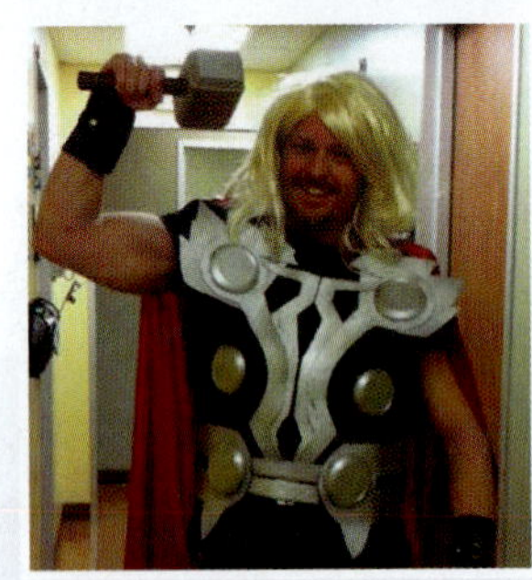

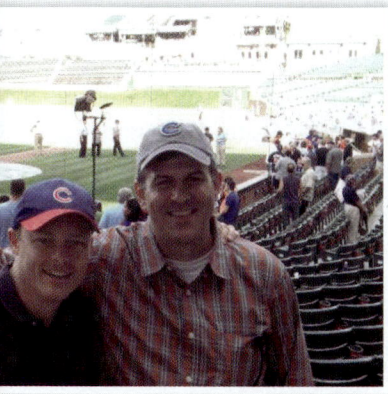

A Note from the Authors on Why They Wrote this Book

This book has its beginning in the friendship that Andy and Steve developed while they both lived in Austin. Andy was beginning his pediatric practice. Steve was completing his doctorate at UT. They had kids the same age and attended the same church. One evening after dinner, while sitting on Andy's back porch, Steve mentioned a new course he had been assigned to teach: Medical Terminology. What started as Steve complaining ended in a game where Andy tried to stump Steve by asking him what various medical words meant. Andy was amazed at how much Steve could figure out just by breaking down words. Steve was astonished to realize that most people–from medical assistants to medical doctors–weren't taught medical language this way. Through this conversation and others like it, Steve and Andy realized three things:

1. Understanding how to break down medical language is an essential skill in the medical field.
2. Having a basic knowledge of the Greek and Latin roots made medical language radically transparent.
3. The current market is lacking a textbook that teaches medical language this way.

This book is their attempt to meet those needs.

How to Use the Book

The Approach

Acquiring Medical Language approaches medical terminology not as words to be memorized but as a language to be learned. If you treat medical terminology as a language and learn how to read terms like sentences, you will be able to communicate clearly as a health care professional and will be a full participant in the culture of medicine. Memorizing definitions is equal to a traveler memorizing a few phrases in another language to help during a brief vacation: It will help a traveler survive for a few days. But if one is going to live in another culture for an extended period of time, learning to speak and understand the language becomes essential.

Acquiring Medical Language teaches students to **break down words into their composite word parts.** Instead of a dictionary full of terms that need to be memorized, a student equipped with groups of roots, prefixes, and suffixes can easily understand a vast amount of medical terminology.

Acquiring Medical Language bridges the gap between the two somewhat disparate fields that make up medical terminology–medicine and second-language acquisition–by providing assistance in language skills to equip health care professionals with the ability to learn and apply a useful skill and not lists of words. It will also equip language professionals with real-world examples that make their knowledge of languages applicable to working in the world of health care.

The process is best illustrated by considering the following word: pneumonoultramicroscopicsilicovolcanoconiosis. Memorizing the definition to words like this would seem like an intimidating task. If you break it into its composite parts, you get:

pneumono / ultra / micro / scopic / silico / volcano / coni / osis
lung extremely small looking sand volcanic dust condition

Through knowledge of roots and word formation, the meaning becomes transparent: "A condition of the lungs caused by extremely small bits of volcanic sand." Instead of having to memorize a long list of even longer words, a student equipped with the knowledge of roots and how to break apart words can tackle–and not be intimidated by–the most complicated sounding medical terms.

Organization and Key Features

Acquiring Medical Language begins with two introductory chapters: Chapter 1, Introduction to Medical Language; and Chapter 2, Introduction to Health Records. Chapters 3 through 13 are dedicated to individual systems of the body and review common roots, words, and abbreviations for each system.

1. **"Card-Based" Approach:** Each chapter opens with a section on word parts for that particular body system. Students are introduced to roots via pages with illustrations of body systems surrounded by "cards" containing the names of body parts, specific word roots related to those parts, a few examples containing the roots, as well as some interesting facts to make the information more memorable. The student is exposed to all relevant information (the root, its meaning, its use) and sees how each root relates to the other roots in the context of the body system, without ever needing to turn the page.

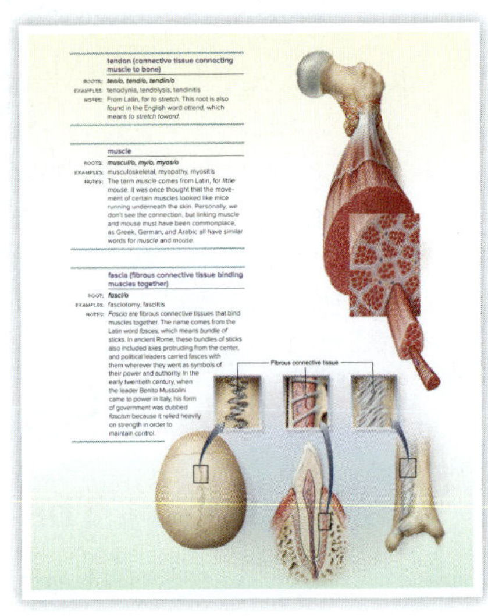

2. **SOAP Note Organization:** After the student is introduced to the important roots for the chapter using "cards," the medical terms relevant to the body system are presented using the SOAP note as an organizational framework. *SOAP* is an acronym used by many health care professionals to help organize the diagnostic process (SOAP is explained more fully in Chapter 2). The terms will be divided under the following headings:

S Subjective: Patient History, Problems, Complaints

O Objective: Observation and Discovery

A Assessment: Diagnosis and Pathology

P Plan: Treatments and Therapies

The SOAP note method is a fundamental way of thinking about the language of health care. By building this approach into the framework of the pedagogy, *Acquiring Medical Language* prepares future health care professionals to speak the language of medicine.

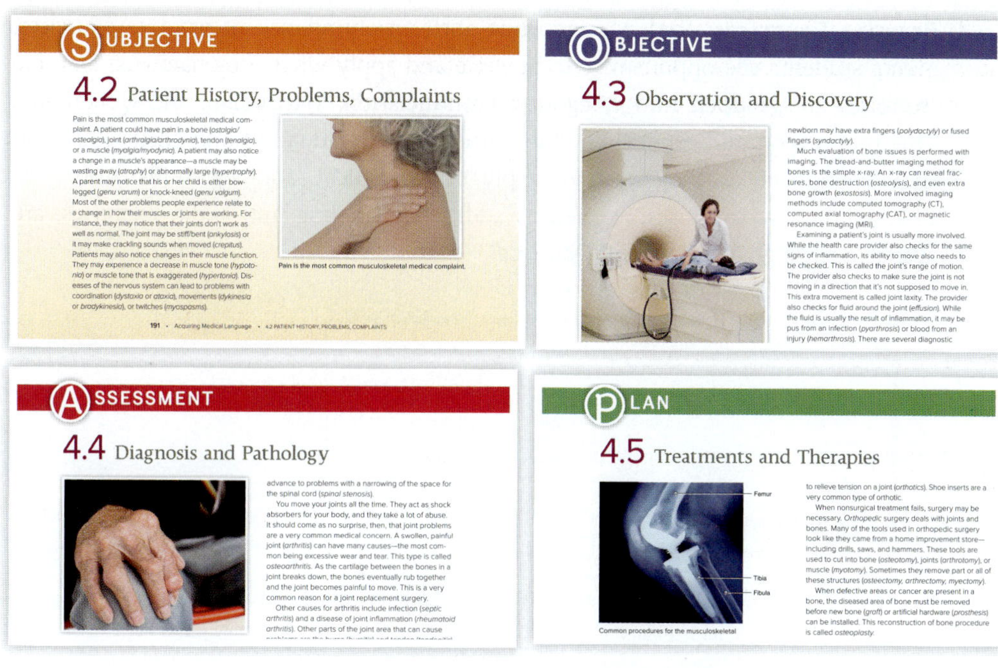

SUBJECTIVE

4.2 Patient History, Problems, Complaints

Pain is the most common musculoskeletal medical complaint. A patient could have pain in a bone (*ostalgia/ostealgia*), joint (*arthralgia/arthrodynia*), tendon (*tenalgia*), or a muscle (*myalgia/myodynia*). A patient may also notice a change in a muscle's appearance—a muscle may be wasting away (*atrophy*) or abnormally large (*hypertrophy*). A parent may notice that his or her child is either bow-legged (*genu varum*) or knock-kneed (*genu valgum*). Most of the other problems people experience relate to a change in how their muscles or joints are working. For instance, they may notice that their joints don't work as well as normal. The joint may be stiff/bent (*ankylosis*) or it may make crackling sounds when moved (*crepitus*). Patients may also notice changes in their muscle function. They may experience a decrease in muscle tone (*hypotonia*) or muscle tone that is exaggerated (*hypertonia*). Diseases of the nervous system can lead to problems with coordination (*dystaxia or ataxia*), movements (*dykinesia* or *bradykinesia*), or twitches (*myospasms*).

Pain is the most common musculoskeletal medical complaint.

191 • Acquiring Medical Language • 4.2 PATIENT HISTORY, PROBLEMS, COMPLAINTS

OBJECTIVE

4.3 Observation and Discovery

newborn may have extra fingers (*polydactyly*) or fused fingers (*syndactyly*).

Much evaluation of bone issues is performed with imaging. The bread-and-butter imaging method for bones is the simple x-ray. An x-ray can reveal fractures, bone destruction (*osteolysis*), and even extra bone growth (*exostosis*). More involved imaging methods include computed tomography (CT), computed axial tomography (CAT), or magnetic resonance imaging (MRI).

Examining a patient's joint is usually more involved. While the health care provider also checks for the same signs of inflammation, its ability to move also needs to be checked. This is called the joint's range of motion. The provider also checks to make sure the joint is not moving in a direction that it's not supposed to move in. This extra movement is called joint laxity. The provider also checks for fluid around the joint (*effusion*). While the fluid is usually the result of inflammation, it may be pus from an infection (*pyarthrosis*) or blood from an injury (*hemarthrosis*). There are several diagnostic

ASSESSMENT

4.4 Diagnosis and Pathology

advance to problems with a narrowing of the space for the spinal cord (*spinal stenosis*).

You move your joints all the time. They act as shock absorbers for your body, and they take a lot of abuse. It should come as no surprise, then, that joint problems are a very common medical concern. A swollen, painful joint (*arthritis*) can have many causes—the most common being excessive wear and tear. This type is called *osteoarthritis*. As the cartilage between the bones in a joint breaks down, the bones eventually rub together and the joint becomes painful to move. This is a very common reason for a joint replacement surgery.

Other causes for arthritis include infection (*septic arthritis*) and a disease of joint inflammation (*rheumatoid arthritis*). Other parts of the joint area that can cause

PLAN

4.5 Treatments and Therapies

Common procedures for the musculoskeletal

to relieve tension on a joint (*orthotics*). Shoe inserts are a very common type of orthotic.

When nonsurgical treatment fails, surgery may be necessary. *Orthopedic* surgery deals with joints and bones. Many of the tools used in orthopedic surgery look like they came from a home improvement store—including drills, saws, and hammers. These tools are used to cut into bone (*osteotomy*), joints (*arthrotomy*), or muscle (*myotomy*). Sometimes they remove part or all of these structures (*osteectomy, arthrectomy, myectomy*).

When defective areas or cancer are present in a bone, the diseased area of bone must be removed before new bone (*graft*) or artificial hardware (*prosthesis*) can be installed. This reconstruction of bone procedure is called *osteoplasty*.

3. **Realistic Medical Histories:** *Acquiring Medical Language* incorporates realistic medical histories in reviewing each chapter's material to expose students to what they can expect in the real world. The student is given an example of an electronic health care record and is asked a series of questions. Though it is not expected that everything in the record will be intelligible to them, the goal is to expose students to the context in which they will see medical terminology. This process will encourage students not to feel intimidated by the prospect of seeing words they are unfamiliar with. We have seen this help students glean information from the chart by using the skills they are acquiring in translating medical terminology.

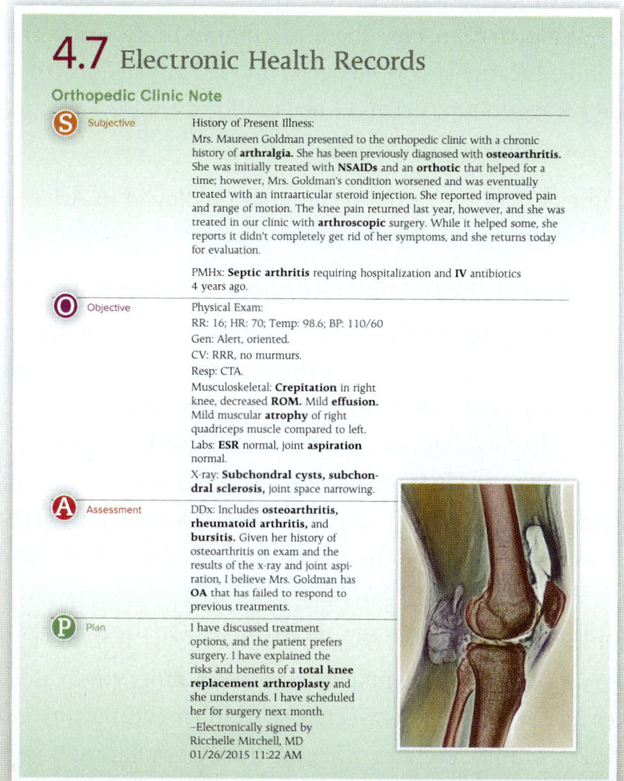

4.7 Electronic Health Records

Orthopedic Clinic Note

S Subjective

History of Present Illness:

Mrs. Maureen Goldman presented to the orthopedic clinic with a chronic history of **arthralgia.** She has been previously diagnosed with **osteoarthritis.** She was initially treated with **NSAIDs** and an **orthotic** that helped for a time; however, Mrs. Goldman's condition worsened and was eventually treated with an intraarticular steroid injection. She reported improved pain and range of motion. The knee pain returned last year, however, and she was treated in our clinic with **arthroscopic** surgery. While it helped some, she reports it didn't completely get rid of her symptoms, and she returns today for evaluation.

PMHx: **Septic arthritis** requiring hospitalization and **IV** antibiotics 4 years ago.

O Objective

Physical Exam:

RR: 16; HR: 70; Temp: 98.6; BP: 110/60

Gen: Alert, oriented.

CV: RRR, no murmurs.

Resp: CTA.

Musculoskeletal: **Crepitation** in right knee, decreased **ROM.** Mild **effusion.** Mild muscular **atrophy** of right quadriceps muscle compared to left.

Labs: **ESR** normal, joint **aspiration** normal.

X-ray: **Subchondral cysts, subchondral sclerosis,** joint space narrowing.

A Assessment

DDx: Includes **osteoarthritis, rheumatoid arthritis,** and **bursitis.** Given her history of osteoarthritis on exam and the results of the x-ray and joint aspiration, I believe Mrs. Goldman has **OA** that has failed to respond to previous treatments.

P Plan

I have discussed treatment options, and the patient prefers surgery. I have explained the risks and benefits of a **total knee replacement arthroplasty** and she understands. I have scheduled her for surgery next month.

–Electronically signed by
Ricchelle Mitchell, MD
01/26/2015 11:22 AM

4. **Practice Exercises:** Each section ends with an abundance of practice exercises, giving students the opportunity to practice and apply what they have just learned. Exercises are grouped into categories: Pronunciation, Translation, and Generation. This progression and repetition allows students to gradually build their skills–and their confidence–as they learn to apply their medical language skills. Abundant Chapter Review exercises, as well as additional labeling and audio exercises, are available through McGraw-Hill Connect®.

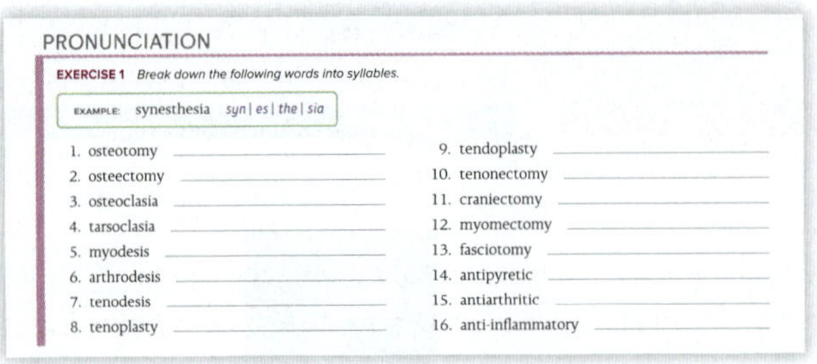
PRONUNCIATION

EXERCISE 1 *Break down the following words into syllables.*

EXAMPLE: synesthesia *syn | es | the | sia*

1. osteotomy
2. osteectomy
3. osteoclasia
4. tarsoclasia
5. myodesis
6. arthrodesis
7. tenodesis
8. tenoplasty
9. tendoplasty
10. tenonectomy
11. craniectomy
12. myomectomy
13. fasciotomy
14. antipyretic
15. antiarthritic
16. anti-inflammatory

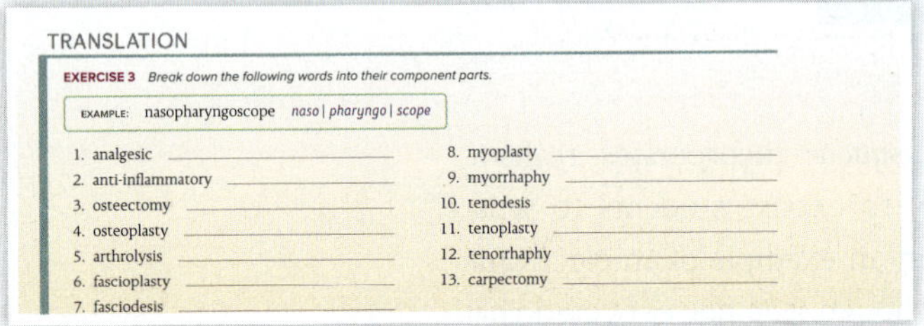
TRANSLATION

EXERCISE 3 *Break down the following words into their component parts.*

EXAMPLE: nasopharyngoscope *naso | pharyngo | scope*

1. analgesic
2. anti-inflammatory
3. osteectomy
4. osteoplasty
5. arthrolysis
6. fascioplasty
7. fasciodesis
8. myoplasty
9. myorrhaphy
10. tenodesis
11. tenoplasty
12. tenorrhaphy
13. carpectomy

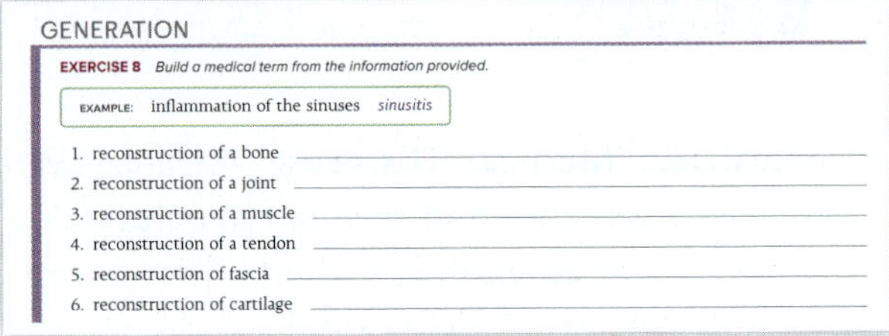
GENERATION

EXERCISE 8 *Build a medical term from the information provided.*

EXAMPLE: inflammation of the sinuses *sinusitis*

1. reconstruction of a bone
2. reconstruction of a joint
3. reconstruction of a muscle
4. reconstruction of a tendon
5. reconstruction of fascia
6. reconstruction of cartilage

To the Instructor

To teach medical terminology as a language, we adopt techniques employed in second-language acquisition. This helps students not just learn the roots, but also adopt a way of thinking and speaking that enables them to communicate using the language of medicine. Cognitive and educational psychologists divide language instruction techniques into two primary categories: contextualized ("real-world" exercises) and decontextualized (academic/grammar exercises).

Using this framework, some of the techniques employed in *Acquiring Medical Language* include:

1. **Contextualized language techniques ("real-world" exercises)**
   a. *Link new language to old language.* Pointing out instances of medical terms or roots in everyday use enables the students to connect new information they are studying with information they already possess.
   b. *Use new language in context.* Using the "card" system to introduce the root words enables students to understand word parts in the context of larger body systems and in relation to other word parts. Using realistic medical charts enables students to see the terms they use not as lists but as parts of a system of communication.
2. **Decontextualized language techniques (academic/grammar exercises)**
   a. *Use repetition.* The students are exposed to roots, prefixes, and suffixes multiple times and in multiple ways. Roots are changed by the addition of prefixes or suffixes. Familiar prefixes and suffixes are applied to new roots. This way, the word components are continuously reinforced.

b. *Use translation.* Students are asked to provide literal definitions of medical terms, which provides practice in breaking down words into their component parts and determining their meaning.

c. *Use generation.* Students are asked to produce medical terms based on the literal definition provided. Though this is only an academic exercise, such practice reinforces material learned by reversing the cognitive process of translation.

d. *Challenge.* Students will be exposed to a handful of longer-than-average terms and asked to break them down into component parts and translate them. A key part of teaching any language is helping students feel comfortable with–not intimidated by–new material. One method is by periodically challenging them to tackle situations that may at first appear overwhelming.

In addition to providing innovative approaches to learning medical terminology, McGraw-Hill Education knows how much effort it takes to prepare for a new course. Through focus groups, symposia, reviews, and conversations with instructors like you, we have gathered information about the materials you need to facilitate successful courses. We are committed to providing you with high-quality, accurate instructor support.

Digital Resources

Knowing the importance of flexibility and digital learning, McGraw-Hill Education has created multiple assets to enhance the learning experience no matter what the class format: traditional, online, or hybrid. This product is designed with digital solutions to help instructors and students be successful.

A one-stop spot to present, deliver, and assess digital assets available from McGraw-Hill Education: McGraw-Hill Connect® Medical Terminology

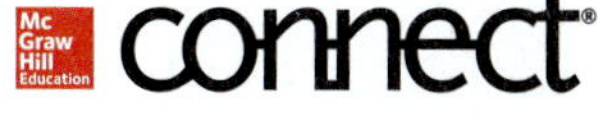

McGraw-Hill Connect Medical Terminology provides online presentation, assignment, and assessment solutions. It connects your students with the tools and resources they'll need to achieve success. With Connect you can deliver assignments, quizzes, and tests online. A robust set of questions and activities–including all of the end-of-section and end-of-chapter questions, additional labeling exercises focused on anatomy and physiology, audio exercises, and interactives–are presented and aligned with the text's learning outcomes. As an instructor, you can edit existing questions and author entirely new problems. Connect enables you to track individual student performance–by question, by assignment, or in relation to the class overall–with detailed grade reports. You can integrate grade reports easily with Learning Management Systems (LMSs) such as Blackboard, Desire2Learn, or eCollege–and much more. Connect also provides students with 24/7 online access to an eBook. This media-rich version of the textbook is available through the McGraw-Hill Connect platform and allows seamless integration of text, media, and assessments. To learn more, visit **connect.mheducation.com**.

A single sign-on with Connect and your Blackboard course—McGraw-Hill Education and Blackboard—for a premium user experience

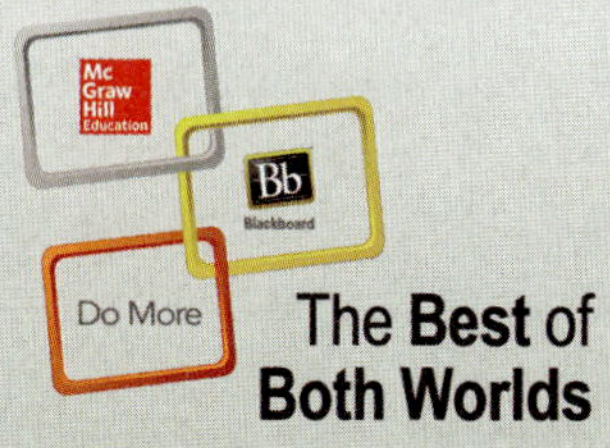

Blackboard, the web-based course management system, has partnered with McGraw-Hill Education to better allow students and faculty to use online materials and activities to complement face-to-face teaching. Blackboard features exciting social learning and teaching tools that foster active learning opportunities for students. You'll transform your closed-door classroom into communities where students remain connected to their educational experience 24 hours a day. This partnership allows you and your students access to McGraw-Hill Connect and Create right from within your Blackboard course–all with a single sign-on. Not only do you get single sign-on with Connect and Create, but you also get deep integration of McGraw-Hill Education content and content engines right in Blackboard. Whether you're choosing a book for your course or building Connect assignments, all the tools you need are right where you want them–inside Blackboard. Gradebooks are now seamless. When a student completes an integrated Connect assignment, the grade for that assignment automatically (and instantly) feeds into your Blackboard grade center. McGraw-Hill Education and Blackboard can now offer you easy access to industry-leading technology and content, whether your campus hosts it or we do. Be sure to ask your local McGraw-Hill Education representative for details.

Still want a single sign-on solutions but using another learning management system?

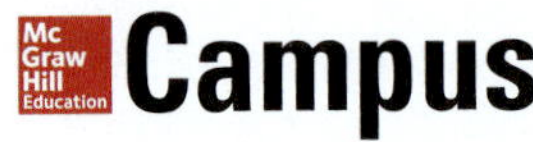

See how **McGraw-Hill Campus** makes the grade by offering universal sign-on, automatic registration, gradebook synchronization, and open access to a multitude of learning resources–all in one place. MH Campus supports Active Directory, Angel, Blackboard, Canvas, Desire2Learn, eCollege, IMS, LDAP, Moodle, Moodlerooms, Sakai, Shibboleth, WebCT, BrainHoney, Campus Cruiser, and Jenzibar eRacer. Additionally, MH Campus can be easily connected with other authentication authorities and LMSs. Visit **http://mhcampus.mhhe.com/** to learn more.

At-a-glance analysis on your class's progress: Connect Insight

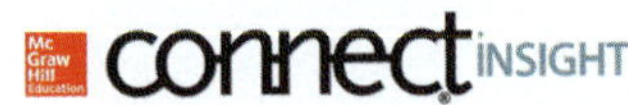

Connect Insight is the first and only analytics tool of its kind, which highlights a series of visual data displays–each framed by an intuitive question–to provide at-a-glance information regarding how your class is doing. As an instructor or administrator, you receive an instant, at-a-glance view of student performance on five key insights. It puts real-time analytics in your hands so you can take action early and keep struggling students from falling behind. It also allows you to be empowered with a more valuable, transparent, and productive connection between you and your students. Available on demand wherever and whenever it's needed, Connect Insight travels from office to classroom!

Create a textbook organized the way you teach: McGraw-Hill Education Create

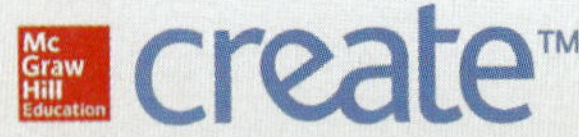

With **Create,** you can easily rearrange chapters, combine material from other content sources, and quickly upload content you have written, such as your course syllabus or teaching notes. Find the content you need in Create by searching through thousands of leading McGraw-Hill Education textbooks. Arrange your book to fit your teaching style. Create even allows you to personalize your book's appearance by selecting the cover and adding your name, school, and course information. Order a Create book and you'll receive a complimentary print review copy in 3 to 5 business days or a complimentary electronic review copy (eComp) via e-mail in minutes. Go to **www.mcgrawhillcreate.com** today and register to experience how Create empowers you to teach your students your way.

Record and distribute your lectures for multiple viewing: My Lectures—Tegrity

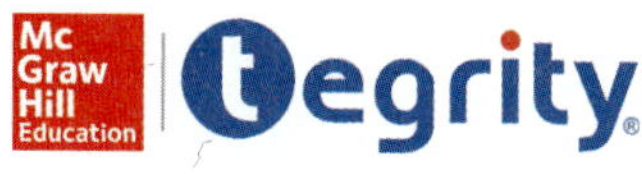

McGraw-Hill Tegrity records and distributes your class lecture with just a click of a button. Students can view it anytime and anywhere via computer, iPod, or mobile device. It indexes as it records your PowerPoint presentations and anything shown on your computer, so students can use keywords to find exactly what they want to study. Tegrity is available as an integrated feature of **McGraw-Hill Connect Medical Terminology** and as a stand-alone product.

Learning at the speed of you: the LearnSmart Advantage Suite

New from McGraw-Hill Education, **LearnSmart Advantage** is a series of adaptive learning products fueled by LearnSmart, the most widely used and intelligent adaptive learning resource proven to improve learning since 2009. Developed to deliver demonstrable results in boosting grades, increasing course retention, and strengthening memory recall, the LearnSmart Advantage series spans the entire learning process from course preparation through final exams. LearnSmart Advantage also provides the first and only adaptive reading experience in SmartBook. Distinguishing what students know from what they don't, and honing in on concepts they are most likely to forget, each product in the series helps students study smarter and retain more knowledge. A smarter learning experience for students coupled with valuable reporting tools for instructors, and available in hundreds of course areas, LearnSmart Advantage is advancing learning like no other products in higher education today. Go to **www.LearnSmartAdvantage.com** for more information.

LearnSmart is one of the most effective and successful adaptive learning resources available on the market today and is now available for *Acquiring Medical Terminology*. More than 2 million students have answered over 1.5 billion questions in LearnSmart since 2009, making it the most widely used and intelligent adaptive study tool that's proven to strengthen memory recall, keep students in class, and boost grades. Studies show that students using LearnSmart are 13 percent more likely to pass their classes and are 35 percent less likely to drop out. This revolutionary learning resource is available only from McGraw-Hill Education. See the power of LearnSmart for yourself by trying it today at **http://learnsmartadvantage.com/trial**.

SmartBook is the first and only adaptive reading experience available today. SmartBook personalizes content for each student in a continuously adapting reading experience. Reading is no longer a passive and linear experience, but an engaging and dynamic one where students are more likely to master and retain important concepts, coming to class better prepared. Valuable reports provide instructors insight as to how students are progressing through textbook content, and are useful for shaping in-class time or assessment. As a result of the adaptive reading experience found in SmartBook, students are more likely to retain knowledge, stay in class, and get better grades. This revolutionary technology is available only from McGraw-Hill Education and for hundreds of courses–including *Acquiring Medical Terminology*–as part of the LearnSmart Advantage series.

Best-in-class digital support

Based on feedback from our users, McGraw-Hill Education has developed Digital Success Programs that will provide you and your students the help you need, when you need it.

- Training for Instructors: Get ready to drive classroom results with our **Digital Success Team**–ready to provide in-person, remote, or on-demand training as needed.

- Peer Support and Training: No one understands your needs like your peers. Get easy access to knowledgeable digital users by joining our **Connect Community,** or speak directly with one of our **Digital Faculty Consultants,** who are instructors using McGraw-Hill Education digital products.
- Online Training Tools: Get immediate anytime, anywhere access to modular tutorials on key features through our **Connect Success Academy.**

Get started today. Learn more about McGraw-Hill Education's Digital Success Programs by contacting your local sales representative or visiting **http://connect.customer.mheducation.com/start.**

Need help? Contact the McGraw-Hill Education Customer Experience Group (CXG)

Visit the CXG website at **www.mhhe.com/support**. Browse our FAQs (frequently asked questions) and product documentation and/or contact a CXG representative.

Additional Instructor Resources

- **Instructor's Manual** with course overview, lesson plans, answers for end-of-section exercises, sample syllabi, and more.
- **PowerPoint Presentations** for each chapter, containing teaching notes correlated to learning outcomes. Each presentation seeks to reinforce key concepts and provide an additional visual aid for students.
- **Test Bank** and answer key for use in class assessment. The comprehensive test bank includes a variety of question types, with each question linked directly to a learning outcome from the text. Questions are also tagged with relevant topic, Bloom's Taxonomy level, and difficulty level. The test bank is available in Connect, and Word and EZ Test versions are also available.

A Note from the Authors: To the Student

The purpose of this program is to equip you with foundational skills as you prepare for a career in health and medicine. As you enter the culture of medicine, you will need to speak the language to understand what is going on around you and to be understood by your colleagues and patients. Though learning medical language can seem a daunting task, it is our hope that this program reduces some of the anxiety that accompanies learning any new language. We hope this program shows you how clear the language of medicine is to understand as you begin to master some key concepts. As you get started, here are some helpful words of advice:

1. *Don't panic.* Immersing yourself in any new language can be intimidating. On occasion you will probably feel overwhelmed, like you are being bombarded with information you don't understand and don't know how to make sense of. Start by trying not to panic. Things always look intimidating when you begin. The water is always coldest when you first jump in. You will get used to it. Be patient. Follow the steps.

2. *Eat the elephant.* Do you know how to eat an elephant? One bite at a time. One of the easiest ways to keep from panicking is to break down things into easily digestible chunks. Don't focus on the total amount of information you have to learn; rather, focus on the bite in front of you.
3. *Practice makes permanent.* The easiest way to master medical language is to practice. You readily absorb what you are repeatedly exposed to. So practice. Repeat. Do it again. The more you do it, the more you will be able to do it, and the more you will enjoy doing it.
4. *Build bridges.* Medical language is everywhere: on TV shows, in the news, in your own life. Look for it. See if you can figure out the meaning of words you hear. Build connections between what you are learning and the world you live in. See how often you encounter these words. The more you practice it, the more it will be burned into your memory.

In addition to providing innovative approaches to learning medical terminology, McGraw-Hill Education wants to provide the materials you need in order to be successful. We are committed to providing you with high-quality, accurate resources.

Connect: Get connected and be successful!

McGraw-Hill Connect is an easy-to-use learning tool that enables your instructor to create and deliver assignments online and automatically collect the results from you. Connect is also a great tool to complete practice assignments to help you study, prepare for exams, and track your performance. You'll get instant feedback on how you're doing during and after the assignment is completed.

Your instructor will give you a web address, which you'll use to register, access your course section, and view your assignments. Setting up your Connect account is simple and takes only a few minutes. This same account can also be used to access other course assignments if you have other instructors who are using Connect.

LearnSmart: A proven tool to improve your grades!

Everyone learns differently, but when it comes to school, we all have similar goals: to get better grades and retain more knowledge. That's why McGraw-Hill Education created the LearnSmart Advantage suite of products–the most widely used adaptive education tools available today.

LearnSmart Advantage was designed to help students like you make the most effective use of your study time and achieve academic success. The suite of adaptive learning products, including LearnSmart and SmartBook, helps you get a baseline understanding of what you know–and what you don't–and then builds a personalized plan for success.

Student support

Need help? Contact the McGraw-Hill Education Customer Experience Group (CXG). Visit the CXG website at **www.mhhe.com/support**. Browse our FAQs (frequently asked questions) and product documentation and/or contact a CXG representative.

Acknowledgments

Suggestions have been received from faculty and students throughout the country. This is vital feedback that is relied on for product development, especially in a first edition. Each person who has offered comments and suggestions has our thanks. The efforts of many people are needed to develop and improve a product. Among these people are the reviewers and consultants who point out areas of concern, cite areas of strength, and make recommendations for change. In this regard, the following instructors provided feedback that was enormously helpful in preparing the book and related products.

Survey Respondents

Many instructors participated in surveys to help guide the early development of the product.

Kim Bell, RHIA
Edgecombe Community College

Dorisann Halvorsen Brandt, MSPT
Greenville Technical College

Christine Chiappini-Williamson, PhD
Stark State College

Pamela Claybaker
Nashville State Community College

Kari Johnson Cook, MSRS, RT (R)
Northwestern State University

Ellen Stoehr Gallavan, RN, BSN, MA
Lansing Community College

Diana Gardner, MBA-HM, CPC, CMPE
Florence-Darlington Technical College

Jackie Gordon, CMA, NCPT, BS
South Suburban College

Susan Harrison, RN
William Rainey Harper College

Lisa Nowak
Waukesha County Technical College

Nancy Owens, RN, DNP
Somerset Community College

Susan Reading-Martin, MS, RN, CS, FNP, ARNP-BC
Western Nebraska Community College

Julie Schumacher, EdD, RD, LDN
Heartland Community College

Valentina Spencer Holder, RHIA, MEd
Pitt Community College

Susan Sykes Berry, RN, BSN, MLS, MA
University of Missouri-Kansas City

Manuscript Reviewers

Multiple instructors reviewed the manuscript while it was in development, providing valuable feedback that directly impacted the product.

Carole Berube, MA, MSN, BSN, RN
Bristol Community College

Cynthia Boles, CMA, MAN, MSHA
Bradford School-Pittsburgh

Mary Ellen Camier, CFS, MS, PhD
University of Maine

Amanda Campbell, MAT
Dorsey Business School

Steven Carlo, AAS, EMT-I, CI/C, BS
Erie Community College-North Campus

Christine Christensen, CCA
Williston State College

Janie Corbitt, RN, MLS
Central Georgia Technical College

Kelly Coreas, RRT, RRT-NPS, BSRT, MSHS
Mt. San Antonio College

Gerard Cronin, CCA, CCS-P, DC, BS
Salem Community College

Colleen Croxall, BA, MSHA, PhD
Eastern Michigan University

Heather Drake, ADN, BSN
Southern West Virginia Community and Technical College

Sally Erdel, BSN, CNE, MS, RN
Bethel College

Connie Erdmann, MS, CT (ASCP)
Utah Valley University

Robert E. Fanger, BS, MSEd
Del Mar College

Savanna Garrity, MPA
Madisonville Community College

Le'Nita Gilliam, BA, CET, CMA, CPT
Lansdale School of Business

Mandi N. Haynes, BSISM, RT (R), ARRT
South Arkansas Community College

Dolly R. Horton, CMA, MEd
AB Tech Community College

Judy Hurtt, MEd
East Central Community College

Cecelia Jacob, MA, MS
Southwest Tennessee Community College

Mark Jaffe, MHA, DPM
Nova Southeastern University

Susan Jaros, RN, MSN, CNP
Owens Community College

Patti Kalvelage, MS, OTR/L
Governors State University

Judith Karls, RN, BSN, MSEd
Madison Area Technical College

Barbara Klomp, BA, RT (R)
Macomb Community College

Jennifer Lame, RHIT, MPH
Southwest Wisconsin Technical College

Joseph K. LeJeune, CPFT, RRT, MS
University of Arkansas Community College at Hope

Cynthia Lowes, ADN, BSN
Southern West Virginia Community and Technical College

Wanda MacLeod, AHI, CMAA
Ross Medical Education Center

Michelle Maguire McDaniel, HCC, BA, CMA, LPN
Ivy Tech Community College

Amie L. Mayhall, MBA, CCA
Olney Central College

Wilsetta McClain, CPT, RMA, NCICS, PhD
Baker College of Auburn Hills

Charlotte Susie Myers, MA
University of Iowa

Alice Noblin, CCS, PBT, PHN
University of Central Florida

Martha Olson, BSN, MS, RN
Iowa Lakes Community College

Tina Paduhovich, BA
Yorktowne Business Institute

Sally Pestana, BS, MT/PBT
Kapiolani Community College

Tammie Petersen, RNC-OB, BSN
Austin Community College

Stephen Picca, MD
Mandl School, the College of Allied Health

Rose M. Powell, PhD, RN
Stephen F. Austin State University

Adrienne Reaves, RMA
Westwood College

LuAnn Reicks, BC, BS, BSN, MSN, RN
Iowa Central Community College

Lisa Ritchie, EdD, RD, LD
Harding University

Lorinda G. Sipe, MS, RD
Front Range Community College

Angela Stahler, AAS, BS, RMA
Lincoln Technical Institute

Charlene Thiessen, MEd, CMT
Gateway Community College

Judy Truempler, RHIT
Idaho State University

Helen Weeks, MA, RMA
Henry Ford Community College

Kari Williams, BS, DC
Front Range Community College

Lori Warren Woodard, CCP, CPC, MA, RN, CPC-I, CLNC
Spencerian College

Technical Editing/Accuracy Panel

A panel of instructors completed a technical edit and review of the content in the book page proofs to verify its accuracy.

Denise Dedeaux, MBA
Fayetteville Technical Community College

Suzee Gay, LPN
Pinnacle Career Institute

Lori Hogue, CMA, RMA, CPT, LPT, LME
Mohave Community College

Sheila Newberry, PhD, RHIT
St. Petersburg College

Brian Spence, BSRS, RT(R)
Tarrant County College

Barbara Westrick, AAS, CMA (AAMA), CPC
Ross Medical Education Center

Digital Tool Development

Special thanks to the instructors who helped with the development of Connect, LearnSmart, and SmartBook.

Jim Hutchins, PhD
Weber State University

Carrie Mack, AS, CMA
Branford Hall Career Institute

Brian Spence, BSRS, RT(R),
Tarrant County College

Acknowledgments from the Authors

We would like to thank the following individuals who helped develop, critique, and shape our textbook, our digital materials, and our other ancillaries. We are grateful for the efforts of our team at McGraw-Hill Education who made all of this come together. We would especially like to thank Chad Grall, director of health professions; William Mulford, brand manager; Jessica Dimitrijevic, product developer; Harper Christopher, executive marketing manager; Marianne Musni, Pat Frederickson, and Sherry Kane, content project managers; Srdjan Savanovic, senior designer; Susan Culbertson, buyer; Katherine Ward, digital product analyst; and Lori Hancock, content licensing specialist.

Acknowledgments from Steven L. Jones

Above all, I am grateful for the love and support of my family: my wife, Tamber, and our four daughters, Bethany, Rachel, Hannah, and Madelyn. I am also grateful for the support of the colleagues and friends at the universities I have taught at while completing this project. At the University of Texas, I would like to thank Karl Galinsky, my academic mentor; Lesley Dean-Jones, who first introduced me to medical terminology pedagogy; and Stephen White, who first gave me the opportunity to teach Medical Terminology. At Baylor University, I would like to thank Alden Smith for encouraging me to pursue this unusual academic project. At Houston Baptist University, I am grateful for the support of Robert Sloan, president; Christopher Hammons, dean of the School of Humanities; Jeffrey Green, dean of the School of Christian Thought; and the encouragement of my colleagues Micah Mattix, Evan J. Getz, Timothy A. Brookins, and Michael Bordelon.

Acknowledgments from Andrew Cavanagh

I am most thankful for the loving support of my wife, Ashley, and children, Katie and Nathaniel. I owe a great debt of gratitude to my mother, Katherine Cavanagh, who worked tirelessly to provide for me as I grew up and passed on to me her admirable work ethic. I would also like to thank John Blevins for fostering my love of medicine and pediatrics and for being a great role model. I would like to thank Caughman Taylor and the entire residency training program at Palmetto Health Richland, University of South Carolina, for their amazing teaching and dedication to the lives of the residents. I would like to thank Norman Chenven and Walter Kuhl of Austin Regional Clinic for giving me the opportunity to practice medicine in a great city, and for allowing me to take on the rewarding endeavor of writing.

Introduction to Medical Language

1

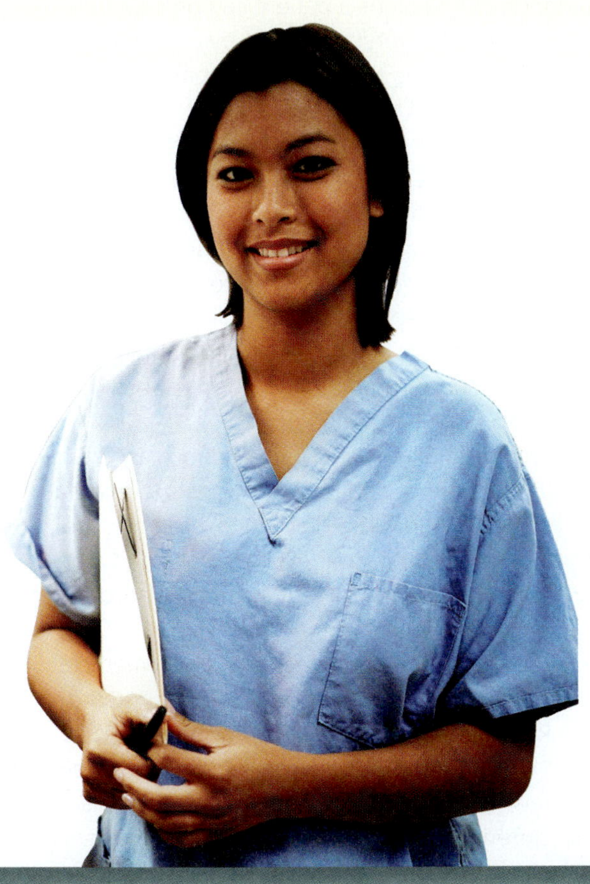

learning outcomes

Upon completion of this chapter, you will be able to:

1.1 Summarize the purpose of **medical language.**

1.2 Summarize the origins of **medical language.**

1.3 Summarize the principles of **medical language.**

1.4 Summarize how to pronounce terms associated with **medical language.**

1.5 Identify the parts used to build **medical language.**

1.6 Summarize how to put together **medical terms.**

1.7 Describe how **medical terms** are translated.

Introduction

You've probably had conversations with people who like to use big words. Maybe you've responded with a blank expression and a sarcastic phrase—something like, "Say it in English, please!" This happens all the time in health care practices.

When a patient comes in for treatment, he or she is often bombarded with unfamiliar words. The patient leaves bewildered, wondering what the health care professional just said. Sometimes patients do get up the courage to ask what it all means and health care professionals explain in simpler terms. And patients wonder, "Well, why couldn't you have just said that in the first place? Why did you have to use all those big words?"

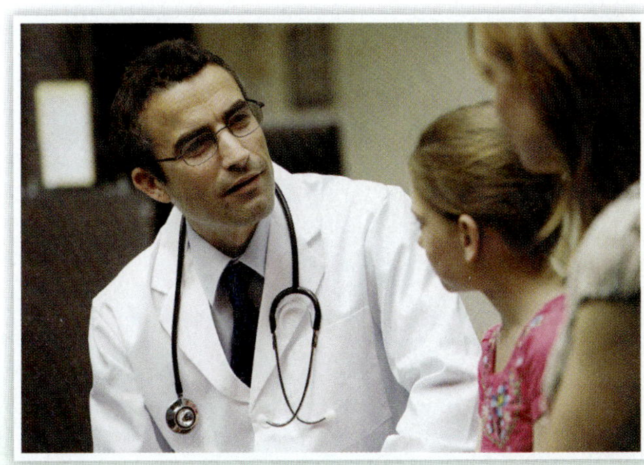

Talking with a doctor, nurse, or other health care professional can sometimes be bewildering or confusing.

1.1 The Purpose of Medical Language

Why Is Medical Language Necessary?

"Why did you have to use all those big words?" is a good question. Why is medical language necessary? Following are a few reasons why medical language is both necessary and useful.

First, medical language allows health care professionals to be **clear.** Ours is a multicultural society. Many languages are spoken, each with their own words for illnesses and body parts. By using medical language, health care professionals are able to communicate and understand one another clearly, no matter what their first language is.

Second, medical language allows health care professionals to communicate **quickly.** Think about how this works in English. Instead of saying "a tall thing in the yard with green leaves," we just use the word "*tree.*" Instead of saying "a meal made up of a few slices of meat and cheese, topped with lettuce, mustard, and mayonnaise, and placed between two slices of bread," we just say "*sandwich.*" Instead of having to use valuable time describing the symptoms of a disease or the findings of an examination, a health care professional uses medical language in order to be clear and easily understandable to other health care professionals.

Third, medical language allows health care professionals to **comfort** patients. This reason might seem kind of odd, but it is true. When patients first enter a health care facility, they often don't feel well and are a little confused and worried about what is going on. Using medical language reassures patients that the health care professionals know what is going on and are in control. Sometimes a patient can be calmed and reassured that everything is OK by a health care professional repeating the same symptoms the patient reported—in medical language.

For example, one of us once saw a doctor about a rapid heart rate. The doctor was very reassuring—it was just "tachycardia." The doctor, however, didn't know he was talking to someone who was familiar with medical language. *Tachycardia* breaks down to *tachy* (fast, as in a car's *tachometer* reports the engine's revolutions per minute) + *card* (heart) + *ia* (condition). It literally means *fast heart condition.* The doctor was just repeating what he had heard.

Here's another example. Once, a young boy was sick and his doctors performed a series of tests to find out what was wrong. After receiving the test reports, the boy's parents were reassured. The doctor's had diagnosed their child with an "idiopathic blood disorder." The diagnosis was enough for them.

Because the doctor had attached a fancy medical term to their son's condition, the parents figured the doctors knew what was wrong and how to treat it. In truth, the doctor hadn't told them anything. *Idiopathic* breaks down to *idio* (private or alone) + *pathic* (disease or suffering). It literally means *suffering alone.* The boy's condition was something the doctors had never seen before.

Medical language enables health care professionals to communicate quickly and easily no matter what their specific speciality or native language.

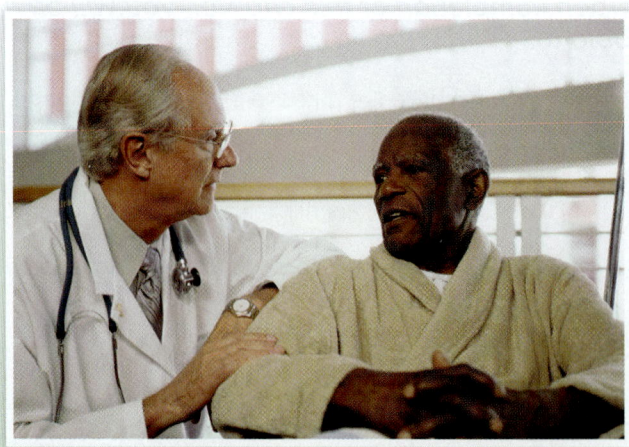

Medical language is able to reassure patients that health care professionals know what is going on and are in control.

Learning Outcome 1.1 Exercises

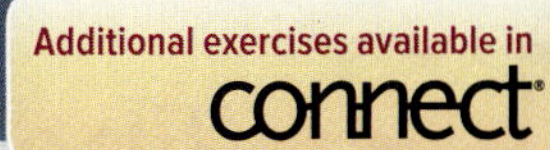
Additional exercises available in
connect

EXERCISE 1 *Multiple-choice questions. Select the correct answer.*

1. Which of the following is NOT a reason why medical language is necessary and useful?
   a. Medical language allows health care professionals to be clear.
   b. Medical language allows health care professionals to comfort patients.
   c. Medical language allows health care professionals to communicate quickly.
   d. Medical language allows health care professionals to intimidate their patients.
2. Medical language allows health care professionals to be clear because
   a. few people really understand medical terminology, so at least everyone is speaking the same way
   b. health care professionals are in control of the situation and don't want to scare patients with a language that they could understand
   c. we live in a multicultural society with a variety of languages, and medical language is a way of speaking the same way about the same thing despite your native language
   d. none of these
3. Medical language allows health care professionals to communicate quickly because
   a. it is a quick way to speak to other health care professionals without taking the time to describe symptoms or examine findings
   b. the patients are usually baffled by the terminology and do not ask additional questions
   c. words with many syllables always communicate more information than words with few syllables
   d. none of these
4. Medical language allows health care professionals to comfort patients because
   a. it communicates a sense that the health care professionals are in control of the situation
   b. it lets the patients know that the health care professionals are not caught off guard by the symptoms at hand
   c. it lets the patients know that the health care professionals know what is going on
   d. all of these

1.2 The Origins of Medical Language

Where Does It Come From?

Medical language is made up primarily (but not exclusively) of words taken from two ancient languages: Greek and Latin. Other words creep in from other sources, but Greek and Latin serve as the foundation of medical language.

Some of these other sources include:

Eponyms. The word *eponym* is derived from the Greek words *epi* (upon) + *onyma* (name). It literally means *to put your name on something.* Thus, an eponym is a word formed by including the name of the person who discovered or invented whatever is being described. Sometimes, in the case of diseases, an eponym is named in honor of the disease's first or most noteworthy diagnosed victim.

This reminds us of a great old joke.

A doctor says to a patient, "I have good news and bad news. Which do you want first?"

The patient responds, "The good news."

The doctor replies, "Well, you are about to have a disease named after you."

One famous eponym is Lou Gehrig's disease. The neurological disease was named after the famous New York Yankee first baseman who suffered from the disease. The disease's scientific name is *amyotrophic lateral sclerosis.*

Acronyms. The word *acronym* is derived from the Greek words *acro* (high, end) + *onyma* (name). It literally means *to make a name with the ends.* Thus, an acronym is a word made up of the first letters of each of the words that make up a phrase. One example is the diagnostic imaging process called **m**agnetic **r**esonance **i**maging, or MRI. Remember that acronyms are just shorthand—you still need to know what the words mean.

Modern languages. Frequently, words from modern languages creep into the vocabulary of health care professionals. These words tend to come from whatever language happens to be most commonly spoken by the majority of health care professionals. In centuries past, German or French were the most common languages, so they were the foundation of many medical terms. Currently, the fastest-growing and most-used language in the world is English. Thus, English has also contributed a fair number of medical terms.

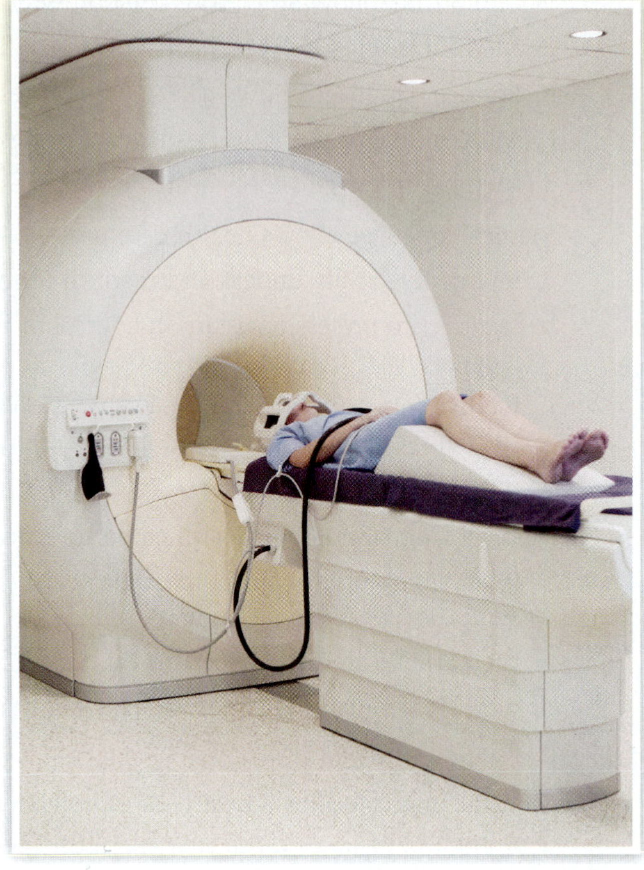

MRI, which stands for ***m**agnetic **r**esonance **i**maging,* is an example of an acronym.

Why Greek and Latin?

Although the three previously mentioned categories have contributed a significant number of words to the language of medicine, Greek and Latin make up its foundation and backbone. Even *eponym* and *acronym* were derived from Greek! But why are Greek and Latin so prevalent? There are at least three reasons why.

Reason 1: The foundations of Western medicine were in ancient Greece and Rome. The first people to systematically study the human body and develop theories about health and disease were the ancient Greeks. The Hippocratic Oath, the foundation of modern medical ethical codes, is named after and was possibly composed by a man named Hippocrates who lived in Greece from about

460 BC to about 370 BC. Hippocrates is widely considered to be the father of Western medicine.

The development of the health care profession began in ancient Greece and continued in ancient Rome. There, Galen, who lived from AD 129 to about AD 217, made some of the greatest advancements of our understanding of the human body, how disease affects it, and how drugs work.

Medical advances began to occur with greater frequency during the scientific revolution, adding to an already existing body of knowledge based on ancient Greek and Latin. In fact, some of the oldest terms have been in use for more than 2,000 years, such as terms for the skin, because these body parts were more easily viewed and studied.

Reason 2: Latin was the global language of the scientific revolution. The scientific revolution took place from the sixteenth through the eighteenth century. It was a time of enormous discoveries in physics, biology, chemistry, and human anatomy. This period saw a rapid increase in human knowledge thanks to the scientific method, which is a set of techniques developed in this period and still in use today using observation and experimentation for developing, testing, and proving or disproving hypotheses.

Medical research involving many different subjects, people, and places occurred all over Europe. To allow people from England, Italy, Spain, Poland, and elsewhere to talk with one another, Latin became the language of scholarly discussion. It was already the common language of the Holy Roman Empire and Catholic Church, so many people already knew it well.

By using Latin to record and spread news of their discoveries, scientists of this time were able to share their new knowledge beyond the borders of their countries. At the same time, the number of medical words that sprang from Latin grew.

Reason 3: Dead languages don't change. "Fine," you think. "The language of medicine is based on Greek and Latin. But why do we keep using it? No one speaks either of these languages anymore. Why don't we just use English?"

The reason we keep using Greek and Latin is exactly that—no one speaks them anymore. All spoken languages change over time. Take the English word *green,* for instance, and its non-color-related meaning. In the past 20 or so years, the word *green* has become understood to mean *environmentally responsible,* as in the phrase *green energy.* Before that, the term was widely understood to mean something different: *immature or inexperienced,* such as "I just started this job, so I am still a little *green.*" Dead languages, which aren't spoken anymore, have an advantage because they don't change. There is no worry that words will change their meaning over time.

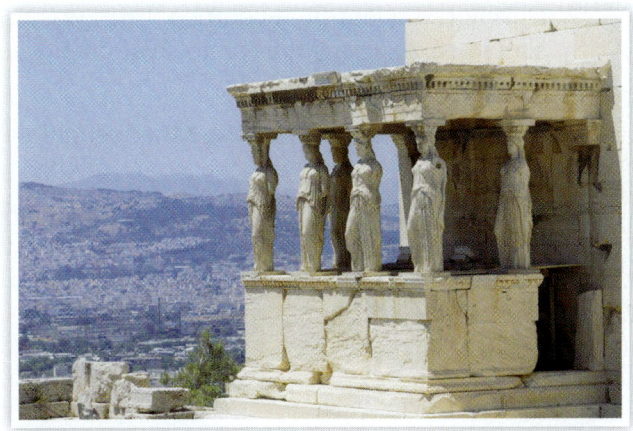

The foundations of Western medicine were laid in Greece and Rome.

Learning Outcome 1.2 Exercises

EXERCISE 1 *True or false questions. Indicate true answers with a T and false answers with an F.*

1. Medical language is made up primarily, but not exclusively, of words taken from two ancient languages: Greek and Latin. ____
2. Some other sources of medical language include eponyms, acronyms, and modern languages. ____
3. An example of an eponym is a medical term named after a famous patient who had the disease. ____
4. *MRI* is an example of an eponym. ____
5. Acronyms are used to say things more quickly. ____
6. Greek and Latin provide the basis of the language of medicine because Western medicine has its foundations in the Greek and Roman cultures. ____
7. The first people to systematically study the human body and develop theories about health and disease were the ancient Greeks. ____
8. Even though German was the global language of the scientific revolution, the Catholic Church forced all academics to use Latin, a language unknown to most people. ____
9. During the scientific revolution, Latin was used as the language of scholarly discussion in order to allow people across Europe to share their knowledge more quickly despite their different native languages. ____
10. A dead language is a language that people do not like to hear or speak anymore because it is no longer useful to a society. ____
11. Latin and Greek provide an excellent basis for medical terminology because dead languages do not change. ____

1.3 The Principles of Medical Language

How Does It Work?

Don't think of medical language as words to be memorized. Instead, they are sentences to be translated.[1]

Each medical word is a description of some aspect of health care. Think of it this way: If you were taking a trip to another country, you might try to memorize a few key words or phrases. It might be useful to know how to say common things like "Where is the bathroom?" or "How much does this cost?" But if you were going to live in that country for a while, you wouldn't just try to memorize a few stock phrases, you would try to learn the language so you could understand what other people were saying.

The same is true of medical language. If you understand the way the language works, you will be able not only to know the meaning of a few individual words, but also to break down and understand words you have never seen before, and even generate words on your own.

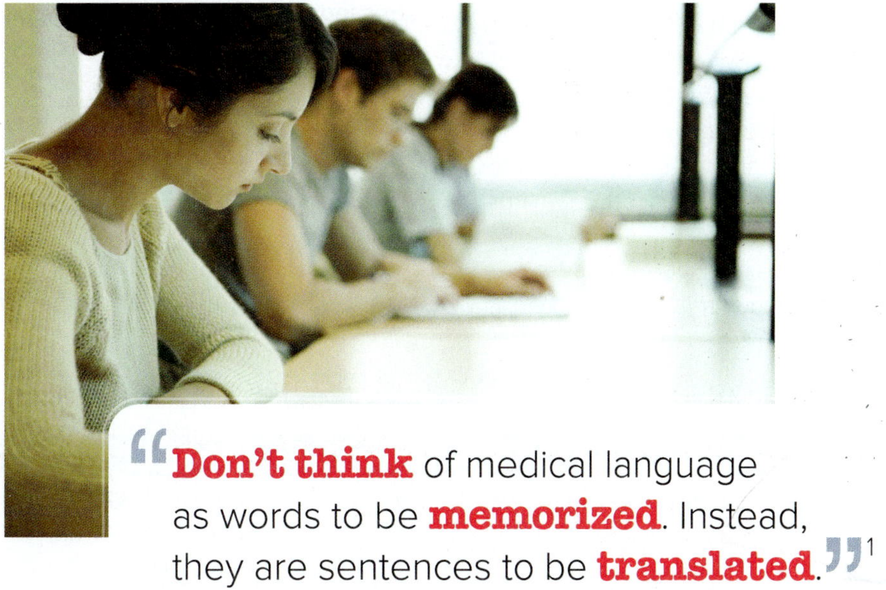

"**Don't think** of medical language as words to be **memorized**. Instead, they are sentences to be **translated**."[1]

[1] For more on this concept, see Lesley A. Dean-Jones, "Teaching Medical Terminology as a Classics Course," *Classical Journal* 93 (1998): 290–96.

1.4 How to Pronounce Terms Associated with Medical Language

The first step in learning any language is learning correct pronunciation. Like any other language, knowing and understanding medical terminology is useless unless you pronounce the terms correctly. With medical terms, the matter is complicated by two facts: First, many of the words come from foreign languages (and not just any foreign languages, but foreign languages no one speaks anymore). Second, some of the words are really long.

You probably have noticed the way native speakers of other languages pronounce certain letters differently. Think of the word *tortilla.* It takes a bit of experience with Spanish to know that two *l*s placed together (*ll*) is pronounced like a *y.* You say *tor-TEE-yah,* not *tor-TILL-ah.* The Spanish word for yellow, *amarillo,* follows this rule. It is pronounced ah-mah-REE-yoh. But the Texas town of the same name is pronounced very differently: am-ah-RIL-oh.

The same is true for medical language. The best way to learn terms is by encountering them in context. Once you get a little experience with the language, you will pick up the unique ways that certain letters are pronounced. In the meantime, below you will find a chart of some commonly mispronounced letters.

Syllable Emphasis

Every medical term is constructed from syllables. Another thing that can affect the way words are pronounced is which syllable or syllables should be stressed, or emphasized. You must always make sure to put the emphasis on the right syllable.

For example, consider that last phrase: *Put the emphasis on the right syllable.* The correct way to pronounce it would be:

PUT the EM-fah-sis on the RAIT SIL-ah-bul.

It would sound funny to say:

PUT the em-FAH-sis on the RAIT si-LAH-bul.

Letter	Sound	Example
c (before *a, o, u*)	k	*cardiac* (KAR-dee-ak) *contra* (KON-trah) *cut* (KUT)
c (before e, *i, y*)	s	*cephalic* (seh-FAL-ik) *cilium* (SIL-ee-um) *cyst* (SIST)
ch	k	*chiropractor* (KAI-roh-PRAK-tor)
g (before *a, o, u*)	g	*gamma* (GAM-ah) *goiter* (GOI-ter) *gutta* (GUT-tah)
g (before e, *i, y*)	j	*genetic* (jeh-NEH-tik) *giant* (JAI-int) *biology* (bai-AW-loh-jee)
ph	f	*pharmacy* (FAR-mah-see)
pn	n	*pneumonia* (noo-MOHN-yah)
pt (initial)	t	*pterigium* (tir-IH-jee-um)
rh, rrh	r	*rhinoplasty* (RAI-noh-PLAS-tee) *hemorrhage* (HEH-moh-rij)
x (initial)	z	*xeroderma* (ZER-oh-DER-mah)

Knowing which syllable to emphasize can seem tricky, but is actually pretty easy. Usually, for the sake of emphasis, the only syllables that you need to focus on are these last three syllables. So, starting at the end of the word, count back three syllables.

Although they are not terribly important to know, there are names for the various syllables in a word. The last syllable is called the *ultima,* which means *last.* The second-to-last syllable is called the *penult,* which means *almost the last.* The prefix *pen-* means *almost.* Think of the word *peninsula,* which is a body of land with water on three sides. The word literally translates to *almost an island.*

The third-to-last syllable is called the *antepenult.* The literal translation of this word is one of our favorites. *Ante-* means *before,* so *antepenult* means *the one before the one that is almost the last.* When it comes to emphasizing the right syllable, the basic rule is this: In most words, the emphasis usually falls on the third-to-last syllable (the *antepenult,* if you are keeping track).

> *Cardiac* is split into three syllables: car / di / ac.
>
> Count backward three syllables from the end of the word to figure out which syllable gets emphasized: *car.*
>
> Therefore, the word is pronounced **KAR** / dee / ak.

> *Cardiology* is split into five syllables: car / di / o / lo / gy.
>
> Count backward three syllables from the end of the word to figure out which syllable gets emphasized: *o.*
>
> Therefore, the word is pronounced kar / dee / **AW** / loh / jee.

It gets tricky when a word remains unchanged except for the addition or subtraction of only a few letters. Two good examples are the words *colonoscopy* and *colonoscope.*

> *Colonoscopy* is split into five syllables: co / lon / o / sco / py.
>
> Count backward three syllables from the end of the word to figure out which syllable gets emphasized: *o.*
>
> Therefore, the word is pronounced koh / lon / **AW** / skoh / pee.

> *Colonoscope* is split into four syllables: co / lon / o / scope.
>
> Count backward three syllables from the end of the word to figure out which syllable gets emphasized: *lon.*
>
> Therefore, the word is pronounced koh / **LAWN** / oh / skohp.

Notice how easy it is to spot the pronunciation change if you focus on counting backward from the end of the word?

As with any rule, there are countless exceptions and technicalities. That said, the easiest way to master pronunciation is not to learn countless rules, but instead to *practice pronouncing words.* Learn this one rule—let's call it the three-syllable rule—and make sure you take note of the pronunciations offered throughout the chapters. Don't just read them silently! Pronounce the words out loud. The more times you practice saying a word, the more comfortable and natural you will feel when you have to use it for real.

But make sure you are pronouncing correctly. Practice does *not* make perfect; practice makes permanent. Whatever you do over and over will be cemented in your brain, so make sure you do it right. *Perfect* practice makes perfect.

Learning Outcome 1.4 Exercises

EXERCISE 1 *Identify the correct pronunciation for the underlined syllable.*

EXAMPLE: thora**co**centesis *answer: koh (the c is hard because it is followed by an o)*
thora**cen**tesis *answer: sin (the c is soft because it is followed by an* ***i****)*

		a.	b.
_____	1. **gut**	a. jut	b. gut
_____	2. di**git**	a. jit	b. git
_____	3. **gag** reflex	a. jag	b. gag
_____	4. dermatolo**gy**	a. jee	b. gee
_____	5. **ge**neticist	a. jen	b. gen
_____	6. **go**nad	a. joh	b. goh
_____	7. colla**gen**	a. jen	b. gen
_____	8. **phar**macist	a. par	b. far
_____	9. **cu**ticle	a. kyoo	b. suh
_____	10. **cor**nea	a. kor	b. sor
_____	11. **cath**eter	a. kath	b. sath
_____	12. on**co**logy	a. kaw	b. saw
_____	13. geneti**cist**	a. kist	b. sist
_____	14. pharma**cist**	a. kist	b. sist
_____	15. **cys**tic fibrosis	a. kis	b. sis
_____	16. **cho**lera	a. kawl	b. chohl
_____	17. psy**cho**sis	a. koh	b. choh
_____	18. pneumato**cele**	a. keel	b. seel
_____	19. **rheu**matoid arthritis	a. roo	b. rhee-yoo
_____	20. **pneu**matocele	a. noo	b. puh-noo
_____	21. **pter**ion	a. tir	b. puh-tir
_____	22. **xer**osis	a. zer	b. ex-er
_____	23. en**cepha**litis	a. kep	b. sef
_____	24. **cirrho**sis	a. kir-hoh	b. sir-oh

EXERCISE 2 *Break down the following words into syllables.*

EXAMPLE: synesthesia *syn | es | the | sia*

1. digit ____________________
2. gonad ____________________
3. cholera ____________________
4. cornea ____________________

5. cuticle ______
6. catheter ______
7. collagen ______
8. anemia ______
9. oncology ______
10. optometry ______
11. rheumatoid ______
12. geneticist ______
13. dermatology ______
14. psychotherapist ______

EXERCISE 3 *Indicate which syllable is emphasized when pronounced.*

EXAMPLE: bronchitis bron**chi**tis

1. cholera ______
2. cornea ______
3. cuticle ______
4. catheter ______
5. collagen ______
6. anemia ______
7. oncology ______
8. optometry ______
9. rheumatoid ______
10. geneticist ______
11. dermatology ______
12. psychotherapist ______

1.5 Parts Used to Build Medical Language

Just as any language has nouns, verbs, and adjectives, the language of medicine is made up of three main building blocks: roots, suffixes, and prefixes. Medical language is constructed by combining a root with a suffix and often a prefix.

Root—foundation or subject of the term

Suffix—ending that gives essential meaning to the term

Prefix—added to the beginning of a term when needed to further modify the root

Common Roots

A root is the foundation of any medical term. Roots function like nouns in the language of medicine. It is the base, or subject, of a word—it is what the word is about. Most roots refer to things like body parts, organs, and fluids.

There are a few types of roots in medical language. In the roots that follow, notice that a slash divides the last letter for the rest of the word (as in *arthr/o*). The final letter in these roots is called a *combining vowel*; these are discussed in detail later in the chapter. For now, just know that the final letter occurs in some words and not in others. Whenever possible, the examples provided include words that have, and some that don't have, the combining vowel. Don't worry about what the example words mean. This is just to get you used to seeing the roots in context.

Some meanings have only one potential root.

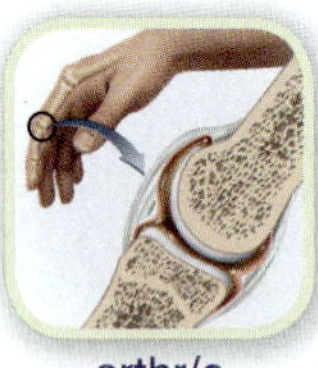

arthr/o

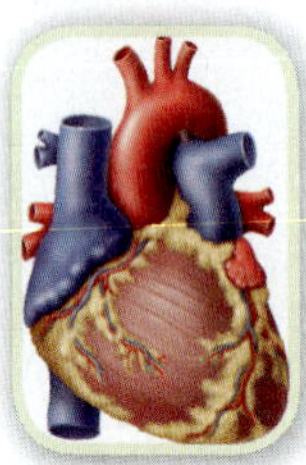

cardi/o

Root	Definition	Examples
arthr/o AR-throh	joint	*arthroscope, arthritis*
cardi/o KAR-dee-oh	heart	*cardiology, pericardium*
enter/o EN-ter-oh	small intestine	*enteropathy, dysentery*
gastr/o GAS-tro	stomach	*gastrointestinal, gastritis*
hepat/o he-PAH-toh	liver	*hepatology, hepatitis*
neur/o NUR-oh	nerve	*neurology, neuralgia*

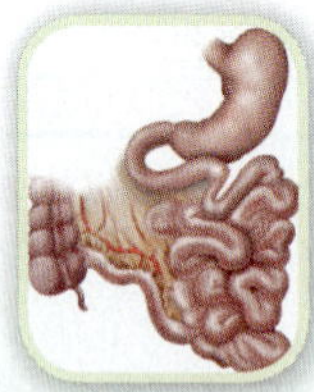

enter/o

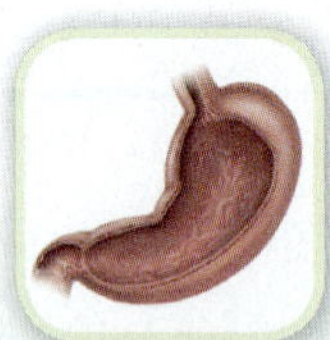

gastr/o

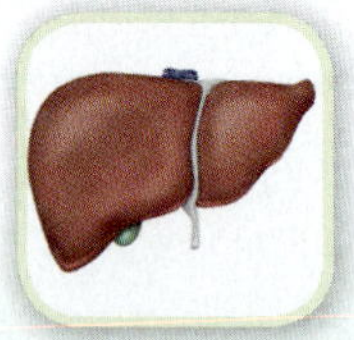

hepat/o

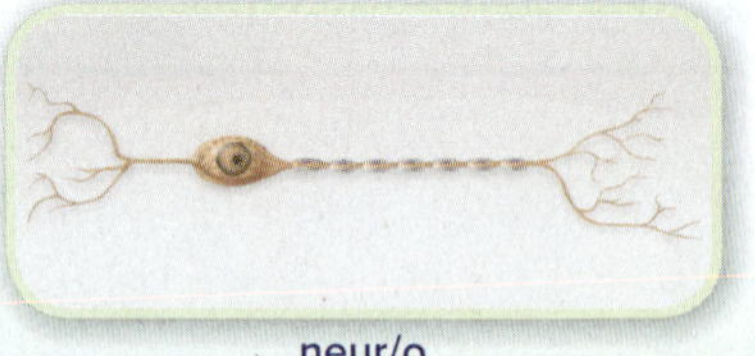

neur/o

Some meanings have a few similar-sounding potential roots. Why? Some suffixes just sound better when attached to another root. Look at the examples in the chart below and switch the roots around—*hematorrhage* and *hemoma.* The meanings are the same, but they sure sound funny.

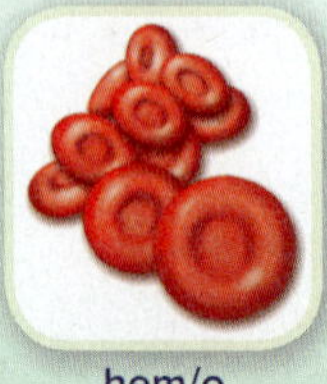

hem/o

Root	Definition	Examples
hem/o HEE-moh	blood	*hemorrhage*
hemat/o heh-MAH-toh		*hematoma*

Some meanings have a couple of potential roots that are completely different but mean the same thing. This is because one word comes from Greek and the other comes from Latin. Normally, however, one of the roots is much more commonly used than the other. As shown below, *myo* is used much more often than *musculo*.

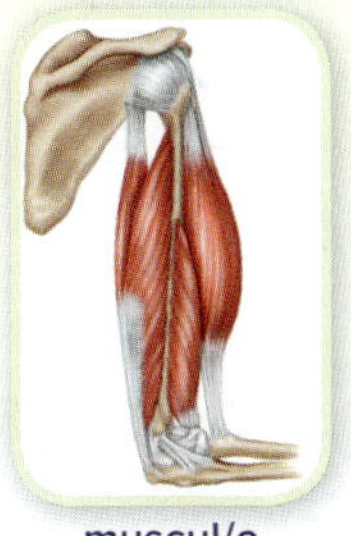
musccul/o

Root	Definition	Examples
my/o MAI-oh	muscle	*myocardial, myalgia*
muscul/o MUS-kyoo-loh		*musculoskeletal, muscular*

Some meanings have several potential roots that mean the same thing. Some are similar, and some are completely different. These are basically a combination of the two previous categories. These meanings each have a couple of similar roots *as well as* at least one root from Greek and one from Latin.

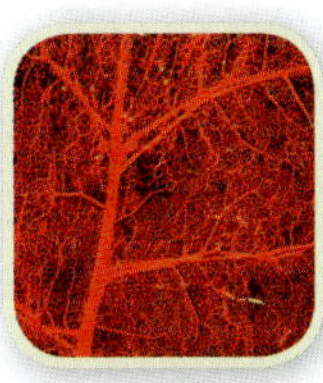
angi/o

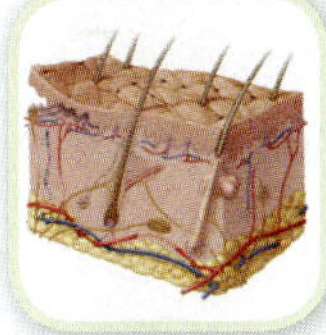
derm/o

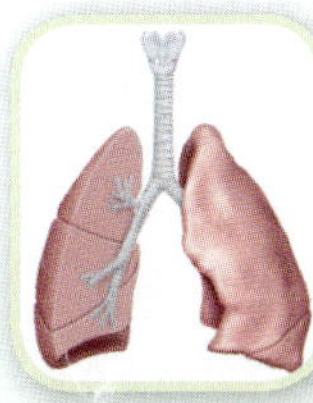
pneum/o

Root	Definition	Examples
angi/o AN-gee-oh	vessel (most commonly refers to blood vessel, but can also refer to other types of vessels as well)	*angioplasty, angiectomy*
vas/o VAS-oh		*vasospasm, vasectomy*
vascul/o VAS-kyoo-loh		*vasculopathy, vasculitis*
derm/o DER-moh	skin	*dermoscopy, dermis*
dermat/o der-MAT-oh		*dermatology, dermatitis*
cutane/o kyoo-TAY-nee-oh		*subcutaneous*
pneum/o NOO-moh	lung	*pneumotomy*
pneumon/o noo-MAW-noh		*pneumonia, pneumonitis*
pulmon/o PUL-maw-noh		*pulmonologist, cardiopulmonary*

Question: Why doesn't each meaning have only one potential root?
Answer: The main reason multiple roots are available is to provide *options*. Some suffixes simply sound better or are easier to say when they are combined with one root rather than another.

GENERAL PURPOSE ROOTS

This list contains roots that will recur often in multiple chapters. It is important to learn these roots now.

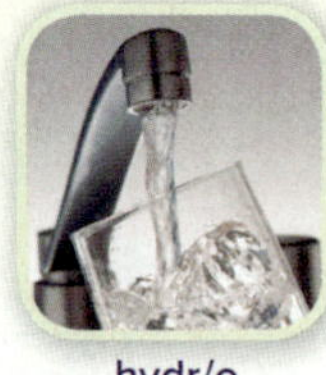
hydr/o

Root	Definition	Examples
gen/o JIN-oh	creation, cause	*pathogenic*
hydr/o HAI-droh	water	*hydrophobia, dehydration*
morph/o MOR-foh	change	*morphology*
myc/o MAI-koh	fungus	*dermatomycosis*
necr/o NEK-roh	death	*necrosis*
orth/o OR-thoh	straight	*orthodontist*
path/o PAH-thoh	suffering, disease	*pathology*
phag/o FAY-goh	eat	*aphagia*
plas/o PLAS-oh	formation	*hyperplasia*
py/o PAI-oh	pus	*pyorrhea, pyemia*
scler/o SKLEH-roh	hard	*scleroderma*
sten/o STIH-noh	narrowing	*stenosis*
troph/o TROH-foh	nourishment, development	*trophology, hypertrophy*
xen/o ZEE-noh	foreign	*xenograft*
xer/o ZEH-roh	dry	*xerosis, xerasia*

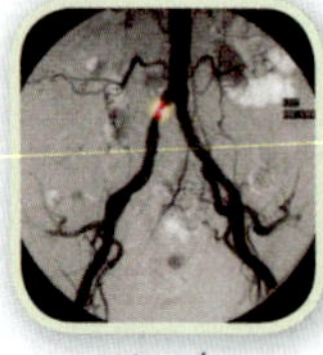
sten/o

Common Suffixes

A *suffix* is a word part placed at the end of a word. The word *suffix* literally means *to attach (fix) after or below (sub, which if you say it fast starts to sound like* suff). As roots function as nouns, so suffixes function as verbs in the language of medicine. They describe something the root is doing, or something that is happening to the root.

There are many types of suffixes in medical language. in general, they can be divided into two basic groups: simple and complex.

SIMPLE SUFFIXES

These suffixes (as their name suggests) are basic and are used to turn a root into a complete word.

Adjective. These suffixes turn the root they follow into an adjective. Thus, they all mean *pertaining to,* or something similar to that.

Suffix	Definition	Examples
-ac ak	pertaining to	*cardiac*
-al al		*skeletal*
-ar ar		*muscular*
-ary ar-ee		*pulmonary*
-eal ee-al		*esophageal*
-ic ik		*medic*
-tic tik		*neurotic*
-ous us		*subcutaneous*

Noun. All these suffixes turn the root they are added to into nouns.

Suffix	Definition	Examples
-ia ee-ah	condition	*pneumonia*
-ism iz-um		*autism*
-ium ee-um	tissue, structure	*pericardium*
-y ee	condition, procedure	*hypertrophy*

Diminutive. When added to a root, these suffixes transform a term's meaning to a smaller version of the root. In English, for example, the suffix *-let* is diminutive. A *booklet* is a *little book.* In Spanish, the suffix *-ita* is diminutive. *Señora* is the Spanish word for *lady,* so *señorita* therefore means *little lady.*

Suffix	Definition	Examples
-icle ik-el	small	*ventricle*
-ole ohl		*arteriole*
-ule yool		*pustule*
-ula yoo-lah		*uvula*

COMPLEX SUFFIXES

Complex suffixes aren't necessarily more difficult to understand than simple suffixes. They just have more parts. Sometimes, these suffixes are referred to as compound or combination suffixes because the suffixes themselves are put together from other suffixes, roots, and prefixes.

Following is an example.

The suffix *-y* means *condition* or *procedure*. When combined with *tom/o*, a root meaning *to cut*, the result is the complex suffix *-tomy*, which means *a cutting procedure* or *incision*.

tom/o (cut) + *-y* (process) = *-tomy* = a cutting procedure or incision

But you can take it a step further. If you add the prefix *ec-* to *-tomy*, you will create the complex suffix *-ectomy*, which means *to cut out* or *to surgically remove something*.

ec- (out) + *tom/o* (cut) + *-y* (process) = *-ectomy* = a cutting out procedure or surgical removal

Following are some lists of some categories of complex suffixes. Some complex suffixes are professional terms.

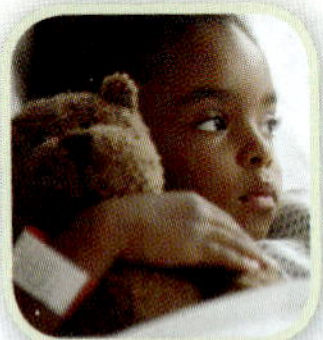

-iatrics (pediatrics)

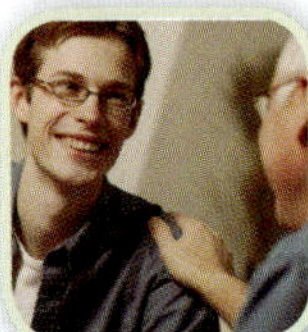

-logist (psychologist)

Suffix	Definition	Examples
-iatrics ee-AH-triks	medical science	*pediatrics*
-iatry AI-ah-tree		*psychiatry*
-iatrist EE-ah-trist	specialist in medicine of	*psychiatrist*
-ist ist	specialist	*dentist*
-logist loh-jist	specialist in the study of	*psychologist*
-logy loh-jee	study of	*psychology*

Some complex suffixes describe symptoms, diseases, or conditions that are either mentioned by patients or diagnosed by health professionals.

symptoms, diseases, and conditions

Suffix	Definition	Examples
-algia AL-jah	pain	*myalgia*
-dynia DAI-nee-ah		*gastrodynia*
-cele SEEL	hernia (a bulging of tissue into an area where it doesn't belong)	*hydrocele*
-emia EE-mee-ah	blood condition	*leukemia*
-iasis AI-ah-sis	presence of	*lithiasis*
-itis AI-tis	inflammation	*arthritis*
-lysis lih-sis	loosen, break down	*hemolysis*
-malacia mah-LAY-shah	abnormal softening	*osteomalacia*
-megaly MEH-gah-lee	enlargement	*hepatomegaly*
-oid OYD	resembling	*keloid*

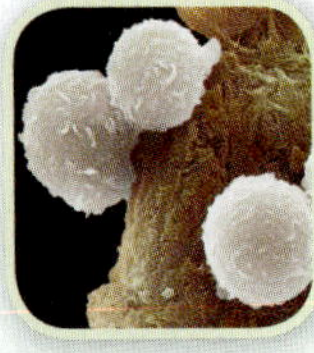

-emia (leukemia)

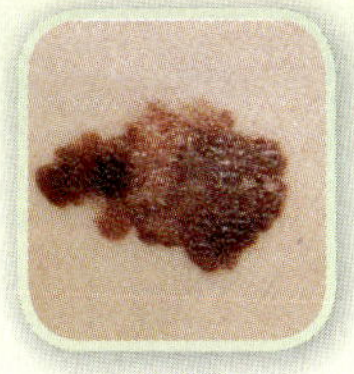
-oma (melanoma)

symptoms, diseases, and conditions *continued*

Suffix	Definition	Examples
-oma OH-mah	tumor	*melanoma*
-osis OH-sis	condition	*thrombosis*
-pathy pah-thee	disease	*myopathy*
-penia PEE-nee-ah	deficiency	*leukopenia*
-ptosis puh-TOH-sis	drooping	*nephroptosis*
-rrhage RIJ	excessive flow	*hemorrhage*
-rrhagia RAY-jee-ah		*menorrhagia*
-rrhea REE-ah	flow	*diarrhea*
-rrhexis REK-sis	rupture	*metrorrhexis*
-spasm SPAZ-um	involuntary contraction	*myospasm*

Some complex suffixes describe tests and treatments performed by health professionals. Although it is convenient to place tests and treatments in the same category and label them as "procedures," it is important to distinguish between the two. A *test* is a *procedure done to gain more information in order to diagnose a problem.* A *treatment* is a *process done after a diagnosis to fix a problem.*

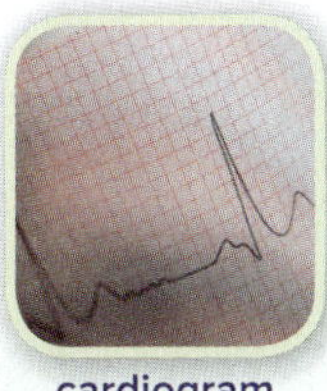
cardiogram

tests

Suffix	Definition	Examples
-centesis sin-TEE-sis	puncture	*amniocentesis*
-gram gram	written record	*cardiogram*
-graph graf	instrument used to produce a record	*cardiograph*
-graphy grah-fee	process of recording	*cardiography*
-meter mee-ter	instrument used to measure	*cephalometer*
-metry meh-tree	process of measuring	*cephalometry*
-scope skohp	instrument used to look	*arthroscope*
-scopy skoh-pee	process of looking	*arthroscopy*

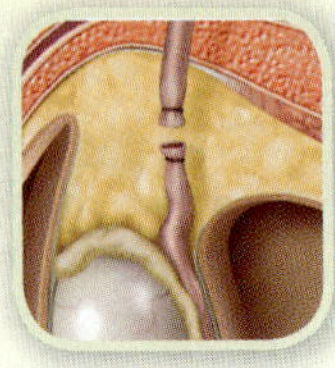

vasectomy

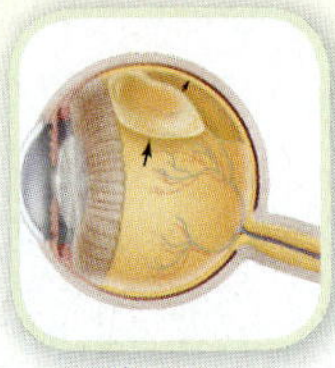

retinopexy

treatments

Suffix	Definition	Examples
-desis DEE-sis	binding, fixation	*arthrodesis*
-ectomy EK-toh-mee	removal	*vasectomy*
-pexy PEK-see	surgical fixation	*retinopexy*
-plasty PLAS-tee	reconstruction	*rhinoplasty*
-rrhaphy rah-fee	suture	*herniorrhaphy*
-stomy stoh-mee	creation of an opening	*colostomy*
-tomy toh-mee	incision	*dermotomy*

SINGULARS AND PLURALS

In English, the most common way to turn a word from singular to plural is to add an "s." The plural of *bag* is *bags,* for example. But there are other ways too. The plural of *goose* is *geese*. The plural of *mouse* is *mice*. The plural of *ox* is *oxen*. The plural of *sheep* is *sheep*.

The same is true for medical terms. Because medical words come from different languages, singular words become plural in a variety of ways.

Singular	Plural	Examples	
-a	*-ae*	*vertebra* *larva*	*vertebrae* *larvae*
-ax	*-aces*	*thorax*	*thoraces*
-ex	*-ices*	*cortex*	*cortices*
-ix	*-ices*	*appendix*	*appendices*
-is	*-es*	*neurosis* *diagnosis*	*neuroses* *diagnoses*
-ma	*-mata*	*sarcoma* *carcinoma*	*sarcomata* *carcinomata*
-on	*-a*	*spermatozoon* *ganglion*	*spermatozoa* *ganglia*
-um	*-a*	*datum* *bacterium* *ovum*	*data* *bacteria* *ova*
-us	*-i*	*nucleus* *alveolus* *thrombus*	*nuclei* *alveoli* *thrombi*
-y	*-ies*	*biopsy* *myopathy*	*biopsies* *myopathies*

Common Prefixes

A *prefix* is a word part placed at the beginning of a word. The word *prefix* literally means *to attach (fix) before (pre)*. Prefixes function like adjectives in the language of medicine. They supply additional information as needed. In the same way that not every sentence has an adjective, not every medical term has a prefix.

There are many types of prefixes in medical language. Following are a few examples.

NEGATION PREFIXES

Some prefixes negate things:

negation

Prefix	Meaning	Examples
a- ay	not	*aphasia*
an- an		*anemia*
anti- AN-tee	against	*antibiotics*
contra- KON-trah		*contraceptive*
de- dee	down, away from	*dehydration*

TIME OR SPEED PREFIXES

Some prefixes describe time or speed:

time/speed

Prefix	Meaning	Examples
ante- an-tee	before	*antepartum*
pre- pree		*precondition*
pro- proh	before, on behalf of	*probiotic*
brady- brah-dih	slow	*bradycardia*
tachy- tak-ih	fast	*tachycardia*
post- pohst	after	*postpartum*
re- ree	again	*rehabilitation*

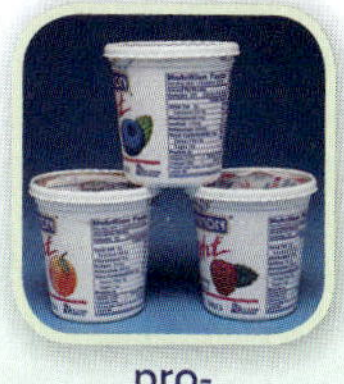

pro-
(probiotic)

DIRECTION OR POSITION PREFIXES

Some prefixes describe direction or position:

direction/position		
Prefix	**Meaning**	**Examples**
ab- ab	away	*abduct*
ad- ad	toward	*adrenaline*
circum- sir-kum	around	*circumcision*
peri- per-ee		*pericardium*
dia- dai-ah	through	*diagnostic*
trans- tranz		*translate*
e- eh	out	*evoke*
ec- ek		*ectopic*
ex- eks		*exhale*
ecto- ek-toh	outside	*ectoderm*
exo- ek-soh		*exoskeleton*
extra- eks-trah		
en- en	in, inside	*enema*
endo- en-doh		*endocrine*
intra- in-trah		*intravenous*
epi- eh-pee	upon	*epididymus*
sub- sub	beneath	*subcutaneous*
inter- in-ter	between	*intercostal*

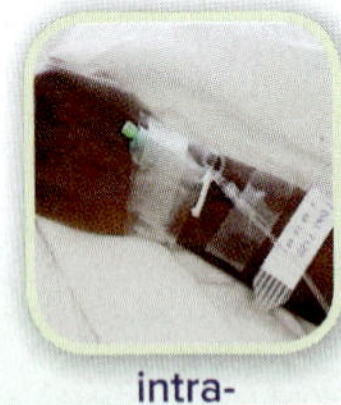
intra-
(intravenous)

SIZE OR QUANTITY PREFIXES

Some prefixes describe size or quantity:

size/quantity

Prefix	Meaning	Examples
bi- bai	two	*bilateral*
hemi- heh-mee	half	*hemiplegia*
semi- seh-mee		*semilunar*
hyper- hai-per	over	*hyperthermia*
hypo- hai-poh	under	*hypothermia*
macro- mak-roh	large	*macrotia*
micro- mai-kroh	small	*microdontia*
mono- maw-noh	one	*monocyte*
uni- yoo-nee		*unisex*
oligo- aw-lih-goh	few	*oligomenorrhea*
pan- pan	all	*pancytopenia*
poly- pawlee	many	*polygraph*
multi- mul-tee		*multicellular*

GENERAL PREFIXES

Some prefixes are general:

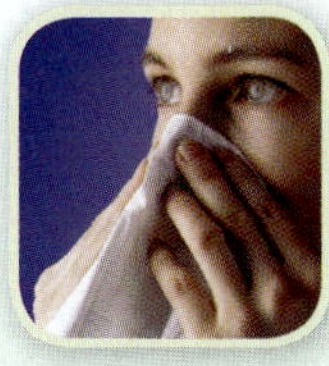

con-
(congestion)

other

Prefix	Meaning	Examples
con- kon	with, together	*congestion*
syn- sin		*syndrome*
sym- sim		*symmetry*
dys- dis	bad	*dysentery*
eu- yoo	good	*euphoria*

Learning Outcome 1.5 Exercises

EXERCISE 1 *Match the root on the left with its definition on the right.*

____	1. neur/o	a.	heart
____	2. cardi/o	b.	joint
____	3. arthr/o	c.	liver
____	4. gastr/o	d.	nerve
____	5. hepat/o	e.	small intestine
____	6. enter/o	f.	stomach

EXERCISE 2 *Translate the following roots.*

1. neur/o ____________
2. cardi/o ____________
3. arthr/o ____________
4. gastr/o ____________
5. hepat/o ____________
6. enter/o ____________

EXERCISE 3 *Underline and define the root in the following terms.*

1. cardiology ____________
2. neurology ____________
3. gastroscope ____________
4. arthroscopy ____________
5. enterology ____________
6. hepatology ____________

EXERCISE 4 *Identify the roots for the following definitions.*

1. heart ____________
2. joint ____________
3. nerve ____________
4. stomach ____________
5. liver ____________
6. small intestine ____________

EXERCISE 5 *Match the root on the left with its definition on the right. Some definitions will be used more than once.*

____	1. muscul/o	a.	blood
____	2. dermat/o	b.	blood vessel
____	3. derm/o	c.	lung
____	4. vascul/o	d.	muscle
____	5. vas/o	e.	skin
____	6. pneumon/o		
____	7. pneum/o		
____	8. pulmon/o		
____	9. my/o		
____	10. angi/o		
____	11. hemat/o		
____	12. hem/o		
____	13. cutane/o		

Learning Outcome 1.5 Exercises

EXERCISE 6 *Translate the following roots.*

1. muscul/o
2. dermat/o
3. derm/o
4. vascul/o
5. vas/o
6. pneumon/o
7. pneum/o
8. pulmon/o
9. my/o
10. angi/o
11. hemat/o
12. hem/o
13. cutane/o

EXERCISE 7 *Underline and define the root in the following terms.*

1. muscular
2. vascular
3. pulmonary
4. dermatology
5. hematology
6. myospasm
7. vasospasm
8. angiogram
9. dermopathy
10. hemostatic
11. percutaneous
12. vasectomy
13. pneumonectomy
14. cardiomyopathy (2 roots)
15. cardiopulmonary (2 roots)

EXERCISE 8 *Identify the roots for the following definitions.*

1. muscle (2 roots)
2. blood (2 roots)
3. skin (3 roots)
4. lung (3 roots)
5. blood vessel (3 roots)

Learning Outcome 1.5 Exercises

EXERCISE 9 *Match the root on the left with its definition on the right.*

____	1. gen/o	a.	change
____	2. necr/o	b.	creation, cause
____	3. xer/o	c.	death
____	4. morph/o	d.	dry
____	5. troph/o	e.	eat
____	6. plas/o	f.	foreign
____	7. sten/o	g.	formation
____	8. phag/o	h.	narrowing
____	9. xen/o	i.	nourishment, development

EXERCISE 10 *Translate the following roots.*

1. hydr/o ____________________
2. orth/o ____________________
3. necr/o ____________________
4. myc/o ____________________
5. py/o ____________________
6. xer/o ____________________
7. path/o ____________________
8. scler/o ____________________
9. phag/o ____________________
10. xen/o ____________________

EXERCISE 11 *Underline and define the roots in the following terms.*

1. morphology ____________________
2. dysplasia ____________________
3. hypertrophic ____________________
4. teratogenic ____________________
5. mycosis ____________________
6. craniostenosis ____________________
7. angiosclerosis (2 roots) ____________________
8. pyarthrosis (2 roots) ____________________

Learning Outcome 1.5 Exercises

EXERCISE 12 *Identify the roots for the following definitions.*

1. water ______
2. creation, cause ______
3. pus ______
4. straight ______
5. fungus ______
6. suffering, disease ______
7. hard ______
8. formation ______

EXERCISE 13 *Match the suffix on the left with its definition on the right. Some definitions will be used more than once.*

______	1. -ium	a.	condition
______	2. -icle	b.	pertaining to
______	3. -ous	c.	tissue, structure
______	4. -ac	d.	small
______	5. -ia		
______	6. -eal		

EXERCISE 14 *Translate the following suffixes.*

1. -y ______
2. -ism ______
3. -al ______
4. -ic, -tic ______
5. -ar, -ary ______
6. -ole, -ule, -ula ______

EXERCISE 15 *Break down the following words into their component parts.*

EXAMPLE: nasopharyngoscope *naso | pharyngo | scope*

1. cardiac ______
2. gastric ______
3. neurotic ______
4. skeletal ______
5. esophageal ______
6. muscular ______
7. pulmonary ______
8. cutaneous ______
9. arteriole ______
10. pneumonia ______
11. cardiovascular ______

Learning Outcome 1.5 Exercises

EXERCISE 16 *Underline and define the suffix in the following terms.*

1. cardiac ____________
2. gastric ____________
3. neurotic ____________
4. skeletal ____________
5. esophageal ____________
6. muscular ____________
7. pulmonary ____________
8. cardiovascular ____________
9. cutaneous ____________
10. arteriole ____________
11. ventricle ____________
12. pustule ____________
13. uvula ____________
14. pneumonia ____________
15. autism ____________
16. pericardium ____________
17. hypertrophy ____________

EXERCISE 17 *Translate the following terms.*

ROOTS: skelet/o *skeleton*	esophag/o *esophagus*	arteri/o *artery*

1. cardiac ____________
2. gastric ____________
3. neurotic ____________
4. skeletal ____________
5. esophageal ____________
6. muscular ____________
7. pulmonary ____________
8. cutaneous ____________
9. arteriole ____________
10. pneumonia ____________
11. cardiovascular ____________

Learning Outcome 1.5 Exercises

EXERCISE 18 *Identify the suffixes for the following definitions.*

1. tissue, structure ________________
2. condition, process ________________
3. condition (three possible options) ________________
4. small or any suffix that makes the root a diminutive, or smaller version of the root (choose three of the four possible options) ________________
5. pertaining to (or any suffix that makes a root into an adjective) (choose four of the eight possible options) ________________

EXERCISE 19 *Match the suffix on the left with its definition on the right. Some definitions will be used more than once.*

e	1. -logy	a. medical science
d	2. -logist	b. specialist
e	3. -ist	c. specialist in the medicine of
c	4. -iatrist	d. specialist in the study of
a.	5. -iatry	e. study of
a	6. -iatrics	f. medicine of

EXERCISE 20 *Translate the following suffixes.*

1. -logy ________________
2. -logist ________________
3. -ist ________________
4. -iatrist ________________
5. -iatry ________________
6. -iatrics ________________

EXERCISE 21 *Break down the following words into their component parts.*

EXAMPLE: sinusitis *sinus | itis*

1. cardiology ________________
2. cardiologist ________________
3. pathology ________________
4. pathologist ________________
5. psychology ________________
6. psychologist ________________
7. dentist ________________
8. psychiatry ________________
9. psychiatrist ________________
10. pediatrics ________________

Learning Outcome 1.5 Exercises

EXERCISE 22 *Underline and define the suffix in the following terms.*

1. cardiology ______________________
2. cardiologist ______________________
3. pathology ______________________
4. pathologist ______________________
5. psychology ______________________
6. psychologist ______________________
7. dentist ______________________
8. psychiatry ______________________
9. psychiatrist ______________________
10. pediatrics ______________________

EXERCISE 23 *Fill in the blanks.*

EXAMPLE: cardiologist *specialist in the study of the heart*

1. *psychiatry:* ______________________ of the mind (*psych/o* = *mind*)
2. *psychiatrist:* ______________________ of the mind (*psych/o* = *mind*)
3. *psychology:* ______________________ of the mind (*psych/o* = *mind*)
4. *psychologist:* ______________________ of the mind (*psych/o* = *mind*)

EXERCISE 24 *Identify the suffixes for the following definitions.*

1. specialist ______________________
2. specialist in the study of ______________________
3. study of ______________________
4. specialist in the medicine of ______________________
5. medical science (two suffixes) ______________________

EXERCISE 25 *Match the suffix on the left with its definition on the right. Some definitions will be used more than once.*

___g___	1. -oid	a. deficiency
___f___	2. -iasis	b. drooping
___d___	3. -cele	c. flow
___a___	4. -penia	d. hernia
___c___	5. -rrhea	e. loosen, break down
___e___	6. -lysis	f. presence of
___b___	7. -ptosis	g. resembling
___h___	8. -rrhexis	h. rupture

Learning Outcome 1.5 Exercises

EXERCISE 26 *Translate the following suffixes.*

1. -spasm ____________________
2. -megaly ____________________
3. -oma ____________________
4. -emia ____________________
5. -itis ____________________
6. -osis ____________________
7. -pathy ____________________
8. -algia ____________________
9. -dynia ____________________
10. -malacia ____________________
11. -rrhage, -rrhagia ____________________

EXERCISE 27 *Break down the following words into their component parts.*

EXAMPLE: sinusitis *sinus | itis*

1. myospasm ____________________
2. myopathy ____________________
3. cardiomegaly ____________________
4. gastritis ____________________
5. gastralgia ____________________
6. gastrodynia ____________________
7. gastromalacia ____________________
8. hematoma ____________________
9. hemolysis ____________________
10. hemorrhage ____________________
11. stenosis ____________________

EXERCISE 28 *Underline and define the suffix in the following terms.*

1. myospasm ____________________
2. myopathy ____________________
3. cardiomegaly ____________________
4. gastritis ____________________
5. gastralgia ____________________
6. gastrodynia ____________________
7. gastromalacia ____________________
8. hematoma ____________________
9. melanoma ____________________
10. hemolysis ____________________
11. hemorrhage ____________________
12. hydrocele ____________________
13. leukopenia ____________________
14. stenosis ____________________

Learning Outcome 1.5 Exercises

EXERCISE 29 *Translate the following terms.*

1. myospasm ______________________
2. myopathy ______________________
3. cardiomegaly ______________________
4. gastritis ______________________
5. gastralgia ______________________
6. gastrodynia ______________________
7. gastromalacia ______________________
8. hematoma ______________________
9. hemolysis ______________________
10. hemorrhage ______________________
11. stenosis ______________________

EXERCISE 30 *Identify the suffixes for the following definitions.*

1. tumor ______________________
2. resembling ______________________
3. blood condition ______________________
4. presence of ______________________
5. deficiency ______________________
6. hernia ______________________
7. drooping ______________________
8. flow ______________________
9. rupture ______________________

EXERCISE 31 *Match the suffix on the left with its definition on the right. Some definitions will be used more than once.*

	Suffix		Definition
b	1. -meter	a.	instrument used to look
e	2. -metry	b.	instrument used to measure
a	3. -scope	c.	instrument used to produce a record
d	4. -scopy	d.	process of looking
c	5. -graph	e.	process of measuring
f	6. -graphy	f.	process of recording
h	7. -gram	g.	puncture
g	8. -centesis	h.	written record

EXERCISE 32 *Translate the following suffixes.*

1. -meter ______________________
2. -metry ______________________
3. -scope ______________________
4. -scopy ______________________
5. -graph ______________________
6. -graphy ______________________
7. -gram ______________________
8. -centesis ______________________

Learning Outcome 1.5 Exercises

EXERCISE 33 *Break down the following words into their component parts.*

EXAMPLE: sinusitis *sinus | itis*

1. audiogram ______
2. audiograph ______
3. audiometer ______
4. gastroscope ______
5. audiography ______
6. audiometry ______
7. gastroscopy ______
8. ovariocentesis ______

EXERCISE 34 *Underline and define the suffix in the following terms.*

1. audiogram ______
2. audiograph ______
3. audiometer ______
4. gastroscope ______
5. audiography ______
6. audiometry ______
7. gastroscopy ______
8. ovariocentesis ______

EXERCISE 35 *Translate the following terms.*

ROOTS: audio *sound* ovario *ovary*

1. audiogram ______
2. audiograph ______
3. audiometer ______
4. gastroscope ______
5. audiography ______
6. audiometry ______
7. gastroscopy ______
8. ovariocentesis ______

EXERCISE 36 *Identify the suffixes for the following definitions.*

1. instrument used to look ______
2. process of looking ______
3. instrument used to measure ______
4. process of measuring ______
5. written record ______
6. instrument used to produce a record ______
7. process of recording ______
8. puncture ______

Learning Outcome 1.5 Exercises

EXERCISE 37 *Match the suffix on the left with its definition on the right.*

d	1. -plasty	a. binding
c	2. -tomy	b. creation of an opening
e	3. -ectomy	c. incision
b	4. -stomy	d. reconstruction
f	5. -pexy	e. removal
a	6. -desis	f. surgical fixation
g	7. -rrhaphy	g. suture

EXERCISE 38 *Translate the following suffixes.*

1. -plasty ______
2. -tomy ______
3. -ectomy ______
4. -stomy ______
5. -pexy ______
6. -desis ______
7. -rrhaphy ______

EXERCISE 39 *Break down the following words into their component parts.*

EXAMPLE: sinusitis *sinus | itis*

1. myodesis ______
2. myorrhaphy ______
3. gastropexy ______
4. myoplasty ______
5. gastrectomy ______
6. tracheotomy ______
7. tracheostomy ______

EXERCISE 40 *Underline and define the suffix in the following terms.*

1. myoplasty ______
2. tracheotomy ______
3. tracheostomy ______
4. gastrectomy ______
5. gastropexy ______
6. myodesis ______
7. myorrhaphy ______

Learning Outcome 1.5 Exercises

EXERCISE 41 *Translate the following terms.*

ROOTS: trache/o *trachea*

1. myoplasty ______
2. tracheotomy ______
3. tracheostomy ______
4. gastrectomy ______
5. gastropexy ______
6. myodesis ______
7. myorrhaphy ______

EXERCISE 42 *Identify the suffixes for the following definitions.*

1. reconstruction ______
2. removal ______
3. incision ______
4. creation of an opening ______
5. surgical fixation ______
6. binding ______
7. suture ______

EXERCISE 43 *Match the singular suffix on the left with the suffix that will make the same term plural on the right. Some plural suffixes will be used more than once.*

	Singular	Plural
b	1. -ax	a. -a
f	2. -ix	b. -aces
f	3. -ex	c. -ae
h	4. -ma	d. -es
d	5. -is	e. -i
c	6. -a	g. -ies
a	7. -um	f. -ices
a	8. -on	h. -mata
g	9. -y	
e	10. -us	

Learning Outcome 1.5 Exercises

EXERCISE 44 *Indicate whether the suffix is singular or plural.*

1. -aces ____
2. -ices ____
3. -ax ____
4. -ex ____
5. -ix ____
6. -ma ____
7. -mata ____
8. -on ____
9. -um ____
10. -ae ____
11. -i ____
12. -y ____
13. -is ____
14. -es ____
15. -us ____
16. -ies ____

EXERCISE 45 *Underline the suffix in the following terms and indicate whether the term is singular or plural.*

EXAMPLE: bacteri<u>um</u> *singular (suffix -um is singular)*

1. appendix ____
2. appendices ____
3. cortex ____
4. cortices ____
5. thorax ____
6. thoraces ____
7. myopathy ____
8. myopathies ____
9. vertebra ____
10. vertebrae ____
11. ganglion ____
12. ganglia ____
13. carcinoma ____
14. carcinomata ____
15. ova ____
16. ovum ____
17. nucleus ____
18. nuclei ____
19. diagnosis ____
20. diagnoses ____
21. biopsy ____
22. thrombus ____
23. spermatozoon ____
24. larvae ____
25. sarcoma ____
26. neuroses ____
27. bacteria ____

Learning Outcome 1.5 Exercises

EXERCISE 46 *Match the prefix on the left with its definition on the right. Some definitions will be used more than once.*

d	1. pre-	a.	after
a	2. post-	b.	again
b	3. re-	c.	against
c	4. contra-	d.	before
c	5. anti-	e.	before, on behalf of
e	6. pro-	f.	down, away from
f	7. de-	g.	fast
h	8. a-	h.	not
h	9. an-	i.	slow
h	10. ante-		
g	11. tachy-		
i	12. brady-		

EXERCISE 47 *Translate the following prefixes.*

1. pre- ____________
2. post- ____________
3. re- ____________
4. contra- ____________
5. anti- ____________
6. pro- ____________
7. de- ____________
8. a- ____________
9. an- ____________
10. ante- ____________
11. tachy- ____________
12. brady- ____________

EXERCISE 48 *Break down the following words into their component parts.*

> **EXAMPLE:** sinusitis *sinus | itis*

1. bradypnea ____________
2. tachypnea ____________
3. apnea ____________
4. prenatal (3 parts: prefix, root, suffix) ____________
5. postnatal (3 parts: prefix, root, suffix) ____________
6. antibiotic (3 parts: prefix, root, suffix) ____________
7. probiotic (3 parts: prefix, root, suffix) ____________

Learning Outcome 1.5 Exercises

EXERCISE 49 *Underline and define the prefix in the following terms.*

1. prenatal ______
2. postnatal ______
3. antepartum ______
4. probiotic ______
5. antibiotic ______
6. contraceptive ______
7. dehydration ______
8. rehabilitation ______
9. bradypnea ______
10. tachypnea ______
11. apnea ______

EXERCISE 50 *Select the correct prefix option for each given translation.*

EXAMPLE: hypoglycemia: *(hypo-)* over/under + *(glyc)* sugar + *(-emia)* blood condition
dysmenorrhea: *(dys-)* not/bad + *(meno)* menstruation + *(-rrhea)* discharge

1. *bradypnea: (brady-)* fast/slow + *(pnea)* breathing
2. *tachypnea: (tachy-)* fast/slow + *(pnea)* breathing
3. *apnea: (a-)* again/not + *(pnea)* breathing
4. *antepartum: (ante-)* after/before + *(partum)* birth
5. *postpartum: (post-)* after/before + *(partum)* birth
6. *amenorrhea: (a-)* not/again + *(meno)* menstruation + *(-rrhea)* discharge
7. *prenatal: (pre-)* after/before + *(nat/o)*birth + *(-al)* condition/pertaining to
8. *probiotic: (pro-)* against/on behalf of + *(bio)* life + *(-tic)* condition/pertaining to
9. *antibiotic: (anti-)* against/on behalf of + *(bio)* life + *(-tic)* condition/pertaining to

EXERCISE 51 *Identify the prefixes for the following definitions.*

1. again ______
2. after ______
3. slow ______
4. fast ______
5. down, away from ______
6. before, on behalf of ______
7. before (2 prefixes) ______
8. not (2 prefixes) ______
9. against (2 prefixes) ______

Learning Outcome 1.5 Exercises

EXERCISE 52 *Match the prefix on the left with its definition on the right. Some definitions will be used more than once.*

______	1. ab-	a.	away
______	2. ad-	b.	toward
______	3. peri-	c.	around
______	4. trans-	d.	through
______	5. ec-	e.	out
______	6. ecto-	f.	outside
______	7. extra-	g.	in, inside
______	8. en-	h.	upon
______	9. intra-	i.	beneath
______	10. epi-	j.	between
______	11. sub-		
______	12. inter-		

EXERCISE 53 *Translate the following prefixes.*

1. sub- ______
2. inter- ______
3. circum- ______
4. dia- ______
5. ab- ______
6. ad- ______
7. epi- ______
8. e-, ec-, ex- ______
9. ecto-, exo-, extra- ______
10. en-, endo-, intra- ______

EXERCISE 54 *Break down the following words into their component parts.*

EXAMPLE: sinusitis *sinus | itis*

1. exhale ______
2. ectoderm ______
3. exoskeleton ______
4. subcutaneous ______
5. epicardium (3 parts) ______
6. pericardium (3 parts) ______
7. transdermal (3 parts) ______
8. intradermal (3 parts) ______
9. epidermal (3 parts) ______
10. extravascular (3 parts) ______
11. pericarditis (3 parts) ______

Learning Outcome 1.5 Exercises

EXERCISE 55 *Underline and define the prefix in the following terms.*

1. transdermal ______
2. exhale ______
3. extravascular ______
4. circumcision ______
5. pericardium ______
6. pericarditis ______
7. subcutaneous ______
8. exoskeleton ______
9. ectoderm ______
10. ectopic ______
11. intercostal ______
12. intravenous ______
13. intradermal ______
14. epidermal ______
15. epicardium ______
16. endometrium ______
17. abduct ______
18. evoke ______
19. diuresis ______
20. enuresis ______

EXERCISE 56 *Translate the following terms.*

1. ectoderm ______
2. exoskeleton ______
3. subcutaneous ______
4. epicardium (3 parts) ______
5. pericardium (3 parts) ______
6. transdermal (3 parts) ______
7. intradermal (3 parts) ______
8. epidermal (3 parts) ______
9. extravascular (3 parts) ______
10. pericarditis (3 parts) ______

Learning Outcome 1.5 Exercises

EXERCISE 57 *Identify the prefixes for the following definitions.*

1. beneath ______
2. between ______
3. upon ______
4. away ______
5. toward ______
6. around (2 prefixes) ______
7. through (2 prefixes) ______
8. in, inside (3 prefixes) ______
9. out (3 prefixes) ______
10. outside (3 prefixes) ______

EXERCISE 58 *Match the prefix on the left with its definition on the right. Some definitions will be used more than once.*

______	1. bi-	a. all
______	2. uni-	b. few
______	3. multi-	c. half
______	4. micro-	d. large
______	5. macro-	e. many
______	6. mono-	f. one
______	7. poly-	g. over
______	8. hyper-	h. small
______	9. hemi-	i. two
______	10. hypo-	j. under
______	11. pan-	
______	12. oligo-	

EXERCISE 59 *Translate the following prefixes.*

1. bi- ______
2. uni- ______
3. multi- ______
4. micro- ______
5. macro- ______
6. mono- ______
7. poly- ______
8. hyper- ______
9. hemi- ______
10. hypo- ______
11. pan- ______
12. oligo- ______

Learning Outcome 1.5 Exercises

EXERCISE 60 *Break down the following words into their component parts.*

EXAMPLE: sinusitis *sinus | itis*

ROOTS: cephal/o *head* cyt/o *cell* nephr/o *kidney* pnea *breathing* uria *urine condition*

1. unisex ______
2. monocyte ______
3. oliguria ______
4. polyuria ______
5. hyperpnea ______
6. hypopnea ______
7. macrocephaly (3 parts) ______
8. microcephaly (3 parts) ______
9. pancytopenia (3 parts) ______
10. heminephrectomy (3 parts) ______

EXERCISE 61 *Underline and define the prefixes in the following terms.*

1. unilateral ______
2. bilateral ______
3. monocyte ______
4. oliguria ______
5. polyuria ______
6. polygraph ______
7. hyperpnea ______
8. hypopnea ______
9. macrocephaly ______
10. microcephaly ______
11. pancytopenia ______
12. heminephrectomy ______
13. panhypopituitarism (2 prefixes) ______

EXERCISE 62 *Translate the following terms.*

ROOTS: cephal/o *head* cyt/o *cell* nephr/o *kidney* pnea *breathing* uria *urine condition*

1. monocyte ______
2. oliguria ______
3. polyuria ______
4. hyperpnea ______
5. hypopnea ______
6. polygraph ______
7. macrocephaly ______
8. microcephaly ______
9. pancytopenia ______
10. heminephrectomy ______

Learning Outcome 1.5 Exercises

EXERCISE 63 *Identify the prefixes for the following definitions.*

1. large __________
2. small __________
3. over __________
4. under __________
5. two __________
6. all __________
7. few __________
8. one (2 prefixes) __________
9. many (2 prefixes) __________
10. half (2 prefixes) __________

EXERCISE 64 *Match the prefix on the left with its definition on the right. Some definitions will be used more than once.*

____	1. syn-	a. bad
____	2. sym-	b. good
____	3. con-	c. with, together
____	4. dys-	
____	5. eu-	

EXERCISE 65 *Translate the following prefixes.*

1. syn- __________
2. sym- __________
3. con- __________
4. dys- __________
5. eu- __________

EXERCISE 66 *Break down the following words into their component parts.*

EXAMPLE: sinusitis *sinus | itis*

ROOTS: dactyl/o *finger* pnea *breathing*

1. dyspnea __________
2. eupnea __________
3. symmetry __________
4. congenital (3 parts) __________
5. syndactyly (3 parts) __________

Learning Outcome 1.5 Exercises

EXERCISE 67 *Underline and define the prefix in the following terms.*

1. congenital ______
2. congestion ______
3. dysuria ______
4. dyspnea ______
5. eupnea ______
6. euthyroid ______
7. syndrome ______
8. symmetry ______

EXERCISE 68 *Translate the following terms.*

ROOTS: dactyl/o *finger* pnea *breathing*

1. dyspnea ______
2. eupnea ______
3. syndactyly ______
4. congenital ______
5. symmetry ______

EXERCISE 69 *Identify the prefixes for the following definitions.*

1. bad ______
2. good ______
3. with, together (3 prefixes) ______

1.6 How to Put Together Medical Terms

Putting It All Together

Now you know about roots, suffixes, and prefixes. There's an additional piece that often goes unnoticed: the *combining vowel.* Take the root *cardio,* which means *heart.* That *o* on the end is optional. It is used when needed to make it easier to combine this root with other word parts. But if it is not needed, it can go away.

So when we say that a word part like *cardio* is a root, we're not speaking precisely. Technically, *cardio* is called a combining form. A *combining form* is a combination of a root with a combining vowel.

So in the example above:

cardi would be the root (which doesn't change)

o would be the combining vowel (which can come or go as needed)

cardi/o would be the combining form (the slash is there to help you tell the difference between the root and combining vowel)

Note: O is by far the most common combining vowel. The letter i is a distant second.

Do Use a Combining Vowel

To join a root to any suffix beginning with a consonant:

splen/o spleen
-megaly enlargement

Root	CV	Suffix	Word	Definition
splen	o	-megaly	splenomegaly	enlargement of the spleen

To join two roots together:

hepat/o liver

Root	CV	Root	CV	Suffix	Word	Definition
hepat	o	splen	o	-megaly	hepatosplenomegaly	enlargement of the liver and spleen

To join two roots together ***even when*** *the second root begins with a vowel:*

gastr/o stomach
enter/o intestine
-logy study of

Root	CV	Root	CV	Suffix	Word	Definition
gastr	o	enter	o	-logy	gastroenterology	study of the stomach and intestine

Don't Use A Combining Vowel

To join a root to a suffix that begins with a vowel:

hepat/o liver
splen/o spleen
cardi/o heart
-ectomy surgical removal
-itis inflammation

Root	CV	Suffix	Word	Definition
hepat		-itis	hepatitis	inflammation of the liver
splen		-ectomy	splenectomy	surgical removal of the spleen
cardi		-itis	carditis	inflammation of the heart

Note: In the last word, the root ends with the same letter that begins the suffix (*cardi* + *itis*). In cases like this, you do not use a combining vowel, and you also drop the final vowel of the root.

Learning Outcome 1.6 Exercises

EXERCISE 1 *Indicate whether the following terms include a combining vowel by underlining the combining vowel.*

EXAMPLE: Root — Word
splen/o — *splenomegaly CV (suffix begins with a consonant)*
splenectomy no CV (suffix begins with a vowel)

ROOTS: cardi/o

1. carditis ____________
2. cardiology ____________
3. cardiomegaly ____________
4. cardiomyopathy ____________
5. cardiovascular ____________
6. bradycardia ____________
7. endocardium ____________
8. pericardiocentesis ____________

EXERCISE 2 *Indicate whether a combining vowel is necessary, and explain why or why not.*

EXAMPLE: Root — Suffix — Combining Vowel?
splen/o — *-megaly* — ☒ *Yes (suffix begins with a consonant)*
☐ *No*

Root	Suffix	Combining Vowel?
1. cardi/o	-gram	☐ Yes ____________ ☐ No ____________
2. gastr/o	-scope	☐ Yes ____________ ☐ No ____________
3. cardi/o	-logist	☐ Yes ____________ ☐ No ____________
4. cardi/o	-megaly	☐ Yes ____________ ☐ No ____________
5. gastr/o	-ic	☐ Yes ____________ ☐ No ____________
6. gastr/o	-dynia	☐ Yes ____________ ☐ No ____________
7. cardi/o	-itis	☐ Yes ____________ ☐ No ____________
8. gastr/o	-itis	☐ Yes ____________ ☐ No ____________
9. cardi/o + my/o	-tomy	☐ Yes ____________ ☐ No ____________
10. gastr/o + esophag/o	-al	☐ Yes ____________ ☐ No ____________

Learning Outcome 1.6 Exercises

EXERCISE 3 *Build a medical term from the information provided.*

EXAMPLE:	Root	Suffix	Term
	splen/o	*-megaly*	*splenomegaly*

Root	Suffix	Term
1. cardi/o	-gram	
2. gastr/o	-scope	
3. cardi/o	-logist	
4. cardi/o	-megaly	
5. gastr/o	-ic	
6. gastr/o	-dynia	
7. cardi/o	-itis	
8. gastr/o	-itis	
9. cardi/o + my/o	-tomy	
10. gastr/o + esophag/o	-al	

1.7 How Medical Terms Are Translated

Think of Medical Terms as Sentences

You can usually figure out the definition of a term by interpreting the

- suffix first
- then the prefix (if one is present)
- then the root or roots

How to translate:

1. Read the word.
2. Say the word out loud.
3. Break the word into parts (suffixes, roots, and prefixes).
4. Translate the parts.
5. Reassemble the pieces into a statement.

Example:

arthritis

1. Read the word:	arthritis
2. Say the word out loud:	ar-THRAI-tis
3. Break the word into parts (suffixes, roots, prefixes):	arthr / itis
4. Translate the parts:	joint / inflammation
5. Reassemble the pieces into one statement:	inflammation of the joint

Here's how this would look in a chart:

Term	Word Analysis
1. arthritis	**3.** arthr / itis
2. ar-THRAI-tis	**4.** joint/inflammation
5. Definition inflammation of the joint	

Some examples are shown to allow you to see the process at work. Don't worry about trying to learn the words themselves right now. They will be taught in later chapters. Right now, focus on getting comfortable with looking at medical terms, breaking them down, and then translating them. The biggest problem people have with medical terms is that they are intimidated by how long or how foreign they look. But if you don't panic and follow these five simple steps, you will be surprised at how quickly you will become comfortable with the language.

Group 1. This group is made up of relatively simple words. Most have just one root and one suffix and the definition is easily deduced from the word analysis.

Term	Word Analysis
angiectomy an-jee-EK-toh-mee	angi / ec / tomy vessel / out / incision
Definition surgical removal of a vessel	
arthritis ar-THRAI-tis	arthr / itis joint / inflammation
Definition inflammation of the joint	
cardiology kar-dee-AW-loh-jee	cardio / logy heart / study of
Definition study of the heart	
hepatitis heh-pah-TAI-tis	hepat / itis liver / inflammation
Definition inflammation of the liver	
myalgia mai-AL-jah	my / algia muscle / pain
Definition pain of muscle	
osteotomy AWS-tee-AW-toh-mee	osteo / tomy bone / incision
Definition incision into a bone	

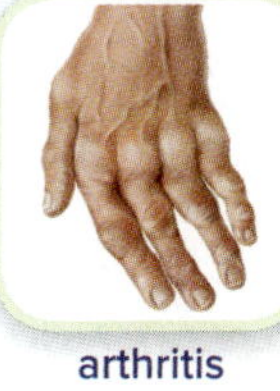
arthritis

Group 2. This group of words contains a little more complex words. The words in this section are made up of at least three parts—either multiple roots or a prefix, root, and suffix.

Term	Word Analysis
angiosclerosis AN-jee-oh-skleh-ROH-sis **Definition** hardening of a blood vessel	angio / scler / osis vessel / hard / condition
cardiopulmonary KAR-dee-oh-PUL-mon-AR-ee **Definition** pertaining to the heart and lungs	cardio / pulmon / ary heart / lung / pertaining to
dermatomycosis der-MAH-toh-mai-KOH-sis **Definition** skin condition caused by fungus	dermato / myc / osis skin / fungus / condition
dysentery dis-en-TER-ee **Definition** bad intestine condition **NOTE:** Another name for severe diarrhea.	dys / enter / y bad / intestine / condition
hepatosplenomegaly heh-PAH-toh-SPLEH-noh-MEH-gah-lee **Definition** enlargement of the liver and spleen	hepato / spleno / megaly liver / spleen / enlargement
hyperplasia hai-per-PLAY-zhah **Definition** overformation condition	hyper / plas / ia over / formation / condition
hypoglycemia hai-poh-glai-SEE-mee-ah **Definition** condition characterized by low sugar in the blood (low blood sugar)	hypo / glyc / emia under / sugar / blood condition
osteocarcinoma AW-stee-oh-KAR-sih-NOH-mah **Definition** bone cancer tumor	osteo / carcin / oma bone / cancer / tumor
osteomyelitis AW-stee-oh-MAI-eh-LAI-tis **Definition** inflammation of the bone marrow	osteo / myel / itis bone / marrow / inflammation
pericardium peh-ree-KAR-dee-um **Definition** tissue around the heart	peri / card / ium around / heart / tissue

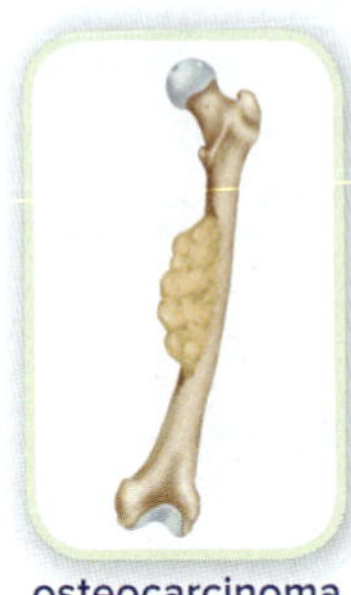
osteocarcinoma

Learning Outcome 1.7 Exercises

EXERCISE 1 *Underline and define the root in the following terms.*

1. cardiology ____________________
2. arthritis ____________________
3. carditis ____________________
4. osteitis ____________________
5. hepatitis ____________________
6. arthralgia ____________________
7. myalgia ____________________
8. ostealgia ____________________
9. myotomy ____________________
10. osteotomy ____________________
11. arthrectomy ____________________
12. hepatectomy ____________________
13. angiectomy ____________________
14. ostectomy ____________________
15. myectomy ____________________

EXERCISE 2 *Underline and define the suffix in the following terms.*

1. cardiology ____________________
2. arthritis ____________________
3. carditis ____________________
4. osteitis ____________________
5. hepatitis ____________________
6. arthralgia ____________________
7. myalgia ____________________
8. ostealgia ____________________
9. myotomy ____________________
10. osteotomy ____________________
11. arthrectomy ____________________
12. hepatectomy ____________________
13. angiectomy ____________________
14. ostectomy ____________________
15. myectomy ____________________

Learning Outcome 1.7 Exercises

EXERCISE 3 *Fill in the blanks.*

EXAMPLE:	Term	Word Analysis
	arthritis	*arthr/itis*
	ar-THRAI-tis	*joint inflammation*

Term	Word Analysis
1. cardiology	cardio / logy heart / ______
2. carditis	card / itis heart / ______
3. osteitis	oste / itis bone / ______
4. hepatitis	hepat / itis liver / ______
5. arthalgia	arth / algia joint / ______
6. myalgia	my / algia muscle / ______
7. ostealgia	oste / algia bone / ______
8. myotomy	myo / tomy muscle / ______
9. osteotomy	osteo / tomy bone / ______
10. arthrectomy	arthr / ec / tomy joint / ___ / ______
11. hepatectomy	hepat / ec / tomy liver / ___ / ______
12. angiectomy	angi / ec / tomy vessel / ___ / ______
13. ostectomy	ost / ec / tomy bone / ___ / ______
14. myectomy	my / ec / tomy muscle / ___ / ______

EXERCISE 4 *Translate the following terms.*

EXAMPLE: sinusitis *inflammation of the sinuses*

1. cardiology ______
2. arthritis ______
3. carditis ______
4. osteitis ______

Learning Outcome 1.7 Exercises

5. hepatitis ______
6. arthralgia ______
7. myalgia ______
8. ostealgia ______
9. myotomy ______
10. osteotomy ______
11. arthrectomy ______
12. hepatectomy ______
13. angiectomy ______
14. ostectomy ______
15. myectomy ______

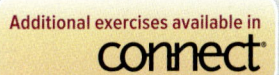

Chapter Review exercises, along with additional practice items, are available in Connect!

review of prefixes, roots, and suffixes

Prefixes	Roots	Suffixes
a- = not	**angi/o** = blood vessel	**-ac** = pertaining to
ab- = away	**arthr/o** = joint	**-al** = pertaining to
ad- = toward	**cardi/o** = heart	**-algia** = pain
an- = not	**derm/o, dermat/o** = skin	**-ar, -ary** = pertaining to
ante- = before	**enter/o** = small intestine	**-cele** = hernia
anti- = against	**gastr/o** = stomach	**-centesis** = puncture
bi- = two	**gen/o** = generation, cause	**-desis** = binding
brady- = slow	**hem/o, hemat/o** = blood	**-dynia** = pain
circum- = around	**hepat/o** = liver	**-eal** = pertaining to
con- = with, together	**hydr/o** = water	**-ectomy** = removal
contra- = against	**morph/o** = change	**-emia** = blood condition
de- = down, away from	**muscul/o** = muscle	**-gram** = written record
dia- = through	**my/o** = muscle	**-graph** = instrument used to produce a record
dys- = bad	**myc/o** = fungus	**-graphy** = process of recording
e- = out	**necr/o** = death	**-ia** = condition
ec- = out	**neur/o** = nerve	**-iasis** = presence of
ecto- = outside	**orth/o** = straight	**-iatrics** = medical science
en- = in, inside	**path/o** = suffering, disease	**-iatrist** = specialist in medicine of
endo- = in, inside	**phag/o** = eat	**-iatry** = medical science
epi- = upon	**plas/o** = formation	**-ic** = pertaining to
eu- = good	**pneum/o, pneumon/o** = lung	**-icle** = small
ex- = out	**pulmon/o** = lung	**-ism** = condition

review of prefixes, roots, and suffixes *continued*

Prefixes	Roots	Suffixes
exo- = outside	**py/o** = pus	**-ist** = specialist
extra- = outside	**scler/o** = hard	**-itis** = inflammation
hemi- = half	**sten/o** = narrowing	**-ium** = tissue, structure
hyper- = over	**troph/o** = nourishment, development	**-logist** = specialist in the study of
hypo- = under	**vas/o, vascul/o** = blood vessel	**-logy** = study of
inter- = between	**xen/o** = foreign	**-lysis** = loosen, break down
intra- = in, inside	**xer/o** = dry	**-malacia** = abnormal softening
macro- = large		**-megaly** = enlargement
micro- = small		**-meter** = instrument used to measure
mono- = one		**-metry** = process of measuring
multi- = many		**-oid** = resembling
oligo- = few		**-ole** = small
pan- = all		**-oma** = tumor
peri- = around		**-osis** = condition
poly- = many		**-ous** = pertaining to
post- = after		**-pathy** = disease
pre- = before		**-penia** = deficiency
pro- = before, on behalf of		**-pexy** = surgical fixation
re- = again		**-plasty** = reconstruction
semi- = half		**-ptosis** = drooping
sub- = beneath		**-rrhage, -rrhagia** = excessive flow
sym- = with, together		**-rrhaphy** = suture
syn- = with, together		**-rrhea** = flow
tachy- = fast		**-rrhexis** = rupture
trans- = through		**-scope** = instrument used to look
uni- = one		**-scopy** = process of looking
		-spasm = involuntary contraction
		-stomy = creation of an opening
		-tic = pertaining to
		-tomy = incision
		-ula, -ula = small
		-y = condition, process

Introduction to Health Records

2

Introduction

Medical records save lives. The information they contain can be critical in patient care. For example, documentation of a patient's allergy to a medication can prevent an adverse, potentially fatal, outcome. Whether found in a paper chart or an electronic health record (EHR), the information contained in a patient's records serves as a roadmap to his or her health history detailing previous illnesses and treatments, continuing medical problems, history of family illnesses, and any current medications. These data provide a clearer picture of the best route to take in future treatment of the patient. With an increasingly busy and time-constrained patient culture, seeking care in multiple places such as emergency rooms and urgent care clinics has become more commonplace. This further fuels the need for thorough documentation, because it is the bedrock of solid communication among health care providers.

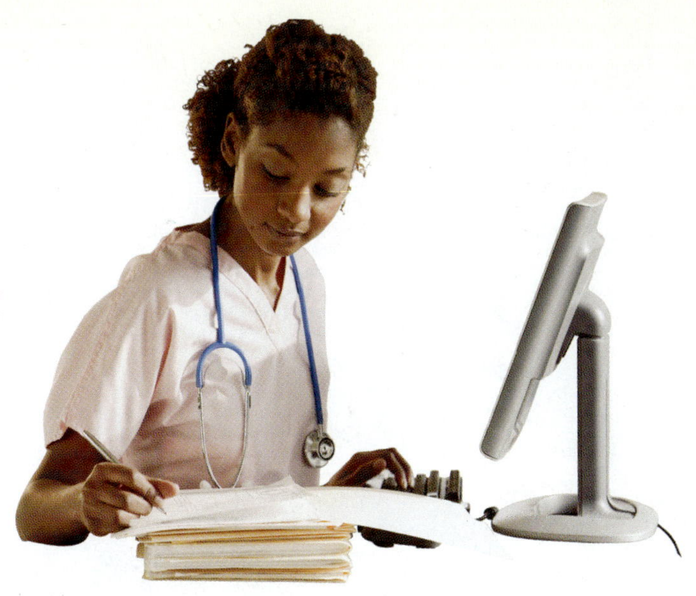

Medical records are an indispensable component of medicine, so it is prudent to be well acquainted with their general layout. There are countless types of medical documents or records in medicine, from routine wellness visits to hospital discharge summaries. Even x-ray reports are medical notes. To the untrained eye, the layout or sheer volume of information of a medical note may be intimidating. In reality, most medical notes share a consistent, logical organization or layout as well as characteristic language. We addressed the concept of medical language in the first chapter and it will be the main focus of this textbook. In this chapter we discuss the organization or layout of medical documents. Having a good grasp on the general flow of medical notes allows for successful navigation through the different elements of a patient's chart so you may find any relevant details you seek.

learning outcomes

Upon completion of this chapter, you will be able to:

2.1 Summarize the **SOAP method.**

2.2 Identify the types of **health records.**

2.3 Use common terms on **health records.**

2.4 Use **abbreviations** associated with health care facilities, patient care, and prescriptions.

2.5 Become familiar with different types of **health records.**

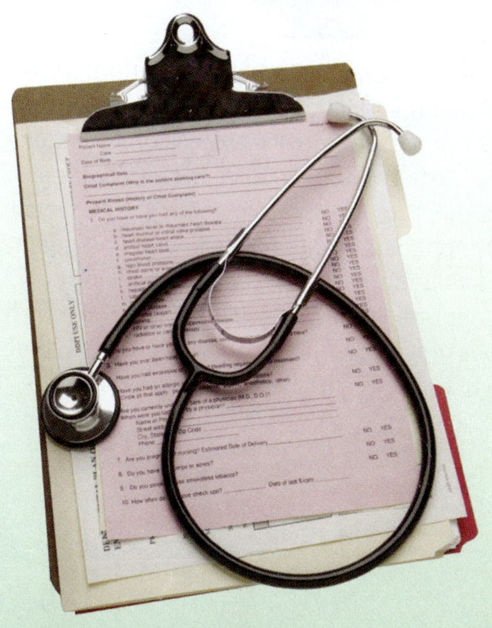

2.1 The SOAP Method

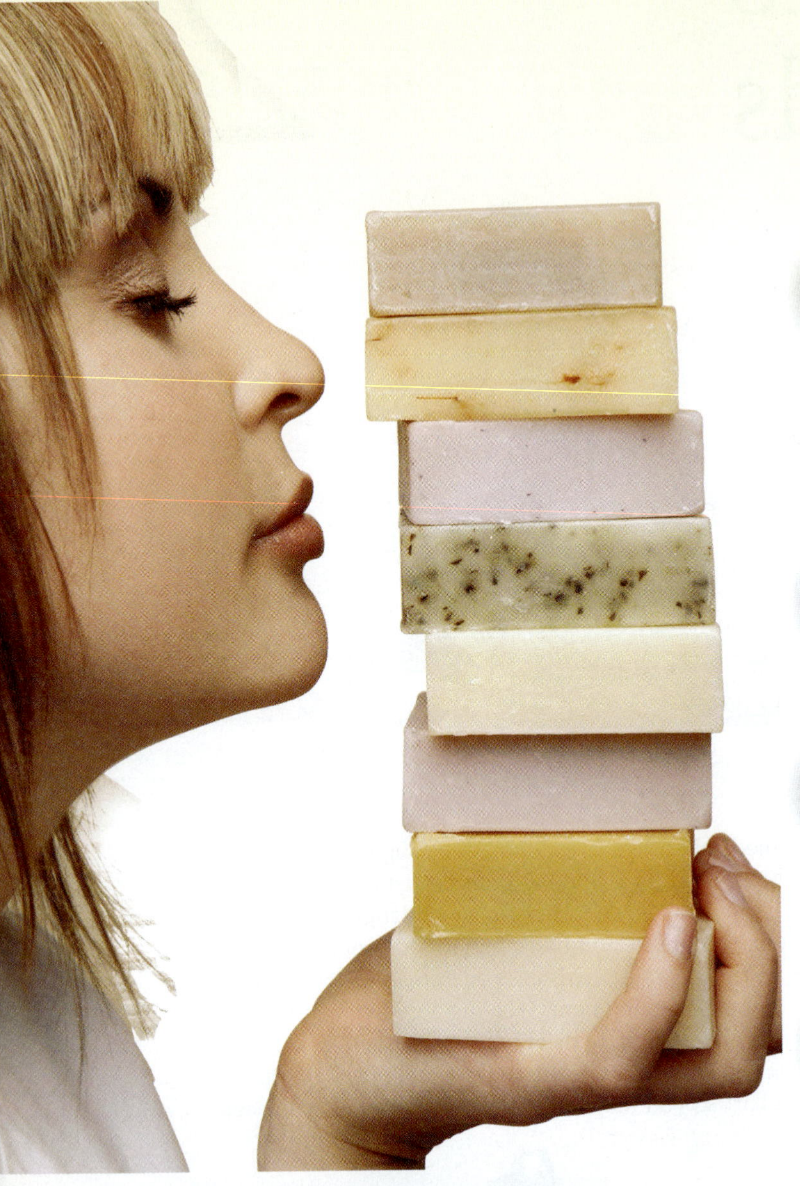

Diagnostic work in medicine is very similar to the investigative work of a detective. By collecting data and using deductive reasoning, a health care provider can make the most accurate assessment of the patient's problem.

Medical notes share a consistent pattern in their organization and layout. This pattern reflects the thought process of health professionals in general. Patient visits typically revolve around addressing a problem. Providers employ a logical approach to solving these problems. In its most rudimentary form, this pattern is presented as what is known as a SOAP note. *SOAP* is an acronym that stands for the four general parts of a medical note: **S**ubjective, **O**bjective, **A**ssessment, and **P**lan.

S The first part of the note is the **subjective** part. It is subject to how a patient experiences and personally describes his or her problem as well as personal and family medical histories. Put simply, it is the problem in the patient's own words. The subjective data include the duration of the problem, the quality of the problem, and any exacerbating or relieving factors for that problem.

O The next step in the investigative process involves collecting **objective** data. Objective data comprise the patient's physical exam, any laboratory findings, and imaging studies performed at the visit.

A Upon gathering all the pertinent information, the health care provider formulates a logical analysis. This is known as the **assessment.** An assessment could be a diagnosis, an identification of a problem, or a list of possibilities for the diagnosis which is known as a differential diagnosis.

P The provider then formulates a **plan,** or a course of action consistent with his or her assessment. The plan could be a treatment with medicine or a procedure. It could also consist of collecting further data to help arrive at a more accurate diagnosis.

The process of collecting subjective history, gathering objective data, formulating an assessment, and developing an action plan is repeated in every health care visit across all disciplines of medicine. It is the baseline of thought in medicine. Consequently, health care records reflect this thought process.

Learning Outcome 2.1 Exercises

EXERCISE 1 *Multiple-choice questions. Select the correct answer.*

1. The *S* in *SOAP* stands for
   a. scrutinize
   b. studies
   c. subjective
   d. survey
2. The *O* in *SOAP* stands for
   a. objective
   b. opinion
   c. order
   d. outline
3. The *A* in *SOAP* stands for
   a. action
   b. appraisal
   c. arrangement
   d. assessment
4. The *P* in *SOAP* stands for
   a. plan
   b. procedure
   c. prognosis
   d. purpose
5. A SOAP note is
   a. a pattern used in writing medical notes
   b. a way of thinking
   c. all of these
   d. none of these
6. A *diagnosis* is
   a. a list of possible causes of the patient's problem or complaint
   b. ordering of more labs
   c. the identification of the actual problem
   d. treatment with medicine or a procedure
7. A *differential diagnosis* is
   a. a list of possible causes of the patient's problem or complaint
   b. ordering of more labs
   c. the identification of the actual problem
   d. treatment with medicine or a procedure

EXERCISE 2 *Match the part of the medical SOAP note on the left with its description on the right.*

_____	1. subjective	a. cause of the problem
_____	2. objective	b. treatment with medicine or a procedure
_____	3. assessment	c. a description of the problem in the patient's own words
_____	4. plan	d. data collected to assist in understanding the nature of the problem

Learning Outcome 2.1 Exercises

EXERCISE 3 *Identify the part of the SOAP note in which the following information would be found.*

EXAMPLE: Ordering of additional lab work to help arrive at the cause *P (Plan)*

1. scheduling of a surgery ________
2. past medical history, family history ________
3. a diagnosis ________
4. patient's description of the problem or complaint ________
5. treatment with medicine ________
6. an identification of the cause of the problem or complaint ________
7. lab results ________
8. determination of how long the patient has suffered from the same complaint ________
9. information forms provided by the patient prior to the appointment ________
10. initial imaging studies (for example, an x-ray) ________
11. differential diagnosis ________
12. ordering of more tests or images ________
13. the patient's exam ________
14. list of possible causes that fit the description of the patient's problem ________

EXERCISE 4 *Give an example of what would be found in each part of the SOAP note.*

1. S–Subjective ________
2. O–Objective ________
3. A–Assessment ________
4. P–Plan ________

2.2 Types of Health Records

From an office setting to the hospital to the operating room, patients receive medical care in many different environments. Consequently, medical documentation of these visits demonstrates differences in their length and format. Regardless of these differences, medical notes continue to follow the same progression, starting from the subjective and ending with the plan. Even radiology and pathology reports exhibit this trend.

Medical records are routinely scoured to find specific information, such as:

- "What medicine did the cardiologist prescribe for the patient?"
- "When is the patient supposed to follow up?"
- "What did the patient have?"

In these instances, subheadings can serve as helpful guideposts. The following table features some common subheadings and their meanings.

The following are descriptions and examples of common types of health care records. As you will notice, they are not complete. The intention is to illustrate how charts are organized. Do not allow yourself to be distracted by any medical terms you have yet to learn. The notes are purposefully color-coded to help emphasize their segment in the SOAP format. The different sections of each note are color-coded in the following manner:

- Subjective: blue
- Objective: red
- Assessment: yellow
- Plan: green (*Note:* Sometimes assessment and plan run together; these instances appear in light green.)

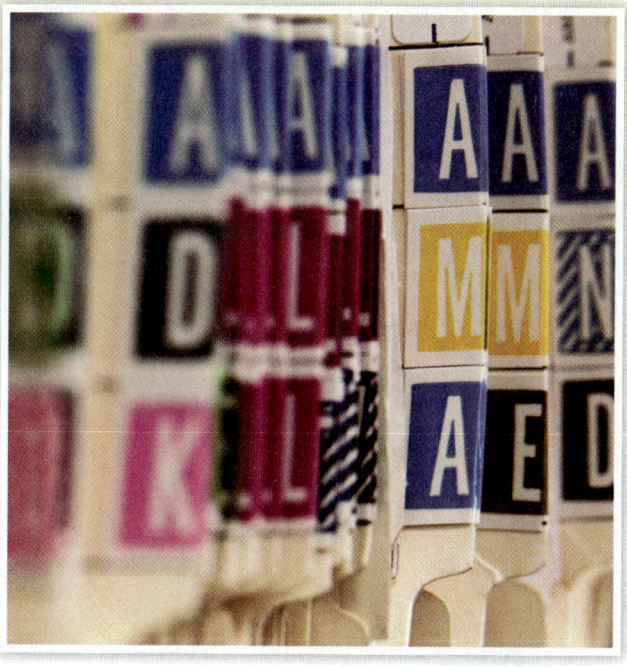

Health records play a vital role in helping organize and document a patient's medical history.

sections of a health record	description
Chief complaint	The main reason for the patient's visit
History of present illness	The story of the patient's problem
Review of systems	Description of individual body systems in order to discover any symptoms not directly related to the main problem
Past medical history	Other significant past illnesses, like high blood pressure, asthma, or diabetes
Past surgical history	Any of the patient's past surgeries
Family history	Any significant illnesses that run in the patient's family
Social history	A record of habits like smoking, drinking, drug abuse, and sexual practices that can impact health

Example Note #1: Clinic Note

Anytime a health care professional sees a patient in an office setting, he or she must document the visit. These notes can be handwritten, dictated, or electronic, or they may involve simply circling the correct words or checking boxes on a template. Regardless of how they are done, these notes always follow the SOAP method. For new patients, there is generally more information in the chart. The SOAP notes for subsequent visits are often more streamlined.

The following is an example of a doctor's office SOAP note.

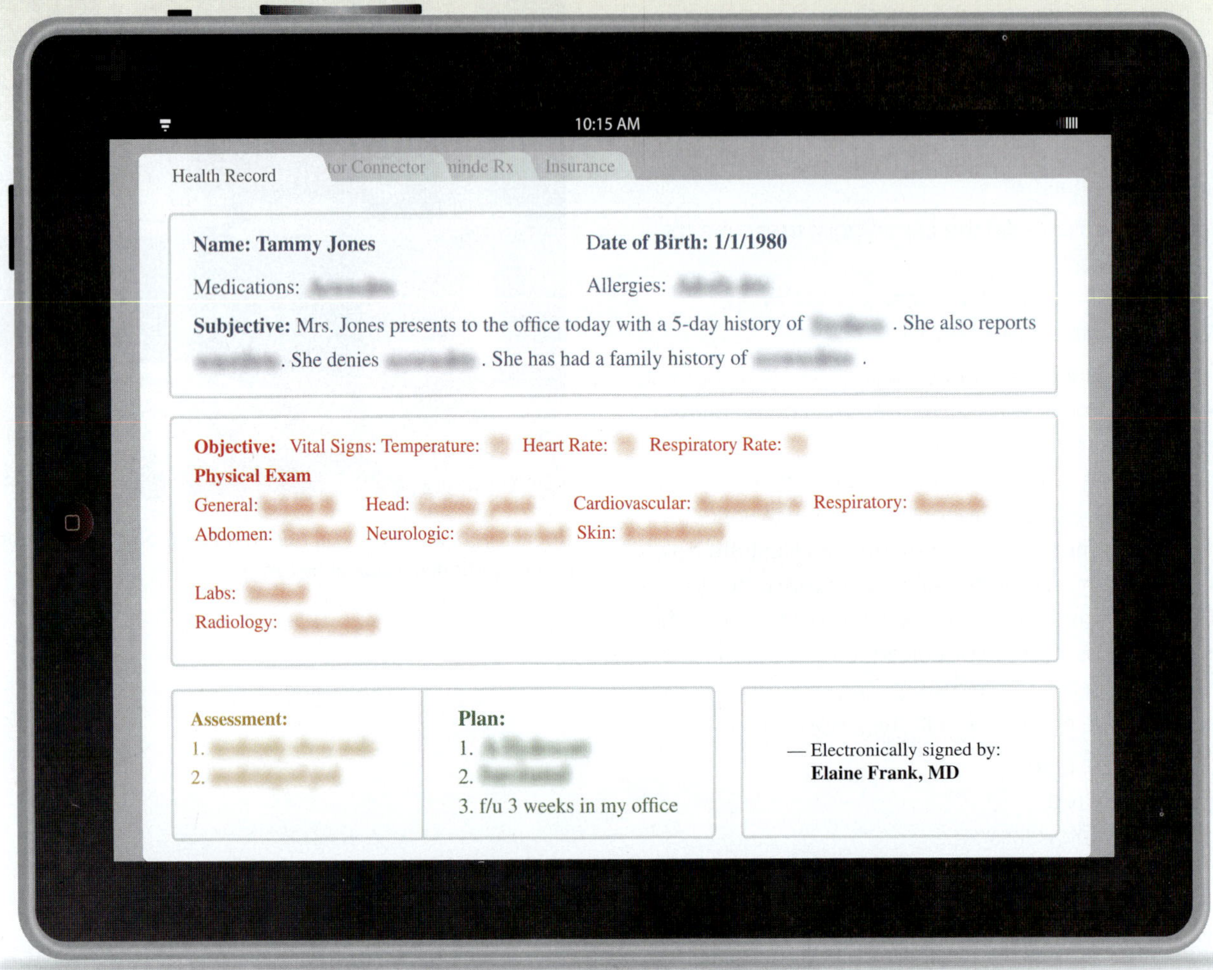

Example Note #2: Consult Note

A note from a visit to a specialist or consultant can take two general types of approaches. The most common format is a note similar to the clinic note. Sometimes, however, the specialist may prefer to write the note in the form of a letter to the primary care provider. Even though the example below is in the form of a letter, you should be able to clearly see the SOAP format.

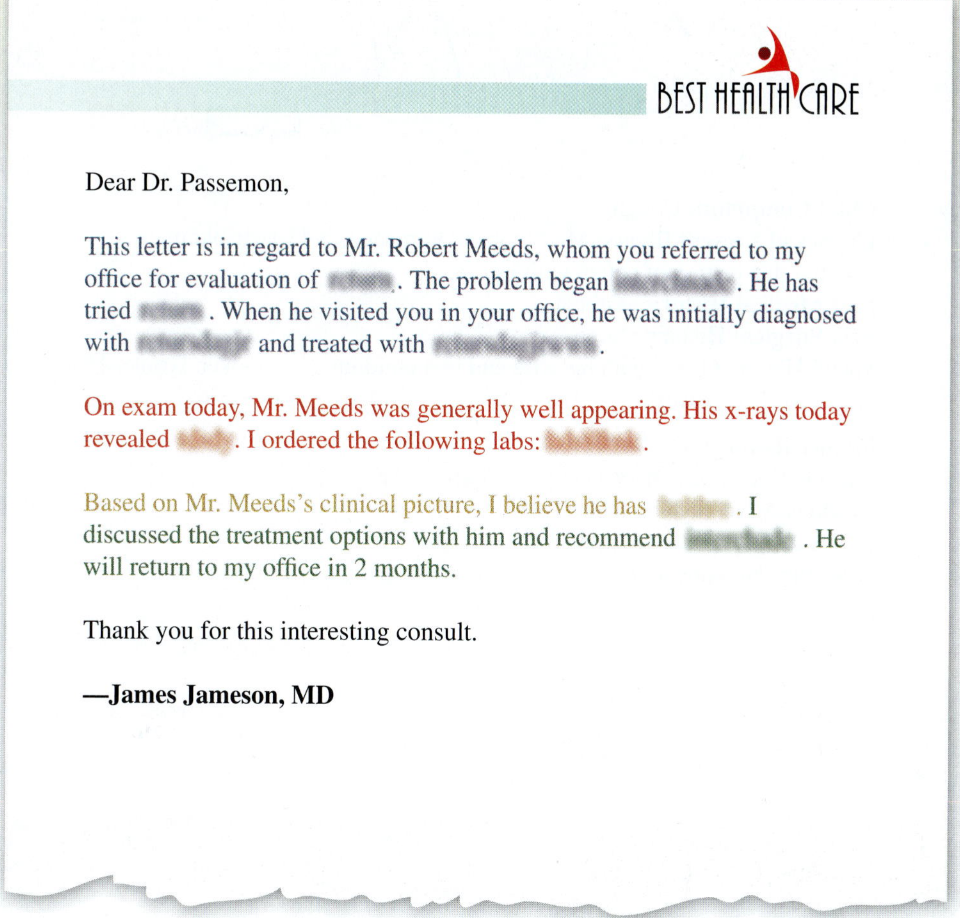

BEST HEALTH CARE

Dear Dr. Passemon,

This letter is in regard to Mr. Robert Meeds, whom you referred to my office for evaluation of [illegible]. The problem began [illegible]. He has tried [illegible]. When he visited you in your office, he was initially diagnosed with [illegible] and treated with [illegible].

On exam today, Mr. Meeds was generally well appearing. His x-rays today revealed [illegible]. I ordered the following labs: [illegible].

Based on Mr. Meeds's clinical picture, I believe he has [illegible]. I discussed the treatment options with him and recommend [illegible]. He will return to my office in 2 months.

Thank you for this interesting consult.

—James Jameson, MD

Example Note #3: Emergency Department Note

Patients seen in emergency departments and urgent care clinics are almost always new to the medical staff. Obtaining a good patient history from an emergency department patient is very important, as information about that patient's past is critical to getting a correct diagnosis in the present. One unique part of these notes is the emergency department (ED) course, which explains what happened to the patient during his or her stay in the ED. The ED course is a mixture of any completed diagnostic tests, the patient assessment, and a plan for the patient that unfolds over time.

CLINIC CORNER

Chief Complaint: Cough.
History of Present Illness: Mr. Stephen Dufresne is a 43-year-old male with a 3-day history of cough with .
Past Medical History: Asthma.
Past Surgical History: None.
Social History: Lives with his wife and two children. Nonsmoker. Drinks 4 glasses of wine a week.

Family History:
Father: Deceased at 68 years of age from stroke.
Mother: Alive, high blood pressure.
Medications: Albuterol, prn.
Allergies: No known drug allergies.

Physical Exam:
Vital Signs: Temperature: Heart Rate: Respiratory Rate:
General:
Head:
Cardiovascular:
Respiratory:
Abdomen:
Neurologic:
Skin:

Emergency Department Course:
Mr. Dufresne arrived to the emergency department in no apparent distress. A chest x-ray showed . We treated him with oxygen and . After two treatments of albuterol, he improved. He was diagnosed with and treated with .

Disposition:
Discharged to home, with follow-up in 3 days with his PCP.

—Christine Christenson, MD

Example Note #4: Admission Summary

Upon admittance to the hospital, patients must provide a medical history and receive a physical exam. Afterward, the attending medical professional writes a detailed admission summary. Detailed admission summaries are usually thorough notes that are very heavy on the subjective and objective parts, because the idea of the summary is to assemble all the facts in one place to help direct the entire hospital course.

- The assessment, which usually describes the thought process behind a patient's diagnosis and a list of possible causes for the patient's problem, is known as a *differential diagnosis.*
- The plan portion of the summary usually involves further testing, as well as care for the patient.

In a problem-based approach, the assessment and plan portions of the summary will be placed together. In such an approach, the patient's problems are numbered. After each number, the problems are described. The description is followed with a plan of what will be done about the problems.

Occasionally, a hospital team will send a courtesy letter to the patient's primary care provider (PCP). This letter can be similar to an admission note, but is usually briefer.

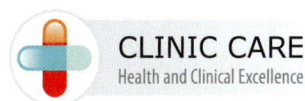

SUBJECTIVE

Chief Complaint: Chest pain.

History of Present Illness: Mr. William Burns is a 45-year-old male with a 2-month history of [illegible].
Review of Systems: Positive for [illegible].
Medications: None.
Allergies: No known drug allergies.
Past Medical History: [illegible].
Past Surgical History: Tonsillectomy/adenoidectomy at 3 years of age.
Social History: 1-pack-per-day smoker, social alcohol intake, divorced. Denies risky sexual behavior.
Family History: Father passed away at [illegible].

OBJECTIVE

Vital Signs: Temp: [illegible] Heart Rate: [illegible] Respiratory Rate: [illegible] Blood Pressure: [illegible]

Physical Exam:

General: [illegible]
Head: [illegible]
Cardiovascular: [illegible]
Respiratory: [illegible]
Abdomen: [illegible]
Neurologic: [illegible]
Skin: [illegible]

Labs: [illegible]

Imaging: [illegible]

Assessment/Plan:

1. **Chest Pain:** The differential diagnosis includes [illegible].
2. **Elevated Blood Sugar:** He did have a large meal [illegible].

—Madison Ginger, MD

Example Note #5: Discharge Summary

A discharge summary note details when and why a patient was admitted. It includes how the patient felt when admitted, what happened during the patient's stay in the hospital, and what kind of follow-up the patient will have. Sometime, the hospital course description of a discharge summary will be broken down into body systems.

A discharge summary can break from the general SOAP pattern in one significant way: Often, the note will lead with the diagnoses—both the initial and also the final—because medical professionals want the most important information to come first. In all other respects it is similar to an emergency department note—but the discharge summary documents a longer stay in the hospital.

CLINIC CARE
Health and Clinical Excellence

DATE OF ADMISSION:
DATE OF DISCHARGE:

ADMISSION DIAGNOSIS:

1.
2.

DISCHARGE DIAGNOSIS:

1.

DISCHARGE CONDITION: Stable

CONSULTATIONS: Pulmonology

PROCEDURES:

1.
2.

LABS:

IMAGING: Chest x-ray

HPI:

Ms. Regina Klebs is a 28-year-old woman admitted to hospital from the ED with pneumonia. She initially presented with .

HOSPITAL COURSE:

Ms. Klebs was admitted to the hospital and placed on oxygen and IV antibiotics.

DISCHARGE PHYSICAL EXAMINATION:

Vital Signs: Temperature: Heart Rate: Respiratory Rate:

Physical Exam:

General:
Head:
Cardiovascular:
Respiratory:
Abdomen:
Neurologic:
Skin:

ACTIVITY: No restrictions.
DIET:
MEDS: Topical penicillin antibiotic ointment.
FOLLOW-UP: Appointment—PCP (Dr. Primo) in 1 week.

—Francis Jerome, MD

Example Note #6: Operative Report

After each surgery, the surgeon completes an operative report that documents in detail the procedure that was performed, the events that transpired during the surgery, and the patient's outcome from the surgery. As with a discharge summary, the diagnosis is presented at the beginning of the note.

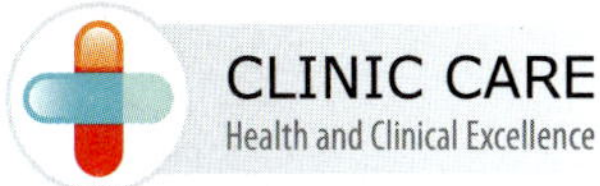

Preoperative Diagnosis: Appendicitis
Postoperative Diagnosis: Appendicitis

Procedure: Appendectomy
Anesthesia: General

Indication: The patient, Wallace Simpson, is a 25-year-old man with acute onset of abdominal pain and fever.

Operative Findings: The patient had a grossly inflamed appendix and local peritonitis.

Description of Procedure: Mr. Simpson was brought to the operating room with suspected appendicitis. Mr. Simpson tolerated the procedure well.

Disposition: Mr. Simpson was sent to the PACU in stable condition.

—James Cutter, MD

Example Note #7: Daily Hospital Note/Progress Note

Every day that a patient is in the hospital, a health care professional must see him or her and document the visit. Usually, the subjective part of these daily hospital notes focuses on how the patient's condition has changed since the previous note. Often, the note's assessment and plan sections will be put together, as with an admission note.

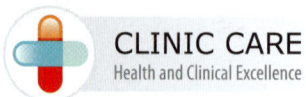

Subjective:

Since yesterday, the patient, Mrs. Penelope Gates, has vomited 3 times.

Objective:

Vital Signs: Temp: [illegible] Heart Rate: [illegible] Respiratory Rate: [illegible]
Intake: [illegible] Output: [illegible]

Physical Exam:

General: [illegible]
Head: [illegible]
Cardiovascular: [illegible]
Respiratory: [illegible]
Abdomen: [illegible]
Neurologic: [illegible]
Skin: [illegible]
Labs: [illegible]

Assessment/Plan:

1. Acute gastroenteritis: No change. Continue IV fluids.
2. Metabolic acidosis: Noticed this AM on lab work. We will begin the patient on [illegible].

—Harry Harrison, MD

Example Note #8: Radiology Report

A radiology report note explains the reason for ordering a radiologic image, how the image was performed, what was seen on the image, and the reviewing radiologist's assessment. Sometimes the note provides a recommendation as well. When a recommendation is provided, it is usually a recommendation for a different type of image, or a request to repeat the same image in a certain time frame.

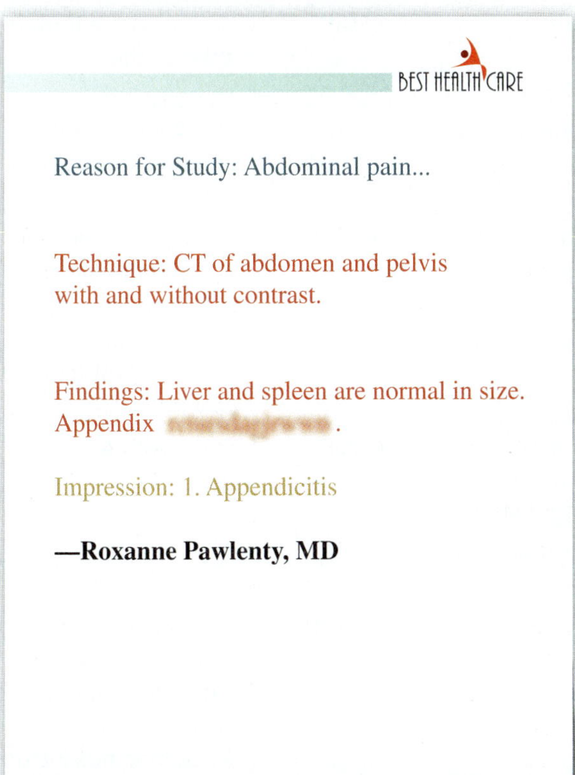

Example Note #9: Pathology Report

A pathology report note mirrors the same style as the radiology note. This note mentions the reason for the study, what was seen in detail, and the assessment.

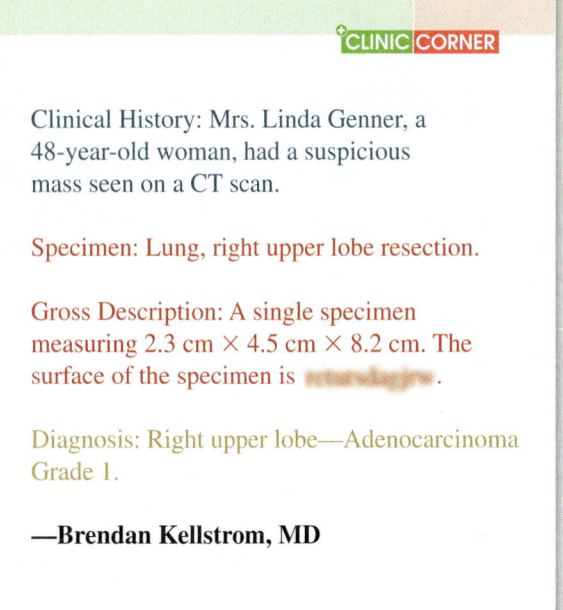

Example Note #10: Prescription

This type of note doesn't follow the SOAP note format—because it *is* the plan. A prescription form has a structure all its own:

- The first line is for the name and strength of the medicine. In the name blank, the health care professional may write either the generic name of the actual medicine (for example, ibuprofen) or a name brand (for example, Advil).
- The second line, marked "Sig," contains the patient's instructions. On the prescription form, these instructions are written in medical language; it is the pharmacist's job to translate these instructions into lay terms for the patient.
- The third line, usually marked "Dispense," tells the pharmacist how much medicine to give the patient.
- The fourth line mentions how many refills are available for the prescription.
- The prescription form's last line is for the health care provider's signature (either written or electronic). It usually includes a box the health care provider can check to indicate whether the prescribed medication must be a brand name (instead of generic). Please note that with the increasing use of electronic medical records, the use of certain, specific medical terms (such as *BID* or *QHS*) are becoming less common in prescriptions. Nonetheless, it is important to be familiar with these terms as they have not completely disappeared.

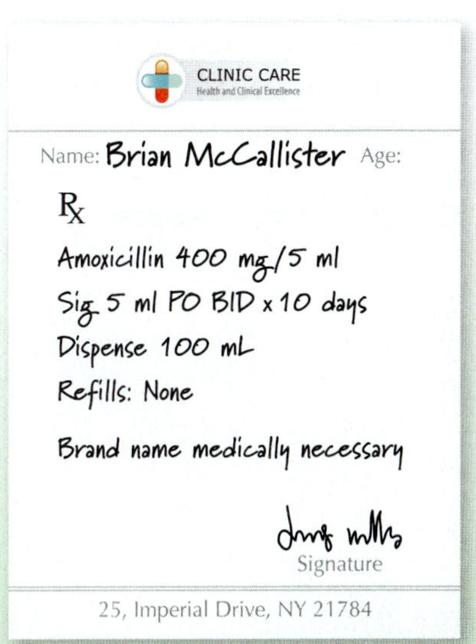

summary of health record notes

	Author	Location	Purpose	Format and Order	Unique Features
1. Clinic note	Medical professional	Clinic	Documents a visit	SOAP	New patient: Includes more history, separate form Repeat patient: Streamlined note
2. Consult note	Physician; usually a specialist	Clinic or hospital	Provides an expert opinion on a more challenging problem	SOAP	Can be in the form of a letter to the PCP
3. Emergency department note	ED medical staff	Emergency department	Documents an emergency department visit	SOAP	The A includes the emergency department course
4. Admission summary	Hospital medical professional	Hospital	Documents the admission of a patient to the hospital	SO A/P	S, O = Very thorough A = Differential diagnosis P = Further testing and care A + P = Problem-based approach
5. Discharge summary	Medical professional	Hospital	Describes when and why the patient was admitted; documents a longer stay	ASOP	Starts with A
6. Operative report	Surgeon		Documents a surgery in detail	ASOP	
7. Daily hospital note/ progress note	Medical professional	Inpatient health care facility	Documents daily hospital visit	SO A/P	S—Focuses on how patient's condition has changed since the previous note A—Sometimes includes a differential diagnosis
8. Radiology report	Radiologist		Explains reason for image, how image was performed, what was seen on image, radiologist's assessment; sometimes a recommendation	SOA	Usually includes only S, O, and A, but may include a P if it recommends that further studies should be performed
9. Pathology report	Pathologist		Provides reasons for test, what was seen on the test, and an assessment	SOA	
10. Prescription	Medical professional		Provides directions for a medication	P	1. Medicine's name 2. Instructions for patient 3. How much medicine should be given 4. Refills, if any 5. Health care professional's signature and whether generic substitution is allowed

Learning Outcome 2.2 Exercises

EXERCISE 1 *Match the health record type on the left with its description on the right.*

______ 1. prescription

______ 2. radiology report

______ 3. pathology report

______ 4. daily hospital note/progress note

______ 5. emergency department note

______ 6. admission summary

______ 7. operative report

______ 8. clinic note

______ 9. consult note

______ 10. discharge summary

a. documents a patient visit in an office setting

b. document sent to a primary physician, usually by a specialist, to give an opinion on a more challenging problem

c. documents a patient's emergency department visit

d. documents a patient's admission to the hospital

e. documents a patient's admission and hospital stay (usually a longer stay)

f. documents a surgery

g. documents a patient's progress during a daily hospital visit

h. documents an imaging procedure by a radiologist

i. documents a pathology procedure

j. a medical professional's directions for a patient's medication

EXERCISE 2 *Match the term on the left with its definition on the right.*

______ 1. past surgical history

______ 2. family history

______ 3. past medical history

______ 4. history of present illness

______ 5. social history

______ 6. chief complaint

______ 7. review of systems

a. the main reason for a visit

b. the story of the patient's problem

c. any symptoms not directly related to the main problem

d. other significant past illnesses, like high blood pressure, asthma, or diabetes

e. any past surgeries

f. any significant illnesses that run in the patient's family

g. mainly health habits, like smoking, drinking, drug use, or sexual practices

EXERCISE 3 *Multiple-choice questions. Select the correct answer.*

1. Which health record does NOT follow the SOAP format?
   a. consult note
   b. daily hospital note
   c. emergency department note
   d. prescription
2. Which type of health record is sometimes found in the form of a letter?
   a. clinic note
   b. consult note
   c. daily hospital note
   d. pathology report

Learning Outcome 2.2 Exercises

3. Select the health records that document a type of procedure:
   a. discharge summary
   b. emergency department note
   c. operative report
   d. pathology report
   e. prescription
   f. radiology report
4. Which health record is NOT routinely used in a hospital or inpatient health care facility?
   a. admission summary
   b. clinic note
   c. discharge summary
   d. emergency department note
   e. progress note
5. Which health record would be used to document a routine pediatric wellness exam?
   a. clinic note
   b. consult note
   c. daily hospital note
   d. operative report
6. In a *problem-based approach*, you
   a. number the problems, describe how the patient's problem has changed, and provide your plan for what to do about the problem
   b. focus on what you are doing wrong and who should take over
   c. try to cause more problems in the patient in the hopes of determining what is really wrong
   d. assume that nothing has been done right so far and redo every test
7. An *emergency department course*
   a. explains what transpired during the patient's stay in the emergency department; it includes any diagnostic tests done, the assessment, and a plan for the patient that unfolds over time
   b. lists the path every patient takes when entering the emergency department for treatment
   c. organizes an emergency department by types of injury
   d. teaches students how to behave in an emergency department

EXERCISE 4 *Identify the author of each of the following types of health records.*

1. pathology report ______________________________
2. operative report ______________________________
3. radiology report ______________________________
4. emergency department note ______________________________
5. consult note ______________________________

Learning Outcome 2.2 Exercises

EXERCISE 5 *Fill in the blanks based on the sample health record.*

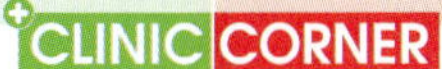

Subjective:

Mrs. Allison Voxenhead is here for a follow-up visit for her schizophrenia. At her last visit, she complained of dystonia on her haloperidol. I changed her to a newer antipsychotic medication at that time, and she is here today to follow up the results. Overall, she is improved and has not had any new hallucinations. Her only concern today is recent insomnia for the past week. She noticed the insomnia started when she began a new job, and she says that learning her new job has been stressful. She has been anxious at night, and that has made it hard for her to sleep.

Objective:

General: Flat affect. Nonagitated. Mood is not dysphoric. Alert, oriented.
HEENT: Pupils equal, round, and reactive to light. Tonsils normal size.
Resp: Clear to auscultation.
CV: RRR without murmur, gallop, rubs.
Neuro: Normal movement. No dyskinesia. Normal tone.

Assessment:

1. Schizophrenia: stable on new medication regimen.
2. Insomnia likely related to new job stress.

Plan:

1. I will begin her short term on an anxiolytic.
2. Continue antipsychotic.
3. Follow-up visit in 2 months.
4. Continue following with psychologist.

Electronically signed by:
Dale Philbert, PA 03/04/2015 9:30 AM

1. The health record type is: ______________________
2. The patient's name is: ______________________
3. The author of the health record is: ______________________
4. The patient has been diagnosed with: ______________________ and ______________________
5. The format of the health record is: ______________________

Learning Outcome 2.2 Exercises

EXERCISE 6 *Based on the sample health record, fill in the blanks and label parts as noted in Question #5 that follows.*

BEST HEALTH CARE

Dear Dr. Childs,

Thank you for referring Mr. Juan Samuels to my office. I saw him on March 3, 2014. Mr. Samuels has a 4-month history of increasing pain in his right distal femur. He first noticed pain after being kicked in the leg at a soccer game. He was evaluated in your office 3 weeks later for persistent pain. There was a soft tissue mass in his distal femur that was tender to touch. An x-ray was performed to rule out a fracture or chronic osteomyelitis. The x-ray showed both osteolysis of the metaphysis and periosteal new bone formation. Labs were drawn, including CBC, CPK, and ESR. Mr. Samuels was referred to my office for further evaluation of the concerning x-ray findings.

5(a) Health Record Part ______

On exam, Mr. Samuels was a pleasant young man, well developed, well nourished, and in no acute distress. His lungs were clear, and his heart was regular in rate and rhythm. No murmurs were heard. His right leg reveals a significant soft tissue mass over his distal femur on the right. The mass is tender. He did not have any knee effusion. I reviewed the labs and x-ray. His findings were consistent with osteosarcoma.

5(b) Health Record Part ______

I discussed the next steps with the patient and family, including staging the tumor and scheduling a biopsy to confirm the diagnosis. I discussed the surgery with the patient and his family present in the office. His tumor will likely require tumor resection with partial ostectomy of the femur with osteoplasty.

I discussed the benefits of a metal endoprosthesis versus an allograft for the osteoplasty.

5(c) Health Record Part ______

Mr. Samuels is scheduled to return to my office in 1 week after his biopsy to discuss the results.

Thank you for this interesting consult.

—Tara Sanchez, MD, FAAOS

1. The health record type is: ______________________________
2. The patient's name is: ______________________________
3. The author of the health record is: ______________________________
4. Some of the patient's symptoms (reason for the visit) include: ______________________________
5. In the blanks alongside the sample, label the correct parts of the health record using the letter associated with each section.

   S–Subjective A–Assessment

   O–Objective P–Plan

Learning Outcome 2.2 Exercises

EXERCISE 7 *Based on the sample health record, fill in the blanks and label parts as noted in Question #4 that follows.*

CLINIC CORNER

Discharge Summary

Patient Name: Decker Woolsey

DATE OF ADMISSION: 1/1/15
DATE OF DISCHARGE: 1/4/15

ADMISSION DIAGNOSIS:
1. Hypotonia
2. Scoliosis

4(a) Health Record Part ______

DISCHARGE DIAGNOSIS:
1. Muscular dystrophy
2. Scoliosis

4(b) Health Record Part ______

DISCHARGE CONDITION:
Stable

4(c) Health Record Part ______

CONSULTATIONS:
Neurology
Cardiology
Orthopedic surgery

4(d) Health Record Part ______

PROCEDURES:
1. Electromyography
2. Muscle biopsy

4(e) Health Record Part ______

LABS:
CBC, CMP, CPK, ESR

4(f) Health Record Part ______

IMAGING:
None

4(g) Health Record Part ______

HPI:
Decker Woolsey is an 8-year-old boy admitted directly to the pediatric floor for a workup of chronic progressive hypotonia. His parents report they have noticed progressive weakness. Decker has had increasing difficulty running, jumping, and climbing stairs. Decker's parents initially thought his problems were due to his asthma, but they noticed he also had a waddling gait. They took him to their PCP, who referred him for evaluation. On admission, the patient denied any history of myalgia, arthrodynia, or dystaxia. His problem appeared limited to muscle tone.

4(h) Health Record Part ______

HOSPITAL COURSE:
NEURO: On admission exam, the patient was found to have mild lumbar lordosis, pseudohypertrophy of his calf muscles, and a waddling gait.He did not have any genu varum or genu valgus. No hyporeflexia was noted. The initial concern was a muscular dystrophy. Given a family history of polymyositis, that was considered as well. His labs were consistent with muscular dystrophy.

-1-

CLINIC CORNER

An electromyography showed myopathic changes. A muscle biopsy was then performed to help distinguish which of the muscular dystrophies the patient had. The results are pending.
CV: Cardiology was consulted, given the strong risk for developing cardiomyopathy.
RESP: No problems occurred throughout hospital stay. Education was given about breathing exercises and the respiratory problems that are frequently seen later on with this condition.
ORTHO: Orthopedic surgery was consulted for his scoliosis.
SOCIAL: Much of the hospital stay focused on patient education.

4(i) Health Record Part ______

DISCHARGE PHYSICAL EXAMINATION:

Temp 98.6 RR 24 HR 86 BP 100/64
Gen: WDWN. Alert.
CV: RRR.
RESP: CTA.
NEURO: Hypotonia of legs (strength 3/5 bilaterally). Waddling gait. Using assistance to get up from seated position. Normal reflexes. Marked enlargement of calves.

4(j) Health Record Part ______

ACTIVITY:

No restrictions. Referral to PT on discharge. First appointment is next week.

4(k) Health Record Part ______

DIET:

Calcium/vit D supplement to prevent osteoporosis.

4(l) Health Record Part ______

MEDS:

Glucocorticoid.

4(m) Health Record Part ______

FOLLOW-UP:

Appointments:
PCP: Dr. Bening in 1 week
Neurology: Dr. Schwarz in 2 weeks
Cardiology: Dr. Benitez in 6 months
Orthopedic: Dr. Jawarz in 6 months

4(n) Health Record Part ______

-2-

1. The health record type is: ______________________
2. The patient's name is: ______________________
3. This health record was written at a(n): ______________________
4. In the blanks alongside the sample, label the correct parts of the health record using the letter associated with each section.

   S–Subjective   A–Assessment

   O–Objective   P–Plan

Learning Outcome 2.2 Exercises

EXERCISE 8 *Based on the sample health record, fill in the blanks, select the correct response, or label parts as noted in Question #3 that follows.*

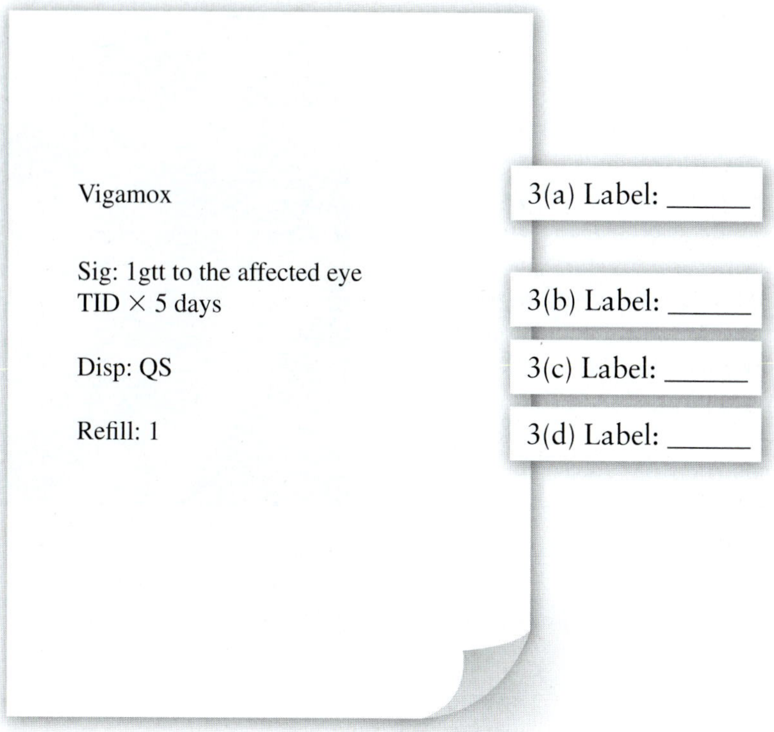

Vigamox
3(a) Label: ______
Sig: 1gtt to the affected eye
TID × 5 days
3(b) Label: ______
Disp: QS
3(c) Label: ______
Refill: 1
3(d) Label: ______

1. The health record type is: ______________________________
2. Which part of the SOAP note is included in this health record (select the correct choice)?
   a. S–Subjective
   b. O–Objective
   c. A–Assessment
   d. P–Plan
3. In the blanks alongside the sample, label the correct parts of the health record using the letter associated with each section.
   a. name and strength of the medicine
   b. patient instructions
   c. how much medicine to give the patient
   d. refill information

2.3 Common Terms on Health Records

Your Future Second-Nature Words

Just as various sports have their own special words, such as *rebound, home run,* and *touchdown,* health records have special words that are essential to know. While the main purpose of this book is to help you use the roots of ancient words to break down medical words, you must also know many commonly used medical words that are not necessarily based on ancient languages.

When you have been working in the medical field long enough, these words will become second nature to you. You will use them so often that they will become part of your normal vocabulary. This chapter will introduce you to those terms so you will be better able to understand the stories told in health records.

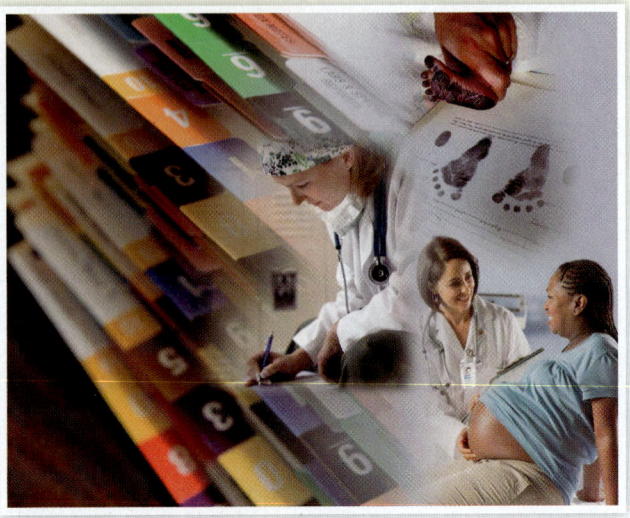

Just like any other specialized field, medicine has a whole host of words that sound strange the first time but become second nature the more you use them.

Subjective

As you recall, the subjective section of a health record tells the patient's personal story of his or her health issue. It includes things such as:

- the main reason for the health visit
- the description of his or her problem
- the timing of the problem
- previous medical problems or surgeries
- family health problems that might relate
- current medications and allergies

In describing the chief concern, you may include when the problem began, the severity, any associated problems, and whether anything seems to make the problem better or worse.

general subjective terms

Term	Definition
acute ah-KYOOT	it just started recently or is a sharp, severe symptom
chronic KRAH-nik	it has been going on for a while now
exacerbation ek-SAS-er-BAY-shun	it is getting worse
abrupt ah-BRUPT	all of a sudden
febrile FEH-brail	to have a fever
afebrile AY-FEH-brail	to not have a fever
malaise mah-LAYZ	not feeling well
progressive proh-GREH-siv	more and more each day
symptom SIM-tom	something a patient feels
noncontributory NON-kon-TRIH-byoo-TOR-ee	not related to this specific problem
lethargic lah-THAR-jik	a decrease in level of consciousness; in a medical record, this is generally an indication that the patient is really sick
genetic/hereditary jih-NEH-tik, hah-REH-dih-TEH-ree	it runs in the family

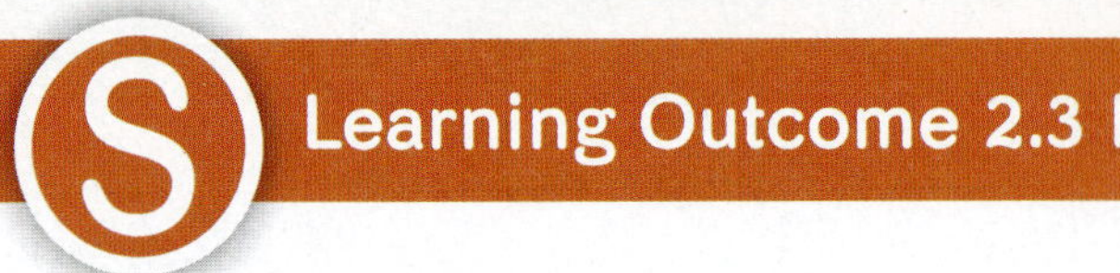

Learning Outcome 2.3 Exercises

PRONUNCIATION

EXERCISE 1 *Break down the following words into syllables.*

EXAMPLE: synesthesia *syn | es | the | sia*

1. abrupt ____________
2. hereditary ____________
3. afebrile ____________
4. exacerbation ____________
5. noncontributory ____________

EXERCISE 2 *Indicate which syllable is emphasized when pronounced.*

EXAMPLE: bronchitis bronchitis (emphasized syllable underlined: "chi")

1. progressive ____________
2. lethargic ____________
3. genetic ____________
4. febrile ____________

EXERCISE 3 *Match the term on the left with its definition on the right.*

	Term		Definition
____	1. symptom	a.	something a patient feels
____	2. progressive	b.	a decrease in the level of consciousness
____	3. chronic	c.	symptoms recently began
____	4. febrile	d.	symptoms have been present for a while
____	5. afebrile	e.	to have a fever
____	6. acute	f.	not feeling well
____	7. malaise	g.	to not have a fever
____	8. lethargic	h.	more and more each day

EXERCISE 4 *Translate the following terms.*

1. genetic ____________
2. noncontributory ____________
3. hereditary ____________
4. abrupt ____________
5. chronic ____________
6. lethargic ____________
7. exacerbation ____________
8. malaise ____________
9. afebrile ____________

EXERCISE 5 *Identify the medical term from the definition provided.*

1. a problem that runs in the family ____________
2. unrelated to the specific problem ____________
3. a problem that recently began ____________
4. all of a sudden ____________
5. more and more each day ____________
6. a problem that is getting worse ____________
7. something a patient feels ____________
8. to not have a fever ____________

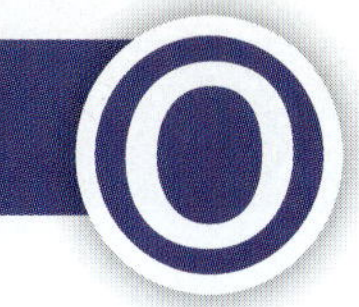

Objective

The objective part of a health record tells about the data collected during the health care provider's interaction with the patient. What does the provider notice about the patient when he or she examines the patient closely? How does the patient look, sound, feel, smell? It also includes any extra data obtained by tests done in a laboratory or by special images of the patient's body.

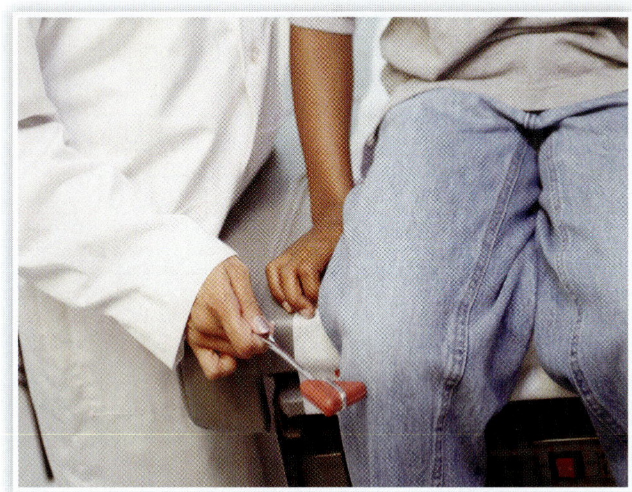

One piece of objective information is measuring a patient's muscle reflexes.

general objective terms

Term	Definition
alert ah-LERT	able to answer questions; responsive; interactive
oriented OR-ee-EN-ted	being aware of who he or she is, where he or she is, and the current time; a patient who is aware of all three is "oriented × 3"
marked MARKT	it really stands out
unremarkable un-ree-MARK-ah-bul	another way of saying normal
auscultation aw-skul-TAY-shun	to listen
percussion per-KUH-shun	to hit something and listen to the resulting sound or feel for the resulting vibration; drums are a percussion instrument
palpation pal-PAY-shun	to feel

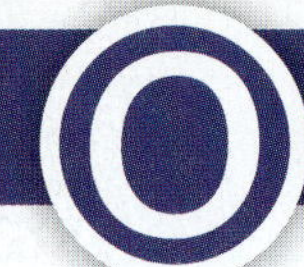

Learning Outcome 2.3 Exercises

EXERCISE 6 *Break down the following words into syllables.*

EXAMPLE: synesthesia *syn | es | the | sia*

1. oriented ______________________
2. auscultation ______________________
3. marked ______________________

EXERCISE 7 *Indicate which syllable is emphasized when pronounced.*

EXAMPLE: bronchitis bronchitis

1. alert ______________________
2. unremarkable ______________________
3. palpation ______________________

EXERCISE 8 *Match the term on the left with its definition on the right.*

	Term		Definition
______	1. unremarkable	a.	able to answer questions; responsive; interactive
______	2. alert	b.	able to identify one's name and location, the time of day, and the date
______	3. marked	c.	something that really stands out
______	4. percussion	d.	normal
______	5. oriented	e.	to listen
______	6. auscultation	f.	to feel
______	7. palpation	g.	to hit something and listen to the sound or feel for the vibration

EXERCISE 9 *Translate the following terms.*

1. marked ______________________
2. unremarkable ______________________
3. percussion ______________________
4. oriented ______________________
5. auscultation ______________________
6. palpation ______________________

EXERCISE 10 *Identify the medical term from the definition provided.*

1. to listen ______________________
2. to feel ______________________
3. normal ______________________
4. something that really stands out ______________________
5. able to answer questions; responsive; interactive ______________________
6. to hit something and listen to the sound or feel for the vibration ______________________

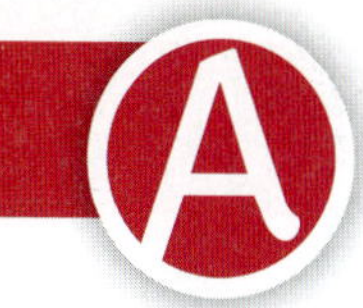

Assessment

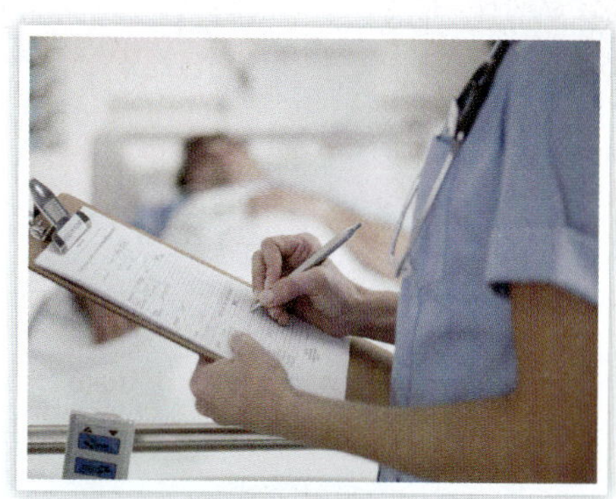

Once the facts from the patient are recorded and data about the patient are collected, it is time to put it all together to reach a conclusion on the nature of the problem. This is known as the diagnosis. Sometimes one exact problem is not so obvious at first. In these cases, a health care provider may list the most likely causes, called a differential diagnosis. In addition to a diagnosis, the provider may offer other opinions, like severity of the problem and the chances for improvement.

general assessment terms

Term	Definition
impression im-PREH-shun	another way of saying assessment
diagnosis DAI-ag-NOH-sis	what the health care professional thinks the patient has
differential diagnosis dih-fer-EN-shal DAI-ag-NOH-sis	a list of conditions the patient may have based on the symptoms exhibited and the results of the exam
benign beh-NAIN	safe
malignant mah-LIG-nant	dangerous; a problem
degeneration dee-jin-er-AY-shun	to be getting worse
etiology ee-tee-AW-loh-jee	the cause
remission reh-MIH-shun	to get better or improve; most often used when discussing cancer; *remission* does not mean cure
idiopathic ih-dee-oh-PA-thik	no known specific cause; it just happens
localized LOH-kah-LAIZD	stays in a certain part of the body
systemic/generalized sih-STEM-ik, jin-er-ah- LAIZD	all over the body (or most of it)
morbidity mor-BID-ih-tee	the risk for being sick
mortality mor-TA-lih-tee	the risk for dying
prognosis prawg-NOH-sis	the chances for things getting better or worse
occult ah-KULT	hidden
pathogen PATH-oh-jin	the organism that causes the problem
lesion LEE-shun	diseased tissue
recurrent ree-KUR-ent	to have again
sequelae seh-KWEL-ah	a problem resulting from a disease or injury
pending PEN-ding	waiting for

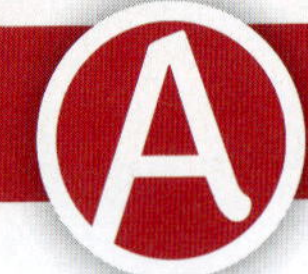

Learning Outcome 2.3 Exercises

EXERCISE 11 *Break down the following words into syllables.*

EXAMPLE: synesthesia *syn | es | the | sia*

1. localized ______
2. diagnosis ______
3. differential diagnosis ______
4. degeneration ______
5. idiopathic ______
6. generalized ______
7. lesion ______
8. recurrent ______

EXERCISE 12 *Indicate which syllable is emphasized when pronounced.*

EXAMPLE: bronchitis bronchitis

1. impression ______
2. malignant ______
3. remission ______
4. systemic ______
5. morbidity ______
6. mortality ______
7. pathogen ______
8. prognosis ______
9. pending ______

EXERCISE 13 *Match the term on the left with its definition on the right.*

	Term		Definition
______	1. degeneration	a.	assessment
______	2. differential diagnosis	b.	what the health care professional thinks the patient has
______	3. diagnosis	c.	a list of conditions the patient may have based on the symptoms exhibited and the results of the exam
______	4. impression	d.	to be getting worse
______	5. remission	e.	the cause
______	6. mortality	f.	to get better or improve; most often used when discussing cancer; does not mean *cure*
______	7. prognosis	g.	no known specific cause; it just happens
______	8. morbidity	h.	the risk for being sick
______	9. pathogen	i.	the risk for dying
______	10. idiopathic	j.	the chances for things getting better or worse
______	11. etiology	k.	the organism that causes the problem
______	12. sequelae	l.	a problem resulting from a disease or injury

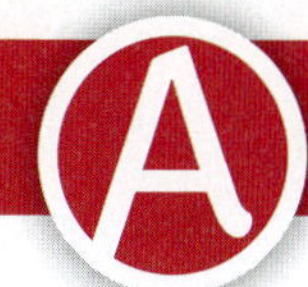

Learning Outcome 2.3 Exercises

EXERCISE 14 *Translate the following terms.*

1. systematic ____________
2. generalized ____________
3. localized ____________
4. occult ____________
5. lesion ____________
6. recurrent ____________
7. pending ____________
8. benign ____________
9. malignant ____________
10. impression ____________
11. degeneration ____________
12. remission ____________
13. pathogen ____________
14. sequelae ____________

EXERCISE 15 *Identify the medical term from the definition provided.*

1. safe ____________
2. dangerous; a problem ____________
3. stays in a certain part of the body ____________
4. all over the body ____________
5. a list of things that the patient may have, based on symptoms and exam ____________
6. what the medical professional thinks the patient may have ____________
7. the cause ____________
8. no known specific cause ____________
9. the chances for things to get better or worse ____________
10. risk for being sick ____________
11. risk for dying ____________
12. hidden ____________
13. diseased tissue ____________
14. to have again ____________
15. waiting for ____________

Plan

In the health record, the plan lays out what the provider recommends to do about the patient's current health status. This may include medicine or home remedies, help from another health provider, surgery, or even waiting to see if the problem will improve on its own. Sometimes the plan is for more data collection to be done in the future to help figure out the true cause of the problem.

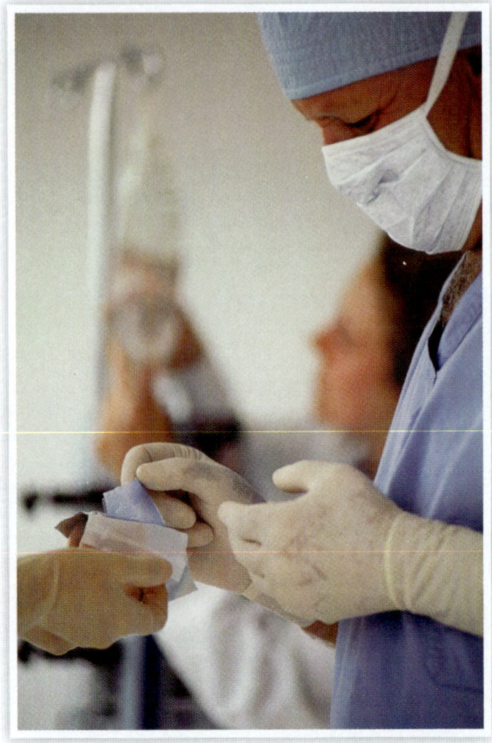

Once an assessment has been made, a course of action is decided upon. This plan can include everything from observation to medication and surgery.

general plan terms

Term	Definition
disposition dis-poh-ZIH-shun	what happened to the patient at the end of the visit; often used at the end of ED notes to reference where the patient went after the visit (home, the ICU, normal hospital bed)
discharge DIS-charj	literally, to *unload*; it has two meanings: 1. to send home (to unload the patient from the health care setting to home) 2. fluid coming out of a part of the body (your body unloading a fluid)
prophylaxis PROH-fuh-LAK-sis	preventive treatment
palliative PA-lee-ah-tiv	treating the symptoms, but not actually getting rid of the cause
observation OB-zer-VAY-shun	watch, keep an eye on
reassurance ree-ah-SHUR-ants	to tell the patient that the problem is not serious or dangerous
supportive care suh-POR-tiv kehr	to treat the symptoms and make the patient feel better
sterile STEH-ril	extremely clean, germ-free conditions; especially important during medical procedures and surgery

Learning Outcome 2.3 Exercises

EXERCISE 16 *Break down the following words into syllables.*

EXAMPLE: synesthesia *syn | es | the | sia*

1. discharge ______
2. disposition ______
3. observation ______
4. reassurance ______
5. supportive care ______

EXERCISE 17 *Match the term on the left with its definition on the right.*

	Term		Definition
____	1. sterile	a.	what happens to the patient at the end of the visit
____	2. observation	b.	to send home
____	3. disposition	c.	preventive treatment
____	4. discharge	d.	treating the symptoms but not actually getting rid of the cause
____	5. reassurance	e.	keep an eye on
____	6. supportive care	f.	to tell the patient that the problem is not serious or dangerous
____	7. prophylaxis	g.	to treat the symptoms and make the patient feel better
____	8. palliative	h.	extremely clean, germ-free conditions; especially important during medical procedures and surgery

EXERCISE 18 *Translate the following terms.*

1. reassurance ______
2. sterile ______
3. discharge ______
4. observation ______
5. disposition ______
6. supportive care ______
7. palliative ______
8. prophylaxis ______

EXERCISE 19 *Identify the medical term from the definition provided.*

1. to send home ______
2. to keep an eye on ______
3. extremely clean, germ-free conditions ______
4. what happens to the patient at the end of the visit ______
5. preventive treatment ______
6. to treat the symptoms to make the patient feel better ______
7. treating the symptoms but not actually getting rid of the cause ______
8. to tell the patient that the problem is not serious/dangerous ______

Body Planes and Orientation

In giving directions, being more specific leads to more accurate results. The same goes for describing parts of the body. Often, the words used to describe directions in the body are opposites, such as north and south. Following is more information about these body specific opposites.

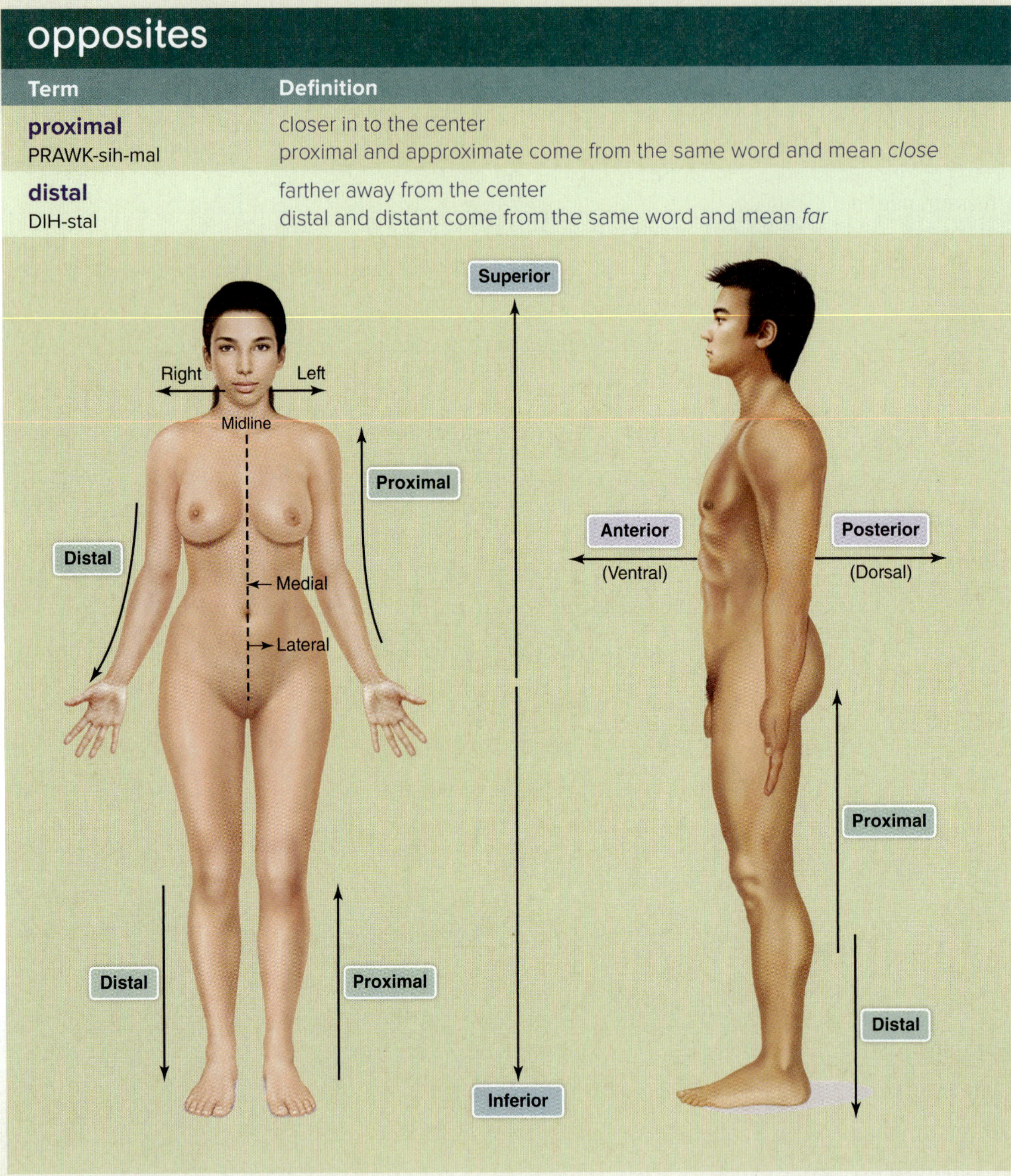

opposites

Term	Definition
proximal PRAWK-sih-mal	closer in to the center proximal and approximate come from the same word and mean *close*
distal DIH-stal	farther away from the center distal and distant come from the same word and mean *far*

opposites *continued*

lateral LA-ter-al	out to the side think of a quarterback lateraling a football to a running back
medial MEE-dee-al	toward the middle like the median of a highway
ventral/antral/ anterior VEN-tral/AN-tral/ an-TIH-ree-or	the front the word *ventral* means *stomach*
dorsal/posterior DOR-sal/ poh-STIH-roh-or	the back a dorsal fin on a shark is on its back
cranial KRAY-nee-al	toward the top
caudal KOW-dal	toward the bottom from Latin, for *tail*

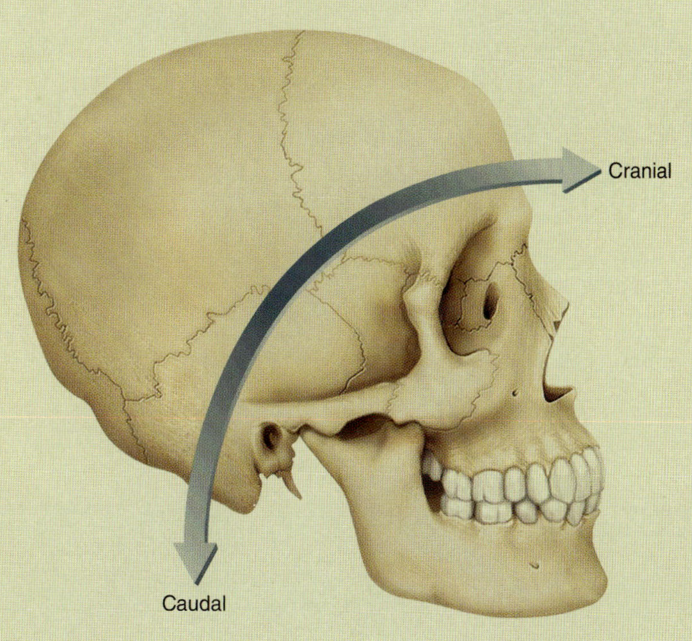

superior soo-PIH-ree-or	above
inferior in-FIH-ree-or	below

opposites *continued*

prone PROHN	lying down on belly
supine SOO-pain	lying down on back

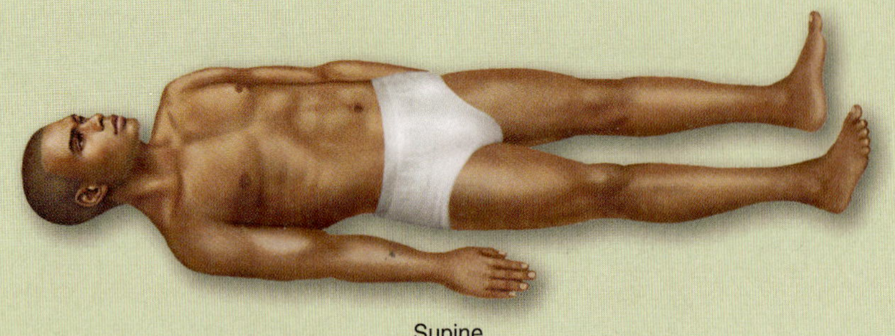
Supine

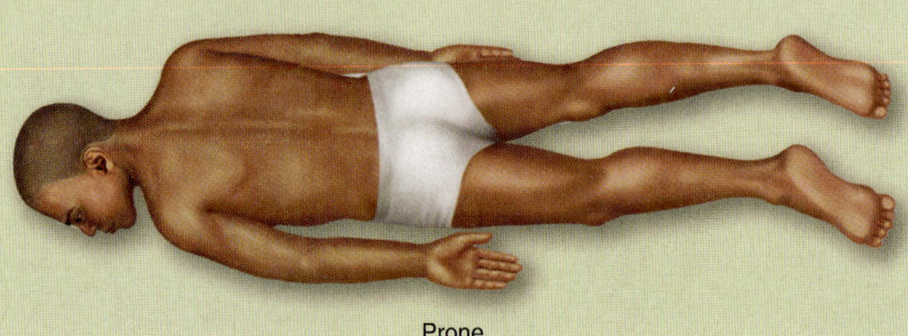
Prone

contralateral KON-trah-LA-ter-al	opposite side
ipsilateral IP-sih-LA-ter-al	same side

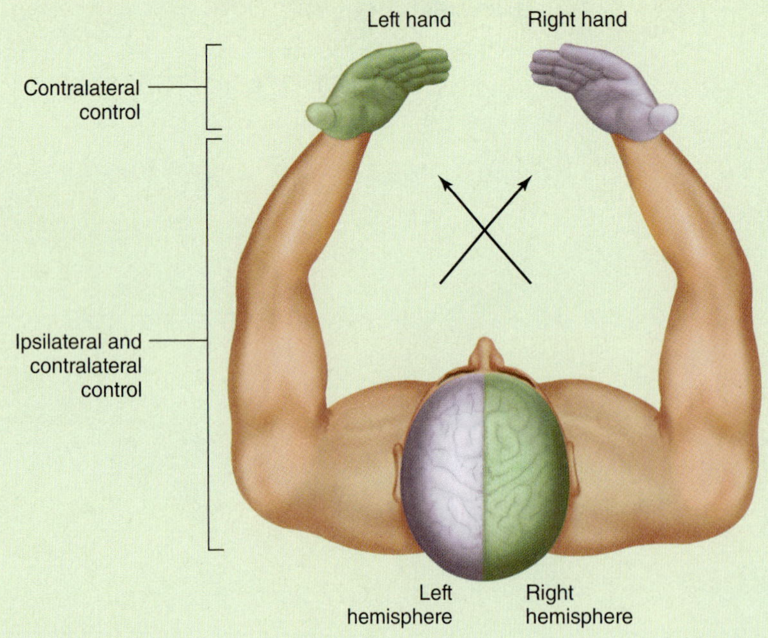

opposites *continued*

Term	Definition
unilateral YOO-nih-LA-teral	one side
bilateral BAI-LA-ter-al	both sides

Unilateral Bilateral

Term	Definition
dorsum DOR-sum	the top of the hand or foot
plantar PLAN-tar	the sole of the foot
palmar PAL-mar	the palm of the hand

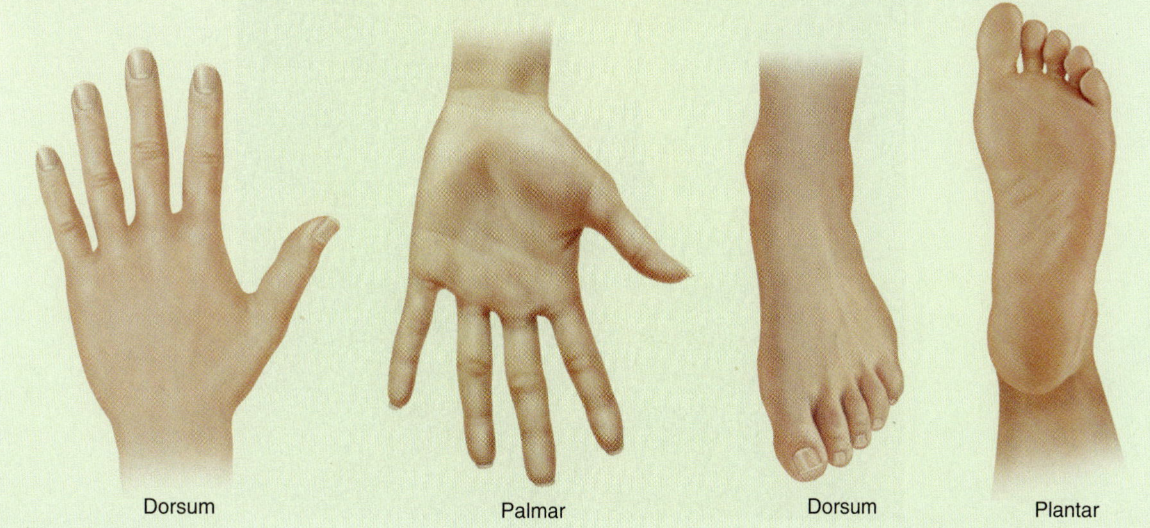

BODY PLANES

Another way of looking at the body is through the three dimensions: right to left (sagittal), front to back (coronal), and top to bottom (transverse). This is especially important in radiology. For instance, a CT scan is actually a series of layered images along one of these dimensions.

body planes

Term	Definition
sagittal SA-jih-tal	divides the body in slices right to left *sagitta* is Latin for *arrow*; think of this as dividing the body in half, as if someone shot an arrow through it.
coronal kah-ROH-nal	divides the body into slices from front to back *corona* is Latin for *crown*; this plane divides the body in half from the top of the head down
transverse tranz-VERS	divides the body from top to bottom

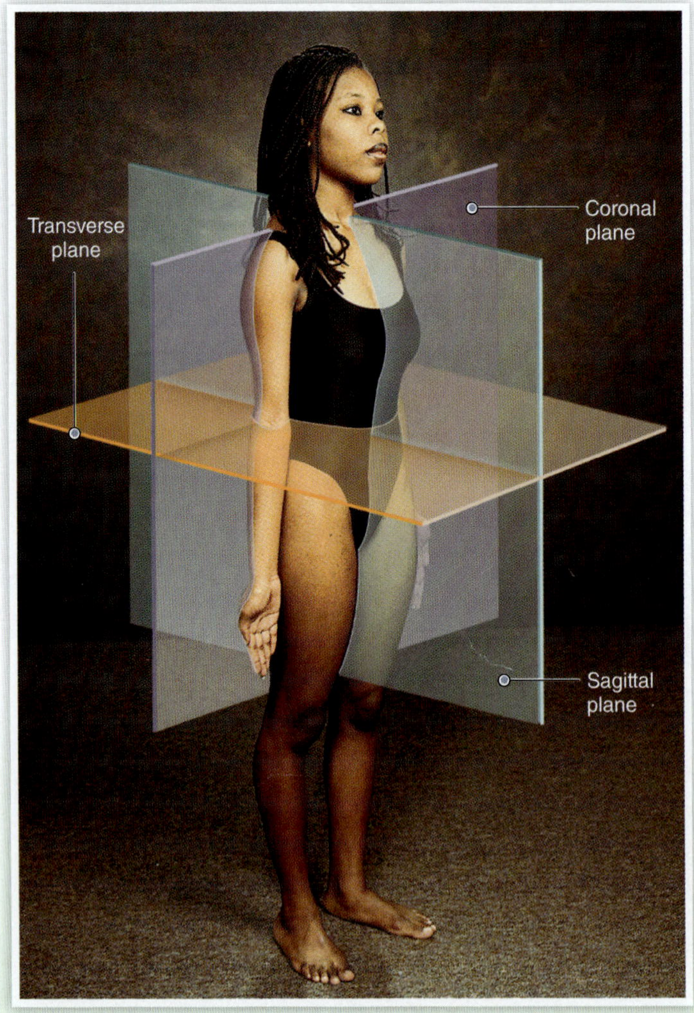

Learning Outcome 2.3 Exercises

EXERCISE 20 *Break down the following words into syllables.*

EXAMPLE: synesthesia syn / es / the / sia

1. prone ______
2. lateral ______
3. contralateral ______
4. ipsilateral ______
5. unilateral ______
6. bilateral ______
7. posterior ______
8. superior ______
9. inferior ______
10. cranial ______

EXERCISE 21 *Indicate which syllable is emphasized when pronounced.*

EXAMPLE: bronchitis bronchitis

1. proximal ______
2. distal ______
3. ventral ______
4. antral ______
5. dorsal ______
6. dorsum ______
7. plantar ______
8. palmar ______
9. coronal ______
10. transverse ______

EXERCISE 22 *Match the term on the left with its definition on the right.*

h	1. bilateral	a. the back
e	2. contralateral	b. the front
f	3. ipsilateral	c. lying down on the belly
g	4. unilateral	d. lying down on the back
i	5. transverse	e. opposite side
a	6. dorsal	f. same side
c	7. prone	g. one side
k	8. coronal	h. both sides
d	9. supine	i. divides the body from top to bottom
b	10. antral	j. divides the body in slices right to left
j	11. sagittal	k. divides the body in slices from front to back

Learning Outcome 2.3 Exercises

EXERCISE 23 *Translate the following terms.*

1. posterior ______________________
2. cranial ______________________
3. caudal ______________________
4. superior ______________________
5. plantar ______________________
6. palmar ______________________
7. transverse ______________________
8. sagittal ______________________
9. contralateral ______________________
10. ventral ______________________

EXERCISE 24 *Identify the medical term from the definition provided.*

1. farther away from the center ______________________
2. closer in to the center ______________________
3. out to the side ______________________
4. toward the middle ______________________
5. toward the top ______________________
6. the top of the hand or foot ______________________
7. one side ______________________
8. divides the body in slices from front to back ______________________
9. lying down on the back ______________________
10. below ______________________

EXERCISE 25 *Identify the opposite for the given term.*

EXAMPLE: cranial *caudal*

1. proximal ______________________
2. lateral ______________________
3. ventral ______________________
4. anterior ______________________
5. inferior ______________________
6. prone ______________________
7. ipsilateral ______________________
8. bilateral ______________________
9. palmar ______________________

2.4 Abbreviations

Abbreviations Associated with Health Care Facilities

With more than 82 million people worldwide now sending text messages on a regular basis, it's no wonder that phrases like "LOL," "JK," and "OMG" have become commonly understood abbreviations. Why do people use them? Efficiency.

This love affair with abbreviations was going on in the world of medicine long before text messaging, mobile phones, and even computers arrived on the scene. Whether that's because it is more efficient to cut down a word to a few letters or because it makes these terms somehow seem more important, acronyms and abbreviations are commonplace in health records.

These abbreviations refer to various types of treatment facilities within the medical profession.

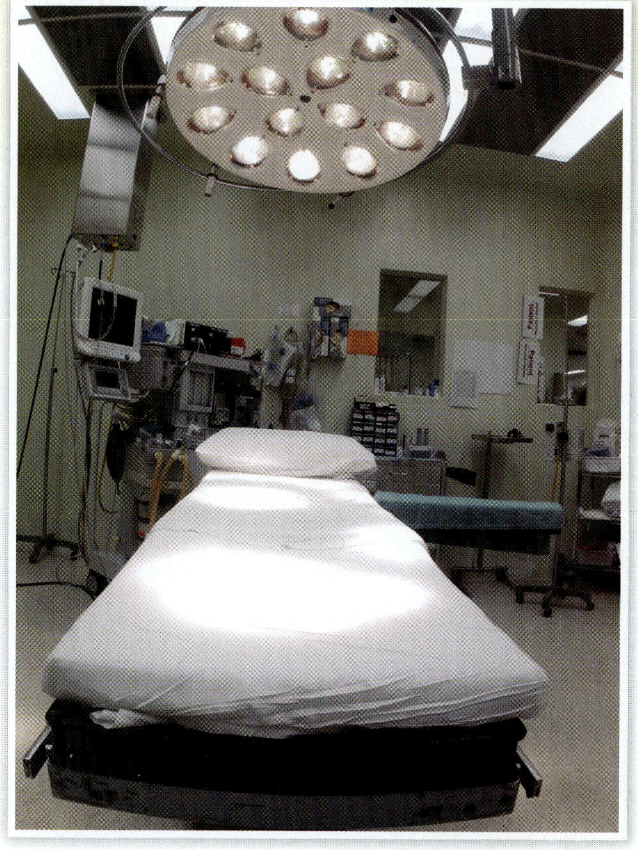

Abbreviations are used to describe a wide variety of health care facilities.

health care facility abbreviations

Abbreviation	Definition
CCU	coronary care unit
ECU	emergency care unit
ER	emergency room
ED	emergency department
ICU	intensive care unit
PICU	pediatric intensive care unit
NICU	neonatal intensive care unit
SICU	surgical intensive care unit
PACU	postanesthesia care unit
L&D	labor and delivery
OR	operating room
post-op	after surgery
pre-op	before surgery

Learning Outcome 2.4 Exercises

EXERCISE 1 *Match the abbreviation on the left with its definition on the right.*

_______ 1. pre-op	a.	coronary care unit
_______ 2. post-op	b.	emergency room
_______ 3. ER	c.	emergency department
_______ 4. ICU	d.	intensive care unit
_______ 5. ED	e.	neonatal intensive care unit
_______ 6. CCU	f.	surgical intensive care unit
_______ 7. L&D	g.	labor and delivery
_______ 8. NICU	h.	after surgery
_______ 9. SICU	i.	before surgery

EXERCISE 2 *Translate the following abbreviations.*

1. ER ________________
2. OR ________________
3. ICU ________________
4. PICU ________________
5. NICU ________________
6. SICU ________________
7. CCU ________________
8. ECU ________________
9. PACU ________________

EXERCISE 3 *Identify the abbreviation given the information provided.*

1. after surgery ________________
2. before surgery ________________
3. emergency department ________________
4. labor and delivery ________________
5. operating room ________________
6. emergency care unit ________________
7. pediatric intensive care unit ________________
8. post-anesthesia care unit ________________

Abbreviations Associated with Patient Care

These abbreviations are typical of the ones found on patient charts and other health records.

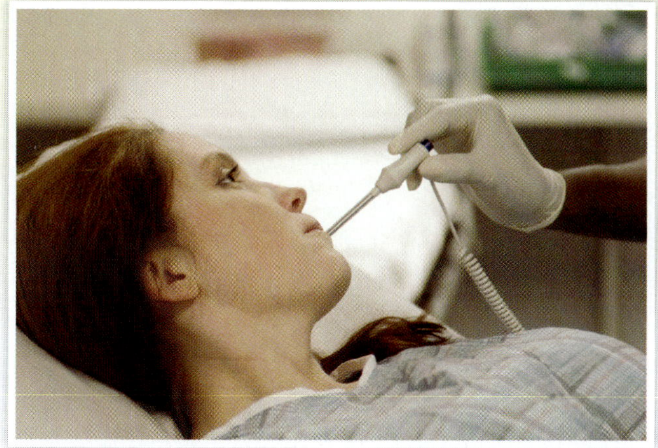

Temperature is one of the many common pieces of information that is abbreviated on health records.

symbols

Abbreviation	Definition
♂	male
♀	female
(R)	right
(L)	left
(B)	bilateral (both sides)
↑	increased
↓	decreased

abbreviations common on health records

Abbreviation	Definition
VS	vital signs
T	temperature
BP	blood pressure
HR	heart rate
RR	respiratory rate
Ht	height
Wt	weight
BMI	body mass index (measurement of body fat based on height and weight)
I/O	intake/output: the amount of fluids a patient has taken in (by IV or mouth) and produced (usually just urine output)
Dx	diagnosis
DDx	differential diagnosis
Tx	treatment
Rx	prescription
H&P	history and physical
Hx	history
CC	chief complaint (the main reason for the visit)
HPI	history of present illness (the story of the symptoms)

abbreviations common on health records *continued*

ROS	review of systems (anything else not directly related to the chief complaint)
PMHx	past medical history
FHx	family history
PE	physical exam
Pt	patient
y/o	years old
h/o	history of
PCP	primary care provider
f/u	follow-up

abbreviations used for symptoms or exam findings

Abbreviation	Definition
SOB	while it may mean something outside of medicine, here, it means *shortness* of breath **NOTE:** Because of the negative non-medical meaning, it has been suggested that SOB is should be replaced by other abbreviations like SOA (shortness of air).
PERRLA	pupils are equal, round, and reactive to light and accommodation
NAD	no acute distress (the patient does not display any intense symptoms)
RRR	regular rate and rhythm (description of a normal heart on exam)
CTA	clear to auscultation (description of normal sounding lungs)
WDWN	well developed, well nourished (the patient is growing or has grown appropriately and does not appear to be malnourished)
A&O	alert and oriented (the patient can answer questions and is aware of what's going on)
WNL	within normal limits
NOS	not otherwise specified
NEC	not elsewhere classified **NOTE:** NOS and NEC are catch-alls for diagnoses that don't quite fit any specific cause (for example, "rash NOS")

abbreviations associated with orders and administering medicine

Abbreviation	Definition
PO	per os. (by mouth)
NPO	nil per os. (nothing by mouth)
PR	per rectum (anal)
IM	intramuscular
SC	subcutaneous (under the skin)
IV	intravenous
CVL	central venous line
PICC	peripherally inserted central catheter
Sig	instructions short for *signa*, from Latin, for *label*
ad lib	as desired

Learning Outcome 2.4 Exercises

EXERCISE 4 *Translate each of the following abbreviations or symbols.*

1. (R) ____________________
2. (L) ____________________
3. ↓ ____________________
4. VS ____________________
5. T ____________________
6. BP ____________________
7. HR ____________________
8. RR ____________________
9. Dx ____________________
10. DDx ____________________
11. Tx ____________________
12. HPI ____________________
13. h/o ____________________
14. PMHx ____________________
15. FHx ____________________
16. Pt ____________________
17. PCP ____________________
18. f/u ____________________
19. NAD ____________________
20. RRR ____________________
21. NOS ____________________
22. ad lib ____________________

EXERCISE 5 *Match the abbreviation on the left with its definition on the right.*

	Abbreviation		Definition
i	1. CC	a.	the patient is growing or has grown properly; is well developed and nourished
g	2. I/O	b.	description of a normal heart on an exam
j	3. ROS	c.	description of normal-sounding lungs
l	4. PO	d.	the patient does not look extremely sick
a	5. WDWN	e.	follow-up
h	6. BMI	f.	catch-all for diagnoses that don't quite fit any specific cause
f	7. NEC /NOS	g.	the amount of fluid a patient has taken in (by IV or mouth) and produced (usually just urine output)
e	8. f/u	h.	measurement of body fat based on height and weight
k	9. NPO	i.	the main reason for the visit
d	10. NAD (No acute distress)	j.	anything else not necessarily directly related to the chief complaint
c	11. CTA	k.	nothing by mouth
m	12. SC	l.	by mouth
b	13. RRR	m.	under the skin

Learning Outcome 2.4 Exercises

EXERCISE 6 *Identify the abbreviation or symbol from the information provided.*

1. body mass index ____________
2. years old ____________
3. shortness of breath ____________
4. clear to auscultation ____________
5. well developed, well nourished ____________
6. ♂ ____________
7. ♀ Female
8. intake/output ____________
9. CC ____________
10. per *os* (by mouth) ____________
11. *nil per os* (nothing by mouth) ____________
12. subcutaneous ____________
13. within normal limits ____________
14. increased ____________
15. pupils are equal, round, and reactive to light and accommodation ____________
16. history and physical ____________
17. physical exam ____________
18. PR ____________
19. follow-up ____________
20. intramuscular ____________
21. peripherally inserted central catheter ____________
22. central venous line ____________

EXERCISE 7 *Multiple-choice questions. Select all correct answers that apply.*

1. Select the abbreviations common on health records.
   a. A&O
   b. Ht
   c. Hx
   d. IV
   e. ROS
   f. Rx
   g. Sig
   h. Wt
2. Select the abbreviations used for symptoms or exam findings.
   a. A&O
   b. Ht
   c. Hx
   d. IV
   e. ROS
   f. Rx
   g. Sig
   h. Wt
3. Select the abbreviations associated with order and administering medicine.
   a. A&O
   b. Ht
   c. Hx
   d. IV
   e. ROS
   f. Rx
   g. Sig
   h. Wt
4. Which abbreviation means *both sides?*
   a. B
   b. BS
   c. SOB
   d. SC

Abbreviations Associated with Prescriptions

The following abbreviations are typical of those found on prescriptions.

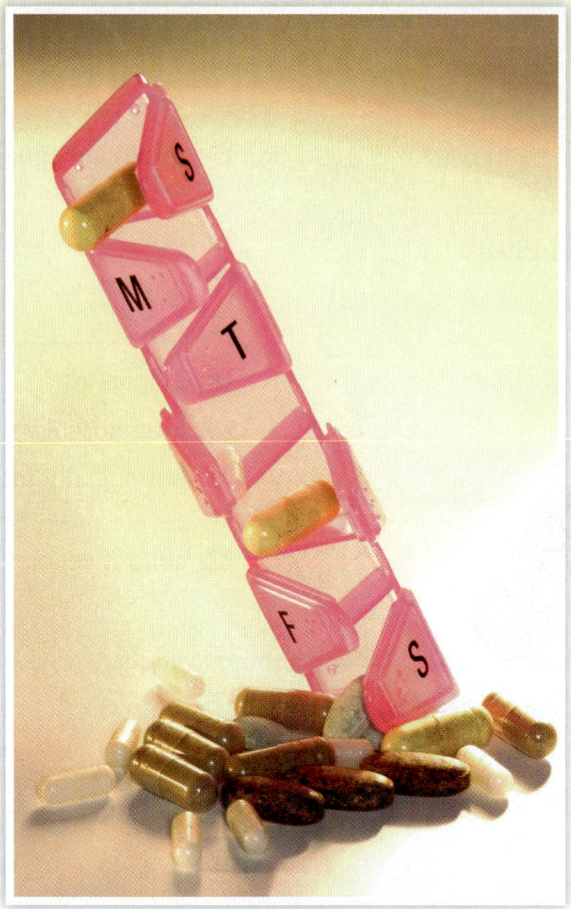

Prescriptions are a major area where doctors use abbreviations.

prescription abbreviations

Abbreviation	Definition
BID	twice daily, from the Latin phrase *bis in die,* which means "two in a day"
TID	three times daily, from the Latin phrase *ter in die,* which means "three in a day"
QD*	daily, from the Latin phrase *quaque die,* which means "each day"
QID*	four times daily, from the Latin phrase *quater in die,* which means "four in a day"
QHS	at night, from the Latin phrase *quaque hora somni,* which means "each night at the hour of sleep"
AC	before meals, from the Latin phrase *ante cibum,* which means "before food"
PC	after meals, from the Latin phrase *post cibum,* which means "after food"
prn	as needed, from the Latin phrase *per re nata,* which means "as the need arises"

*** The abbreviations *QD* and *QID* are now prohibited in many health care settings because they are easily confused. We've included mention of them in case you come across them, but we *do not* encourage their use.**

Learning Outcome 2.4 Exercises

EXERCISE 8 *Match the term on the left with its definition on the right.*

______ 1. AC	a. daily
______ 2. BID	b. twice daily
______ 3. PC	c. three times daily
______ 4. prn	d. four times daily
______ 5. QD	e. before meals
______ 6. QHS	f. after meals
______ 7. QID	g. as needed
______ 8. TID	h. at night

EXERCISE 9 *Translate the following terms.*

1. BID ______________________________
2. TID ______________________________
3. AC ______________________________
4. PC ______________________________
5. prn ______________________________
6. QD ______________________________
7. QID ______________________________
8. QHS ______________________________

EXERCISE 10 *Identify the medical abbreviation from the information provided.*

1. before meals ______________________________
2. after meals ______________________________
3. at night ______________________________
4. as needed ______________________________
5. daily ______________________________
6. twice daily ______________________________
7. three times daily ______________________________
8. four times daily ______________________________

2.5 Electronic Health Records

Clinic Note

To help you become more familiar with health records, we will include cases at the end of every chapter. Following each case, you will be able to do exercises about the cases to help you practice your medical language skills. Now that you are more familiar with many general medical words and abbreviations, let's reexamine some of the records you saw earlier in the chapter.

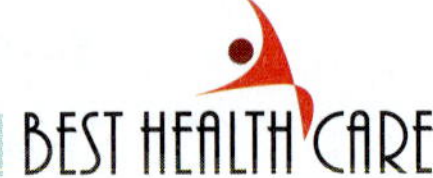

Name: Tammy Jones Date of Birth: 1/1/1980
Medications: Flovent **BID**; Albuterol **prn**; Singulair **QDay**
Allergies: **NKDA**

Subjective:

Mrs. Jones presents to the office today with a 5-day history of wheezing. She has been using her albuterol at home, but she noticed an **acute** increase in her coughing and wheezing 2 days ago. She also reports **progressively** worse congestion, sneezing, and a runny nose. These **symptoms** have also increased in the past 2 days. She has been **afebrile**. She denies chest pain or difficulty breathing.

Objective:

Vital Signs: **T**: 98.8 **HR**: 72 **RR**: 24 **BP**: 118/72 **Pulse Ox**: 92% on room air

Physical Exam:

Gen: **WDWN.**
HEENT: PERRLA, lips slightly dry.
CV: RRR, no murmurs.
Resp: Wheezing heard **bilaterally** on **auscultation.**
Abd: Soft, nontender.
Skin: Good capillary refill.
Imaging: Chest x-ray: Mild hyperinflation. No opacities.

Assessment:

1. Asthma **exacerbation**
2. Allergies

Plan:

1. Steroids **PO** x 3 days.
2. Continue albuterol **Q4-6 hours prn wheezing.**
3. **Supportive care** for the allergies, including over-the-counter antihistamines.
4. **F/u** 3 weeks in my office.

—Signed electronically by: **Elaine Frank, MD**

Learning Outcome 2.5 Exercises

EXERCISE 1 *Match the term on the left with its definition on the right.*

_____	1. symptom	a.	well developed, well nourished
_____	2. progressive	b.	pupils are equal, round, and reactive to light and accommodation
_____	3. acute	c.	to listen
_____	4. auscultation	d.	symptoms just started
_____	5. afebrile	e.	more and more each day
_____	6. exacerbation	f.	something the patient feels
_____	7. PERRLA	g.	to not have a fever
_____	8. WDWN	h.	the symptoms are getting worse

EXERCISE 2 *Fill in the blanks.*

1. The name of the patient is: _____________________
2. The author of this health record is: _____________________
3. The patient's temperature is: _____________________
4. The patient's heart rate is: _____________________
5. The patient's respiratory rate is: _____________________
6. The patient's blood pressure is: _____________________

EXERCISE 3 *True or false questions. Indicate true answers with a T and false answers with an F.*

1. The patient has had a fever. _____
2. Two days ago the patient's coughing and wheezing suddenly increased. _____
3. The patient has an irregular heart rate and rhythm. _____
4. The patient has wheezing on both sides of her body. _____
5. As part of the patient's plan, she will take steroids by mouth for 3 days. _____

EXERCISE 4 *Multiple-choice questions. Select the correct answer.*

1. The patient takes Flovent
   - a. once a day
   - b. twice a day
   - c. three times a day
   - d. as needed
2. The patient takes albuterol
   - a. once a day
   - b. twice a day
   - c. three times a day
   - d. as needed
3. The patient takes Singulair
   - a. once a day
   - b. twice a day
   - c. three times a day
   - d. as needed
4. The term that means *to treat the symptoms and make the patient feel better* is
   - a. discharge
   - b. palliative
   - c. reassurance
   - d. supportive care

Consult Note

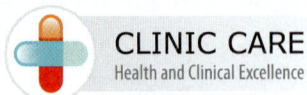

Dear Dr. Passemon,

This letter is in regard to Mr. Robert Meeds, whom you referred to my office for evaluation of chronic arthralgia. The problem began about 2 years ago. He has tried over-the-counter NSAIDs with some relief, but his condition slowly deteriorated. When he saw you in your office, he was initially diagnosed with osteoarthritis and treated with naproxen. This helped for a while, but over the past 2 months the pain has worsened.

4(a) Health Record Part ______

On exam today, Mr. Meeds was generally well appearing. His heart was regular in rate and rhythm, without murmurs, and his lungs were clear to auscultation. His knee exam showed mild edema of the left knee. It was not erythematous, tender, or warm to touch. His x-rays today showed osteophytes and joint space narrowing. His labs were normal.

4(b) Health Record Part ______

Based on Mr. Meeds's clinical picture, I believe he has osteoarthritis and is failing current medical management. I discussed the treatment options with him and recommend intraarticular injection of steroids. He will return to my office in 2 months.

4(c) Health Record Part ______

Thank you for this interesting consult.

—James Jameson, MD

Learning Outcome 2.5 Exercises

EXERCISE 5 *Based on the sample health record, fill in the blanks and label parts as noted in Question #4 that follows.*

1. The patient's name is: ______________________________
2. The author of the health record is: ______________________________
3. The name of the doctor who referred the patient is: ______________________________
4. In the blanks alongside the sample, label the correct parts of the health record using the letter associated with each section.

   S–Subjective

   O–Objective

   A–Assessment

   P–Plan

Emergency Department Note

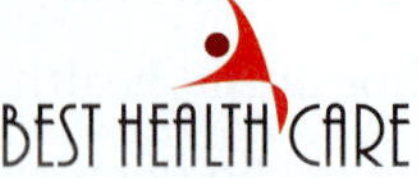

Chief Complaint: Cough

History of Present Illness: Mr. Stephen Dufresne is a 43-year-old male with a 3-day history of cough with wheezing. He has used his inhaler of albuterol but noticed the prescription had expired 3 years ago. The inhaled treatments were mildly effective, but his wheezing returned after 2 hours. He has not been febrile. He does report a runny nose, congestion, and mild headache. He has not had any shortness of breath or chest pain.

PMHx: Asthma.
Past Surgical History: None.
Social History: Lives with his wife and two children. Nonsmoker. Drinks 4 glasses of wine a week.
FHx:
Father: Deceased at 68 years of age from stroke.
Mother: Alive, high blood pressure.

6(a) Health Record Part ______

Medications: Albuterol, prn.

6(b) Health Record Part ______

Allergies: No known drug allergies.

6(c) Health Record Part ______

Physical Exam:

VS: T: 98.8 HR: 80 RR: 28
Gen: WDWN. Mild respiratory distress.
HEENT: TMs normal. Nasal passage patent with clear discharge. mucous membranes moist and pink.
CV: RRR without murmur.
Resp: Wheezing throughout. Fair air entry. Minimal nasal flaring. Mild retractions.
Abdomen: Soft, nontender.
Skin: Pink, good cap refill.

6(d) Health Record Part ______

Emergency Department Course:

Mr. Dufresne arrived to the ER in no apparent distress. A chest x-ray showed mild hyperinflation of his lungs and peribronchial cuffing. No focal infiltrates were noted. We treated him with oxygen and bronchodilators via nebulizer. He also recieved IV steroids. After two treatments of albuterol, he improved. He was no longer in distress. His lungs were clear. He was diagnosed with acute asthma exacerbation and treated wtih oral steroids and a new inhaler of asthma.

6(e) Health Record Part ______

Disposition:

Discharged to home, with follow-up in three days with his PCP.

6(f) Health Record Part ______

—Christine Christenson, MD

Learning Outcome 2.5 Exercises

EXERCISE 6 *Match the abbreviation on the left with its definition on the right.*

h	1. IV	a. past medical history
g	2. ER	b. chief complaint
i	3. PCP	c. well developed, well nourished
b	4. CC	d. family history
d.	5. FHx	e. respiratory rate
a	6. PMHx	f. regular rate and rhythm
c	7. WDWN	g. emergency room
e	8. RR	h. intravenous
f	9. RRR	i. primary care physician

EXERCISE 7 *Based on the sample health record, fill in the blanks and label parts as noted in Question #6 that follows.*

1. The patient's name is: ____________________
2. The patient's temperature is: ____________________
3. The patient's heart rate is: ____________________
4. The patient's respiratory rate is: ____________________
5. The author of this health record is: ____________________
6. In the blanks alongside the sample, label the correct parts of the health record using the letter associated with each section.

   S–Subjective

   O–Objective

   A–Assessment

   P–Plan

EXERCISE 8 *True or false questions. Indicate true answers with a T and false answers with an F.*

1. The patient has not had a fever. __________
2. Along with wheezing and a mild headache, the patient has had SOB. __________
3. Mr. Dufresne was diagnosed with asthma that just started recently and was getting worse. __________
4. The patient was sent home. __________

Admission Note

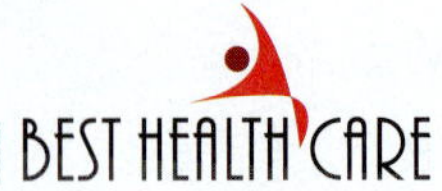

Chief Complaint: Chest pain

5(a) Health Record Part ______

HPI: Mr. William Burns is a 45-year-old male with a 2 day h/o chest pain. The pain is worse when lying **supine**, begins **medially,** and travels down the **lateral** part of his left arm. He has also had mild **SOB.** He took over-the-counter pain medicine, which helped some at first, but now he has **recurrent** pain.
ROS: Positive for **malaise** for 3 days prior to admission. He has not had any coughing, fever, or fainting.
Medications: None.
Allergies: No known drug allergies.
PMHx: Malignant lung mass 5 years ago removed surgically and treated with chemotherapy. His cancer is now in **remission.**
Past Surgical Hx: Tonsillectomy/adenoidectomy at 3 years of age. Tumor removal as above.
Social Hx: 1-pack-per-day smoker. Social alcohol intake. Divorced. Denies sexually risky behavior.
FHx: Father passed away at 40 y/o from unknown **etiology.**

5(b) Health Record Part ______

Vital Signs: Temp: 99.0 HR: 80 RR: 20 BP: 140/92

5(c) Health Record Part ______

Physical Exam

General: NAD. Alert.
HEENT: WNL. Normal fundoscopic exam.
CV: RRR with no murmurs. No carotid bruits.
Resp: Clear to auscultation.
Abd: **WNL.**

5(d) Health Record Part ______

Labs: Elevated glucose: 180. Cardiac enzymes **pending.**

5(e) Health Record Part ______

Imaging: Chest x-ray: **nml.**

5(f) Health Record Part ______

Assessment/Plan

1. Chest pain: The **differential diagnosis** includes heart attack, pneumonia, recurrent lung cancer, and muscular soreness. We will admit him for **observation** while his labs are pending. We will treat him with **supportive care,** including pain relievers.
2. Elevated blood sugar: He did have a large meal prior to coming to the emergency department. We will check his blood sugars **QAC, QPC,** and **QHS.**

5(g) Health Record Part ______

—Madison Ginger, MD

Learning Outcome 2.5 Exercises

EXERCISE 9 *Match the term on the left with its definition on the right.*

_______	1. remission	a. to have again
_______	2. observation	b. not feeling well
_______	3. pending	c. dangerous; a problem
_______	4. recurrent	d. most often used to refer to cancer when it gets better; not the same as a cure
_______	5. malignant	e. cause
_______	6. malaise	f. waiting on
_______	7. etiology	g. to keep an eye on

EXERCISE 10 *Based on the sample health record, fill in the blanks and label parts as noted in Question #5 that follows.*

1. The health record type is: ______________________________
2. The patient's name is: ______________________________
3. The author of this medical note is: ______________________________
4. This health record was written at a(n): ______________________________
5. In the blanks alongside the sample, label the correct parts of the health record using the letter associated with each section.

   S-Subjective

   O-Objective

   A-Assessment

   P-Plan
6. Using the data recorded at the patient's discharge physical examination, fill in the following blanks.
   a. The patient's temperature is: ______________________________
   b. The patient's heart rate is: ______________________________
   c. The patient's respiratory rate is: ______________________________
   d. The patient's blood pressure is: ______________________________

EXERCISE 11 *Translate the following abbreviations.*

1. Hx ______________________________
2. PMHx ______________________________
3. FHx ______________________________
4. y/o ______________________________
5. h/o ______________________________
6. CC ______________________________
7. SOB ______________________________
8. HPI ______________________________
9. ROS ______________________________

Learning Outcome 2.5 Exercises

10. NAD ________________

11. WNL ________________

12. RRR ________________

EXERCISE 12 *Multiple-choice questions. Select the correct answer.*

1. Mr. Burns's pain
   a. begins in the middle of his chest and travels out to the side
   b. begins in the middle of his chest and travels toward the middle of his left arm
   c. begins on the side of his chest and moves toward the middle
   d. begins on the side of his chest and moves down his left arm
2. Based on the patient's symptoms and exams, the chest pain may be caused by
   a. heart attack or recurrent lung cancer
   b. pneumonia
   c. muscular soreness
   d. all of these
   e. none of these
3. Supportive care is intended to
   a. treat the symptoms, but not get rid of the cause
   b. help the patient feel better
   c. prevent the patient from getting sick
   d. monitor the patient to make sure the symptoms do not get worse

EXERCISE 13 *True or false questions. Indicate true answers with a T and false answers with an F.*

1. The patient's father died from lung cancer. ________
2. The patient was admitted to monitor his chest pain while waiting for the lab results. ________
3. The patient had been feeling well prior to admission to the hospital. ________
4. The patient's chest pain is worse when he is lying on his back. ________
5. The patent's lung cancer has been cured. ________
6. The patient looked very ill when he was admitted to the hospital. ________

Discharge Summary

CLINIC CORNER

Patient Name: Regina Klebs

DATE OF ADMISSION: 01/18/2015
DATE OF DISCHARGE: 01/30/2015

4(a) Health Record Part ______

ADMISSION DIAGNOSIS:

1. Pneumonia
2. Respiratory distress

4(b) Health Record Part ______

DISCHARGE DIAGNOSIS:

1. Pneumonia—resolved
2. Cellulitis—resolved

4(c) Health Record Part ______

DISCHARGE CONDITION:

Stable

4(d) Health Record Part ______

CONSULTATIONS:

Pulmonology

4(e) Health Record Part ______

PROCEDURES:

None

LABS:

Blood culture:	1/20/2015 positive for *Staph aureus* 1/24/2015 negative

4(f) Health Record Part ______

Imaging:

Chest x-ray:	1/18/2015: right upper lobe pneumonia 1/24/2015: improving pneumonia 1/30/2015: normal

4(g) Health Record Part ______

HPI:

Ms. Regina Klebs is a 28-year-old woman admitted to hospital from the emergency department with pneumonia. She initially presented with coughing, fever, and shortness of breath. In the **ER,** she had mildly low oxygen levels and was in **acute distress.** A chest x-ray showed a pneumonia in the right upper lobe. She was admitted for oxygen and **IV** antibiotics.

4(h) Health Record Part ______

HOSPITAL COURSE:

Ms. Klebs was admitted to the hospital and placed on oxygen and IV antibiotics. Her status improved until day 3 of her hospitalization, when her conditions **abruptly degenerated.** She was noted as **febrile** and **lethargic.** She had a **marked** increased in pain at her IV site and it was red and tender to **palpation.** A culture was sent and came back positive. She was transferred to the **ICU.**

-1-

continued

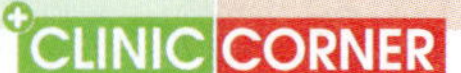

A **PICC** line was placed and she was given IV antibiotics. Her condition quickly improved and she was transferred back to the hospital floor. After completing her course of antibiotics, she was discharged to home. Given the risk of significant **morbidity** with her type of infection, we sent her home with **prophylactic topical** antibiotics to put in the nostrils of all her family members.

4(i) Health Record Part ______

DISCHARGE PHYSICAL EXAMINATION:

VS: T: 98.6 **HR:** 64 **RR:** 20 **BP:** 112/74 **Pulse Ox:** 94% on room air

4(j) Health Record Part ______

PE:

Gen: **Alert and oriented. NAD.**
HEENT: PERRLA. Mucous membranes moist.
CV: **RRR,** no murmurs.
Resp: **CTA.**
Abd: Soft, nontender.
Skin: Mild redness to the **proximal** third of the **ventral** side of the right forearm, where the IV site had been. Improving from previous exams.

4(k) Health Record Part ______

ACTIVITY:

No restrictions.

DIET:

Normal.

MEDS:

Topical antibiotic ointment to the nostrils of family members **TID** x 5 days.

FOLLOW-UP:
Appointment—**PCP** (Dr. Primo) in 1 week.

4(l) Health Record Part ______

—Francis Jerome, MD

-2-

Learning Outcome 2.5 Exercises

EXERCISE 14 *Based on the sample health record, fill in the blanks and label parts as noted in Question #4 that follows.*

1. The health record type is: ____________________
2. The patient's name is: ____________________
3. This health record was written at a(n): ____________________
4. In the blanks alongside the sample, label the correct parts of the health record using the letter associated with each section.

   S–Subjective

   O–Objective

   A–Assessment

   P–Plan
5. Using the data recorded at the patient's discharge physical examination, fill in the following blanks.
   a. The patient's temperature is: ____________________
   b. The patient's heart rate is: ____________________
   c. The patient's respiratory rate is: ____________________
   d. The patient's blood pressure is: ____________________
6. The patient's primary care physician is: ____________________
7. The patient was transferred to the ICU, which stands for ____________________.
8. The patient's heart had RRR, which means ____________________ and ____________________.
9. The patient's respiratory exam was CTA, or ____________________ to auscultation.

EXERCISE 15 *Match the term on the left with its definition on the right.*

______	1. discharge	a.	what the patient has
______	2. diagnosis	b.	to have a fever
______	3. marked	c.	a decrease in level of consciousness
______	4. lethargic	d.	something that really stands out
______	5. febrile	e.	to feel
______	6. auscultation	f.	peripherally inserted central catheter
______	7. palpation	g.	literally, *to unload;* to send home
______	8. morbidity	h.	the risk for being sick
______	9. PICC	i.	pupils are equal, round, and reactive to light and accommodation
______	10. PERRLA	j.	to listen

EXERCISE 16 *True or false questions. Indicate true answers with a T and false answers with an F.*

1. The patient was admitted to the hospital from the ER. __________
2. The patient was admitted for oxygen and oral antibiotics. __________
3. The patient was A&O upon discharge, without any acute distress. __________
4. The patient's family will be given medication 3 times a day for 5 days. __________

Learning Outcome 2.5 Exercises

EXERCISE 17 *Multiple-choice questions. Select the correct answer.*

1. The record indicates that Ms. Klebs was in *acute distress* in the emergency department. This means that her distress
   a. was getting worse
   b. had been going on for a while
   c. started recently
   d. was unrelated to her chief complaint
2. The record indicates that Ms. Klebs's condition *abruptly degenerated,* which means it
   a. suddenly got better
   b. suddenly got worse
   c. got better over time
   d. got worse over time
3. The record indicates that the hospital discharged the patient with *prophylactic topical antibiotics* to put in the nostrils of all her family members. These topical antibiotics are intended to
   a. treat the symptoms but not the actual cause of the illness
   b. prevent an illness
   c. treat the symptoms of an illness to make a patient feel better
   d. create a clean, germ-free environment
4. The record indicates the patient has "mild redness to the *proximal* third of the *ventral* side of the right forearm where the IV site had been." The redness is located on which part of her forearm?
   a. the front, closer to the center
   b. the front, farther away from the center
   c. the back, closer to the center
   d. the back, farther away from the center

Operative Report

CLINIC CORNER

Preoperative Diagnosis: Appendicitis
Postoperative Diagnosis: Appendicitis

3(a) Health Record Part ______

Procedure: Appendectomy
Anesthesia: General

3(b) Health Record Part ______

Indication: The patient, Wallace Simpson, is a 25-year-old man with acute onset of abdominal pain and fever.
Operative Findings: The patient had a grossly inflamed appendix and local peritonitis.

3(c) Health Record Part ______

Description of Procedure: Mr. Simpson was brought to the operating room for suspected appendicitis. He was intubated and placed under general anesthesia. He was prepped and wrapped in sterile technique. A transverse incision was made in right lower quadrant over McBurney's point. Further incision was made through the underlying fascia and the abdominal muscles were separated. The appendix was located and noted to be grossly abnormal. The appendix was dissected, ligated, and sutured. The area was irrigated with normal saline. The cecum was inspected. The peritoneum and fascia were sutured, as well as the skin incision. The wound was cleaned and bandaged with benzoin and steristrips. All gauze and instruments were accounted for.

Disposition: Mr. Simpson was sent to the PACU in stable condition.

3(d) Health Record Part ______

—James Cutter, MD

EXERCISE 18 *Based on the sample health record, fill in the blanks and label parts as noted in Question #3 that follows.*

1. The health record type is: ______________________________
2. The author of this health record is: ______________________________
3. In the blanks alongside the sample, label the correct parts of the health record using the letter associated with each section.

   S–Subjective

   O–Objective

   A–Assessment

   P–Plan
4. The patient was transferred to the PACU, which stands for ______________________________ ______________ ______________ ______________.

Daily Hospital Note/Progress Note

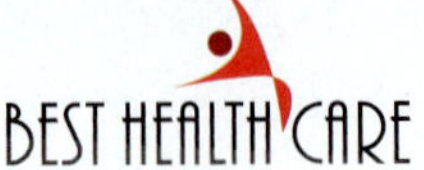

Subjective:

Since yesterday, the patient, Penelope Gates, has vomited 3 times, but she has experienced no vomiting in the past 6 hours. The emesis was not bloody or bilious. She also had 5 episodes of nonbloody, nonmucoid diarrhea in the past 24 hours. She has been afebrile and is without other complaints.

Objective:

Vital Signs: **T**: 99.0 **HR**: 100 **RR**: 24 **Intake:** 1500 ml **Output**: 1200 ml

Physical Exam:

General: Tired but responsive and alert.
HEENT: PERRLA, TMs normal, mucous membranes slightly dry and pink.
CV: RRR without murmurs, gallops, or rubs.
Respiratory: CTA without wheezes, rales, or rhonchi.
Abdomen: Soft, nondistended. Minimal generalized tenderness. Normoactive bowel sounds.
Skin: Pink, warm, and dry.
Labs: Na 139. Cl 120 CO2 14. K 3.8 BUN 15 Cr. 0.4 Glc 100

Assessment/Plan:

1. Acute gastroenteritis: No change. Continue IV fluids. Will give another dose of ondansetron. If patient has no vomiting for 4 hours, then we will advance diet as tolerated. If the patient tolerates it well, will decrease IVF accordingly.
2. Metabolic acidosis: Noticed this AM on lab work. We will begin the patient on sodium bicarbonate.

—Harry Harrison, MD

Learning Outcome 2.5 Exercises

EXERCISE 19 *Fill in the blanks based on the sample health record.*

1. The health record type is: ____________________
2. This health record was written at a(n): ____________________
3. The author of this health record is: ____________________
4. Using the data recorded at the patient's discharge physical examination, fill in the following blanks.
   a. The patient's temperature is: ____________________
   b. The patient's heart rate is: ____________________
   c. The patient's respiratory rate is: ____________________
   d. The patient's I/O is: ____________________

EXERCISE 20 *Translate the following terms.*

1. T ____________________
2. HR ____________________
3. RR ____________________
4. I/O ____________________
5. PERRLA ____________________
6. RRR ____________________
7. CTA ____________________
8. IV ____________________

EXERCISE 21 *True or false questions. Indicate true answers with a T and false answers with an F.*

1. The patient has been without fever. ________
2. The patient vomited 3 times on the day of the report. ________
3. The physician decided to begin IV fluids. ________
4. Before declaring the patient CTA, the physician first listened to the lungs to see how they sounded. ________
5. The patient's gasteroenteritis is getting worse. ________

Radiology Report

CLINIC CORNER

Reason for Study: Abdominal pain.

Technique: CT of abdomen and pelvis with and without contrast.

Findings: Liver and spleen are normal in size. Appendix measures 9 mm in diameter. Appendicolith noted with thickening of the appendix wall. Kidneys, adrenal glands, pancreas, and gallbladder are unremarkable.

Impression: 1. Appendicitis

—Roxanne Pawlenty, MD

EXERCISE 22 *Multiple-choice questions. Select the correct answer.*

1. Dr. Pawlenty is most likely a
   a. cardiologist
   b. pathologist
   c. radiologist
   d. surgeon
2. The CT was ordered because the patient had
   a. abdominal pain
   b. prophylaxis
   c. sequelae
   d. history of appendicitis
3. What technique was used in this study?
   a. CT of abdomen with contrast
   b. CT of abdomen with and without contrast
   c. CT of abdomen and pelvis with contrast
   d. CT of abdomen and pelvis with and without contrast
4. The Findings section of the report would be considered which part of a SOAP note?
   a. S–Subjective
   b. O–Objective
   c. A–Assessment
   d. P–Plan
5. The liver and spleen are
   a. exacerbated
   b. febrile
   c. marked
   d. unremarkable
6. The kidneys and gallbladder
   a. are exacerbated
   b. are larger than normal
   c. are normal
   d. require further testing
7. The impression of appendicitis is considered which part of a SOAP note?
   a. S–Subjective
   b. O–Objective
   c. A–Assessment
   d. P–Plan

Pathology Report

BEST HEALTH CARE

Clinical History: Mrs. Linda Genner, a 48-year-old woman, had a suspicious mass seen on a CT scan.

Specimen: Lung, right upper lobe resection.

Gross description: A single specimen measuring 2.3 cm x 4.5 cm x 8.2 cm. The surface of the specimen is smooth, red, and pearly. 1 cm bronchial margin. No invasion of surrounding pleura.

Diagnosis: Right upper lobe: Adenocarcinoma Grade 1.

—Brendan Kellstrom, MD

3(a) Health Record Part ______

3(b) Health Record Part ______

3(c) Health Record Part ______

EXERCISE 23 *Based on the sample health record, fill in the blanks and label parts as noted in Question #3 that follows.*

1. The health record type is: ________________________________

2. The author of this health record is: ________________________________

3. In the blanks alongside the sample, label the correct parts of the health record using the letter associated with each section.

   S–Subjective

   O–Objective

   A–Assessment

   P–Plan

Prescription

CLINIC CORNER

Albuterol inhaler

Sig: 2-3 puffs inhaled q-4hours prn wheezing

Disp: 1

Refill: 2

3(a) Health Record Part ______

3(b) Health Record Part ______

3(c) Health Record Part ______

3(d) Health Record Part ______

EXERCISE 24 *Based on the sample health record, fill in the blanks and label parts as noted in Question #3 that follows.*

1. The health record type is: ________________________________

2. Which part of the SOAP note is included in this health record (select one)?
   a. S–Subjective
   b. O–Objective
   c. A–Assessment
   d. P–Plan

3. Label the parts of the health record with
   a. name and strength of the medicine
   b. patient instructions
   c. how much medicine to give the patient
   d. refill information

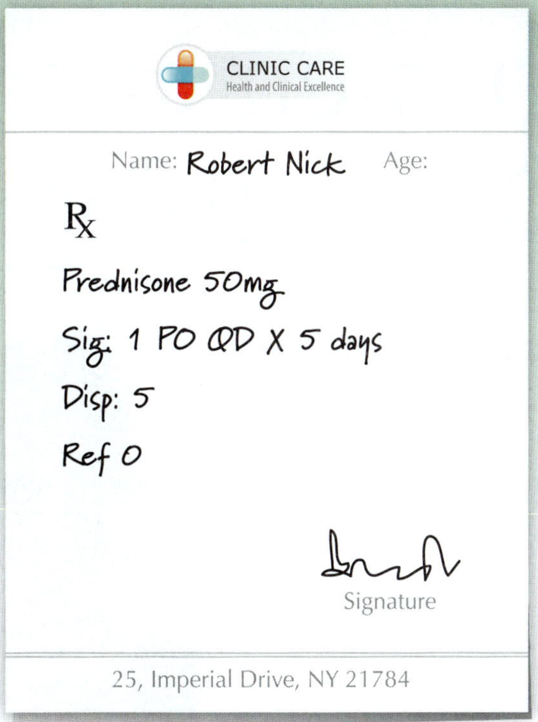

CLINIC CARE
Health and Clinical Excellence
Name: Robert Nick
Age:
Rx
Prednisone 50mg
Sig: 1 PO QD X 5 days
Disp: 5
Ref 0
Signature
25, Imperial Drive, NY 21784

EXERCISE 25 *Multiple-choice questions. Select the correct answer.*

1. This is a
   a. prescription
   b. part of the plan for a patient
   c. instructions for the pharmacist
   d. all of these
   e. none of these
2. The first line is the
   a. name of the medication
   b. strength of the medication
   c. name and strength of the medication
   d. pharmacist instructions
3. The abbreviation *Sig*
   a. means the instructions for the patient
   b. means the instructions for the pharmacist
   c. is short for *signa,* from Latin, for label
   d. means the instructions for the patient and is short for *signa,* from Latin for label
   e. means the instructions for the pharmacist and is short for *signa,* from Latin for label
4. The patient will take the medication
   a. 5 pills a day by mouth
   b. 4 times a day by mouth
   c. daily by mouth for 5 days
   d. 4 times daily by mouth for 5 days
5. The pharmacist will dispense how many pills?
   a. 1
   b. 5
   c. 20
   d. 25

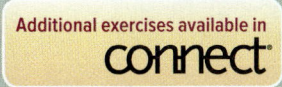

Additional practice items are available in Connect!

The Integumentary System–Dermatology 3

Introduction and Overview of Dermatology

For thousands of years, walls of earth, wood, or stone surrounded cities. These outside walls defined the city boundaries. More importantly, they protected the city's inhabitants. By limiting access to the inside of the city and offering a strategic point of attack, walls deterred would-be invaders. In addition, walls provided a convenient vantage point to view the surrounding countryside. In effect, the walls offered protection and surveillance.

Skin serves a similar function as city walls. As an outer protective barrier, skin is the first line of defense from germs and irritants. It also serves as the body's first point of contact with its surroundings.

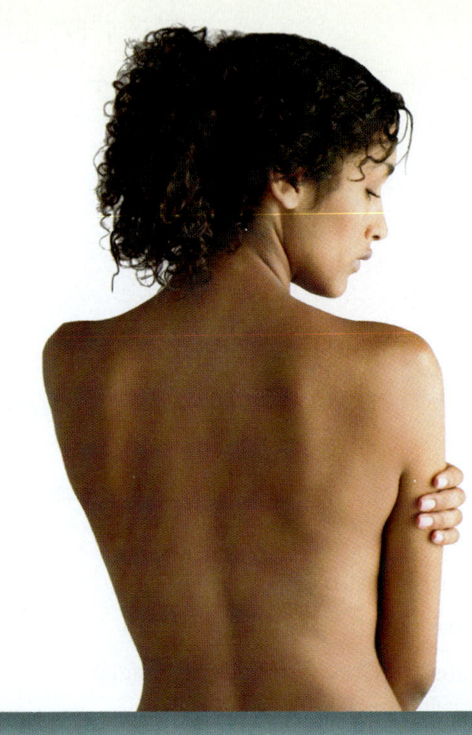

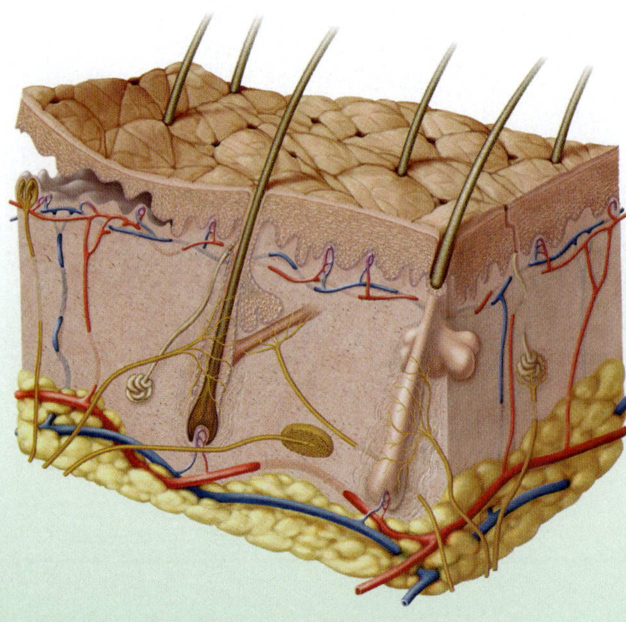

Your skin is your largest organ. It serves as your body's first point of contact with its surroundings.

learning outcomes

Upon completion of this chapter, you will be able to:

- **3.1** Identify the **roots/word parts** associated with the **integumentary system.**
- (S) **3.2** Translate the **Subjective** terms associated with the **integumentary system.**
- (O) **3.3** Translate the **Objective** terms associated with the **integumentary system.**
- (A) **3.4** Translate the **Assessment** terms associated with the **integumentary system.**
- (P) **3.5** Translate the **Plan** terms associated with the **integumentary system.**
- **3.6** Use **abbreviations** associated with the **integumentary system.**
- **3.7** Distinguish terms associated with the **integumentary system** in the context of **electronic health records.**

3.1 Word Parts of the Integumentary System

Word Parts Associated with the Anatomy of the Integumentary System

At first glance, the skin appears to be very simple—just a thin layer of tissue covering our bodies. However, the truth is that the **integumentary system** (*the skin*) is very complex. Your skin (roots: *cutaneo/dermo*) has many structures, each of which has its own special job.

The outermost layer, the one that is visible, is the **epidermis**. It is made of large cells that look like the scales of a fish under the microscope. The term **squamous cell** refers to this scaly appearance.

Under the epidermis lies a deeper layer known as the **dermis**. This layer, which is much thicker than the epidermis, has fewer cells and more thick fibers to give the skin strength and flexibility. The dermis is also home to hair follicles, nerves, and glands.

- Hair follicles are the roots of your hair (*pilo/tricho*). The follicles anchor the hair to the skin and provide nourishment to it.
- The nerves of the dermis detect fine pressure, deep pressure, temperature, and pain. The vast network of nerves in your skin makes it the largest sensory organ in your body.
- The skin has two types of glands, which are groups of cells that release fluid. Sweat glands (*hidro*) release sweat to rid the body of waste and to cool the body. Sebaceous glands (*sebaceo*) secrete oil as a natural moisturizer for the skin and hair.

At the ends of your fingers and toes are nails, specialized tissue made of a hard substance (*keratin*). Your nails (*onycho/ungo*) protect your fingers and toes and provide a good base for movement.

fat

ROOTS: ***adip/o, lip/o, steat/o***

EXAMPLES: adipocyte, lipoma, steatosis

NOTES: Next time you are offered a fatty food, you can tell the person who is offering it that you try to avoid *adipogenic* foods.

skin

ROOTS: ***cutane/o, derm/o, dermat/o***

EXAMPLES: subcutaneous, epidermal, dermatology

NOTES: A patient once sought medical treatment for a rash around the mouth. When the health care professional diagnosed her with *perioral dermatitis,* the patient thought to herself, "Duh! You just said the same thing I said—just in a different language." Think about it: What does *perioral dermatitis* mean? You can break it down easily: *peri* = around, *oral* = mouth, *dermat* = skin, and *itis* = inflammation.

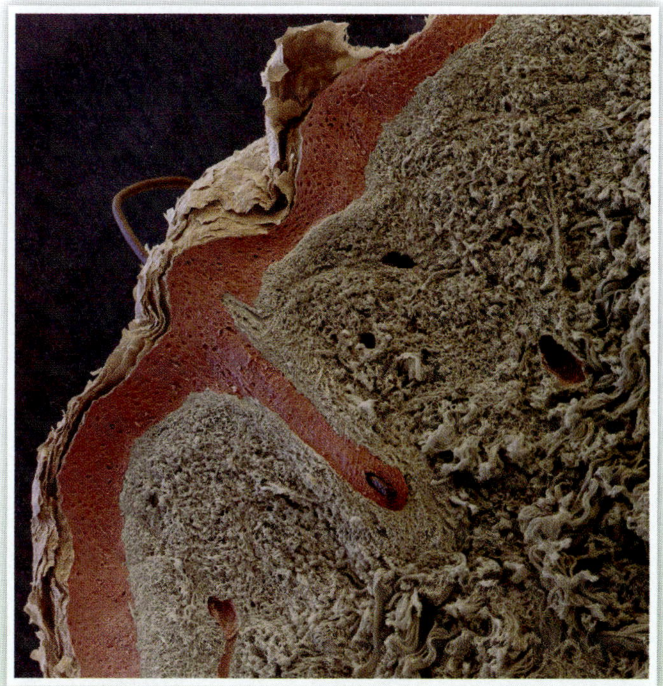

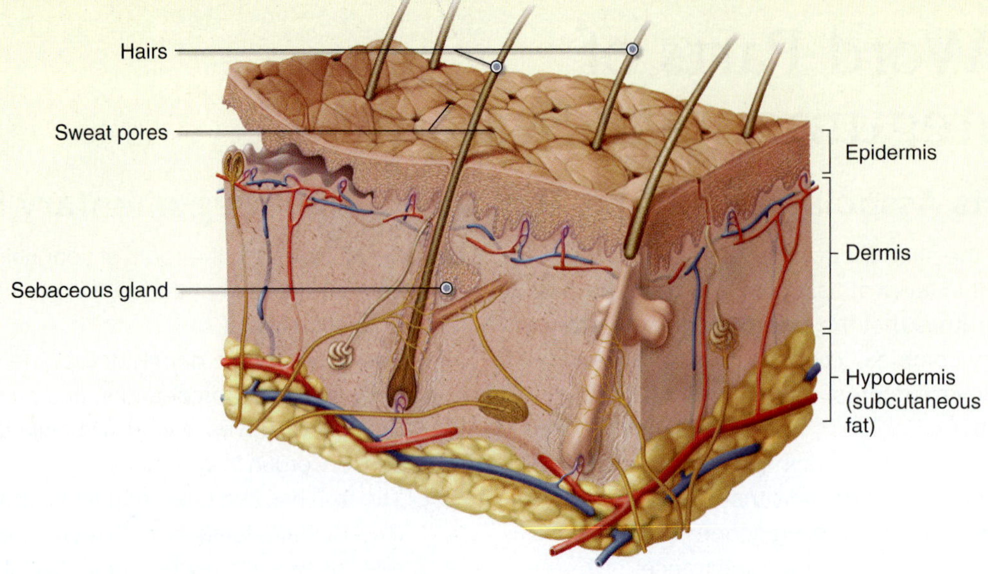

Structure of the Skin.

hair

ROOTS: ***pil/o, trich/o***

EXAMPLES: piloid, atrichosis

NOTES: The word *caterpillar* is believed to come from two Latin words: *catta,* meaning *cat,* and *pila,* meaning *hair*; thus, *caterpillar,* meaning *hairy cat.* Have you ever had split ends? If you do, you can always ask your hairstylist for a treatment for your *schizotrichia.*

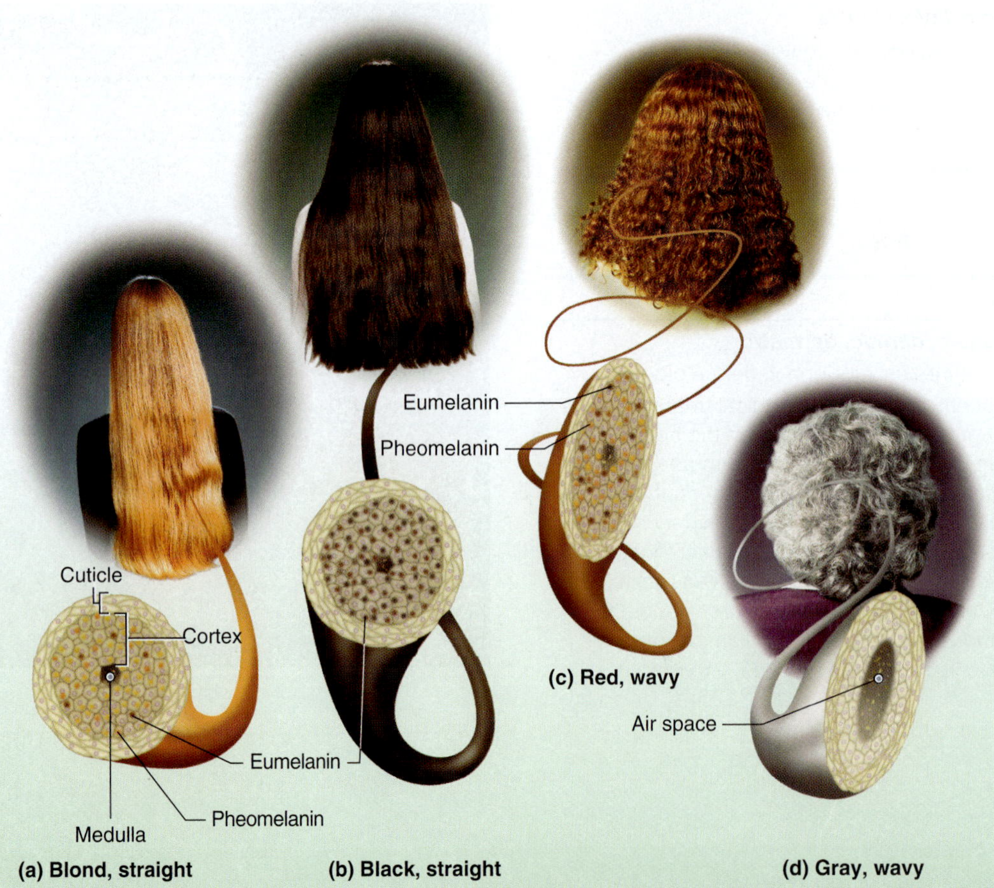

sweat

ROOT: ***hidr/o***

EXAMPLES: hyperhidrosis, hypohidrosis

NOTES: Humans have gone to great lengths to keep the environment cool—inventing air conditioning and fans, for example—which suggests that humans do not like to get sweaty. But if you didn't have the ability to sweat, your body would have a very hard time regulating its temperature. In fact, *hypohidrosis,* which means a lack of sweat, can be a sign that something is wrong.

Unlike humans, dogs cannot sweat. Instead, they pant—their bodies are cooled by the air passing over their moist tongues.

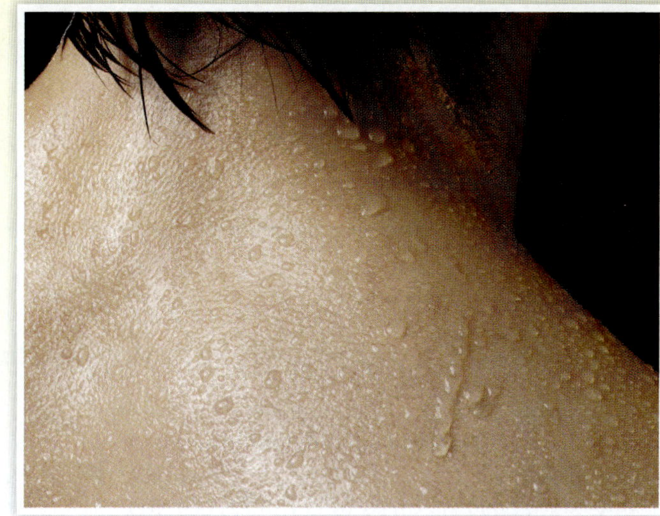

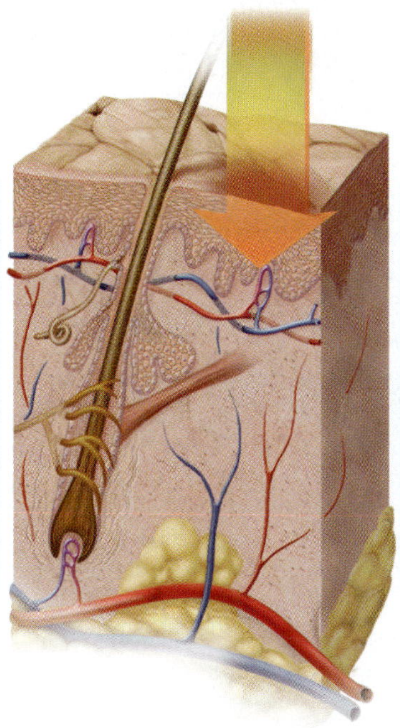

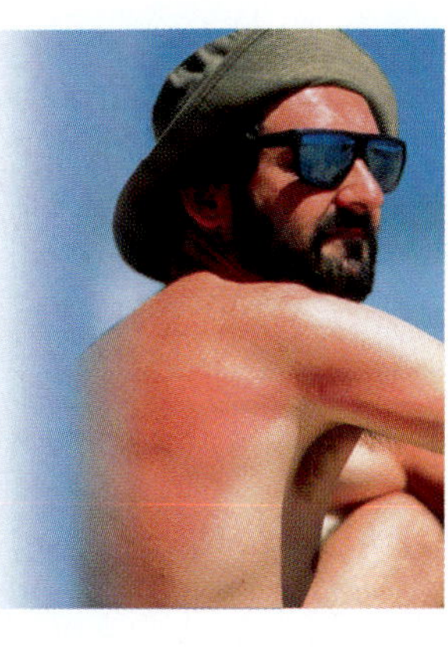

scale

ROOT: ***squam/o***

EXAMPLE: squamous layer

NOTES: Have you ever gotten a sunburn that led to peeling skin? Have you ever removed the scales from a fresh fish before cooking it? Either process can be referred to as *desquamation*, a Latin word meaning *to remove the scales from a fish.*

nail

ROOTS: ***onych/o, ungu/o***

EXAMPLES: onychalgia, subungual

NOTES: Have you noticed that it is time to trim your nails? Excuse yourself to take care of that task by telling your friends you need to step outside to *exungulate.* If the situation is more complicated, and there is a broken nail, you can mention that you have diagnosed yourself with *onychoclasis.*

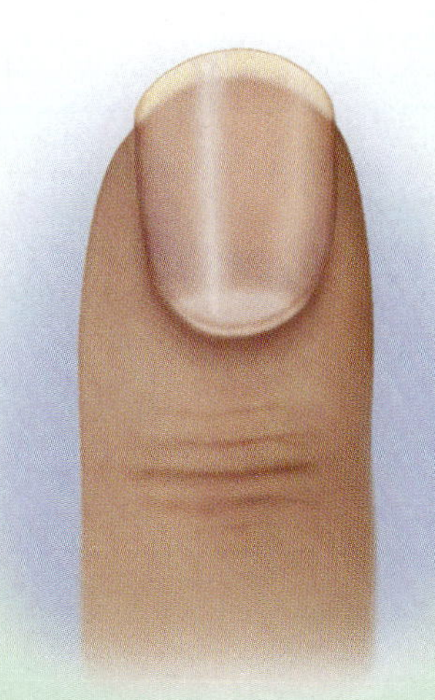

oil

ROOTS: ***seb/o, sebace/o***

EXAMPLES: sebolith, pilosebaceous

NOTES: Later, when you learn more about the ears, you will learn the root *cerumen*, which refers to ear wax. Actually, *cerumen* is just sebum that is produced in the ears.

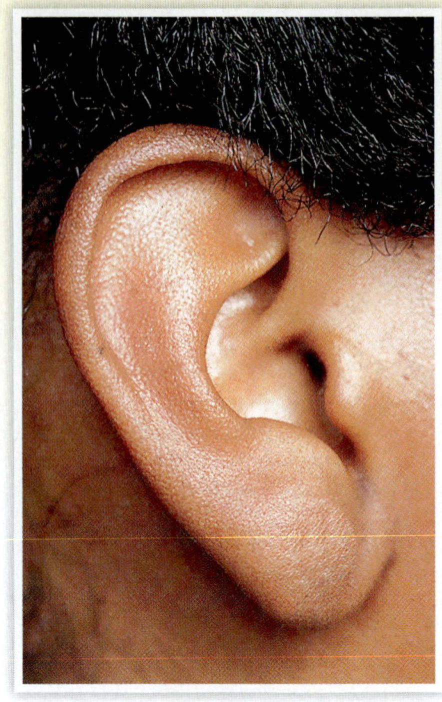

Word Parts Associated with Pathology—Change

Skin abnormalities are generally categorized into two groups: unusual skin texture and unusual skin color. Problems with skin texture can present as scaliness (*ichthyo-*), hardness or horniness (*kerato-*), thickness (*pachyo-*), dryness (*xero-*), or wrinkled appearance (*rhytido-*). Of course, skin tones differ from person to person and ethnicity to ethnicity, but certain prefixes are used to describe abnormal skin conditions: whiteness (*leuko-*), redness (*erythro-*), yellowness (*xantho-*), and blackness (*melano-*).

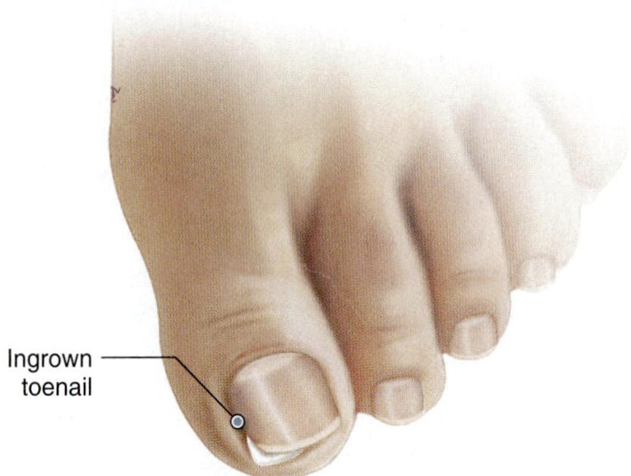

hidden

ROOT: ***crypt/o***

EXAMPLE: onychocryptosis

NOTES: A person who specializes in breaking codes and deciphering secret messages is called a *cryptolinguist. Onychocryptosis* is an ingrown, or hidden, toenail.

The word *crypt* used by itself can refer to a room or vault hidden beneath the floor. It is usually associated with a chamber in which corpses are placed, whether it is located in a church (generally beneath the floor) or a mausoleum (generally above ground).

scaly

ROOT: ***ichthy/o***

EXAMPLE: ichthyosis

NOTES: The root *ichthyo* comes from the Greek word *ichthus*, meaning *fish*. A person who studies fish is called an *ichthyologist*. If you like to eat fish, you are an *ichthyophagist*. In dermatology, the word refers to scalelike changes in the skin.

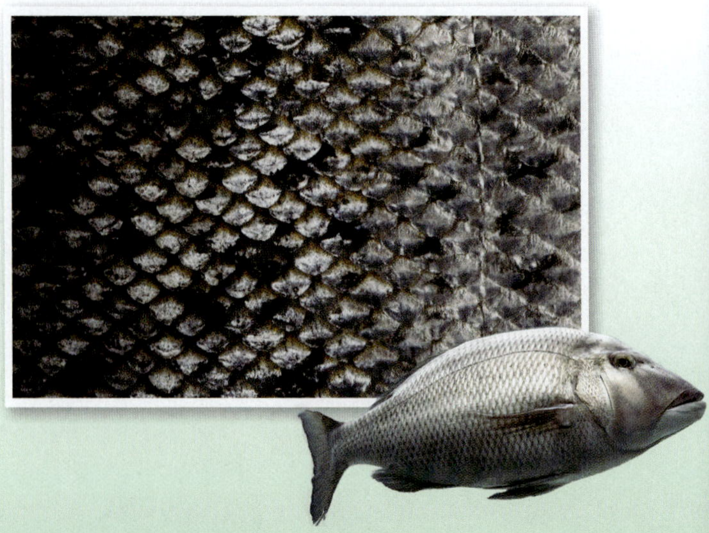

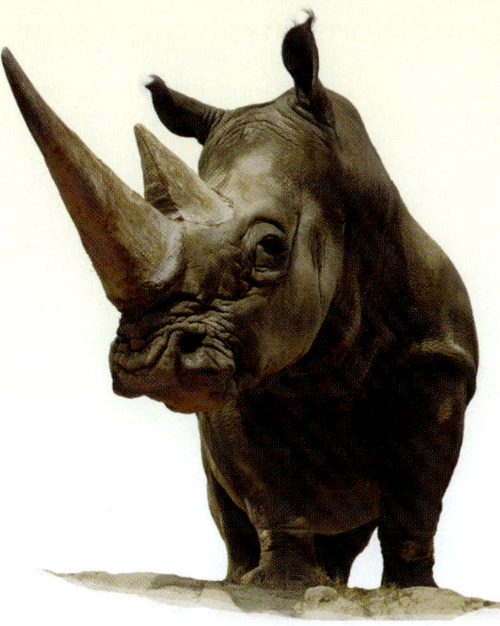

hard, horny

ROOT: ***kerat/o***

EXAMPLES: keratosis, keratoderma

NOTES: The *rhinoceros* is so named because it has a *horn* on its *nose*. The dinosaur *Triceratops* was so named because of the three (*tri*) horns (*kerat*) on its head.

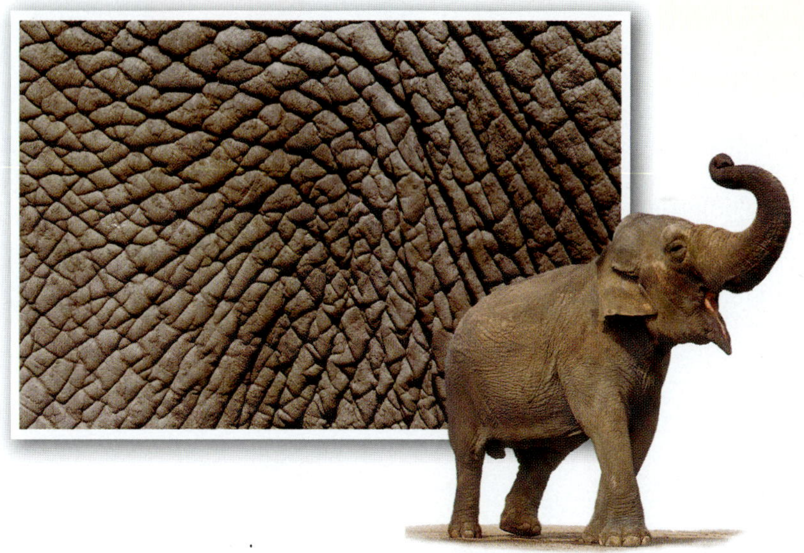

thick

ROOT: ***pachy/o***

EXAMPLES: pachyderma

NOTES: Elephants are referred to as *pachyderms* because of their thick (*pachy*) hides (*derm*).

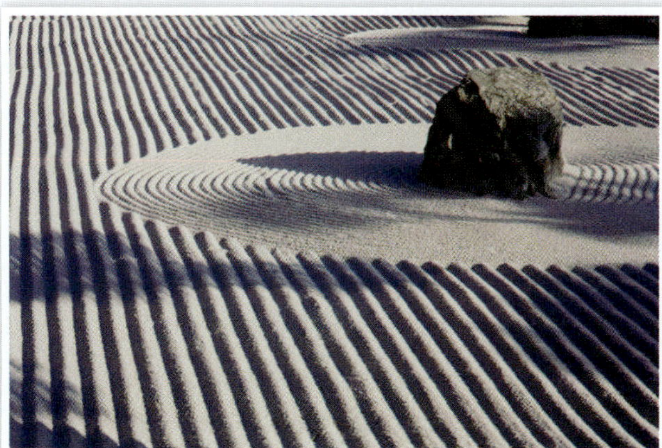

dry

ROOT: ***xer/o***

EXAMPLE: xeroderma

NOTES: People who live in dry or desert regions often forgo lawns and instead use *xeriscaping*, which means landscaping using plants that require little water. Because grounds that are xeriscaped are typically rocky and brown, some think this type of landscaping is spelled *zeroscaping*—and the fact that the *x* is pronounced like a *z* probably does not help.

wrinkle

ROOT: ***rhytid/o***

EXAMPLE: rhytidoplasty

NOTES: Some people are not afraid of getting old; they are instead afraid of *looking* old. People who simply fear getting wrinkles have *rhytiphobia*. Notice that the *-do* dropped off the root when it combined with *-phobia*. The reason is that *rhytiphobia* is easier to say than *rhytidophobia*. In fact, try saying *rhytidophobia* quickly a total of 20 times. By the end, you will probably drop that *-do* sound.

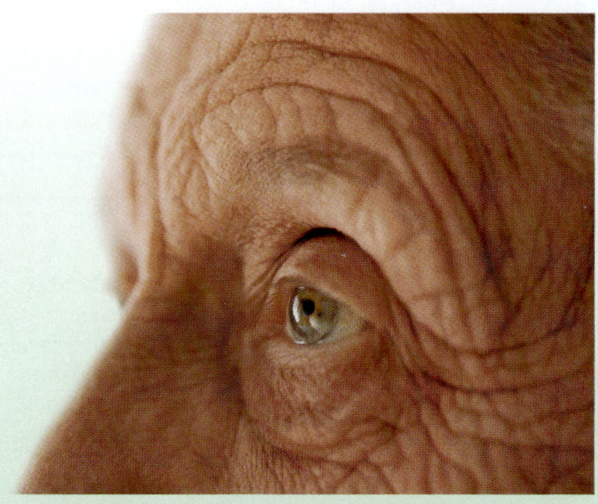

Word Parts Associated with Pathology—Skin Conditions Involving Color

One important aspect of diagnosing skin conditions is noting changes. This section gives the roots that refer to the most commonly occurring changes in skin color.

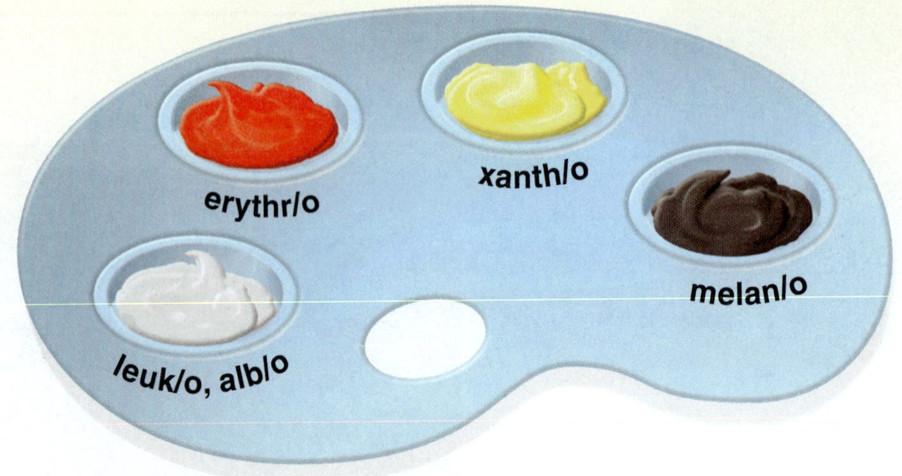

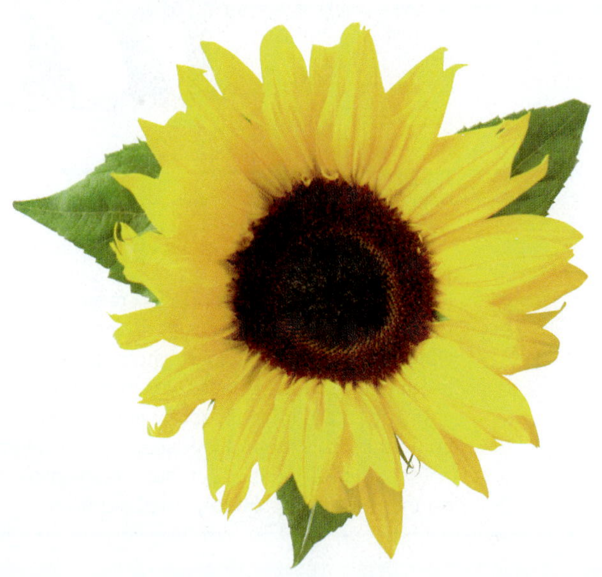

yellow

ROOT: ***xanth/o***

EXAMPLE: xanthoderma

NOTES: If you are unable to see the color yellow, you may have *axanthopsia*.

red

ROOT: ***erythr/o***

EXAMPLE: erythroderma

NOTES: *Erythroderma* is a redness of the skin. The Red Sea, a sea that separates Africa from Egypt, was originally called the Erythraen (or Red) Sea. The country Eritrea, which lies on the Red Sea between the Sudan and Ethiopia, gets its name from this ancient moniker for the sea.

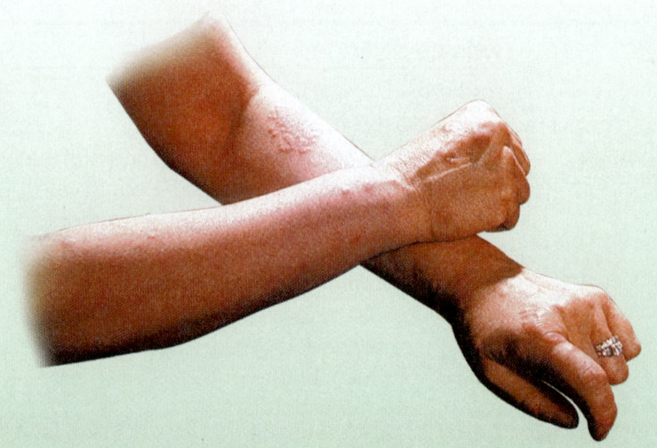

white

ROOTS: ***leuk/o, alb/o***

EXAMPLES: leukoderma, albinism

NOTES: A person with white hair has *leukotrichia.* A complete lack of skin pigment is known as *albinism.*

The *albatross* is a white seabird. Its name is derived in part from a need to distinguish it from a black seabird called the *frigate bird.*

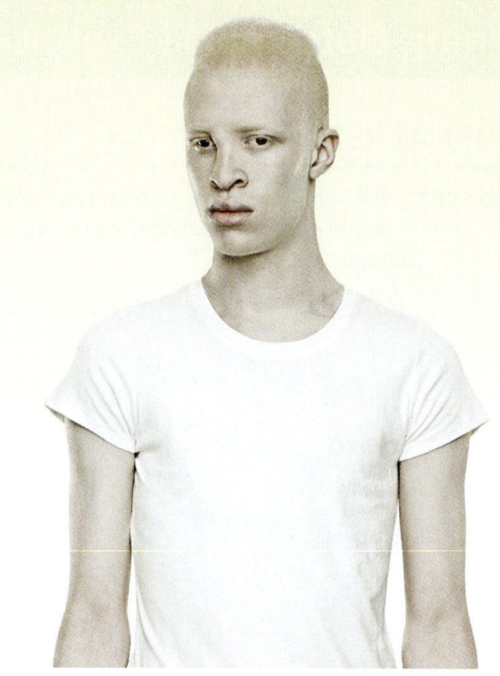

black

ROOT: ***melan/o***

EXAMPLE: melanoma

NOTES: Ancient Greeks thought that the human body was filled with four substances they called *humors:* bile (*chole*), black bile (*melan chole*), phlegm (*phlegma*), and blood (*sanguis*). According to this system, a healthy person must have all four humors in perfect balance. If a person was sick, an imbalance of the humors was to blame, and a physician's goal was to figure out which humor was too plentiful and which was insufficient. *Bloodletting* was developed to help rid the body of excess blood. The word *melancholy* also comes from belief in a balance of the humors, because it was believed that a person who was sad or depressed had too much black bile.

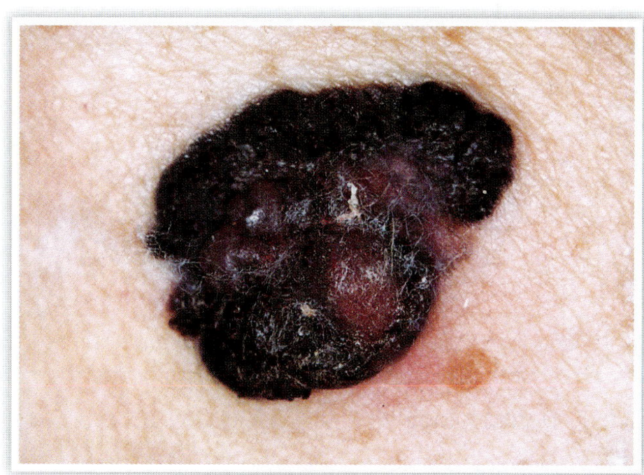

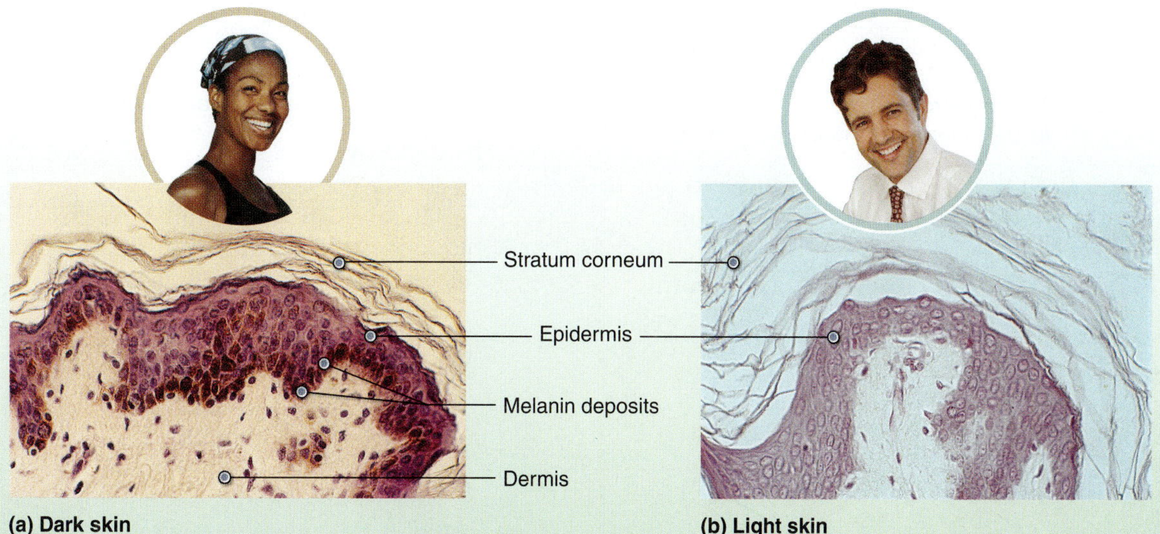

(a) Dark skin **(b) Light skin**

The differences in skin color are caused by the varying levels of melanin deposited in the basal layer. Picture (a) has heavy deposits while picture (b) contains little visible melanin in the basal layer.

Learning Outcome 3.1 Exercises

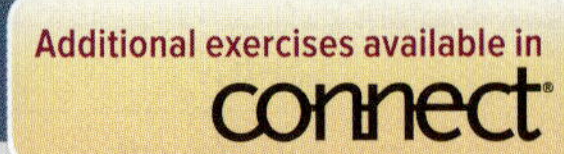
Additional exercises available in
connect

TRANSLATION

EXERCISE 1 *Match the root on the left with its definition on the right. Some definitions will be used more than once.*

a	1. lip/o	a. fat
b	2. derm/o	b. skin
b	3. dermat/o	c. hair
d	4. hidr/o	d. sweat
f	5. squam/o	e. nail
a	6. adip/o	f. scale
b	7. cutane/o	g. oil
g	8. seb/o	
c	9. pil/o	
a	10. steat/o	
g	11. sebace/o	
c	12. trich/o	
e	13. onych/o	
e	14. ungu/o	

EXERCISE 2 *Translate the following roots.*

1. derm/o ______
2. lip/o ______
3. cutane/o ______
4. squam/o ______
5. adip/o ______
6. dermat/o ______
7. seb/o ______
8. pil/o ______
9. hidr/o ______
10. ungu/o ______
11. steat/o ______
12. sebace/o ______
13. trich/o ______
14. onych/o ______

EXERCISE 3 *Break down the following words into their component parts and translate.*

EXAMPLE: sinusitis *sinus | itis* *inflammation of the sinuses*

1. dermatology ______
2. lipoma ______
3. steatosis ______
4. epidermal ______
5. subungual ______
6. subcutaneous ______
7. onychalgia ______

EXERCISE 4 *Match the root on the left with its definition on the right.*

a	1. crypt/o	a. hidden
e	2. xer/o	b. scaly
c	3. kerat/o	c. hard, horny
d	4. pachy/o	d. thick
b	5. ichthy/o	e. dry
f	6. rhytid/o	f. wrinkle

EXERCISE 5 *Translate the following roots.*

1. hard, horny ______
2. scaly ______
3. hidden ______

Learning Outcome 3.1 Exercises

EXERCISE 6 *Break down the following words into their component parts and translate.*

EXAMPLE: sinusitis *sinus | itis* *inflammation of the sinuses*

1. ichthyosis ____________________
2. keratosis ____________________
3. xeroderma ____________________
4. pachyderma ____________________

EXERCISE 7 *Identify the roots for the following definitions.*

1. dry ____________________
2. hard, horny ____________________
3. hidden ____________________
4. scaly ____________________
5. thick ____________________
6. wrinkle ____________________

EXERCISE 8 *Build a medical term from the information provided.*

1. wrinkled skin ____________________
2. dry skin ____________________
3. dry conditions ____________________

EXERCISE 9 *Match the root on the left with its definition on the right. Some definitions will be used more than once.*

c.	1. alb/o	a. black
a	2. melan/o	b. red
c	3. leuk/o	c. white
b.	4. erythr/o	d. yellow
d.	5. xanth/o	

EXERCISE 10 *Translate the following roots.*

1. melan/o ____________________
2. leuk/o ____________________
3. alb/o ____________________
4. xanth/o ____________________
5. erythr/o ____________________

EXERCISE 11 *Break down the following words into their component parts and translate.*

EXAMPLE: sinusitis *sinus | itis* *inflammation of the sinuses*

1. leukoderma ____________________
2. xanthoderma ____________________
3. erythroderma ____________________
4. melanoma ____________________

GENERATION

EXERCISE 12 *Identify the roots for the following definitions.*

1. skin (3 roots) ____________________
2. fat (3 roots) ____________________
3. sweat (1 root) ____________________
4. scale (1 root) ____________________
5. oil (2 roots) ____________________
6. hair (2 roots) ____________________
7. nail (2 roots) ____________________

Learning Outcome 3.1 Exercises

EXERCISE 13 *Build a medical term from the information provided.*

1. inflammation of the skin ____________________
2. inflammation of fat tissue ____________________
3. nail disease ____________________
4. pertaining to the skin ____________________

EXERCISE 14 *Identify the roots for the following definitions*

1. white (2 roots) ____________________
2. black (1 root) ____________________
3. red (1 root) ____________________
4. yellow (1 root) ____________________

EXERCISE 15 *Build a medical term from the information provided*

1. red skin ____________________
2. white skin ____________________
3. yellow skin ____________________

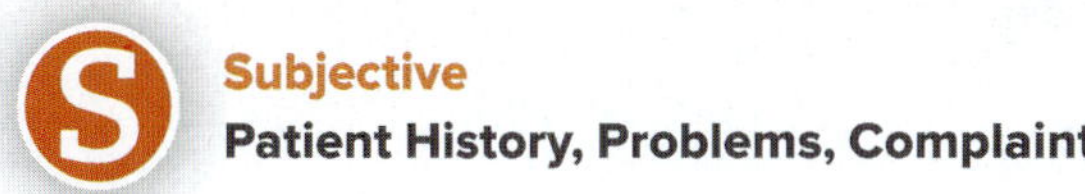

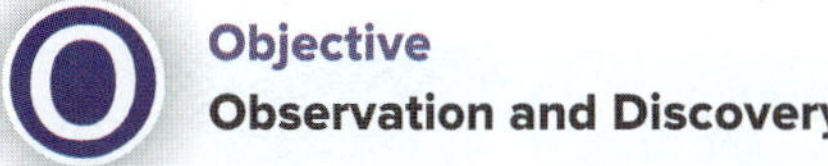

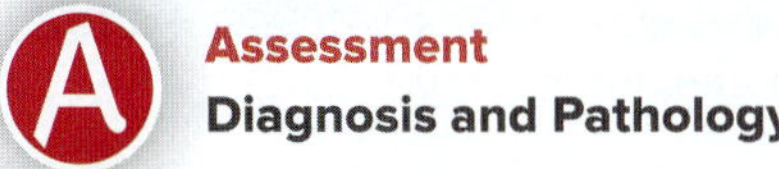

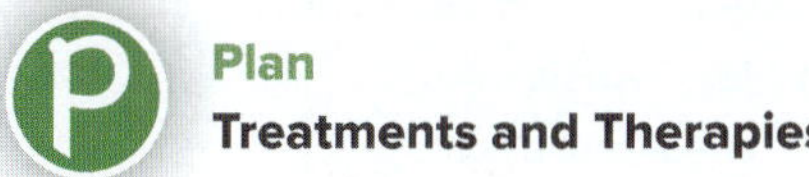

This section contains medical terms built from the roots presented in the previous section. The purpose of this section is to expose you to words used in dermatology that are built from the word roots you learned earlier in the chapter.

The focus of this book is to teach you the process of learning roots and translating them in context. Each term is presented with the correct pronunciation followed by a word analysis that breaks down the word into its component parts, a definition that provides a literal translation of the word, and supplemental information (if the literal translation deviates from its medical use).

The terms are organized using a health care professional's SOAP note (see Chapter 2) as a model.

SUBJECTIVE

3.2 Patient History, Problems, Complaints

The most common reason a person seeks medical care in relation to his or her skin is a new rash. The rash may be painful (*dermatalgia/dermatodynia*) or itchy (*pruritus*). The rash may appear as hives (*urticaria*) or as an oily secretion (*seborrhea*). The rash may be very dry (*xerosis*) or very wet (*macerate*). Patients may also notice that they are producing too much sweat (*hyperhidrosis*) or not enough sweat (*anhidrosis*).

Sometimes the patient's concern is change in normal skin color. These color changes may involve a loss of pigment (*depigmentation*) or darkening of the skin (*hypermelanosis*). Some people lack pigment altogether, as in *albinism*.

Another reason a patient might consult a dermatologist is problems with the hair. Hair falls under the responsibility of a dermatologist because the hair follicles are embedded in the skin. The most common hair complaint for men is hair loss (*alopecia*), but it occurs in women as well. Another hair problem is too much hair (*hypertrichosis*).

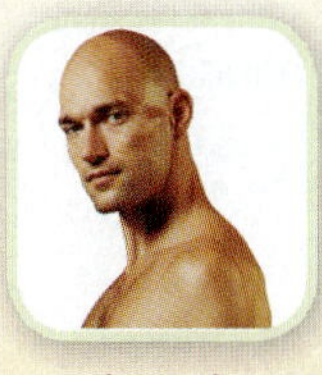
alopecia

dermatological terms

Term	Word Analysis
abrasion uh-BRAY-zhun **Definition** scraping away of skin	ab / rasion away / scrape
albinism AL-bin-ism **Definition** lack of pigment in skin causing patient to look white	albin / ism white / condition
albino al-BAY-noh **Definition** a person afflicted with albinism	albino
alopecia a-loh-PEE-sha **Definition** baldness	from Greek, for *fox*
anhidrosis an-ih-DROH-sis **Definition** lack of sweating	an / hidr / osis no / sweat / condition

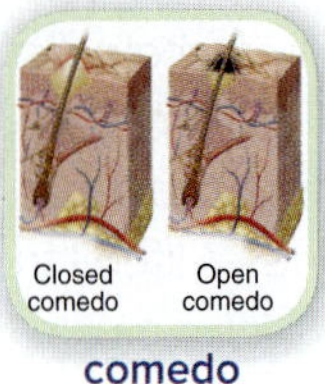

comedo

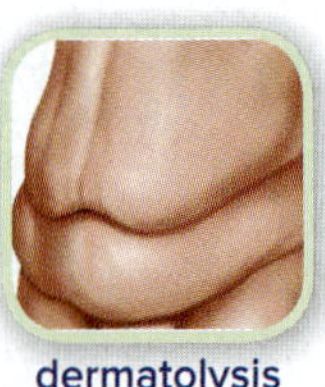
dermatolysis

dermatological terms *continued*

Term	Word Analysis
comedo koh-MEE-doh **Definition** a hair follicle that is plugged with sebum (black head, white head)	from Latin, for *to eat up*
cyanidrosis sai-yan-ih-DROH-sis **Definition** blue sweat	cyan / idr / osis blue / sweat / condition
depigmentation DE-pig-men-TAY-shun **Definition** loss of pigmentation	de / pigment / ation away / pigment / condition
dermatalgia der-mah-TAL-jah **Definition** skin pain	dermat / algia skin / pain
dermatodynia der-MA-toh-DAI-nee-ah **Definition** skin pain	dermato / dynia skin / pain
dermatolysis der-mah-TAW-lis-is **Definition** loose skin	dermato / lysis skin / loose
erythema eh-rih-THEE-ma **Definition** redness	from Greek, for *redness*
erythroderma eh-RIH-throh-DER-ma **Definition** red skin	erythro / derma red / skin
hemathidrosis heh-mat-ih-DROH-sis **Definition** sweating blood	hemat / hidr / osis blood / sweat / condition
hidropoiesis hih-droh-poh-EE-sis **Definition** the formation of sweat	hidro / poiesis sweat / formation
hyperhidrosis hai-per-hih-DROH-sis **Definition** excessive sweating	hyper / hidr / osis over / sweat / condition
hyperkerotosis hai-per-ker-ah-TOH-sis **Definition** excessive growth of horny skin	hyper / kerat / osis over / horny / condition
hypermelanosis hai-per-mel-an-OH-sis **Definition** excessive melanin in the skin	hyper / melan / osis over / black / condition
hyperpigmentation hai-per-pig-men-TAY-shun **Definition** excessive pigment in the skin	hyper / pigment / ation over / pigment / condition
hypohidrosis hai-poh-hih-DROH-sis **Definition** diminished sweating	hypo / hidr / osis under / sweat / condition

3.2 Patient History, Problems, Complaints

dermatological terms *continued*

leukoderma

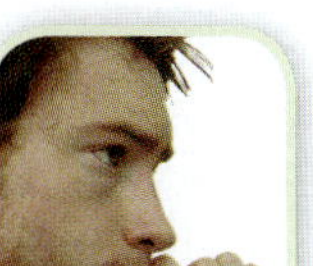

onychophagia

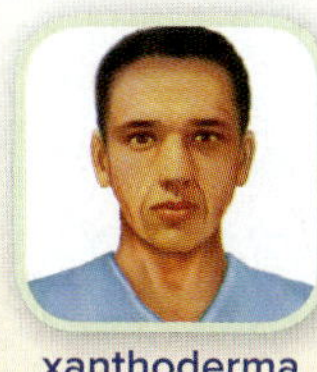

xanthoderma

Term	Word Analysis
hypomelanosis hai-poh-mel-an-OH-sis **Definition** diminished melanin in the skin	hypo / melan / osis under / black / condition
hypopigmentation hai-poh-pig-men-TAY-shun **Definition** diminished pigment in the skin	hypo / pigment / ation under / pigment / condition
leukoderma loo-koh-DER-mah **Definition** white skin	leuko / derma white / skin
macerate MAS-ir-ayt **Definition** to soften the skin	from Latin, for to make soft
onychophagia aw-nih-koh-FAY-jah **Definition** eating or biting the nails	onycho / phag / ia nail / eat / condition
pruritus prur-AI-tis **Definition** an itch NOTE: The ending on this word is easily confused with *-itis*.	from Latin, for *itching*
rhytidermia rih-tih-DER-mee-ah **Definition** wrinkled skin NOTE: Because *rhytid-* ends with a *d* and *-dermia* starts with one, the two combined into one.	rhyti / dermia wrinkle / skin
sebopoiesis see-boh-poh-EE-sis **Definition** formation of oil (sebum)	sebo / poiesis oil / formation
seborrhea seh-boh-REE-ah **Definition** discharge of oil (sebum)	sebo / rrhea oil / discharge
trichomegaly tri-koh-MEG-ah-lee **Definition** abnormally thick hair	tricho / megaly hair / enlargement
urticaria ur-tih-KAR-ee-ah **Definition** swollen raised itchy areas of the skin	from Latin, for *burning nettle*
xanthoderma zan-thoh-DER-mah **Definition** yellow skin	xantho / derma yellow / skin
xeroderma zeh-roh-DER-mah **Definition** dry skin	xero / derma dry / skin
xerosis ze-ROH-sis **Definition** condition of dryness	xer / osis dry / condition

Learning Outcome 3.2 Exercises

PRONUNCIATION

EXERCISE 1 *Indicate which syllable receives emphasis when pronounced.*

EXAMPLE: bronchitis bron**chi**tis

1. albinism ______
2. anhidrosis ______
3. dermatolysis ______
4. dermatalgia ______
5. erythema ______
6. hyperhidrosis ______
7. hyperpigmentation ______
8. macerate ______
9. pruritus ______
10. hyperkerotosis ______
11. rhytidermia ______
12. trichomegaly ______
13. urticaria ______
14. xerosis ______

TRANSLATION

EXERCISE 2 *Break down the following words into their component parts.*

EXAMPLE: nasopharyngoscope *naso | pharyngo | scope*

1. leukoderma ______
2. rhytidermia ______
3. hidropoiesis ______
4. anhidrosis ______
5. dermatolysis ______
6. hyperkeratosis ______
7. hypohidrosis ______
8. hypopigmentation ______
9. hyperpigmentation ______
10. sebopoiesis ______
11. xeroderma ______
12. depigmentation ______

Learning Outcome 3.2 Exercises

EXERCISE 3 *Underline and define the word parts from this chapter in the following terms.*

1. dermatalgia ______________________
2. albinism ______________________
3. onychophagia ______________________
4. seborrhea ______________________
5. trichomegaly ______________________
6. xerosis ______________________
7. hyperhidrosis ______________________
8. hypomelanosis ______________________
9. xanthoderma (2 roots) ______________________
10. erythroderma (2 roots) ______________________
11. hypermelanosis ______________________
12. hemathidrosis ______________________
13. cyanidrosis ______________________

EXERCISE 4 *Match the term on the left with its definition on the right.*

Response	Term	Definition
b	1. albino	a. scraping away of skin
d	2. erythema	b. a person with a lack of skin pigment, causing the person to look completely white
c	3. alopecia	c. baldness
a.	4. abrasion	d. redness
e.	5. macerate	e. to soften the skin
h.	6. comedo	f. an itch
f	7. pruritus	g. swollen, raised, itchy areas of the skin
g	8. urticaria	h. a follicle plugged with sebum (black head, white head)

EXERCISE 5 *Translate the following terms as literally as possible.*

EXAMPLE: nasopharyngoscope *an instrument for looking at the nose and throat*

1. albinism ______________________
2. xerosis ______________________
3. leukoderma ______________________
4. rhytidermia ______________________
5. seborrhea ______________________
6. depigmentation ______________________
7. hypomelanosis ______________________
8. hypopigmentation ______________________
9. trichomegaly ______________________
10. erythema ______________________
11. erythroderma ______________________
12. hyperhidrosis ______________________
13. hyperkeratosis ______________________

Learning Outcome 3.2 Exercises

GENERATION

EXERCISE 6 *Build a medical term from the information provided.*

EXAMPLE: inflammation of the sinuses *sinusitis*

1. yellow skin ______________
2. dry skin ______________
3. loose skin ______________
4. skin pain ______________
5. no sweat condition ______________
6. nail eating ______________
7. oil formation ______________
8. sweat formation ______________
9. under sweat condition ______________
10. over black condition ______________
11. over pigment condition ______________
12. blue sweat condition ______________
13. blood sweat condition ______________

EXERCISE 7 *Multiple-choice questions. Select the correct answer.*

1. From the Latin, meaning *to eat up*, which term describes a hair follicle plugged with sebum (black head, white head)?
   a. abrasion
   b. comedo
   c. macerate
   d. pruritus
2. A person with albinism has what color skin?
   a. black
   b. red
   c. yellow
   d. white
3. Which term means *to soften the skin*?
   a. abrasion
   b. comedo
   c. macerate
   d. pruritus
4. *Pruritus* describes
   a. an itch
   b. soft skin
   c. scraped skin
   d. dry skin
5. Which term comes from the Latin, meaning *burning nettle*, and describes swollen, raised, itchy areas of the skin?
   a. pruritus
   b. urticaria
   c. albinism
   d. comedo
6. Select all terms below that have roots that mean *skin*.
   a. anhidrosis
   b. albinism
   c. cyanidrosis
   d. dermatolysis
   e. erythema
   f. hemathidrosis
   g. hypohidrosis
   h. leukoderma
   i. rhytidermia
   j. xanthoderma
   k. xeroderma
   l. xerosis
7. Select all terms below that have roots meaning *sweat*.
   a. anhidrosis
   b. albinism
   c. cyanidrosis
   d. dermatolysis
   e. erythema
   f. hemathidrosis
   g. hypohidrosis
   h. leukoderma
   i. rhytidermia
   j. xanthoderma
   k. xeroderma
   l. xerosis
8. Select all terms below that have roots meaning *white*.
   a. anhidrosis
   b. albinism
   c. cyanidrosis
   d. dermatolysis
   e. erythema
   f. hemathidrosis
   g. hypohidrosis
   h. leukoderma
   i. rhytidermia
   j. xanthoderma
   k. xeroderma
   l. xerosis

OBJECTIVE

3.3 Observation and Discovery

A very specific language applies to rashes. This allows medical professionals to tell one another about rashes even when the patient is not present or no photo is available. These descriptions relate to the location, size, color, texture, and filling of the rash or its pustules, and they also describe whether the rash is flat or raised.

Usually, skin conditions are first described by their location. If the rash is limited to a specific area, it is *localized*. If the rash is all over the body, it is called a *generalized* rash. Some rashes begin in one area and spread to another. Rashes that start from the middle and work their way outward are *centrifugal*. Rashes that spread from the outside inward are *centripetal*.

Small bumps (under 1 cm) are called *papules*. When they become larger—specifically over 1 cm—they are called *nodules*. If they are large and flat like a plateau, they are known as *plaques*.

What is inside the rash is important as well. Small bumps (less than 1 cm) filled with clear fluid are called *vesicles*. If the bumps are filled with pus, they are known as *pustules*. A larger vesicle, such as a blister, is called a *bulla*, and larger pustules are called *abscesses*. Small, flat spots, such as freckles, are known as *macules*. Larger macules are *patches*.

Some skin findings are actually caused by blood vessels of the skin or just below the skin. Too many blood vessels formed in one area can cause a mass called a *cherry angioma*. A heavy concentration of blood vessels that is flat but still visible is called a *telangiectasia*. Small bruises under the skin are *petechiae*. Larger bruises are known as *ecchymosis*.

Diagnostic procedures in dermatology are limited. If the skin is being *cultured* for infection, it is being sampled to see if it harbors bacteria (culture and sensitivity), a virus, or a fungus. The most common diagnostic procedure is a *skin biopsy*. Many skin conditions can only be clearly distinguished from one another when examined under a microscope. Thus, the skin biopsy is a mainstay of dermatology. A skin biopsy can involve removal of the entire lesion. It can also be *excisional*, which means removal of a part of the lesion. It can be removed with a slice of the blade (a *shave biopsy*), or it can be punched out using a device similar to the hole punches used for paper.

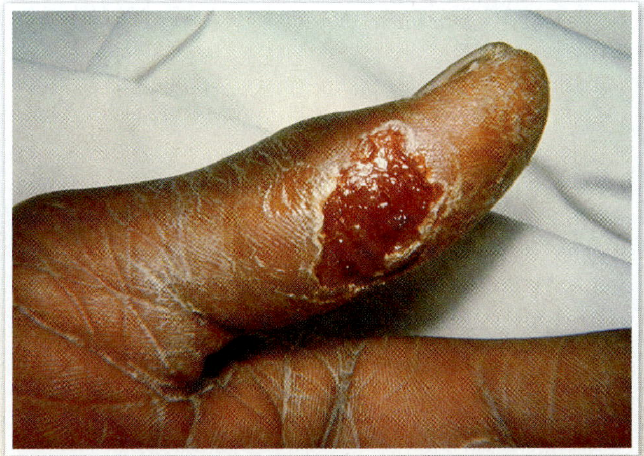

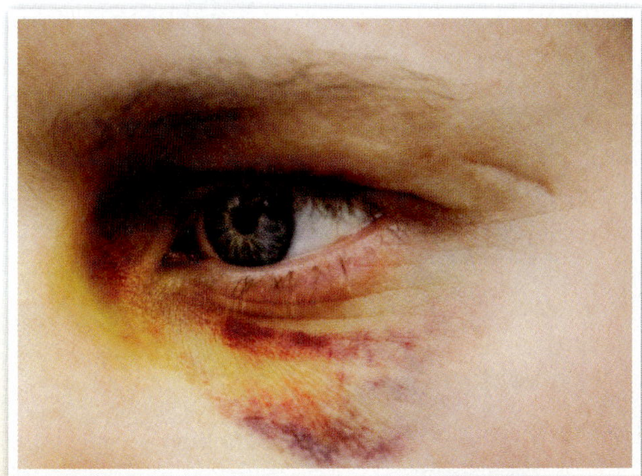

Common skin conditions observed by doctors include abscesses and black eyes.

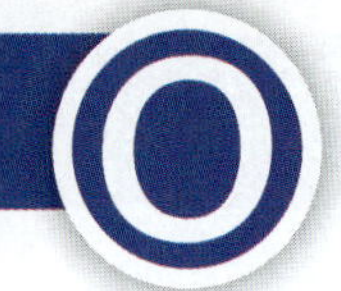

3.3 Observation and Discovery

primary lesions

Term	Word Analysis
Flat, Nonpalpable	
macule, macula (freckle) MA-kyool, MAW-koo-lah **Definition** small, flat discolored area	from Latin, for *spot or stain*
patch (vitiligo) pach (vih-tih-LAI-goh) **Definition** larger, flat discolored area	
Elevated, Palpable, Solid-Mass	
papule PA-pyool **Definition** a small solid mass	from Latin, for *pimple*
plaque PLAK **Definition** a solid mass on the surface of the skin	
nodule NAWD-jyool **Definition** a solid mass that extends deeper into the skin	
tumor TOO-mur **Definition** a larger solid mass	
Elevated, Fluid-Filled	
vesicle VEH-sih-kul **Definition** a smaller blister	ves / icle bladder / little
bulla BUL-lah **Definition** a larger blister	from Latin, for *bubble*
pustule PUS-tyool **Definition** a pus-filled blister	from Latin, for *little blister*
abscess AB-ses **Definition** a localized collection of pus in the body NOTE: The reason this word means *going away* is because in ancient times, it was believed that the harmful humors of the body would "go away" from the body via pus leaking from an abscess.	ab / scess away / go

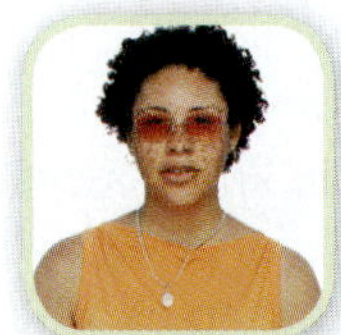

macule, macula (freckle)

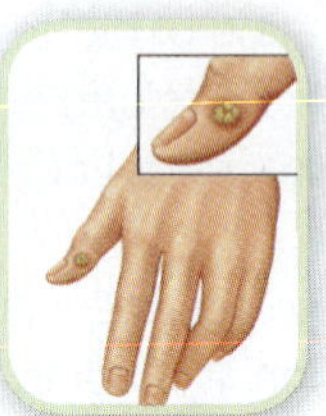

papule

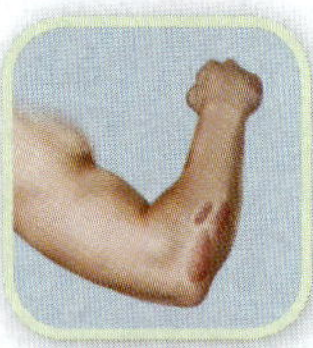

plaque

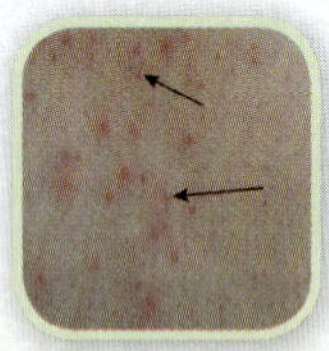

pustule

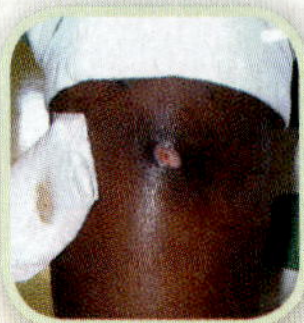

abscess

3.3 Observation and Discovery

secondary lesions

Term	Word Analysis
Loss of Skin Surface	
erosion ee-ROH-zhun **Definition** loss of skin **NOTE:** The root *ros* is where we get the word *rodent* because they gnaw on everything	e / rosion away / gnaw/eat
ulcer UL-sir **Definition** a sore	from Latin, for *sore*
excoriation eks-kor-ee-A-shun **Definition** a scratch	ex / cori / ation out / skin / condition
fissure FIH-zhur **Definition** a crack in the skin	from Latin, for a *split* or *divide*
Material on Skin Surface	
scale SKAYL **Definition** skin flaking off	
crust krust **Definition** a dried substance (i.e., blood, pus) on the skin	

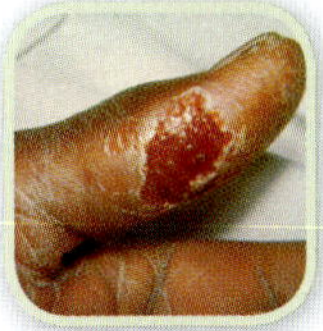

ulcer

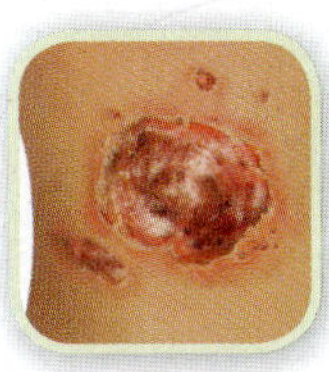

crust

vascular lesions

Term	Word Analysis
vascular lesion VAS-kyoo-lar LEE-zhun **Definition** wounds related to blood vessels	vascular lesion blood vessel wound
cherry angioma CHEH-ree an-gee-OH-mah **Definition** a small blood vessel tumor	angi / oma blood vessel / tumor
telangiectasia (spider angioma) tel-an-jee-ek-TAY-zhuh **Definition** the overexpansion of the end of a blood vessel; sometimes called a *spider angioma* because of how it looks on the skin	tel / angi / ectasia end / blood vessel / expansion

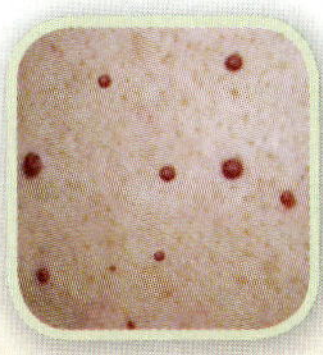

cherry angioma

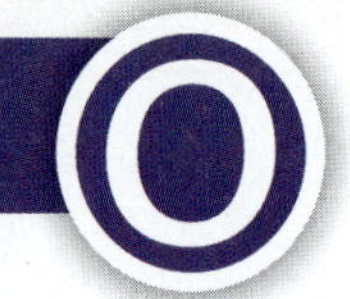

3.3 Observation and Discovery

vascular lesions *continued*

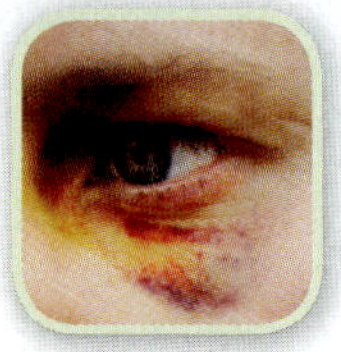
petechiae

Term	Word Analysis
petechia puh-TEE-kee-yah **Definition** a small bruise	from Latin, for *freckle* or *spot*
ecchymosis eh-kih-MOH-sis **Definition** a larger bruise	from Greek, for to *pour out*

scar formations

Term	Word Analysis
cicatrix (plural: cicatrices) SIK-ah-triks **Definition** scar	from Latin, for *scar*
keloid KEE-loid **Definition** overgrowth of scar tissue	kel / oid tumor / resembling

epidermal tumors

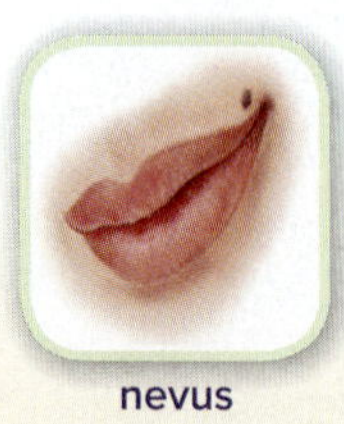
nevus

Term	Word Analysis
epidermal tumors eh-pi-DER-mal TOO-murs **Definition** tumors on the skin	epi / derm / al tumor upon / skin / pertaining to tumor
nevus NEE-vus **Definition** mole	from Latin, for *birthmark* or *mole*
dysplastic nevus dis-PLAS-tic NEE-vus **Definition** a mole with bad changes/formations (often precancerous)	dys / plastic nevus bad / formation mole
verucca vah-ROO-kah **Definition** wart	from Latin, for *wart*

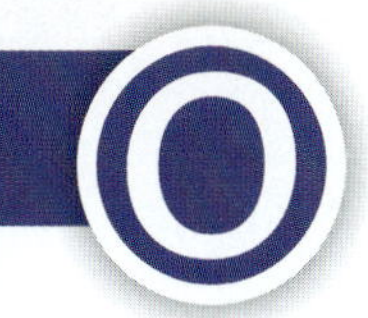

3.3 Observation and Discovery

diagnostic procedures

Term	Word Analysis
culture and sensitivity (C&S) KUL-chur and sin-sih-TIV-ih-tee **Definition** growing microorganisms in isolation in order to determine which drugs it might respond to	
biopsy (Bx) BAI-op-see **Definition** removal of tissue in order to examine it (with your own two eyes)	bi / ops / y two / eye / procedure
excisional biopsy ek-SIH-zhun-al **Definition** removal of an entire lesion for examination (to cut it out)	ex / cision / al out / cut / pertaining to
incisional biopsy in-SIH-zhun-al **Definition** removal of a portion of a lesion for examination (to cut into it)	in / cision / al in / cut / pertaining to
dermatoscope dir-MA-toh-SKOHP **Definition** instrument used to look at the skin	dermato / scope skin / instrument to look
dermoscopy der-MAW-skoh-pee **Definition** procedure for looking at the skin **Note:** The root changes from *dermato to derm* when the suffix changes from *-scope* to *-scopy*. This is unusual, but whoever came up with these terms decided that different roots sounded better—and we agree.	dermo / scop / y skin / look / procedure

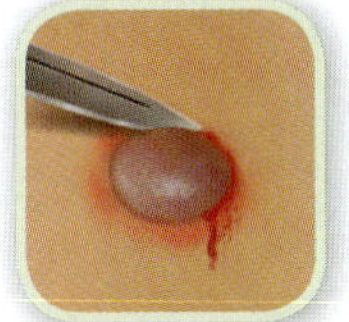
excisional biopsy

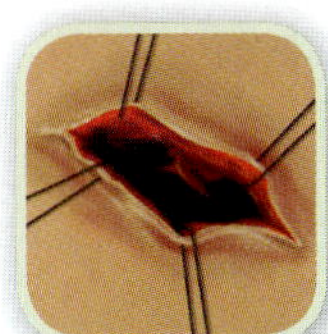
incisional biopsy

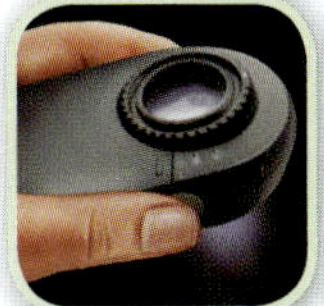
dermoscopy

pathological findings/terms

Term	Word Analysis
adipocele a-dih-poh-SEEL **Definition** a hernia filled with fatty tissue **NOTE:** *cele* originally means *tumor* or *swelling* but is frequently used to refer to types of hernia.	adipo / cele fat / tumor / hernia
dermatofibroma der-MA-toh-fai-BROH-mah **Definition** a fibrous skin tumor	dermato / fibr / oma skin / fiber / tumor
erythrocyanosis eh-RITH-roh-SAI-an-OH-sis **Definition** a red and/or blue discoloration of the skin	erytho / cyan / osis red / blue / condition
keratogenic keh-RA-toh-jen-ik **Definition** causing horny tissue development	kerato / gen / ic horny / creation / pertaining to

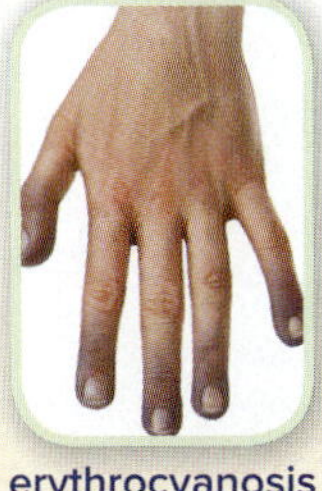
erythrocyanosis

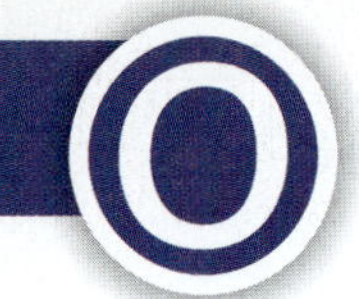

3.3 Observation and Discovery

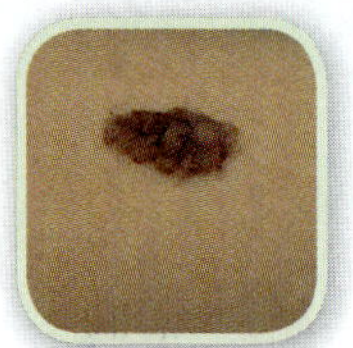

keratosis

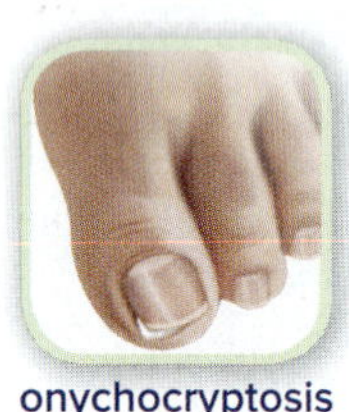

onychocryptosis

pathological findings/terms *continued*

Term	Word Analysis
keratosis KEH-rah-TOH-sis **Definition** horny tissue condition	kerat / osis horny / condition
necrosis neh-KROH-sis **Definition** tissue death	necr / osis death / condition
onychia oh-NIK-ee-ah **Definition** a nail condition	onych / ia nail / condition
onychocryptosis AW-nih-koh-krip-TOH-sis **Definition** an ingrown nail	onycho / crypt / osis nail / hidden / condition
onycholysis AW-nih-KAWL-is-is **Definition** the loss of a nail	onycho / lysis nail / loose
onychomalacia AW-nih-koh-mah-LAY-shah **Definition** abnormal softening of a nail	onycho / malac / ia nail / softness / condition
onychopathy aw-nik-AW-pah-thee **Definition** nail disease	onycho / pathy nail / disease
onychophagia aw-nih-koh-FAY-jah **Definition** eating (biting) the nail	onycho / phag / ia nail / eat / condition
pachyderma pa-kih-DER-mah **Definition** tough skin	pachy / derma thick / skin
paronychia par-aw-NIH-kee-ah **Definition** a condition of the tissue around a nail **NOTE:** The prefix *para-* has been modified here to *par-* because the root that follows it begins with a vowel.	par / onych / ia around / nail / condition
steatoma STAY-ah-TOH-ma **Definition** a fatty tumor	steat / oma fat / tumor
xanthoma zan-THOH-mah **Definition** a yellow tumor	xanth / oma yellow / tumor

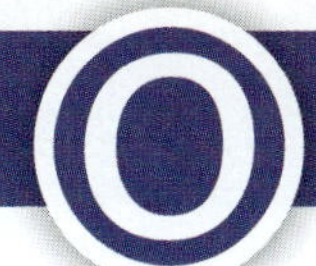

Learning Outcome 3.3 Exercises

PRONUNCIATION

EXERCISE 1 *Indicate which syllable receives emphasis when pronounced.*

EXAMPLE: bronchitis bron**chi**tis

1. vitiligo ______
2. papule ______
3. nodule ______
4. vesicle ______
5. pustule ______
6. excoriation ______
7. angioma ______
8. telangiectasia ______
9. petechia ______
10. ecchymosis ______
11. dysplastic nevus ______
12. verucca ______
13. excisional ______
14. dermatofibroma ______
15. keratogenic ______
16. keratosis ______
17. onychia ______
18. onycholysis ______
19. onychopathy ______
20. pachyderma ______

TRANSLATION

EXERCISE 2 *Break down the following words into their component parts.*

EXAMPLE: nasopharyngoscope *naso | pharyngo | scope*

1. excisional biopsy ______
2. incisional biopsy ______
3. dysplastic nevus ______
4. telangiectasia ______
5. biopsy ______
6. keratosis ______
7. necrosis ______
8. onychocryptosis ______
9. onychopathy ______
10. pachyderma ______
11. dermatoscope ______

EXERCISE 3 *Underline and define the word parts from this chapter in the following terms.*

1. epidermal tumor ______
2. adipocele ______
3. dermatofibroma ______
4. erythocyanosis ______
5. keratogenic ______
6. onychia ______
7. onycholysis ______
8. onychomalacia ______
9. onychophagia ______
10. paronychia ______
11. steatoma ______
12. xanthoma ______

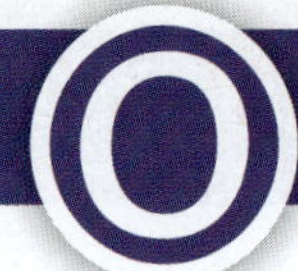

Learning Outcome 3.3 Exercises

EXERCISE 4 *Match the term on the left with its definition on the right.*

Term	Definition
____ 1. tumor	a. freckle; small, flat discolored area
____ 2. abscess	b. larger, flat discolored area
____ 3. pustule	c. from Latin, for *pimple*, a small solid mass
____ 4. culture and sensitivity	d. a solid mass on the surface of the skin
____ 5. nodule	e. a solid mass that extends deeper into the skin
____ 6. patch (vitiligo)	f. a larger solid mass
____ 7. plaque	g. a small blister
____ 8. vesicle	h. a large blister
____ 9. macule	i. a pus-filled blister
____ 10. papule	j. a localized collection of pus in the body
____ 11. bulla	k. diagnostic procedure in dermatology

EXERCISE 5 *Match the term on the left with its definition on the right.*

Term	Definition
____ 1. ulcer	a. a small bruise
____ 2. erosion	b. a large bruise
____ 3. petechia	c. a small blood vessel tumor
____ 4. scale	d. a crack in the skin
____ 5. crust	e. loss of skin
____ 6. cherry angioma	f. skin flaking off
____ 7. fissure	g. a sore
____ 8. keloid	h. dried substance (i.e., blood, pus) on the skin
____ 9. verucca	i. a scratch
____ 10. nevus	j. scar
____ 11. cicatrix	k. overgrowth of scar tissue
____ 12. ecchymosis	l. mole
____ 13. excoriation	m. wart

EXERCISE 6 *Translate the following terms as literally as possible.*

> EXAMPLE: nasopharyngoscope *an instrument for looking at the nose and throat*

1. vesicle ____________________
2. abscess ____________________
3. erosion ____________________
4. keloid ____________________
5. epidermal tumor ____________________
6. dysplastic nevus ____________________
7. biopsy ____________________
8. incisional biopsy ____________________
9. dermatofibroma ____________________
10. erythocyanosis ____________________
11. keratosis ____________________
12. necrosis ____________________
13. onychocryptosis ____________________
14. onycholysis ____________________
15. pachyderma ____________________

Learning Outcome 3.3 Exercises

GENERATION

EXERCISE 7 *Build a medical term from the information provided.*

EXAMPLE: inflammation of the sinuses *sinusitis*

1. nail condition ______
2. nail disease ______
3. fat tumor (2 terms) ______
4. to cut it out ______
5. pertaining to horny tissue creation ______
6. nail softness condition ______
7. yellow tumor ______
8. eating the nail ______
9. procedure to look at the skin ______
10. (over) expansion of the end of a blood vessel ______
11. a condition of the tissue around the nail ______
12. blood vessel tumor ______

EXERCISE 8 *Multiple-choice questions. Select the correct answer(s).*

1. Select all terms below that refer to flat, nonpalpable lesions.
   a. abscess
   b. bulla
   c. macule (freckle)
   d. nodule
   e. papule
   f. patch
   g. plaque
   h. pustule
   i. tumor
   j. vesicle
   k. vitiligo
2. Select all terms below that refer to elevated, palpable, solid-mass lesions.
   a. abscess
   b. bulla
   c. macule (freckle)
   d. nodule
   e. papule
   f. patch
   g. plaque
   h. pustule
   i. tumor
   j. vesicle
   k. vitiligo
3. Select all terms below that refer to elevated, fluid-filled lesions.
   a. abscess
   b. bulla
   c. macule (freckle)
   d. nodule
   e. papule
   f. patch
   g. plaque
   h. pustule
   i. tumor
   j. vesicle
   k. vitiligo
4. Which flat, nonpalpable lesion is the smallest?
   a. macule
   b. papule
   c. patch
   d. vitiligo
5. Which elevated, palpable, solid-mass lesion is the largest?
   a. papule
   b. plaque
   c. nodule
   d. tumor
6. Which elevated, fluid-filled lesion is pus-filled?
   a. bulla
   b. plaque
   c. pustule
   d. vesicle
7. Select all terms below that refer to lesions involving the loss of skin surface.
   a. crust
   b. erosion
   c. excoriation
   d. fissure
   e. scale
   f. ulcer
8. Select all terms below that refer to lesions involving material on the skin surface.
   a. crust
   b. erosion
   c. excoriation
   d. fissure
   e. scale
   f. ulcer
9. Select all terms below that refer to vascular lesions.
   a. cherry angioma
   b. cicatrix
   c. dysplastic nevus
   d. ecchymosis
   e. keloid
   f. nevus
   g. petechia
   h. telangiectasia
   i. verucca

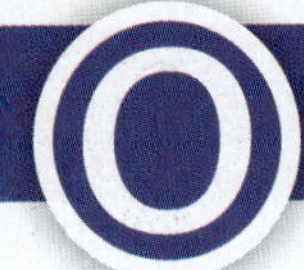

Learning Outcome 3.3 Exercises

10. Select all terms below that refer to scar formation.
    a. cherry angioma
    b. cicatrix
    c. dysplastic nevus
    d. ecchymosis
    e. keloid
    f. nevus
    g. petechia
    h. telangiectasia
    i. verucca
11. Select all terms below that refer to epidermal tumors.
    a. cherry angioma
    b. cicatrix
    c. dysplastic nevus
    d. ecchymosis
    e. keloid
    f. nevus
    g. petechia
    h. telangiectasia
    i. verucca
12. Which diagnostic procedure involves growing microorganisms in order to determine what drugs it might respond to best?
    a. biopsy
    b. culture and sensitivity
    c. excisional biopsy
    d. incisional biopsy
13. Rashes that start from the middle and work their way outward are __________.
    a. centrifugal
    b. centripetal
    c. generalized
    d. localized
14. Rashes that spread from the outside inward are __________.
    a. centrifugal
    b. centripetal
    c. generalized
    d. localized
15. If the rash is limited to a specific area, it is a __________ rash.
    a. centrifugal
    b. centripetal
    c. generalized
    d. localized
16. If the rash is all over the body, it is a __________ rash.
    a. centrifugal
    b. centripetal
    c. generalized
    d. localized

EXERCISE 9 *Define the following terms.*

1. macule __________
2. vitiligo __________
3. patch __________
4. papule __________
5. plaque __________
6. nodule __________
7. tumor __________
8. bulla __________
9. pustule __________
10. ulcer __________
11. excoriation __________
12. fissure __________
13. scale __________
14. crust __________
15. petechia __________
16. ecchymosis __________
17. cicatrix __________
18. verucca __________
19. nevus __________

3.4 Diagnosis and Pathology

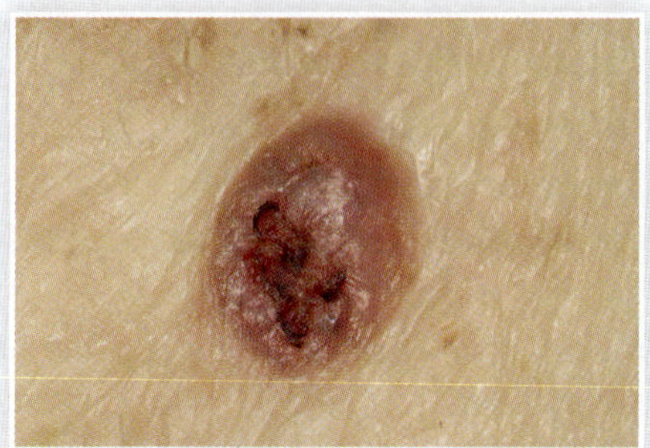
Basal cell carcinoma

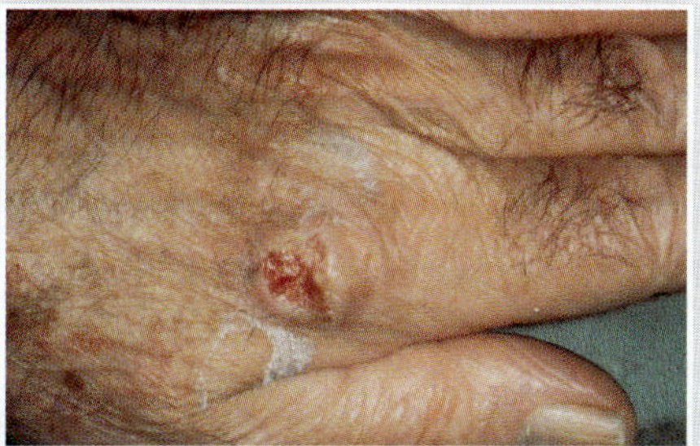
Squamous cell carcinoma

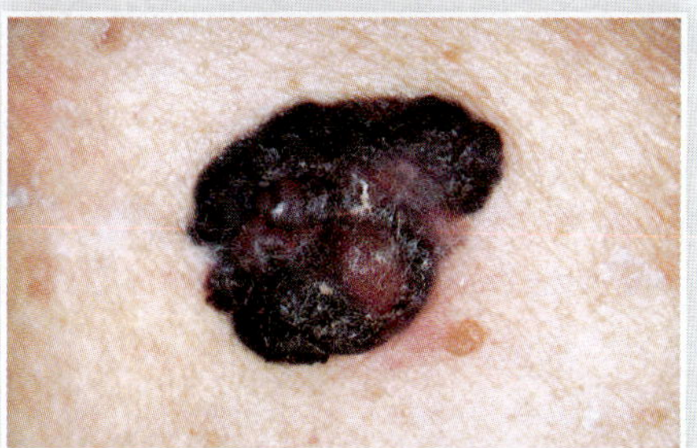
Malignant melanoma

Skin problems are fairly limited in variety. For the most part, skin problems are infections, inflammations, tumors, or changes in the skin. Bacterial infections of the skin can be a small yellow crust, like *impetigo*, or a more extensive one, like *cellulitis*, which invades deeper layers of skin.

Other skin structures may be infected by bacteria as well: *Hidradenitis* is an infection of the sweat glands in the skin. *Acne* is similar. It is an infection of the *sebaceous* glands that commonly occurs in puberty because of the increase in hormones. Skin can be infected with a fungus (*mycosis*), and fingernails and toenails can also be infected with a fungus (*onychomycosis*). Nail infections typically require a long course of treatment.

Skin may be inflamed without being infected. *Dermatitis* is a general term for skin inflammation that does not indicate its cause. *Actinic dermatitis* is a skin condition related to sun exposure. *Seborrheic dermatitis* is a scaly red rash common in infants and elderly people.

Most tumors of the skin are related to ultraviolet (UV) exposure from the sun. As a result, dermatologists often spend at least part of their visits with their patients explaining how to avoid sun exposure. Basal cell carcinomas, melanomas, and squamous cell carcinomas are all tumors associated with sun exposure.

- *Basal cell carcinoma*, the most common cancer of the skin, often presents as a round, flesh-colored, and pearly nodule.

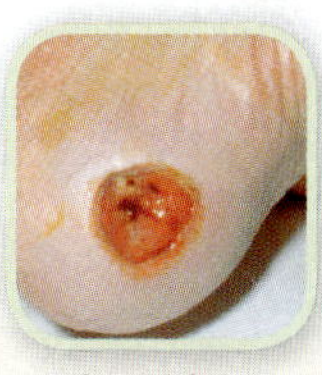
decubitus ulcer

general skin changes

Term	Word Analysis
decubitus ulcer deh-KYOO-bih-tus UL-sir **Definition** bed sore	**de / cubitus ulcer** down / lie sore
dermatosis der-mah-TOH-sis **Definition** skin condition	**dermat / osis** skin / condition
dermopathy der-MAW-pa-thee **Definition** skin disease	**dermo / pathy** skin / disease
eczema EK-zeh-mah **Definition** a red itchy rash that may weep or ooze, then become crusted and scaly	**from Greek, for to** *boil over*

3.4 Diagnosis and Pathology

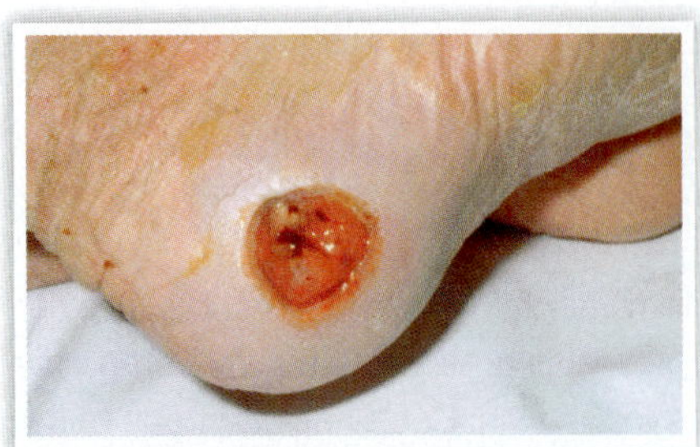

Decubitus ulcer

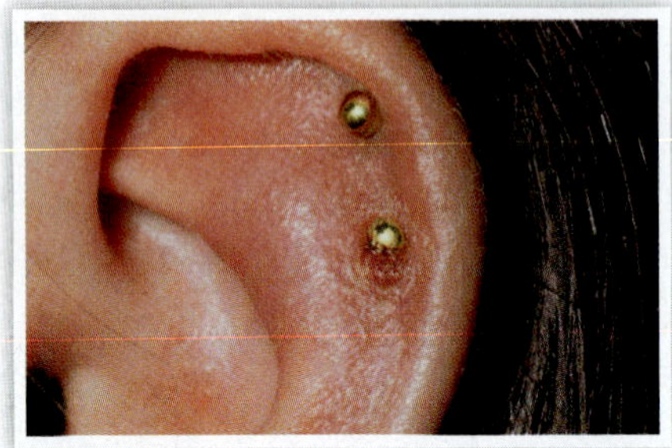

Dermatitis

- While *melanoma*, a cancer of the pigment-producing cells in the skin, is not the most common form of skin cancer, it is responsible for the most deaths. Melanomas are brown in color.
- *Squamous cell carcinoma* can occur anywhere in the skin where squamous cells are found. Squamous cell carcinoma of the skin begins as a small papule but eventually leads to an ulcer.
- *Actinic keratosis* is a precancerous condition also associated with sun exposure.

General skin problems, such as atopic dermatitis, can affect large areas of the body. *Atopic dermatitis* is very sensitive skin that is common in people with allergies and asthma. The skin is very dry and itchy. *Ichthyosis* is a condition that involves the skin becoming very thick and scaly. *A decubitus ulcer* is a large erosion of skin often seen in bedridden people. When the skin is under constant pressure, it can break down and cause an ulcer.

general skin changes *continued*

Term	Word Analysis
atopic dermatitis AY-taw-pik der-mah-TAI-tis **Definition** an unusual inflammation of the skin NOTE: *Atopic* literally means *not in the right place and thus unusual.*	**a / top / ic dermat / itis** not / place / pertaining to skin / inflammation
hypertrichosis HAI-per-trih-KOH-sis **Definition** excessive growth of hair	**hyper / trich / osis** over / hair / condition
ichthyosis ik-thee-OH-sis **Definition** a condition in the skin is dry and scaly resembling fish scales	**ichthy / osis** fish scale / condiion
postpartum alopecia post-PAR-tum al-oh-PEE-shah **Definition** baldness experienced by women after a pregnancy	**post / partum alopecia** after / birth baldness
sclerodermatitis skleh-roh-der-mah-TAI-tis **Definition** inflammation of the skin accompanied by thickening and hardening	**sclero / dermat / itis** hard / skin / inflammation
scleronychia skleh-raw-NIH-kee-ah **Definition** thickening and hardening of the nails	**scler / onych / ia** hard / nail / condition
xanthosis zan-THOH-sis **Definition** yellowing of the skin	**xanth / osis** yellow / condition

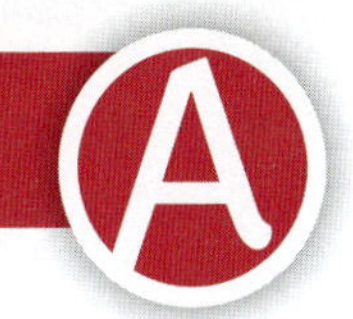

3.4 Diagnosis and Pathology

malignant melanoma

squamous cell carcinoma

tumors

Term	Word Analysis
actinic keratosis ak-TIN-ik keh-rah-TOH-sis **Definition** horny skin condition caused by sun exposure	actin / ic kerat / osis sun ray / pertaining to horny / condition
basal cell carcinoma BAY-zul sell kar-sih-NOH-mah **Definition** cancerous tumor of basal skin cells	basal cell carcin / oma base cell cancer / tumor
hidradenoma hih-drad-eh-NOH-mah **Definition** tumor of the sweat gland	hidr / aden / oma sweat / gland / tumor
malignant cutaneous neoplasm mah-LIG-nant kuh-TAY-nee-us NEE-oh-plaz-um **Definition** a harmful new formation of skin tissue (i.e., skin cancer)	malignant cutane / ous neo / plasm harmful skin / pertaining to new / formation
malignant melanoma ma-LIG-nant meh-lah-NOH-mah **Definition** a harmful tumor of melanin cells	malignant melan / oma bad black / tumor
squamous cell carcinoma SKWAY-mus sell kar-sih-NO-mah **Definition** cancerous tumor of squamous skin cells	squam / ous cell carcin / oma scale / pertaining to cell cancer / tumor

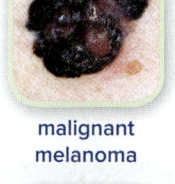

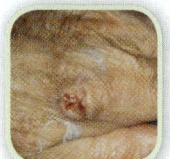

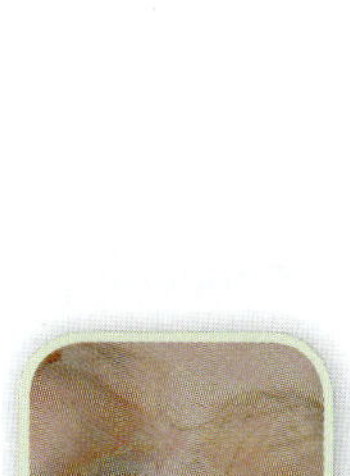

dermatomycosis

infections

Term	Word Analysis
acne vulgaris AK-nee vul-GAR-is **Definition** inflammation of the skin follicles	acne vulgaris acne common
dermatomycosis der-mah-toh-mai-KOH-sis **Definition** a fungal skin condition	dermato / myc / osis skin / fungus / condition
hidradenitis hih-dra-deh-NAI-tis **Definition** inflammation of the sweat glands	hidr / aden / itis sweat / gland / inflammation
impetigo im-peh-TAI-goh **Definition** a highly contagious bacterial infection of the skin	from Latin, for *to attack*
mycodermatitis mai-koh-der-mah-TAI-tis **Definition** inflammation of the skin caused by fungus	myco / dermat / itis fungus / skin / inflammation
mycosis mai-KOH-sis **Definition** a fungal condition	myc / osis fungus / condition

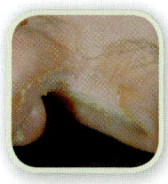

infections *continued*

Term	Word Analysis
onychodystrophy AW-ni-koh-DIS-troh-fee **Definition** poor nourishment (and development) of the nail	onycho / dys / troph / y nail / bad / nourishment / condition
onychomycosis AW-nih-koh-mai-KOH-sis **Definition** a fungal condition of the nail	onycho / myc / osis nail / fungus / condition
trichomycosis trik-koh-mai-KOH-sis **Definition** a fungal condition of the hair	tricho / myc / osis hair / fungus / condition

inflammations

Term	Word Analysis
actinic dermatitis ak-TIN-ik der-mah-TAI-tis **Definition** inflammation of the skin caused by sun exposure	actin / ic dermat / itis sun ray / pertaining to skin / inflammation
dermatitis der-mah-TAI-tis **Definition** inflammation of the skin	dermat / itis skin / inflammation
dermatoconiosis der-ma-toh-COH-nee-oh-sis **Definition** a skin condition caused by dirt	dermato / coni / osis skin / dust / condition
seborrheic dermatitis se-boh-RAY-ik der-mah-TAI-tis **Definition** inflammation of the skin caused by the discharge of oil (sebum)	sebo / rrhe / ic dermat / itis oil / discharge / pertaining to skin / inflammation
steatitis stay-ah-TAI-tis **Definition** inflammation of fat tissue	steat / itis fat / inflammation

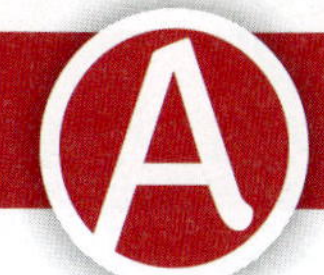

Learning Outcome 3.4 Exercises

PRONUNCIATION

EXERCISE 1 *Indicate which syllable receives emphasis when pronounced.*

EXAMPLE: bronchitis bron**chi**tis

1. actinic ________
2. dermatoconiosis ________
3. dermatomycosis ________
4. onychomycosis ________
5. hidradenitis ________
6. mycodermatitis ________
7. mycosis ________
8. hidradenoma ________
9. dermopathy ________
10. eczema ________
11. sclerodermatitis ________
12. xanthosis ________

TRANSLATION

EXERCISE 2 *Break down the following words into their component parts.*

EXAMPLE: nasopharyngoscope *naso | pharyngo | scope*

1. dermopathy ________
2. mycodermatitis ________
3. mycosis ________
4. onychomycosis ________
5. dermatitis ________
6. dermatoconiosis ________
7. hidradenoma ________
8. malignant melanoma ________
9. dermatosis ________
10. atopic dermatitis ________
11. sclerodermatitis ________

EXERCISE 3 *Underline and define the word parts from this chapter in the following terms.*

1. hidradenitis ________
2. dermatomycosis ________
3. onychodystrophy ________
4. trichomycosis ________
5. actinic dermatitis ________
6. seborrhetic ________
7. steatitis ________
8. keratosis ________
9. squamous cell carcinoma ________
10. scleronychia (2 roots) ________
11. xanthosis ________

EXERCISE 4 *Match the term on the left with its definition on the right.*

____ 1. impetigo
____ 2. acne vulgaris
____ 3. decubitus ulcer
____ 4. eczema
____ 5. postpartum alopecia
____ 6. malignant cutaneous neoplasm
____ 7. ichthyosis
____ 8. actinic keratosis

a. a highly contagious bacterial infection of the skin
b. horny skin condition caused by sun exposure
c. a harmful new formation of skin tissue
d. a skin condition that is dry and scaly
e. baldness experienced by women after a pregnancy
f. a red, itchy rash that may weep or ooze and then become crusted and scaly
g. bed sore
h. common acne

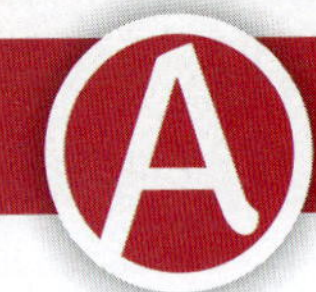

Learning Outcome 3.4 Exercises

EXERCISE 5 *Translate the following terms as literally as possible.*

EXAMPLE: nasopharyngoscope *an instrument for looking at the nose and throat*

1. dermatosis ______
2. mycosis ______
3. steatitis ______
4. mycodermatitis ______
5. sclerodermatitis ______
6. scleronychia ______
7. basal cell carcinoma ______
8. hidradenoma ______
9. ichthyosis ______
10. malignant melanoma ______

GENERATION

EXERCISE 6 *Build a medical term from the information provided.*

EXAMPLE: inflammation of the sinuses *sinusitis*

1. skin disease ______
2. skin inflammation ______
3. sweat gland inflammation ______
4. a fungal condition of the nail ______
5. a fungal condition of the hair ______
6. a fungal condition of the skin ______
7. yellowing of the skin ______
8. an unusual inflammation of the skin ______
9. cancerous tumor of squamous skin cells ______
10. baldness experienced by women after a pregnancy ______

EXERCISE 7 *Multiple-choice questions. Select the correct answer.*

1. *Acne vulgaris* means
   a. common acne
   b. inflammation of the skin follicles
   c. both common acne and inflammation of the skin follicles
   d. neither common acne nor inflammation of the skin follicles

2. Impetigo is a
   a. bacterial infection
   b. fungal infection
   c. viral infection
   d. none of these

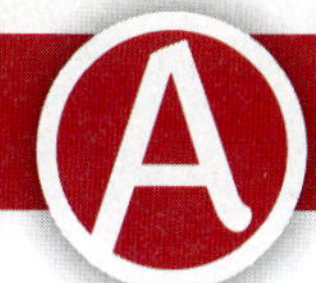

Learning Outcome 3.4 Exercises

3. *Onychodysptrophy* is
   a. poor nourishment (and development) of the nail
   b. a fungal condition of the nail
   c. a bad infection of the nail
   d. inflammation of the nail

4. Inflammation of the skin caused by sun exposure is
   a. dermatoconiosis
   b. seborrheic dermatitis
   c. actinic dermatitis
   d. actinic keratosis

5. A skin condition caused by dirt is
   a. dermatoconiosis
   b. seborrheic dermatitis
   c. actinic dermatitis
   d. actinic keratosis

6. A skin condition caused by the discharge of oil is
   a. dermatoconiosis
   b. seborrheic dermatitis
   c. actinic dermatitis
   d. actinic keratosis

7. A horny skin condition caused by sun exposure is
   a. dermatoconiosis
   b. seborrheic dermatitis
   c. actinic dermatitis
   d. actinic keratosis

8. A *malignant cutaneous neoplasm* is
   a. a harmful new formation of the skin tissue (i.e., skin cancer)
   b. a harmful tumor of melanin cells
   c. a cancerous tumor of squamous skin cells
   d. a tumor of the sweat gland

9. A bed sore is a(n)
   a. ichthyosis
   b. decubitus ulcer
   c. steatitis
   d. scleronychia

10. Eczema is
   a. from Greek, for to *boil over*
   b. from Latin, for to *attack*
   c. from Greek, for *to boil over;* and from Latin, for to attack impetigo
   d. neither from Greek, for *to boil over;* nor from Latin, for to attack

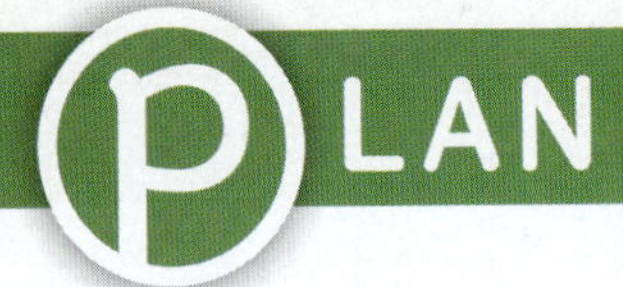

3.5 Treatments and Therapies

There is an old joke in the health community that treatment options in dermatology are very simple: If it's wet, dry it; if it's dry, wet it; and if nothing else works, use steroids. The medicines available in skin care have increased significantly, but they mostly fall in one of a few categories: anti-infection or cleansing (*antibiotics, antiseptics*), anti-immune (*steroids* or related), and anti-itch or allergy (*antihistamines*). In contrast to the limited number of medicines, the field of dermatology employs a variety of types of procedures in eradicating disease. They use chemicals (*chemosurgery* and *chemotherapy*), vacuums (*liposuction*), cold (*cryosurgery*), lasers (*dermabrasion*), and even electricity (*electrosurgery, electrodesiccation*). Of the many different surgical techniques to treat cancer, one of the oldest is Mohs micrographic surgery. The procedure involves removing very thin layers of tissue, examining them under the microscope for cancer, and continuing to remove skin layers until the cancer can no longer be detected. Originally, this technique involved the use of a chemical to "fix" the tissue in place; hence, the original term was *chemosurgery*. Chemicals are no longer used to fix the skin. The newer term, *micrography*, reflects the use of "mapping" out the skin for cancer under the microscope. This procedure and many others still rely on cold, hard steel for cutting, incision and drainage of an abscess, removing all or part of a nail (*onychectomy*), and biopsies still generally rely on the use of a scalpel.

One very challenging and important area of skin surgery is transplanting or grafting new skin in place of old skin. This is needed in areas where skin has been burned, scraped off, or killed. The transplanted skin can come from the patient (*autograft*), another person (*homograft*), or even another species (*heterograft*). While not all health care workers perform such in-depth procedures, most do perform skin-related procedures many times a day—specifically, injections. Inserting a needle into the skin to give medicine is a very routine part of many medical fields.

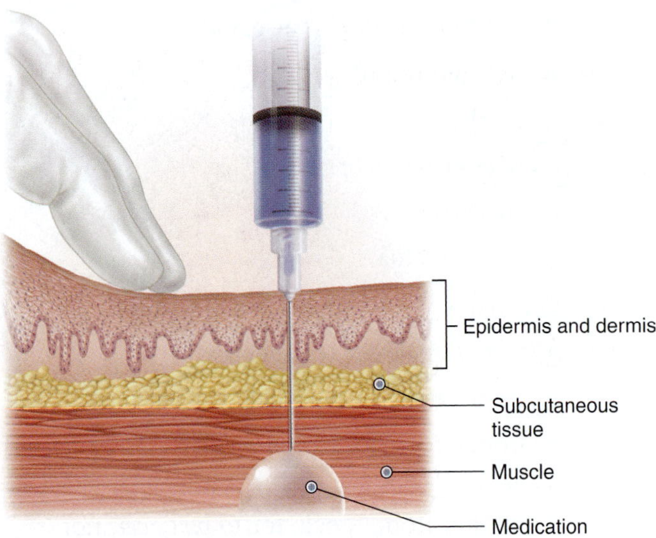

A wide variety of medications are administered via hypodermic needle. As the name suggests, it injects the medicine "beneath (*hypo-*) the skin (*dermic*)."

general terms

Term	Word Analysis
epidermal eh-pih-DER-mal **Definition** pertaining to the skin	**epi / derm / al** upon / skin / pertaining to
hypodermic hai-poh-DER-mik **Definition** pertaining to beneath the skin	**hypo / derm / ic** beneath / skin / pertaining to
intradermal in-tra-DER-mal **Definition** pertaining to inside the skin	**intra / derm / al** inside / skin / pertaining to

intradermal

3.5 Treatments and Therapies

general terms *continued*

Term	Word Analysis
percutaneous per-kyoo-TAY-nee-us **Definition** pertaining to through the skin	per / cutane / ous through / skin / pertaining to
subcutaneous sub-kyoo-TAY-nee-us **Definition** pertaining to beneath the skin	sub / cutane / ous beneath / skin / pertaining to
transdermal trans-DER-mal **Definition** pertaining to through the skin	trans / derm / al through / skin / pertaining to

procedures

Term	Word Analysis
chemosurgery KEE-moh-SIR-juh-ree **Definition** removal of tissue that has been destroyed using chemicals	chemo / surgery chemical / surgery
chemotherapy KEE-moh-THEH-rah-pee **Definition** treatment using chemicals	chemo / therapy chemical / treatment
cryosurgery KRAI-oh-SIR-juh-ree **Definition** destruction of tissue through freezing	cryo / surgery cold / surgery
dermabrasion der-mah-BRAY-zhun **Definition** rubbing or scraping away the outer surface of skin	derm / ab / rasion skin / away / rub
electrocauterization e-LEK-troh-KAW-ter-ai ZAY-shun **Definition** using electricity to destroy tissue by burning it	electro / cauteriz / ation electricity / burn / process
electrodesiccation e-LEK-troh-deh-sih-KAY-shun **Definition** using electricity to destroy tissue by drying it NOTE: That little packet labeled "Do Not Eat" that you sometimes find in packages is called a *desiccant* because it absorbs moisture and keeps the product dry.	electro / desicc / ation electricity / drying / process
incision and drainage (I&D) in-SIH-zhun and DRAY-nij **Definition** to cut into a wound to allow trapped infected liquid to drain	in / cision in / cut

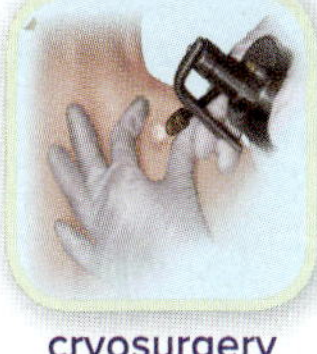
cryosurgery

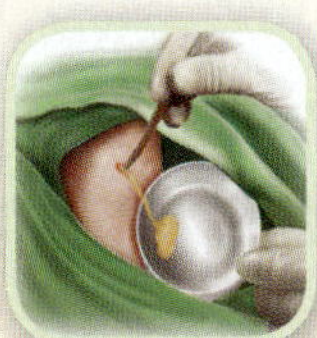
incision and drainage (I&D)

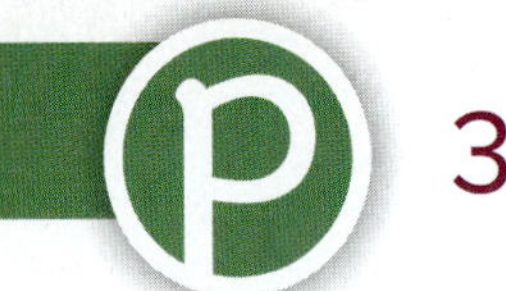

3.5 Treatments and Therapies

procedures *continued*

Term	Word Analysis
lipectomy lih-PEK-toh-mee **Definition** removal of fatty tissue	**lip / ec / tomy** fat / out / cut
liposuction LAI-poh-SUK-shun **Definition** removal of fatty tissue using a vacuum	**lipo / suction** fat / vacuum
onychectomy aw-nik-EK-toh-mee **Definition** remove of a nail	**onych / ec / tomy** nail / out / cut
onychotomy aw-ni-KAW-toh-mee **Definition** incision into a nail	**onycho / tomy** nail / cut
rhytidoplasty rih-tih-doh-PLAS-tee **Definition** reconstruction of wrinkled skin	**rhytido / plasty** wrinkle / reconstruction

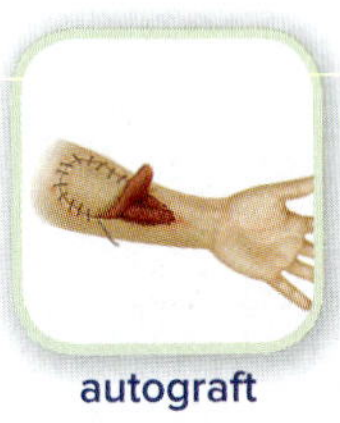

autograft

skin grafting

Term	Word Analysis
autograft AW-toh-GRAFT **Definition** skin transplant taken from a different place on the patient's body	**auto / graft** self / transplant
homograft (allograft) HOH-moh-GRAFT (A-loh-GRAFT) **Definition** skin transplant taken from another member of the patient's species (homo, because it is from a similar species, and allo, because it is from another person)	**homo / graft (allo / graft)** similar / transplant (other / transplant)
heterograft HEH-ter-oh-GRAFT **Definition** skin transplant taken from a species other than the patient's	**hetero / graft** different / transplant
xenograft ZEE-noh-graft **Definition** skin transplant taken from a species other than the patient's **NOTE:** The terms *heterograft* and *xenograft* are interchangeable and mean basically the same thing: *hetero* because it is a different species, and *xeno* because it is a foreign species.	**xeno / graft** foreign / transplant

3.5 Treatments and Therapies

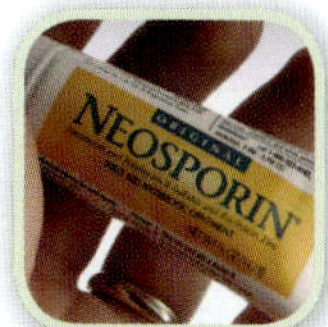

antibiotic

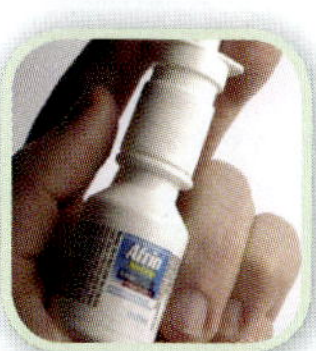
antihistamine

drugs

Term	Word Analysis
anesthetic an-es-THET-ik **Definition** a drug that temporarily blocks sensation	an / esthetic no / sensation
antibiotic an-tai-bai-OH-tk **Definition** a drug that destroys or opposes growth of microorganisms **Note:** The life that the drug is preventing is not the life of the patient but the life of microorganisms; similarly, a drug that encourages the growth of microorganisms (especially in the digestive system) is called a probiotic.	anti / biotic against / life
antihistamine an-tee-HIS-tah-meen **Definition** a drug that opposes the effects of histamine	anti / histamine against / histamine
antipruritic an-tee-pruh-RIH-tik **Definition** a drug that prevents or relieves itching	anti / pruritic against / itching
antiseptic an-tee-SEP-tik **Definition** a drug that prevents sepsis (rotting of flesh) by killing microorganisms	anti / septic against / rotting

Learning Outcome 3.5 Exercises

PRONUNCIATION

EXERCISE 1 *Indicate which syllable receives emphasis when pronounced.*

EXAMPLE: bronchitis bron**chi**tis

1. dermabrasion ______
2. lipectomy ______
3. onychectomy ______
4. onychotomy ______
5. xenograft ______
6. epidermal ______
7. transdermal ______
8. percutaneous ______
9. hypodermic ______
10. intradermal ______
11. antihistamine ______
12. antipruritic ______

TRANSLATION

EXERCISE 2 *Break down the following words into their component parts.*

EXAMPLE: nasopharyngoscope *naso | pharyngo | scope*

1. incision ______
2. autograft ______
3. homograft ______
4. allograft ______
5. heterograft ______
6. xenograft ______
7. intradermal ______
8. transdermal ______
9. chemosurgery ______
10. chemotherapy ______
11. cryosurgery ______
12. liposuction ______
13. onychotomy ______

EXERCISE 3 *Underline and define the word parts from this chapter in the following terms.*

1. dermabrasion ______
2. lipectomy ______
3. hypodermic ______
4. onychectomy ______
5. rhytidoplasty ______
6. epidermal ______
7. percutaneous ______
8. subcutaneous ______

EXERCISE 4 *Match the term on the left with its definition on the right.*

h 1. anesthetic
b 2. antibiotic
d 3. antihistamine
f 4. antipruritic
e 5. antiseptic
a 6. electrocauterization
g 7. electrodesiccation
c 8. incision and drainage (I&D)

a. using electricity to destroy tissue by burning it
b. a drug that destroys or opposes growth of microorganisms
c. to cut into a wound to allow infected liquid to drain
d. a drug that opposes the effects of histamine
e. a drug that prevents sepsis (rotting of flesh) by killing microorganisms
f. a drug that prevents or relieves itching
g. using electricity to destroy tissue by drying it
h. a drug that temporarily blocks sensation

Learning Outcome 3.5 Exercises

EXERCISE 5 *Translate the following terms as literally as possible.*

EXAMPLE: nasopharyngoscope *an instrument for looking at the nose and throat*

1. chemosurgery ______
2. cryosurgery ______
3. dermabrasion ______
4. electrocauterization ______
5. incision ______
6. liposuction ______
7. onychotomy ______
8. rhytidoplasty ______
9. homograft ______
10. allograft ______
11. heterograft ______
12. xenograft ______

GENERATION

EXERCISE 6 *Build a medical term from the information provided.*

EXAMPLE: inflammation of the sinuses *sinusitis*

1. pertaining to upon the skin ______
2. pertaining to beneath the skin (use *cutaneo*) ______
3. pertaining to inside the skin ______
4. pertaining to through the skin (2 terms) ______
5. pertaining to beneath the skin (use *dermo*) ______
6. chemical treatment ______
7. removing fatty tissue ______
8. removing a nail ______
9. using electricity to destroy tissue by drying it ______
10. skin transplant taken from a different place on the patient's body ______

EXERCISE 7 *Describe the purpose of the following drugs.*

1. anesthetic ______
2. antibiotic ______
3. antihistamine ______
4. antipruritic ______
5. antiseptic ______

3.6 Abbreviations

Abbreviations provide medical professionals with a shorthand for writing words that commonly occur in their field. In dermatology, these abbreviations can refer to things ranging from procedures (C&S), to common diagnoses (AK), or even to mnemonic devices for remembering steps in analysis (ABCDE).

integumentary system abbreviations

Abbreviation	Definition
ABCDE	asymmetry, border, color, diameter, evolving
AK	actinic keratosis
BCC	basal cell carcinoma
Bx	biopsy
C&S	culture and sensitivity
decub	decubitus ulcer
derm	dermatology
EAHF	eczema, asthma, hay fever
FS	frozen section
ID	intradermal
SC	subcutaneous
SCC	squamous cell carcinoma
SQ	subcutaneous
subcut	subcutaneous
TD	transdermal
XP	xeroderma pigmentosa

Learning Outcome 3.6 Exercises

TRANSLATION

EXERCISE 1 *Define the following abbreviations.*

1. derm ________
2. C&S ________
3. subcut ________
4. SC ________
5. decub ________
6. ID ________
7. TD ________
8. FS ________
9. XP ________
10. ABCDE ________
11. EAHF ________

EXERCISE 2 *Give the abbreviations for the following terms.*

1. biopsy ________
2. dermatology ________
3. asymmetry, border, color, diameter, evolving ________
4. culture and sensitivity ________
5. frozen section ________
6. eczema, asthma, hay fever ________
7. xeroderma pigmentation ________
8. basal cell carcinoma ________
9. squamous cell carcinoma ________
10. actinic keratosis ________

EXERCISE 3 *Match the root on the left with its definition on the right.*

e.	1. ID	a. bed sore
h.	2. C&S	b. transdermal; through the skin
i	3. Bx	c. cancerous tumor of squamous skin cells
b.	4. TD	d. cancerous tumor of basal cells
g	5. SC	e. intradermal; within the skin
c.	6. SCC	f. horny skin condition caused by sun exposure
f.	7. AK	g. subcutaneous; below the skin
d.	8. BCC	h. growing microorganisms in isolation in order to determine which drugs it might respond best to
a.	9. decub	i. removal of tissue in order to examine it

3.7 Electronic Health Records

Consult Note

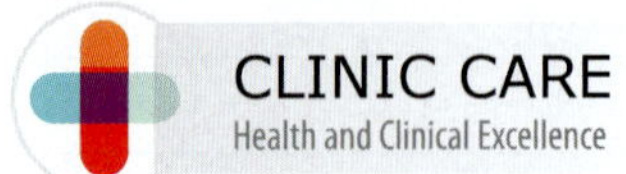

Reason for Consult: Rash

I had the pleasure of seeing your patient in my clinic. As you know, Mr. Skein is a 39-year-old male with a chronic history of **atopic dermatitis.** His atopic dermatitis was well controlled with **topical corticosteroids** until 3 weeks ago, when he developed a new rash consisting of **vesicles** overlying the areas of xerosis on his extremities. He was initially diagnosed with **impetigo** and treated with topical antibiotic therapy. He returned in 1 week without any improvement and was put on **oral** antibiotics at that time. He has now come to my office for a second opinion.

Mr. Skein reports mild pain and **pruritus,** but denies fever/chills, wheezing, or **edema** of his extremities. He has had a recent cold sore prior to the new rash. Except for a case of **tinea pedis** and **tinea corporis,** Mr. Skein's dermatological history is unremarkable.

The physical exam showed **erythematous, xerotic patches** in his flexural creases of his elbows and knees as well as the extensor surface of his legs. He has numerous **hemorrhagic crusts** and **vesicles,** along with scattered excoriations and erosions. The rest of the exam was unremarkable except mild scalp **alopecia.**

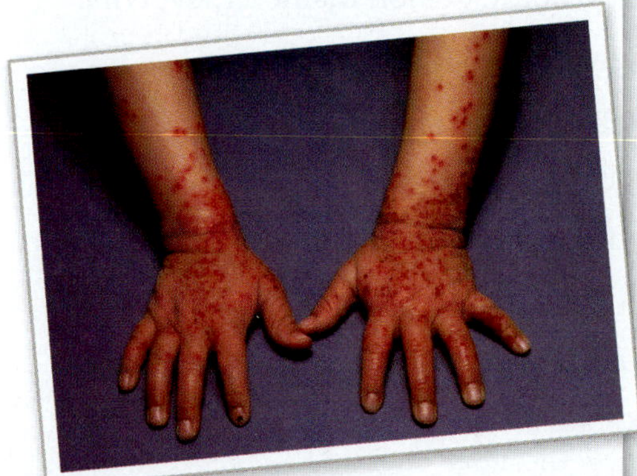

Laboratory testing with viral culture confirmed the diagnosis of **eczema herpeticum.** I treated him with oral antiviral medicine and he will follow up in my office in 2 weeks.

Thank you for this interesting consult.

Sincerely,
Robertra Mandel, MD

Learning Outcome 3.7 Exercises

EXERCISE 1 *Match the term on the left with its definition on the right.*

______	1. atopic dermatitis	a.	swollen, raised, itchy areas of the skin
______	2. vesicle	b.	loss of skin
______	3. xerosis	c.	a small blister
______	4. impetigo	d.	larger, flat discolored areas
______	5. antibiotic	e.	a drug that destroys or opposes the growth of microorganisms
______	6. pruritus	f.	condition of dryness
______	7. patch	g.	a scratch
______	8. crust	h.	baldness
______	9. excoriation	i.	an unusual inflammation of the skin
______	10. erosion	j.	a highly contagious bacterial infection of the skin
______	11. alopecia	k.	a red, itchy rash that may weep or ooze, then become crusted and scaly
______	12. eczema	l.	dried substance (i.e., blood, pus) on the skin

EXERCISE 2 *Fill in the blanks.*

1. The patient has a history of ______________________ (an unusual inflammation of the skin).
2. The new rash consisted of vesicles overlying the areas of *xerosis* (give definition: ______________________ ______________________).
3. Mr. Skein reports mild pain and ______________________ (swollen, raised, itchy areas of the skin).
4. The physical exam shows *xerotic* ______________________ (larger, flat discolored areas).
5. The patient had mild scalp *alopecia* (give definition: ______________________).

EXERCISE 3 *True or false questions. Indicate true answers with a T and false answers with an F.*

1. The patient did respond to topical antibiotic therapy. ______
2. The physical exam showed dry red patches in the creases of his elbows and knees. ______
3. The patient was given an antiviral medication by a shot in the arm. ______

Learning Outcome 3.7 Exercises

EXERCISE 4 *Multiple-choice questions. Select the correct answer.*

1. The patient's new rash consisted of
   a. small blisters
   b. large blisters
   c. warts
   d. moles
2. The initial diagnosis was a highly contagious bacterial infection of the skin called
   a. dermatomycosis
   b. eczema
   c. hyperkeratosis
   d. impetigo
3. The patient's impetigo was treated with a drug that
   a. temporarily blocks sensation
   b. destroys or opposes growth of microorganisms
   c. opposes the effects of histamine
   d. prevents or relieves itching
4. "Physical exam showed erythematous, xerotic patches in his flexural creases of his elbows and knees as well as the extensor surface of his legs." The root of *erythematous* means
   a. black
   b. red
   c. white
   d. yellow

Use the health professional's note "He has numerous hemorrhagic crusts and vesicles along with scattered excoriations and erosions" to answer the following questions:

5. Which symptom is NOT described by the health professional?
   a. localized collection of pus in the body
   b. dried substance (i.e., pus, blood) on the skin
   c. scratches
   d. skin loss
   e. small blisters
6. The patient was diagnosed with *eczema herpticum.* Which of the following symptoms is NOT characteristic of eczema?
   a. erythroderma
   b. pruritus
   c. crusts
   d. ecchymosis

Dermatology Clinic Note

S Subjective

Mrs. Smith is a 53-year-old woman with a 2-year history of worsening rash on her knees and elbows. She has had mild **pruritus,** but otherwise minimal discomfort. She came to my office today because the rash is worsening, and she also has problems with her toenails. She has tried topical moisturizer, which has not helped at all.

Social Hx: 1-pack-per day smoker. Social drinker; 3-4 glasses of wine a week.

Family Hx: Positive for **psoriasis** in mother.

PMHx: **Dermatofibromas** x 3 on legs removed via **cryotherapy** 3 years ago.

Objective

Temp: 98.7; HR: 74; RR: 16; BP: 115/73
Gen: Woman with healthy appearance, alert and oriented.
HEENT: TMs normal. **Xanthochromic**/stained teeth. Mucous membranes moist and pink.
CV: RRR no murmurs.
Resp: CTA.
Skin: **Erythematous papules** and **plaques** with a silver **scale** on the extensor surface of knees, elbows, and back; **onycholysis** of toe nails.

Skin Bx: **Epidermal hyperplasia.**

Assessment

DDx:
1. Rash: **Plaque psoriasis, seborrheic dermatitis, atopic dermatitis.**
2. Onycholysis: Psoriatic vs. **onychomycosis.**

Given that the rash is found on the extensor surface and not the flexural creases, in addition to the presence of a silver scale, I suspected psoriasis. My diagnosis was confirmed with **histologic** appearance on the biopsy.

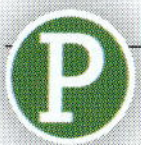

Plan

I will begin her on topical corticosteroids and have her follow up in 2-4 months. For any unresponsive areas I will try **photochemotherapy.** For the patient's onycholysis, I have referred her to a podiatrist **onychectomy.**

–Electronically signed by Joaquin Hernandez, MD

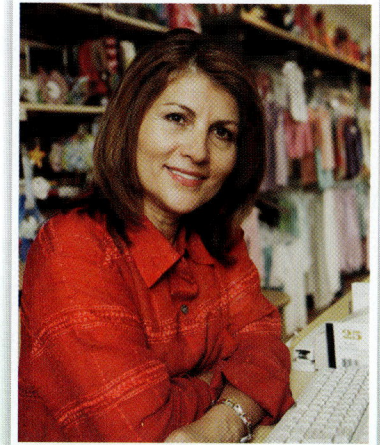

Learning Outcome 3.7 Exercises

EXERCISE 5 *Match the term on the left with its definition on the right.*

i	1. pruritus	a.	skin flaking off
c	2. dermatofibroma	b.	a solid mass on the surface of the skin
f	3. onychectomy	c.	a fibrous skin tumor
h	4. papule	d.	inflammation of the skin caused by the discharge of oil
b	5. plaque	e.	a fungal condition of the nail
a	6. scale	f.	to remove a nail
g	7. onycholysis	g.	the loss of a nail
d	8. seborrheic dermatitis	h.	a small, solid mass
j	9. atopic dermatitis	i.	swollen, raised, and itchy areas of the skin
e	10. onychomycosis	j.	an unusual inflammation of the skin

EXERCISE 6 *Fill in the blanks.*

1. Mrs. Smith has mild ____pruritus____ (swollen, raised, itchy areas of the skin).
2. Mrs. Smith had 3 *dermatofibromas* (define: ________) removed with ________ (treatment using cold).
3. The dermatology assessment showed erythematous *papules* (define: ________) and plaques (define: ________) with a silver ________ (skin flaking off).
4. The health care professional referred Mrs. Smith to a podiatrist *onychectomy* (define: ________).

EXERCISE 7 *True or false questions. Indicate true answers with a T and false answers with an F.*

1. Topical moisturizers have helped Mrs. Smith's worsening pruritus. ____
2. Mrs. Smith is losing her toenails. ____
3. The health professional performed a biopsy. ____
4. Seborrheic dermatitis is inflammation of the nail caused by oil. ____
5. *Atopic dermatitis* is a term to describe routine skin inflammation and is quite common. ____
6. Mrs. Smith has psoriasis. ____

Learning Outcome 3.7 Exercises

EXERCISE 8 *Multiple-choice questions. Select the correct answer.*

1. Mrs. Smith has teeth that are stained
   a. white
   b. black
   c. brown
   d. yellow
2. The papules on Mrs. Smith's skin are *erythematous,* which means they are
   a. red
   b. itchy
   c. raised
   d. blistered
3. *Bx* is an abbreviation for
   a. biopsy
   b. bulla
   c. basal cell
   d. cicatrix
4. Mrs. Smith's biopsy revealed hyperplasia that pertained to
   a. the nail
   b. the skin
   c. the teeth
   d. the rash
5. The root words in *onychomycosis* are *onycho,* meaning *nail,* and *myco,* meaning
   a. fungus
   b. bacteria
   c. virus
   d. tumor

Dermatology Consult Note

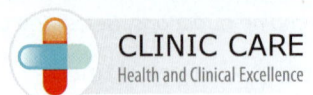

Dermatology Consult

I had the pleasure of seeing your patient John Johnson in my clinic on February 14. Your office referred him to me regarding a rash on sun-exposed areas of his body. He is a 45-year-old landscape architect who spends a large part of his days outdoors. He had noticed several spots on his arms, but did not seek medical care at that time. At his routine physical, his care provider noticed the rash on his arms.

Physical exam revealed a well-developed, well-nourished, fair-skinned male. His heart was regular in rate and rhythm. His lungs were clear. His mucous membranes were moist and pink. His skin exam was significant for papules of **hyperkeratosis** with surrounding **erythema.** A few of the lesions are **hyperpigmented.** He has larger patches on his scalp.

A skin biospy performed in my office confirmed the diagnosis of **actinic keratosis (AK).** After explaining the results to Mr. Johnson, I recommended **cryotherapy** for the smaller lesions on his arms and **dermabrasion** for his scalp lesions. I explained to Mr. Johnson that **AK** can lead to **squamous cell carcinoma** and taught him about the risks of sun exposure, including further AKs and **melanoma.**

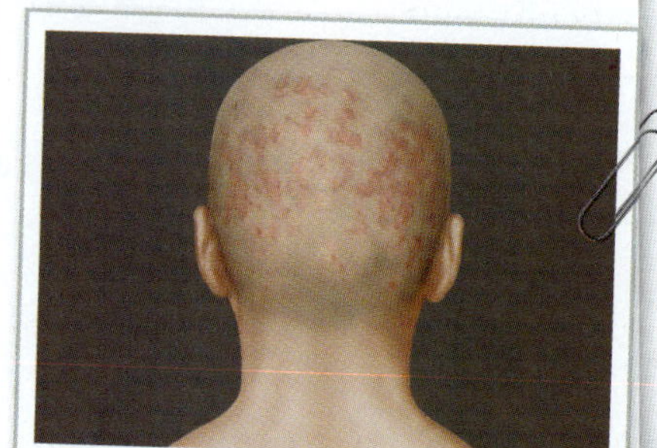

Thank you for this interesting consult.

— James Skinner, MD

EXERCISE 9 *Match the term on the left with its definition on the right.*

____ 1. papule		a. horny skin condition caused by sun exposure
____ 2. hyperkeratosis		b. redness
____ 3. erythema		c. removal of tissue in order to examine it
____ 4. hyperpigmented		d. excessive growth of horny skin
____ 5. patch		e. treatment of the skin using cold
____ 6. biopsy		f. actinic keratosis
____ 7. actinic keratosis		g. a small, solid mass
____ 8. cryotherapy		h. larger, flat discolored area
____ 9. dermabrasion		i. tumor of melanin cells
____ 10. AK		j. excessive pigment in the skin
____ 11. squamous cell carcinoma		k. cancerous tumor of squamous skin cells
____ 12. melanoma		l. rubbing or scraping away the outer surface of skin

Learning Outcome 3.7 Exercises

EXERCISE 10 *Fill in the blanks.*

1. The patient's skin exam was significant for ________________ (small, solid masses) of *hyperkeratosis* (excessive growth of ________________ skin) with surrounding *erythema* (define: ________________).

2. He has larger ________________ (larger, flat discolored areas) on his scalp.

3. *Actinic* ________________ is a horny skin condition caused by ________________.

EXERCISE 11 *Multiple-choice questions. Select the correct answer.*

1. A few of Mr. Johnson's lesions are *hyperpigmented,* which means
   a. excessive pigmentation
   b. underpigmentation
   c. loss of pigmentation
   d. creation of pigmentation

2. *Actinic keratosis* is
   a. inflammation of the skin caused by sun exposure
   b. horny skin condition caused by sun exposure
   c. a harmful new formation of the skin tissue (i.e., skin cancer)
   d. common acne

3. The diagnosis of actinic keratosis was confirmed by performing
   a. biopsy
   b. cryotherapy
   c. dermabrasion
   d. C&S

4. Which treatment option was NOT recommended for the patient?
   a. biopsy
   b. treatment using cold
   c. rubbing or scraping away the outer surface of skin
   d. corticosteroids

5. The root word in *squamous* means
   a. scaly
   b. dry
   c. oily
   d. yellow

6. The root word in *melanoma* means
   a. white
   b. black
   c. yellow
   d. red

Quick Reference

quick reference glossary of roots

Root	Definition	Root	Definition	Root	Definition
adip/o	fat	**kerat/o**	hard, horny	**sebace/o**	oil
alb/o	white	**leuk/o**	white	**seb/o**	oil
crypt/o	hidden	**lip/o**	fat	**squam/o**	scale
cutane/o	skin	**melan/o**	black	**steat/o**	fat
dermat/o	skin	**onych/o**	nail	**trich/o**	hair
derm/o	skin	**pachy/o**	thick	**ungu/o**	nail
erythr/o	red	**pil/o**	hair	**xanth/o**	yellow
hidr/o	sweat	**rhytid/o**	wrinkle	**xer/o**	dry
ichthy/o	scaly				

quick reference glossary of terms

Terms	Definition
abrasion	a scraping away of skin
abscess	a localized collection of pus in the body
acne vulgaris	common acne; an inflammation of the skin follicles
actinic dermatitis	inflammation of the skin caused by sun exposure
actinic keratosis	horny skin condition caused by sun exposure
adipocele	a hernia filled with fatty tissue
albinism	lack of pigment in skin causing patient to look white
albino	a person afflicted with albinism
allograft	see *homograph*
alopecia	baldness
anesthetic	a drug that temporarily blocks sensation
anhidrosis	lack of sweating
antibiotic	a drug that destroys or opposes the growth of microorganisms
antihistamine	a drug that opposes the effects of histamine
antipruritic	a drug that prevents or relieves itching
antiseptic	a drug that prevents sepsis (rotting of flesh) by killing microorganisms

quick reference glossary of terms *continued*

Root	Definition
atopic dermatitis	an unusual inflammation of the skin (*atopic* usually means *not in the right place*)
autograft	skin transplant taken from a different place on the patient's body
basal cell carcinoma	cancerous tumor of basal skin cells
biopsy	removal of tissue in order to examine it
bulla	from Latin, for *bubble*; a larger blister
chemosurgery	removal of tissue that has been destroyed using chemicals
chemotherapy	treatment using chemicals
cherry angioma	a small blood vessel tumor
cicatrix (plural *cicatrices*)	from Latin, for *scar;* a scar
comedo	from Latin, for *to eat up*; a hair follicle plugged with sebum (black head, white head)
crust	dried substance (i.e., blood, pus) on the skin
cryosurgery	destruction of tissue through freezing
culture & sensitivity	growing microorganisms in isolation in order to determine which drugs it might respond to
cyanidrosis	blue sweat
decubitus ulcer	bed sore
depigmentation	loss of skin pigmentation
dermabrasion	rubbing or scraping away the outer surface of skin
dermatitis	inflammation of the skin
dermatoconiosis	a skin condition caused by dirt
dermatofibroma	a fibrous skin tumor
dermatolysis	loss of skin
dermatomycosis	a fungal skin condition
dermatoscope	instrument used to look at the skin
dermatosis	skin condition
dermopathy	skin disease
dermoscopy	procedure for looking at the skin
dysplastic nevus	a mole with bad changes/formations (often precancerous)
ecchymosis	from Greek, for *to pour out*; a larger bruise
eczema	from Greek, for *to boil over*; a red, itchy rash that may weep or ooze, then become crusted and scaly

quick reference glossary of terms *continued*

Root	Definition
electrocauterization	using electricity to destroy tissue by burning it
electrodesiccation	using electricity to destroy by drying it
epidermal	pertaining to the skin
epidermal tumor	tumors on the skin
erosion	loss of skin
erythema	from Greek, for *redness*; redness
erythrocyanosis	a red and/or blue discoloration of the skin
erythroderma	red skin
excisional biopsy	removal of an entire lesion for examination (to cut it out)
excoriation	a scratch
fissure	from Latin, for a *split* or *divide;* a crack in the skin
hemathidrosis	sweating blood
heterograft (xenograft)	skin transplant taken from a species other than the patient's (*hetero* because it is a different species; *xeno* because it is a foreign species)
hidradenitis	inflammation of the sweat glands
hidradenoma	tumor of the sweat gland
hidropoiesis	the formation of sweat
homograft (allograft)	skin transplant taken from another member of the patient's species (*homo* because it is from a similar species; *allo* because it is from another person)
hyperhidrosis	excessive sweating
hyperkeratosis	excessive growth of horny skin
hypermelanosis	excessive melanin in the skin
hyperpigmentation	excessive pigment in the skin
hypodermia	pertaining to beneath the skin
hypohidrosis	diminished sweating
hypomelanosis	diminished melanin in the skin
hypopigmentation	diminished pigment in the skin
ichthyosis	a condition in the skin that is dry and scaly resembling fish scales
impetigo	from Latin, for *to attack;* a highly contagious bacterial infection of the skin
incision and drainage (I&D)	to cut into a wound to allow trapped infected liquid to drain
incisional biopsy	removal of a portion of a lesion for examination (to cut into)

quick reference glossary of terms *continued*

Root	Definition
intradermal	pertaining to inside the skin
keloid	overgrowth of scar tissue
keratogenic	causing horny tissue development
keratosis	horny tissue condition
leukoderma	white skin
lipectomy	removal of fatty tissue
liposuction	removal of fatty tissue using a vacuum
macerate	from Latin, for *to make soft;* to soften the skin
macule	from Latin, for *spot* or *stain;* small, flat, discolored area (freckle)
malignant cutaneous neoplasm	a harmful new formation of the skin tissue (i.e., skin cancer)
malignant melanoma	a harmful tumor of melanin cell
mycodermatitis	inflammation of the skin caused by fungus
mycosis	fungus condition
necrosis	tissue death
nevus	from Latin, for *birthmark* or *mole*; a mole
nodule	a solid mass that extends deeper into the skin
oncyhomalacia	abnormal softening of a nail
onychectomy	remove a nail
onychia	a nail condition
onychocryptosis	an ingrown nail
onychodystrophy	poor nourishment (and development) of the nail
onycholysis	the loss of a nail
onychomycosis	a fungal condition of the nail
onychopathy	nail disease
onychophagia	eating (biting) the nail

quick reference glossary of terms *continued*

Root	Definition
onychotomy	incision into a nail
pachyderma	tough skin
papule	from Latin, for *pimple;* a small, solid mass
paronychia	a condition of the tissue around a nail
patch (vitiligo)	larger, flat discolored area
percutaneous	pertaining to through the skin
petechia	from Latin, for *freckle* or *spot;* a small bruise
plaque	a solid mass on the surface of the skin
postpartum alopecia	baldness experienced by women after a pregnancy
pruritus	from Latin, for *burning nettle;* swollen, raised, itchy areas of the skin
pustule	from Latin, for *little blister;* a pus-filled blister
rhytidoplasty	reconstruction of wrinkled skin
scale	skin flaking off
sclerodermatitis	inflammation of the skin accompanied by thickening and hardening
scleronychia	thickening and hardening of the nails
seborrheic dermatitis	inflammation of the skin caused by the discharge of oil (sebum)
spider angioma	see *telangiectasia*
squamous cell carcinoma	cancerous tumor of squamous skin cells
steatitis	inflammation of fat tissue
steatoma	a fatty tumor
subcutaneous	pertaining to beneath the skin
telangiectasia (spider angioma)	the overexpansion of the blood vessel, sometimes called a spider angioma because of how it looks on the skin
transdermal	pertaining to through the skin
trichomycosis	a fungal condition of the hair
tumor	a larger solid mass
ulcer	from Latin, for *sore;* a sore

quick reference glossary of terms *continued*

Root	Definition
vascular lesion	wounds related to blood vessels
verucca	from Latin, for *wart;* a wart
vesicle	from Latin, for *little bladder;* a small blister
vitiligo	see *patch*
xanthoderma	yellow skin
xanthoma	a yellow tumor
xanthosis	yellowing of the skin
xenograft	see *heterograft*
xeroderma	dry skin
xerosis	condition of dryness

review of terms by roots

Root	Term(s)
adip/o	adipocele
alb/o	albinism albino
crypt/o	onychocryptosis
cutane/o	malignant cutaneous neoplasm percutaneous subcutaneous

review of terms by roots *continued*

Root	Term(s)	
derm/o, dermat/o	actinic dermatitis	epidermal
	atopic dermatitis	epidermal
	dermabrasion	erythroderma
	dermatitis	hypodermia
	dermatoconiosis	intradermal
	dermatofibroma	leukoderma
	dermatolysis	mycodermatitis
	dermatomycosis	pachyderma
	dermatoscope	sclerodermatitis
	dermatosis	seborrheic dermatitis
	dermopathy	transdermal
	dermoscopy	xeroderma
erythr/o	erythema	
	erythrocyanosis	
	erythroderma	
hidr/o	anhidrosis	hidradenoma
	cyanidrosis	hidropoiesis
	hemathidrosis	hyperhidrosis
	hidradenitis	hypohidrosis
ichthy/o	ichthyosis	
kerat/o	actinic keratosis	
	hyperkeratosis	
	keratogenic	
	keratosis	
leuk/o	leukoderma	
lip/o	lipectomy	
	liposuction	

review of terms by roots *continued*

Root	Term(s)	
melan/o	hypermelanosis	
	hypomelanosis	
	malignant melanoma	
onych/o	onychomalacia	onychopathy
	onychectomy	onychophagia
	onychia	onychophagia
	onychocryptosis	onychotomy
	onychodystrophy	paronychia
	onycholysis	scleronychia
	onychomycosis	
pachy/o	pachyderma	
rhytid/o	rhytidoplasty	
seb/o	seborrheic dermatitis	
squam/o	squamous cell carcinoma	
steat/o	steatitis	
	steatoma	
trich/o	trichomycosis	
xanth/o	xanthoderma	
	xanthoma	
	xanthosis	
xer/o	xeroderma	
	xerosis	

other terms

abrasion	fissure
abscess	heterograft
acne vulgaris	homograft
allograft	hyperpigmentation
alopecia	hypopigmentation
anesthetic	impetigo
antibiotic	incision and drainage
antihistamine	incisional biopsy
antipruritic	keloid
antiseptic	macerate
autograft	macule
basal cell carcinoma	mycosis
biopsy	necrosis
bulla	nevus
chemosurgery	nodule
chemotherapy	papule
cherry angioma	patch
cicatrix	petechia
comedo	plaque
crust	postpartum alopecia
cryosurgery	pruritus
culture & sensitivity	pustule
decubitus ulcer	scale
depigmentation	spider angioma
dysplastic nevus	telangiectasia
ecchymosis	tumor
eczema	ulcer
electrocauterization	vascular lesion
electrodesiccation	verucca
erosion	vesicle
excisional biopsy	vitiligo
excoriation	xenograft

The Musculoskeletal System–Orthopedics 4

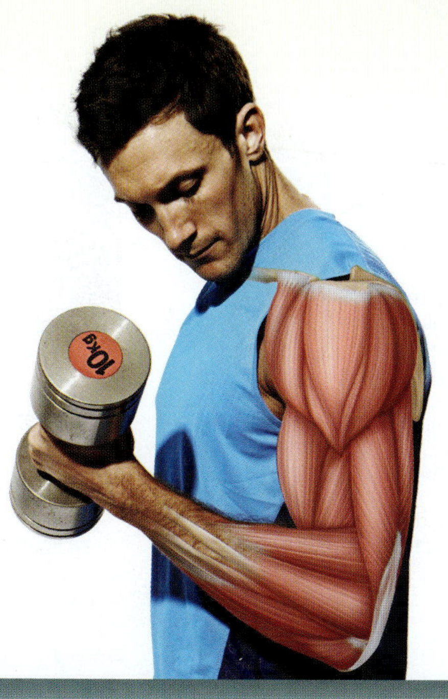

learning outcomes

Upon completion of this chapter, you will be able to:

4.1 Identify the **roots/word parts** associated with the **musculoskeletal system.**

S **4.2** Translate the **Subjective** terms associated with the **musculoskeletal system.**

O **4.3** Translate the **Objective** terms associated with the **musculoskeletal system.**

A **4.4** Translate the **Assessment** terms associated with the **musculoskeletal system.**

P **4.5** Translate the **Plan** terms associated with the **musculoskeletal system.**

4.6 Use **abbreviations** associated with the **musculoskeletal system.**

4.7 Distinguish terms associated with the **musculoskeletal system** in the context of **electronic health records.**

Introduction and Overview of the Musculoskeletal System

Think of a crane at a construction site. It's an impressive piece of machinery. All the parts work together to move some very heavy objects.

Your body, specifically your musculoskeletal system, is also an amazing machine. All the parts work just right to allow you to make big movements, like lifting a heavy box, and fine movements, like writing a note on the box.

Continuing the crane analogy, your bones are like the metal fused together to make the framework of the crane. Like the metal, your bones are strong and sturdy. They make the framework of your body. This framework supports your body and protects your internal organs. Your bones are lighter than the steel of a crane, but like steel, they are incredibly strong.

Unlike steel, however, your bones are living organs. They can grow, maintain themselves, and even self-repair.

If you look at a crane up close, you'll notice that the framework is not one solid piece. Instead, it is made up of many smaller pieces that are welded, bolted, or hinged together. Some connection points are immobile, while others allow movement. Your joints are the connection points in your body. They keep the parts together and allow for movement so the crane can actually move things.

The crane couldn't move anything without any power, though. Your muscles are the workhorses of your musculoskeletal system. They act as powerful movers and stabilizers. Some muscles, like those in your thighs, are thick and strong, while others, like those in your hands, are smaller and are made for delicate movements. In fact, the muscles of your eyes are at work even now as you read these words. Together, your bones, joints, and muscles move you, protect you, and give your body support.

4.1 Word Parts of the Musculoskeletal System

Bones

Bones start as cartilage. Blood vessels penetrate the cartilage and bone cells (*osteocytes*) begin the process of replacing the cartilage model with actual bone. This process begins well before you are born and does not finish until puberty ends. Many bones harden from the center outward. Some bones, however, grow at special growth centers called the epiphyseal plate (also known as the growth plate). This growth center lies in the metaphysis area between the end of the bone (*epiphysis*) and the long shaft of the bone (*diaphysis*).

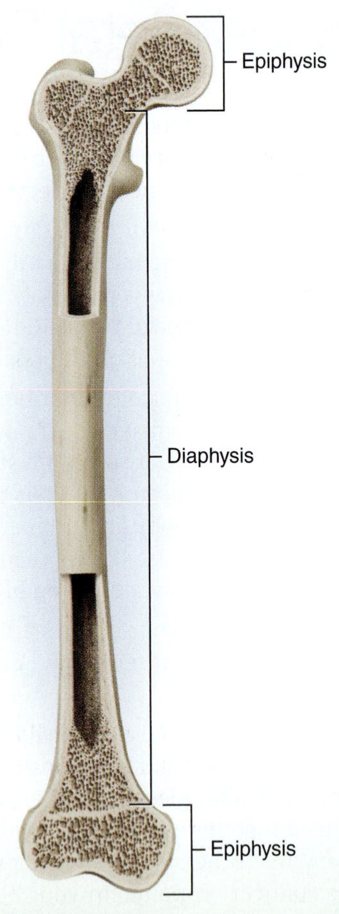

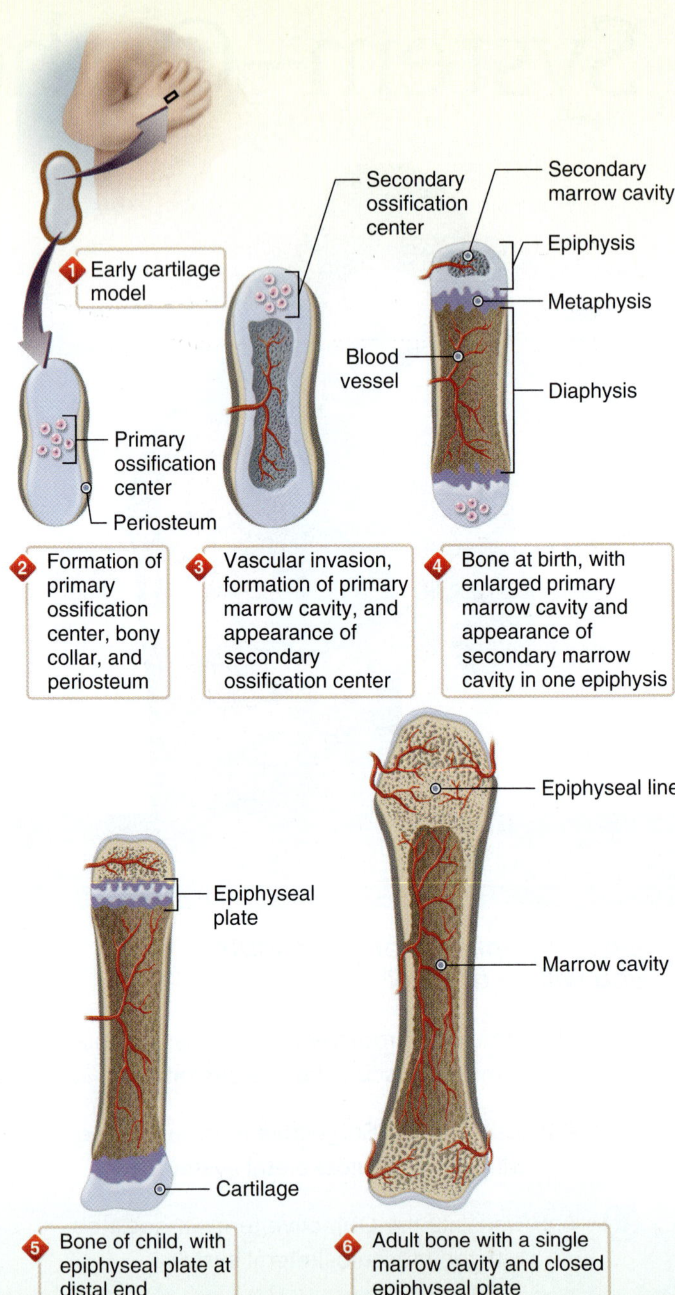

growth

SUFFIX: ***-physis***

EXAMPLES: epiphysis, diaphysis, metaphysis

NOTES: *Physics* is the study of matter, energy, and motion. You might think that a subject like quantum physics is completely disconnected from health care, but *physics* comes from a Greek word meaning *growth* and once referred to the study of nature and living things. The Greek term is also the root of the terms *physical* and *physician.*

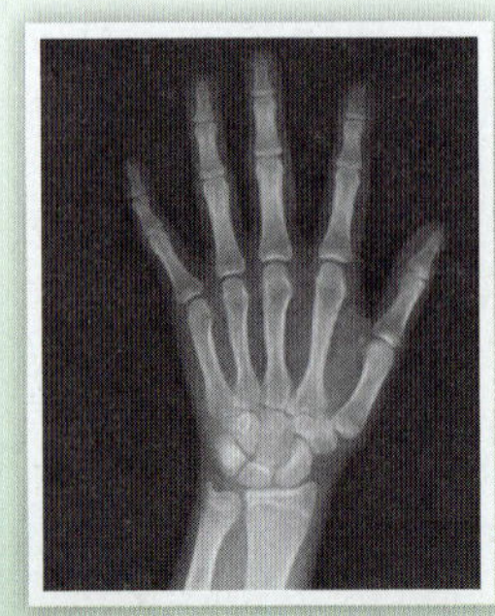

The Skeleton

Your bones make up the framework of your body—your skeleton. Like any good design, your skeleton has a specific layout. The bones in the middle of the skeleton are called the *axial* part of your skeleton. Your skull (*cranio*) is attached to your spine.

Your spine is made of many smaller bones (*vertebra*) that connect together. They protect your spinal cord, a very fragile and important body structure. Your spine has four sections: the neck section (*cervical*), chest/upper back section (*thoracic*), and lower back (*lumbar* and *sacral*). Your ribs (*costo*) attach to the vertebra of the thoracic section.

Your arms and legs branch off both sides of this central part of the skeleton. Your upper arm (*brachio*) leads to the two bones of your forearm (*radius* and *ulna*), then to your wrist (*carpe*), and finally to your fingers (*phalanges*). Your legs begin with your thigh bone (*femur*), work down to the two shin bones (*tibia* and *fibula*), move on to your ankle (*tarsal*), and ultimately reach your toes (*phalanges* again, just like the fingers).

---

bone

ROOT: ***oste/o***

EXAMPLES: osteopathy, periosteum

NOTES: At birth, you had over 300 bones, but no kneecaps. As a full-grown adult, you now have 206 bones including two kneecaps—a net loss of at least 96 bones. A human's neck also contains the same number of bones as a giraffe's.

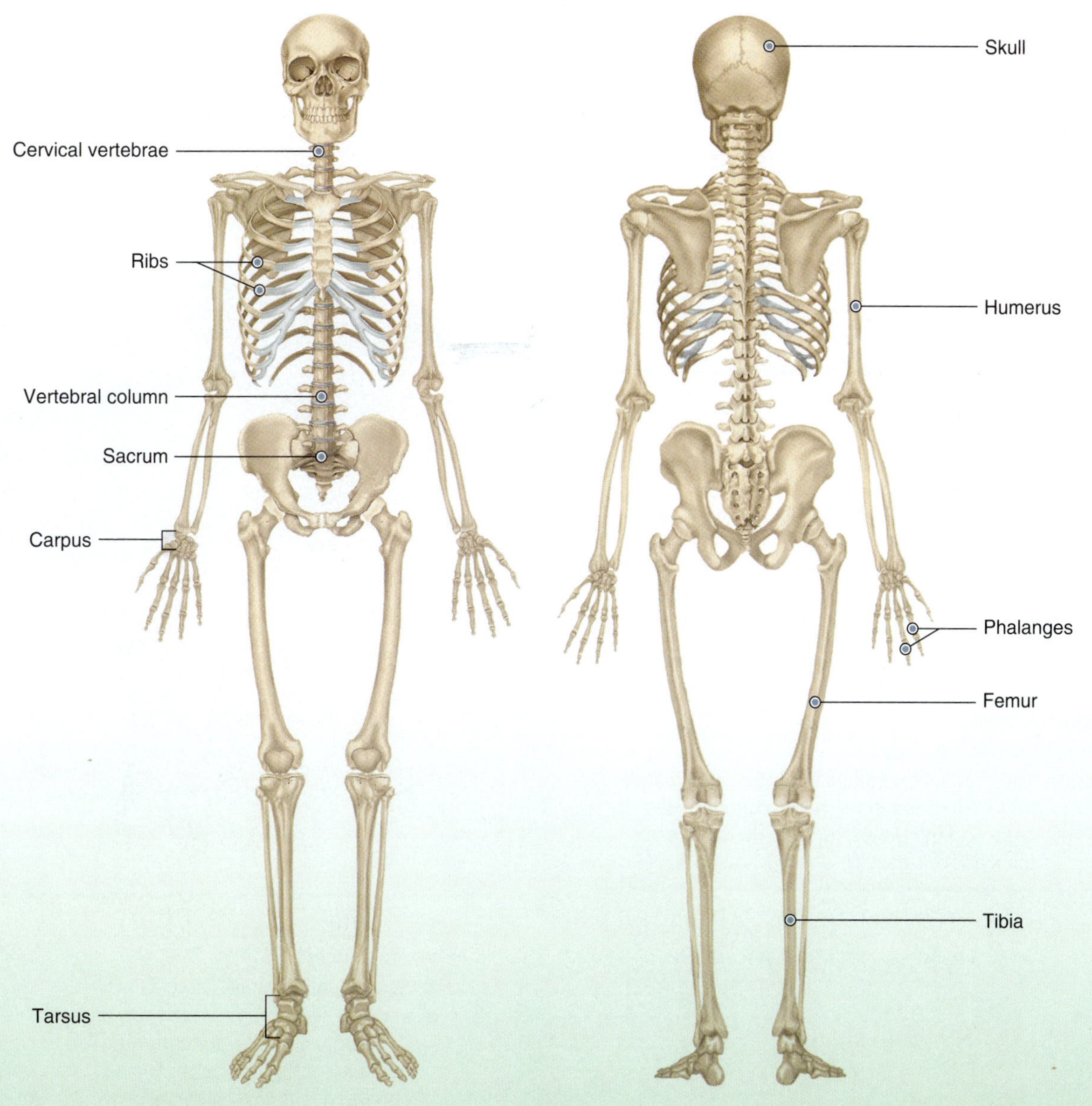

head, skull

ROOT: ***crani/o***

EXAMPLES: craniometer, craniomalacia

NOTES: The term *migraine* comes from the word *hemicrania,* meaning *half the head.* The term reflects the fact that most migraines are localized in half the patient's head.

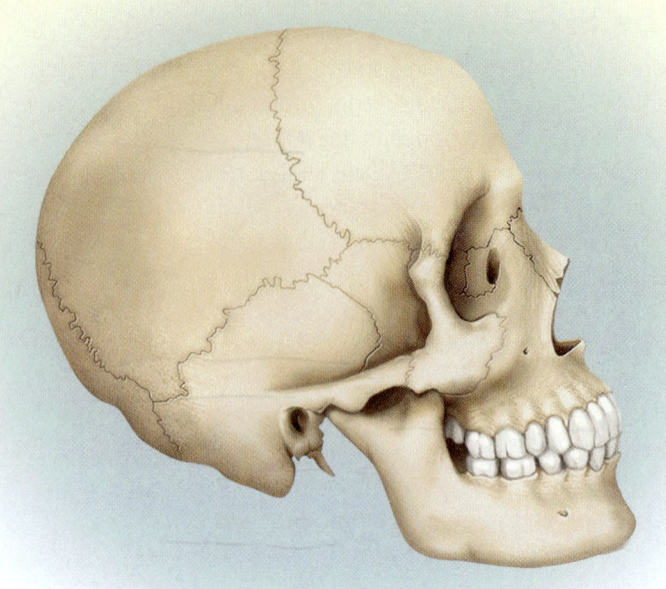

neck

ROOT: ***cervic/o***

EXAMPLES: cervical spine, cervicitis

NOTES: Remember: When a *c* is followed by *a, o,* or *u,* it is pronounced hard like a *k.* When followed by *e* or *i,* it is pronounced soft like an *s.* Therefore, the two example words above are pronounced SIR-vih-kal and SIR-vih-SAI-tis.

vertebra

ROOT: ***spondyl/o***

EXAMPLES: invertebrate, spondylitis

NOTES: *Vertebra* comes from Latin, for *to turn.* It is called this because the spine was once thought of as the hinge or center around which all other bones turned.

loin, lower back

ROOT: ***lumb/o***

EXAMPLES: lumbar, lumbodynia

NOTES: The root *lumbo* comes from the Latin *lumbo,* for *loin.* It refers to the region between the rib cage and the pelvis, but frankly, it makes us think about steak.

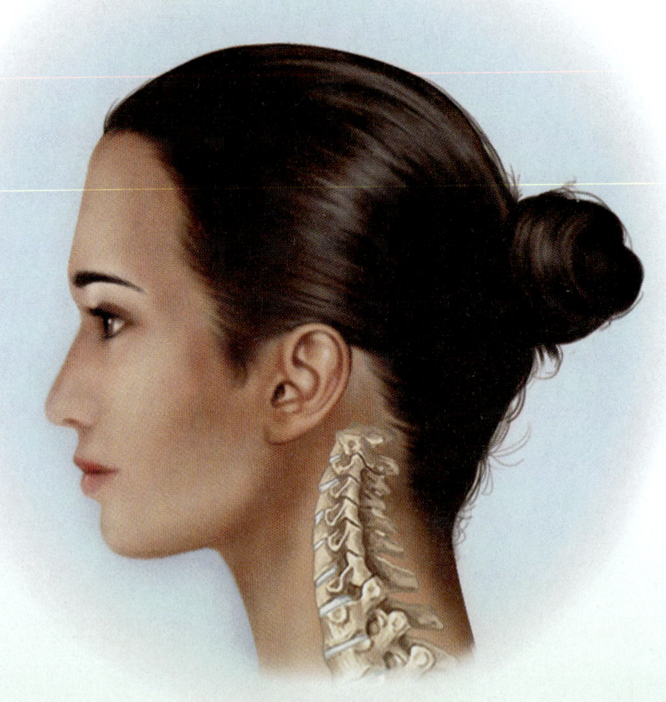

arm

ROOT: ***brachi/o***

EXAMPLES: brachiocephalic, brachialgia

NOTES: The term *brace,* which comes from this word, originally referred to armor used to cover a knight's upper arm. This root can also be seen in the word *embrace,* which literally means *to put someone in your arms.*

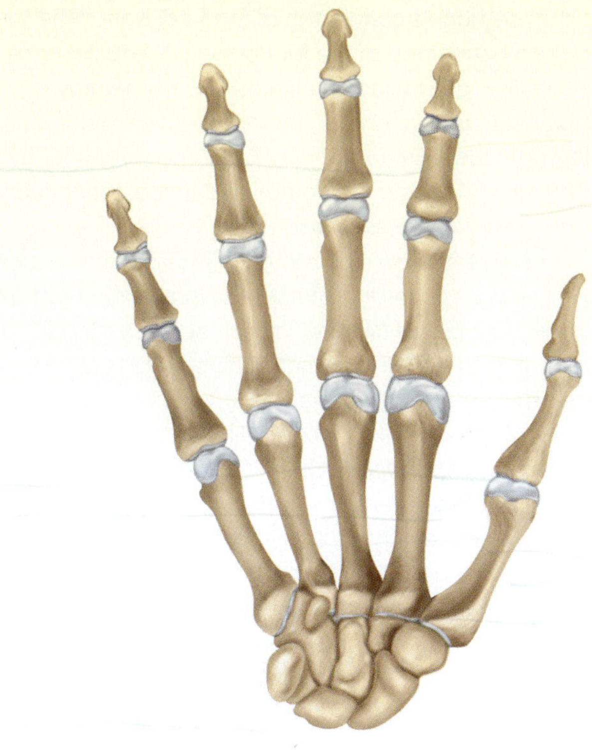

finger

ROOT: ***dactyl/o***

EXAMPLES: adactyly, dactylalgia

NOTES: The flying dinosaur called the pterodactyl gets its name from *ptero* (winged) + *dactly* (fingers), which obviously literally means *winged fingers*.

wrist

ROOT: ***carp/o***

EXAMPLES: carpectomy, metacarpal

NOTES: The *carpal tunnel* is the area in the wrist where the nerves enter the hand. Repetitive motions using the wrist can cause the nerve to swell, press against the walls of the carpal tunnel, and result in numbness in the hand; this condition is called *carpal tunnel syndrome*.

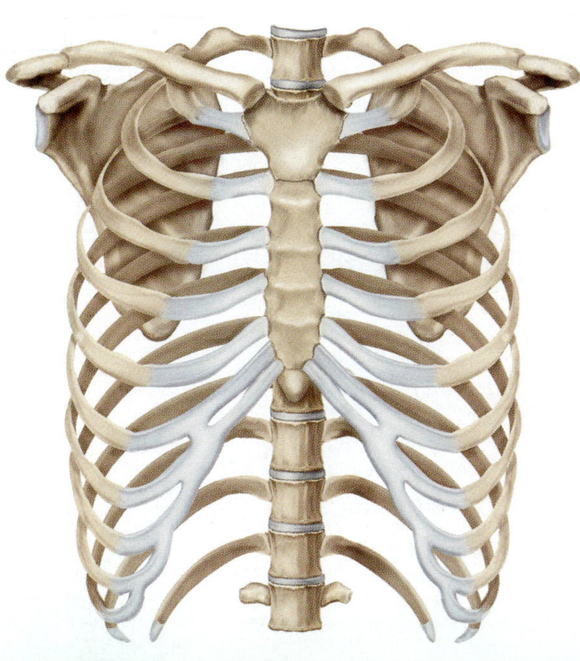

rib

ROOT: ***cost/o***

EXAMPLES: costectomy, intercostal

NOTES: The English word *coast* comes from this word. Think of a country's coasts as its ribs or sides. Also, the word *accost,* which means *to come alongside someone,* comes from this word.

femur (thighbone)

ROOT: ***femor/o***

EXAMPLES: femoral artery

NOTES: The femur is the strongest bone in the human body (nonetheless, a hyena can bite right through it—*ouch*). The femur makes up about a fourth of a person's overall height.

ankle

ROOT: ***tors/o***

EXAMPLES: tarsitis, tarsalgia

NOTES: The root *tarso* comes from the Latin word *tarsus,* which can refer to the ankle or in general to the entire foot. But what makes this truly intriguing is that the word *tarsus* in Latin was derived from the Latin word *terra,* which means *earth.* The foot was called the *tarsus* because it is the body part that touches the *terra* most.

tibia (shinbone)

ROOT: ***tibi/o***

EXAMPLES: tibiaglia

NOTES: The term *tibia* originally meant *pipe* or *flute.* Evidently, the person who named this bone thought the shinbone bore a resemblance to this instrument.

Joints

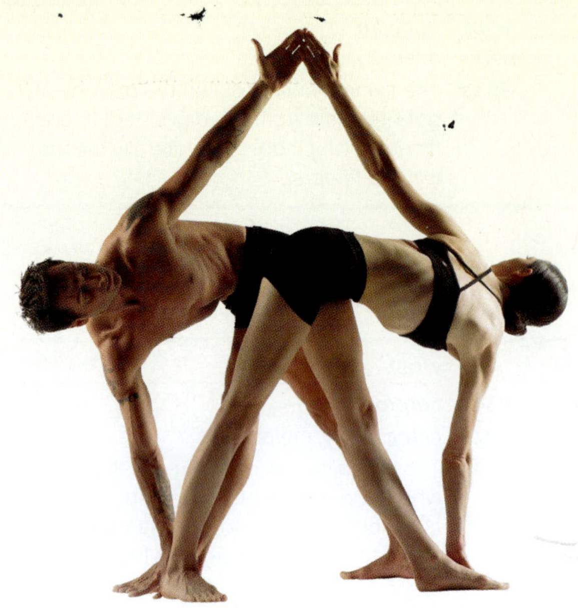

"The toe bone's connected to the heel bone. The heel bone's connected to the foot bone . . ." and so it goes. While it doesn't exactly reflect the way anatomy is taught in medical school, the old children's song has the right idea. Every bone in the body except the hyoid bone is connected to another, and these connection points are known as *joints*.

Not all joints allow movement. For example, the bones in your skull are bound together tightly. Usually when we think of joints, we picture the moving ones, because after all, these are the ones that we hurt when participating in sports or that cause problems in older age.

Moving joints allow motions like bending and rotating. When a joint bends, it's called *flexion*. When it straightens, it's called *extension*. *Abduction* is the widening of a joint to move parts away from the body. The term *adduction* means just the opposite—during adduction, the joint narrows to bring parts back toward the body.

Moving joints often have surrounding support tissues to absorb shock, keep the bones aligned, and keep the bones moving smoothly. *Tendons* hold muscle to bone. *Ligaments* hold bone to bone. *Cartilage* surrounds bones at the joints and allows smooth movement among them. Under many tendons lie sacs of fluid, known as *bursae*, that help keep muscles and bones moving smoothly as well.

cartilage

ROOT: ***chondr/o***

EXAMPLES: chondritis, chondrodynia

NOTES: People who always think they are sick are called *hypochondriacs*. This term comes from *hypo-* (beneath) + *chondro* (cartilage—here specifically referring to the ribs) and reflected an ancient belief that such thoughts came from deep within the rib cage.

joint

ROOT: ***arthr/o***

EXAMPLES: arthritis, arthroscopic surgery

NOTES: Insects, spiders, scorpions, and shellfish belong to the animal family known as *arthropods*. This term comes from *arthro* (joint) + *pod* (feet) and refers to their segmented limbs. If you have ever eaten crab legs, you know exactly what I mean.

bursa

ROOT: ***burs/o***

EXAMPLES: bursitis, bursectomy

NOTES: A *bursa* is a small fluid-filled sac found near the body's joint. Bursae reduce friction and act as cushions. The word comes from the Greek word meaning *purse* or *bag*. In some places, the treasurer of an organization is called a *bursar* because he handles the purse. Also, to be *reim**burs**ed* means to have money *put back in your purse*.

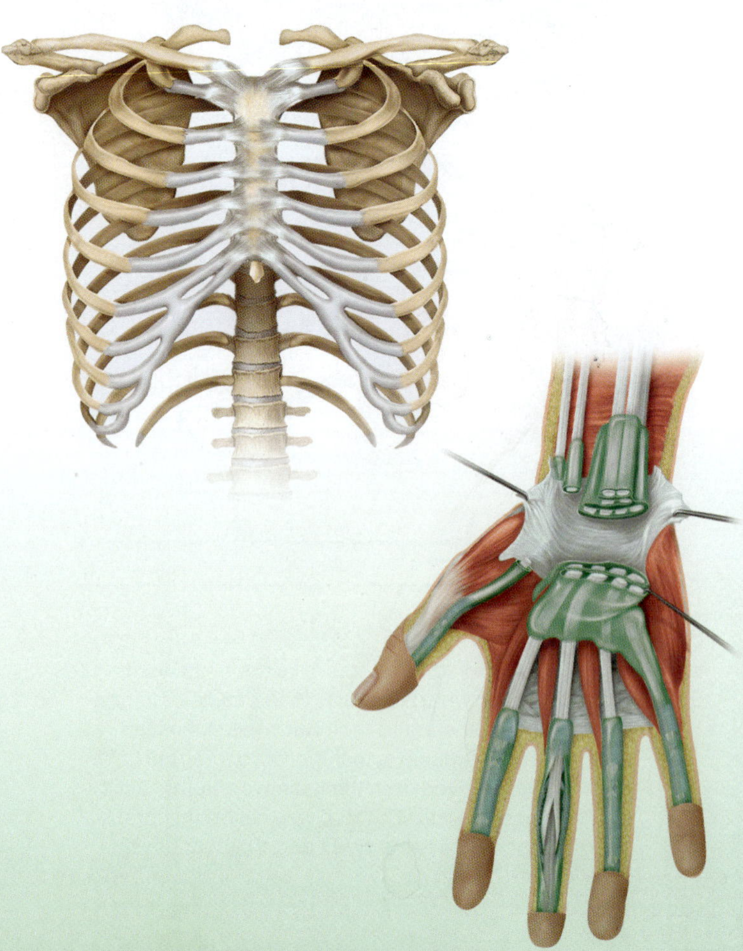

Muscles

Think of a thick rope. Unlike a piece of string, it is not one strand but numerous strands bundled together. This design makes the rope much stronger. Your skeletal muscles are similar, as they are a collection of thousands of muscle fibers bundled together. The bundles are grouped together to form a muscle.

The muscle is encased in a thick membrane called *fascia*. The fascia helps keep the muscle together. Muscles attach to bones. If they didn't, they wouldn't be very useful. Their job is to move the bones, after all. Muscles attach to bones via *tendons*, which are thick bands of connective tissue.

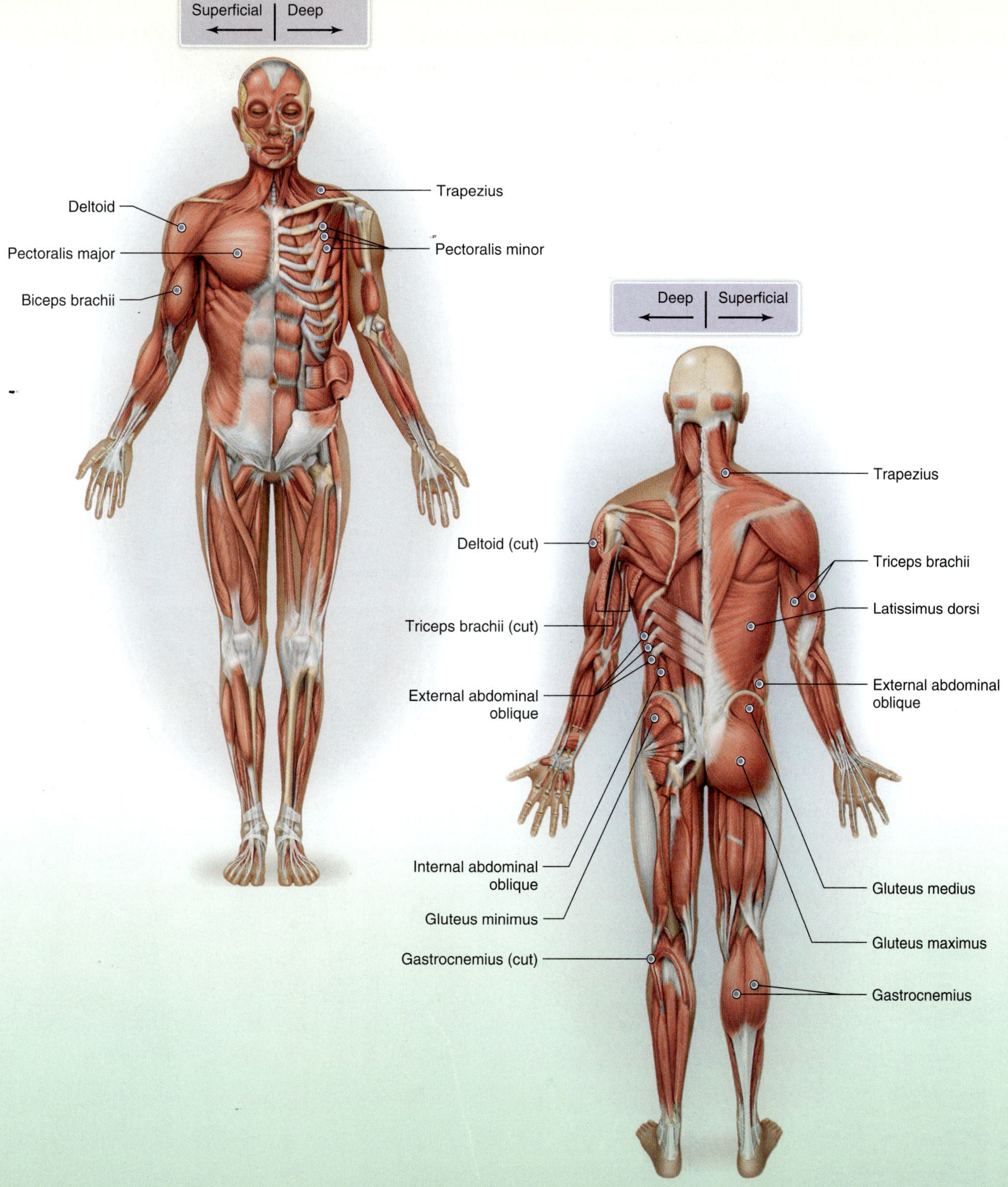

tendon (connective tissue connecting muscle to bone)

ROOTS: ***ten/o, tend/o, tendin/o***

EXAMPLES: tenodynia, tendolysis, tendinitis

NOTES: From Latin, for *to stretch.* This root is also found in the English word *attend,* which means *to stretch toward.*

muscle

ROOTS: ***muscul/o, my/o, myos/o***

EXAMPLES: musculoskeletal, myopathy, myositis

NOTES: The term *muscle* comes from Latin, for *little mouse.* It was once thought that the movement of certain muscles looked like mice running underneath the skin. Personally, we don't see the connection, but linking muscle and mouse must have been commonplace, as Greek, German, and Arabic all have similar words for *muscle* and *mouse.*

fascia (fibrous connective tissue binding muscles together)

ROOT: ***fasci/o***

EXAMPLES: fasciotomy, fasciitis

NOTES: *Fascia* are fibrous connective tissues that bind muscles together. The name comes from the Latin word *fasces,* which means *bundle of sticks.* In ancient Rome, these bundles of sticks also included axes protruding from the center, and political leaders carried fasces with them wherever they went as symbols of their power and authority. In the early twentieth century, when the leader Benito Mussolini came to power in Italy, his form of government was dubbed *fascism* because it relied heavily on strength in order to maintain control.

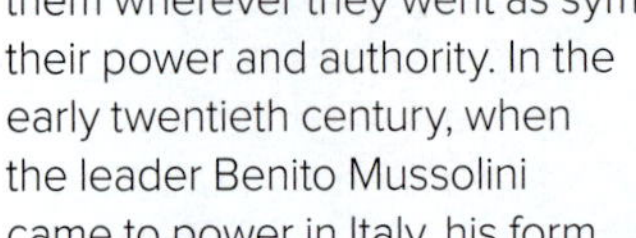

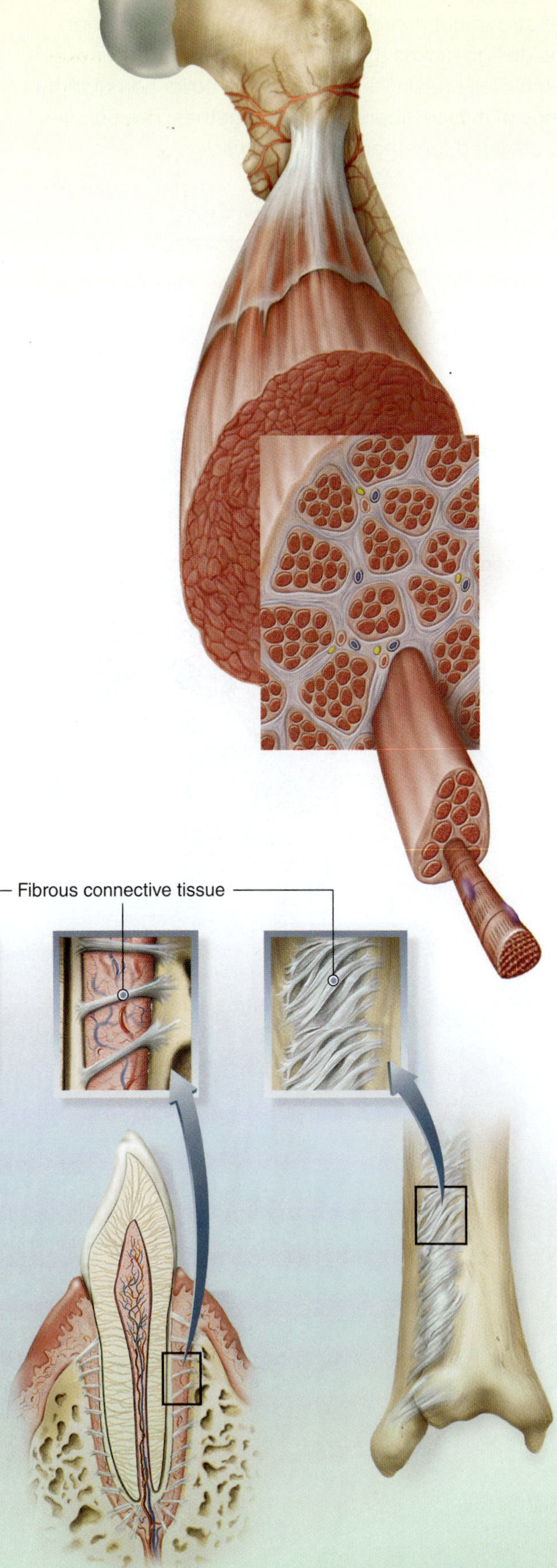

Motion

Usually when you think about your muscles, you think of movement (*kinesio*). While this is a very important part of what they do, they're also hard at work when they're not moving. Your muscles not only move you, they also support you.

This constant holding together—the built-in strength of your muscles—is your muscles' tone (*tono*). Without any muscle tone, your body would be completely limp. Your muscles require input from your nervous system to move and coordinate (*taxo*). If you have problems transferring this input from the nervous system, you may suffer from partial paralysis (*paresis*) or complete paralysis (*plegia*).

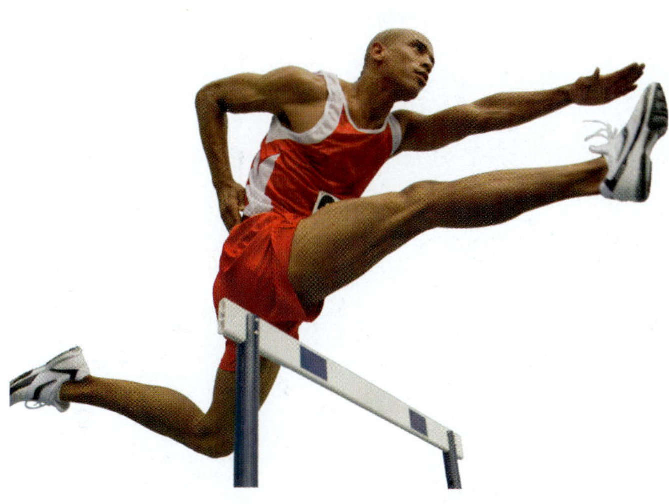

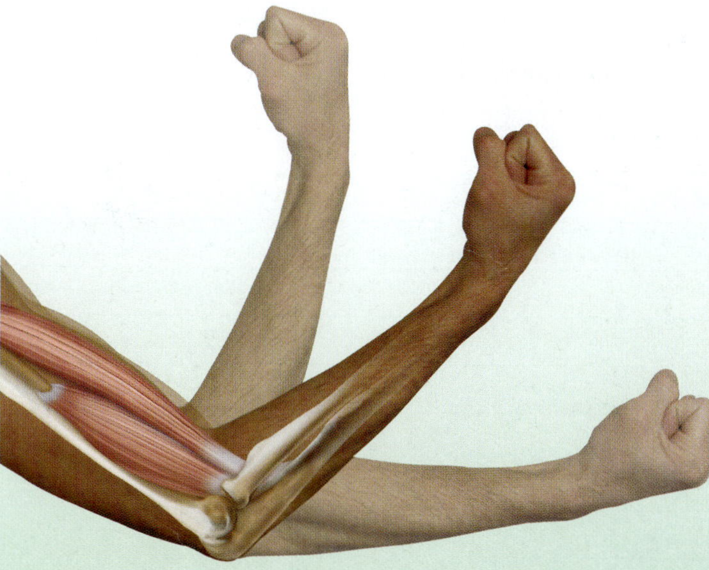

tone, tension

ROOT: ***ton/o***

EXAMPLES: dystonia, tonograph

NOTES: *Tonic* is a word for a medicinal drink. This term was used because medicinal drinks were once thought to restore a person's good muscle tone.

Today, tonic water still has medicinal value. Although some people think tonic water is simply another name for carbonated soda water, tonic is actually a form of carbonated soda water in which quinine, a drug used to treat malaria, has been dissolved. Tonic water was developed to treat people who lived in tropical areas, where malaria is often prevalent.

movement, motion

ROOTS: ***kinesi/o* (also sometimes *kinet/o*)**

EXAMPLES: kinesiology, hyperkinesia, kinetic energy

NOTES: *Akinetopsia* (pronounce ah-KEE-no-TOP-see-ah) comes from the roots *a* (no) + *kinet* (movement) + *opsia* (vision) and refers to a condition where a patient can see an object if it is still, but is unable to see it if it is moving.

arrangement, order, coordination

ROOT: ***tax/o***

EXAMPLES: ataxia, hypotaxia

NOTES: *Syntax* is an English grammar term made up of the roots *syn* (together) + *tax* (arrangement) and refers to the study of the way words are arranged in a sentence.

Taxidermy, which comes from *taxo* (arrange) + *dermy* (skin), refers to the practice of removing and displaying the head and skin of an animal killed during a hunt.

The arrangement of military forces before a battle is called *tactics*.

stiff, bent

ROOT: ***ankyl/o***

EXAMPLES: ankylosis, ankylodactyly

NOTES: This root comes from a Greek word meaning *hooked* or *bent*. The word came to mean *stiff* because if something stays bent, it must be stiff. Your ankle got its name because it bends. People who fish are called *anglers* because they use hooks.

Learning Outcome 4.1 Exercises

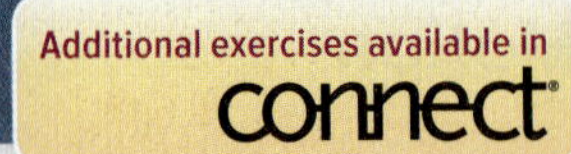
Additional exercises available in
connect

TRANSLATION

EXERCISE 1 *Match the word part on the left with its definition on the right.*

f	1. crani/o	a. ankle
c	2. oste/o	b. arm
g	3. lumb/o	c. bone
j	4. femor/o	d. finger
h	5. cervic/o	e. growth
d	6. dactyl/o	f. head, skull
i	7. cost/o	g. loin, lower back
l	8. carp/o	h. neck
a	9. tars/o	i. rib
b	10. brachi/o	j. thighbone
k	11. spondyl/o	k. vertebra
e	12. -physis	l. wrist

EXERCISE 2 *Translate the following word parts.*

1. femor/o __________
2. crani/o __________
3. oste/o __________
4. cervic/o __________
5. lumb/o __________
6. dactyl/o __________
7. -physis __________
8. brachi/o __________
9. tars/o __________
10. carp/o __________
11. spondyl/o __________

EXERCISE 3 *Break down the following words into their component parts and translate.*

EXAMPLE: sinusitis *sinus | itis* *inflammation of the sinuses*

1. costalgia __________
2. tibialgia __________
3. cervicodynia __________
4. osteodynia __________
5. carpectomy __________
6. tarsectomy __________
7. spondylomalacia __________
8. craniomalacia __________

Learning Outcome 4.1 Exercises

EXERCISE 4 *Match the word part on the left with its definition on the right. Some definitions will be used more than once.*

b	1. burs/o	a.	arrangement, order, coordination
g	2. muscul/o	b.	bursa
e	3. arthr/o	c.	cartilage
j	4. ten/o, tend/o, tendin/o	d.	fibrous connective tissue binding muscles together fascia
k	5. ton/o	e.	joint
g	6. my/o, myos/o	f.	movement, motion
f	7. kinesi/o	g.	muscle
h	8. -plegia	h.	paralysis
c	9. chondr/o	i.	stiff, bent
i	10. ankyl/o	j.	tendon
a	11. tax/o	k.	tone, tension
d	12. fasci/o		

EXERCISE 5 *Translate the following word parts.*

1. ankyl/o ____________________
2. arthr/o ____________________
3. burs/o ____________________
4. chondr/o ____________________
5. fasci/o ____________________
6. kinesi/o ____________________
7. muscul/o ____________________
8. my/o, myos/o ____________________
9. -plegia ____________________
10. tax/o ____________________
11. ten/o, tend/o, tendin/o ____________________
12. ton/o ____________________

EXERCISE 6 *Break down the following words into their component parts and translate.*

EXAMPLE: sinusitis *sinus | itis* *inflammation of the sinuses*

1. fasciitis ____________________
2. tenalgia ____________________
3. arthralgia ____________________
4. myodynia ____________________
5. chondroma ____________________
6. hypertonia ____________________
7. hyperkinesia ____________________
8. bursotomy ____________________
9. ankylosis ____________________

Learning Outcome 4.1 Exercises

GENERATION

EXERCISE 7 *Identify the word parts for the following definitions.*

1. tibia ______
2. growth ______
3. thighbone ______
4. arm ______
5. head, skull ______
6. loin, lower back ______
7. ankle ______
8. neck ______
9. finger ______
10. rib ______

EXERCISE 8 *Build a medical term from the information provided.*

1. bone inflammation ______
2. wrist inflammation ______
3. finger inflammation ______
4. inflammation of the vertebra ______
5. removal of a rib ______

EXERCISE 9 *Identify the word parts for the following definitions.*

1. tendon (3 roots) ______
2. bursa ______
3. tone, tension ______
4. joint ______
5. fascia ______
6. movement, motion ______
7. muscle (3 roots) ______
8. paralysis ______
9. stiff, bent ______
10. arrangement, order, coordination ______
11. cartilage ______

EXERCISE 10 *Build a medical term from the information provided.*

1. inflammation of the tendon ______
2. inflammation of the bursa ______
3. joint inflammation ______
4. incision into fascia ______
5. decrease in muscle tone or tightness ______
6. decrease in muscle movement or activity ______
7. softening of a muscle ______
8. abnormal softening of the cartilage ______

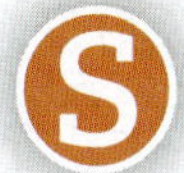

Subjective

Patient History, Problems, Complaints

Bones

Joints

Muscles

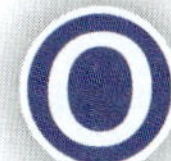

Objective

Observation and Discovery

Diagnostic procedures

Spinal curvatures

Bones

Joints

Muscles

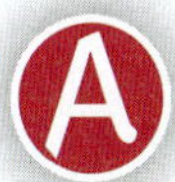

Assessment

Diagnosis and Pathology

Bones

Joints

Muscles

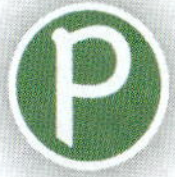

Plan

Treatments and Therapies

Drugs

Bones

Joints

Muscles

This section contains medical terms built from the roots presented in the previous section. The purpose of this section is to expose you to words used in the musculoskeletal system that are built from the word roots presented earlier. The focus of this book is to teach you the process of learning roots and translating them in context. Each term is presented with the correct pronunciation, followed by a word analysis that breaks down the word into its component parts, a definition that provides a literal translation of the word, as well as supplemental information if the literal translation deviates from its medical use.

The terms are organized using a health care professional's SOAP note (first introduced in Chapter 2) as a model.

SUBJECTIVE

4.2 Patient History, Problems, Complaints

Pain is the most common musculoskeletal medical complaint. A patient could have pain in a bone (*ostalgia/ostealgia*), joint (*arthralgia/arthrodynia*), tendon (*tenalgia*), or a muscle (*myalgia/myodynia*). A patient may also notice a change in a muscle's appearance—a muscle may be wasting away (*atrophy*) or abnormally large (*hypertrophy*). A parent may notice that his or her child is either bow-legged (*genu varum*) or knock-kneed (*genu valgum*). Most of the other problems people experience relate to a change in how their muscles or joints are working. For instance, they may notice that their joints don't work as well as normal. The joint may be stiff/bent (*ankylosis*) or it may make crackling sounds when moved (*crepitus*). Patients may also notice changes in their muscle function. They may experience a decrease in muscle tone (*hypotonia*) or muscle tone that is exaggerated (*hypertonia*). Diseases of the nervous system can lead to problems with coordination (*dystaxia* or *ataxia*), movements (*dykinesia* or *bradykinesia*), or twitches (*myospasms*).

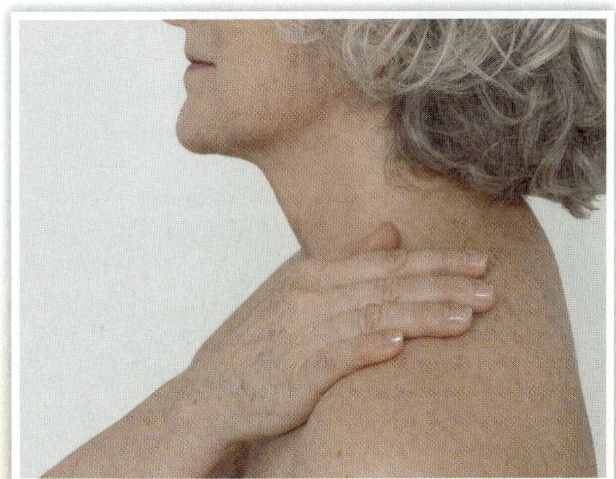

Pain is the most common musculoskeletal medical complaint.

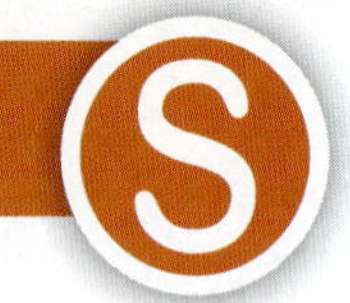

4.2 Patient History, Problems, Complaints

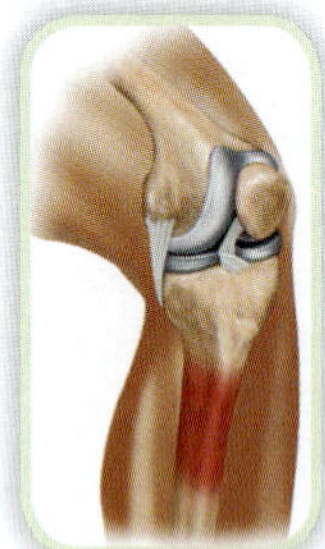
ostalgia

bones

Term	Word Analysis
costalgia kaws-TAL-jah **Definition** rib pain	cost / algia rib / pain
metatarsalgia meh-tah-tar-SAL-jah **Definition** pain in the bones of the foot	meta / tars / algia after / ankle / pain
ostalgia aws-TAL-jah **Definition** bone pain	ost / algia bone / pain
ostealgia aws-tee-AL-jah **Definition** bone pain	oste / algia bone / pain
osteodynia aws-tee-oh-DAI-nee-ah **Definition** bone pain	osteo / dynia bone / pain
spondylodynia spawn-dih-loh-DAI-nee-ah **Definition** vertebra pain	spondylo / dynia vertebra / pain
tibialgia tih-bee-AL-ja **Definition** tibia (shin) pain	tibi / algia tibia / pain

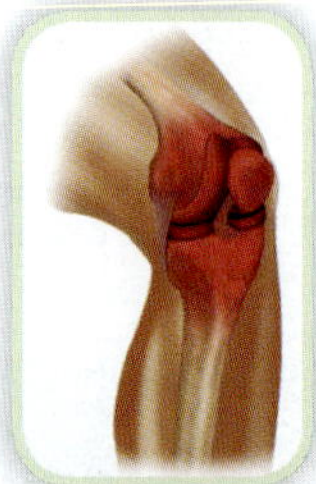
arthrodynia

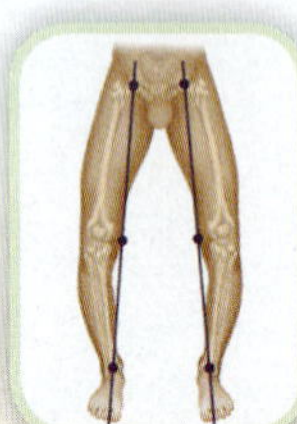
genu valgum

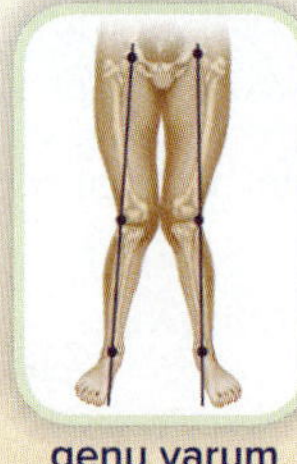
genu varum

joints

Term	Word Analysis
ankylosis an-kih-LOH-sis **Definition** joint stiffness	ankyl / osis stiff / condition
arthralgia ar-THRAL-jah **Definition** joint pain	arthr / algia joint / pain
arthrodynia ar-throh-DAI-nee-ah **Definition** joint pain	arthro / dynia joint / pain
cervicodynia sir-vih-koh-DAI-nee-ah **Definition** neck pain	cervico / dynia neck / pain
crepitation kreh-pih-TAY-shun **Definition** a crackling sound heard in joints	from Latin, for *rattle* or *creaking*
genu valgum JEH-noo VAL-gum **Definition** bow-legged	genu valgum knee bowed out
genu varum JEH-noo VAH-rum **Definition** knock-kneed	genu varum knee pointed in

muscles

Term	Word Analysis
bradykinesia bray-dih-kih-NEE-zhah **Definition** slow movement	brady / kinesia slow / movement
dyskinesia dis-kih-NEE-zhah **Definition** inability to control movement	dys / kinesia bad / movement
dystaxia dis-TAK-see-ah **Definition** poor coordination	dys / taxia bad / coordination
dystonia dis-TOH-nee-ah **Definition** poor muscle tone	dys / tonia bad / muscle tone
graphospasm gra-foh-SPAZ-um **Definition** writer's cramp	grapho / spasm write / involuntary contraction
hyperkinesia hai-per-kih-NEE-zhah **Definition** increase in muscle movement or activity	hyper / kinesia over / movement
hypertonia hai-per-TOH-nee-yah **Definition** increased muscle tone or tightness	hyper / tonia over / muscle tone
hypokinesia hai-poh-kih-NEE-zhah **Definition** decrease in muscle movement or activity	hypo / kinesia under / movement
hypotonia hai-poh-TOH-nee-yah **Definition** decrease in muscle tone or tigtness	hypo / tonia under / muscle tone
myalgia mai-AL-jah **Definition** muscle pain	my / algia muscle / pain
myasthenia mai-as-THEH-nee-ah **Definition** muscle weakness	my / asthenia muscle / weakness
myodynia mai-oh-DAI-nee-ah **Definition** muscle pain	myo / dynia muscle / pain
myospasm mai-oh-SPAZ-um **Definition** muscle spasm	myo / spasm muscle / involuntary contraction
tenalgia ten-AL-jah **Definition** tendon pain	ten / algia tendon / pain

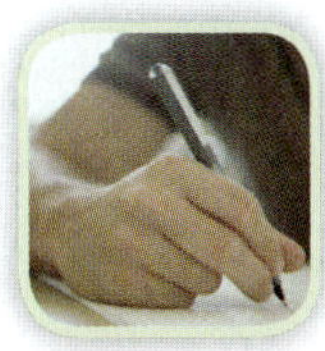

graphospasm

Learning Outcome 4.2 Exercises

PRONUNCIATION

EXERCISE 1 *Break down the following words into syllables.*

EXAMPLE: synesthesia *syn | es | the | sia*

1. ostealgia ______
2. cervicodynia ______
3. bradykinesia ______
4. dyskinesia ______
5. dystaxia ______
6. hypokinesia ______
7. tenalgia ______
8. metatarsalgia ______
9. genu varum ______
10. myodynia ______

EXERCISE 2 *Indicate which syllable is emphasized when pronounced.*

EXAMPLE: bronchitis bron**chi**tis

1. ostalgia ______
2. tibialgia ______
3. costalgia ______
4. arthralgia ______
5. myalgia ______
6. ankylosis ______
7. myospasm ______
8. crepitation ______
9. arthrodynia ______
10. hyperkinesia ______

TRANSLATION

EXERCISE 3 *Break down the following words into their component parts.*

EXAMPLE: nasopharyngoscope *naso | pharyngo | scope*

1. ostealgia ______
2. arthralgia ______
3. myospasm ______
4. myasthenia ______
5. bradykinesia ______
6. graphospasm ______

EXERCISE 4 *Underline and define the word parts from this chapter in the following terms.*

1. tenalgia ______
2. tibialgia ______
3. ostalgia ______
4. myalgia ______
5. costalgia ______
6. metatarsalgia ______
7. myodynia ______
8. osteodynia ______

Learning Outcome 4.2 Exercises

9. arthrodynia ______
10. spondylodynia ______
11. cervicodynia ______
12. ankylosis ______
13. dyskinesia ______
14. dystaxia ______
15. dystonia ______

EXERCISE 5 *Match the term on the left with its definition on the right.*

	Term		Definition
g	1. crepitation	a.	increase in muscle movement or activity
e	2. genu valgum	b.	increased muscle tone or tightness
f	3. genu varum	c.	decrease in muscle movement or activity
a	4. hyperkinesia	d.	decrease in muscle tightness
b	5. hypertonia	e.	bow-legged
c	6. hypokinesia	f.	knock-kneed
d	7. hypotonia	g.	from Latin, for *rattle* or *creaking;* a crackling sound heard in joints

EXERCISE 6 *Translate the following terms as literally as possible.*

EXAMPLE: nasopharyngoscope *an instrument for looking at the nose and throat*

1. dystonia ______
2. dyskinesia ______
3. hyperkinesia ______
4. hypertonia ______
5. metatarsalgia ______
6. myasthenia ______
7. graphospasm ______
8. ankylosis ______

Learning Outcome 4.2 Exercises

GENERATION

EXERCISE 7 *Build a medical term from the information provided.*

EXAMPLE: inflammation of the sinuses *sinusitis*

1. tendon pain ____________
2. tibia (shin) pain ____________
3. rib pain ____________
4. vertebra pain ____________
5. neck pain ____________
6. muscle spasm ____________
7. decrease in muscle movement ____________
8. decrease in muscle tone ____________
9. slow movement ____________
10. poor coordination ____________

EXERCISE 8 *Multiple-choice questions. Select the correct answer(s).*

1. Select the terms that mean *bone pain.*
   a. arthralgia
   b. myalgia
   c. ostalgia
   d. ostealgia
   e. arthrodynia
   f. myodynia
   g. osteodynia
2. Select the terms that mean *joint pain.*
   a. arthralgia
   b. myalgia
   c. ostalgia
   d. ostealgia
   e. arthrodynia
   f. myodynia
   g. osteodynia
3. Select the terms that mean *muscle pain.*
   a. arthralgia
   b. myalgia
   c. ostalgia
   d. ostealgia
   e. arthrodynia
   f. myodynia
   g. osteodynia
4. Which of the following terms comes from Latin, for *rattle* or *creaking?*
   a. crepitation
   b. genu varum
   c. genu valgum
   d. kyphosis
5. A person whose knees point inward has which of the following conditions?
   a. crepitation
   b. genu varum
   c. genu valgum
   d. kyphosis
6. A person whose knees are curved outward (bowed) has which of the following conditions?
   a. crepitation
   b. genu varum
   c. genu valgum
   d. kyphosis

OBJECTIVE

4.3 Observation and Discovery

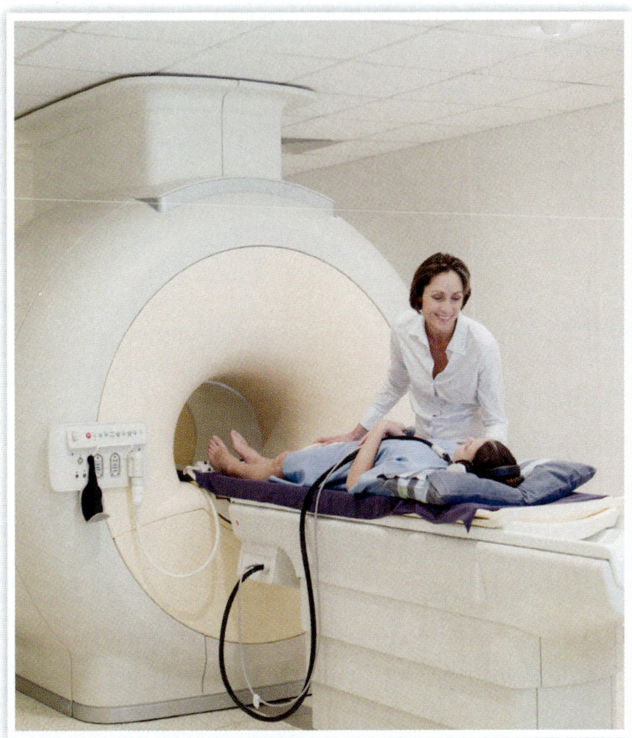

Evaluation of bone issues is commonly performed with imaging, including MRI (magnetic resonance imaging)

When a patient with musculoskeletal problems is evaluated, the physical exam is very important. The exam of the muscles and bones focuses mainly on typical signs of inflammation: redness, swelling, heat, and pain. Any of these symptoms can indicate that an infection or inflammation is present.

There are not many skills that are specific to evaluating bones. Patients with fractured bones may present with a limp or pain upon touching or pressure. A newborn may have extra fingers (*polydactyly*) or fused fingers (*syndactyly*).

Much evaluation of bone issues is performed with imaging. The bread-and-butter imaging method for bones is the simple x-ray. An x-ray can reveal fractures, bone destruction (*osteolysis*), and even extra bone growth (*exostosis*). More involved imaging methods include computed tomography (CT), computed axial tomography (CAT), or magnetic resonance imaging (MRI).

Examining a patient's joint is usually more involved. While the health care provider also checks for the same signs of inflammation, its ability to move also needs to be checked. This is called the joint's range of motion. The provider also checks to make sure the joint is not moving in a direction that it's not supposed to move in. This extra movement is called joint laxity. The provider also checks for fluid around the joint (*effusion*). While the fluid is usually the result of inflammation, it may be pus from an infection (*pyarthrosis*) or blood from an injury (*hemarthrosis*). There are several diagnostic procedures specific to the joints. To get a better view, the health care provider can inject dye into the joint and perform an MRI. This specialized MRI is called an *MR angiogram*. Other means of investigating a joint include injecting a needle and collecting fluid to send to the lab (*arthrocentesis*) or even using a camera-like device to look inside the joint (*arthroscope*).

Examining muscles often means checking how they work. The function of muscles can be evaluated by checking their muscle tone (*myotonia*) or strength. A more involved way to check this is electromyography. In this procedure, two needles are inserted into a muscle to measure the muscle activity.

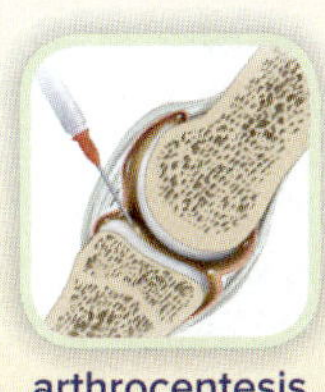

arthrocentesis

diagnostic procedures

Term	Word Analysis
arthrocentesis ar-throh-sin-TEE-sis **Definition** puncture of a joint	**arthro / centesis** joint / puncture
arthrogram AR-throh-gram **Definition** visual record of a joint	**arthro / gram** joint / record

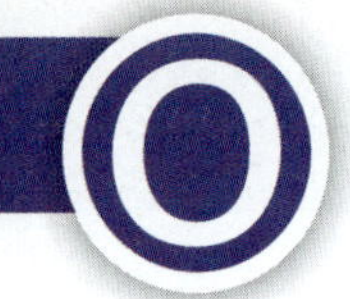

4.3 Observation and Discovery

diagnostic procedures *continued*

Term	Word Analysis
arthrography ar-THRAW-grah-fee **Definition** procedure used to examine a joint	arthro / graph / y joint / recording / process
arthroscope AR-throh-skohp **Definition** instrument for looking into a joint	arthro / scope joint / instrument to look
arthroscopy ar-THRAW-skoh-pee **Definition** procedure of looking into a joint	arthro / scopy joint / procedure to look
computed axial tomography (CAT or CT) kom-PYOO-ted AK-see-al taw-MAW-grah-fee **Definition** imaging procedure using a computer to produce cross sections along an axis	axi / al tomo / graphy axis / pertaining to cut / recording procedure
electromyogram eh-lek-troh-MAI-o-gram **Definition** a record of the electrical activity of a muscle	electro / myo / gram electricity / muscle / record
electromyography eh-LEK-troh-mai-AW-grah-fee **Definition** procedure for measuring the electrical activity of a muscle	electro / myo / graphy electricity / muscle / recording procedure
myography mai-AW-grah-fee **Definition** procedure for studying muscles	myo / graphy muscle / recording procedure
osteometry aw-stee-AW-meh-tree **Definition** procedure for measuring bone	osteo / metry bone / measurement

arthroscopy

kyphosis

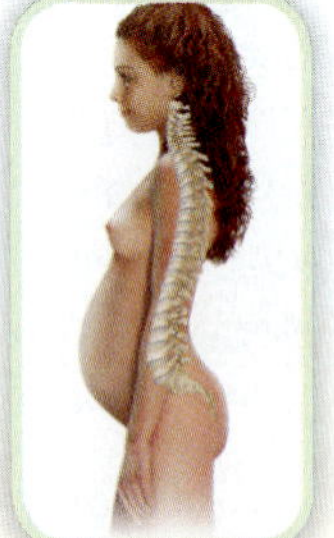

lordosis

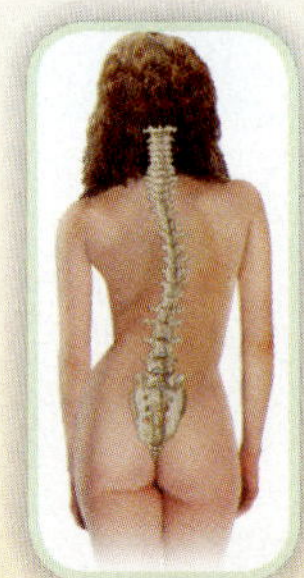

scoliosis

spinal curvatures

Term	Word Analysis
kyphosis kai-FOH-sis **Definition** humped back; abnormal forward curvature of the upper spine	kyph / osis bent / condition
lordosis lor-DOH-sis **Definition** sway back; abnormal forward curvature of the lower spine	lord / osis bent backward / condition
scoliosis SKOH-lee-OH-sis **Definition** crooked back; abnormal lateral curvature of the spine	scoli / osis crooked / condition

bones

Term	Word Analysis
carpitis kar-PAI-tis **Definition** wrist inflammation	carp / itis wrist / inflammation
craniomalacia kray-nee-oh-mah-LAY-shah **Definition** softening of the skull	cranio / malacia skull / softening
exostosis ek-saw-STOH-sis **Definition** an abnormal growth of bone out of another bone	ex / ost / osis out / bone / condition
fracture FRAK-shur **Definition** a bone break	from Latin, for *break*
osteodystrophy aw-stee-oh-DIH-stroh-fee **Definition** poor bone development	osteo / dys / trophy bone / bad / nourishment
osteolysis aw-stee-AW-lih-sis **Definition** bone loss	osteo / lysis bone / loss
osteonecrosis aw-stee-oh-nih-KROH-sis **Definition** death of bone	osteo / necr / osis bone / death / condition
osteosclerosis aw-stee-oh-skleh-ROH-sis **Definition** abnormal hardening of bone	osteo / scler / osis bone / hardening / condition

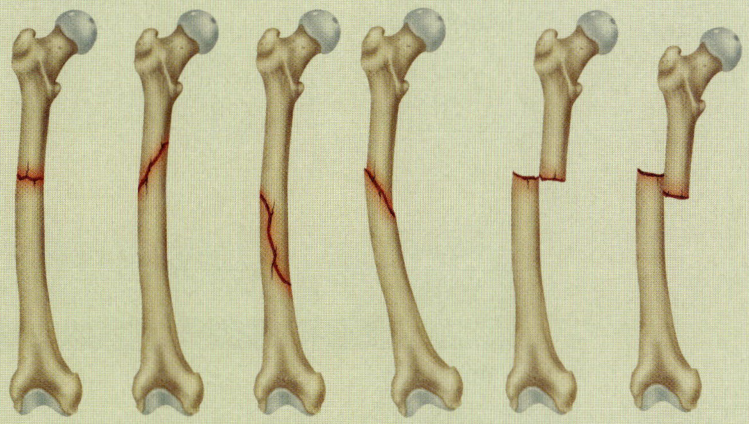

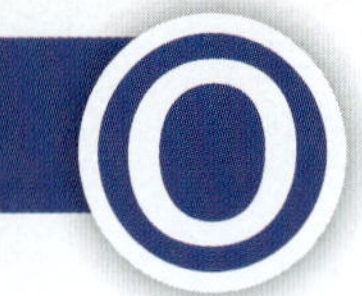

4.3 Observation and Discovery

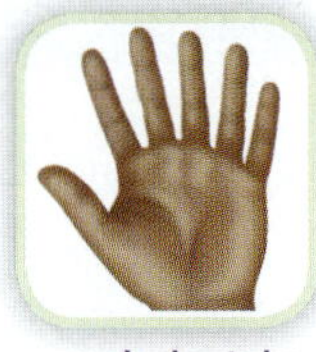
polydactyly

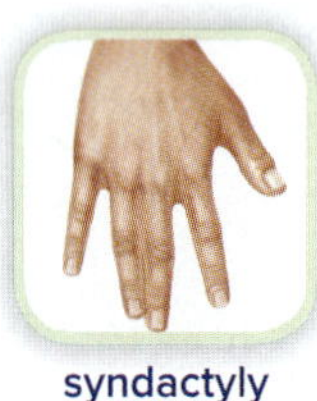
syndactyly

bones *continued*

Term	Word Analysis
polydactyly paw-lee-DAK-tih-lee **Definition** having more than the normal number of fingers (or toes)	poly / dactyl / y many / finger / condition
spondylitis spawn-dih-LAI-tis **Definition** vertebra inflammation	spondyl / itis vertebra / inflammation
spondylomalacia spawn-dih-loh-mah-LAY-shah **Definition** softening of the vertebra	spondylo / malacia vertebra / softening
syndactyly sin-DAK-tih-lee **Definition** fusion (sometimes called webbing) of fingers (or toes)	syn / dactly / y together / finger / condition
tarsoptosis tar-sawp-TOH-sis **Definition** flat feet	tarso / ptosis ankle / drooping condition

joints

Term	Word Analysis
bursolith BIR-soh-lith **Definition** a stone in a bursa	burso / lith bursa / stone
effusion ee-FYOO-zhun **Definition** fluid build-up NOTE: The prefix on *effusion* is actually *ex-*; the *x* turns to an *f* when followed by an *f*. Why? Say *exfusion* 10 times. Most people slur *exfusion* into *effusion* because it is easier to say.	ef / fusion out / pour
hemarthrosis hee-mar-THROH-sis **Definition** blood in a joint	hem / arthr / osis blood / joint / condition
hydrarthrosis hai-drar-THROH-sis **Definition** water (fluid) in a joint	hydr / arthr / osis water / joint / condition
pyarthrosis pai-ar-THROH-sis **Definition** pus in a joint	py / arthr / osis pus / joint / condition

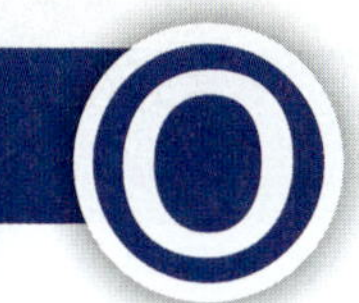

4.3 Observation and Discovery

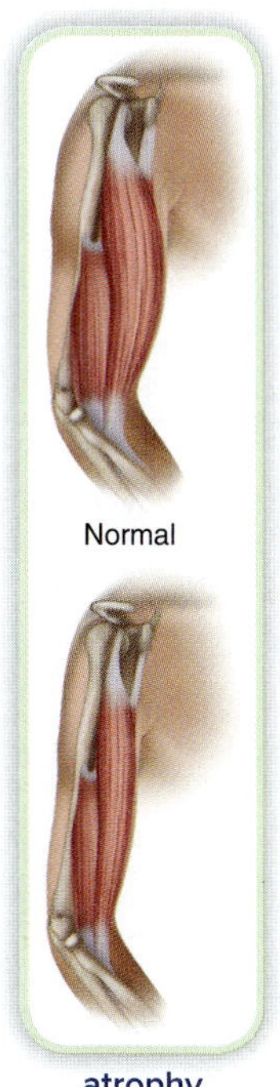

atrophy

muscles

Term	Word Analysis
atrophy A-troh-fee	a / trophy no / nourishment
Definition underdevelopment, decrease, or loss of muscle tissue	
hypertrophy hai-PER-troh-fee	hyper / trophy over / nourishment
Definition overdevelopment of muscle tissue	
myocele MAI-oh-seel	myo / cele muscle / hernia
Definition hernia of muscle tissue	
myolysis mai-AW-lih-sis	myo / lysis muscle / loss
Definition loss of muscle tissue	
myomalacia mai-oh-mah-LAY-shah	myo / malacia muscle / softening
Definition softening of a muscle	
myosclerosis mai-oh-skleh-ROH-sis	myo / scler / osis muscle / hardening / condition
Definition hardening of a muscle	
myotasis mai-AW-tah-sis	myo / tasis muscle / expansion
Definition stretching of a muscle **Note:** The *-tasis* suffix appears as -ectasis in blood vessels (*angiectasis*) and lungs (*bronchiectasis*).	
myotonia mai-oh-TOH-nee-ah	myo / tonia muscle / tone
Definition muscle tone	

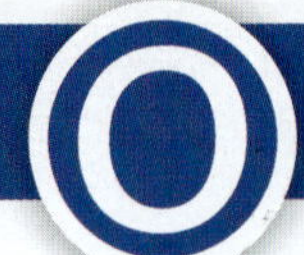

Learning Outcome 4.3 Exercises

PRONUNCIATION

EXERCISE 1 *Break down the following words into syllables.*

EXAMPLE: synesthesia *syn | es | the | sia*

1. bursolith ______
2. myolysis ______
3. tarsoptosis ______
4. hydrarthrosis ______
5. arthrography ______
6. osteometry ______
7. exostosis ______
8. polydactyly ______
9. osteosclerosis ______
10. myosclerosis ______
11. spondylomalacia ______

EXERCISE 2 *Indicate which syllable is emphasized when pronounced.*

EXAMPLE: bronchitis bron**chi**tis

1. atrophy ______
2. effusion ______
3. arthroscope ______
4. arthroscopy ______
5. lordosis ______
6. craniomalacia ______
7. osteolysis ______
8. spondylitis ______
9. osteodystrophy ______
10. pyarthrosis ______
11. myotasis ______
12. myomalacia ______
13. electromyography ______

TRANSLATION

EXERCISE 3 *Break down the following words into their component parts.*

EXAMPLE: nasopharyngoscope *naso | pharyngo | scope*

1. arthrogram ______
2. arthroscope ______
3. myocele ______
4. myography ______
5. electromyography ______
6. spondylomalacia ______
7. arthrocentesis ______
8. myolysis ______
9. osteolysis ______
10. osteonecrosis ______
11. osteosclerosis ______
12. myosclerosis ______
13. hydrarthrosis ______
14. polydactyly ______
15. exostosis ______

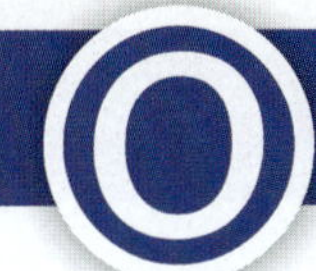

Learning Outcome 4.3 Exercises

EXERCISE 4 *Underline and define the word parts from this chapter in the following terms.*

1. carpitis ______
2. spondylitis ______
3. bursolith ______
4. arthroscopy ______
5. arthrography ______
6. myomalacia ______
7. craniomalacia ______
8. osteometry ______
9. myotasis ______
10. syndactyly ______
11. tarsoptosis ______
12. osteodystophy ______
13. electromyogram ______
14. hemarthrosis ______
15. pyarthrosis ______
16. myotonia (2 roots) ______

EXERCISE 5 *Match the term on the left with its definition on the right.*

e	1. fracture	a.	imaging procedure using a computer to produce cross sections along an axis
g	2. atrophy	b.	humped back; abnormal forward curvature of the upper spine
d	3. scoliosis	c.	sway back; abnormal forward curvature of the lower spine
a	4. computed axial tomography	d.	crooked back; abnormal lateral curvature of the spine
h	5. hypertrophy	e.	from Latin, for *break;* a bone break
f	6. effusion	f.	fluid build-up
c	7. lordosis	g.	underdevelopment, decrease, or loss of muscle tissue
b	8. kyphosis	h.	overdevelopment of muscle tissue

EXERCISE 6 *Translate the following terms as literally as possible.*

EXAMPLE: nasopharyngoscope *an instrument for looking at the nose and throat*

1. osteonecrosis ______
2. syndactyly ______
3. bursolith ______
4. myotasis ______
5. hydrarthrosis ______
6. hemarthrosis ______
7. pyarthrosis ______
8. tarsoptosis ______
9. kyphosis ______
10. lordosis ______
11. scoliosis ______

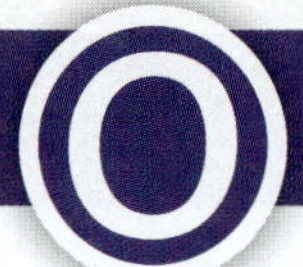

Learning Outcome 4.3 Exercises

GENERATION

EXERCISE 7 *Build a medical term from the information provided.*

EXAMPLE: inflammation of the sinuses *sinusitis*

1. wrist inflammation ______
2. vertebra inflammation ______
3. softening of the skull ______
4. softening of a muscle ______
5. softening of the vertebra ______
6. muscle tone ______
7. many finger condition ______
8. instrument for looking into a joint ______
9. procedure of looking into a joint ______
10. procedure for measuring bone ______

EXERCISE 8 *Multiple-choice questions. Select the correct answer(s).*

1. Select the terms that pertain to bone.
   - a. fracture
   - b. exostosis
   - c. arthrocentesis
   - d. myography
   - e. arthrography
   - f. electromyogram
   - g. electromyography
   - h. atrophy
   - i. hypertrophy
   - j. osteodystrophy
2. Select the terms that pertain to joints.
   - a. fracture
   - b. exostosis
   - c. arthrocentesis
   - d. myography
   - e. arthrography
   - f. electromyogram
   - g. electromyography
   - h. atrophy
   - i. hypertrophy
   - j. osteodystrophy
3. Select the terms that pertain to muscle.
   - a. fracture
   - b. exostosis
   - c. arthrocentesis
   - d. myography
   - e. arthrography
   - f. electromyogram
   - g. electromyography
   - h. atrophy
   - i. hypertrophy
   - j. osteodystrophy
4. What does the abbreviation *CAT* stand for?
   - a. chondro-arthrodysplasia tenotomy
   - b. computed axial tomography
   - c. computed arthrography telectasia
   - d. chondro-axial tomography
5. Which of the following terms means *fluid build-up?*
   - a. affusion
   - b. effusion
   - c. effision
   - d. exfusure

EXERCISE 9 *Briefly describe the difference between each pair of terms.*

1. osteolysis, myolysis ______
2. osteosclerosis, myosclerosis ______
3. arthrogram, myogram ______
4. arthrocele, myocele ______

ASSESSMENT

4.4 Diagnosis and Pathology

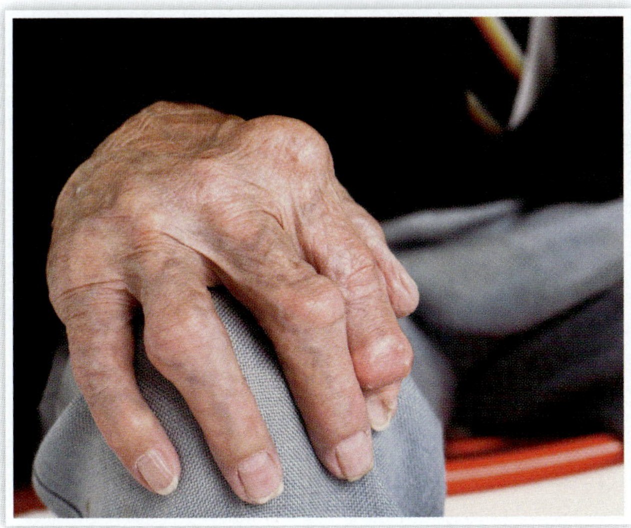

As mentioned earlier, fractures are a common reason why patients see health care providers. Fractures are more common in people with weaker bones. Bone loss (*osteopenia*) can be related to age or to a diet that is deficient in calcium. Osteopenia leads to soft bones in children (*osteomalacia*) or weak, frail bones in adults (*osteoporosis*). Some patients suffer from infections of the bone (*osteomyelitis*), a serious illness that often requires hospitalization.

The vertebral column of bones is susceptible to injury. Gymnasts, football players, or weight lifters who bend their backs too far can suffer small stress fractures of their vertebra (*spondylolysis*). If the fracture is severe, the vertebrae can slip onto one another (*spondylolisthesis*). A very serious version of this condition can advance to problems with a narrowing of the space for the spinal cord (*spinal stenosis*).

You move your joints all the time. They act as shock absorbers for your body, and they take a lot of abuse. It should come as no surprise, then, that joint problems are a very common medical concern. A swollen, painful joint (*arthritis*) can have many causes—the most common being excessive wear and tear. This type is called *osteoarthritis*. As the cartilage between the bones in a joint breaks down, the bones eventually rub together and the joint becomes painful to move. This is a very common reason for a joint replacement surgery.

Other causes for arthritis include infection (*septic arthritis*) and a disease of joint inflammation (*rheumatoid arthritis*). Other parts of the joint area that can cause problems are the bursa (*bursitis*) and tendon (*tendonitis*). These are not usually caused by an injury; instead, they are a result of normal wear and tear over time.

Unusual inflammatory conditions also affect the muscles. Muscles can become inflamed individually (*myositis*) or in groups (*polymyositis*). Sometimes this can involve the skin as well (*dermatomyostis*). General problems with all the muscles are called *myopathies*. *Myasthenia gravis and muscular dystrophy* are two of the most common types of myopathy.

Like any system in the body, the musculoskeletal system can develop tumors. Tumors can develop in the bones (*osteosarcoma, osteocarcinoma, osteochondroma*) or they can spread to the bones from other parts of the body. Your muscles can get tumors (*myoma*) as well—one example is an *osteosarcoma.*

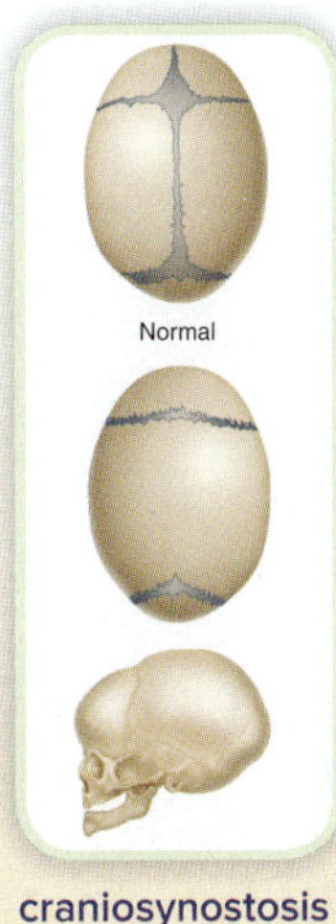

craniosynostosis

bones

Term	Word Analysis
ankylosing spondylitis an-kih-LOH-sing spawn-dih-LAI-tis **Definition** a stiffening inflammation of the vertebrae	ankylos / ing spondyl / itis stiffen / causing vertebra / inflammation
chondro-osteodystrophy KAWN-droh-AW-stee-oh-DIH-stroh-fee **Definition** poor development of bones and cartilage	chondro / osteo / dys / trophy cartilage / bone / bad / nourishment
craniosynostosis KRAY-nee-oh-SIN-aw-STOH-sis **Definition** the premature fusing of the skull bones	cranio /syn / ost / osis skull / together / bone / condition

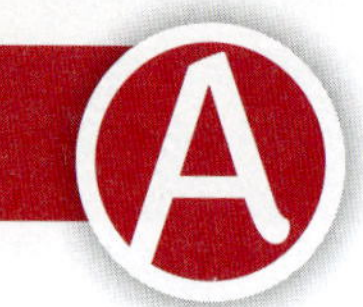

4.4 Diagnosis and Pathology

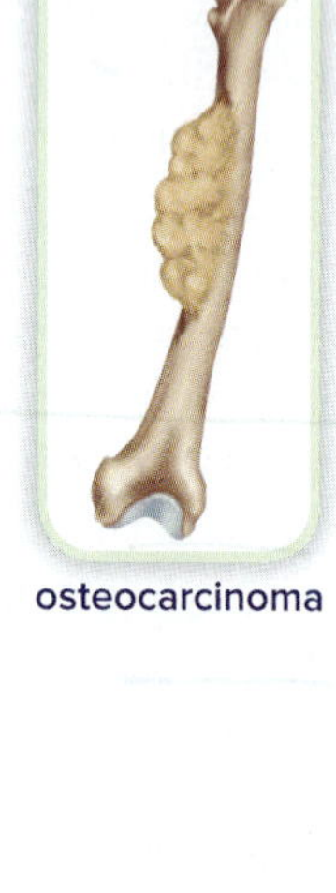

osteocarcinoma

bones *continued*

Term	Word Analysis
dactylitis DAK-tih-LAI-tis **Definition** finger inflammation	**dactyl / itis** finger / inflammation
hypertrophic spondylitis HAI-per-TROH-fik spon-dih-LAI-tis **Definition** overdevelopment of the vertebrae causing inflammation	**hyper / trophic spondyl / itis** over / nourishment vertebra / inflammation
osteitis AW-stee-AI-tis **Definition** bone inflammation	**oste / itis** bone / inflammation
osteocarcinoma AW-stee-oh-KAR-sih-NOH-mah **Definition** bone cancer tumor	**osteo / carcin / oma** bone / cancer / tumor
osteochondritis AW-stee-oh-kon-DRAI-tis **Definition** inflammation of bone and cartilage	**osteo / chondr / itis** bone / cartilage / inflammation
osteochondroma AW-stee-oh-kon-DROH-mah **Definition** a tumor made up of bone and cartilage, also known as an exostosis made up of cartilage	**osteo / chondr / oma** bone / cartilage / tumor
osteogenesis imperfecta AW-stee-oh-JIN-eh-sis IM-per-FEK-tah **Definition** a disease in which the bones do not develop correctly, also known as *brittle bone disease*	**osteo / genesis im / perfecta** bone / creation not / complete
osteomalacia AW-stee-oh-mah-LAY-shah **Definition** softening of the bone	**osteo / malacia** bone / softening
osteomyelitis AW-stee-oh-MAI-eh-LAI-tis **Definition** inflammation of the bone and bone marrow	**osteo / myel / itis** bone / marrow / inflammation
osteopathy AW-stee-AW-pah-thee **Definition** bone disease	**osteo / pathy** bone / disease
osteopenia AW-stee-oh-PEE-nee-yah **Definition** reduction in bone volume	**osteo / penia** bone / deficiency
osteoporosis AW-stee-oh-por-OH-sis **Definition** loss of bone density	**osteo / por / osis** bone / pore / condition
osteosarcoma AW-stee-oh-sar-KOH-mah **Definition** cancerous tumor arising out of bone cells	**osteo / sarc / oma** bone / flesh / tumor

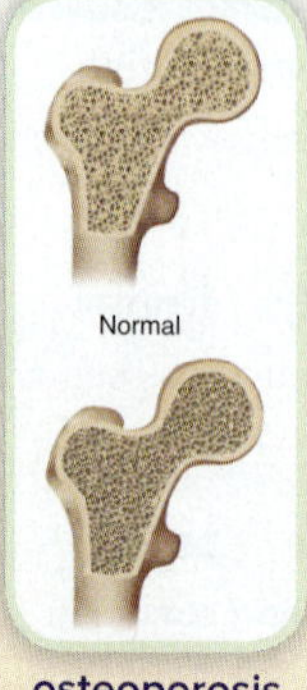

osteoporosis

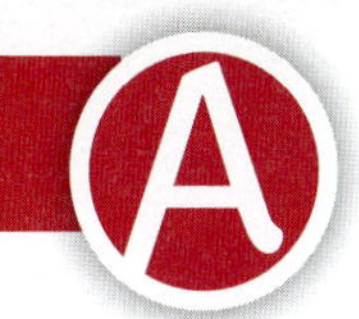

4.4 Diagnosis and Pathology

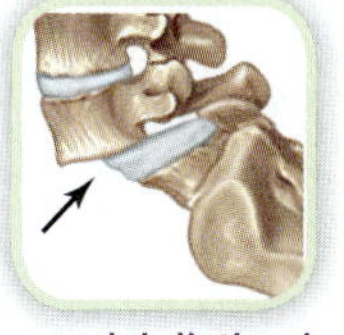
spondylolisthesis

bones *continued*

Term	Word Analysis
spinal stenosis SPAI-nal stih-NOH-sis **Definition** abnormal narrowing of the spine	spinal sten / osis spine narrow / condition
spondyloarthropathy SPAWN-dih-loh-ar-THRAW-pah-thee **Definition** joint disease of the vertebrae	spondylo / arthro / pathy vertebra / joint / disease
spondylolisthesis SPAWN-dih-loh-lis-THEE-sis **Definition** the slipping or dislocation of a vertebra	spondylo / listhesis vertebra / slipping
spondylolysis SPAWN-dih-LO-li-sis **Definition** loss of vertebra structure	spondylo / lysis vertebra / loss
spondylosis SPAWN-dih-LOH-sis **Definition** vertebra condition	spondyl / osis vertebra / condition

rheumatoid arthritis

joints

Term	Word Analysis
arthritis ar-THRAI-tis **Definition** joint inflammation	arthr / itis joint / inflammation
rheumatoid arthritis ROO-mah-toyd ar-THRAI-tis **Definition** inflammation of the joints; it is called *rheumatoid* because its symptoms resemble those of rheumatic fever	rheumat / oid arthr / itis rheumatic fever / resembling joint / inflammation
septic arthritis SEP-tik ar-THRAI-ti **Definition** inflammation of the joint caused by infection	septic arthr / itis rotting joint / inflammation
osteoarthritis AW-stee-oh-ar-THRAI-tis **Definition** inflammation of the joints, specifically those that bear weight	osteo / arthr / itis bone / joint / inflammation
arthrocele AR-throh-seel **Definition** hernia of a joint	arthro / cele joint / hernia

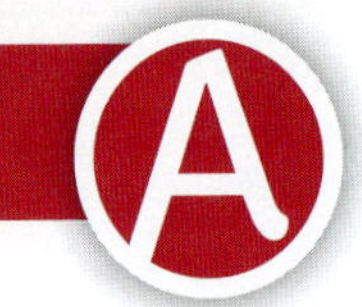

4.4 Diagnosis and Pathology

joints *continued*

Term	Word Analysis
arthrodysplasia AR-throh-dis-PLAY-zhah **Definition** abnormal joint development	arthro / dys / plasia joint / bad / formation
arthropathy ar-THRAW-pah-thee **Definition** joint disease	arthro / pathy joint / disease
arthrosclerosis AR-throh-skleh-ROH-sis **Definition** hardening of the joints	arthro / scler / osis joint / hardening / condition
bursitis bur-SAI-tis **Definition** inflammation of the bursa	burs / itis bursa / inflammation
bursopathy bur-SAW-pah-thee **Definition** disease of the bursa	burso / pathy bursa / disease
subluxation sub-luk-SAY-shun **Definition** partial dislocation of a joint	sub / luxation beneath / dislocation

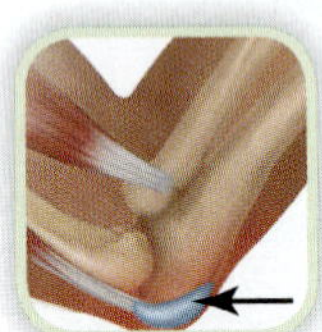
bursitis

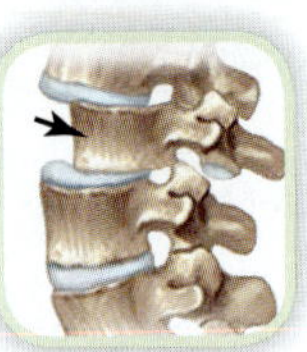
subluxation

muscles

Term	Word Analysis
achondroplasia AY-kawn-droh-PLAY-zhah **Definition** a defect in the formation of cartilage	a / chondro / plasia no / cartilage / formation
chondroma kawn-DROH-mah **Definition** a tumor-like growth of cartilage tissue	chondr / oma cartilage / tumor
chondromalacia KAWN-droh-mah-LAY-shah **Definition** abnormal softening of the cartilage	chondro / malacia cartilage / softening
costochondritis KAW-stoh-kawn-DRAI-tis **Definition** inflammation of the cartilage of the rib	costo / chondr / itis rib / cartilage / inflammation
fasciitis FA-shee-AI-tis **Definition** inflammation of the fascia	fasci / itis fascia / inflammation

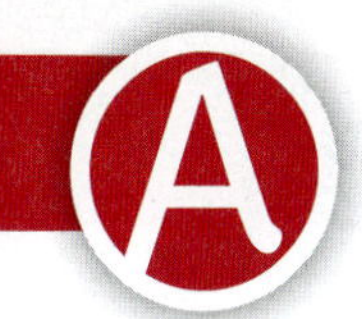

4.4 Diagnosis and Pathology

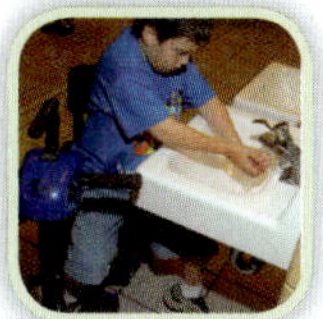

muscular dystrophy

muscles *continued*

Term	Word Analysis
muscular dystrophy MUS-kyoo-lar DIS-troh-fee **Definition** disorder characterized by poor muscle development	muscul / ar dys / trophy muscle / pertaining to bad / nourishment
myoclonus MAI-oh-KLAWN-us **Definition** violent muscle contraction	myo / clonus muscle / turmoil
myopathy mai-AW-pah-thee **Definition** muscle disease	myo / pathy muscle / disease
myasthenia MAI-as-THEE-nee-ah **Definition** muscle weakness	my / asthenia muscle / weakness
myofasciitis MAI-oh- FA-shee-AI-tis **Definition** inflammation of muscle and fascia	myo / fasci / itis muscle / fascia / inflammation
myoma mai-OH-mah **Definition** a muscle tumor	my / oma muscle / tumor
myosarcoma MAI-oh-sar-KOH-mah **Definition** a cancerous muscle tumor	myo / sarc / oma muscle / flesh / tumor
myositis MAI-oh-SAI-tis **Definition** muscle inflammation	myos / itis muscle / inflammation
necrotizing fasciitis NEH-kroh-TAI-zing FA-shee-AI-tis **Definition** inflammation of the fascia causing the death of tissue	necrot / izing fasci / itis death / causing fascia / inflammation
polymyositis PAW-lee-MAI-oh-SAI-tis **Definition** inflammation of multiple muscles	poly / myos / itis many / muscle / inflammation
tardive dyskinesia TAR-div DIS-kin-EE-zhah **Definition** condition characterized by the loss of muscle control	tardive dys / kines / ia slow bad / movement / condition
tendinitis TEN-dih-NAI-tis **tendonitis** TEN-dah-NAI-tis **Definition** tendon inflammation **NOTE:** These words are both accepted spellings for the same condition.	tendin / itis tendon / inflammation tendon / itis tendon / inflammation

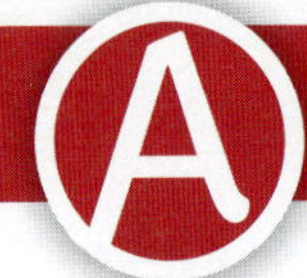

Learning Outcome 4.4 Exercises

PRONUNCIATION

EXERCISE 1 *Break down the following words into syllables.*

EXAMPLE: synesthesia *syn | es | the | sia*

1. myositis ______
2. myasthenia ______
3. polymyositis ______
4. osteopenia ______
5. osteoarthritis ______
6. osteomalacia ______
7. osteomyelitis ______
8. osteochondritis ______
9. osteochondroma ______
10. spondylosis ______
11. spondylolysis ______
12. spondylolisthesis ______
13. arthrodysplasia ______
14. arthrosclerosis ______
15. achondroplasia ______
16. craniosynostosis ______

EXERCISE 2 *Indicate which syllable is emphasized when pronounced.*

EXAMPLE: bronchitis bron**chi**tis

1. arthritis ______
2. osteitis ______
3. bursitis ______
4. myoma ______
5. chondroma ______
6. arthropathy ______
7. bursopathy ______
8. myopathy ______
9. subluxation ______

TRANSLATION

EXERCISE 3 *Break down the following words into their component parts.*

EXAMPLE: nasopharyngoscope *naso | pharyngo | scope*

1. myopathy ______
2. myoclonus ______
3. polymyositis ______
4. myofasciitis ______
5. arthrocele ______
6. arthropathy ______
7. arthritis ______
8. bursitis ______
9. hypertrophic spondylitis ______
10. chondroma ______
11. osteoarthritis ______
12. osteochondritis ______
13. osteomyelitis ______
14. osteosarcoma ______
15. osteocarcinoma ______
16. chondro-osteodystrophy ______

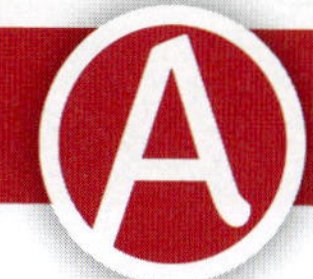

Learning Outcome 4.4 Exercises

EXERCISE 4 *Underline and define the word parts from this chapter in the following terms.*

1. bursopathy ______
2. fasciitis ______
3. dactylitis ______
4. osteitis ______
5. tendinitis ______
6. tendonitis ______
7. myositis ______
8. rheumatoid arthritis ______
9. myoma ______
10. muscular dystrophy ______
11. osteomalacia ______
12. osteopenia ______
13. osteogenesis imperfecta ______
14. osteochondroma (2 roots) ______
15. chondromalacia ______
16. myasthenia ______
17. spondylolisthesis ______
18. spondylolysis ______
19. tardive dyskinesia ______
20. costochondritis (2 roots) ______
21. craniosynostosis (2 roots) ______
22. ankylosing spondylitis (2 roots) ______

EXERCISE 5 *Match the term on the left with its definition on the right.*

____	1. achondroplasia	a.	bone disease
____	2. arthrodysplasia	b.	loss of bone density
____	3. arthrosclerosis	c.	abnormal narrowing of the spine
____	4. myosarcoma	d.	joint disease of the vertebrae
____	5. necrotizing fasciitis	e.	vertebrate condition
____	6. osteopathy	f.	inflammation of the joints caused by infection
____	7. osteoporosis	g.	abnormal joint development
____	8. septic arthritis	h.	hardening of the joints
____	9. spinal stenosis	i.	a defect in the formation of cartilage
____	10. spondylosis	j.	inflammation of the fascia causing the death of tissue
____	11. spondyloarthropathy	k.	partial dislocation of a joint
____	12. subluxation	l.	a cancerous muscle tumor

EXERCISE 6 *Translate the following terms as literally as possible.*

EXAMPLE: nasopharyngoscope *an instrument for looking at the nose and throat*

1. tendinitis ______
2. tendonitis ______
3. arthropathy ______
4. bursopathy ______
5. spinal stenosis ______
6. polymyositis ______
7. craniosynostosis ______
8. tardive dyskinesia ______
9. osteogenesis imperfecta ______
10. osteomyelitis ______
11. osteoporosis ______
12. spondylolisthesis ______
13. arthrodysplasia ______
14. subluxation ______
15. achondroplasia ______

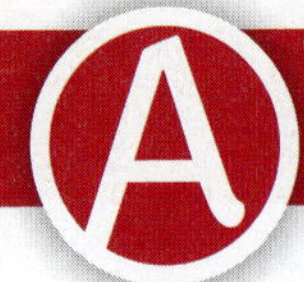

Learning Outcome 4.4 Exercises

GENERATION

EXERCISE 7 *Build a medical term from the information provided.*

EXAMPLE: inflammation of the sinuses *sinusitis*

1. inflammation of the bursa ____________
2. inflammation of the fascia ____________
3. finger inflammation ____________
4. inflammation of the cartilage and rib ____________
5. a stiffening inflammation of the vertebrae ____________
6. overdevelopment (*trophic*) vertebrae inflammation ____________
7. joint hardening condition ____________
8. bone disease ____________
9. bone deficiency ____________
10. muscle weakness ____________

EXERCISE 8 *Multiple-choice questions. Select the correct answer(s).*

1. Select the terms that have the root meaning *muscle*.
   a. osteitis
   b. arthritis
   c. myositis
   d. myofasciitis
   e. osteoarthritis
   f. osteochondritis
2. Select the terms that have the root meaning *joint*.
   a. osteitis
   b. arthritis
   c. myositis
   d. myofasciitis
   e. osteoarthritis
   f. osteochondritis
3. Select the terms that have the root meaning *cartilage*.
   a. osteitis
   b. arthritis
   c. myositis
   d. myofasciitis
   e. osteoarthritis
   f. osteochondritis
4. Select the terms that have the root meaning *bone*.
   a. osteitis
   b. arthritis
   c. myositis
   d. myofasciitis
   e. osteoarthritis
   f. osteochondritis
5. *Necrotizing fasciitis* is
   a. inflammation of the fascia causing the regeneration of muscle
   b. inflammation of muscle causing the death of tissue
   c. a disease of the fascia causing abnormal tissue growth
   d. inflammation of the fascia causing the death of tissue
6. A violent muscle contraction is called
   a. myotonic
   b. myoclonus
   c. myodysplasia
   d. muscular dystrophy
7. A disorder characterized by poor muscle development is known as
   a. myotonic
   b. myoclonus
   c. myodysplasia
   d. muscular dystrophy

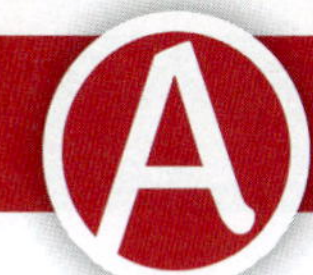

Learning Outcome 4.4 Exercises

EXERCISE 9 *Match the term on the left with its definition on the right*

____	1. rheumatoid arthritis	a.	bone cancer tumor
____	2. arthrocele	b.	a tumor made up of bone and cartilage
____	3. septic arthritis	c.	a cancerous muscle tumor
____	4. myoma	d.	cancerous tumor arising out of bone cells
____	5. myosarcoma	e.	inflammation of the joints, the symptoms of which resemble rheumatic fever
____	6. osteosarcoma	f.	inflammation of the joint caused by infection
____	7. osteocarcinoma	g.	poor development of bones and cartilage
____	8. chondroma	h.	muscle tumor
____	9. osteochondroma	i.	hernia of a joint
____	10. chondroosteodystrophy	j.	a tumor-like growth of cartilage tissue

EXERCISE 10 *Briefly describe the difference between each pair of terms.*

1. osteomalacia, chondromalacia ____________________
2. spondyloarthropathy, myopathy ____________________
3. spondylolysis, spondylosis ____________________

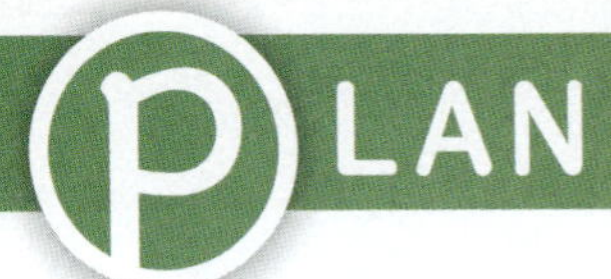

4.5 Treatments and Therapies

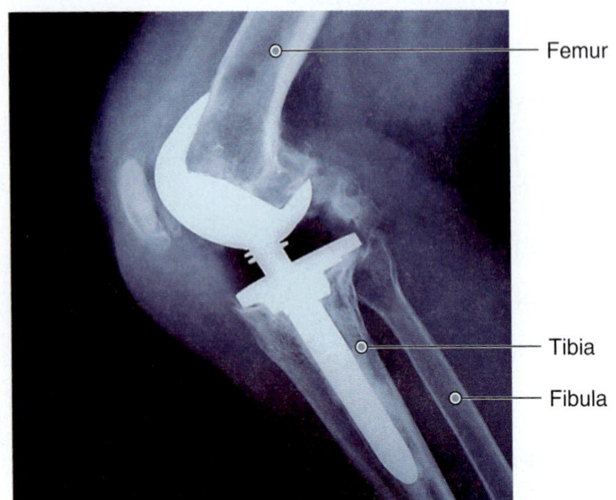

Common procedures for the musculoskeletal system include knee and hip replacements.

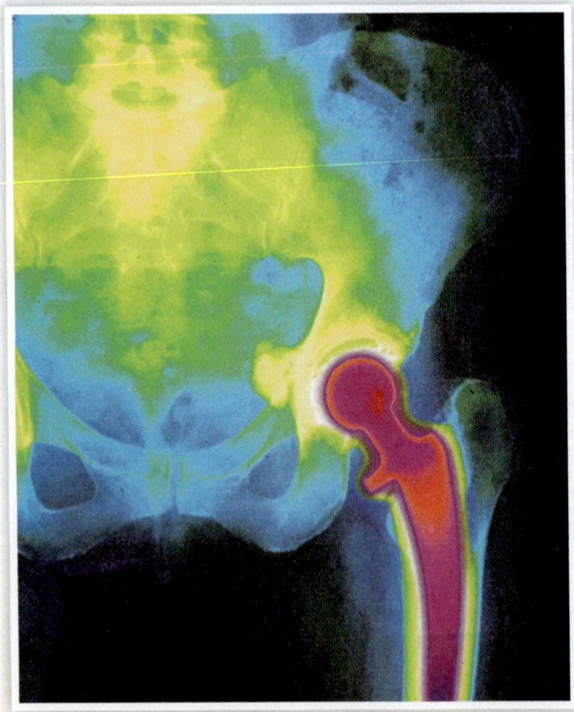

The medicines used to treat musculoskeletal problems are designed to decrease pain (*analgesic*) or inflammation (*anti-inflammatory*). The most commonly used medicines for both are known as nonsteroidal anti-inflammatory drugs (NSAIDs). Ibuprofen is a common example of this type of medicine. Other nonsurgical treatments include doing *physical therapy,* in which patients exercise and stretch in order to heal injuries, or wearing a device used to relieve tension on a joint (*orthotics*). Shoe inserts are a very common type of orthotic.

When nonsurgical treatment fails, surgery may be necessary. *Orthopedic* surgery deals with joints and bones. Many of the tools used in orthopedic surgery look like they came from a home improvement store—including drills, saws, and hammers. These tools are used to cut into bone (*osteotomy*), joints (*arthrotomy*), or muscle (*myotomy*). Sometimes they remove part or all of these structures (*osteectomy, arthrectomy, myectomy*).

When defective areas or cancer are present in a bone, the diseased area of bone must be removed before new bone (*graft*) or artificial hardware (*prosthesis*) can be installed. This reconstruction of bone procedure is called *osteoplasty.*

Similar procedures exist for joints. Sometimes, removal of a diseased joint (*arthrectomy*) is necessary, followed by a reconstruction of the joint with a prosthesis (*arthroplasty*). These are common treatments for diseased knees and hips. A less aggressive surgery for fixing diseased joints, *chondroplasty,* involves fixing the bad cartilage of a joint. It is very common in athletes and older patients with chronic osteoarthritis.

Not all orthopedic surgery involves complete reconstruction of a bone or joint. Sometimes something that has snapped must be repaired, as in a tendon repair (*tenorrhaphy*) or a muscle repair (*myorrhaphy*). Other times, new attachments must be made. This can involve attaching leftover muscle to bone (*myodesis*) after an amputation or fixing two bones surrounding a joint (*arthrodesis*). While the latter procedure results in immobility of the joint, it may be necessary to relieve pain.

Correcting fractures are among the most common problems encountered when working with bones. Sometimes, the fractured bones end up out of place. Putting them back in place is known as *reduction.* Often, a fracture can be reduced without surgery (*closed reduction*), but sometimes the problem must be corrected surgically (*open reduction*). Once a fracture is corrected, it may need to be held in place with hardware (*fixation*). When hardware is installed inside the body, the procedure is referred to as *internal fixation.* Often, this involves drilling a metal plate into bones and affixing it to the bones with screws. When hardware is installed outside the body, the procedure is referred to as *external fixation.*

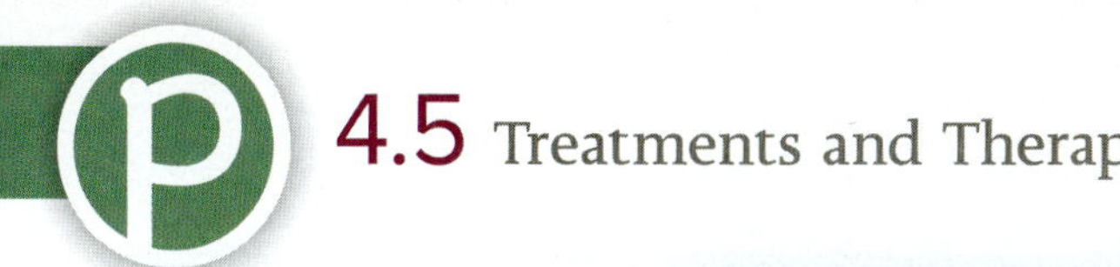

4.5 Treatments and Therapies

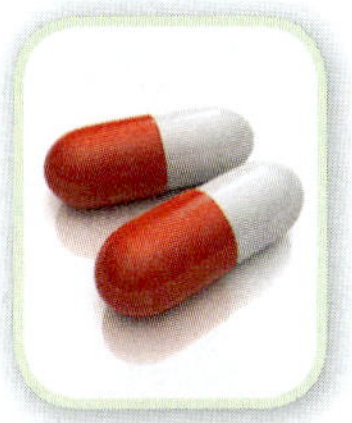

analgesic

drugs

Term	Word Analysis
analgesic A-nal-JEE-zik **Definition** a drug that relieves pain	an / alge / sic no / pain / agent
antiarthritic AN-tee-ar-THRIH-tik **Definition** a drug that opposes joint inflammation	anti / arthri / tic against / joint (pain) / agent
anti-inflammatory AN-tee-in-FLA-mah-TOR-ee **Definition** a drug that opposes inflammation	anti / inflammatory against / inflammation
antipyretic AN-tee-pir-ih-tik **Definition** a drug that opposes fever	anti / pyre / tic against / fever / agent

bones

Term	Word Analysis
carpectomy kar-PEK-toh-mee **Definition** removal of all or part of the wrist	carp / ectomy wrist / removal
costectomy kaws-TEK-toh-mee **Definition** removal of a rib	cost / ectomy rib / removal
craniectomy KRAY-nee-EK-toh-mee **Definition** removal of a portion of the skull	crani / ectomy skull / removal
craniotomy KRAY-nee-AW-toh-mee **Definition** removal of a portion of the skull NOTE: The difference between a craniectomy and a craniotomy is whether or not the piece of bone is replaced. After a craniotomy, the piece of bone that was removed to allow surgical access to the brain is replaced. In a craniectomy, the piece of bone is not replaced.	cranio / tomy skull / incision
external fixation EKS-tir-nal fik-SAY-shun **Definition** the fixation of a fractured bone from the outside (i.e., using casts, splints, stabilizers, etc.) NOTE: Though external fixation refers to things attached outside the body, things like stabilizers often require surgery to attach.	external fix / ation outside fix / procedure
internal fixation IN-tir-nal fik-SAY-shun **Definition** the fixation of a fractured bone from the inside (i.e., using screws, pins, plates, and so on)	internal fix / ation inside fix / procedure

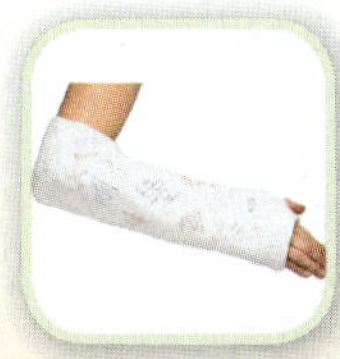

external fixation

4.5 Treatments and Therapies

bones *continued*

Term	Word Analysis
closed reduction klohzd ree-DUK-shun **Definition** returning bones to their proper position without the use of surgery	closed re / duc / tion closed back / lead / procedure
open reduction OH-pen ree-DUK-shun **Definition** returning bones to their proper position through the use of surgery	open re / duc / tion open back / lead / procedure
metacarpectomy MEH-tah-kar-PEK-toh-mee **Definition** removal of a bone in the hand	meta / carp / ectomy after / wrist / removal
orthotics or-THAW-tiks **Definition** a device that aids in the straightening or stabilizing of a part of the body	ortho / tics straight / agent
ostectomy aws-TEK-toh-mee **Definition** removal of a bone	ost / ectomy bone / removal
osteectomy aws-tee-EK-toh-mee **Definition** removal of a bone	oste / ectomy bone / removal
osteoclasia AWS-tee-oh-KLAY-zhah **Definition** the surgical breaking of a bone (often done to remedy a deformity)	osteo / clasia bone / breaking
osteoplasty AWS-tee-oh-PLAS-tee **Definition** reconstruction of a bone	osteo / plasty bone / reconstruction
osteotomy AWS-tee-AW-toh-mee **Definition** incision into a bone	osteo / tomy bone / incision
prosthesis praws-THEE-sis **Definition** a device that is added to a body to replace a missing part or lost function	pros / thesis toward / place
spondylosyndesis SPAWN-dih-loh-sin-DEE-sis **Definition** fusing together of multiple vertebrae	spondylo / syn / desis vertebra / together / binding
sternotomy stir-NAW-toh-mee **Definition** incision into the sternum	sterno / tomy sternum / incision
tarsectomy tar-SEK-toh-mee **Definition** removal of all or a portion of the ankle	tars / ectomy ankle / removal
tarsoclasia TAR-soh-KLAY-zhah **Definition** surgical fracture of the ankle (i.e., to treat clubfoot)	tarso / clasia ankle / breaking

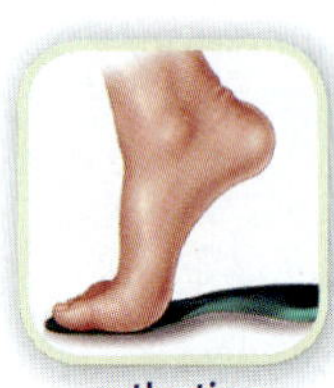
orthotics

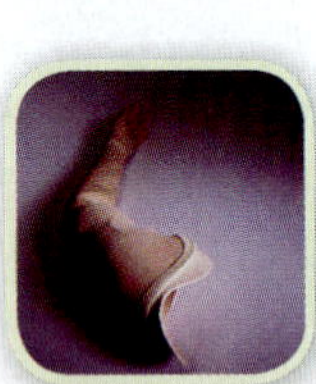
prosthesis

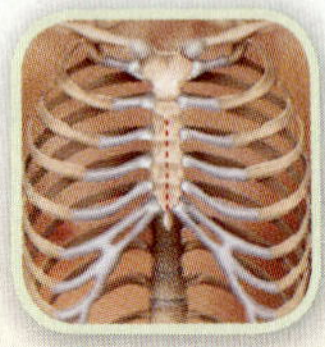
sternotomy

4.5 Treatments and Therapies

joints

Term	Word Analysis
arthrectomy ar-THREK-toh-mee **Definition** removal of a joint	arthr / ectomy joint / removal
arthroclasia AR-throh-KLAY-zhah **Definition** the therapeutic breaking of a joint to allow for increased mobility	arthro / clasia joint / breaking
arthrodesis AR-throh-DEE-sis **Definition** surgical fixation of a joint	arthro / desis joining / binding
arthrolysis ar-THRAW-lih-sis **Definition** loosening a stiff joint	arthro / lysis joint / loose
arthroplasty AR-throh-PLAS-tee **Definition** reconstruction of a joint	arthro / plasty joint / reconstruction
arthrotomy ar-THRAW-toh-mee **Definition** incision into a joint	arthro / tomy joint / incision
bursectomy bir-SEK-toh-mee **Definition** removal of a bursa	burs / ectomy bursa / removal
bursotomy bir-SAW-toh-mee **Definition** incision into a bursa	burso / tomy bursa / incision
chondrectomy kawn-DREK-toh-mee **Definition** removal of cartilage	chondr / ectomy cartilage / removal
chondroplasty KAWN-droh-PLAS-tee **Definition** reconstruction of cartilage	chondro / plasty cartilage / reconstruction

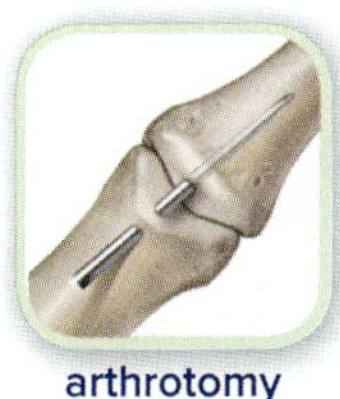
arthrotomy

4.5 Treatments and Therapies

muscles

Term	Word Analysis
fasciectomy FA-shee-EK-toh-mee **Definition** removal of fascia	fasci / ectomy fascia / removal
fasciodesis FA-shoh-DEE-sis **Definition** binding of fascia	fascio / desis fascia / binding
fascioplasty FA-shoh-PLAS-tee **Definition** reconstruction of fascia	fascio / plasty fascia / reconstruction
fasciorrhaphy fah-SHOR-ah-fee **Definition** suturing of fascia	fascio / rrhaphy fascia / suture
fasciotomy FA-shee-AW-toh-mee **Definition** incision into fascia	fascio / tomy fascia / incision
myectomy mai-EK-toh-mee **Definition** removal of muscle	my / ectomy muscle / removal
myodesis MAI-oh-DEE-sis **Definition** binding of a muscle	myo / desis muscle / binding
myomectomy MAI-oh-MEK-toh-mee **Definition** removal of a muscle tumor **NOTE:** It is easy to miss the *oma* root in this word because the *o* looks like it belongs with *myo* and the *a* gets swallowed up by *ectomy*. The *m* is your clue. Don't just read over it—it needs to be explained.	my / om / ectomy muscle / tumor / removal
myoplasty MAI-oh-PLAS-tee **Definition** muscle reconstruction	myo / plasty muscle / reconstruction
myorrhaphy mai-OR-ah-fee **Definition** muscle suture	myo / rrhaphy muscle / suture
myotomy mai-AW-toh-mee **Definition** incision into muscle	myo / tomy muscle / incision

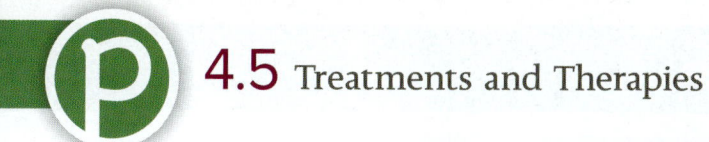

muscles *continued*

Term	Word Analysis
tendectomy ten-DEK-toh-mee **Definition** removal of a tendon	tend / ectomy tendon / removal
tendoplasty TEN-doh-PLAS-tee **Definition** reconstruction of a tendon	tendo / plasty tendon / reconstruction
tenodesis TEN-oh-DEE-sis **Definition** binding of a tendon	teno / desis tendon / binding
tenolysis ten-AW-lih-sis **Definition** freeing/loosening a tendon	teno / lysis tendon / loosen
tenonectomy TEN-oh-NEK-toh-mee **Definition** removal of a tendon	tenon / ectomy tendon / removal
tenoplasty TEN-oh-PLAS-tee **Definition** reconstruction of a tendon	teno / plasty tendon / reconstruction
tenorrhaphy ten-OR-ah-fee **Definition** suture of a tendon	teno / rrhaphy tendon / suture
tenotomy ten-AW-toh-mee **Definition** incision into a tendon	teno / tomy tendon / incision

Learning Outcome 4.5 Exercises

PRONUNCIATION

EXERCISE 1 *Break down the following words into syllables.*

EXAMPLE: synesthesia *syn | es | the | sia*

1. osteotomy ______
2. osteectomy ______
3. osteoclasia ______
4. tarsoclasia ______
5. myodesis ______
6. arthrodesis ______
7. tenodesis ______
8. tenoplasty ______
9. tendoplasty ______
10. tenonectomy ______
11. craniectomy ______
12. myomectomy ______
13. fasciotomy ______
14. antipyretic ______
15. antiarthritic ______
16. anti-inflammatory ______

EXERCISE 2 *Indicate which syllable is emphasized when pronounced.*

EXAMPLE: bronchitis bron**chi**tis

1. orthotics ______
2. prosthesis ______
3. myotomy ______
4. tenotomy ______
5. bursotomy ______
6. sternotomy ______
7. arthrotomy ______
8. carpectomy ______
9. chondrectomy ______
10. bursectomy ______
11. myectomy ______
12. tendectomy ______
13. costectomy ______
14. ostectomy ______
15. tarsectomy ______
16. arthrectomy ______
17. arthrolysis ______
18. tenolysis ______
19. fasciorrhaphy ______

TRANSLATION

EXERCISE 3 *Break down the following words into their component parts.*

EXAMPLE: nasopharyngoscope *naso | pharyngo | scope*

1. analgesic ______
2. anti-inflammatory ______
3. osteectomy ______
4. osteoplasty ______
5. arthrolysis ______
6. fascioplasty ______
7. fasciodesis ______
8. myoplasty ______
9. myorrhaphy ______
10. tenodesis ______
11. tenoplasty ______
12. tenorrhaphy ______
13. carpectomy ______

Learning Outcome 4.5 Exercises

EXERCISE 4 *Underline and define the word parts from this chapter in the following terms.*

1. myodesis ______________________
2. arthrodesis ______________________
3. arthroplasty ______________________
4. tendoplasty ______________________
5. chondroplasty ______________________
6. bursectomy ______________________
7. costectomy ______________________
8. craniectomy ______________________
9. tenonectomy ______________________
10. metacarpectomy ______________________
11. myomectomy ______________________
12. fasciorrhaphy ______________________
13. tarsoclasia ______________________
14. osteoclasia ______________________
15. tenolysis ______________________
16. spondylosyndesis ______________________

EXERCISE 5 *Match the term on the left with its definition on the right.*

	Term	Definition
____	1. arthrectomy	a. incision into a bone
____	2. arthrotomy	b. incision into a bursa
____	3. bursotomy	c. incision into a joint
____	4. carpectomy	d. incision into a muscle
____	5. chondrectomy	e. incision into a tendon
____	6. craniotomy	f. incision into fascia
____	7. fasciectomy	g. incision into the skull
____	8. fasciotomy	h. incision into the sternum
____	9. myectomy	i. removal of a bone
____	10. myotomy	j. removal of a joint
____	11. ostectomy	k. removal of a tendon
____	12. osteotomy	l. removal of all or a portion of the ankle
____	13. sternotomy	m. removal of all or part of the wrist
____	14. tarsectomy	n. removal of cartilage
____	15. tendectomy	o. removal of fascia
____	16. tenotomy	p. removal of muscle

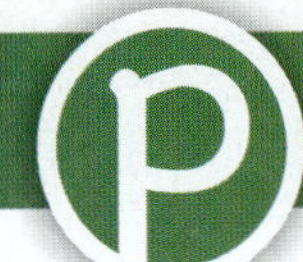

Learning Outcome 4.5 Exercises

EXERCISE 6 *Match the term on the left with its definition on the right.*

g 1. arthroclasia
e 2. closed reduction
a 3. external fixation
b 4. internal fixation
f 5. open reduction
c 6. orthotics
d 7. prosthetics

a. the fixation of a fractured bone from the outside
b. the fixation of a fractured bone from the inside
c. a device that aids in the straightening or stabilizing of a part of the body
d. a device that is added to a body to replace a missing part or lost function
e. returning bones to their proper position without the use of surgery
f. returning bones to their proper position through the use of surgery
g. the therapeutic breaking of a joint to allow for increased mobility

EXERCISE 7 *Translate the following terms as literally as possible.*

EXAMPLE: nasopharyngoscope *an instrument for looking at the nose and throat*

1. bursotomy ______
2. fasciotomy ______
3. myotomy ______
4. tenotomy ______
5. osteotomy ______
6. sternotomy ______
7. ostectomy ______
8. osteectomy ______
9. tendectomy ______
10. tenonectomy ______
11. metacarpectomy ______
12. arthrodesis ______
13. fasciodesis ______
14. myodesis ______
15. tenodesis ______
16. spondylosyndesis ______
17. tenoplasty ______
18. tendoplasty ______
19. analgesic ______
20. antiarthritic ______
21. anti-inflammatory ______
22. antipyretic ______

Learning Outcome 4.5 Exercises

GENERATION

EXERCISE 8 *Build a medical term from the information provided.*

EXAMPLE: inflammation of the sinuses *sinusitis*

1. reconstruction of a bone ______
2. reconstruction of a joint ______
3. reconstruction of a muscle ______
4. reconstruction of a tendon ______
5. reconstruction of fascia ______
6. reconstruction of cartilage ______
7. removal of a bursa ______
8. removal of a tendon ______
9. removal of fascia ______
10. removal of a rib ______
11. removal of all or part of the ankle ______
12. removal of all or part of the wrist ______
13. removal of cartilage ______
14. breaking of a bone ______
15. breaking of a joint ______
16. breaking of an ankle ______
17. suture of a muscle ______
18. suturing of fascia ______
19. suture of a tendon ______

EXERCISE 9 *Briefly describe the difference between each pair of terms.*

1. arthrolysis, tenolysis ______
2. arthrectomy, arthrotomy ______
3. myectomy, myomectomy ______
4. external fixation, internal fixation ______
5. closed reduction, open reduction ______
6. craniectomy, craniotomy ______
7. orthotics, prosthesis ______

4.6 Abbreviations

Abbreviations provide a shorthand way of referring to things that either recur often or are too long to write out. When dealing with bones, joints, and muscles, these abbreviations can refer to everything from observational findings (Hx, ROM), to specific body parts (PCL, MCL), diagnoses (CTS, RA), and treatments (THR, ORIF).

musculoskeletal system abbreviations

Abbreviation	Definition
Hx	history
Fx	fracture
Tx	traction or treatment
ACL	anterior cruciate ligament
MCL	medial collateral ligament
LCL	lateral collateral ligament
PCL	posterior cruciate ligament
C1–C7	cervical (of the neck) vertebrae
T1–T12	thoracic (of the chest) vertebrae
L1–L5	lumbar (of the loin) vertebrae
S1–S5	sacral vertebrae
CTS	carpal tunnel syndrome
EMG	electromyogram
FROM	full range of motion
MD	muscular dystrophy
NSAID	nonsteroidal anti-inflammatory drug
OA	osteoarthritis
ORIF	open reduction internal fixation
PT	physical therapy
RA	rheumatoid arthritis
RICE	rest, ice, compression, elevation
ROM	range of motion
THR	total hip replacement
TKR	total knee replacement
WB	weight bearing
WBAT	weight bearing as tolerated

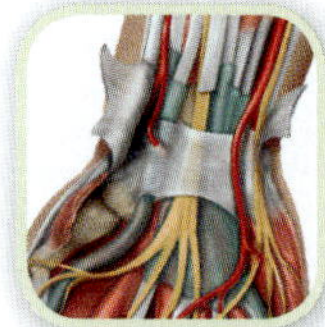

CTS

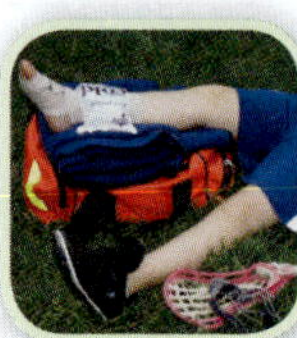

RICE

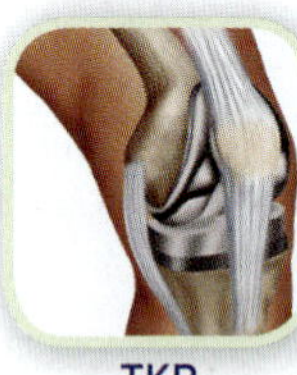

TKR

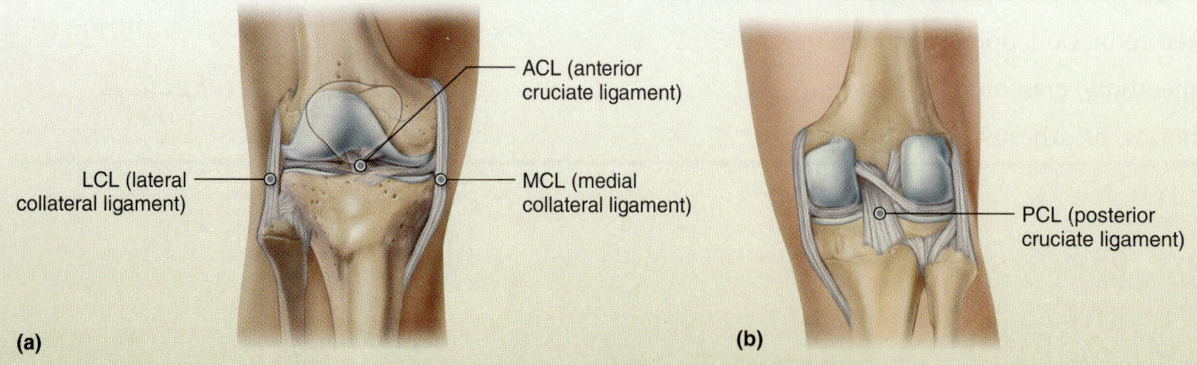

Ligaments of the knee (a) anterior and lateral ligaments (b) posterior ligaments

Learning Outcome 4.6 Exercises

TRANSLATION

EXERCISE 1 *Define the following abbreviations.*

1. Hx ______
2. EMG ______
3. FROM ______
4. ROM ______
5. C1-C7 ______
6. T1-T12 ______
7. L1-L5 ______
8. CTS ______
9. Fx ______
10. OA ______
11. RA ______
12. NSAID ______
13. PT ______
14. TKR ______

EXERCISE 2 *Give the abbreviations for the following definitions.*

1. anterior cruciate ligament ACL
2. lateral collateral ligament LCL
3. medial collateral ligament MCL
4. posterior cruciate ligament PCL
5. muscular dystrophy MD
6. open reduction internal fixation ORIF
7. rest, ice, compression, elevation RICE
8. total hip replacement THR
9. traction Tx
10. weight bearing as tolerated WBAT

EXERCISE 3 *Multiple-choice questions. Select the correct answer.*

1. C1-C7 refer to the vertebrae of the
   - a. neck
   - b. chest/upper back
   - c. lower back
   - d. sacrum
2. T1-T12 refer to the vertebrae of the
   - a. neck
   - b. chest/upper back
   - c. lower back
   - d. sacrum

Learning Outcome 4.6 Exercises

3. L1-L5 refer to the vertebrae of the

   a. neck
   b. chest/upper back
   c. lower back
   d. sacrum

4. An NSAID is a(n)

   a. anti-inflammatory
   b. steroid
   c. antipyretic
   d. antiarthritic

5. What is the abbreviation for a record of the electrical activity of a muscle?

   a. EAM
   b. EMG
   c. RAM
   d. EEG

6. Select the procedures that would require surgery.

   a. ORIF
   b. PT
   c. RICE
   d. THR
   e. TKR

7. Select the procedures that do NOT require surgery.

   a. ORIF
   b. PT
   c. RICE
   d. THR
   e. TKR

8. RICE means

   a. rheumatic internal chondrectomy
   b. rest, ice, compression, elevation
   c. range in circular electromyograms
   d. risk for internal fixation and elevation

9. A patient with OA has

   a. inflammation of the bones
   b. inflammation of the joints
   c. inflammation of the joints, specifically those that bear weight
   d. inflammation of the joints and bones

10. Which of the following acronyms does NOT refer to a part of the body?

    a. ACL
    b. LCL
    c. MCL
    d. C1-C7
    e. T1-T12
    f. L1-L5
    g. M1-M9

4.7 Electronic Health Records

Orthopedic Clinic Note

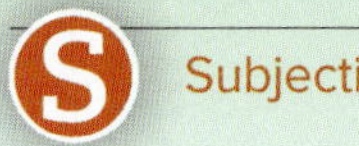

Subjective

History of Present Illness:

Mrs. Maureen Goldman presented to the orthopedic clinic with a chronic history of **arthralgia.** She has been previously diagnosed with **osteoarthritis.** She was initially treated with **NSAIDs** and an **orthotic** that helped for a time; however, Mrs. Goldman's condition worsened and was eventually treated with an intraarticular steroid injection. She reported improved pain and range of motion. The knee pain returned last year, however, and she was treated in our clinic with **arthroscopic** surgery. While it helped some, she reports it didn't completely get rid of her symptoms, and she returns today for evaluation.

PMHx: **Septic arthritis** requiring hospitalization and **IV** antibiotics 4 years ago.

Objective

Physical Exam:

RR: 16; HR: 70; Temp: 98.6; BP: 110/60

Gen: Alert, oriented.

CV: RRR, no murmurs.

Resp: CTA.

Musculoskeletal: **Crepitation** in right knee, decreased **ROM.** Mild **effusion.** Mild muscular **atrophy** of right quadriceps muscle compared to left.

Labs: **ESR** normal, joint **aspiration** normal.

X-ray: **Subchondral cysts, subchondral sclerosis,** joint space narrowing.

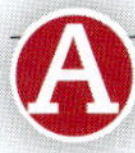

Assessment

DDx: Includes **osteoarthritis, rheumatoid arthritis,** and **bursitis.** Given her history of osteoarthritis on exam and the results of the x-ray and joint aspiration, I believe Mrs. Goldman has **OA** that has failed to respond to previous treatments.

Plan

I have discussed treatment options, and the patient prefers surgery. I have explained the risks and benefits of a **total knee replacement arthroplasty** and she understands. I have scheduled her for surgery next month.

–Electronically signed by
Ricchelle Mitchell, MD
01/26/2015 11:22 AM

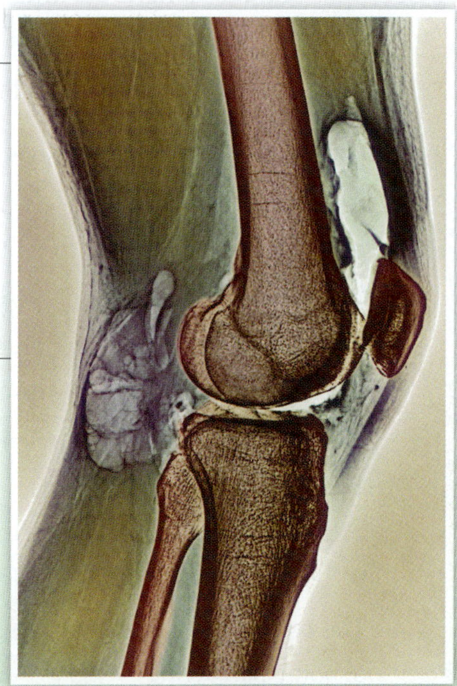

Learning Outcome 4.7 Exercises

EXERCISE 1 *Match the term on the left with its definition on the right.*

______	1. ROM	a.	underdevelopment, decrease, or loss of muscle tissue
______	2. atrophy	b.	procedure of looking into a joint
______	3. osteoarthritis	c.	beneath the cartilage
______	4. arthroplasty	d.	reconstruction of a joint
______	5. arthroscopy	e.	range of motion
______	6. subchondral	f.	inflammation of the joints, specifically those that bear weight

EXERCISE 2 *Fill in the blanks.*

1. Mrs. Goldman was previously diagnosed with ______________ (abbreviation for inflammation of the joints, specifically those that bear weight).
2. Along with ______________ (nonsteroidal anti-inflammatory drugs), she was given an *orthotic* (give definition: ____ ______________________________________).
3. Upon evaluation, Mrs. Goldman's right knee had a noticeable creaking sound, or ______________ ______________ , as well as mild *effusion* (give definition: ______________________).

EXERCISE 3 *True or false questions. Indicate true answers with a T and false answers with an F.*

1. Mrs. Goldman has a chronic history of bone pain. ______
2. Mrs. Goldman was initially treated with nonsteroidal anti-inflammatory drugs. ______
3. After the intraarticular steroid injection, Mrs. Goldman reported improved arthralgia and ROM. ______
4. Mrs. Goldman was previously hospitalized for joint inflammation caused by infection. ______
5. Mrs. Goldman's right quadricep muscle had an unusual new growth. ______
6. Mrs. Goldman's x-ray revealed hardening of the cartilage. ______
7. After understanding the risks involved, Mrs. Goldman has agreed to a TKR joint reconstruction. ______

EXERCISE 4 *Multiple-choice questions. Select the correct answer.*

1. *Arthroscopic surgery* is
   a. closed reduction
   b. external fixation
   c. surgery on a bone
   d. surgery on a joint
2. *Septic arthritis* requires which of the following forms of treatment?
   a. antibiotics
   b. prosthesis
   c. osteectomy
   d. myomectomy
3. The term *subchondral* means
   a. beneath the cartilage
   b. beneath the knee
   c. beneath the joint
   d. beneath the muscle
4. The term *arthrostenosis* means
   a. joint narrowing
   b. muscle narrowing
   c. joint hardening
   d. muscle hardening

Discharge Summary

Patient Name: Decker Macmillan

Date of Admission: 1/1/15
Date of Discharge: 1/4/15

Admission Diagnosis
1. **Hypotonia**
2. **Lordosis**

Discharge Diagnosis
1. Muscular **dystrophy**
2. Scoliosis

Discharge Condition: Stable
Consultations: Neurology, cardiology, orthopedic surgery

Procedures
1. **Electromyography**
2. **Muscle biopsy**

Labs: CBC, CMP, CPK, ESR
Imaging: None

HPI
Decker Macmillan is an 8-year-old boy admitted directly to the pediatric floor for workup of chronic progressive **hypotonia.** His parents report they have noticed progressive weakness. Decker has had increasing difficulty running, jumping, and climbing stairs. His parents initially thought his problems were due to his asthma, but they noticed that he also had a waddling gait. They took him to their primary care provider, who referred him for evaluation. On admission, Decker denied any history of **myalgia, arthrodynia,** or **dystaxia.** His problem appeared limited to muscle tone.

Hospital Course
Neuro: On admission exam, Decker was found to have mild **lumbar lordosis, pseudohypertrophy** of his calf muscles, and a waddling gait. He did not have any **genu varum** or **genu valgus.** No **hyporeflexia** was noted. The initial concern was a muscular dystrophy. Given a family history of **polymyositis,** that was considered as well. Decker's labs were consistent with muscular dystrophy. An **electromyography** showed **myopathic** changes. A muscle biopsy was then performed to help distinguish which of the muscular dystrophies the patient has. The results are pending.

CV: Cardiology was consulted, given the strong risk for developing **cardiomyopathy.**

Resp: No problems were seen throughout the hospital stay. Decker was educated in performing on breathing exercises and also about the respiratory problems often seen later on in the condition.

Ortho: Orthopedic surgery was consulted for Decker's scoliosis.

Social: Much of the hospital stay focused on patient education.

Discharge Physical Examination
Temp: 98.6; RR: 24; HR: 86; BP: 100/64
Gen: WDWN. Alert.
CV: RRR.
Resp: CTA.
Neuro: Hypotonia of legs (strength 3/5 bilaterally). Waddling gait. Using assistance to get up from seated position. Normal reflexes. Marked enlargement of calves.

Activity: No restrictions. Referral to **PT** on discharge. First appointment is next week.
Diet: Calcium/vit. D supplement to prevent **osteoporosis.**
Meds: Glucocorticoid.

Follow-Up Appointments
- Primary care provider: Dr. Klim in 1 week.
- Neurology: Dr. Willis in 2 weeks.
- Cardiology: Dr. Chatham in 6 months.
- Orthopedic: Dr. Pye in 6 months.

Learning Outcome 4.7 Exercises

EXERCISE 5 *Match the term on the left with its definition on the right.*

______	1. osteoporosis	a. decrease in muscle tone
______	2. electromyography	b. crooked back; abnormal lateral curvature of the spine
______	3. scoliosis	c. disorder characterized by poor muscle development
______	4. myalgia	d. procedure for measuring the electrical activity of a muscle
______	5. muscular dystrophy	e. muscle tone
______	6. myotonia	f. muscle pain
______	7. hypotonia	g. joint pain
______	8. arthrodynia	h. poor coordination
______	9. dystaxia	i. loss of bone density

EXERCISE 6 *Fill in the blanks.*

1. Decker's discharge diagnosis included ______________ (abbreviation for *muscular dystrophy*).
2. Decker did not have any *genu valgum* (give definition: ______________________________) or *genu varum* (give definition: ______________________________).
3. Due to Decker's family history, ______________________________ (inflammation of multiple muscles) was considered in the diagnosis.
4. A(n) ______________________________ (abbreviation for *electromyography*) showed *myopathic* (pertaining to ______________________________) changes.
5. The patient will be referred to PT (give definition: ______________________________).

EXERCISE 7 *True or false questions. Indicate true answers with a T and false answers with an F.*

1. The patient's muscle tone suddenly began to decrease, which is why he is being referred for an evaluation. ____________
2. The patient's problems appear limited to myotonia. ____________
3. The patient denies any joint or muscle pain. ____________
4. The patient has a family history of muscular dystrophy. ____________
5. Calcium and vitamin D supplements were recommended to boost muscle development. ____________

EXERCISE 8 *Multiple-choice questions. Select the correct answer.*

1. Decker's admission diagnosis included
   a. decrease in muscle tone and abnormal forward curvature of the lower spine
   b. decrease in muscle tone and abnormal forward curvature of the upper spine
   c. increase in muscle tone and abnormal forward curvature of the lower spine
   d. increase in muscle tone and abnormal forward curvature of the upper spine
2. Procedures performed on the patient included
   a. EAG and muscle Fx
   b. EEG and muscle Bx
   c. EKG and muscle Fx
   d. EMG and muscle Bx

Learning Outcome 4.7 Exercises

3. The patient does NOT have a history of
   a. poor coordination
   b. muscle pain
   c. joint pain
   d. all of these
   e. none of these
4. The term *lumbar lordosis* means
   a. abnormal forward curvature of the lower spine
   b. abnormal forward curvature of the upper spine
   c. abnormal lateral curvature of the lower spine
   d. abnormal lateral curvature of the upper spine
5. *Pseudohypertrophia* is a medical term derived from the combining form *pseudo*, meaning *false*, and *hypertrophia*, meaning
   a. underdevelopment of muscle
   b. overdevelopment of muscle
   c. poor muscle coordination
   d. decrease in muscle movement or activity
6. *Cardiomyopathy* is a disease of
   a. the muscles of the heart
   b. the growth of the heart
   c. the bursa of the heart
   d. the joints of the heart

Orthopedic Consult Note

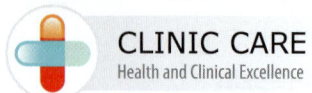

Re: Sam Samuels

Dear Dr. Childs,

Thank you for referring Mr. Samuels to my office. I saw him on March 3, 2015. Mr. Samuels has a 4-month history of increasing pain in his right **distal femur.** He first noticed pain after being kicked in the leg at a soccer game and was evaluated in your office 3 weeks later for persistent pain. There was a soft tissue mass in his distal femur that was tender to touch. An x-ray was performed to rule out a **fracture** or **chronic osteomyelitis.** The x-ray showed both **osteolysis** of the **metaphysis** and **periosteal** new bone formation. Labs were drawn including CBC, CPK, and ESR. He was referred to my office for further evaluation of the x-ray findings.

On exam, Mr. Samuels was a pleasant young man, well developed and well nourished, and in no acute distress. His lungs were clear and heart was regular in rate and rhythm. No murmurs were heard. Examination of his right leg revealed a significant soft tissue mass over his distal femur on the right. The mass was tender. He did not have any knee **effusion.** I reviewed the labs and x-ray. His findings were consistent with **osteosarcoma.**

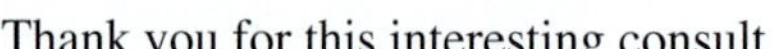

I discussed the next steps with Mr. Samuels and his family, including staging the tumor and scheduling a biopsy to confirm the diagnosis. I discussed the surgery with Mr. Samuels and his family in the office. His tumor will likely require tumor resection with partial **ostectomy** of the femur with **osteoplasty.** I discussed the benefits of a metal **endoprosthesis** versus an **allograft** for the osteoplasty. Mr. Samuels is scheduled to return to my office 1 week following his biopsy to discuss the results.

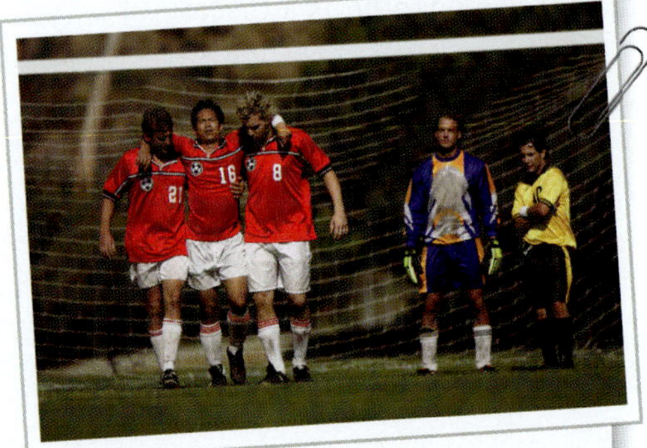

Thank you for this interesting consult.

—Phyllis Sanchez, MD, FAAOS

Learning Outcome 4.7 Exercises

EXERCISE 9 *Match the term on the left with its definition on the right.*

____	1. effusion	a.	bone pain
____	2. ostalgia	b.	a device that is added to a body to replace a missing part or lost function
____	3. ostectomy	c.	inflammation of the bone and bone marrow
____	4. osteoplasty	d.	bone loss
____	5. osteomyelitis	e.	fluid build-up
____	6. osteosarcoma	f.	cancerous tumor arising out of bone cells
____	7. osteolysis	g.	removal of a bone
____	8. prosthesis	h.	reconstruction of a bone

EXERCISE 10 *Fill in the blanks.*

1. An x-ray was performed to rule out ______________ (bone break) or chronic *osteomyelitis* (give definition: ______________________________________).
2. Mr. Samuels did not have any fluid build-up in his knee, which is also known as ______________.
3. The labs and x-ray findings were consistent with an *osteosarcoma* (give definition: ______________________________________).
4. The patient's tumor will likely require tumor resection with partial *ostectomy* (give definition: ______________________) and ______________________ (reconstruction of the bone).

EXERCISE 11 *Multiple-choice questions. Select the correct answer.*

1. Mr. Samuels has a 4-month history of
   a. progressive ostealgia in his femur
   b. acute ostealgia in his femur
   c. progressive myalgia in his femur
   d. acute myalgia in his femur
2. *Osteomyelitis* is
   a. inflammation of the bone and muscle
   b. inflammation of the bone and bone marrow
   c. disease of the bone and muscle
   d. disease of the bone and bone marrow
3. The root word of *periosteal* is
   a. bone
   b. muscle
   c. cartilage
   d. joints
4. An *osteosarcoma* is
   a. a tumor made up of bone and cartilage
   b. a tumor arising from the cartilage of the vertebrae
   c. a tumor arising from bone cells
   d. a benign mass
5. The patient's tumor will likely require
   a. partial removal of the bone
   b. complete removal of the bone
   c. an incision into the bone
   d. closed reduction
6. The term *endoprosthesis* is created by combining the prefix *endo-*, meaning *within*, and *prosthesis*, which is a device that
   a. is added to a body to replace a missing part or lost function
   b. aids in the straightening or stabilizing of a part of the body
   c. is used to internally fix a broken bone (i.e., screw, pin, plate)
   d. is used to externally immobilize a fractured bone (i.e., cast or splint)

Additional exercises available in connect®

Chapter Review exercises, along with additional practice items, are available in Connect!

Quick Reference

quick reference glossary of roots

Root	Definition	Root	Definition
ankyl/o	stiff, bent	**kinesi/o**	movement, motion
arthr/o	joint	**lumb/o**	loin, lower back
brachi/o	arm	**muscul/o**	muscle
burs/o	bursa (a small fluid-filled sac found near the body's joint)	**my/o, myos/o**	muscle
carp/o	wrist	**oste/o**	bone
cervic/o	neck	**-physis**	growth
chondr/o	cartilage	**spondyl/o**	vertebra
cost/o	rib	**tars/o**	ankle
crani/o	head, skull	**tax/o**	arrangement, order, coordination
dactyl/o	finger	**ten/o, tend/o, tendin/o**	tendon
fasci/o	fascia (fibrous connective tissue binding muscles together)	**tibi/o**	tibia (shinbone)
femor/o	femur (thighbone)	**ton/o**	tone, tension

quick reference glossary of terms

Term	Definition
achondroplasia	a defect in the formation of cartilage
analgesic	a drug that relieves pain
ankylosing spondylitis	a stiffening inflammation of the vertebrae
ankylosis	joint stiffness
antiarthritic	a drug that opposes joint inflammation
anti-inflammatory	a drug that opposes inflammation
antipyretic	a drug that opposes fever
arthrodysplasia	abnormal joint development
arthralgia	joint pain

quick reference glossary of terms *continued*

Term	Definition
arthritis	joint inflammation
arthrocele	hernia of a joint
arthrocentesis	puncture of a joint
arthroclasia	the therapeutic breaking of a joint to allow for increased mobility
arthrodesis	the surgical fixation of a joint
arthrodynia	joint pain
arthrectomy	removal of a joint
arthrogram	visual record of a joint
arthrography	procedure used to examine a joint
arthrolysis	loosening a stiff joint
arthropathy	joint disease
arthroplasty	reconstruction of a joint
arthrosclerosis	hardening of the joints
arthroscope	instrument for looking into a joint
arthroscopy	procedure of looking into a joint
arthrotomy	incision into a joint
atrophy	underdevelopment, decrease, or loss of muscle tissue
bradykinesia	slow movement
bursectomy	removal of a bursa
bursitis	inflammation of the bursa
bursolith	a stone in a bursa
bursopathy	disease of the bursa
bursotomy	incision into a bursa
carpectomy	removal of all or part of the wrist
carpitis	wrist inflammation
cervicodynia	neck pain
chondrectomy	removal of cartilage
chondroma	a tumor-like growth of cartilage tissue
chondromalacia	abnormal softening of the cartilage
chondro-osteodystrophy	poor development of bones and cartilage

quick reference glossary of terms *continued*

Term	Definition
chondroplasty	reconstruction of cartilage
closed reduction	returning bones to their proper position without the use of surgery
computed axial tomography (CAT or CT)	imaging procedure using a compuer to produce cross sections along an axis
costalgia	rib pain
costectomy	removal of a rib
costochondritis	inflammation of the cartilage of the rib
craniectomy	removal of a portion of the skull (bone is not replaced)
craniomalacia	softening of the skull
craniosynostosis	the premature fusing of the skull bones
craniotomy	removal of a portion of the skull (bone is later replaced)
crepitation	from Latin, for *rattle* or *creaking;* a crackling sound heard in joints
dactylitis	finger inflammation
dyskinesia	inability to control movement
dystaxia	poor coordination
dystonia	poor muscle tone
effusion	fluid build-up
electromyogram	record of the electrical activity of a muscle
electromyography	procedure for measuring the electrical activity of a muscle
exostosis	an abnormal growth of bone out of another bone
external fixation	a fixation of a fractured bone from the outside (i.e., using a cast or splint)
fasciectomy	removal of fascia
fasciitis	inflammation of the fascia
fasciodesis	binding of fascia
fascioplasty	reconstruction of fascia
fasciorrhaphy	suturing of fascia
fasciotomy	incision into fascia
fracture	from Latin, for *break;* a bone break
genu valgum	bow-legged

quick reference glossary of terms *continued*

Term	Definition
genu varum	knock-kneed
graphospasm	writer's cramp
hemarthrosis	blood in a joint
hydrarthrosis	water (fluid) in a joint
hyperkinesia	increase in muscle movement or activity
hypertonia	increased muscle tone or tightness
hypertrophic spondylitis	overdevelopment of the vertebrae causing inflammation
hypertrophy	overdevelopment of muscle tissue
hypokinesia	decrease in muscle movement or activity
hypotonia	decrease in muscle tone or tightness
internal fixation	the fixation of a fractured bone from the inside (i.e., using screws, pins, plates, etc.)
kyphosis	humped back—abnormal forward curvature of the upper spine
lordosis	sway back—abnormal forward curvature of the lower spine
metacarpectomy	removal of a bone of the hand
metatarsalgia	pain in the bones of the foot
muscular dystrophy	disorder characterized by poor muscle development
myalgia	muscle pain
myasthenia	muscle weakness
myectomy	removal of muscle
myocele	hernia of muscle tissue
myoclonus	violent muscle contraction
myodesis	binding of muscle
myodynia	muscle pain
myofasciitis	inflammation of the muscle and fascia
myography	procedure for studying muscles
myolysis	loss of muscle tissue
myoma	a muscle tumor

quick reference glossary of terms *continued*

Term	Definition
myomalacia	softening of a muscle
myomectomy	removal of a muscle tumor
myopathy	muscle disease
myoplasty	muscle reconstruction
myorrhaphy	muscle suture
myosarcoma	a cancerous muscle tumor
myosclerosis	hardening of a muscle
myositis	muscle inflammation
myospasm	muscle spasm
myotasis	stretching of a muscle
myotomy	incision into muscle
myotonia	muscle tone
necrotizing fasciitis	inflammation of the fascia causing the death of tissue
open reduction	returning bones to their proper position through the use of surgery
orthotics	a device that aids in the straightening or stabilizing of a part of the body
ostalgia	bone pain
ostealgia	bone pain
ostectomy	removal of a bone
osteectomy	removal of a bone
osteitis	bone inflammation
osteoarthritis	inflammation of the joints, specifically those that bear weight
osteocarcinoma	bone cancer tumor
osteochondritis	inflammation of bone and cartilage
osteochondroma	a tumor made up of bone and cartilage
osteodynia	bone pain
osteodystrophy	poor bone development
osteogenesis imperfecta	a disease in which the bones do not develop correctly; also known as *brittle bone disease*
osteolysis	bone loss
osteomalacia	softening of the bone
osteometry	procedure for measuring bone
osteomyelitis	inflammation of the bone and bone marrow
osteonecrosis	death of bone

quick reference glossary of terms *continued*

Term	Definition
osteopathy	bone disease
osteopenia	reduction in bone volume
osteoplasty	reconstruction of a bone
osteoporosis	loss of bone density
osteosarcoma	cancerous tumor arising out of bone cells
osteosclerosis	abnormal hardening of bone
osteotomy	incision into a bone
polydactyly	having more than the normal number of fingers (or toes)
polymyositis	inflammation of multiple muscles
prosthesis	a device that is added to a body to replace a missing part or lost function
pyarthrosis	pus in a joint
rheumatoid arthritis	inflammation of the joint is called rheumatoid because its symptoms resemble those of rheumatic fever
scoliosis	crooked back, or abnormal lateral curvature of the spine
septic arthritis	inflammation of the joint caused by infection
spinal stenosis	abnormal narrowing of the spine
spondylitis	inflammation of the vertebra
spondyloarthropathy	joint disease of the vertebrae
spondylolisthesis	the slipping or dislocation of a vertebra
spondylolysis	loss of vertebra structure
spondylomalacia	softening of the vertebra
spondylonia	vertebra pain
spondylosis	vertebra condition
spondylosyndesis	fusing together of multiple vertebrae
sternotomy	incision into the sternum
subluxation	partial dislocation of a joint
syndactyly	fusion (sometimes called webbing) of fingers or toes
tardive dyskinesia	condition characterized by the loss of muscle control
tarsectomy	removal or all or a portion of the ankle
tarsoclasia	the surgical fracture of the ankle (i.e., to treat clubfoot)
tarsoptosis	flat feet
tenalgia	tendon pain
tendectomy	removal of a tendon

quick reference glossary of terms *continued*

Term	Definition
tendonitis	tendon inflammation
tendoplasty	reconstruction of a tendon
tenodesis	binding of a tendon
tenolysis	freeing/loosening a tendon
tenonectomy	removal of a tendon
tenoplasty	reconstruction of a tendon
tenorrhaphy	suture of a tendon
tenotomy	incision into a tendon
tibialgia	tibia (shin) pain

review of terms by roots

Root	Term(s)	
ankyl/o	ankylosing spondylitis ankylosis	
arthr/o	antiarthritic arthrectomy arthralgia arthritis arthrocele arthrocentesis arthroclasia arthrodesis arthrodynia arthrodysplasia arthrogram arthrography arthrolysis	arthropathy arthroplasty arthrosclerosis arthroscope arthroscopy arthrotomy hemarthrosis hydrarthrosis osteoarthritis pyarthrosis rheumatoid arthritis septic arthritis spondyloarthropathy
burs/o	bursectomy bursitis bursolith	bursopathy bursotomy
carp/o	carpectomy carpitis	metacarpectomy
cervic/o	cervicodynia	
chondr/o	achondroplasia costochondritis chondrectomy chondroma chondromalacia	chondro-osteodystrophy chondroplasty osteochondritis osteochondroma

review of terms by roots *continued*

Root	Term(s)	
cost/o	costalgia costectomy	costochondritis
crani/o	craniectomy craniomalacia	craniosynostosis craniotomy
dactyl/o	dactylitis polydactyly	syndactyly
fasci/o	fasciectomy fasciitis fasciodesis fascioplasty	fasciorrhaphy fasciotomy myofasciitis necrotizing fasciitis
kinesi/o	bradykinesia dyskinesia hyperkinesia	hypokinesia tardive dyskinesia
muscul/o	muscular dystrophy	
my/o **myos/o**	electromyogram electromyography myalgia myasthenia myectomy myocele myoclonus myodesis myodynia myofasciitis myography myospasm myotasis myotomy	myolysis myoma myomalacia myomectomy myopathy myoplasty myorrhaphy myosarcoma myosclerosis myositis myotonia polymyositis
oste/o	chondro-osteodystrophy craniosynostosis exostosis ostalgia ostealgia ostectomy osteectomy osteitis osteoarthritis osteocarcinoma osteochondritis osteochondroma osteodynia osteodystrophy	osteogenesis imperfecta osteolysis osteomalacia osteometry osteomyelitis osteonecrosis osteopathy osteopenia osteoplasty osteoporosis osteosarcoma osteosclerosis osteotomy

review of terms by roots *continued*

Root	Term(s)	
spondyl/o	ankylosing spondylitis hypertrophic spondylitis spondylitis spondyloarthropathy spondylodynia	spondylolisthesis spondylolysis spondylomalacia spondylosis spondylosyndesis
tars/o	metatarsalgia tarsectomy	tarsoclasia tarsoptosis
tax/o	dystaxia	
ten/o **tend/o** **tendin/o**	tenalgia tendectomy tendinitis tendonitis tendoplasty tenodesis tenolysis	tenonectomy tenoplasty tenorrhaphy tenotomy
tibi/o	tibialgia	
ton/o	dystonia hypertonia	hypotonia myotonia

other terms

analgesic
anti-inflammatory
antipyretic
atrophy
closed reduction
computed axial tomography (CAT or CT)
crepitation
effusion
external fixation
fracture
genu valgum
genu varum
graphospasm
hypertrophy
internal fixation
open reduction
orthotics
prosthesis
spinal stenosis
sternotomy
subluxation

The Nervous System–Neurology and Psychiatry

5

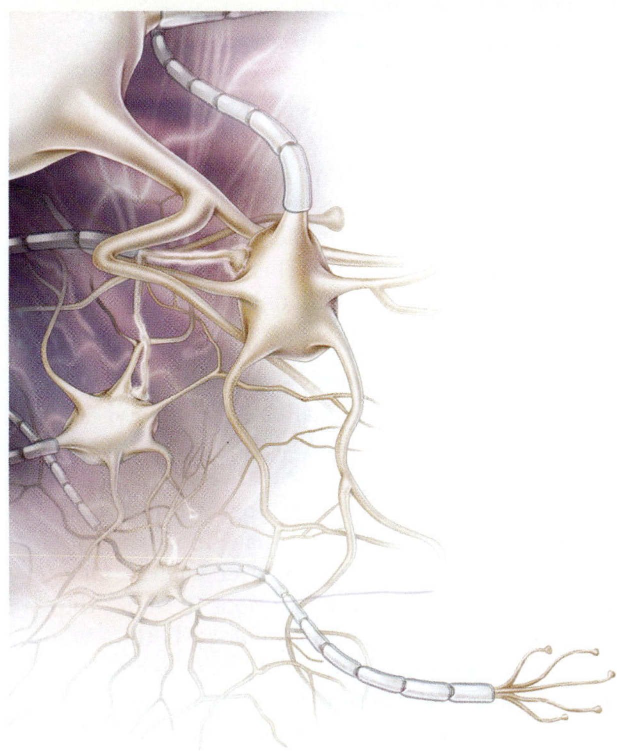

Introduction and Overview of the Nervous System

One of our defining characteristics is our ability to think. Aristotle distinguished humans as "rational animals." French philosopher René Descartes famously remarked, "I think, therefore I am." Thinking is one of the most important parts of what makes us who we are. Our knowledge, perception, and response to the world around us are due to the center of thought in our body: the nervous system. More than just the center of conscious thought, the nervous system is always at work gathering information from the world around us, deciding what to do about it, and telling the rest of the body how to respond. It functions as the body's command center for data processing, thought, and action for the

learning outcomes

Upon completion of this chapter, you will be able to:

5.1 Identify the **roots/word parts** associated with the **nervous system.**

S **5.2** Translate the **Subjective** terms associated with the **nervous system.**

O **5.3** Translate the **Objective** terms associated with the **nervous system.**

A **5.4** Translate the **Assessment** terms associated with the **nervous system.**

P **5.5** Translate the **Plan** terms associated with the **nervous system.**

5.6 Use **abbreviations** associated with the **nervous system.**

5.7 Distinguish terms associated with the **nervous system** in the context of **electronic health records.**

conglomerate of many cells, organs, and systems that make up the human body. Thanks to the nervous system, the body acts as a coordinated team reacting to its surroundings with alacrity and precision. The nervous system serves as the body's communications network, coordinating data reception with appropriate reaction.

This network is comprised of two parts: the peripheral nervous system and central nervous system. The peripheral nervous system collects data. It receives information such as temperature, pain, light, and pressure from its surroundings. As quickly as it receives input, it transmits it to an analytic center via special conduits known as nerves. The unified collection of cells in the brain and spine are known as the central nervous system. The central nervous system processes the details and formulates a response. Commands are directed back to the appropriate body parts via nerves. This constant progression of receiving, reasoning, and reacting repeats itself continuously as we go about our daily lives.

The nervous system handles both voluntary and involuntary action of the body. In addition, we associate the brain and nervous system with conscious thought and actions. The voluntary command of the body's actions is known as the somatic nervous system. Most often, this voluntary system involves the relationship of the nervous system with the skeletal muscular system. Nerves detect input from the surroundings and send this specific information to the central nervous system for processing. These incoming nerves are called afferent neurons or nerves. The person chooses how to respond and the central nervous system directs the body how to respond through signals sent by efferent neurons. Often these are commands sent to muscles. The signal travels down the nerve through an electric current and connects to the muscle at a special connection point (the neuromuscular junction). This voluntary observation and response represents a small part of the work of the nervous system. The central nervous system also directs the involuntary actions of the body, things that our body does without our conscious choice or awareness. This background control is called the autonomic nervous system and encompasses everything from the beating of our heart, to sweating, to digesting food.

The central nervous system also possesses supporting structures to protect and maintain itself. The skull serves as a dense external layer to protect the brain from common injury. The body also produces cerebrospinal fluid, which surrounds the brain and spinal cord and acts as a shock absorber cushioning them from injury. The brain consumes 20 to 25 percent of the body's oxygen. This huge need for oxygen necessitates a rich blood supply. Nearly 20 percent of the blood pumped from the heart is sent to the brain. This demand is met through an extensive network of blood vessels.

But the brain is more than the neurological controller of the human body's physical processes. What we see, hear, and feel affects our general perception of the world around us. We don't just move and react. We behave. We are more than just digestion, heartbeats, and breathing. We have emotions, opinions, and beliefs. We have more than brains. We have minds we call psyche (Greek for *mind*). These more complex functions fit under the umbrella of psychiatry and psychology, both of whose roots come from the Greek word *psyche*, which means *mind* or *soul*. These fields deal with problems in our perceptions, emotions, and behavior.

5.1 Word Parts of the Nervous System

Word Parts Associated with the Structure of the Nervous System

Your sensory system—specifically your eyes, ears, nose, and skin—collects data from your surroundings and sends the information to your brain (*encephalo*) by wires known as nerves (*neuro*). Your brain then makes sense of the data and determines the appropriate action. Then it sends out the action plan to the rest of the body via a web of nerves.

Together, your brain and the collecting/acting nerves make up your nervous system. The nerves that send and receive signals from the brain are collectively known as the peripheral nervous system.

Your brain and spinal cord (*myelo*) are called the central nervous system. The brain has several sections (*lobes*) and is divided in two halves (*hemispheres*). The largest portion of your brain is the cerebrum. Under the cerebrum is the *cerebellum*, which controls things like coordination of movements. Your central nervous system is fragile and needs a protective membrane (*meninges*). The tough outer layer is known as the *dura*.

brain

ROOTS: ***cerebr/o, encephal/o***

EXAMPLES: cerebropathy, cerebrospinal, encephalitis, encephalogram

NOTES: The encephalo root comes from *en* (inside) and *cephalus* (head) and literally means *the stuff inside your head.*

cerebellum

ROOT: ***cerebell/o***

EXAMPLES: cerebellar, cerebellitis

NOTES: This word is just the word *cerebrum* (brain) plus a diminutive suffix. It means *the little brain.* It refers to the region of the brain that controls voluntary movements and looks somewhat like a little version of the whole brain.

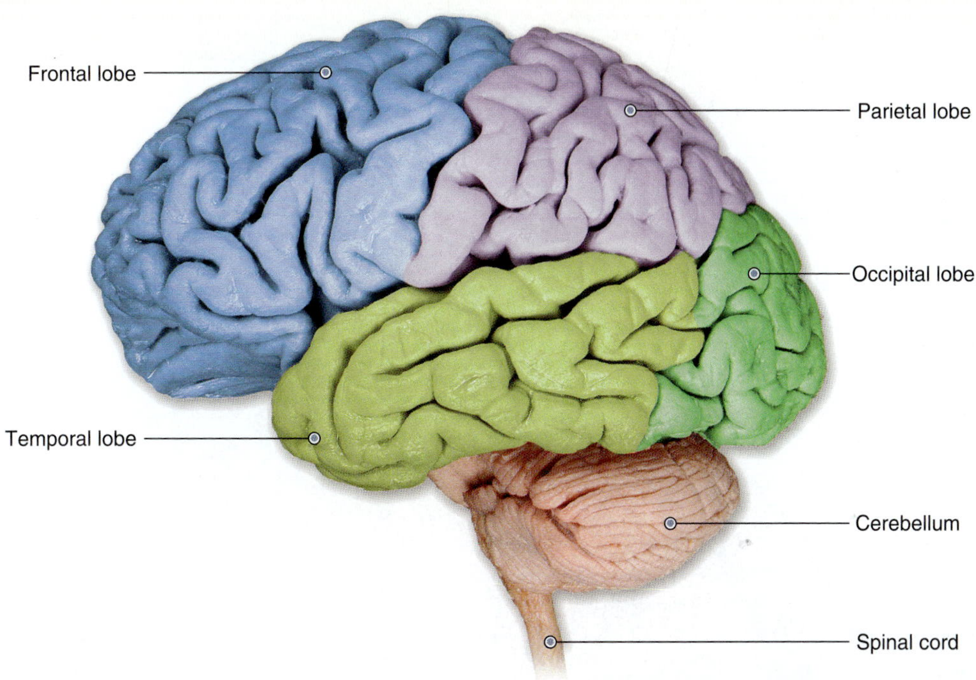

lobe

ROOT: ***lob/o***

EXAMPLES: lobotomy, lobectomy

NOTES: The term *lobotomy* is commonly used as a word meaning *a brain operation that changes one's personality.* In reality, the term means *incision into a lobe.* Lobes are smaller subdivisions of any organ—including the brain, liver, lungs, and, of course, the ears.

The connection between the term *lobotomy* and personality changes probably started with Phineas Gage, a railroad worker in the mid-1800s, who lost a large piece of his brain's frontal lobe in a railroad explosion.

Gage's job was to pack holes full of explosives in order to blast away rock. On one occasion, while Gage was packing a hole, the explosives ignited and sent a rod that was more than 1 inch thick and more than 3 feet long through the front of his skull. Surprisingly, Gage recovered, but he had a much more reserved personality.

This led doctors to understand the role the front lobe of the brain plays in human personality and was the genesis of the use of the term *lobotomy*—which Gage accidentally performed on himself—to describe a brain operation used to make a person more sedate and controlled.

head

ROOT: ***cephal/o***

EXAMPLES: microcephaly, macrocephaly

NOTES: The scientific term for octopus, squid, and other sea creatures that are made up of a head and tentacles is *cephalopod*—-literally head (*cephalo*) + feet (*pod*).

head, skull

ROOT: ***crani/o***

EXAMPLES: craniometer, craniomalacia

NOTES: The term *migraine* comes from the word *hemicranias*, meaning *half the head*. It reflects the fact most migraines are localized on half the patient's head.

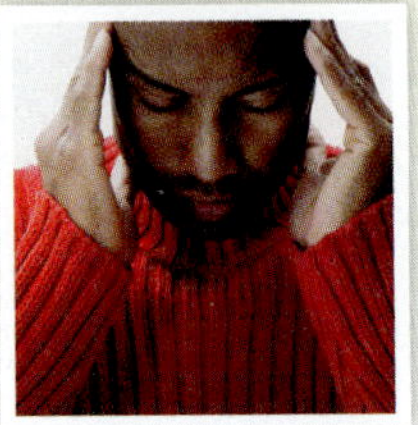

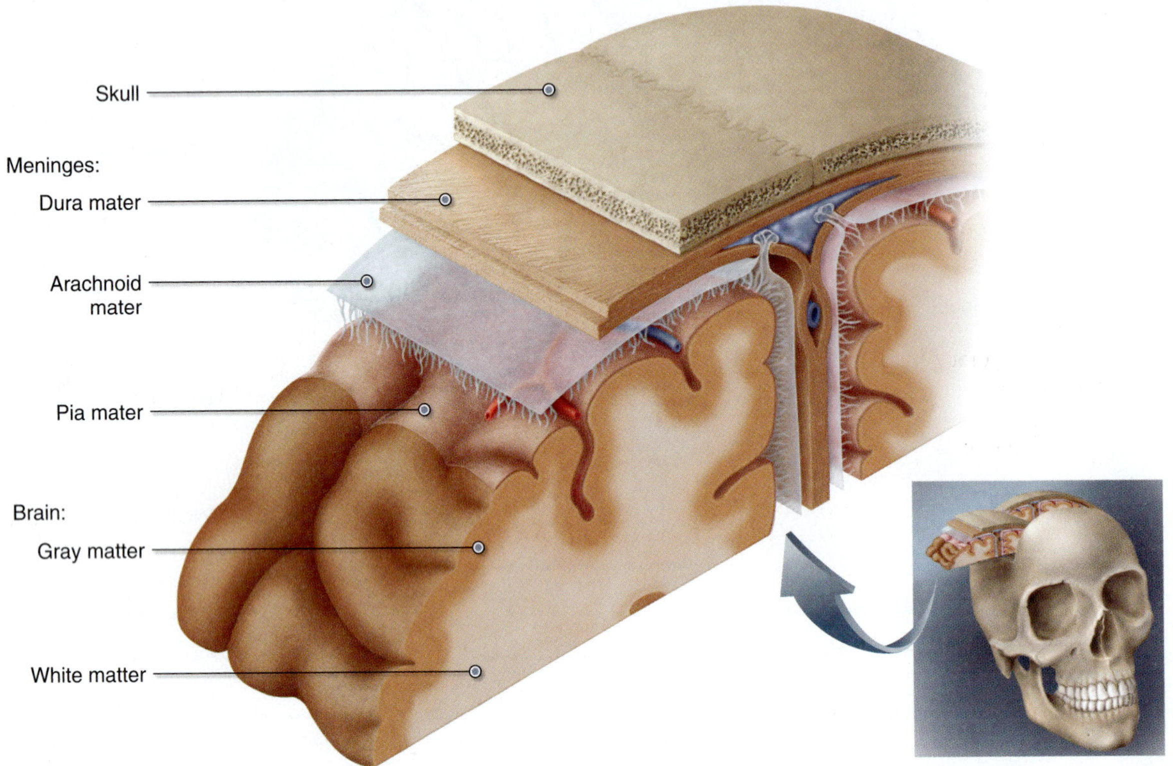

meninges (membrane surrounding the brain and spinal cord)

ROOTS: ***mening/o, meningi/o***

EXAMPLES: meningitis, meningopathy

NOTES: When the letter *g* is followed by an *e* or an *i*, it is pronounced soft (like *j* in *jar*): men-in-JAI-tis. When the letter *g* is followed by an *a*, *o*, or *u*, it is pronounced hard (like *g* in *gas*): men-in-GOH-pah-thee

dura (tough outer membrane surrounding the brain and spinal cord)

ROOT: ***dur/o***

EXAMPLES: epidural, subdural hematoma

NOTES: This root literally means *hard*. The full name of the membrane it refers to is *dura mater cerebri*, which translates to *the tough mother of the brain*. Words like *endurance* and *durable* come from the same word.

nerve

ROOT: ***neur/o***

EXAMPLES: neuralgia, neuropathy

NOTES: *Neuron* comes from a Greek word meaning *tendon* or *string*. In ancient times, when people first began examining brains, they thought neurons looked like string.

nerve bundle

ROOT: ***gangli/o***

EXAMPLES: ganglion, gangliitis

NOTES: According to Galen, a doctor in ancient Rome, the term *ganglion* means *knot* and could refer to anything gathered up into a ball, which is what Galen thought nerve tissue coming out of the brain looked like.

spinal cord, bone marrow

ROOT: ***myel/o***

EXAMPLES: myelitis, myelodysplasia

NOTES: This root comes from a Greek word meaning *the innermost part* and is used in medicine to refer to two different things—bone marrow and the spinal cord. But if you think about it, it makes sense, as both are in the innermost part of something else. Bone marrow is in the center of bones. The spinal cord is in the center of the spine.

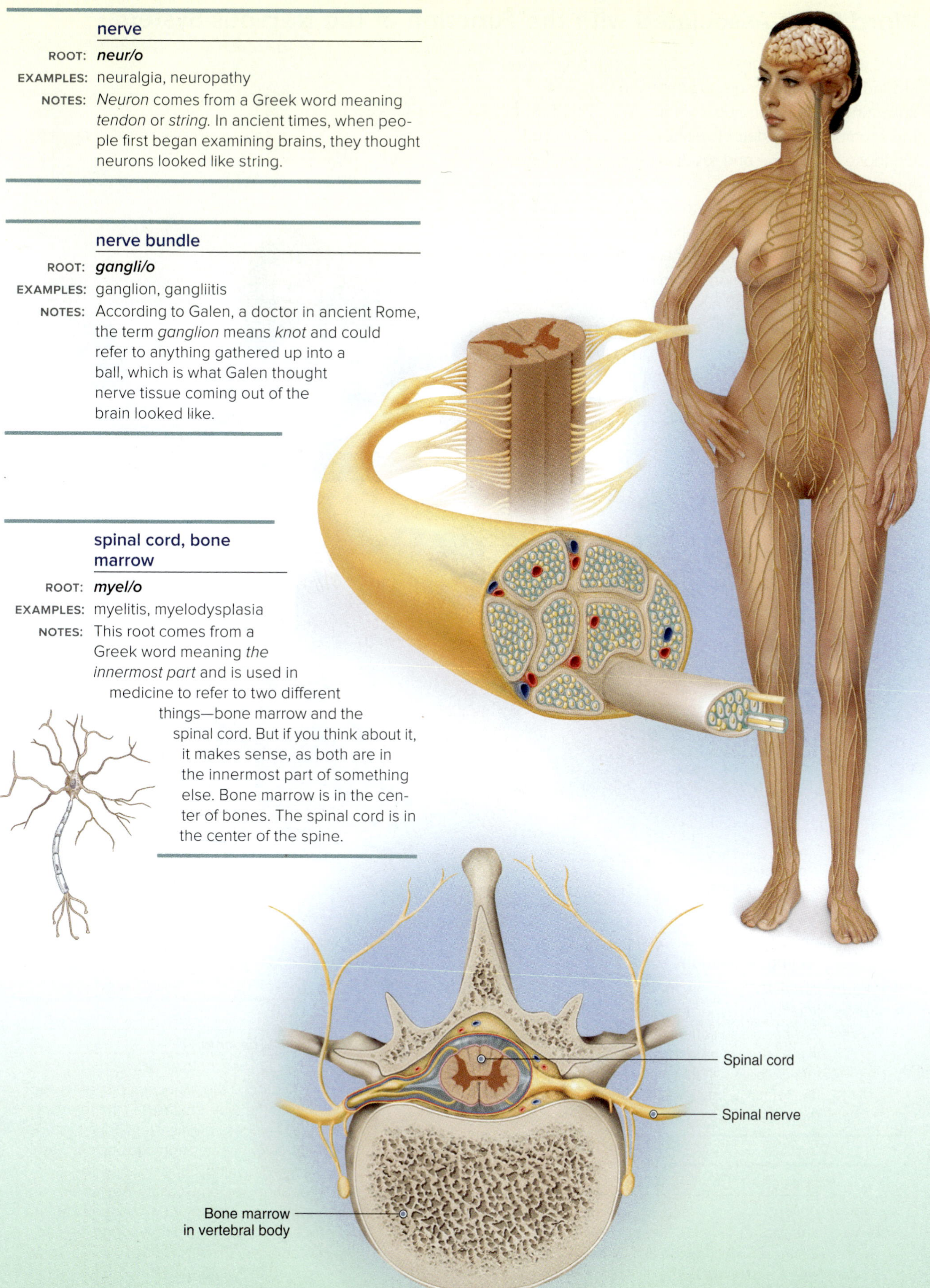

Word Parts Associated with the Function of the Nervous System

While your brain is constantly responding to the world around you, there is more to your mind than just collecting and responding to information. This is where the example of the detective show can go only so far. On those shows, the end result is generally the same—arresting a criminal.

Not all of the data that go to your brain lead to a specific action, though. Much of what you see, hear, and feel affects your general perception of the world around you. It affects your emotions, opinions, or beliefs.

Neurology focuses on actions. The more complex functions often fit under the umbrella of what we call *psyche* (from Greek, for *mind*). We don't just move and react. We *behave*. This is the realm of psychiatry and psychology. These fields of study deal with problems in human perceptions, emotions, and behavior.

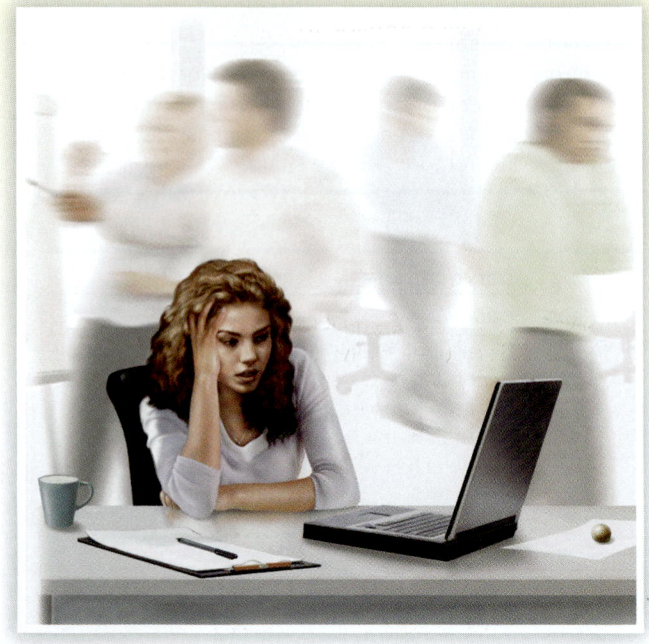

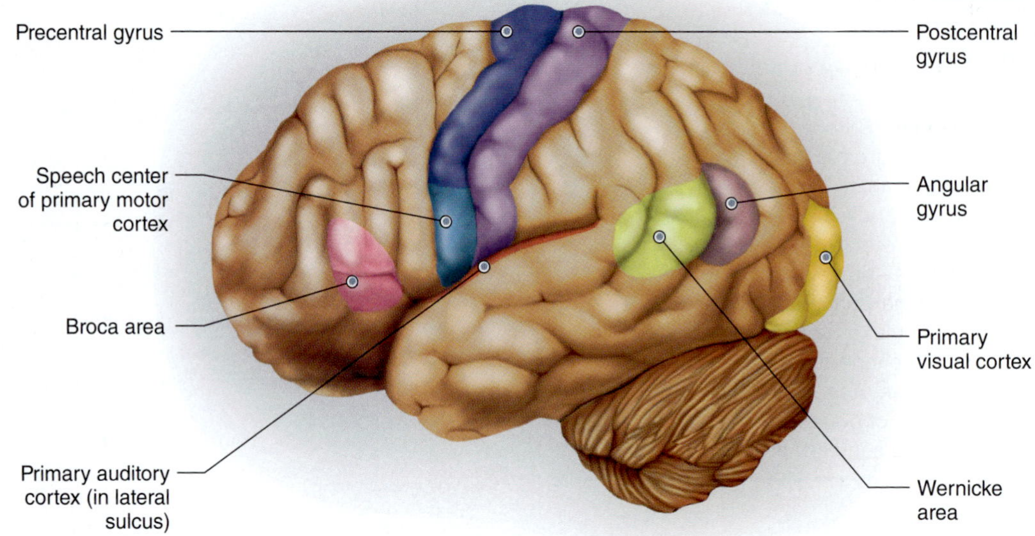

feeling, sensation

ROOT: ***esthesi/o***

EXAMPLES: anesthesia, hyperesthesia

NOTES: *Esthetics* (also sometimes spelled *aesthetics*) is the study of art and philosophy as it pertains to beauty. What makes something beautiful? Can you measure beauty? Is beauty really in the eye of the beholder?

speech

ROOT: ***phas/o***

EXAMPLE: aphasia

NOTES: If a friend is talking too fast, perhaps he or she is stricken with the disease *tachyphasia*.

mind

ROOTS: ***phren/o, psych/o***

EXAMPLES: phrenetic, psychology

NOTES: In addition to the mind, *phren/o* can also refer to the diaphragm (as in the term *phrenospasm,* a fancy medical term for a hiccup). The reason comes from the ancient Greek view of the mind. Early on, the Greeks thought of the chest as the seat of emotion and reason. As that view changed and the location of the mind moved from the chest to the brain, this term for *mind* began to be applied to both areas of the body.

"You don't know what you've got until it's gone." It's a catchy phrase used in country songs and fortune cookies, and it also applies to the brain. Much of neurology and psychiatry deals with loss of function. A break from reality (*schizo*), a loss of speaking (*phaso*), the inability to feel (*esthesio*)—thinking about each of these conditions helps you appreciate the functions of your brain. When your mind can't keep your fears (*phobo*) or passions (*mania*) at a healthy level, they can cause problems as well. Even fears and obsessions provide a glimpse of the subtler jobs your brain performs.

sleep

ROOTS: ***somn/o, somn/i, hypn/o***

EXAMPLES: somnography, insomnia, hypnosis

NOTES: Someone who walks while sleeping is experiencing *somnambulation,* which comes from the words *somno* (sleep) + *ambulo* (walk).

know

ROOT: ***gnosi/o***

EXAMPLES: agnosia, diagnosis, prognosis

NOTES: Frequently, people who have had a limb amputated report feeling or sensing the missing limb. Such an experience is called *autosomatognosis,* from *auto* (self) + *somato* (body) + *gnosis* (know).

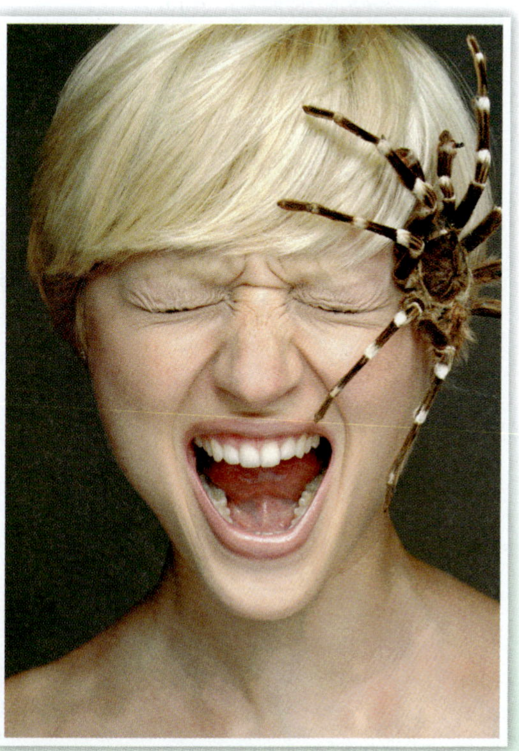

excessive desire

SUFFIX: ***-mania***

EXAMPLES: pyromania, kleptomania

NOTES: Because of the commonly used psychological term *manic-depressive,* some people mistakenly assume that *manic* refers to a type of depression. "He doesn't just have depression, he has *manic* depression." On the contrary—it actually refers to the exact opposite state. Manic-depression is characterized by intense swings of emotion. At times, sufferers are extremely energetic (the *manic* state) and at other times, they are extremely sad (the *depressed* state). Because of these swings in mood, people with this condition are sometimes referred to as being *bipolar,* because their personality is always swinging from one extreme (pole) to the other.

excessive fear or sensitivity

SUFFIX: ***-phobia***

EXAMPLES: photophobia, hydrophobia

NOTES: Phobias can refer to actual symptoms or anxieties. For example, hydrophobia is a main symptom of rabies. *Agoraphobia,* which is the fear of being outdoors or in public spaces and comes from the Greek word *agora,* meaning *marketplace*, is common in people who have experienced major traumatic accidents.

Consider these interesting phobias:

- ablutophobia—the fear of taking a bath
- acrophobia—the fear of heights
- alektorophobia—the fear of chickens
- arachnophobia—the fear of spiders
- cynophobia—the fear of dogs
- dendrophobia—the fear of trees
- gynophobia—the fear of women
- ichthyphobia—the fear of fish
- nyctophobia—the fear of night
- phobophobia—the fear of being afraid
- triskaidekaphobia—the fear of the number 13

slight or partial paralysis

SUFFIX: ***-paresis***

EXAMPLE: hemiparesis

NOTES: *Paresis* comes from Greek, for *to let go,* or *to slacken;* it is used in health care to refer not to complete loss of sensation or control but instead to a partial or isolated form of paralysis.

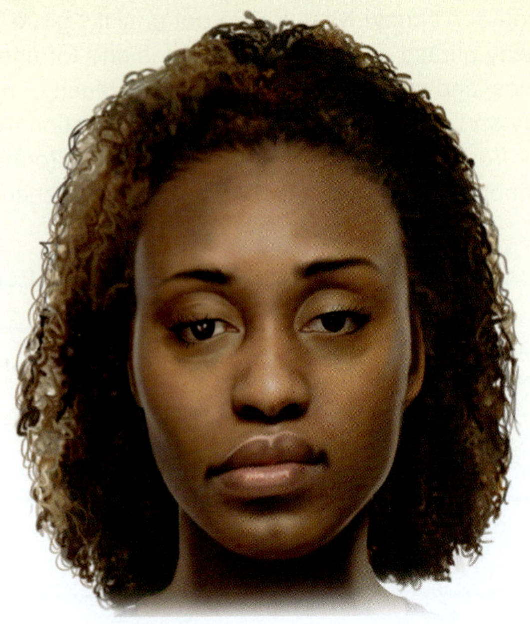

muscle tone, tension, pressure

ROOT: ***ton/o***

EXAMPLES: dystonia, tonograph

NOTES: *Tonic* is used to refer to a medicinal drink. The term was used because these drinks were once thought to restore a person to good muscle *tone.* Today's tonic water still has medicinal value. Though some people think *tonic water* is simply another name for carbonated soda water, tonic is actually a form of carbonated soda water in which quinine, a drug used to treat malaria, has been dissolved. Tonic water was developed for consumption by people living in tropical areas, where malaria is commonplace.

movement, motion

ROOT: ***kinesi/o (also sometimes kinet/o)***

EXAMPLES: kinesiology, hyperkinesia, kinetic energy

NOTES: *Akinetopsia* (pronounced ah-KEE-no-TOP-see-ah), which comes from the roots *a* (no) + *kinet* (movenment) + *opsia* (vision), refers to a condition where a patient can see an object if it is still but is unable to see it if it is moving.

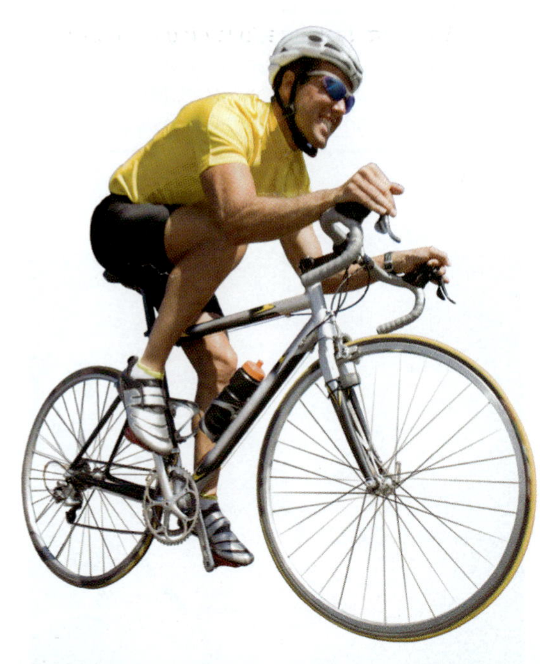

arrangement, order, coordination

ROOT: ***tax/o***

EXAMPLES: ataxia, hypotaxia

NOTES: *Syntax* is an English grammar term made up of the prefix *syn* (together) and the root *tax* (arrangement). It refers to the study of the way words are arranged in a sentence. *Taxidermy,* which comes from *taxo* (arrange) and *dermy* (skin), refers to the practice of removing and displaying the head and skin of an animal killed during a hunt. The arrangement of military forces before a battle is called *tactics.*

paralysis

SUFFIX: ***-plegia***

EXAMPLE: quadriplegia

NOTES: *Plegia* is from Greek, for *to strike.* So a word like *thermoplegia* doesn't mean *heat paralysis;* instead, it means *heat stroke.*

weakness

SUFFIX: ***-asthenia***

EXAMPLES: myasthenia, phonasthenia

NOTES: Several years back, reports surfaced that a cat in a very rural region of China had spontaneously grown wings. Upon examination by a vet, the cat was diagnosed with a skin condition that causes the skin along the back to become loose and then harden into flat, winglike protrusions. The term for this is *feline* (cat) *cutaneous* (skin) *asthenia* (weakness).

Learning Outcome 5.1 Exercises

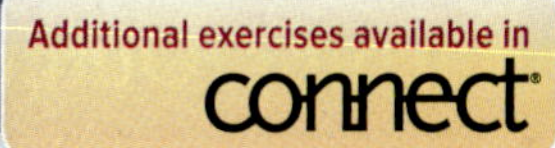

TRANSLATION

EXERCISE 1 *Match the word part on the left with its definition on the right. Some definitions will be used more than once.*

____	1. mening/o	a.	head
____	2. cerebell/o	b.	cerebellum
____	3. neur/o	c.	brain
____	4. crani/o	d.	head, skull
____	5. cerebr/o	e.	tough outer membrane surrounding the brain and spinal cord
____	6. lob/o	f.	nerve bundle
____	7. encephal/o	g.	meninges; membrane surrounding the brain and spinal cord
____	8. cephal/o	h.	nerve
____	9. gangli/o	i.	lobe
____	10. myel/o	j.	spinal cord
____	11. dur/o		

EXERCISE 2 *Translate the following word parts.*

1. crani/o ____________________
2. cerebr/o ____________________
3. cerebell/o ____________________
4. cephal/o ____________________
5. encephal/o ____________________
6. mening/o, meningi/o ____________________
7. neur/o ____________________
8. dur/o ____________________
9. myel/o ____________________
10. gangli/o ____________________

EXERCISE 3 *Break down the word into its component parts and translate.*

EXAMPLE: sinusitis *sinus | itis* *inflammation of the sinuses*

1. cerebral ____________________
2. epidural ____________________
3. meningitis ____________________
4. myelitis ____________________
5. cerebellitis ____________________
6. cephalalgia ____________________
7. neuralgia ____________________
8. lobotomy ____________________
9. craniotomy ____________________
10. encephalopathy ____________________

Learning Outcome 5.1 Exercises

EXERCISE 4 *Match the word part on the left with its definition on the right. Some definitions will be used more than once.*

_____	1. psych/o		a. weakness
_____	2. somn/o		b. feeling, sensation
_____	3. -phobia		c. know
_____	4. -mania		d. sleep
_____	5. ton/o		e. movement, motion
_____	6. kinesi/o		f. excessive desire
_____	7. hypn/o		g. slight or partial paralysis
_____	8. -plegia		h. speech
_____	9. -paresis		i. excessive fear or sensitivity
_____	10. esthesi/o		j. mind
_____	11. gnosi/o		k. arrangement, order, coordination
_____	12. phas/o		l. muscle tone, tension
_____	13. tax/o		m. paralysis
_____	14. -asthenia		
_____	15. phren/o		

EXERCISE 5 *Translate the following word parts.*

1. kinesi/o _______________
2. -phobia _______________
3. -mania _______________
4. -paresis _______________
5. somn/o _______________
6. phren/o _______________
7. tax/o _______________

EXERCISE 6 *Break down the following words into their component parts and translate.*

EXAMPLE: sinusitis *sinus | itis* *inflammation of the sinuses*

1. psychology _______________
2. hypnotic _______________
3. anesthetic _______________
4. dystonia _______________
5. aphasia _______________
6. neurasthenia _______________
7. monoplegia _______________

Learning Outcome 5.1 Exercises

GENERATION

EXERCISE 7 *Underline and define the word parts from this chapter in the following terms.*

1. cerebral thrombosis ________________
2. subdural hematoma ________________
3. lobectomy ________________
4. craniosclerosis ________________
5. encephalocele ________________
6. ganglioma ________________
7. meningioma ________________
8. cephalodynia ________________
9. myelodysplasia ________________
10. neuropharmacology ________________

EXERCISE 8 *For the following words, identify and translate the word parts from this chapter.*

1. hyperkinesia ________________
2. pyromania ________________
3. hydrophobia ________________
4. schizophrenia ________________
5. psychosomatic ________________
6. somnambulism ________________
7. hemiparesis ________________
8. myasthenia ________________

EXERCISE 9 *Build a medical term from the information provided.*

1. incision into the brain (use *cerebral*) ________________
2. incision into the skull ________________
3. incision into a nerve ________________
4. inflammation of the ganglion ________________
5. inflammation of the dura ________________
6. inflammation of the cerebellum ________________
7. hernia of the meninges ________________
8. hernia of the spinal cord ________________
9. hernia of the brain (use *encephalo*) ________________
10. large head (use *cephalo*) ________________

EXERCISE 10 *Build a medical term from the information provided.*

1. pertaining to muscle tone ________________
2. half paralysis (use *-plegia*) ________________
3. bad feeling (use *dys-*) ________________
4. bad speaking condition ________________
5. no coordination condition ________________
6. sleep agent (use *hypno*) ________________

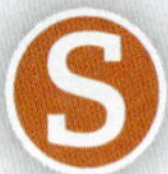

Subjective

Patient History, Problems, Complaints

Impairments

Pain

Paralysis

Sensation/feeling

Phobia/mania

Objective

Observation and Discovery

Diagnostic procedures

Structure

Function

Professional terms

Seizure

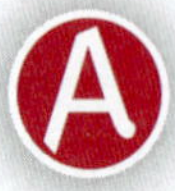

Assessment

Diagnosis and Pathology

Structure

Function

Plan

Treatments and Therapies

Anesthesia

Drugs

Surgical procedures

This section contains medical terms built from the roots presented in the previous section. The purpose of this section is to expose you to words used in neurology that are built from the word roots presented earlier. The focus of this book is to teach you the process of learning roots and translating them in context. Each term is presented with the correct pronunciation, followed by a word analysis that breaks down the word into its component parts, a definition that provides a literal translation of the word, as well as supplemental information if the literal translation deviates from its medical use.

The terms are organized using a health care professional's SOAP note (first introduced in Chapter 2) as a model.

SUBJECTIVE

5.2 Patient History, Problems, Complaints

When someone comes to a health care professional with neurological complaints, the complaint will usually fall into problems with either the peripheral or central nervous system. Some patients with peripheral nervous system complaints have problems with the signals being sent to the brain. Their brains may be sending painful signals (*neuralgia, causalgia*) or their brains could have problems receiving sensations (*hyperesthesia, dysesthesia*). Other problems with the peripheral nervous system relate to interruptions in receiving signals from the brain or spinal cord, which could lead to partial or complete paralysis. Central nervous system problems can affect the entire body, as with fainting (*syncope*). Other problems can be more focused, such as problems with speaking (*aphasia, dysphasia*) and reading (*dyslexia*).

The most common psychiatric complaints health care professionals see deal with emotions, such as

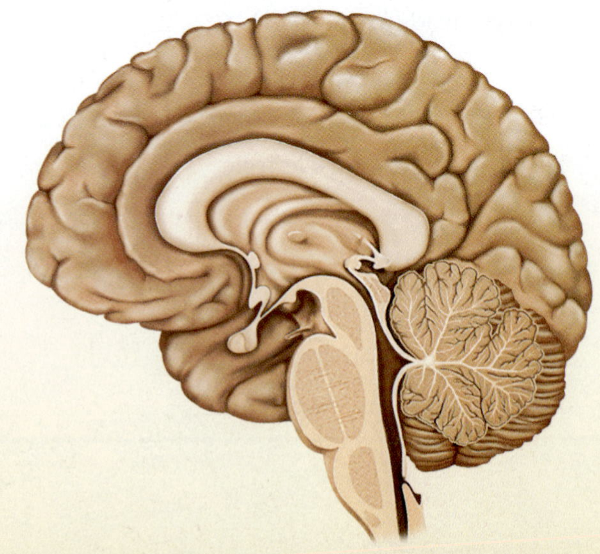

A sagittal cross section of the brain showing the cerebrum, cerebellum, brain stem, and other supporting structures.

depression and anxiety. Other common complaints may include concerns over erratic behaviors, abnormal fears *(phobias)*, or unhealthy obsessions *(manias)*. When a patient enters a sudden state of confusion or abrupt loss of awareness of his or her surroundings, it is *delirium*. When it is a more permanent loss in orientation and thinking ability, it is *dementia*.

impairments

Term	Word Analysis
aphasia ah-FAY-zhah **Definition** inability to speak	a / phas / ia not / speaking / condition
ataxia ah-TAK-see-ah **Definition** lack of coordination	a / tax / ia no / coordination / condition
catatonia KAT-ah-TOH-nee-ah **Definition** condition characterized by reduced muscle tone	cata / ton / ia down / muscle / tone
delirium deh-LEER-ee-um **Definition** brief loss of mental function	from Latin, for *to plow outside the furrow;* perhaps translates to *go off the tracks*
dementia da-MEN-chah **Definition** loss/decline in mental function	de / ment / ia down / mind / condition
dyskinesia dis-kih-NEE-zhah **Definition** difficulty moving	dys / kines / ia bad / movement / condition
dyslexia dis-LEK-see-ah **Definition** difficulty reading	dys / lex / ia bad / reading / condition
dysphasia dis-FAY-zhah **Definition** difficulty speaking	dys / phas / ia bad / speaking / condition
dystonia dis-TOH-nee-ah **Definition** condition characterized by involuntary muscle movements	dys / ton / ia bad / muscle tone / condition
insomnia in-SOM-nee-ah **Definition** inability to sleep	in / somn / ia not / sleeping / condition
myoclonus mai-AWK-loh-nus **Definition** muscle twitching	myo / clonus muscle / turmoil
myospasm MAI-oh-spaz-um **Definition** involuntary muscle contraction	myo / spasm muscle / involuntary contraction

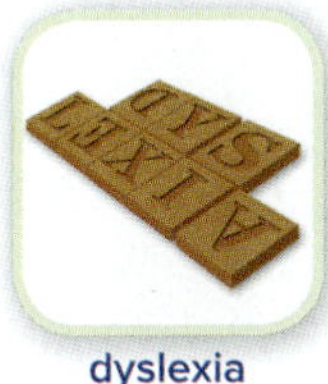
dyslexia

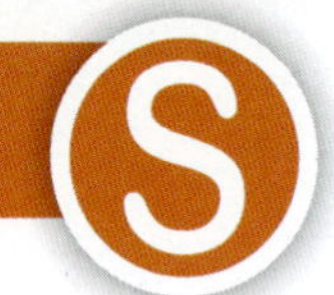

5.2 Patient History, Problems, Complaints

impairments *continued*

Term	Word Analysis
neurasthenia NUR-as-THEN-ee-ah **Definition** nerve weakness	neur / asthenia nerve / weakness
somnambulism sawm-NAM-byoo-liz-um **Definition** sleep walking	somn / ambul / ism sleep / walk / condition
syncope SIN-koh-pee **Definition** fainting; losing consciousness due to temporary loss of blood flow to brain	from Greek, for *contraction* or *cut off*

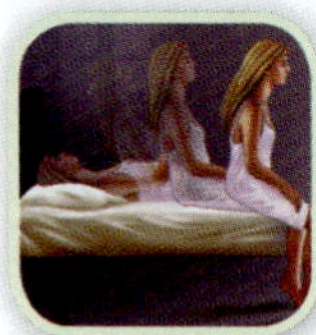

somnambulism

pain

Term	Word Analysis
cephalalgia SEH-ful-AL-jah **Definition** head pain	cephal / algia head / pain
cephalodynia SEH-fah-loh-DAI-nee-ah **Definition** head pain	cephalo / dynia head / pain
encephalalgia in-SE-ful-AL-jah **Definition** brain pain	encephal / algia brain / pain
neuralgia nur-AL-jah **Definition** nerve pain	neur / algia nerve / pain
neurodynia NUR-oh-DAI-nee-ah **Definition** nerve pain	neuro / dynia nerve / pain

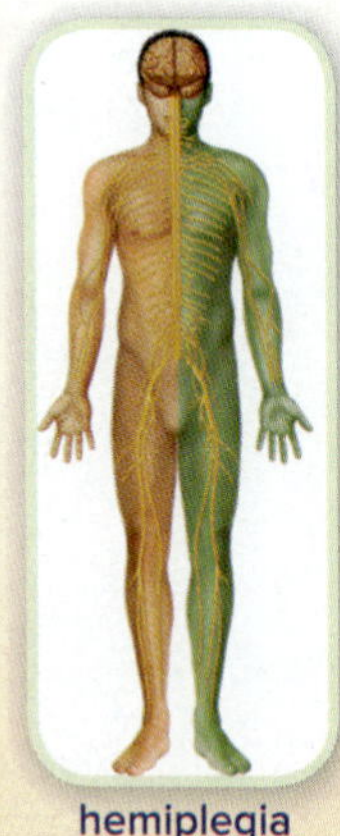

hemiplegia

paralysis

Term	Word Analysis
hemiparesis HEH-mee-puh-REE-sis **Definition** partial paralysis on half the body	hemi / paresis half / partial paralysis
hemiplegia HEH-mee-PLEE-jah **Definition** paralysis on half the body	hemi / plegia half / paralysis

5.2 Patient History, Problems, Complaints

paralysis *continued*

Term	Word Analysis
monoparesis MAW-noh-puh-REE-sis **Definition** partial paralysis of one limb	mono / paresis one / partial paralysis
monoplegia MAW-noh-PLEE-jah **Definition** paralysis of one limb	mono / plegia one / paralysis
paralysis puh-RAH-lu-sis **Definition** complete loss of sensation and motor function	from Greek, for *to disable*
paresis puh-REE-sis **Definition** partial paralysis characterized by varying degrees of sensation and motor function	from Greek, for *to let go*

sensation/feeling

Term	Word Analysis
anosmia an-AWZ-mee-ah **Definition** lack of a sense of smell	an / osm / ia no / smell / condition
causalgia kaw-ZAL-jah **Definition** painful sensation of burning	caus / algia burn / pain
dysesthesia DIS-es-THEE-zhah **Definition** bad feeling	dys / esthesia bad / sensation
hyperesthesia HAI-per-es-THEE-zhah **Definition** increased sensation	hyper / esthesia over / sensation
paresthesia PAR-es-THEE-zhah **Definition** abnormal sensation (usually numbness or tingling in the skin)	par / esthesia beside / sensation
pseudesthesia SOO-des-THEE-zhah **Definition** false sensation	pseud / esthesia false / sensation
synesthesia SIN-es-THEE-zhah **Definition** condition where one sensation is experienced as another	syn / esthesia together / sensation

5.2 Patient History, Problems, Complaints

phobia/mania

Term	Word Analysis
acrophobia AK-roh-FOH-bee-ah **Definition** fear of heights	**acro / phobia** heights / excessive fear
agoraphobia ah-GOR-ah-FOH-bee-ah **Definition** fear of outdoor spaces **NOTE:** *Agora* is Greek for *marketplace*; similar to the Roman *forum*.	**agora / phobia** marketplace / excessive fear
hydrophobia HAI-druh-FOH-bee-ah **Definition** fear of water	**hydro / phobia** water / excessive fear
kleptomania KLEP-toh-MAY-nee-ah **Definition** desire to steal	**klepto / mania** theft / excessive desire
photophobia FOH-toh-FOH-bee-ah **Definition** excessive sensitivity to light **NOTE:** This is an example of *phobia* meaning not just *fear* of but also *sensitivity* to something. Someone with photophobia isn't afraid of light, but rather is extremely sensitive to light.	**photo / phobia** light / excessive sensitivity
pyromania PAI-roh-MAY-nee-ah **Definition** desire to set fire	**pyro / mania** fire / excessive desire

S Learning Outcome 5.2 Exercises

PRONUNCIATION

EXERCISE 1 *Break down the following words into syllables.*

EXAMPLE: synesthesia *syn | es | the | sia*

1. catatonia ____________
2. myoclonus ____________
3. paresthesia ____________
4. neurasthenia ____________
5. photophobia ____________
6. agoraphobia ____________
7. encephalalgia ____________
8. pseudoesthesia ____________

EXERCISE 2 *Indicate which syllable is emphasized when pronounced.*

EXAMPLE: bronchitis bron**chi**tis

1. dystonia ____________
2. ataxia ____________
3. paresis ____________
4. neuralgia ____________
5. causalgia ____________
6. aphasia ____________
7. paralysis ____________
8. anosmia ____________
9. dysphasia ____________
10. somnambulism ____________

TRANSLATION

EXERCISE 3 *Break down the following words into their component parts.*

EXAMPLE: nasopharyngoscope *naso | pharyngo | scope*

1. dementia ____________
2. pseudesthesia ____________
3. synesthesia ____________
4. causalgia ____________
5. pyromania ____________
6. hydrophobia ____________
7. dysphasia ____________
8. myoclonus ____________
9. dyslexia ____________
10. neuralgia ____________

EXERCISE 4 *Underline and define the word parts from this chapter in the following terms.*

1. neurasthenia ____________
2. neurodynia ____________
3. cephalalgia ____________
4. encephalalgia ____________
5. dyskinesia ____________
6. dysesthesia ____________
7. paresthesia ____________
8. kleptomania ____________
9. agoraphobia ____________

Learning Outcome 5.2 Exercises

10. photophobia ______________________________
11. monoparesis ______________________________
12. monoplegia ______________________________
13. aphasia ______________________________
14. ataxia ______________________________
15. insomnia ______________________________
16. catatonia ______________________________
17. myospasm ______________________________

EXERCISE 5 *Match the term on the left with its definition on the right.*

____	1. paralysis	a.	head pain
____	2. delirium	b.	brief loss of mental function
____	3. insomnia	c.	increased sensation
____	4. acrophobia	d.	fear of heights
____	5. cephalodynia	e.	fainting; losing consciousness due to temporary loss of blood flow to the brain
____	6. anosmia	f.	partial paralysis on half the body
____	7. syncope	g.	paralysis on half the body
____	8. hyperesthesia	h.	inability to sleep
____	9. dystonia	i.	condition characterized by involuntary movements
____	10. hemiplegia	j.	from Greek, for *to disable;* complete loss of sensation and motor function
____	11. paresis	k.	from Greek, for *to let go;* partial paralysis characterized by varying degrees of sensation and motor function
____	12. hemiparesis	l.	lack of a sense of smell

EXERCISE 6 *Translate the following terms as literally as possible.*

> EXAMPLE: nasopharyngoscope *an instrument for looking at the nose and throat*

1. aphasia ______________________________
2. catatonia ______________________________
3. somnambulism ______________________________
4. myoclonus ______________________________
5. cephalodynia ______________________________
6. encephalalgia ______________________________
7. monoplegia ______________________________
8. monoparesis ______________________________

9. neurodynia ____________________
10. pseudesthesia ____________________
11. synesthesia ____________________
12. hydrophobia ____________________
13. pyromania ____________________

GENERATION

EXERCISE 7 *Multiple-choice questions. Select the correct answer(s).*

1. The main categories for nerve complaints are
   a. peripheral and central nervous system problems
   b. central nervous system and psychiatric problems
   c. peripheral and psychiatric problems
   d. autonomic and pyramidal problems
2. Select the terms that pertain to peripheral nerve problems.
   a. sending painful signals to the brain (*algia*)
   b. problems receiving sensation (*esthesia*)
   c. excessive desire (*manio*)
   d. problems speaking (*phaso*)
   e. abnormal fear (*phobo*)
   f. paralysis (*plegia*)
3. Select the terms that pertain to central nervous system problems.
   a. sending painful signals to the brain (*algia*)
   b. problems receiving sensation (*esthesia*)
   c. excessive desire (*manio*)
   d. problems speaking (*phaso*)
   e. abnormal fear (*phobo*)
   f. paralysis (*plegia*)
4. Select the terms that pertain to psychiatric problems.
   a. sending painful signals to the brain (*algia*)
   b. problems receiving sensation (*esthesia*)
   c. excessive desire (*manio*)
   d. problems speaking (*phaso*)
   e. abnormal fear (*phobo*)
   f. paralysis (*plegia*)

Learning Outcome 5.2 Exercises

EXERCISE 8 *Build a medical term from the information provided.*

EXAMPLE: inflammation of the sinuses *sinusitis*

1. bad speaking condition ______
2. no coordination condition ______
3. bad muscle tone condition ______
4. bad feeling ______
5. increased sensation ______
6. not sleeping condition ______
7. difficulty moving ______
8. involuntary muscle contraction ______
9. nerve weakness ______
10. partial paralysis on half the body ______
11. paralysis on half the body ______
12. fear of outdoor spaces ______
13. excessive sensitivity to light ______
14. desire to steal ______

EXERCISE 9 *Multiple-choice questions. Select the correct answer.*

1. Which of the following means *fear of heights?*
   a. hydrophobia
   b. agoraphobia
   c. acrophobia
   d. photophobia
2. Which of the following literally means *beside sensation* and normally refers to numbness or tingling in the skin?
   a. dysesthesia
   b. hyperesthesia
   c. paresthesia
   d. pseudesthesia
   e. synesthesia
3. Which of the following is a painful sensation of burning?
   a. causalgia
   b. cephalalgia
   c. pyromania
   d. anosmia
4. A person who lacks a sense of smell has
   a. ataxia
   b. anosmia
   c. syncope
   d. dyskinesia

EXERCISE 10 *Briefly describe the difference between each pair of terms.*

1. paralysis, paresis ______
2. neuralgia, cephalalgia ______
3. dementia, delirium ______
4. dyslexia, dyskinesia ______

OBJECTIVE

5.3 Observation and Discovery

When a health care professional sees a patient with a neurologic or psychiatric problem, the exam is often quite involved. The neurologic exam involves checking the patient's muscle strength and coordination, sensation, and reflexes. A reflex is a muscle contraction that bypasses the brain. When certain tendons are tapped, an impulse flows directly to the spinal cord, which sends a quick command to the nearby muscle to contract. Checking sensation involves studying afferent nerve paths, which are the paths that lead from the peripheral to the central nervous system. Strength and coordination check efferent pathways, the pathways that lead from the brain to the peripheral nerves. Psychiatric evaluation is very involved, because it depends on extensive questions and history to help discover the root of the patient's problem.

The most common lab work done in the evaluation of the neurologic system focuses on testing a patient's cerebrospinal fluid, which is obtained via lumbar puncture. This is a procedure in which a needle is gently inserted between the vertebrae of the lower spine and a small amount of fluid is drawn and evaluated for signs of infection and other types of inflammation.

Imaging the brain is commonly performed to evaluate for bleeding after an injury, to determine the presence of diseased brain tissue, and to look for brain tumors. The most common imaging technique is the computed tomography (CT) scan, which is complex type of x-ray. The benefit of a CT is its speed. When a more detailed view is needed, or when the cerebellum is of special importance, a magnetic resonance image (MRI) is beneficial. Ultrasounds can be used to assess blood circulation to the brain and monitor the speed of the blood passing through the vessels, helpful in detecting both blockages and bleeding. For a more involved view of the vessels, dye can be injected into the bloodstream and an MRI performed. This special image is known as magnetic resonance angiography (MRA). Another type of image utilizing dye is a myelogram, in which an x-ray of the spine is completed after dye is injected into the vertebrae. Another very common procedure for analyzing the electric function of the brain is an electroencephalogram (EEG). An EEG is not exactly an image of the brain; electrodes are placed around the skull and the brain's electric currents are monitored. This is the most effective means to detect seizure activity in the brain.

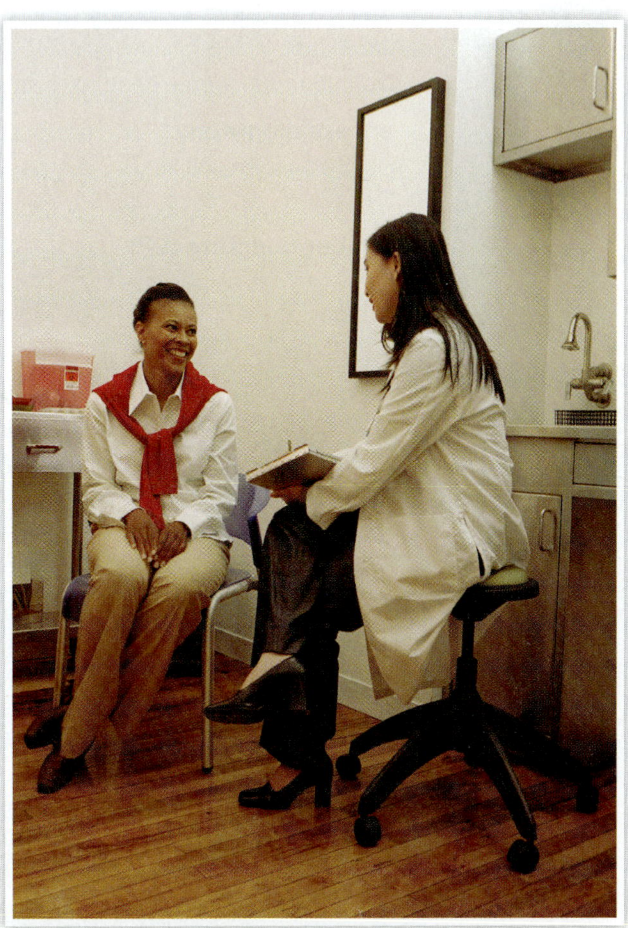

Two of the most common ways of obtaining data to be used in diagnosing neurological or psychiatric disorders involve patient interview and imaging.

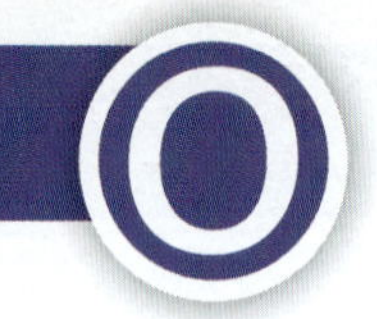

5.3 Observation and Discovery

diagnostic procedures

Term	Word Analysis
cerebral angiography sih-REE-bral AN-gee-AW-grah-fee **Definition** procedure used to examine blood vessels in the brain	cerebr / al — angio / graph / y brain / pertaining to — vessel / writing / procedure
echoencephalography EH-koh-in-SEH-fah-LAW-grah-fee **Definition** procedure used to examine the brain using sound waves	echo / encephalo / graph / y echo / brain / writing / procedure
electroencephalography (EEG) eh-LEK-troh-in-SEH-fah-LAW-grah-fee **Definition** procedure used to examine the electrical activity of the brain	electro / encephalo / graph / y electricity / brain / writing / procedure
encephalography in-SEH-fah-LOH-grah-fee **Definition** procedure for studying the brain	encephalo / graph / y brain / writing / procedure
lumbar puncture (LP) LUM-bar PUNK-chir **Definition** inserting a needle into the lumbar region of the spine in order to collect spinal fluid, commonly called a "spinal tap"	lumb / ar — puncture lower back / pertaining to
magnetic resonance angiography (MRA) mag-NET-ik REH-zawn-ants AN-gee-AW-grah-fee **Definition** procedure used to examine blood vessels	angio / graph / y vessel / writing / procedure
myelogram MAI-el-oh-gram **Definition** image of the spinal cord, usually done using x-ray	myelo / gram spinal cord / record
positron emission tomography (PET) scan PAWZ-ih-trawn ee-MISH-un taw-MAW-gra-fee **Definition** an imaging procedure that uses radiation (positrons) to produce cross sections of the brain	e / mission tomo / graph / y out / send cut / writing / procedure
transcranial Doppler sonography tranz-KRAY-nee-al DAW-plir saw-NAW-gra-fee **Definition** an imaging technique that produces an image of the brain using sound waves sent through the skull	trans / cranial Doppler sono / graph / y through / skull Doppler sound / writing / procedure

electroence-phalography (EEG)

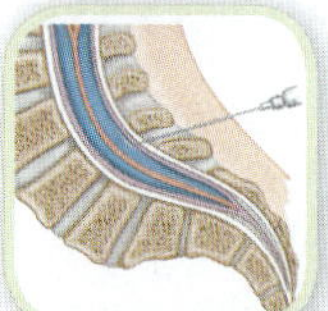

lumbar puncture (LP)

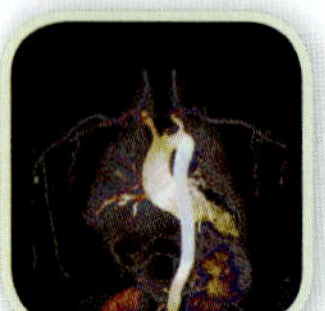

magnetic resonance angiography (MRA)

structure

Term	Word Analysis
cerebellitis ser-eh-bell-AI-tis **Definition** inflammation of the cerebellum	cerebell / itis cerebellum / inflammation
cerebral atrophy seh-REE-bral A-troh-fee **Definition** wasting away of brain tissue	cerebr / al — a / trophy brain / pertaining to — no / nourishment
duritis dur-AI-tis **Definition** inflammation of the dura	dur / itis dura / inflammation

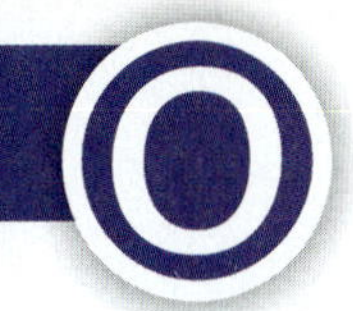

5.3 Observation and Discovery

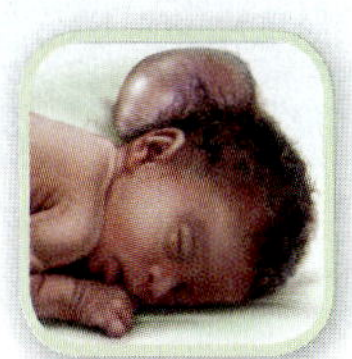

encephalocele

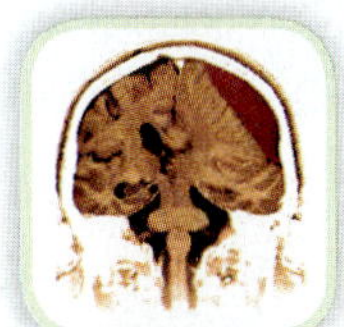

subdural hematoma

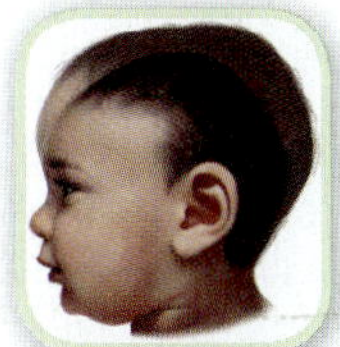

microcephaly

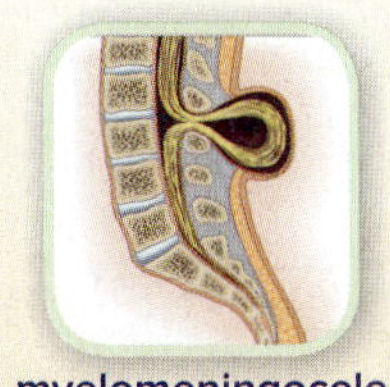

myelomeningocele

structure *continued*

Term	Word Analysis
encephalocele en-SEF-ah-loh-SEEL **Definition** hernia of the brain (normally through a defect in the skull)	encephalo / cele brain / hernia
hematoma HEE-mah-TOH-mah **Definition** a tumor-like mass made up of blood	hemat / oma blood / tumor
cranial hematoma KRAY-nee-al HEE-mah-TOH-mah **Definition** a hematoma beneath the skull	crani / al hemat / oma skull / pertaining to blood / tumor
epidural hematoma EH-pi-DIR-al HEE-mah-TOH-mah **Definition** a hematoma located on top of the dura	epi / dur / al hemat / oma upon / dura / pertaining to blood / tumor
intracerebral hematoma IN-trah-se-REE-bral HEE-mah-TOH-mah **Definition** a hematoma located inside the brain	intra / cerebr / al hemat / oma inside / brain / pertaining to blood / tumor
subdural hematoma sub-DIR-al HEE-mah-TOH-mah **Definition** a hematoma located beneath the dura	sub / dur / al hemat / oma beneath / dura / pertaining to blood / tumor
macrocephaly MA-kroh-SEH-fah-lee **Definition** abnormally large head	macro / cephal / y large / head / condition
microcephaly MAI-kroh-SEH-fah-lee **Definition** abnormally small head	micro / cephal / y small / head / condition
meningocele meh-NIN-goh-seel **Definition** a hernia of the meninges	meningo / cele meninges / hernia
myelocele MAI-el-oh-SEEL **Definition** a hernia of the spinal cord	myelo / cele spinal cord / hernia
myelomalacia MAI-el-oh-mah-LAY-shah **Definition** abnormal softening of the spinal cord	myelo / malacia spinal cord / softening
myelomeningocele MAI-el-oh-meh-NIN-goh-seel **Definition** a hernia of the spinal cord and meninges	myelo / meningo / cele spinal cord / meninges / hernia
neuritis nir-AI-tis **Definition** nerve inflammation	neur / itis nerve / inflammation

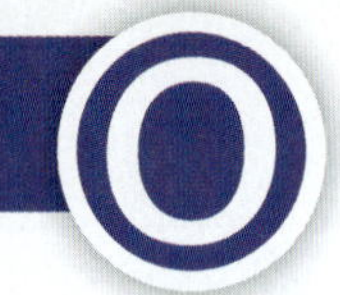

5.3 Observation and Discovery

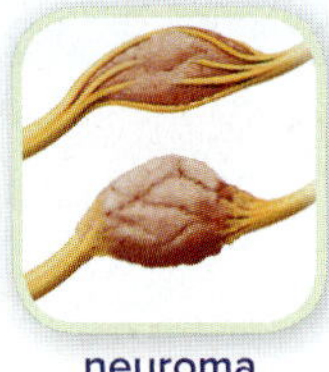
neuroma

structure *continued*

Term	Word Analysis
neuroma nir-OH-mah **Definition** a nerve tumor	neur / oma nerve / tumor
neurosclerosis NIR-oh-skleh-ROH-sis **Definition** hardening of nerves	neuro / scler / osis nerve / hardening / condition
polyneuritis PAW-lee-nir-AI-tis **Definition** inflammation of multiple nerves	poly / neur / itis many / nerve / inflammation

function

Term	Word Analysis
agnosia AG-noh-zhah **Definition** inability to comprehend	a / gnos / ia not / knowledge / condition
apathy A-pah-thee **Definition** lack of emotion	a / path / y no / suffering / condition
atopognosis AY-top-aw-GNOH-sis **Definition** inability to locate a sensation	a / topo / gnosis no / place / knowledge
hyperkinesia HAI-per-kin-EE-shah **Definition** increase in muscle movement or activity	hyper / kines / ia over / movement / condition
neurasthenia NIR-as-THEN-ee-ah **Definition** nerve weakness	neur / asthenia nerve / weakness
neuroglycopenia NIR-oh-GLAI-koh-PEE-nee-ah **Definition** deficiency of sugar that interferes with normal brain activity	neuro / glyco / penia nerve / sugar / deficiency
nystagmus nih-STAG-mus **Definition** involuntary back and forth eye movements	from Greek, for *to nod*
prosopagnosia PRAW-soh-pag-NOH-zhah **Definition** inability to recognize faces	prosop / a / gnos / ia face / no / knowledge / condition

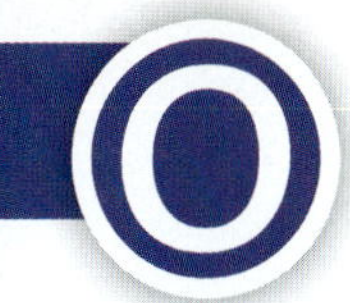

5.3 Observation and Discovery

professional terms

Term	Word Analysis
anesthesiologist A-neh-STHEE-zee-AW-loh-jist	an / esthesio / log / ist no / sensation / study / specialist
Definition doctor who specializes in anesthesiology	
afferent nerve A-fir-ent nirv	af / ferent nerve toward / carry
Definition a nerve that carries impulses toward the central nervous system **NOTE:** The prefix *af-* is actually *ad- (toward)*, like in *admit* or *address*. When *ad-* is added to *-ferent*, the word *adferent* changes to *afferent*—it's just easier to easier to say.	
efferent nerve EH-fir-ent nirv	ef / ferent nerve away / carry
Definition a nerve that carries impulses away from the central nervous system **NOTE:** The prefix *ef-* is actually *ex- (out or away)*, like in *exit*. When added to *-ferent*, it changes for the same reasons as described for *afferent*.	
neurogenic NIR-oh-JIN-ik	neuro / gen / ic nerve / creation / pertaining to
Definition originating from/created by nerves	
psychogenic SAI-koh-JIN-ik	psycho / gen / ic mind / creation / pertaining to
Definition originating in/created by the mind	
psychiatrist sai-KAI-ah-trist	psych / iatr / ist mind / treatment / specialist
Definition doctor who specializes in treatment of the mind	
psychiatry sai-KAI-ah-tree	psych / iatr / y mind / treatment / specialty
Definition branch of medicine that focuses on the treatment of the mind	
psychologist sai-KAW-loh-jist	psycho / log / ist mind / study / specialist
Definition doctor who specializes in the study of the mind.	
psychology sai-KAW-loh-jee	psycho / log / y mind / study / specialty
Definition branch of medicine that focuses on the study of the mind **NOTE:** The chief differences between a psychologist and a psychiatrist are their training and approach; a psychologist has a PhD and normally uses psychotherapy, and a psychiatrist has an MD or a DO and can prescribe medication.	
psychosomatic SAI-koh-soh-MA-tik	psycho / somat / ic mind / body / pertaining to
Definition pertaining to the relationship between the body and the mind	

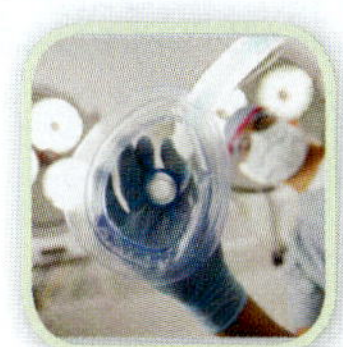

anesthesiologist

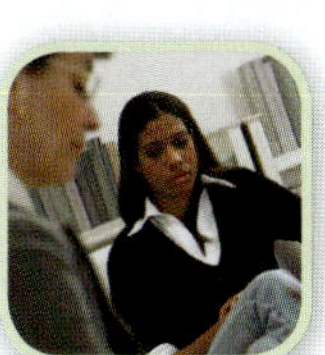

psychiatrist

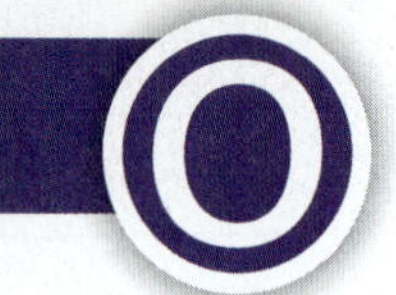

5.3 Observation and Discovery

seizure

Term	Word Analysis
idiopathic IH-dee-oh-PAH-thik **Definition** having no known cause or origin **NOTE:** *idio-* means *private* and comes from the Greek word *idiotes*, meaning *private person*. Greeks were such social people that anybody who kept to themselves was called an *idiot*.	idio / path / ic private / disease / pertaining to
interictal IN-ter-IK-tal **Definition** time between seizures	inter / ictal between / seizure
postictal post-IK-tal **Definition** time after a seizure	post / ictal after / seizure
preictal pree-IK-tal **Definition** time before a seizure	pre / ictal before / seizure
tonic TAW-nik **Definition** pertaining to muscle tone (normally weak or unresponsive)	ton / ic muscle / pertaining to
clonus CLAH-nis **Definition** muscle spasm or twitching	from Greek, for *violent*
tonic-clonic seizure TAW-nik CLAH-nik SEE-zhir **Definition** a seizure characterized by both a tonic and a clonic phase	ton / ic — clon / ic muscle / pertaining to — spasm / pertaining to

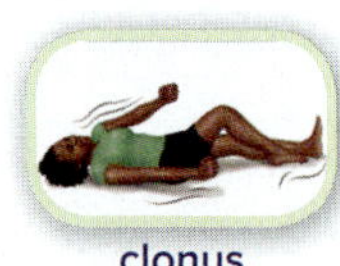

clonus

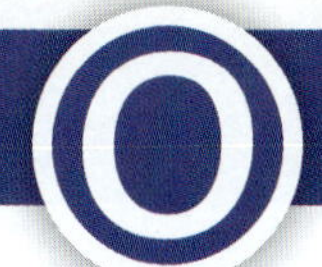

Learning Outcome 5.3 Exercises

PRONUNCIATION

EXERCISE 1 *Break down the following words into syllables.*

EXAMPLE: synesthesia *syn | es | the | sia*

1. preictal ______
2. interictal ______
3. afferent nerve ______
4. efferent nerve ______
5. macrocephaly ______
6. microcephaly ______
7. hematoma ______
8. myelocele ______
9. neurogenic ______
10. psychogenic ______
11. hyperkinesia ______
12. neurasthenia ______
13. neuroglycopenia ______
14. prosopagnosia ______
15. encephalography ______
16. psychosomatic ______

EXERCISE 2 *Indicate which syllable is emphasized when pronounced.*

EXAMPLE: bronchitis bron**chi**tis

1. tonic ______
2. clonus ______
3. psychiatrist ______
4. psychologist ______
5. neuritis ______
6. myelogram ______
7. agnosia ______

TRANSLATION

EXERCISE 3 *Break down the following words into their component parts.*

EXAMPLE: nasopharyngoscope *naso | pharyngo | scope*

1. neuroma ______
2. tonic ______
3. duritis ______
4. neuritis ______
5. polyneuritis ______
6. myelomalacia ______
7. microcephaly ______
8. psychiatry ______
9. psychology ______
10. psychosomatic ______
11. atopognosis ______
12. cerebral atrophy ______
13. myelomeningocele ______
14. neuroglycopenia ______
15. cranial hematoma ______
16. intracerebral hematoma ______
17. subdural hematoma ______
18. encephalography ______
19. echoencephalography ______

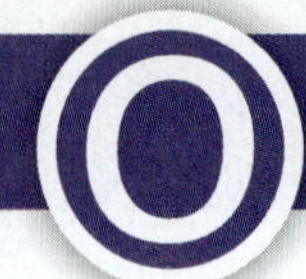

Learning Outcome 5.3 Exercises

EXERCISE 4 *Underline and define the word parts from this chapter in the following terms.*

1. hyperkinesia ____________
2. cerebellitis ____________
3. neurogenic ____________
4. psychogenic ____________
5. psychologist ____________
6. myelocele ____________
7. meningocele ____________
8. encephalocele ____________
9. macrocephaly ____________
10. neurosclerosis ____________
11. agnosia ____________
12. prosopagnosia ____________
13. myelogram ____________
14. cerebral angiography ____________
15. transcranial Doppler sonography ____________
16. neurasthenia (two word parts) ____________
17. epidural hematoma ____________
18. tonic-clonic seizure ____________
19. anesthesiologist ____________
20. electroencephalography ____________

EXERCISE 5 *Match the term on the left with its definition on the right.*

____	1. apathy	a.	inserting a needle into the lumbar (lower back) region of the spine in order to collect spinal fluid
____	2. hematoma	b.	procedure used to examine blood vessels
____	3. idiopathic	c.	an imaging procedure that uses radiation (positrons) to produce cross sections of the brain
____	4. lumbar puncture (LP)	d.	lack of emotion
____	5. postictal	e.	involuntary back and forth eye movements
____	6. preictal	f.	a nerve that carries impulses toward the CNS
____	7. interictal	g.	a nerve that carries impulses away from the CNS
____	8. magnetic resonance angiography (MRA)	h.	time between seizures
____	9. positron emission tomography (PET) scan	i.	time after a seizure
____	10. nystagmus	j.	time before a seizure
____	11. clonus	k.	from Greek, for *violent;* muscle spasm or twitching
____	12. afferent nerve	l.	having no known cause or origin
____	13. efferent nerve	m.	a tumor-like mass made up of blood

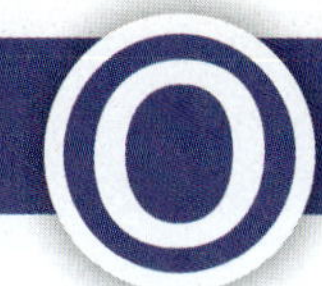

Learning Outcome 5.3 Exercises

EXERCISE 6 *Translate the following terms as literally as possible.*

EXAMPLE: nasopharyngoscope *an instrument for looking at the nose and throat*

1. neuroma ______
2. atopognosis ______
3. encephalocele ______
4. myelocele ______
5. myelomalacia ______
6. polyneuritis ______
7. psychosomatic ______
8. anesthesiologist ______
9. afferent nerve ______
10. efferent nerve ______

GENERATION

EXERCISE 7 *Build a medical term from the information provided.*

EXAMPLE: inflammation of the sinuses *sinusitis*

1. inflammation of the nerves ______
2. inflammation of the cerebellum ______
3. inflammation of the dura ______
4. no knowledge condition ______
5. over movement condition ______
6. pertaining to muscle tone ______
7. a hernia of the meninges ______
8. a hernia of the spinal cord and meninges ______
9. brain writing procedure (use *encephalo*) ______
10. spinal cord record ______
11. nerve weakness ______
12. branch of medicine that focuses on the treatment of the mind ______
13. branch of medicine that focuses on the study of the mind ______

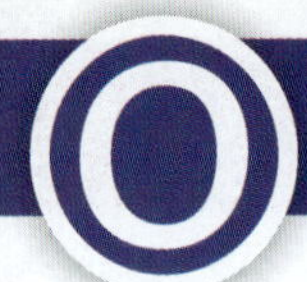

Learning Outcome 5.3 Exercises

EXERCISE 8 *Multiple-choice questions. Select the correct answer(s).*

1. Select the terms that pertain to seizures.
   a. afferent
   b. agnostic
   c. apathetic
   d. clonus
   e. efferent
   f. idiopathic
   g. interictal
   h. tonic-clonic
2. Which diagnostic procedure is used to examine blood vessels in the brain?
   a. cerebral angiography
   b. lumbar puncture
   c. positron emission tomography
   d. transcranial Doppler sonography
3. During a lumbar puncture (LP), the needle is inserted into what part of the body?
   a. arm
   b. brain
   c. heart
   d. spine
4. A person with *apathy* lacks
   a. knowledge/comprehension
   b. emotion
   c. sensation
   d. sleep
5. A person with *prosopagnosia* cannot
   a. comprehend
   b. feel emotion
   c. locate a sensation
   d. recognize faces
6. Which term means *hardening of nerves?*
   a. neuroglycopenia
   b. neurosclerosis
   c. neurasthenia
   d. polyneuritis
7. Which term means *deficiency of sugar that interferes with normal brain activity?*
   a. neuroglycopenia
   b. neurosclerosis
   c. neurasthenia
   d. polyneuritis
8. Which term means *a tumor-like mass made up of blood located beneath the skull?*
   a. cranial hematoma
   b. intracerebral hematoma
   c. subdural hematoma
   d. encephaloma
9. Which term means *a tumor-like mass made up of blood located inside the brain?*
   a. cranial hematoma
   b. intracerebral hematoma
   c. subdural hematoma
   d. encephaloma
10. *Nystagmus* comes from the Greek word meaning
    a. back and forth
    b. repetition
    c. to nod
    d. to jump

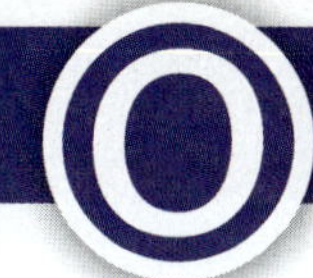

Learning Outcome 5.3 Exercises

EXERCISE 9 *Briefly describe the difference between each pair of terms.*

1. macrocephaly, microcephaly ____________
2. neurogenic, psychogenic ____________
3. psychiatrist, psychologist ____________
4. preictal, postictal ____________
5. afferent nerve, efferent nerve ____________
6. epidural hematoma, subdural hematoma ____________
7. echoencephalography, electroencephalography ____________

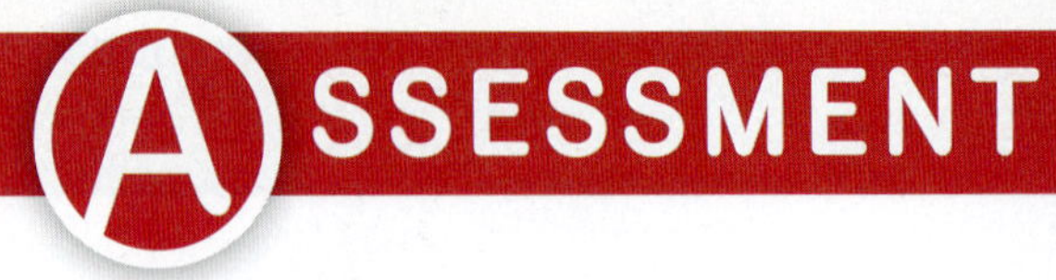

5.4 Diagnosis and Pathology

When assessing a patient with neuropsychiatric problems, it's helpful to determine whether the problem originates from the nervous system (*neurogenic*) or mind (*psychogenic*).

Neurogenic problems may arise from conditions involving the supporting structures, like the skull or blood supply. Disorders of the skull, like premature closure of the bones (*craniosynostosis*), can limit brain growth and lead to pressure on the brain. Increased pressure can also arise from too much fluid around the brain, as seen in hydrocephalus. Pressure in the brain (*intracranial hypertension*) from these conditions can present as headache and vomiting. Disruption of critical blood supply to the brain presents with sudden changes in neurologic function, like slurring of speech. It can happen from a rupture in the blood vessel (*hemorrhagic stroke*) or a blockage cutting off blood supply (*ischemic stroke*). These vascular events constitute a medical emergency.

Problems of the central nervous system may also arise from direct injury or irritation to nerves or brain cells. The symptoms depend on which part of the nervous system is affected. For example, problems involving only the spinal cord, like myelitis or spinal injury, do not cause problems with thought but can lead to muscle weakness or even paralysis. Infections of the tissue surrounding the brain and spinal cord (*meningitis*) cause headache and a stiff neck, while infections of the brain matter (*encephalitis*) lead to generalized dysfunction of the brain, characterized by an altered mental state (*encephalopathy*). Other causes of encephalopathy include prolonged deprivation of oxygen, exposure to toxins, increased pressure in the brain, or chronic injuries. Not all conditions of the brain matter lead to changes in general mental state. Abnormal firing of nerves leads to involuntary changes in muscle tone (*seizure*), and a dysfunction in higher functions like personal interaction and communication is seen in autism.

Nerves can be affected directly by injury or compression, or indirectly through diseases or toxins. Typically, injury or compression will cause a decrease or total loss of function of a single nerve or a group of nerves that exits the spinal cord in the same place. This may lead to pain (*neuralgia*) and/or loss of function (*paresis* or *paralysis*). Diseases such as diabetes and medicines like chemotherapy drugs can be toxic to nerves. Often, this has a greater effect on the nerves that are farther from the brain and spinal cord (*peripheral neuropathy*).

Common psychogenic problems include depression and anxiety. Some people have an inability to control their urges for periods of time, which is known as mania. Most often, these manic phases alternate with bouts of depression, producing a condition known as bipolar disorder or manic-depressive disorder. Some patients have an altered perception of reality known as a psychosis. One of the more common psychotic conditions is schizophrenia. Patients often struggle with distorted perceptions of reality (*delusions*) and may even hear or see things that are not there (*hallucinations*). Furthermore, their thinking patterns are disorganized and emotions are erratic. Another condition characterized by a patient's distorted view of reality occurs in eating disorders. Rather than misunderstanding the world around them, patients with eating disorders such as anorexia and bulimia suffer from an altered perception of their own body.

structure

Term	Word Analysis
Cerebrovascular Accident	
cerebrovascular accident (CVA) seh-REE-broh-VAS-kyoo-lar AK-sih-dent	cerebro / vascul / ar brain / blood vessel / pertaining to
Definition an accident involving the blood vessels of the brain	
stroke STROHK	*stroke*
Definition loss of brain function caused by interruption of blood flow/supply to the brain	

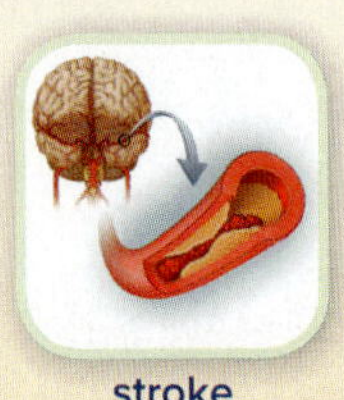
stroke

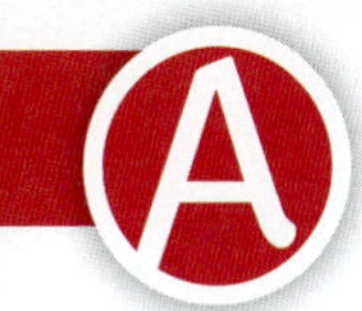

5.4 Diagnosis and Pathology

structure *continued*

Term	Word Analysis
hemorrhagic stroke HEM-oh-RA-jok STROHK	hemo / rrhag / ic blood / excessive bleeding / pertaining to
Definition a stroke where the blood loss is caused by the rupture of a blood vessel	
ischemic stroke ih-SKEE-mik STROHK	isch / em / ic hold back / blood / pertaining to
Definition a stroke where the blood loss is caused by a blockage	
transient ischemic attack (TIA) TRAN-zee-ent ih-SKEE-mik ah-TAK	trans / ient isch / em / ic across / go hold back / blood / pertaining to
Definition a "mini-stroke" caused by the blockage of a blood vessel, which resolves (goes away) within 24 hours	
Cerebrovascular Disease	
cerebrovascular disease seh-REE-broh-VAS-kyoo-lar dih-ZEEZ	cerebro / vascul / ar brain / blood vessel / pertaining to
Definition a disease of the blood vessels of the brain	
cerebral aneurysm seh-REE-bral AN-yir-iz-um	cerebr / al an / eury / sm brain / pertaining to out / wide / condition
Definition the widening or abnormal dilation of a blood vessel in the brain	
Note: In *aneurysm*, the *an-* prefex doesn't come from *a* (not) but from *ana* (meaning up or out). Another word you can see this in is *analysis, ana* (up) + *lysis* (loose). So to *analyze* something means *to break something up and look at the parts.*	
cerebral arteriosclerosis seh-REE-bral ar-TIR-ee-oh-skleh-ROH-sis	cerebr / al arterio / scler / osis brain / pertaining to artery / hardening / condition
Definition the hardening of an artery in the brain	
cerebral atherosclerosis seh-REE-bral A-ther-oh-skleh-ROH-sis	cerebr / al athero / scler / osis brain / pertaining to fatty / hardening / condition
Definition the hardening of an artery in the brain caused by the buildup of fatty plaque	
cerebral embolism seh-REE-bral EM-boh-lih-zum	cerebr / al embol / ism brain / pertaining to stopper / condition
Definition the blockage of a blood vessel in the brain caused by a foreign object (*embolus*) such as fat or bacteria	
Note: *Embolus* is a Greek word meaning *stopper* or *plug.*	
cerebral thrombosis seh-REE-bral throm-BOH-sis	cerebr / al thromb / osis brain / pertaining to clot / condition
Definition the blockage of a blood vessel in the brain caused by a blood clot	
Skull	
craniomalacia KRAY-nee-oh-mah-LAY-shah	cranio / malacia skull / softening
Definition abnormal softening of the skull	
craniosclerosis KRAY-nee-oh-skleh-ROH-sis	cranio / scler / osis skull / hardening / condition
Definition abnormal hardening of the skull	

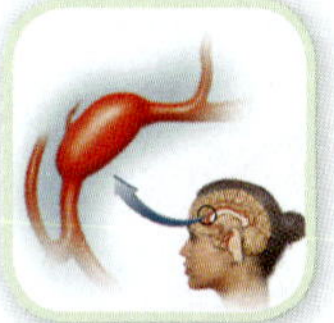
cerebral aneurysm

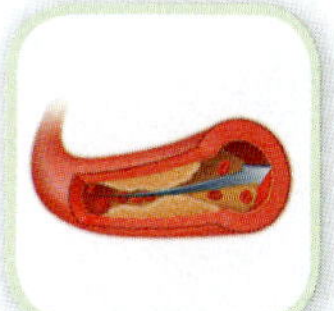
cerebral atherosclerosis

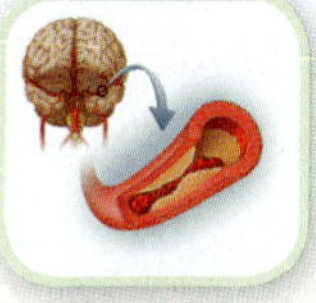
cerebral embolism

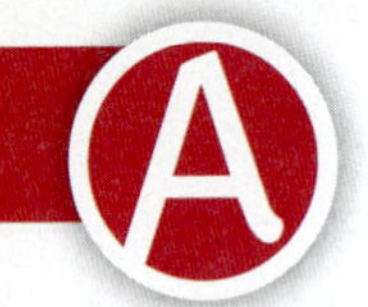

5.4 Diagnosis and Pathology

structure *continued*

Term	Word Analysis
craniostenosis KRAY-nee-oh-steh-NOH-sis **Definition** abnormal narrowing of the skull	cranio / sten / osis skull / narrow / condition
craniosynostosis KRAY-nee-oh-SIN-aw-STOH-sis **Definition** premature fusing of the skull bones	cranio / syn / ost / osis skull / together / bone / condition
hydrocephaly HAI-droh-SEH-fah-lee **Definition** abnormal accumulation of spinal fluid in the brain	hydro / cephal / y water / head / condition
Other	
cerebellitis SEH-rah-bell-AI-tis **Definition** inflammation of the cerebellum	cerebell / itis cerebellum / inflammation
cerebromeningitis seh-REE-broh-MEN-in-JAI-tis **Definition** inflammation of the brain and meninges	cerebro / mening / itis brain / meninges / inflammation
encephalitis in-SEF-ah-LAI-tis **Definition** inflammation of the brain	encephal / itis brain / inflammation
encephalomyelitis in-SEF-ah-loh-MAI-el-AI-tis **Definition** inflammation of the brain and spinal cord	encephalo / myel / itis brain / spinal cord / inflammation
encephalomyeloneuropathy in-SEF-ah-loh-MAI-el-oh-nir-AW-pah-thee **Definition** disease of the brain, spinal cord, and nerves	encephalo / myelo / neuro / pathy brain / spinal cord / nerve / disease
encephalopathy in-SEF-ah-LAW-pah-thee **Definition** disease of the brain	encephalo / pathy brain / disease
encephalopyosis in-SEF-ah-loh-pai-OH-sis **Definition** a pus-filled abscess in the brain	encephalo / py / osis brain / pus / condition
gangliitis GAN-glee-AI-tis **Definition** inflammation of a ganglion	gangli / itis ganglion / inflammation
ganglioma GAN-glee-OH-mah **Definition** ganglion tumor	gangli / oma ganglion / tumor
intracerebral hemorrhage IN-trah-sih-REE-bral HIH-moh-rij **Definition** excessive bleeding inside the brain	intra / cerebr / al hemo / rrhage inside / brain / pertaining to blood / excessive bleeding

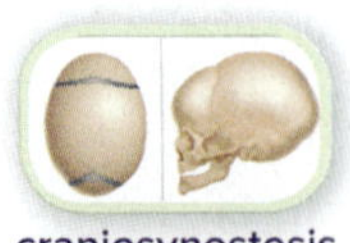
craniosynostosis

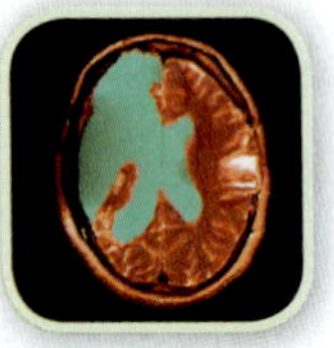
hydrocephaly

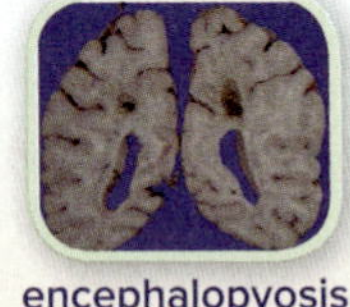
encephalopyosis

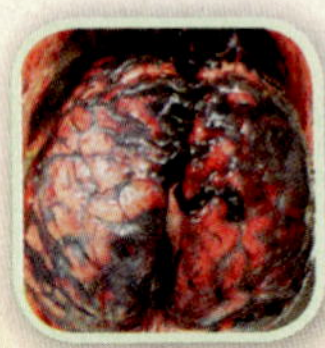
intracerebral hemorrhage

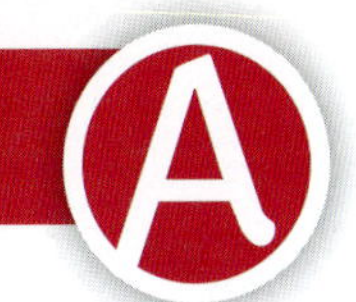

structure *continued*

Term	Word Analysis
meningopathy MEH-nin-GAW-pah-thee **Definition** disease of the meninges	meningo / pathy meninges / disease
meningioma meh-NIN-jee-OH-mah **Definition** tumor of the meninges	meningi / oma meninges / tumor
meningitis MEH-nin-JAI-tus **Definition** inflammation of the meninges	mening / itis meninges / inflammation
meningoencephalitis meh-NIN-goh-in-SEF-ah-LAI-tis **Definition** inflammation of the meninges and brain	meningo / encephal / itis meninges / brain / inflammation
myelitis MAI-el-AI-tis **Definition** inflammation of the spinal cord	myel / itis spinal cord / inflammation
myelodysplasia MAI-el-oh-dis-PLAY-zhah **Definition** defective formation of the spinal cord **NOTE:** Since the root *myelo* can be used for both spinal cord and bone marrow, this term is also used to mean *bad bone marrow formation;* you can tell them apart by considering the context they occur in.	myelo / dys / plas / ia spinal cord / bad / formation / condition
myelopathy MAI-el-AW-pah-thee **Definition** disease of the spinal cord	myelo / pathy spinal cord / disease
neuroarthropathy NIR-oh-ar-THRAW-pah-thee **Definition** disease of the joint associated with nerves	neuro / arthro / pathy nerve / joint / disease
neuroencephalomyelopathy NIR-oh-in-SEF-ah-loh-MAI-el-AW-pah-thee **Definition** disease of the nerves, brain, and spinal cord	neuro / encephalo / myelo / pathy nerve / brain / spinal cord / disease
neuropathy nir-AW-pah-thee **Definition** disease of the nervous system	neuro / pathy nerve / disease
poliomyelitis POH-lee-oh-MAI-el-AI-tis **Definition** inflammation of the gray matter of the spinal cord **NOTE:** This is the full name of the disease known as polio	polio / myel / itis gray / spinal cord / inflammation
polyneuropathy PAW-lee-nir-AW-pah-thee **Definition** disease affecting multiple nerves	poly / neuro / pathy many / nerve / disease

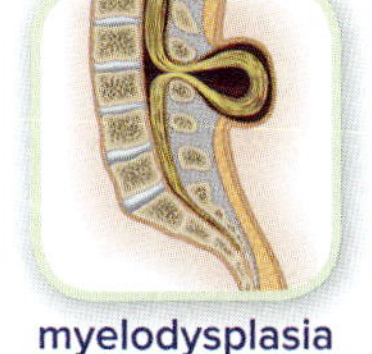
myelodysplasia

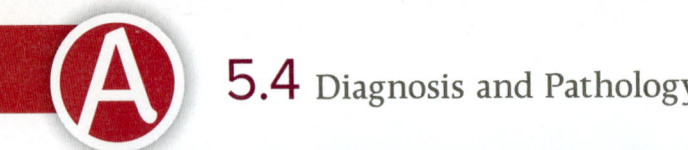

5.4 Diagnosis and Pathology

function

Term	Word Analysis
amyotrophic lateral sclerosis (ALS) a-MAI-aw-TROH-fik LAT-tih-ral skleh-ROH-sis	a / myo / troph / ic lateral scler / osis not / muscle / nourishment / pertaining to side hardening / condition
Definition a degenerative disease of the central nervous system causing loss of muscle control Literally, *the hardening (sclerosis) of the nerve cells on the sides (lateral) of the spine leading to the loss of muscle tissue from disuse.* **Note:** This disease is more commonly known as Lou Gehrig's disease, after the famous baseball player was diagnosed with it in 1939.	
anorexia a-noh-REK-see-ah	an / orex / ia no / appetite / condition
Definition an eating disorder characterized by the patient's refusal to eat	
autism AH-tiz-um	aut / ism self / condition
Definition a psychiatric disorder characterized by withdrawal from communication with others; the patient is focused only on the self	
bulimia boo-LEE-mee-ah	bu / lim / ia ox / hunger / condition
Definition an eating disorder characterized by overeating and usually followed by forced vomiting	
cerebral palsy sih-REE-bral PAL-zee	cerebr / al palsy brain / pertaining to paralysis
Definition paralysis caused by damage to the area of the brain responsible for movement **Note:** palsy is less common word for paralysis	
dysphoria dis-FOR-ee-ah	dys / phor / ia bad / carry / condition
Definition a negative emotional state	
euphoria yoo-FOR-ee-ah	eu / phor / ia good / carry / condition
Definition a positive emotional state	
epilepsy eh-pih-LEP-see	epi / lepsy upon / seize
Definition a disease marked by seizures	
hypomania HAI-poh-MAY-nee-ah	hypo / mania under / excessive anger
Definition a mental state just below mania	
manic depression (bipolar) MAN-ik de-PREH-shun	manic depression excitement depression
Definition a psychiatric disorder characterized by alternating bouts of excitement and depression **Note:** This disease is referred to by the name *bipolar* because the patient fluctuates between two extremes.	
myasthenia mai-as-THEH-nee-ah	my / asthenia muscle / weakness
Definition muscle weakness	

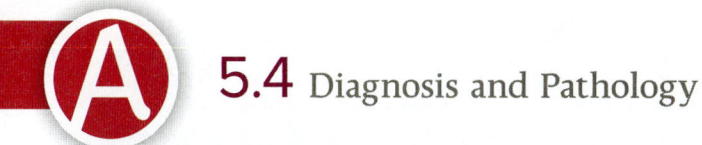

5.4 Diagnosis and Pathology

function *continued*

Term	Word Analysis
narcolepsy NAR-coh-LEP-see	**narco / lepsy** sleep / seize
Definition a disease characterized by sudden, uncontrolled sleepiness	
neurosis neh-ROH-sis	**neur / osis** nerve / condition
Definition a nerve condition	
psychosis sai-KOH-sis	**psych / osis** mind / condition
Definition a mind condition **NOTE:** Both neurosis and psychosis are general terms of psychiatric conditions, but a neurosis doesn't interfere with rational thought or daily functioning; a psychosis involves some sort of break with reality.	
psychopathy sai-KAW-pah-thee	**psycho / pathy** mind / disease
Definition a mental illness	
schizophrenia SKIT-zoh-FREH-nee-ah	**schizo / phren / ia** divide / mind / condition
Definition a mental illness characterized by delusions, hallucinations, and disordered speech **NOTE:** *Schizo* refers to the division in the mind between the mind itself and reality, not the division of the mind into multiple personalities.	

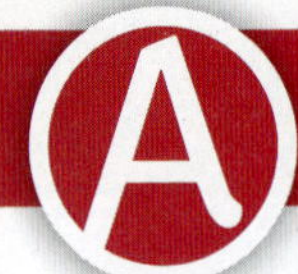

Learning Outcome 5.4 Exercises

PRONUNCIATION

EXERCISE 1 *Break down the following words into syllables.*

EXAMPLE: synesthesia *syn | es | the | sia*

1. gangliitis ______
2. ganglioma ______
3. myelitis ______
4. myelopathy ______
5. myelodysplasia ______
6. meningitis ______
7. myasthenia ______
8. hemorrhagic stroke ______
9. ischemic stroke ______
10. polyneuropathy ______
11. craniomalacia ______
12. craniostenosis ______
13. encephalopathy ______
14. encephalopyosis ______
15. cerebral aneurysm ______
16. cerebral arteriosclerosis ______
17. cerebral atherosclerosis ______

EXERCISE 2 *Indicate which syllable is emphasized when pronounced.*

EXAMPLE: bronchitis bron**chi**tis

1. neuropathy ______
2. anorexia ______
3. autism ______
4. bulimia ______
5. dysphoria ______
6. euphoria ______
7. epilepsy ______
8. neurosis ______
9. psychosis ______
10. psychopathy ______

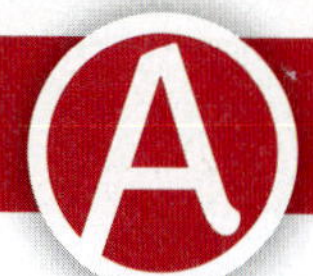

Learning Outcome 5.4 Exercises

TRANSLATION

EXERCISE 3 *Break down the following words into their component parts.*

EXAMPLE: nasopharyngoscope *naso | pharyngo | scope*

1. hypomania ______
2. dysphoria ______
3. euphoria ______
4. psychopathy ______
5. intracerebral ______
6. cerebrovascular ______
7. craniosclerosis ______
8. craniostenosis ______
9. gangliitis ______
10. meningitis ______
11. cerebromeningitis ______
12. encephalitis ______
13. encephalomyelitis ______
14. poliomyelitis ______
15. enchephalopathy ______
16. encephalomyeloneuropathy ______
17. neuroarthropathy ______
18. myelodysplasia ______

EXERCISE 4 *Underline and define the word parts from this chapter in the following terms.*

1. encephalopyosis ______
2. cerebral aneurysm ______
3. cerebral embolism ______
4. craniomalacia ______
5. craniosynostosis ______
6. hydrocephaly ______
7. cerebellitis ______
8. ganglioma ______
9. meningopathy ______
10. meningioma ______
11. meningoencephalitis (2 roots) ______
12. myelitis ______
13. myelopathy ______
14. neuropathy ______
15. polyneuropathy ______
16. amyotrophic lateral sclerosis ______
17. cerebral palsy ______
18. manic depression ______
19. myasthenia ______
20. neurosis ______
21. psychosis ______
22. schizophrenia ______

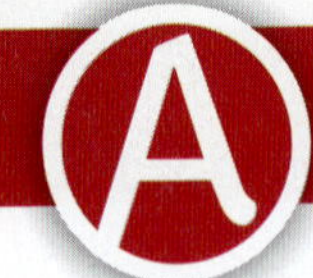

Learning Outcome 5.4 Exercises

EXERCISE 5 *Match the term on the left with its definition on the right.*

_____ 1. autism
_____ 2. bulimia
_____ 3. anorexia
_____ 4. epilepsy
_____ 5. stroke
_____ 6. transient ischemic attack (TIA)
_____ 7. hemorrhagic stroke
_____ 8. narcolepsy
_____ 9. cerebral atherosclerosis
_____ 10. cerebral thrombosis
_____ 11. cerebral arteriosclerosis
_____ 12. cerebrovascular accident (CVA)
_____ 13. ischemic stroke

a. an accident involving the blood vessels of the brain
b. loss of brain function caused by interruption of blood flow/supply to the brain
c. a stroke where the blood loss is caused by the rupture of a blood vessel
d. a stroke where the blood loss is caused by blockage
e. a mini-stroke caused by the blockage of a blood vessel that resolves (goes away) within 24 hours
f. the hardening of an artery in the brain
g. the hardening of an artery in the brain caused by the buildup of fatty plaque
h. the blockage of a blood vessel in the brain caused by a blood clot
i. an eating disorder characterized by overeating and usually followed by forced vomiting
j. an eating disorder characterized by the patient's refusal to eat
k. a psychiatric disorder characterized by the withdrawal from communication with others; the patient is focused only on the self
l. a disease marked by seizures
m. a disease characterized by sudden, uncontrolled sleepiness

EXERCISE 6 *Translate the following terms as literally as possible.*

EXAMPLE: nasopharyngoscope *an instrument for looking at the nose and throat*

1. hypomania _____
2. gangliitis _____
3. meningitis _____
4. meningoencephalitis _____
5. meningopathy _____
6. psychopathy _____
7. encephalopathy _____
8. encephalomyeloneuropathy _____
9. encephalopyosis _____
10. myelodysplasia _____
11. myelopathy _____
12. neuropathy _____

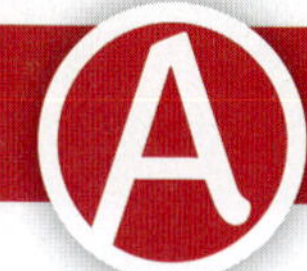

Learning Outcome 5.4 Exercises

13. polyneuropathy ____________________
14. poliomyelitis ____________________
15. dysphoria ____________________
16. euphoria ____________________
17. bulimia ____________________
18. cerebrovascular accident ____________________
19. craniosynostosis ____________________

GENERATION

EXERCISE 7 *Build a medical term from the information provided.*

EXAMPLE: inflammation of the sinuses *sinusitis*

1. ganglion tumor ____________________
2. meninges tumor ____________________
3. inflammation of the spinal cord ____________________
4. inflammation of the cerebellum ____________________
5. inflammation of the brain (*cerebro*) and meninges ____________________
6. inflammation of the brain (use *encephalo*) ____________________
7. inflammation of the brain (*encephalo*) and spinal cord ____________________
8. abnormal narrowing of the skull ____________________
9. literally, *water head condition* ____________________
10. a disease of the blood vessels of the brain ____________________
11. disease of the joint associated with nerves ____________________
12. muscle weakness condition ____________________

EXERCISE 8 *Multiple-choice questions. Select the correct answer.*

1. Anorexia is
   a. a disease marked by seizures
   b. an eating disorder characterized by the patient's refusal to eat
   c. an eating disorder characterized by overeating and usually followed by forced vomiting
   d. a psychiatric disorder characterized by the withdrawal from communication with others
2. Autism is
   a. a disease marked by seizures
   b. an eating disorder characterized by the patient's refusal to eat
   c. an eating disorder characterized by overeating and usually followed by forced vomiting
   d. a psychiatric disorder characterized by the withdrawal from communication with others

A Learning Outcome 5.4 Exercises

3. Epilepsy is
   a. a disease marked by seizures
   b. an eating disorder characterized by the patient's refusal to eat
   c. an eating disorder characterized by overeating and usually followed by forced vomiting
   d. a psychiatric disorder characterized by the withdrawal from communication with others
4. A person who is *narcoleptic* has a disease characterized by sudden, uncontrolled
   a. desire for food
   b. sleepiness
   c. desire for medication
   d. withdrawal into self
5. A person with *cerebral palsy* has paralysis caused by damage to the area of the brain responsible for
   a. emotion
   b. hunger
   c. movement
   d. feeling/sensation
6. A loss of brain function caused by interruption of blood flow/supply to the brain is
   a. stroke
   b. hemorragia
   c. cerebral aneurysm
   d. cerebrovascular disease
   e. intracerebral hemorrhage
7. The widening or abnormal dilation of a blood vessel in the brain is a(n)
   a. stroke
   b. hemorragia
   c. cerebral aneurysm
   d. cerebrovascular disease
   e. intracerebral hemorrhage
8. Excessive bleeding inside the brain is a(n)
   a. stroke
   b. hemorragia
   c. cerebral aneurysm
   d. cerebrovascular disease
   e. intracerebral hemorrhage
9. The common name for this disease is Lou Gehrig's disease.
   a. poliomyelitis
   b. cerebral palsy
   c. encephalomyelitis
   d. amyotrophic lateral sclerosis (ALS)

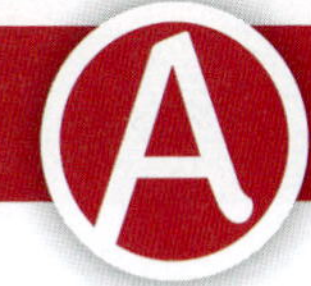

Learning Outcome 5.4 Exercises

10. An alternate term for someone who has *manic depression* is
    a. bipolar
    b. autistic
    c. phrenetic
    d. schizophrenic
11. Which of the following characteristics is *not* displayed by a schizophrenic?
    a. delusions
    b. disordered speech
    c. hallucinations
    d. multiple personalities

EXERCISE 9 *Briefly describe the difference between each pair of terms.*

1. craniomalacia, craniosclerosis ______________________________
2. neurosis, psychosis ______________________________
3. hemorrhagic stroke, ischemic stroke ______________________________
4. ischemic stroke, transient ischemic attack (TIA) ______________________________
5. cerebral arteriosclerosis, cerebral atherosclerosis ______________________________
6. cerebral embolism, cerebral thrombosis ______________________________

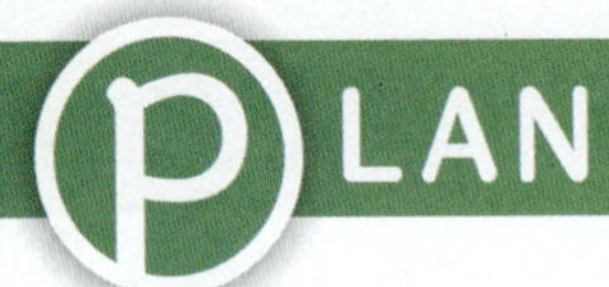

5.5 Treatments and Therapies

There are few medicines that work directly on the neurologic system. The largest class of neurologic medicine works to dull the pain reception from nerves (*anesthetics*). Anesthetics have revolutionized medicine. They may be injected into a small area (*local*), injected into a group of nerves (*epidural*), or even affect the entire body (*general*). In fact, this type of medicine is so critical, there is an entire medical specialty devoted to its use (*anesthesiology*). Another large class of neurologic medicine treats seizures (*anticonvulsants*).

Perhaps one of the fastest-growing areas in drug development has been in the field of psychiatry. There are numerous medicines to treat problems of the mind. Whether they treat depression (*antidepressants*), anxiety (*anxiolytics*), or psychosis (*antipsychotics*), these medicines all work in a similar fashion—by altering the response or availability of the chemicals that allow communication between nerves (*neurotransmitters*). Psychiatric medicines work by increasing or decreasing the activity of specific neurotransmitters that lead to an increase or decrease in activity of certain areas of the brain.

Surgical interventions to treat neurologic disorders can involve direct cutting and cleaning of a partially blocked artery, as in endarterectomy. Treating diseased blood vessels in the brain may also be carried out by less invasive techniques such as radiology guided therapy. In endovascular neurology, medicines are injected into specific areas to cause or destroy clots, depending on the need. Neurosurgery can also be used to treat problems of the nervous system's support structures. These procedures can help remedy skull problems (*cranioplasty*), or to remove part of the vertebral bone (*laminectomy*) or an intervertebral disc (*discectomy*). In cases of hydrocephalus, a special drain can be inserted leading from the brain into another part of the body. Most commonly, the drain is placed in the open area surrounding the inside of the abdomen. This type of shunt is called a ventriculoperitoneal (VP) shunt. Invasive brain surgery may be necessary to remove a tumor, to place a device to monitor the pressure in the brain, to insert a device to treat seizures, or to remove part of a lobe of the brain (*lobectomy*). Nerves have traditionally posed a challenge to repair surgically, but advances are being made that allow for nerves to be reconnected (*neurorrhaphy*).

anesthesia

Term	Word Analysis
anesthetic an-es-THET-ik **Definition** a drug that causes loss of sensation	an / esthetic not / sensation
general anesthetic JIH-nir-al an-es-THET-ik **Definition** anesthetic that causes complete loss of consciousness	general anesthetic
local anesthetic LOH-kal an-es-THET-ik **Definition** anesthetic that does not affect consciousness	local anesthetic
regional anesthetic REE-jih-nal an-es-THET-ik **Definition** anesthetic that is injected into a nerve causing loss of sensation over a particular area	regional anesthetic
topical anesthetic TAW-pih-kal an-es-THET-ik **Definition** local anesthesia applied to the surface of the area to be anesthetized	topical anesthetic
epidural anesthetic eh-pih-DIR-al an-es-THET-ik **Definition** anesthetic applied in the dural region of the spinal cord	epi / dur / al upon / dura

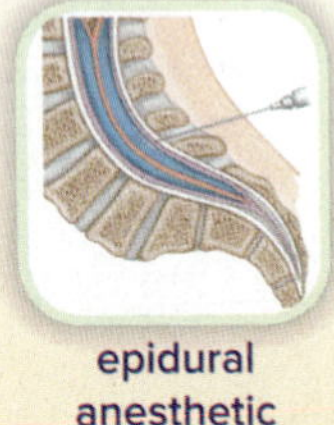

epidural anesthetic

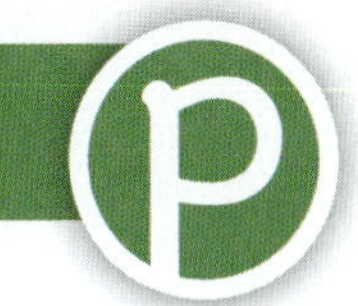

5.5 Treatments and Therapies

drugs

Term	Word Analysis
analgesic an-al-JEE-zik **Definition** a drug that relieves pain	an / alge / sic not / pain / agent
anticonvulsant AN-tee-kon-VUL-sant **Definition** a drug that opposes convulsions	anti / convuls / ant against / convulsion / agent
antidepressant AN-tee-deh-PREH-sant **Definition** a drug that opposes depression	anti / depress / ant against / depression / agent
antipsychotic AN-tee-sai-KAW-tik **Definition** a drug that opposes psychoses	anti / psychot / ic against / psychosis / agent
anxiolytic ANG-zee-oh-LIH-tik **Definition** a drug that lessens anxiety	anxio / lyt / ic anxiety / loss / agent
hypnotic hip-NAWT-ik **Definition** a drug that aids sleep	hypno / tic sleep / agent
neuropharmacology nir-oh-FAR-mah-KAW-loh-jee **Definition** the study of the effects of drugs on the nervous system	neuro / pharmaco / logy nerve / drug / study
psychopharmacology SAI-koh-FAR- mah-KAW-loh-jee **Definition** the study of the effects of drugs on mental processes	psycho / pharmaco / logy mind / drug / study
pyschotropic SAI-koh-TROH-pik **Definition** drugs that are able to turn the mind	psycho / trop / ic mind / turn / agent
thrombolytic THRAWM-boh-LIH-tik **Definition** a drug that dissolves clots	thrombo / lyt / ic clot / loss / agent

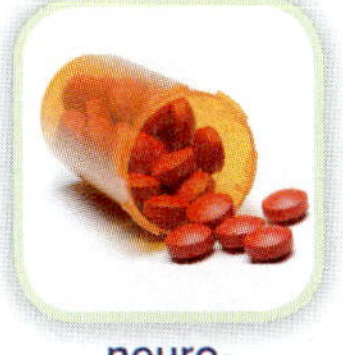
neuro-pharmacology

surgical procedures and treatments

Term	Word Analysis
cerebrotomy sih-ree-BRAW-toh-mee **Definition** incision into the brain	cerebro / tomy brain / incision
chemotherapy KEE-moh-THER-ah-pee **Definition** treatment using chemicals	chemo / therapy chemical / treatment

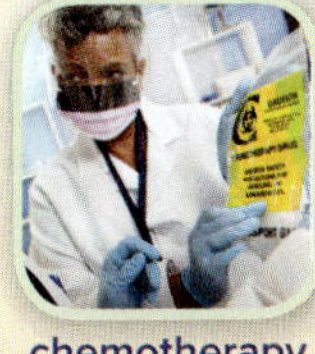
chemotherapy

surgical procedures and treatments *continued*

Term	Word Analysis
craniectomy KRAY-nee-EK-toh-mee **Definition** removal of a piece of the skull	crani / ectomy skull / removal
craniotomy KRAY-nee-AW-toh-mee **Definition** incision into the skull	cranio / tomy skull / incision
endarterectomy EN-dar-tir-EK-toh-mee **Definition** removal of the inside of an artery	end / arter / ectomy inside / artery / removal
endovascular neurosurgery EN-doh-VAS-kyoo-lar NIR-oh-SIR-jir-ee **Definition** surgery on the nervous system performed by entering the body through blood vessels	endo / vascul / ar neuro / surgery inside / vessel / pertaining to nerve / surgery
lobectomy loh-BEK-toh-mee **Definition** removal of a lobe	lob / ectomy lobe / removal
lobotomy loh-BAW-toh-mee **Definition** incision into a lobe	lobo / tomy lobe / incision
neurectomy nir-EK-toh-mee **Definition** removal of a nerve	neur / ectomy nerve / removal
neurolysis nir-AW-lih-sis **Definition** destruction of nerve tissue NOTE: You may wonder why this term is under treatment and not disease; the reason is because one common treatment for chronic nerve pain is to destroy the nerve causing it.	neuro / lysis nerve / loose
neuroplasty NIR-oh-PLAS-tee **Definition** reconstruction of a nerve	neuro / plasty nerve / reconstruction
neurorrhaphy nir-OR-ah-fee **Definition** suturing of a nerve (often the severed ends of a nerve)	neuro / rrhaphy nerve / suture
neurotomy nir-AW-toh-mee **Definition** incision into a nerve	neuro / tomy nerve / incision

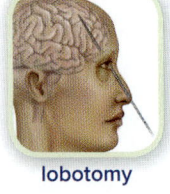

lobotomy

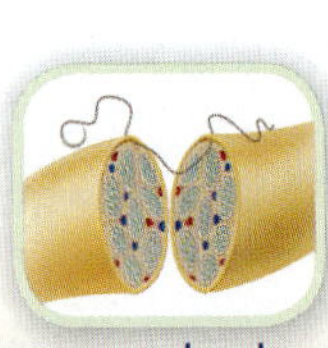

neurorrhaphy

Learning Outcome 5.5 Exercises

PRONUNCIATION

EXERCISE 1 *Break down the following words into syllables.*

EXAMPLE: synesthesia *syn | es | the | sia*

1. anesthetic __________
2. antidepressant __________
3. craniectomy __________
4. craniotomy __________
5. endarterectomy __________
6. neuroplasty __________
7. epidural anesthetic __________
8. thrombolytic __________
9. anticonvulsant __________
10. chemotherapy __________

EXERCISE 2 *Indicate which syllable is emphasized when pronounced.*

EXAMPLE: bronchitis bron**chi**tis

1. hypnotic __________
2. lobotomy __________
3. neurotomy __________
4. cerebrotomy __________
5. lobectomy __________
6. neurectomy __________
7. anxiolytic __________
8. neurolysis __________

TRANSLATION

EXERCISE 3 *Break down the following words into their component parts.*

EXAMPLE: nasopharyngoscope *naso | pharyngo | scope*

1. craniotomy __________
2. lobotomy __________
3. neurotomy __________
4. neurolysis __________
5. neuroplasty __________
6. antipsychotic __________
7. neuropharmacology __________
8. psychopharmacology __________

Learning Outcome 5.5 Exercises

EXERCISE 4 *Underline and define the word parts from this chapter in the following terms.*

1. anesthetic ______________________________
2. epidural ______________________________
3. hypnotic ______________________________
4. psychotropic ______________________________
5. cerebrotomy ______________________________
6. lobectomy ______________________________
7. neurectomy ______________________________
8. craniectomy ______________________________
9. neurorrhaphy ______________________________
10. endovascular neurosurgery ______________________________

EXERCISE 5 *Match the term on the left with its definition on the right.*

e	1. analgesic	a.	anesthetic that causes complete loss of consciousness
f	2. anticonvulsant	b.	anesthetic that does not affect consciousness
g	3. antidepressant	c.	anesthetic that is injected into a nerve, causing loss of sensation over a particular area
h	4. anxiolytic	d.	local anesthesia applied to the surface of the treatment area using chemicals
j	5. chemotherapy	e.	a drug that relieves pain
k	6. endarterectomy	f.	a drug that opposes convulsions
a	7. general anesthetic	g.	a drug that opposes depression
b	8. local anesthetic	h.	a drug that lessens anxiety
c	9. regional anesthetic	i.	a drug that dissolves clots
i	10. thrombolytic	j.	treatment using chemicals
d	11. topical anesthetic	k.	removal of the inside of an artery

EXERCISE 6 *Translate the following terms as literally as possible.*

EXAMPLE: nasopharyngoscope *an instrument for looking at the nose and throat*

1. anesthetic ______________________________
2. craniectomy ______________________________
3. lobotomy ______________________________
4. neurotomy ______________________________
5. neurolysis ______________________________
6. neurorrhaphy ______________________________
7. neuropharmacology ______________________________
8. psychopharmacology ______________________________

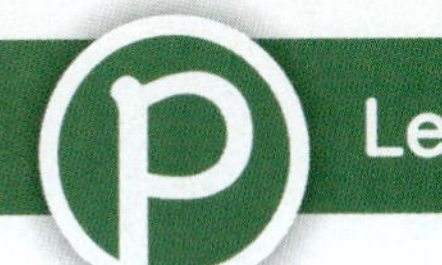

Learning Outcome 5.5 Exercises

GENERATION

EXERCISE 7 *Build a medical term from the information provided.*

EXAMPLE: inflammation of the sinuses *sinusitis*

1. sleep agent ______
2. brain incision ______
3. skull incision ______
4. lobe removal ______
5. nerve removal ______
6. nerve reconstruction ______
7. chemical treatment ______
8. anesthetic applied in the dural region of the spinal cord ______
9. a drug (literally, *agent*) that opposes psychosis ______

EXERCISE 8 *Multiple-choice questions. Select the correct answer.*

1. *Endovascular neurosurgery* is surgery on the nervous system performed by entering the body through
   a. the heart
   b. the spine
   c. nerve tissue
   d. blood vessels
2. A medical professional may recommend which drug to relieve pain?
   a. analgesia
   b. anxiolytic
   c. general anesthetic
   d. thrombolytic
3. The root *trope* in the term *psychotropic* means
   a. to turn
   b. to lessen
   c. to oppose
   d. to remove
4. Which term means *the removal of the inside of an artery*?
   a. endarterectomy
   b. subarterectomy
   c. endarterotomy
   d. subarterotomy

EXERCISE 9 *Briefly describe the difference between each pair of terms.*

1. anticonvulsant, antidepressant ______
2. anxiolytic, thrombolytic ______
3. general anesthetic, local anesthetic ______
4. regional anesthetic, topical anesthetic ______

5.6 Abbreviations

Abbreviations provide medical professionals with a shorthand for writing words that commonly occur in their field. In neurology and psychiatry, these abbreviations can refer to things ranging from procedures (EEG), to common diagnoses (MS), to parts of the system itself (CNS).

nervous system abbreviations

Abbreviation	Definition
ADHD	attention-deficit hyperactivity disorder
ALS	Lou Gehrig's disease (amyotrophic lateral sclerosis)
CNS	central nervous system
CP	cerebral palsy
CSF	cerebrospinal fluid
CVA	cerebrovascular accident
EEG	electroencephalogram
EMG	electromyogram
HD	Huntington's disease
ICP	intracranial pressure
LOC	level of consciousness
LP	lumbar puncture
MRA	magnetic resonance angiography
MS	multiple sclerosis
OCD	obsessive compulsive disorder
PET	positron emission tomography
PNS	peripheral nervous system
SRS	stereotactic radiosurgery
TIA	transient ischemic attack

Learning Outcome 5.6 Exercises

EXERCISE 1 *Define the following abbreviations.*

1. ADHD ____________
2. MS ____________
3. TIA ____________
4. ALS ____________
5. CSF ____________
6. PET ____________
7. LOC ____________
8. ICP ____________
9. PNS ____________
10. CP ____________

EXERCISE 2 *Give the abbreviations for the following definitions.*

1. lumbar puncture ____________
2. central nervous system ____________
3. obsessive compulsive disorder ____________
4. magnetic resonance angiography ____________
5. cerebrovascular accident ____________
6. electromyogram ____________
7. electroencephalogram ____________
8. stereotactic radiosurgery ____________
9. Lou Gehrig's disease ____________
10. Huntington's disease ____________

EXERCISE 3 *Multiple-choice questions. Select the correct answer.*

1. Problems with which part of the body can result in a person having problems sending or receiving signals to the brain?
   a. CNS c. PET
   b. CSF d. PNS
2. Problems with which part of the body can affect the entire body?
   a. CNS c. PET
   b. CSF d. PNS
3. Which of the following medical procedures is used as a treatment or therapy?
   a. EEG c. MRA
   b. LP d. SRS
4. A person who has an accident involving the blood vessels of the brain has a(n)
   a. CVA c. MS
   b. CNS d. PNS
5. A mini-stroke caused by the blockage of a blood vessel that resolves within 24 hours is a(n)
   a. ICP c. ADHD
   b. LOC d. TIA
6. A procedure used to examine the electrical activity of the brain is a(n)
   a. CSF c. EEG
   b. CVA d. EMG

5.7 Electronic Health Records

S Subjective

Mrs. Voxenhead is here for follow-up for her schizophrenia. At her last visit, she complained of dystonia on her haloperidol. I changed her to a newer antipsychotic, and she is here today to follow up the results. Overall, her condition is improved, and she has not had any new hallucinations. Her only concern today is recent insomnia (the past week). She noticed the insomnia started when she began a new job. She says that learning her new job has been stressful. She has been anxious at night, and that has made it hard for her to sleep.

O Objective

General: Flat affect. Nonagitated. Mood is not dysphoric. Alert, oriented.

HEENT: Pupils equal, round, and reactive to light. Tonsils normal size.

Resp: Clear to auscultation.

CV: RRR without murmur, gallop, rubs.

Neuro: Normal movement. No dyskinesia. Normal tone.

A Assessment

1. Schizophrenia: Stable on new medical regimen.
2. Insomnia. Likely related to new job stress.

P Plan

1. I will begin her short term on an anxiolytic.
2. Continue antipsychotic.
3. Follow-up visit in 2 months.
4. Continue following up with psychologist.

–Electronically signed by
Dale Kelly, MD
03/04/2015 9:30 AM

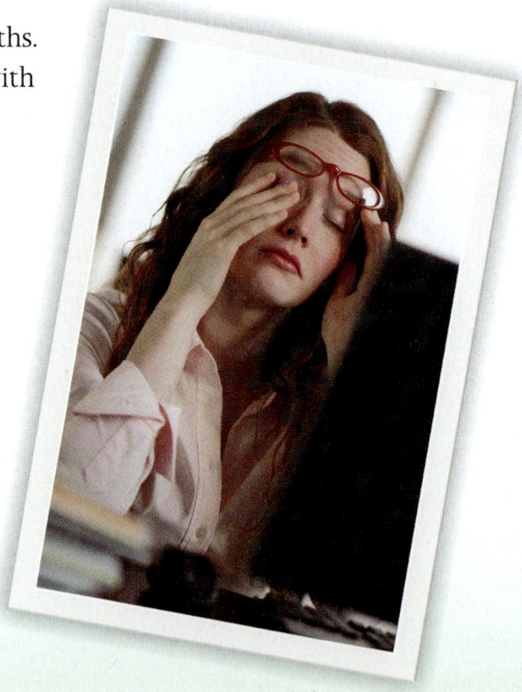

Learning Outcome 5.7 Exercises

EXERCISE 1 *Match the term on the left with its definition on the right.*

	Term		Definition
______	1. schizophrenia	a.	a drug that opposes psychosis
______	2. dystonia	b.	a condition characterized by involuntary muscle movements
______	3. antipsychotic	c.	a mental illness characterized by delusions, hallucinations, and disordered speech
______	4. insomnia	d.	inability to sleep
______	5. dysphoric	e.	a negative emotional state
______	6. dyskinesia	f.	a condition characterized by involuntary muscle movements
______	7. anxiolytic	g.	a drug that lessens anxiety
______	8. psychologist	h.	a doctor who specializes in the study of the mind

EXERCISE 2 *Refer to the document on the previous page and fill in the blanks.*

1. Mrs. Voxenhead is following up on her *schizophrenia* (give definition: ______________________).
2. Her mood is not characterized as ______________________ (negative emotional state).
3. Learning her new job has made Mrs. Voxenhead stressed; this is likely related to her *insomnia* (give definition: ______________________).
4. Mrs. Voxenhead will continue to follow up with a(n) ______________________ (doctor who specializes in the study of the mind).

EXERCISE 3 *True or false questions. Refer to the document on the previous page and indicate true answers with a T and false answers with an F.*

1. The patient suffers from a mental illness characterized by hallucinations. ______
2. Mrs. Voxenhead complained of involuntary muscle movements during her last visit. ______
3. The antipsychotic has helped her sleep much better. ______
4. Mrs. Voxenhead will continue to follow up with a psychopharmacologist. ______

EXERCISE 4 *Multiple-choice questions. Refer to the document on the previous page and select the correct answer.*

1. An *anxiolytic* and *antipsychotic* are both
   a. drugs that lessen and/or oppose
   b. drugs that increase and/or heighten
   c. drugs that remove sensation
2. The plan for treating Mrs. Voxenhead is to
   a. discontinue her antipsychotic and begin an anxiolytic
   b. continue her antipsychotic and begin an anxiolytic
   c. discontinue her anxiolytic and begin an antipsychotic
   d. continue her anxiolytic and begin an antipsychotic
3. The medical professional who wrote the health record for Mrs. Voxenhead is Dale Kelly, MD. Dr. Kelly is a
   a. psychologist
   b. psychiatrist
   c. psychogenist
   d. neuropharmacologist

Emergency Department Visit

Patient Name: Manuel Skayken

Chief Complaint: Confusion, fever.

History of Present Illness:

Manuel Skayken is a 15-year-old boy who presents with a 2-day history of fever to 104°F. He has been more lethargic today and his headache has worsened. He has **photophobia** and his parents are concerned that he is acting abnormally. He is not using his right arm and legs as much as his left. He appears **ataxic** in his gait and has been **hypersomnolent** at home. His parents are concerned that he is not responding to questions normally.

Past Medical History: **Somnambulation,** otherwise noncontributory.

Medications: None.

Allergies: NKDA.

Social History: Lives at home with his parents.

Sophomore in high school. A/B student. Nonsmoker.

Surgical History: None.

Physical Exam:

RR: 30; HR: 98; Temp: 104.2; BP: 88/60

Gen: WDWN. Lethargic.

Confused and disoriented.

HEENT: PERRLA, mild **nystagmus.**

Neck: Stiff.

CV: Mildly fast heart rate. No murmurs.

Resp: Clear.

GI: Normal.

Neuro: CN II-XII grossly intact; DTRs normal.

Hemiparesis: Strength in right arm and leg.

Failed mini-mental status exam.

Emergency Department Course:

Manuel was driven to the emergency room by his parents. On arrival, he appeared very confused, though not agitated. With his encephalopathic picture, we were most worried about **psychotropic** drug abuse or infection. A normal urine drug screen and a CBC with an elevated WBC count were suspicious for infection. Because **encephalitis** and **meningitis** were the main concerns, we performed a **lumbar puncture.** The opening pressure was consistent with elevated **intracranial pressure.** The **CSF** showed an elevated WBC count. The culture is pending. Shortly after his lumbar puncture, Manuel had a tonic-clonic **seizure.** We treated him with an **anticonvulsant** and the seizure stopped. The **electroencephalogram** showed paroxysmal lateral epileptiform discharges (PLEDs), which are characteristic of herpes encephalitis. The pediatric team was called, and they admitted him to the PICU.

Learning Outcome 5.7 Exercises

EXERCISE 5 *Match the term on the left with its definition on the right.*

	Term		Definition
h	1. anticonvulsant	a.	excessive sensitivity to light
d	2. encephalitis	b.	lack of coordination
e	3. meningitis	c.	drugs that are able to turn the mind
g	4. EEG	d.	inflammation of the brain
c	5. psychotropic	e.	inflammation of the meninges
f	6. ICP	f.	intracranial pressure
a	7. photophobia	g.	electroencephalography
b	8. ataxia	h.	a drug that opposes convulsions

EXERCISE 6 *Refer to the document on the previous page and fill in the blanks.*

1. The patient's gait has been ______________________________ (lacking coordination).
2. The root word in *hypersomnolent* is ______________________________ (sleep).
3. Manuel has mild ______________________ (involuntary back and forth eye movements).
4. The root word in *encephalopathic* is *encephalo,* which means ______________________.
5. The term *intracranial* comes from combining ________ (inside) and *cranio,* which means ______.

EXERCISE 7 *True or false questions. Refer to the document on the previous page and indicate true answers with a T and false answers with an F.*

1. Manuel has not been sleeping as much as usual at home. ______
2. The medical professionals worried that Manuel was abusing drugs. ______
3. Because of their concern about encephalitis and meningitis, the health professionals performed an LP. ______
4. In response to his seizure, Manuel was given a thrombolytic. ______

Learning Outcome 5.7 Exercises

EXERCISE 8 *Multiple-choice questions. Select the correct answer.*

1. *Photophobia* is defined as
   a. fear of fire
   b. excessive sensitivity to light
   c. fear of pictures
   d. fear of outdoor spaces
2. A seizure characterized by alternating bouts of muscle spasms and weak or unresponsive muscles is
   a. tonic
   b. clonic
   c. tonic-clonic
   d. ischemic
3. *Hemiparesis* is defined as
   a. partial paralysis on half of the body
   b. complete paralysis on half of the body
   c. partial paralysis of one limb
   d. complete paralysis of one limb
4. The health professionals were concerned about the possibility of which two conditions?
   a. inflammation of the brain and the membrane surrounding the brain and spinal cord
   b. inflammation of the brain and spinal cord
   c. inflammation of the spinal cord and the tough outer membrane surrounding the brain and spinal cord
   d. inflammation of the spinal cord and the membrane surrounding the brain and spinal cord
5. Which procedures were used to assist in the diagnosis and treatment of the patient?
   a. LP, EEG
   b. CSF, EEG
   c. LP, CSF
   d. EEG, LP, ICP
   e. ICP, LP, CSF

Brief Admission Summary Letter

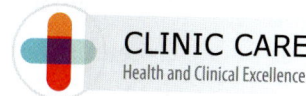

Dear Dr. Dowling,

This letter is to inform you that your patient Sally Chia has been admitted to Bed 4 of the ICU for observation and treatment of recent cerebrovascular accident. As you know, I have been following Mrs. Chia for cerebrovascular disease. She has had two transient ischemic attacks in the past 2 years and underwent a carotid endarterectomy last February. She presented to the ED last night with a sudden onset of left-sided hemiparesis and hyperesthesia. She was also noted to have mild agnosia and aphasia. She was brought to the ED by her husband, who is not sure when the symptoms began. A cerebral CT and CT angiogram showed middle cerebral artery occlusion and ruled out intracranial hemorrhage or hematoma. She was treated with a thrombolytic. Her symptoms have improved.

—I. C. Hilliard, MD

Learning Outcome 5.7 Exercises

EXERCISE 9 *Match the term on the left with its definition on the right.*

b 1. hemiparesis	a. inability to comprehend
a 2. agnosia	b. partial paralysis on half of the body
d 3. hyperesthesia	c. cerebrovascular accident
e 4. aphasia	d. increased sensation
c 5. CVA	e. inability to speak
f 6. TIA	f. a mini-stroke caused by the blockage of a blood vessel that resolves (goes away) within 24 hours

EXERCISE 10 *Fill in the blanks.*

1. Last February, Mrs. Chia underwent a carotid ______________ (removal of the inside of an artery).
2. She was treated with a *thrombolytic* (give definition: ______________).
3. Mrs. Chia's CT scans ruled out *intracranial* (inside the ______________) hemorrhage or ______________ (a tumor-like mass made up of blood).

EXERCISE 11 *True or false questions. Indicate true answers with a T and false answers with an F.*

1. The patient suffered a recent CVA. ________
2. Mrs. Chia has had two TIAs in the past 2 years. ________
3. Dr. Hilliard is writing to Dr. Dowling to inform him that his patient, Mrs. Chia, may have a brain tumor. ________

EXERCISE 12 *Multiple-choice questions. Select the correct answer.*

1. The medical professionals took a CT of her
   - a. brain
   - b. spine
   - c. nerves
   - d. meninges
2. Which symptom was *not* displayed by the patient?
   - a. inability to comprehend
   - b. inability to speak
   - c. increased sensation
   - d. complete paralysis on half of the body
3. A transient ischemic attack is caused by
   - a. blockage of a blood vessel
   - b. inflammation of the blood vessels
   - c. inflammation of the brain
   - d. tumor in the brain
4. Dr. Hilliard has been following the patient for a disease of the blood vessels of the brain, which is called
   - a. cerebrovascular accident
   - b. cerebrovascular disease
   - c. cerebral arteriosclerosis
   - d. cerebral atherosclerosis

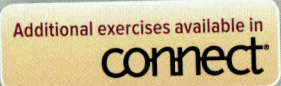

Chapter Review exercises, along with additional practice items, are available in Connect!

Quick Reference

quick reference glossary of roots and suffixes

Term	Definition	Term	Definition
-asthenia	weakness	**-mania**	excessive desire
cephal/o	head	**mening/o, meningi/o**	meninges; membrane surrounding the brain and spinal cord
cerebell/o	cerebellum	**myel/o**	spinal cord, bone marrow
cerebr/o	brain	**neur/o**	nerve
crani/o	head, skull	**-paresis**	slight or partial paralysis
dur/o	tough outer membrane surrounding the brain and spinal cord	**phas/o**	speech
encephal/o	brain	**-phobia**	excessive fear
esthesi/o	feeling, sensation	**phren/o**	mind
gangli/o	nerve bundle	**-plegia**	paralysis
gnosi/o	know	**psych/o**	mind
hypn/o	sleep	**somn/o, somn/i**	sleep
kinesi/o	movement, motion	**tax/o**	arrangement, order, coordination
lob/o	lobe	**ton/o**	muscle tone, tension

quick reference glossary of terms

Term	Definition
acrophobia	fear of heights
afferent nerve	a nerve that carries impulses toward the central nervous system
agnosia	inability to comprehend
agoraphobia	fear of outdoor spaces
amyotrophic lateral sclerosis (ALS)	a degenerative disease of the central nervous system causing loss of muscle control; also known as Lou Gehrig's disease
analgesic	a drug that relieves pain
anesthesiologist	doctor who specializes in anesthesiology
anesthetic	a drug that causes loss of sensation
anorexia	an eating disorder characterized by the patient's refusal to eat
anosmia	lack of a sense of smell
anticonvulsant	a drug that opposes convulsions

quick reference glossary of terms *continued*

Term	Definition
antidepressant	a drug that opposes depression
antipsychotic	a drug that opposes psychosis
anxiolytic	a drug that lessens anxiety
apathy	lack of emotion
aphasia	inability to speak
ataxia	lack of coordination
atopognosis	inability to locate a sensation
autism	a psychiatric disorder characterized by the withdrawal from communication with others. The patient is focused only on the self
bulimia	an eating disorder characterized by overeating and usually followed by forced vomiting
catatonia	condition characterized by reduced muscle tone
causalgia	painful sensation of burning
cephalalgia	head pain
cephalodynia	head pain
cerebellitis	inflammation of the cerebellum
cerebral aneurysm	the widening or abnormal dilation of a blood vessel in the brain
cerebral angiography	procedure used to examine blood vessels in the brain
cerebral arteriosclerosis	the hardening of an artery in the brain
cerebral atherosclerosis	the hardening of an artery in the brain caused by the buildup of fatty plaque
cerebral atrophy	wasting away of brain tissue
cerebral embolism	the blockage of a blood vessel in the brain caused by a foreign object (embolus) such as fat or bacteria
cerebral palsy	paralysis caused by damage to the area of the brain responsible for movement
cerebral thrombosis	the blockage of a blood vessel in the brain caused by a clot
cerebromeningitis	inflammation of the brain and meninges
cerebrotomy	incision into the brain
cerebrovascular accident (CVA)	an accident involving the blood vessels of the brain
cerebrovascular disease	a disease of the blood vessels of the brain
chemotherapy	treatment using chemicals
clonus	muscle spasm or twitching
cranial hematoma	a hematoma beneath the skull
craniectomy	removal of a piece of the skull

quick reference glossary of terms *continued*

Term	Definition
craniomalacia	abnormal softening of the skull
craniosclerosis	abnormal hardening of the skull
craniostenosis	abnormal narrowing of the skull
craniosynostosis	the premature fusing of the skull bones
craniotomy	incision into the skull
delirium	brief loss of mental function
dementia	loss/decline in mental function
duritis	inflammation of the dura
dysesthesia	bad feeling
dyskinesia	difficulty moving
dyslexia	difficulty reading
dysphasia	difficulty speaking
dysphoria	a negative emotional state
dystonia	condition characterized by involuntary muscle movements
echoencephalography	procedure used to examine the brain using sound waves
efferent nerve	a nerve that carries impulses away from the central nervous system
electroencephalography (EEG)	procedure used to examine the electrical activity of the brain
encephalalgia	brain pain
encephalitis	inflammation of the brain
encephalocele	hernia of the brain (normally through a defect in the skull)
encephalography	procedure for studying the brain
encephalomyelitis	inflammation of the brain and spinal cord
encephalomyeloneuropathy	disease of the brain, spinal cord, and nerves
encephalopathy	disease of the brain
encephalopyosis	a pus-filled abscess in the brain
endarterectomy	removal of the inside of an artery
endovascular neurosurgery	surgery on the nervous system performed by entering the body through blood vessels
epidural anesthetic	anesthetic applied in the dural region of the spinal cord
epidural hematoma	a hematoma located on top of the dura
epilepsy	a disease marked by seizures
euphoria	a positive emotional state
gangliitis	inflammation of the ganglion

quick reference glossary of terms *continued*

Term	Definition
ganglioma	ganglion tumor
general anesthetic	anesthetic that causes complete loss of consciousness
hematoma	a tumor-like mass made up of blood
hemiparesis	partial paralysis on half of the body
hemiplegia	paralysis on half the body
hemorrhagic stroke	a stroke where blood loss is caused by the rupture of a blood vessel
hydrocephaly	abnormal accumulation of spinal fluid in the brain
hydrophobia	fear of water
hyperesthesia	increased sensation
hyperkinesia	increase in muscle movement or activity
hypnotic	a drug that aids sleep
hypomania	a mental state just below mania
idiopathic	having no known cause or origin
insomnia	inability to sleep
interictal	time between seizures
intracerebral hematoma	a hematoma located inside the brain
intracerebral hemorrhage	excessive bleeding inside the brain
ischemic stroke	a stroke where blood loss is caused by a blockage
kleptomania	desire to steal
lobectomy	removal of a lobe
lobotomy	incision into a lobe
local anesthetic	any anesthetic that does not affect consciousness
lumbar puncture (LP)	inserting a needle into the lumbar region of the spine in order to collect spinal fluid
macrocephaly	abnormally large head
magnetic resonance angiography (MRA)	procedure used to examine blood vessels
manic depression (bipolar)	a psychiatric disorder characterized by alternating bouts of excitement and depression
meningioma	tumor of the meninges
meningitis	inflammation of the meninges
meningocele	a hernia of the meninges
meningoencephalitis	inflammation of the meninges and brain
meningopathy	disease of the meninges

quick reference glossary of terms *continued*

Term	Definition
microcephaly	abnormally small head
monoparesis	partial paralysis of one limb
monoplegia	paralysis of one limb
myasthenia	condition characterized by muscle weakness
myelitis	inflammation of the spinal cord
myelocele	a hernia of the spinal cord
myelodysplasia	defective formation of the spinal cord
myelogram	image of the spinal cord, usually done using x-ray
myelomalacia	abnormal softening of the spinal cord
myelomeningocele	a hernia of the spinal cord and meninges
myelopathy	disease of the spinal cord
myoclonus	muscle twitching
myospasm	involuntary muscle contraction
narcolepsy	a disease characterized by sudden, uncontrolled sleepiness
neuralgia	nerve pain
neurasthenia	nerve weakness
neurectomy	removal of a nerve
neuritis	nerve inflammation
neuroarthropathy	disease of the joint associated with nerves
neurodynia	nerve pain
neuroencephalomyelopathy	disease of the nerves, brain, and spinal cord
neurogenic	originating from/created by nerves
neuroglycopenia	deficiency of sugar that interferes with normal brain activity
neurolysis	destruction of nerve tissue
neuroma	a nerve tumor
neuropathy	disease of the nervous system
neuropharmacology	the study of the effects of drugs on the nervous system
neuroplasty	reconstruction of a nerve
neurorrhaphy	suturing of a nerve (often the severed ends of a nerve)
neurosclerosis	hardening of nerves
neurosis	a nerve condition
neurotomy	incision into a nerve
nystagmus	involuntary back and forth eye movements

quick reference glossary of terms *continued*

Term	Definition
paralysis	complete loss of sensation and motor function
paresis	partial paralysis characterized by varying degrees of sensation and motor function
paresthesia	abnormal sensation (usually numbness or tingling in the skin)
photophobia	excessive sensitivity to light
poliomyelitis	inflammation of the gray matter of the spinal cord
polyneuritis	inflammation of multiple nerves
polyneuropathy	disease affecting multiple nerves
positron emission tomography (PET) scan	an imaging procedure that uses radiation (positrons) to produce cross sections of the brain
postictal	time after a seizure
preictal	time before a seizure
prosopagnosia	inability to recognize faces
pseudoesthesia	false sensation
psychiatrist	doctor who specializes in treatment of the mind
psychiatry	branch of medicine that focuses on the treatment of the mind
psychogenic	originating in/created by the mind
psychologist	doctor who specializes in the study of the mind
psychology	branch of medicine that focuses on the study of the mind
psychopathy	a mental illness
psychopharmacology	the study of the effects of drugs on mental processes
psychosis	a mind condition (involves some sort of break with reality interfering with rational thought or daily functioning)
psychosomatic	pertaining to the relationship between the body and the mind
psychotropic	drugs that are able to turn the mind
pyromania	desire to set fires
regional anesthesia	anesthetic that is injected into a nerve causing loss of sensation over a particular area
schizophrenia	a mental illness characterized by delusions, hallucinations, and disordered speech
somnambulism	sleep walking
stroke	loss of brain function caused by interruption of blood flow/supply to the brain
subdural hematoma	a hematoma located beneath the dura
syncope	fainting; losing consciousness due to temporary loss of blood flow to the brain
synesthesia	condition where one sensation is experienced as another

quick reference glossary of terms *continued*

Term	Definition
thrombolytic	a drug that dissolves clots
tonic	pertaining to muscle tone (normally weak or unresponsive)
tonic-clonic seizure	a seizure characterized by both a tonic and a clonic phase
topical anesthetic	local anesthesia applied to the surface of the area to be anesthetized
transcranial Doppler sonography	an imaging technique that produces an image of the brain using sound waves sent through the skull
transient ischemic attack (TIA)	a mini-stroke caused by the blockage of a blood vessel that resolves (goes away) within 24 hours

review of terms by roots

Term	Term(s)	
-asthenia	myasthenia neurasthenia	
cephal/o	cephalalgia cephalodynia hydrocephaly	macrocephaly microcephaly
cerebell/o	cerebellitis	
cerebr/o	cerebral aneurysm cerebral angiography cerebral arteriosclerosis cerebral atherosclerosis cerebral embolism cerebral palsy cerebral thrombosis	cerebromeningitis cerebrotomy cerebrovascular accident cerebrovascular disease intracerebral hematoma intracerebral hemorrhage
crani/o	cranial hematoma craniectomy craniomalacia craniosclerosis	craniostenosis craniosynostosis craniotomy transcranial Doppler sonography
dur/o	duritis epidural anesthetic	epidural hematoma subdural hematoma
encephal/o	echoencephalography electroencephalography encephalalgia encephalitis encephalocele encephalography	encephalomyelitis encephalomyeloneuropathy encephalopathy encephalopyosis meningoencephalitis neuroencephalomyelopathy
esthesi/o	anesthesiologist anesthetic dysesthesia epidural anesthetic general anesthetic hyperesthesia	local anesthetic parasthesia pseudesthesia regional anesthetic synesthesia topical anesthetic

review of terms by roots

Term	Term(s)	
gangli/o	gangliitis ganglioma	
gnosi/o	agnosia atopognosis prosopagnosia	
hypn/o	hypnotic	
kinesi/o	hyperkinesia dyskinesia	
lob/o	lobectomy lobotomy	
-mania	hypomania kleptomania	manic depression (bipolar) pyromania
mening/o, meningi/o	cerebromeningitis meningioma meningitis meningocele	meningoencephalitis meningopathy myelomeningocele
myel/o	encephalomyelitis encephalomyeloneuropathy myelitis myelocele myelodysplasia myelogram	myelomalacia myelomeningocele myelopathy neuroencephalomyelopathy poliomyelitis
neur/o	encephalomyeloneuropathy endovascular neurosurgery neuralgia neurasthenia neurectomy neuritis neuroarthropathy neurodynia neuroencephalomyelopathy neurogenic neuroglypenia	neurolysis neuroma neuropathy neuropharmacology neuroplasty neurorrhaphy neurosclerosis neurosis neurotomy polyneuritis polyneuropathy
-paresis	hemiparesis monoparesis	
phas/o	aphasia dysphasia	
-phobia	acrophobia agoraphobia	hydrophobia photophobia
phren/o	schizophrenia	
-plegia	hemiplegia monoplegia	

review of terms by roots

Term	Term(s)	
psych/o	antipsychotic psychiatrist psychiatry psychogenic psychologist psychology	psychopathy psychopharmacology psychosis psychosomatic psychotropic
somn/o	insomnia somnambulism	
tax/o	ataxia	
ton/o	catatonia dystonia	tonic tonic-clonic seizure

other terms

afferent nerve	hematoma
amyotrophic lateral sclerosis (ALS)	hemorrhagic stroke
analgesic	idiopathic
anorexia	interictal
anosmia	ischemic stroke
anticonvulsant	lumbar puncture (LP)
antidepressant	magnetic resonance angiography (MRA)
anxiolytic	myoclonus
apathy	myospasm
autism	narcolepsy
bulimia	nystagmus
causalgia	paralysis
clonus	paresis
delirium	positron emission tomography (PET) scan
dementia	postictal
dyslexia	preictal
dysphoria	stroke
efferent nerve	syncope
endarterectomy	thrombolytic
epilepsy	transient ischemic attack (TIA)
euphoria	

The Sensory System—Ophthalmology and Otolaryngology

6

Introduction and Overview of Sensory Organs

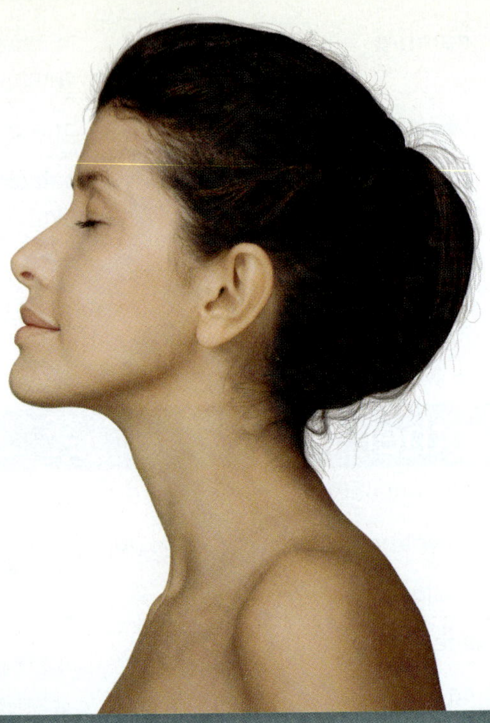

You are standing at a music festival listening to live music. The feeling is electric and the experience is unforgettable. What makes it so memorable? The sound is fantastic, but you could download the music. The sights are great. The band is in top form and everyone around you is excited. However, you could watch and hear it all online. There are distinct smells. Many of them are unpleasant, but for some reason, as part of a whole, they are acceptable. You feel the bass. You sweat as you dance. Overall, the experience is far greater than the parts. Why is that the case? Your brain processes each component of these things and integrates them into a whole. Yet each sense is important in defining the experience. The function of the sensory system is collecting specific details about the surroundings and sending the information on to the central nervous system.

Sensory organs and cells are found throughout your entire body. As mentioned before, your skin is your largest sensory organ. It contains thousands upon thousands of cells sending information to your brain, including information about pain, pressure, and temperature. Your most complex sensory organs, however, are your eyes and ears. They provide you with a wealth of information about the world around you.

learning outcomes

Upon completion of this chapter, you will be able to:

- **6.1** Identify the **roots/word parts** associated with the **sensory system.**
- (S) **6.2** Translate the **Subjective** terms associated with the **sensory system.**
- (O) **6.3** Translate the **Objective** terms associated with the **sensory system.**
- (A) **6.4** Translate the **Assessment** terms associated with the **sensory system.**
- (P) **6.5** Translate the **Plan** terms associated with the **sensory system.**
- **6.6** Use **abbreviations** associated with the **sensory system.**
- **6.7** Distinguish terms associated with the **sensory system** in the context of **electronic health records.**

6.1 Word Parts of the Sensory System

Word Roots Associated with the Eye

OUTER STRUCTURES AND VISION

The eye (*oculo*) is a very valuable but vulnerable organ. There are many protective structures around the eye that help keep it safe and wet. The eye rests in a socket made of seven connecting bones in the skull. This socket is also known as the orbit. Just outside the eye are a set of eyelids (*blepharo*) that protect the eyes from dust and other floating particles in the air. In addition, eyelids aid in keeping the eye moist. It is extremely important for the eye to remain wet. For this reason, there are additional structures that help keep the eye moist. The lacrimal gland is a small gland that sits just above and to the side of the eye. It produces tears that stream across the eye and keep it wet. Finally, the eyes and eyelids are lined with a thin invisible membrane known as the conjunctiva.

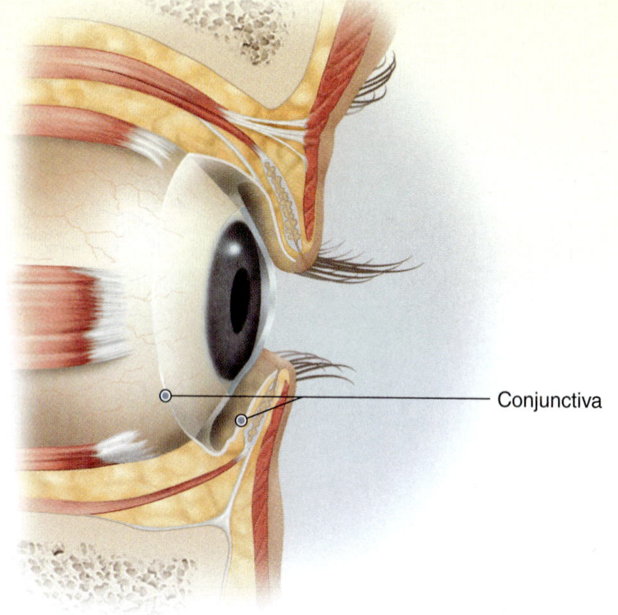

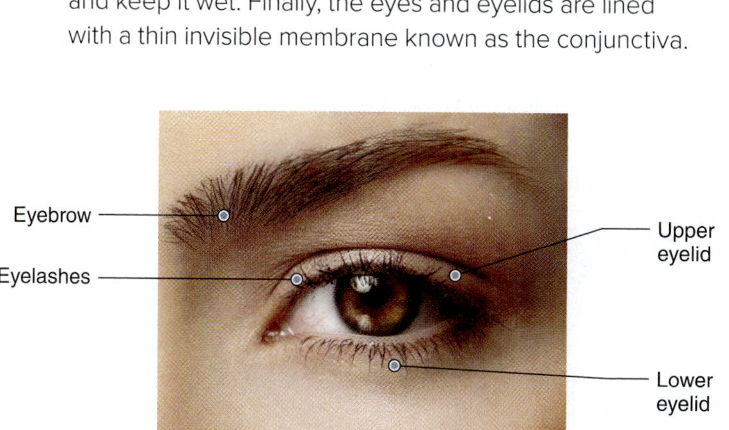

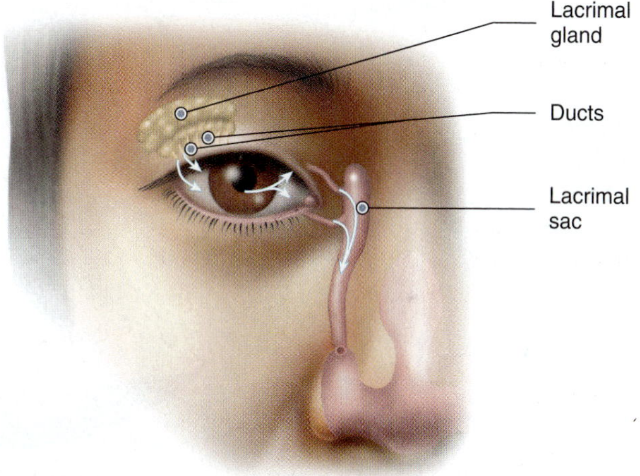

eye

ROOTS: ***ocul/o, ophthalm/o, opt/o***

EXAMPLES: oculopathy, ophthalmologists, optometrist

NOTES: It might sound nitpicky, but *ophthalmo* has two *h*s, not one. Many people think the root is *OPthalmo* but it is actually *OPHthalmo*.

Some people think the word *antler* comes from the Latin phrase *ante ocular,* which means *in front of the eye,* because that is where the horns grow on deer and cows.

vision condition

SUFFIXES: ***-opia, -opsia***

EXAMPLES: hyperopia, akinetopsia

NOTES: Akinetopsia = *a* + *kinet* + *-opsia* = no movement vision condition. It refers to a condition where patients are unable to see objects in motion.

tear

ROOTS: ***lacrim/o, dacry/o***

EXAMPLES: lacrimation, dacryorrhea

NOTES: Often the term *lacrimal* is used interchangeably for the word *tear.* Keep in mind that the lacrimal gland and the tear gland refer to the same thing.

Although it isn't the origin of the term, you may find it easy to remember that *dacryo* means *tear* because it has the word *cry* in the middle of it—daCRYo.

eyelid

ROOT: ***blephar/o***

EXAMPLES: blepharedema, blepharoplasty

NOTES: Blepharoplasty = *blepharo* + *plasty* = surgical reconstruction of the eyelid.

Also, remember that the *ph* is pronounced *f.* The word is ble*ph*aroplasty, *not* bleparoplasty.

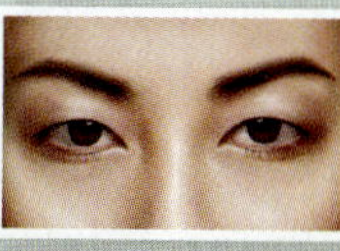

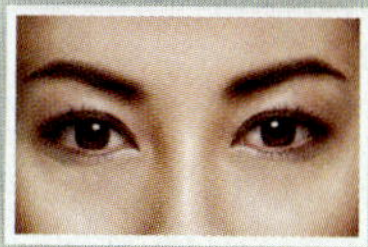

SCLERA AND CORNEA

An eye is like a video camera with three layers. The outermost layer includes the *sclera* and the *cornea*. The *sclera* is the white part of the eye—a dense, protective layer, like the hard shell on the outside of the video camera. The *cornea* is a clear surface in the middle of the eye. Like the glass on a video camera, the cornea protects the lens and begins the work of focusing light to the back of the eye.

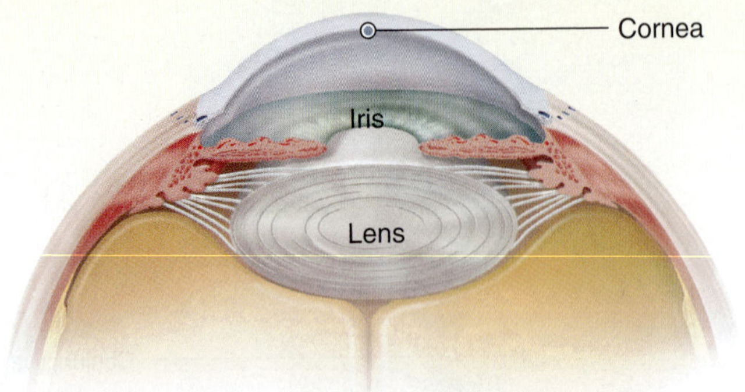

cornea

ROOTS: ***corne/o, kerat/o***

EXAMPLES: corneal transplant, keratitis

NOTES: *Kerato* is a tricky root because it has multiple meanings. In the context of the eye, *kerato* means *cornea*. In the context of the skin, *kerato* refers to a horny texture to the skin. What's the connection? *Kerato* comes from a Greek word meaning *horn* (think of a rhinoCEROS) and *corneo* comes from a Latin word meaning *horn* (think of a CORNUcopia, a horn of plenty). Apparently someone thought the cornea of the eye looked like a horn.

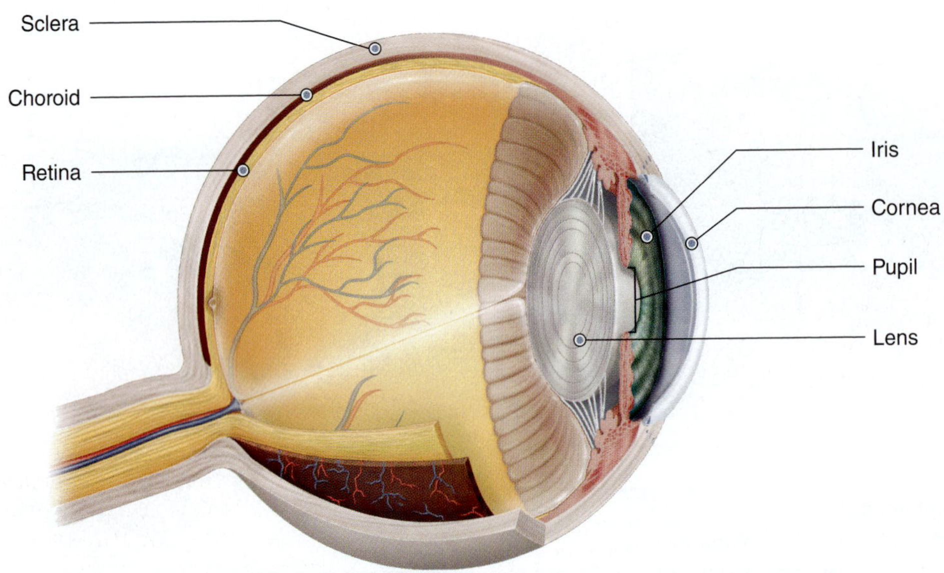

conjunctiva

ROOT: ***conjunctiv/o***

EXAMPLE: conjunctivitis

NOTES: The *conjunctiva* is a clear membrane that covers the sclera and lines the eyelids. The root comes from two Latin words, *con* (with/together) and *junct* (join). Evidently, someone thought it joined the eye to the rest of body.

sclera (the white of the eye)

ROOT: ***scler/o***

EXAMPLE: scleritis

NOTES: Just like *kerato,* sclera has multiple meanings. In other contexts, *sclero* means *hard* and can refer to the abnormal hardening of any tissue or organ. In the eye, it refers to the white, tough, and fibrous protective covering of the eye. Words having to do with the eye use *sclero* in both ways:

phacosclerosis = *phaco* + *scler* + *osis* = an abnormal hardening of the lens

scleromalacia = *sclero* + *malacia* = an abnormal softening of the sclera

CHOROID AND RETINA

The next layer down is the *choroid.* It includes the *lens,* which gathers light and focuses on images in the same way a lens on a camera does. The choroid also includes the *iris* and the *ciliary muscles.*

The iris is what gives eyes their color. By expanding (*dilating*) or shrinking (*constricting*) the pupils, the irises control how much light hits the back of the eye.

The ciliary muscles adjust the shape of the eye and lens to focus on near or far objects. As light passes through the lens, it passes through liquid in the eye (*vitreous*) that bends the light and aims it to the back of the eyeball—all the way to the deepest layer, the *retina,* which is the eye's image processor. The retina helps turn visual stimuli into electric signals. The collected information is then sent to the brain by electric signals along the optic nerve.

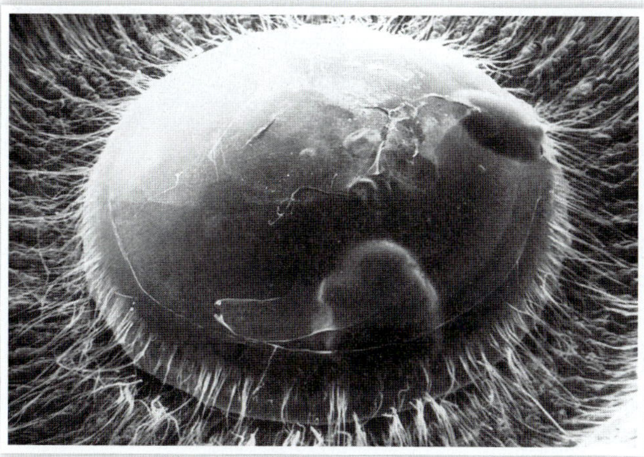

An up-close picture of the eye's lens.

vitreous liquid (also called vitreous humor)

ROOT: ***vitre/o***

EXAMPLES: vitreous liquid, vitrectomy

NOTES: The root *vitreo* means *glass* and refers to the liquid in the eye that helps focus light on the back of the retina.

You're probably more familiar with the root *vitreo* in the term *in vitro fertilization.* This is the scientific word for a test-tube baby, an embryo that is fertilized not in the body but *in vitro,* which means *in a glass tube.*

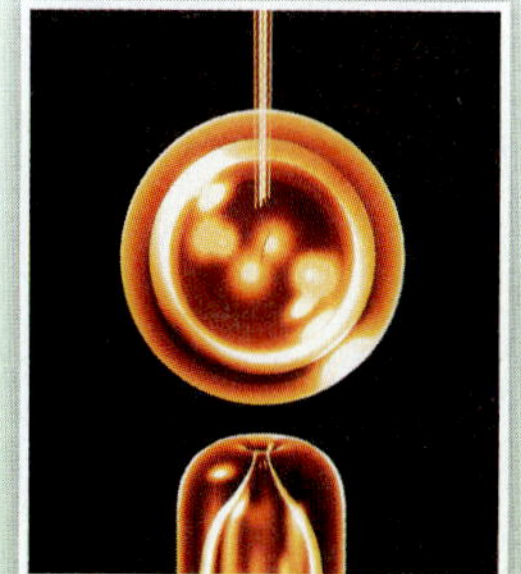

ciliary body

ROOT: ***cycl/o***

EXAMPLE: cycloplegia

NOTES: The ciliary body is a circle of tissue surrounding the lens. One of its primary jobs is to change the shape of the lens of the eye in order to allow the eye to maintain focus, a process called accommodation. Someone who can't read things close up without the help of glasses has ciliary bodies that are unable to sufficiently focus their lenses. When this happens in old age, it is called *presbyopia.*

retina

ROOT: ***retin/o***

EXAMPLES: retinitis, retinoscope

NOTES: *Retina* comes from a word that means *net;* it refers to the netlike pattern of light-sensitive tissue on the inside surface of the eye.

iris

ROOTS: ***ir/o, irid/o***

EXAMPLES: iritis, iridalgia

NOTES: The iris is the colored part of the eye. It is responsible for adjusting the size of the pupil to control the amount of light that enters the eye.

In Greek mythology, Iris was a female messenger of the gods. She was the personification of the rainbow, which is why her name was given to the colored part of the eye.

lens

ROOTS: ***phac/o, phak/o***

EXAMPLES: phacoscope, phakitis

NOTES: *Phaco* is a Greek word meaning *lentil,* a type of bean, which is where we get the word *lens.* Notice that *phaco* can be spelled with a c (*phaco*) or a *k* (*phako*). Because c sounds like *s* before i and e, the *k* sound is used sometimes to be sure the syllable is pronounced hard. For example, *phacitis* could be pronounced fah-SAI-tis. To avoid confusion, the word is sometimes spelled *phakitis* so it is pronounced fah-KAI-tis.

Word Roots Associated with the Ear

THE EAR AND HEARING

Ears work like stereo speakers in reverse. While stereo speakers turn electrical signals into sounds (*acouso, audio*), ears (*auro, oto*) turn sounds into electrical signals. First, they collect sounds. Next, they turn the energy from the sound into movement, and then they convert them again into electrical signals. Last, they send the signals to the brain, where it all gets sorted out into meaning.

ear

ROOTS: ***aur/o, ot/o***

EXAMPLES: aural, otoscope

NOTES: If you learn better by hearing something than by reading it, then you are an *aural learner.* It's easy to confuse *aural* with *oral.* But since *oral* means *mouth,* we guess an oral learner would be someone who learns by eating.

Also, the root *oto* is pronounced OH- toh, not AW-toh. An instrument a doctor uses to look in the ear is called an *otoscope,* which is pronounced OH-toh-skohp, not AW-toh-skohp.

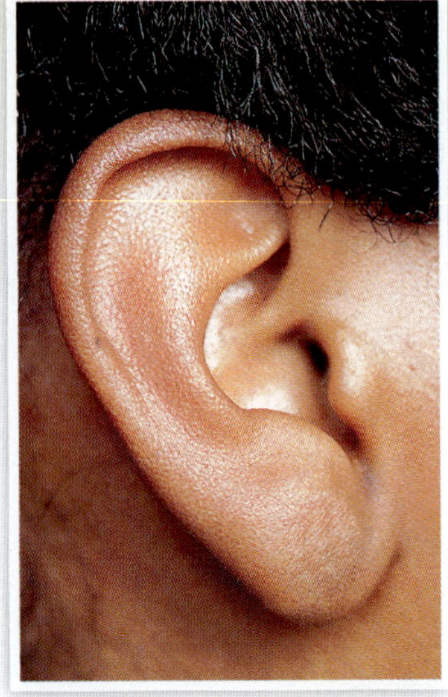

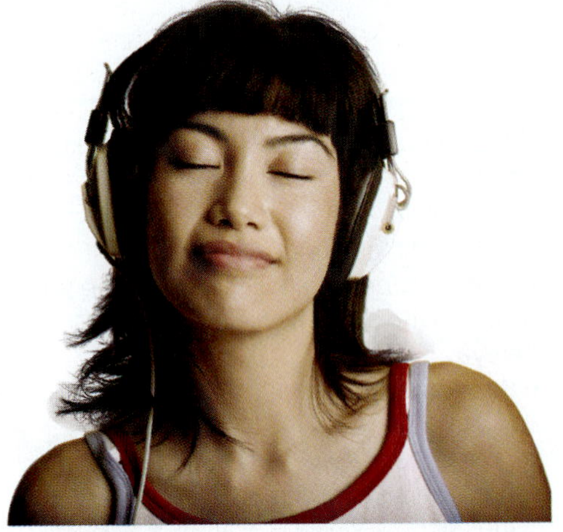

sound, hearing

ROOTS: ***acous/o, audi/o***

EXAMPLES: acoustic, audiogram

NOTES: Sound travels at 768 miles per hour. That's about 12 miles per minute, or about 1 mile every 5 seconds. Light, however, travels a lot faster—186,282 miles per second, which is about 5.6 million miles per minute, or more than 335 million miles per hour. That's why you see a flash of lightning before you hear the thunder.

hearing condition

SUFFIX: ***-acusis***

EXAMPLES: hyperacusis, osteoacusis

NOTES: Have you ever wondered why your voice sounds different to you than it does to other people, or why you seem to sound different when you hear a recording of yourself? That's because of *osteoacusis* (*osteo* + *-acusis* = bone hearing condition). When you speak, your voice passes through the air and hits other people's eardrums. But it reaches your own ear in two very different ways—through the air, as it does for others, but also through the bones of your head, which is why you can hear yourself talk even if you plug your ears. Sound waves travel differently through bone than through air, so your voice sounds different to you than it does to other people.

OUTER/MIDDLE EAR

There are three main divisions of the ear: the outer ear, the middle ear, and the inner ear.

The outer ear includes the *pinna* and the *ear canal.* The pinna is what we first think of when we think about the ear—it's the fleshy part we pierce, tug on, and cover up in the winter. The pinna sits on the mastoid bone of the skull. Its funnel shape helps collect sounds from the air and send it down the ear canal toward the eardrum (*tympanic membrane*).

The eardrum is part of the middle ear and is a very important structure. It turns sound waves into physical energy. To keep the eardrum free from interference, the body protects it from both sides. From the outside, the ear canal produces ear wax (*cerumen*). Despite its gross appearance, ear wax is very helpful—it is a natural antibiotic and also a lubricant that keeps the ear canal moist. On the other side of the eardrum is a drainage system. The middle ear is connected to the nose and throat through a tube (*salpinx*). This tube helps drain the ear of any fluid and keeps the pressure inside the middle ear the same as outside the ear. Your eardrum is attached to three bones that make up the rest of the middle ear. These bones are the *incus, stapes,* and *malleus* (anvil, stirrup, and hammer). When the eardrum moves, these tiny bones move too. They transfer their movement to the inner ear.

ear wax

ROOT: ***cerumin/o***

EXAMPLE: ceruminolysis

NOTES: Remember: *C* is pronounced like an *s* before *e* and *i* and like a *k* before *a, o,* and *u.* So *cerumen* is pronounced SEH-roo-men.

eustachian tube

ROOT: ***salping/o***

EXAMPLE: rhinosalpingitis

NOTES: *Salpingo* is derived from the Latin word *salpinx,* which means *trumpet.* It refers to the long, straight kind used by Roman legions in battle, not the curvy kind with keys that is used today. This is important because *salpingo* is used in two body systems: in the ear, referring to the eustachian tubes, and in the female reproductive system, referring to the fallopian tubes. Both have long, tubelike shapes. And what are eustachian tubes? They connect the middle ear to the throat. Hold your nose, close your mouth, and blow. You'll make your eardrum pop by forcing air into your middle ear through the eustachian tubes. Ear infections occur when the eustachian tubes are prevented from draining fluid out of the middle ear.

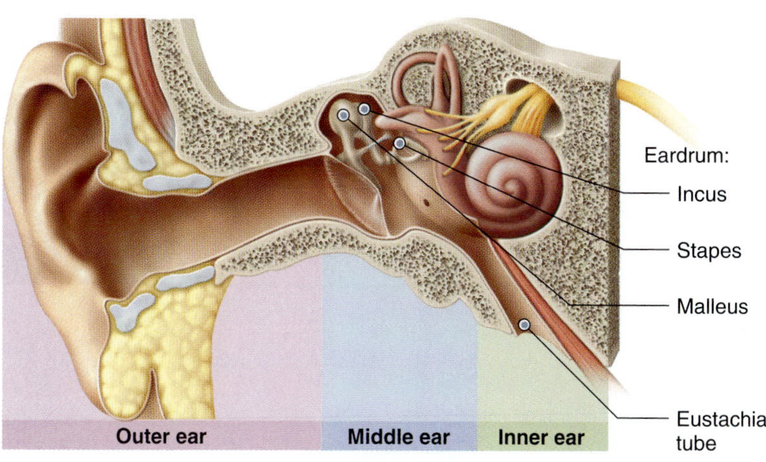

eardrum

ROOTS: ***tympan/o, myring/o***

EXAMPLES: tympanostomy, myringotomy

NOTES: The root *tympano* comes from a Greek word meaning *drum.* Orchestras' big kettle drums are called *tympany,* so *eardrum* is not a bad translation. If you take a peek inside someone's ear sometime, you'll probably agree that it does resemble a drum.

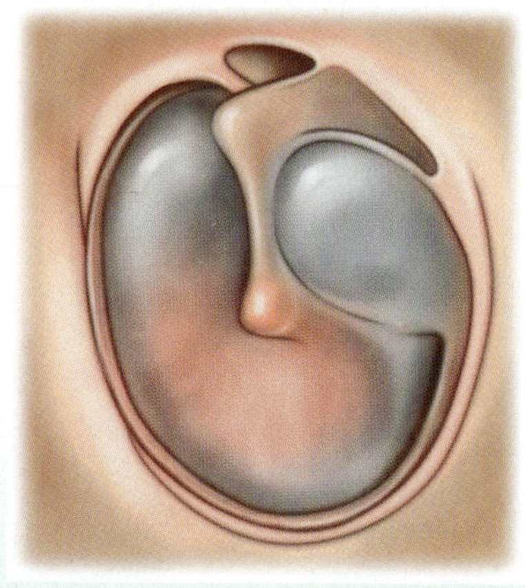

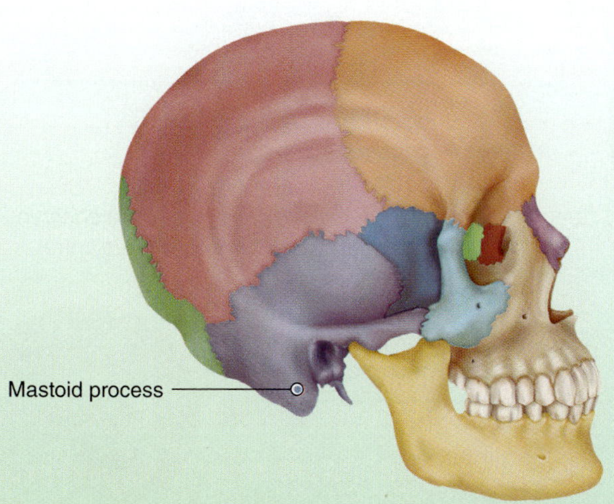

mastoid process

ROOT: ***mastoid/o***

EXAMPLE: mastoiditis

NOTES: Put your hand on the protruding part of your skull behind your ear—that's the mastoid process. It sticks out from the side rear portion of the skull. Its name comes from *mast* (breast) + *oid* (resembling) = resembling a breast.

INNER EAR

The bones of the middle ear are connected to the *cochlea,* a shell-shaped organ in your inner ear (*labyrinth*) filled with fluid and hair. When the *stapes* (pronounced STAY-peez) moves, it presses on the cochlea and causes the fluid to move. Just as the ocean waters move through seaweed, when the fluid moves, the hairs bend. The hairs, which are connected to the nervous system, create an electric signal carried by the *acoustic nerve* to the brain. Finally, the brain receives and processes the electric signals.

The inner ear also has another critical job: helping maintain balance. The *vestibular system* sends information to the brain about the tilt, rotation, and motion of the head. Like the cochlea, it is made up of small canals filled with fluid and hair. These hairs are moved not by sound but by movement and head angle. This helps maintain balance and also allows the brain to coordinate movement with the eyes.

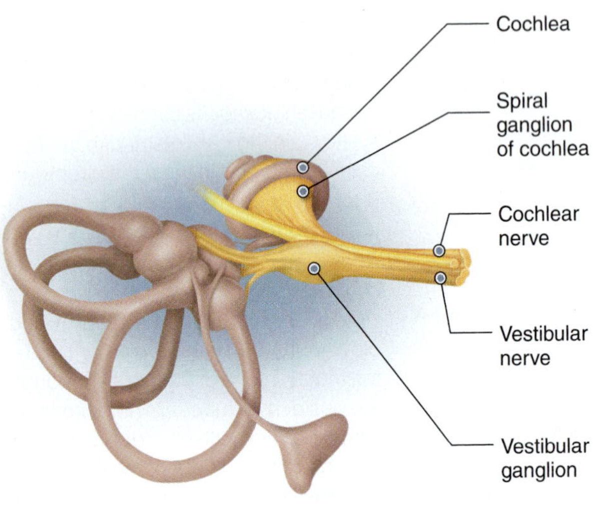

labyrinth

ROOT: ***labyrinth/o***

EXAMPLE: labyrinthitis

NOTES: The *labyrinth* is the innermost part of the ear. It contains two structures: the *cochlea,* which controls hearing, and the *vestibular system,* which controls balance.

The term *labyrinth* comes from Greek mythology. It is the name of an elaborate maze built by King Minos to imprison the Minotaur, a half-man, half-bull creature.

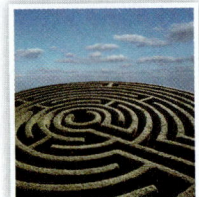

vestibule

ROOT: ***vestibul/o***

EXAMPLE: vestibulitis

NOTES: The term *vestibule* literally means the lobby of a building. Sometimes church lobbies are called vestibules. In medicine, *vestibule* refers to a small space at the beginning of a canal. In the ear, it refers to the area in front of semicircular canals (hence the name); it contains structures that help regulate balance.

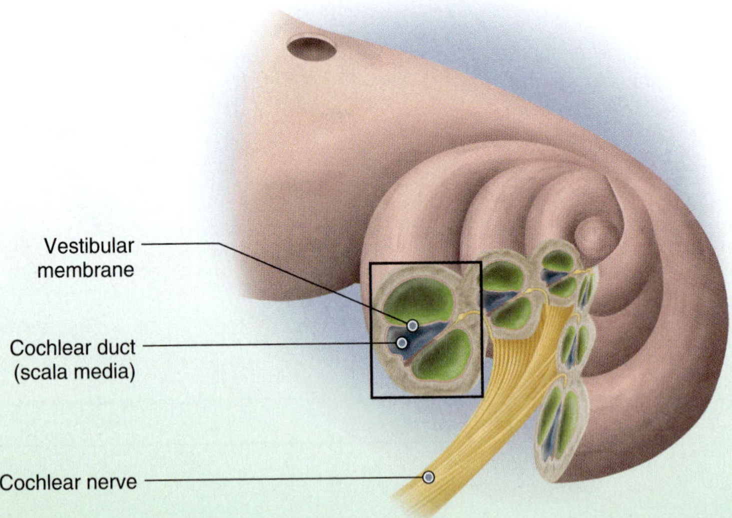

cochlea

ROOT: ***cochle/o***

EXAMPLE: cochleitis

NOTES: From Greek, for *snail shell,* the *cochlea* (pronounced KOH-klee-ah) is a spiral, snail shell–shaped tube in the inner ear that contains hearing receptors.

Learning Outcome 6.1 Exercises

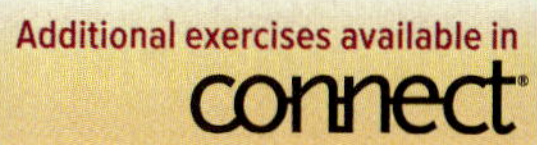

TRANSLATION

EXERCISE 1 *Match the word part on the left with its definition on the right.*

____	1. ophthalm/o	a. eye
____	2. dacry/o	b. eye condition
____	3. -opia	c. eyelid
____	4. blephar/o	d. tear

EXERCISE 2 *Translate the following word parts.*

1. opt/o ____________________
2. ocul/o ____________________
3. -opsia ____________________
4. opthalm/o ____________________
5. blephar/o ____________________
6. dacry/o ____________________
7. lacrim/o ____________________

EXERCISE 3 *Break down the following words into their component parts and translate.*

EXAMPLE: sinusitis *sinus | itis* *inflammation of the sinuses*

1. optic ____________________
2. oculopathy ____________________
3. ophthalmitis ____________________
4. blepharitis ____________________
5. hyperopia ____________________
6. dacryorrhea ____________________

EXERCISE 4 *Match the word part on the left with its definition on the right.*

____	1. retin/o	a. ciliary body
____	2. corne/o	b. conjunctiva
____	3. conjunctiv/o	c. cornea
____	4. scler/o	d. iris
____	5. ir/o	e. lens
____	6. vitre/o	f. retina
____	7. phac/o	g. sclera
____	8. cycl/o	h. vitreous liquid

EXERCISE 5 *Translate the following roots.*

1. corne/o ____________________
2. retin/o ____________________
3. irid/o ____________________
4. conjunctiv/o ____________________
5. ir/o ____________________
6. phac/o ____________________
7. cycl/o ____________________
8. kerat/o ____________________
9. phak/o ____________________

Learning Outcome 6.1 Exercises

EXERCISE 6 *Break down the following words into their component parts and translate.*

> EXAMPLE: sinusitis *sinus | itis* *inflammation of the sinuses*

1. corneal transplant ______
2. conjunctivitis ______
3. iritis ______
4. scleromalacia ______
5. retinopathy ______
6. keratopathy ______
7. cyclotomy ______
8. phacoscope ______
9. iridalgia ______
10. vitrectomy ______
11. sclerokeratitis ______

EXERCISE 7 *Match the word part on the left with its definition on the right. Some definitions will be used more than once.*

______	1. audi/o	a. ear
______	2. -acusis	b. hearing condition
______	3. acous/o	c. sound
______	4. aur/o	
______	5. ot/o	

EXERCISE 8 *Translate the following word parts.*

1. -acusis ______
2. acous/o ______
3. aur/o ______
4. audi/o ______
5. ot/o ______

EXERCISE 9 *Break down the following words into their component parts and translate.*

> EXAMPLE: sinusitis *sinus | itis* *inflammation of the sinuses*

1. audiologist ______
2. hyperacusis ______
3. hypoacusis ______
4. otalgia ______
5. otoscope ______
6. acoustic neuroma ______

Learning Outcome 6.1 Exercises

EXERCISE 10 *Match the word part on the left with its definition on the right.*

a	1. cochle/o	a. cochlea
g	2. vestibul/o	b. eardrum
e	3. labyrinth/o	c. ear wax
f	4. mastoid/o	d. eustachian tube
b	5. myring/o	e. labyrinth
c	6. cerumin/o	f. mastoid process
d	7. salping/o	g. vestibule

EXERCISE 11 *Translate the following word parts.*

1. cochle/o ______
2. mastoid/o ______
3. vestibul/o ______
4. labyrinth/o ______
5. tympan/o ______
6. cerumin/o ______
7. myring/o ______
8. salping/o ______

EXERCISE 12 *Break down the following words into their component parts and translate.*

EXAMPLE: sinusitis *sinus | itis* *inflammation of the sinuses*

1. cochleitis ______
2. labyrinthitis ______
3. vestibulitis ______
4. myringitis ______
5. mastoidalgia ______
6. salpingoscope ______
7. ceruminoma ______
8. tympanometry ______
9. labyrinthectomy ______
10. myringodermatitis ______

GENERATION

EXERCISE 13 *Identify the word parts from this chapter for the following terms.*

1. ambiopia ______
2. ophthalmologist ______
3. blepharospasm ______
4. lacrimation ______
5. oculomycosis ______
6. optomyometer ______
7. hemianopsia ______
8. dacryohemorrhea ______
9. optokinetic ______

EXERCISE 14 *Build a medical term from the information provided.*

1. surgical reconstruction of the eye (use *ocul/o*) ______
2. surgical reconstruction of the eyelid ______
3. disease of the eye (use *ophthalm/o*) ______
4. specialist in measuring the eye (use *opt/o*) ______
5. weak vision condition (use *-opia*) ______
6. tear stone (use *dacry/o*) ______
7. inflammation of the optic nerve ______

Learning Outcome 6.1 Exercises

EXERCISE 15 *Identify the word parts from this chapter for the following terms.*

1. corneal xerosis ________________
2. keratomalacia ________________
3. retinopexy ________________
4. cycloplegia ________________
5. iridemia ________________
6. phacoemulsification ________________
7. aphakia ________________
8. blepharoconjunctivitis ________________
9. sclerokeratoiritis ________________

EXERCISE 16 *Build a medical term from the information provided.*

1. inflammation of the lens (use *phak/o*) ________________
2. inflammation of the conjunctiva ________________
3. inflammation of the cornea (use *kerat/o*) ________________
4. inflammation of the ciliary body and cornea (use *kerat/o*) ________________
5. inflammation of the iris and ciliary body (use *irid/o*) ________________
6. inflammation of the sclera and iris (use *ir/o*) ________________
7. lens softening (use *phac/o*) ________________
8. incision into the retina ________________
9. incision into the sclera ________________

EXERCISE 17 *Identify the word parts from this chapter for the following terms.*

1. otitis media ________________
2. aural ________________
3. audiogram ________________
4. auditory prosthesis ________________
5. pneumatic otoscopy ________________
6. osteoacusis ________________
7. otoneurology ________________

EXERCISE 18 *Build a medical term from the information provided.*

1. pertaining to the ear (use *aur/o*) ________________
2. pertaining to sound/hearing (use *acous/o*) ________________
3. surgical reconstruction of the ear (use *ot/o*) ________________
4. ear hardening condition (use *ot/o*) ________________
5. procedure for looking in the ear (use *ot/o*) ________________
6. procedure for measuring hearing (use *audi/o*) ________________
7. instrument for measuring hearing (use *audi/o*) ________________

Learning Outcome 6.1 Exercises

EXERCISE 19 *Identify the word parts from this chapter for the following terms.*

1. tympanic perforation ______
2. cochlear implant ______
3. mastoidectomy ______
4. ceruminolysis ______
5. vestibular neuritis ______
6. myringomycosis ______
7. salpingopharyngeal ______

EXERCISE 20 *Build a medical term from the information provided.*

1. inflammation of the mastoid ______
2. inflammation of the cochlea ______
3. ear wax condition ______
4. surgical reconstruction of the eardrum (use *myring/o*) ______
5. surgical reconstruction of the eardrum (use *tympan/o*) ______
6. incision into the vestibule ______
7. incision into the labyrinth ______
8. instrument for looking at the eustachian tubes ______

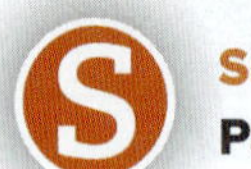

Subjective

Patient History, Problems, Complaints

Eye	Ear
Vision conditions	Hearing conditions
Outer structures and vision	Outer/middle ear
Sclera	Inner ear
Choroid/retina	

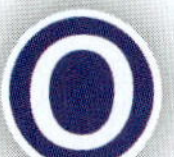

Objective

Observation and Discovery

Eye	Ear
Diagnostic procedures	Diagnostic procedures
Professional terms	Professional terms
Outer structures and vision	Outer ear
Sclera	Middle ear
Choroid/retina	

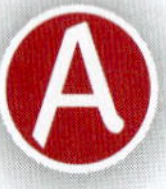

Assessment

Diagnosis and Pathology

Eye	Ear
Outer structures and vision	Outer ear
Sclera	Middle ear
Choroid/retina	Inner ear

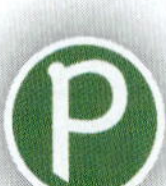

Plan

Treatments and Therapies

Eye	Ear
Outer structures and vision	Outer ear
Sclera	Middle ear
Choroid/retina	Inner ear

This section contains medical terms built from the roots presented in the previous section. The purpose of this section is to expose you to words used in ophthalmology and otolaryngology that are built from the word roots presented earlier. The focus of this book is to teach you the process of learning roots and translating them in context. Each term is presented with the correct pronunciation, followed by a word analysis that breaks down the word into its component parts, a definition that provides a literal translation of the word, as well as supplemental information if the literal translation deviates from its medical use.

The terms are organized using a health care professional's SOAP note (first introduced in Chapter 2) as a model.

SUBJECTIVE

6.2 Patient History, Problems, Complaints

The Eye

When a patient goes to a health clinic for an eye problem, often the problem deals with a change in vision. While many people think of vision problems only in terms of either nearsightedeness (*myopia*) or farsightedness (*hyperopia*), vision problems can also be much more specific in nature. For example, a patient could have blindness in half of her field of vision (*hemianopsia*).

Complaints relating to the tear glands are very common as well. Excessive tearing (*dacrorrhea*) or excessive dryness (*xerophthalmia*) can both cause a patient discomfort.

Patients may also experience problems with their eyelids. An eyelid twitch (*blepharospasm*) is not serious, but it can be very uncomfortable and distracting.

As with any part of the body, patients can experience pain in their eyes. The pain may be generalized

6.2 Patient History, Problems, Complaints

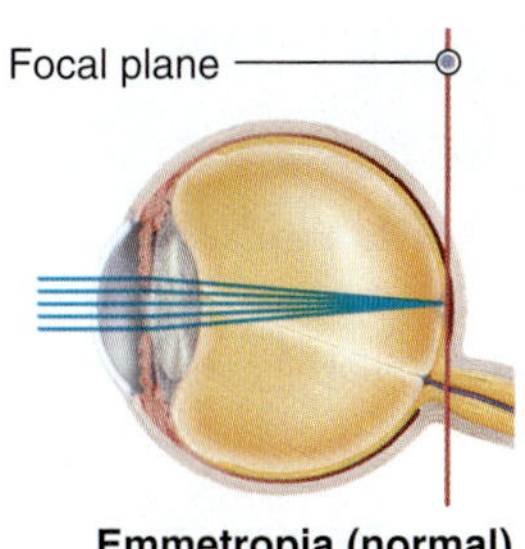

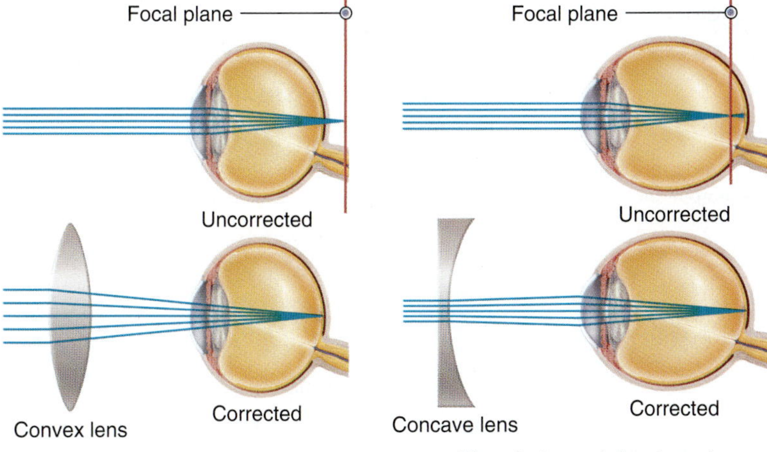

(*ophthmalgia*) or specific to a part of the eye (*iridalgia* or *keratalgia*). Finally, patients may notice that their pupils are either large (*mydriasis*) or small (*miosis*).

The Ear

A change in hearing, like a change in vision, is a common ear complaint. A patient may complain of decreased (*hypoacusis*) or increased (*hyperacusis*) sensitivity to sound. Patients might also complain of ringing in the ears (*tinnitus*). Ear pain (*otalgia/ otodynia*) and discharge (*otorrhea*) are especially common in children with ear infections. Pain in the mastoid (*mastoidalgia*) may indicate a dangerous spread of the ear infection into the mastoid bone. *Vertigo* is a severe form of dizziness that often indicates problems with the patient's inner ear.

eye

Term	Word Analysis
Vision Conditions—Opias	
akinetopsia uh-KEE-nah-TOP-see-ah **Definition** inability to see objects in motion	a / kinet / opsia no / movement / vision condition
ambiopia AM-bee-OH-pee-ah **Definition** double vision	ambi / opia both / vision condition
amblyopia AM-blih-OH-pee-ah **Definition** decreased vision; when it occurs in one eye, it is referred to as *lazy eye*	ambly / opia dull / vision condition
asthenopia AS-then-OH-pee-ah **Definition** weak vision (i.e., eye strain)	asthen / opia weak / vision condition
diplopia dih-PLOH-pee-ah **Definition** double vision	dipl / opia double / vision condition

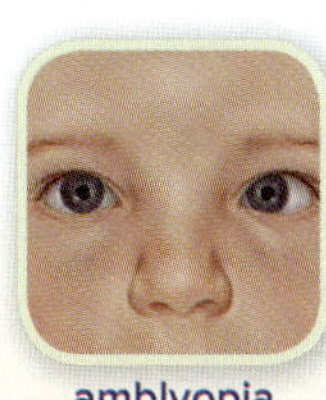
amblyopia

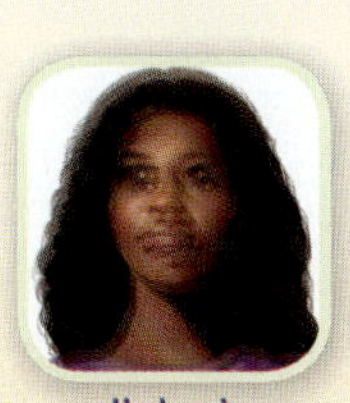
diplopia

6.2 Patient History, Problems, Complaints

eye *continued*

Term	Word Analysis
hemianopsia HEH-mee-an-OP-see-ah **Definition** blindness in half the visual field	**hemi / an / opsia** half / no / vision condition
hyperopia HAI-per-OH-pee-ah **Definition** farsightedness	**hyper / opia** over / vision condition
myopia mai-OH-pee-ah **Definition** nearsightedness **NOTE:** The *my* root in this word is not from *myo* (muscle); instead, it's from another word that means *to shut* that is related to the word at the root of *mystery*—from something that is hidden from view until it is revealed.	**my / opia** shut / vision condition
presbyopia PREZ-bee-OH-pee-ah **Definition** decreased vision caused by old age	**presby / opia** old age / vision condition
scotopia skaw-TOH-pee-ah **Definition** adjustment of the eye to seeing in darkness	**scot / opia** darkness / vision condition
Eye—Outer Structures and Vision	
blepharoplegia BLEF-ah-roh-PLEE-jah **Definition** paralysis of the eyelid	**blepharo / plegia** eyelid / paralysis
blepharospasm BLEF-ah-roh-SPAZ-um **Definition** involuntary contraction of an eyelid	**blepharo / spasm** eyelid / involuntary contraction
dacryoadenalgia DAK-ree-oh-AD-en-AL-jah **Definition** pain in the tear gland	**dacryo / aden / algia** tear / gland / pain
dacryocystalgia DAK-ree-oh -sis-TAL-jah **Definition** pain in the tear sac	**dacryo / cyst / algia** tear / sac / pain
dacryohemorrhea DAK-ree-oh -HIM-oh-REE-ah **Definition** blood in the tears	**dacryo / hemo / rrhea** tear / blood / excessive discharge
dacryorrhea DAK-ree-oh-REE-ah **Definition** excessive tearing	**dacryo / rrhea** tear / excessive discharge
ophthalmalgia awf-thal-MAL-jah **Definition** eye pain	**ophthalm / algia** eye / pain

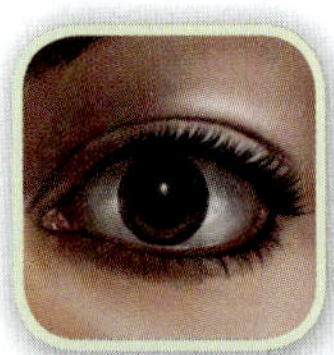
scotopia

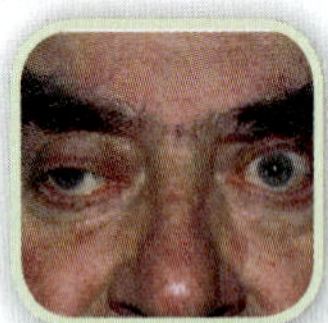
blepharoplegia

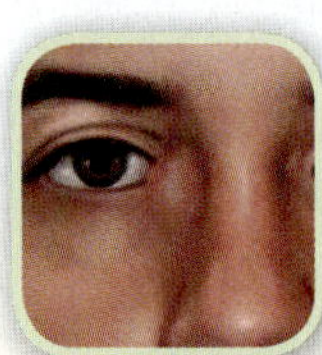
dacryocystalgia

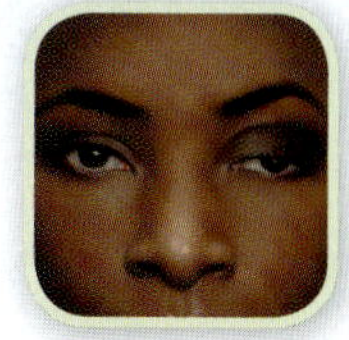
ophthalmoplegia

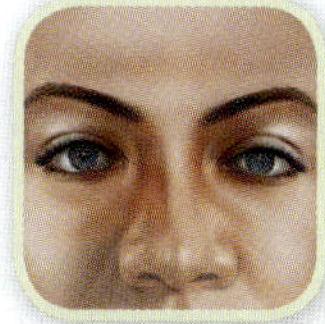
miosis

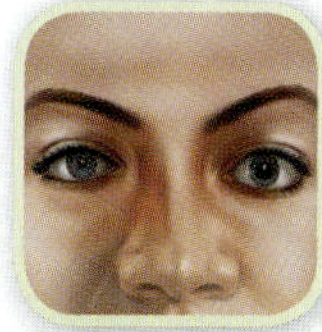
mydriasis

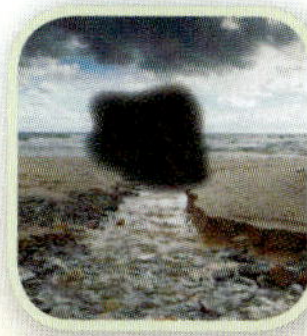
scotoma

eye *continued*

Term	Word Analysis
ophthalmoplegia awf-THAL-moh-PLEE-jah **Definition** eye paralysis	ophthalmo / plegia eye / paralysis
xerophthalmia ZER-off-THAL-mee-ah **Definition** dry eyes	xer / ophthalm / ia dry / eye / condition
Eye—Sclera	
astigmatism ah-STIG-mah-TIZ-um **Definition** vision problem caused by the fact that light rays entering the eye aren't focused on a single point in the back of the eye	a / stigmat / ism no / point / condition
corneal xerosis KOR-nee-al ZER-oh-sis **Definition** dryness of the cornea	corne / al xer / osis cornea / pertaining to dry / condition
keratalgia KEH-rah-TAL-jah **Definition** pain in the cornea	kerat / algia cornea / pain
Eye—Choroid/Retina	
cycloplegia SAI-kloh-PLEE-jah **Definition** paralysis of the ciliary body	cyclo / plegia ciliary body / paralysis
iridalgia IH-rid-AL-jah **Definition** pain in the iris	irid / algia iris / pain
miosis mai-OH-sis **Definition** abnormal contraction of the pupil	from Greek, for *to lessen*
mydriasis mi-DRAI-ah-sis **Definition** abnormal dilation of pupil NOTE: We don't really see the connection—do you?	from Greek, for red-hot metal
scotoma skaw-TOH-mah **Definition** dark spot in the visual field	scot / oma darkness / tumor

6.2 Patient History, Problems, Complaints

ear

Term	Word Analysis
Hearing Conditions—Acuses	
hyperacusis HAI-per-ah-KOO-sis **Definition** excessively sensitive hearing	hyper / acusis over / hearing condition
hypoacusis HAI-poh-ah-KOO-sis **Definition** excessively insensitive hearing	hypo / acusis under / hearing condition
osteoacusis AW-stee-oh-ah-KOO-sis **Definition** hearing through bone	osteo / acusis bone / hearing condition
presbycusis PREZ-bih-KOO-sis **Definition** loss of hearing in old age NOTE: The *a* in *acusis* was swallowed up by the *y* at the end of *presby*. The word is sometimes written as *presbyacusis*, but that's a lot harder to pronounce.	presby / cusis old age / hearing condition
Outer/Middle Ear	
mastoidalgia MAS-toid-AL-jah **Definition** pain in the mastoid	mastoid / algia mastoid / pain
otalgia oh-TAL-jah **Definition** ear pain	ot / algia ear / pain
otodynia OH-toh-DAI-nee-ah **Definition** ear pain	oto / dynia ear / pain
otorrhea OH-toh-REE-ah **Definition** discharge from the ear	oto / rrhea ear / excessive discharge
Inner Ear	
tinnitus tih-NAI-tis **Definition** ringing in the ears	from Latin, for *to ring or jingle*
vertigo VER-tih-goh **Definition** sensation of moving through space (while stationary)	from Latin, for *to whirl around*

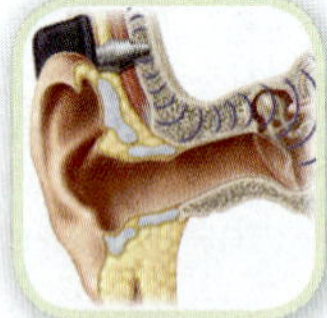
osteoacusis

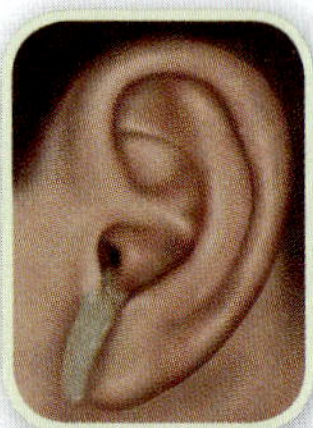
otorrhea

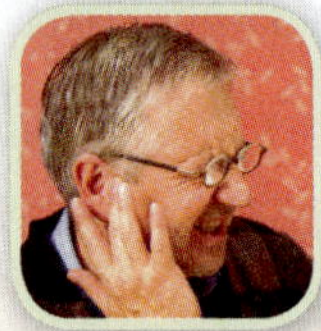
tinnitus

Learning Outcome 6.2 Exercises

PRONUNCIATION

EXERCISE 1 *Break down the following words into syllables.*

EXAMPLE: synesthesia *syn | es | the | sia*

1. ambiopia ______
2. asthenopia ______
3. iridalgia ______
4. hypoacusis ______
5. presbycusis ______
6. blepharospasm ______
7. xerophthalmia ______
8. ophthalmoplegia ______
9. dacryoadenalgia ______
10. dacryohemorrhea ______

EXERCISE 2 *Indicate which syllable is emphasized when pronounced.*

EXAMPLE: bronchitis bron**chi**tis

1. diplopia ______
2. myopia ______
3. miosis ______
4. otalgia ______
5. mydriasis ______
6. scotoma ______
7. tinnitus ______

TRANSLATION

EXERCISE 3 *Break down the following words into their component parts.*

EXAMPLE: nasopharyngoscope *naso | pharyngo | scope*

1. otalgia ______
2. otorrhea ______
3. asthenopia ______
4. hyperopia ______
5. hyperacusis ______
6. osteoacusis ______
7. hemianopsia ______
8. akinetopsia ______
9. blepharospasm ______
10. ophthalmoplegia ______
11. dacryoadenalgia ______
12. dacryocystalgia ______
13. dacryohemorrhea ______
14. xerophthalmia ______

Learning Outcome 6.2 Exercises

EXERCISE 4 *Underline and define the word parts from this chapter in the following terms.*

1. dacryorrhea ____________
2. iridalgia ____________
3. keratalgia ____________
4. mastoidalgia ____________
5. ophthalmalgia ____________
6. otodynia ____________
7. cycloplegia ____________
8. scotopia ____________
9. diplopia ____________
10. myopia ____________
11. hypoacusis ____________
12. corneal xerosis ____________

EXERCISE 5 *Match the term on the left with its definition on the right.*

____	1. vertigo	a.	vision problem caused by the fact that light rays entering the eye aren't focused on a single point in the back of the eye
____	2. astigmatism	b.	abnormal contraction of the pupil
____	3. ambiopia	c.	abnormal dilation of the pupil
____	4. amblyopia	d.	dark spot in the visual field
____	5. presbyopia	e.	decreased vision (when it occurs in one eye, it is referred to as *lazy eye*)
____	6. presbycusis	f.	decreased vision caused by old age
____	7. tinnitus	g.	double vision
____	8. scotoma	h.	loss of hearing in old age
____	9. mydriasis	i.	ringing in the ears
____	10. miosis	j.	the sensation of moving through space (while stationary)

EXERCISE 6 *Translate the following terms as literally as possible.*

EXAMPLE: nasopharyngoscope *an instrument for looking at the nose and throat*

1. otalgia ____________
2. otodynia ____________
3. ophthalmalgia ____________
4. ambiopia ____________
5. diplopia ____________
6. hemianopsia ____________
7. osteoacusis ____________
8. presbycusis ____________
9. akinetopsia ____________
10. corneal xerosis ____________
11. xerophthalmia ____________
12. dacryoadenalgia ____________
13. dacryocystalgia ____________
14. dacryohemorrhea ____________
15. astigmatism ____________

Learning Outcome 6.2 Exercises

GENERATION

EXERCISE 7 *Build a medical term from the information provided.*

EXAMPLE: inflammation of the sinuses *sinusitis*

1. eye paralysis (use *ophthalm/o*) ______
2. paralysis of the ciliary body ______
3. paralysis of the eyelid ______
4. involuntary contraction of an eyelid ______
5. pain in the cornea (use *kerat/o*) ______
6. pain in the mastoid ______
7. pain in the iris ______
8. discharge from the ear (use *ot/o*) ______
9. excessive tearing (use *dacry/o*) ______
10. over vision condition (farsightedness) ______
11. decreased vision caused by old age ______

EXERCISE 8 *Multiple-choice questions. Select the correct answer.*

1. The medical term for nearsightedness is
   a. amblyopia c. myopia
   b. asthenopia d. tinnitus
2. When this condition occurs in one eye, it is known as *lazy eye.*
   a. amblyopia c. myopia
   b. asthenopia d. tinnitus
3. The medical term for *eye strain* is
   a. amblyopia c. myopia
   b. asthenopia d. tinnitus
4. The medical term used to describe *ringing in the ears* is
   a. amblyopia c. myopia
   b. asthenopia d. tinnitus
5. *Vertigo* is a condition of the
   a. inner ear c. inner eye
   b. outer/middle ear d. outer eye

EXERCISE 9 *Briefly describe the difference between each pair of terms.*

1. hyperacusis, hypoacusis ______
2. myopia, hyperopia ______
3. dacryohemorrhea, dacryorrhea ______
4. scotopia, scotoma ______
5. miosis, mydriasis ______

OBJECTIVE

6.3 Observation and Discovery

The Eye

As you might imagine, the physical exam of the eye is mainly limited to visual inspection. Often an eye exam begins with looking at the parts that surround it. An examiner might observe swelling (*blepharedema*) or drooping (*blepharoptosis*) around the eyelids. If pus is draining from the eyelids (*blepharopyorrhea*), that's a strong sign of infection.

After checking the eyelids, a health care professional might examine the position of the eye. An eye bulging from the orbit is known as *exophthalmos,* a condition commonly seen in hyperthyroidism.

The main areas of emphasis when inspecting the eye during a routine exam are the color of the sclera, the size of the pupils, and the movement of the eyes. The sclera of the eye is normally white. The blood vessels of the conjunctiva are normally so small that they are invisible. If the conjunctiva becomes inflamed, the vessels increase in size and the sclera may appear red. If one of the vessels in the conjunctiva ruptures, a small collection of blood may remain. Using a penlight or specialized light for examining eyes (*ophthalmoscope*), an examiner can check the size of a patient's pupils and determine how they react to light. They should constrict when exposed to light (*miosis*) and dilate when the light is dimmed.

Both eyes should work together. Shining a light in one eye should cause both pupils to constrict. The pupils should appear symmetric when looking straight ahead. One eye angled inward (*esotropia*) or outward (*exotropia*) is known as *strabismus.* A jittery, abnormal movement of the eye is called *nystagmus.* This may be a sign of an eye problem or a problem with the nervous system.

Further inspection of the eye may require specialized tools. An ophthalmoscope may be used to examine the back of a patient's eyes. It may show swelling of the optic nerve (*papilledema*). Other tools look at specific parts of the eye (*retinoscope, phacoscope*) or check for the pressure inside the eye (*tonometer*).

The Ear

When a patient presents with an ear problem, a health care professional is likely to first examine the outer part of the ear, including its size (*macrotia/microtia*) and signs of inflammation, like redness and swelling. To inspect the ear canal and eardrum, a special light known as an *otoscope* is needed.

One common finding is an excessive amount of ear wax in the ear (*ceruminosis/cerminoma*) that makes it difficult to see the eardrum. Upon visualizing the eardrum, the examiner looks for signs of fluid behind the ear. If the eardrum is red or bulging outward, an ear infection may be present. If the ear infection is bad enough, the eardrum may burst (*tympanic perforation*). Once the burst eardrum heals, the perforation may leave small, visible scars (*tympanosclerosis*).

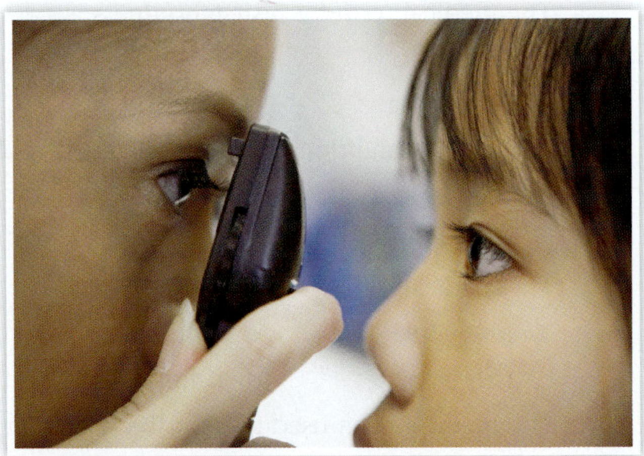

The doctor's primary instruments for observation of the eye and ear are the ophthalmoscope and the otoscope.

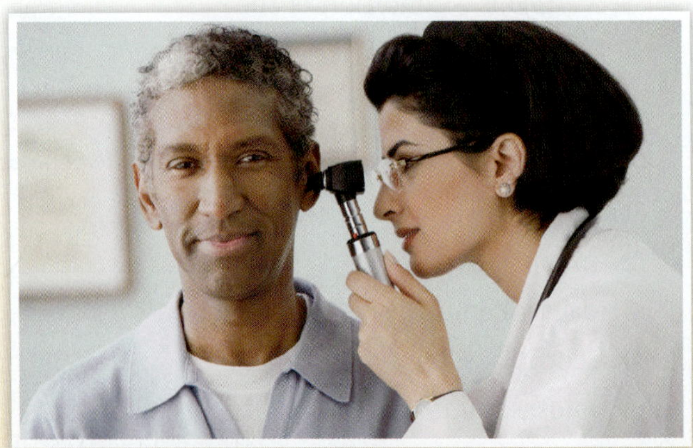

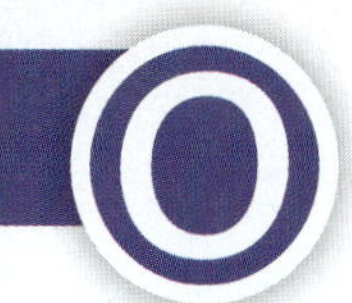

6.3 Observation and Discovery

The visualization of the ear canal and eardrum with an otoscope is called *otoscopy*. While very important, it can be difficult to determine the presence of an ear infection just by looking. If otoscopy alone does not reveal the presence of an ear infection, forcing air into the ear canal to see if it moves the eardrum (*pneumatic otoscopy*) may work.

Other tools to evaluate the ear include the *audiometer*, an instrument commonly used to check a patient's hearing, and the *salpingoscope*, a specialized instrument for examining the tubes that connect the middle ear to the nose and throat.

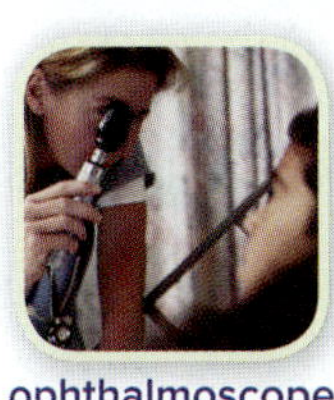
ophthalmoscope

eye

Term	Word Analysis
Diagnostic Procedures	
ophthalmoscope awf-THAL-mah-SKOHP **Definition** instrument for looking at the eye	**ophthalmo / scope** eye / instrument for looking
optomyometer AWP-toh-MAI-oh-MEE-tir **Definition** device used to determine the strength of eye muscles	**opto / myo / meter** eye / muscle / instrument for measuring
phacoscope FAY-koh-SKOHP **Definition** instrument for looking at the lens	**phaco / scope** lens / instrument for looking
retinoscope RET-in-aw-SKOP **Definition** instrument for looking at the retina	**retino / scope** retina / instrument for looking
retinoscopy RET-in-AWS-koh-pee **Definition** procedure for looking at the retina	**retino / scop / y** retina / looking / procedure
tonometer TOH-naw-MEE-tir **Definition** instrument for measuring tension or pressure in the eye (intraocular pressure)	**tono / meter** tension / instrument for measuring
Professional Terms	
binocular bai-NAW-kyoo-lar **Definition** pertaining to both eyes	**bin / ocul / ar** two / eye / pertaining to
iridokinesis IR-ih-doh-kin-EE-sis **Definition** the movement of the iris	**irido / kinesis** iris / movement
lacrimation LAH-krih-MAY-shun **Definition** formation of tears (i.e., crying)	**lacrim / ation** tear / condition
nasolacrimal NAY-zoh-LAH-krih-mal **Definition** pertaining to the nose and tear system	**naso / lacrim / al** nose / tear / pertaining to

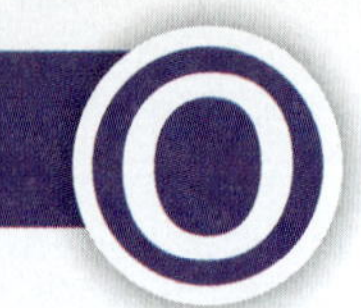

6.3 Observation and Discovery

eye *continued*

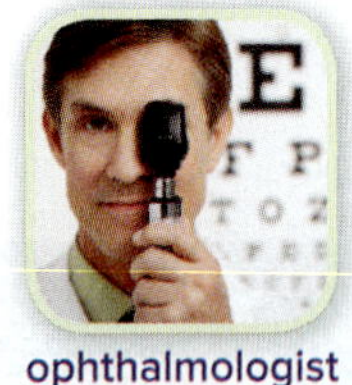
ophthalmologist

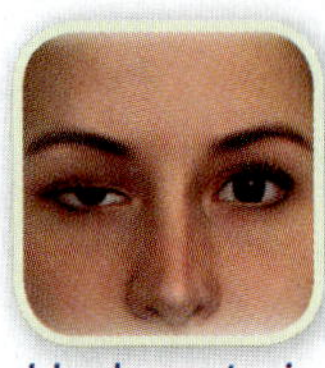
blepharoptosis

Term	Word Analysis
ophthalmic awf-THAL-mik **Definition** pertaining to the eye	ophthalm / ic eye / pertaining to
ophthalmologist AWF-thal-MAW-loh-jist **Definition** eye specialist	ophthalmo / logist eye / specialist
optic AWP-tik **Definition** pertaining to the eye	opt / ic eye / pertaining to
optokinetic AWP-toh-kih-NEH-tik **Definition** pertaining to eye movement	opto / kinet / ic eye / movement / pertaining to
optometrist awp-TAW-meh-trist **Definition** specialist in measuring the eye	opto / metr / ist eye / measure / specialist
retinal REH-tih-nal **Definition** pertaining to the retina	retin / al retina / pertaining to
Outer Structures and Vision	
blepharedema BLEF-ar-eh-DEE-mah **Definition** eyelid swelling	blephar / edema eyelid / swelling
blepharoptosis BLEF-ar-awp-TOH-sis **Definition** drooping eyelid	blepharo / ptosis eyelid / drooping
blepharopyorrhea BLEF-ah-roh-PAI-oh-REE-ah **Definition** discharge of pus from the eyelid	blepharo / pyo / rrhea eyelid / pus / discharge
dacryolith DAK-ree-oh-lith **Definition** hard formation (stone) in the tear system	dacryo / lith tear / stone
dacryopyorrhea DAK-ree-oh-pai-REE-ah **Definition** discharge of pus in tears	dacryo / pyo / rrhea tear / pus / discharge
ectropion ek-TROH-pee-on **Definition** outward turning of the eyelid, away from the eye	ec / tropion out / turn
entropion en-TROH-pee-on **Definition** inward turning of the eyelid, toward the eye	en / tropion in / turn

6.3 Observation and Discovery

eye *continued*

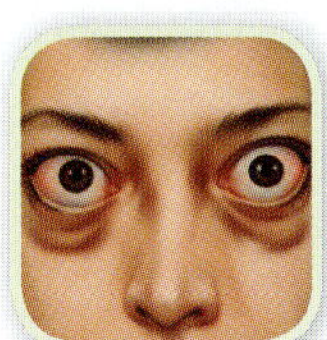
exophthalmus

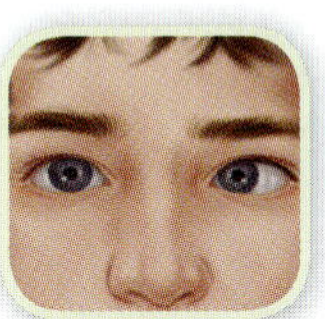
esotropia

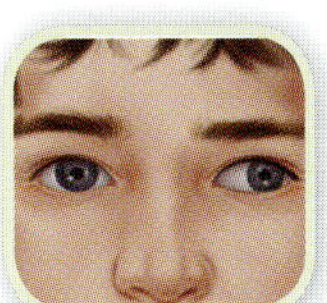
exotropia

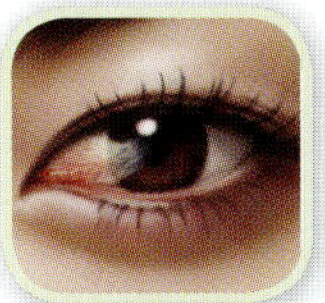
pterygium

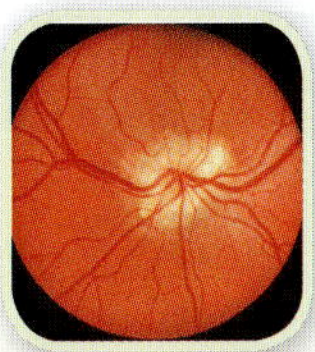
papilledema

Term	Word Analysis
exophthalmus EKS-of-THAL-mus **Definition** protrusion of the eyes out of the eye socket	**ex / ophthalmus** out / eye
nystagmus nih-STAG-mus **Definition** involuntary back-and-forth movement of the eyes	**from Greek, for** *to nod*
strabismus stuh-BIZ-mus **Definition** condition where the eyes deviate when looking at the same object	**from Latin, for** *to squint*
esotropia AY-soh-TROH-pee-ah **Definition** inward turning of the eye, toward the nose	**eso / trop / ia** inward / turn / condition
exotropia EK-soh-TROH-pee-ah **Definition** outward turning of the eye, away from the nose	**exo / trop / ia** outward / turn / condition
Sclera	
keratomalacia ker-AH-toh-mah-LAY-shah **Definition** abnormal softening of the cornea	**kerato / malacia** cornea / softening
pterygium ter-IH-jee-um **Definition** winglike growth of conjunctival tissue extending to the cornea **NOTE:** Think of the pterodactyl, a flying dinosaur whose name means *winged fingers.*	**from Greek, for** *wing*
scleromalacia SKLEH-roh-mah-LAY-shah **Definition** abnormal softening of the sclera	**sclero / malacia** sclera / softening
Choroid/Retina	
papilledema PAH-pil-ah-DEE-mah **Definition** swelling of the optic nerve where it enters the retina **NOTE:** *Papilla* is the term for the place in the back of the eye where the optic nerve enters the retina. It looks like a nipple, so that is what they named it.	**papill / edema** nipple / swelling
phacomalacia FAH-koh-mah-LAY-shah **Definition** abnormal softening of the lens	**phaco / malacia** lens / softening
phacosclerosis FAH-koh-skleh-ROH-sis **Definition** abnormal hardening of the lens	**phaco / scler / osis** lens / hardening / condition

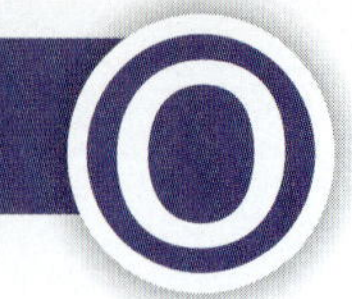

6.3 Observation and Discovery

ear

Term	Word Analysis
Diagnostic Procedures	
audiogram AW-dee-oh-GRAM **Definition** record produced by an audiometer	**audio / gram** hearing / record
audiometer aw-dee-AW-meh-ter **Definition** instrument for measuring hearing	**audio / meter** hearing / instrument for measuring
audiometry aw-dee-AW-meh-tree **Definition** procedure for measuring hearing	**audio / metr / y** hearing / measuring / procedure
otoscope OH-toh-SKOHP **Definition** instrument for looking in the ear	**oto / scope** ear / instrument for looking
otoscopy oh-TAW-skoh-pee **Definition** procedure for examining the ear	**oto / scop / y** ear / looking / procedure
pneumatic otoscopy noo-MA-tik oh-TAW-skoh-pee **Definition** procedure for examining the ear using air **NOTE:** Air is pushed against the eardrum to see how much it moves. Less movement indicates that fluid has built up—an indicator of otitis media.	**pneumat / ic** **oto / scop / y** air / pertaining to ear / looking / procedure
salpingoscope sal-PING-goh-skohp **Definition** instrument for examining the eustachian tubes	**salpingo / scope** eustachian tube / instrument for looking
tympanometry tim-pan-AW-meh-tree **Definition** procedure for measuring the eardrum **NOTE:** In this context, *measurement* is not about size of the eardrum, but about how much it moves.	**tympano / metr / y** eardrum / measuring / procedure
Professional Terms	
audiologist aw-dee-AW-loh-jist **Definition** hearing specialist	**audio / logist** hearing / specialist
aural AW-ral **Definition** pertaining to the ear **NOTE:** This word is easily confused with *oral*.	**aur / al** ear / pertaining to
otolaryngologist OH-toh-LAH-rin-GAW-loh-jist **Definition** specialist in the ear and throat	**oto / laryngo / logist** ear / throat / specialist

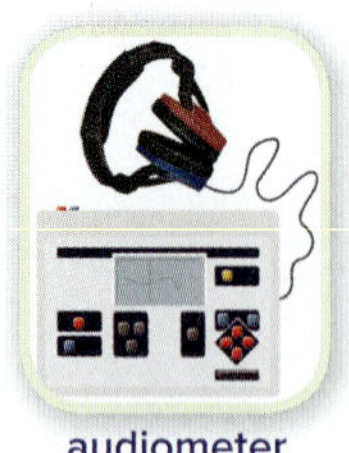
audiometer

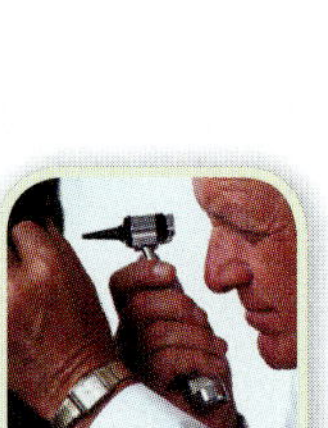
otoscopy

6.3 Observation and Discovery

ear *continued*

Term	Word Analysis
otoneurologist OH-toh-nih-RAW-loh-jist	**oto / neuro / logist** ear / nerve / specialist
Definition specialist in the nerve connections between the ear and brain	
otorhinolaryngologist OH-toh-RAI-noh-LAH-rin-GAW-loh-jist	**oto / rhino / laryngo / logist** ear / nose / throat / specialist
Definition specialist in the ear, nose, and throat	
otosteal oh-TAWS-tee-all	**ot / oste / al** ear / bone / pertaining to
Definition pertaining to the bones of the ear	
salpingopharyngeal sal-PING-goh-fah-RIN-jee-al	**salpingo / pharyng / eal** eustachian tube / throat / pertaining to
Definition pertaining to the eustachian tubes and the throat	
Outer Ear	
ceruminoma seh-ROO-min-OH-mah	**cerumin / oma** ear wax / tumor
Definition benign tumor of the cerumen-secreting glands of the ear	
ceruminosis seh-ROO-min-OH-sis	**cerumin / osis** ear wax / condition
Definition excessive formation of ear wax	
macrotia mah-KROH-shee-ah	**macr / ot / ia** big / ear / condition
Definition abnormally large ears	
microtia mai-KROH-shee-ah	**micr / ot / ia** small / ear / condition
Definition abnormally small ears	
otopyorrhea OH-toh-PAI-oh-REE-ah	**oto / pyo / rrhea** ear / pus / discharge
Definition discharge of pus from the ears	
Middle Ear	
otosclerosis OH-toh-skleh-ROH-sis	**oto / scler / osis** ear / hardening / condition
Definition hearing loss caused by the hardening of the bones of the middle ear	
tympanic perforation tim-PAN-ik per-fer-AY-shun	**tympan / ic** — eardrum / pertaining to **per / for / ation** — through / pierce / condition
Definition tear or hole in the eardrum	
tympanosclerosis tim-PAN-oh-skleh-ROH-sis	**tympano / scler / osis** eardrum / hardening / condition
Definition hardening of the eardrum	

ceruminosis

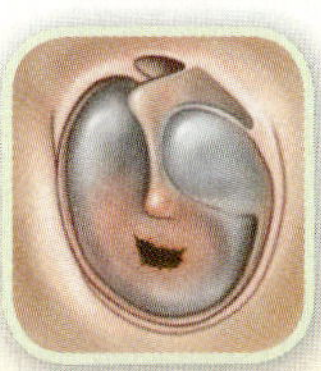

tympanic perforation

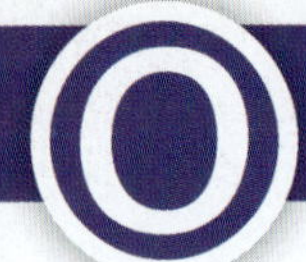

Learning Outcome 6.3 Exercises

PRONUNCIATION

EXERCISE 1 *Break down the following words into syllables.*

EXAMPLE: synesthesia *syn | es | the | sia*

1. esotropia __________
2. retinoscopy __________
3. lacrimation __________
4. otosclerosis __________
5. optokinetic __________
6. nasolacrimal __________
7. scleromalacia __________
8. optomyometer __________
9. iridokinesis __________
10. blepharoptosis __________
11. ceruminoma __________
12. keratomalacia __________
13. papilledema __________
14. otolaryngologist __________
15. tympanosclerosis __________

EXERCISE 2 *Indicate which syllable is emphasized when pronounced.*

EXAMPLE: bronchitis bron**chi**tis

1. retinal __________
2. otoscopy __________
3. dacryolith __________
4. ophthalmic __________
5. audiometer __________
6. audiometry __________
7. audiologist __________
8. ectropion __________
9. entropion __________
10. strabismus __________
11. nystagmus __________
12. macrotia __________
13. microtia __________
14. tympanometry __________

TRANSLATION

EXERCISE 3 *Break down the following words into their component parts.*

EXAMPLE: nasopharyngoscope *naso | pharyngo | scope*

1. audiogram __________
2. audiometer __________
3. aural __________
4. microtia __________
5. optometrist __________
6. optokinetic __________
7. otosclerosis __________
8. phacosclerosis __________
9. tympanosclerosis __________
10. ceruminosis __________
11. nasolacrimal __________
12. blepharoptosis __________
13. blepharopyorrhea __________
14. dacryopyorrhea __________
15. exophthalmus __________
16. otoneurology __________
17. otolaryngologist __________
18. otorhinolaryngologist __________
19. salpingopharyngeal __________

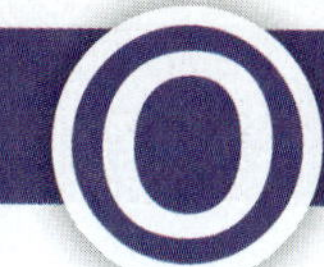

Learning Outcome 6.3 Exercises

EXERCISE 4 *Underline and define the word parts from this chapter in the following terms.*

1. optic ______
2. retinal ______
3. otoscopy ______
4. otosteal ______
5. audiometry ______
6. tympanometry ______
7. ophthalmic ______
8. audiologist ______
9. ophthalmologist ______
10. dacryolith ______
11. retinoscopy ______
12. keratomalacia ______
13. phacomalacia ______
14. scleromalacia ______
15. tonometer ______
16. binocular ______
17. otopyorrhea ______
18. optomyometer ______
19. iridokinesis ______
20. lacrimation ______
21. blepharedema ______
22. ceruminoma ______
23. pneumatic otoscopy ______
24. macrotia ______

EXERCISE 5 *Match the term on the left with its definition on the right.*

b	1. tympanic perforation	a. condition where the eyes deviate when looking at the same object
e	2. papilledema	b. tear or hole in the eardrum
c.	3. pterygium	c. winglike growth of conjunctival tissue extending to the cornea
g	4. exotropia	d. involuntary back-and-forth movement of the eyes
f	5. esotropia	e. swelling of the optic nerve where it enters the retina
h	6. ectropion	f. inward turning of the eye, toward the nose
i	7. entropion	g. outward turning of the eye, away from the nose
d	8. nystagmus	h. inward turning of the eyelid, toward the eye
a	9. strabismus	i. outward turning of the eyelid, away from the eye

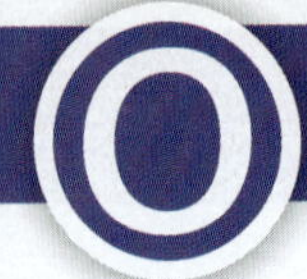

Learning Outcome 6.3 Exercises

EXERCISE 6 *Match the term on the left with its definition on the right.*

______	1. retinoscope	a.	instrument for looking at the eustachian tubes
______	2. otoscope	b.	instrument for looking at the eye
______	3. ophthalmoscope	c.	instrument for looking at the lens
______	4. salpingoscope	d.	instrument for looking at the retina
______	5. phacoscope	e.	instrument for looking in the ear

EXERCISE 7 *Translate the following terms as literally as possible.*

EXAMPLE: nasopharyngoscope *an instrument for looking at the nose and throat*

1. optomyometer ______________________
2. retinoscopy ______________________
3. tonometer ______________________
4. binocular ______________________
5. nasolacrimal ______________________
6. retinal ______________________
7. blepharopyrorrhea ______________________
8. dacryolith ______________________
9. dacryopyorrhea ______________________
10. exophthalmus ______________________
11. audiometer ______________________
12. audiometry ______________________
13. tympanometry ______________________
14. aural ______________________
15. otolaryngologist ______________________
16. otorhinolaryngologist ______________________
17. salpingopharyngeal ______________________
18. ceruminosis ______________________
19. macrotia ______________________
20. otopyorrhea ______________________
21. tympanic perforation ______________________

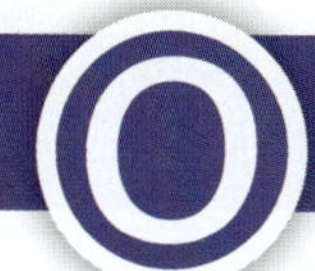

Learning Outcome 6.3 Exercises

GENERATION

EXERCISE 8 *Build a medical term from the information provided.*

EXAMPLE: inflammation of the sinuses *sinusitis*

1. instrument for looking at the eye (use *ophthalm/o*) ______
2. instrument for looking in the ear (use *ot/o*) ______
3. instrument for looking at the lens ______
4. instrument for looking at the retina ______
5. instrument for looking at the eustachian tubes ______
6. abnormal softening of the cornea (use *kerat/o*) ______
7. ear wax tumor ______
8. procedure for looking in the ear (use *ot/o*) ______
9. procedure for looking in the ear using air ______
10. hearing record (use *audi/o*) ______
11. hearing specialist (use *audi/o*) ______
12. ear nerve specialist (use *ot/o*) ______
13. pertaining to the eye (use *ophthalm/o*) ______
14. pertaining to the eye (use *opt/o*) ______
15. pertaining to eye movement (use *opt/o*) ______
16. pertaining to the bones of the ear (use *ot/o*) ______
17. the movement of the iris (use *irid/o*) ______

EXERCISE 9 *Multiple-choice questions. Select the correct answer.*

1. The swelling of the optic nerve where it enters is retina is known as
   - a. nystagmus
   - b. papilledema
   - c. pterygium
   - d. strabismus
2. This term comes from Greek, for *wing*, and describes a winglike growth of conjunctival tissue extending to the cornea.
   - a. lacrimation
   - b. papilledema
   - c. pterygium
   - d. strabismus
3. The medical term for tear formation, or *crying*, is
   - a. lacrimation
   - b. nystagmus
   - c. pterygium
   - d. strabismus
4. A condition where the eyes deviate when looking at the same object is
   - a. lacrimation
   - b. nystagmus
   - c. papilledema
   - d. strabismus
5. Involuntary back-and-forth movement of the eyes is called
   - a. lacrimation
   - b. nystagmus
   - c. papilledema
   - d. pterygium

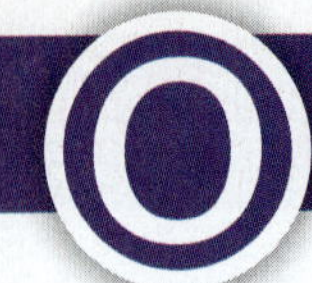

Learning Outcome 6.3 Exercises

EXERCISE 10 *Briefly describe the difference between each pair of terms.*

1. microtia, macrotia ______
2. tympanosclerosis, otosclerosis ______
3. phacomalacia, scleromalacia ______
4. phacomalacia, phacosclerosis ______
5. optometrist, ophthalmologist ______
6. blepharedema, blepharoptosis ______
7. ectropion, entropion ______
8. esotropia, exotropia ______

ASSESSMENT

6.4 Diagnosis and Pathology

The Eye

OUTER STRUCTURES

Structures around the eye often get inflamed. *Blepharitis* is usually caused by a mild bacterial skin infection. *Dacryoadenitis* is inflammation of the tear gland. The cause is not well understood, but it's thought to be an extension of inflammation of the conjunctiva.

More common is inflammation of the tear duct that drains the eye. In infants, this drainage system can be blocked (*dacryostenosis*) and can lead to a mild infection (*dacryocystitis*). Probably the most common eye complaint seen in most doctors' offices is inflammation of the conjunctiva (*conjunctivitis*). This can result from allergies, irritants in the eye, or infection. Infections of the conjunctiva (commonly known as *pink eye*) are usually caused by a virus or bacteria.

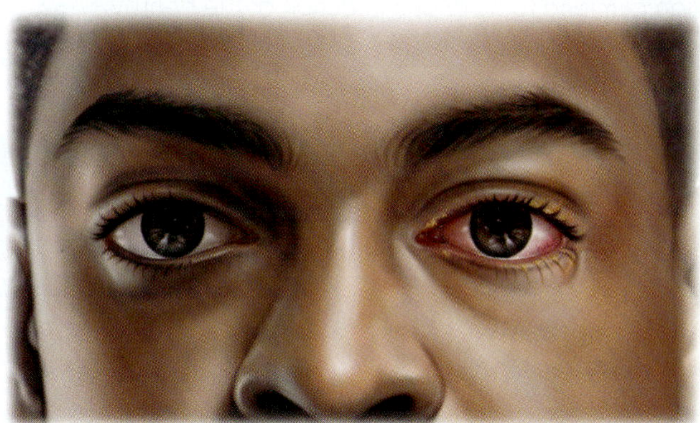

Infections of the conjunctiva are commonly known as pink eye.

OUTER LAYER

The sclera has few general problems—the main one being *scleritis*. This painful, chronic illness is often due to general inflammatory disorders like *rheumatoid arthritis*. Problems with the cornea (*keratopathy*) include scratching from a foreign object (*corneal abrasion*) and inflammation (*keratitis*). Often caused by infection, keratitis is generally a very serious condition.

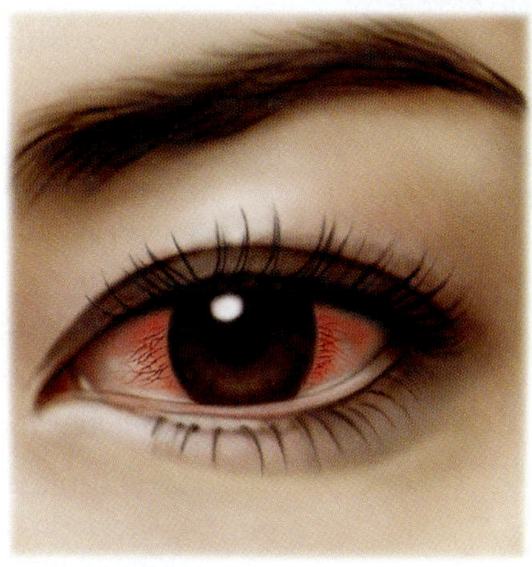

Inflamed blood vessels in the sclera

MIDDLE LAYER

The most common concern of the lens is clouding (*cataract*). The lens may also be undeveloped/absent (*aphakia*). Often aphakia is a result of surgical removal. Iridopathies, or disorders of the iris, include bleeding (*iridemia*). Inflammation of the iris (*iritis*) and iris with extension to the ciliary muscle (*iridocyclitis*) are unusual and painful.

INNER LAYER

The optic nerve is vulnerable to pressure from inside the eye (*glaucoma*) or from the brain; pressure from the brain can lead to swelling of the optic disc (*papilledema*). Like the other parts of the eye, the optic nerve can become inflamed (*optic neuritis*).

The retina can become detached from the blood supply. This emergency situation requires immediate reattachment, or blindness will occur. General retinal damage (*retinopathy*) can result from diabetes or blood disorders. Premature infants sometimes develop retinopathy after receiving oxygen as treatment for a lung disease.

The Ear

Many problems of the outer and middle ear involve infection. Infection of the outer ear (*otitis externa*) is a very common problem in summer, as swimmers often get water trapped in the ear canal. The common term for this illness is *swimmer's ear.* Otitis externa can also result from using a cotton swab to clean out the ears, which can push ear wax down into the ear until it forms a hard mass known as *cerumen impaction.*

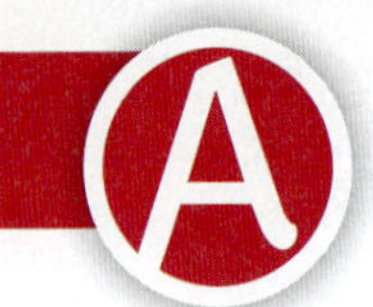

6.4 Diagnosis and Pathology

Infection of the middle ear (*otitis media*) is one of the most common complaints seen in pediatric offices. Occasionally, the eardrum can be so inflamed that it blisters (*bullous myrigitis*). Less commonly, an ear infection can lead to a serious infection of the nearby skull bone (*mastoiditis*).

Inner ear problems manifest as either a loss of hearing (*sensorineural hearing loss*) or *vertigo*. Vertigo arises from inflammation of the inner ear structures (*labyrinthitis*) or the nerve that connects it to the brain (*vestibular neuritis*).

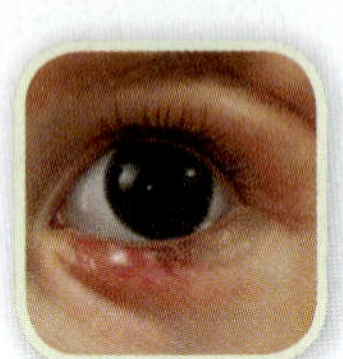

blepharitis

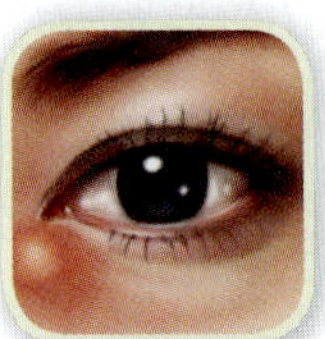

dacryocystitis

eye

Term	Word Analysis
Outer Structures and Vision	
blepharitis BLEF-ah-RAI-tis **Definition** eyelid inflammation	**blephar / itis** eyelid / inflammation
blepharoconjunctivitis BLEF-ah-roh-con-JUNK-tih-VAI-tis **Definition** inflammation of the eyelid and conjunctiva	**blepharo / conjunctiv / itis** eyelid / conjunctiva / inflammation
dacryocystitis DA-kree-oh-sis-TAI-tis **Definition** inflammation of the tear sac	**dacryo / cyst / itis** tear / sac / inflammation
dacryoadenitis DAK-ree-oh-AD-en-AI-tis **Definition** inflammation of the tear gland	**dacryo / aden / itis** tear / gland / inflammation
dacryohemorrhea DAK-ree-oh-HEH-moh-REE-ah **Definition** discharge of blood in tears	**dacryo / hemo / rrhea** tear / blood / discharge
dacryolithiasis DAK-ree-oh-lih-THAI-ah-sis **Definition** presence of hard formations (stones) in the tear system	**dacryo / lith / iasis** tear / stone / presence
dacryostenosis DAK-ree-oh-steh-NOH-sis **Definition** narrowing of the tear duct	**dacryo / sten / osis** tear / narrowing / condition
oculomycosis AW-kyoo-loh-mai-KOH-sis **Definition** fungal eye condition	**oculo / myc / osis** eye / fungus / condition
oculopathy AW-kyoo-LAW-pah-thee **Definition** eye disease	**oculo / pathy** eye / disease
ophthalmatrophy AWF-thal-MAW-troh-fee **Definition** atrophy (wasting away) of the eye	**ophthalm / a / trophy** eye / non / development

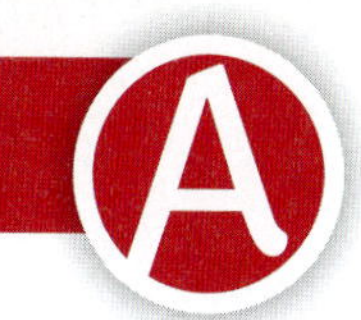

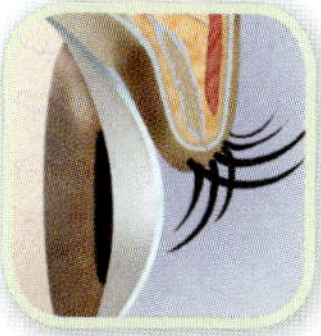
trichiasis

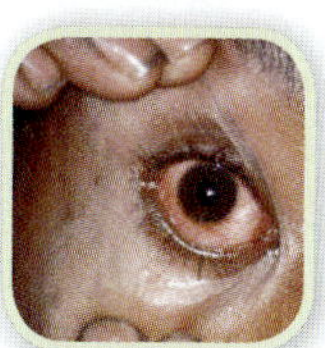
conjunctivitis

eye *continued*	
Term	**Word Analysis**
ophthalmitis AWF-thal-MAI-tis **Definition** inflammation of the eye	ophthalm / itis eye / inflammation
ophthalmomycosis awf-THAL-moh-mai-KOH-sis **Definition** fungal eye condition	ophthalmo / myc / osis eye / fungus / condition
ophthalmomyitis awf-THAL-moh-mai-AI-tis **Definition** inflammation of the eye muscles	ophthalmo / my / itis eye / muscle / inflammation
ophthalmopathy AWF-thal-MOH-pah-thee **Definition** eye disease	ophthalmo / pathy eye / disease
trichiasis trih-KAI-ah-sis **Definition** condition caused by eyelashes growing backward and coming in contact with the eye	trich / iasis hair / presence
Sclera	
conjunctivitis con-JUNK-tih-VAI-tis **Definition** inflammation of the conjunctiva (also known as *pink eye*)	conjunctiv / itis conjunctiva / inflammation
keratitis KEH-rah-TAI-tis **Definition** inflammation of the cornea	kerat / itis cornea / inflammation
keratopathy KEH-rah-TOP-ah-thee **Definition** disease of the cornea	kerato / pathy cornea / disease
sclerectasia SKLER-ek-TAY-zhah **Definition** overexpansion of the sclera	scler / ectas / ia sclera / expansion / condition
scleroiritis SKLER-oh-ai-RAI-tis **Definition** inflammation of the sclera and iris	sclero / ir / itis sclera / iris / inflammation
sclerokeratitis SKLER-oh-KEH-rah-TAI-tis **Definition** inflammation of the sclera and cornea	sclero / kerat / itis sclera / cornea / inflammation
sclerokeratoiritis SKLER-oh-KEH-ra-toh-ai-RAI-tis **Definition** inflammation of the sclera, cornea, and iris	sclero / kerato / ir / itis sclera / cornea / iris / inflammation

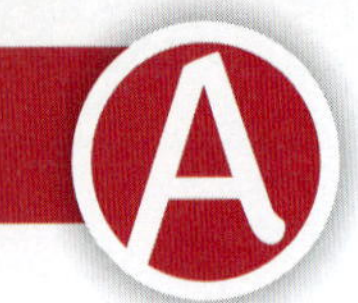

6.4 Diagnosis and Pathology

eye *continued*

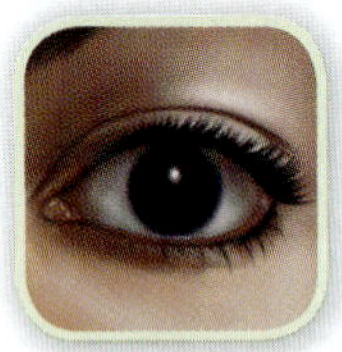
aniridia

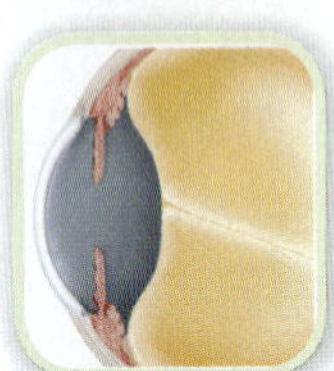
aphakia

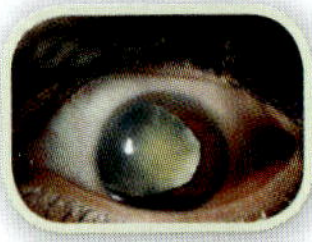
cataract

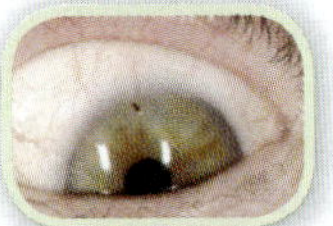
corneal abrasion

Term	Word Analysis
Choroid/Retina	
aniridia AN-ih-RIH-dee-ah **Definition** absence of an iris	an / irid / ia no / iris / condition
aphakia ah-FAY-kee-ia **Definition** absence of a lens **NOTE:** *Phak* is written with a *k* instead of a *c*. Although both are acceptable spellings, some people use a *k* to make sure the word is pronounced ah-FAY-kee-ia instead of ah-FAY-see-ia, which could be confused with other terms.	a / phak / ia no / lens / condition
cataract KAT-ah-RAKT **Definition** opacity (cloudiness) of the lens of the eye	from Latin, for *waterfall*
corneal abrasion KOR-nee-al a-BRAY-zhun **Definition** scratch on the cornea	corne / al — ab / rasion cornea / pertaining to — away / rubbing
cyclokeratitis SAI-cloh-keh-rah-TAI-tis **Definition** inflammation of the ciliary body and cornea	cyclo / kerat / itis ciliary body / cornea / inflammation
endophthalmitis EN-dof-thal-MAI-tis **Definition** inflammation of the inside of the eye (often a complication from intraocular surgery)	end / ophthalm / itis inside / eye / inflammation
iridemia EAR-ih-DEE-mee-ah **Definition** bleeding from the iris	irid / emia iris / blood condition
iridocyclitis EAR-ih-doh-sai-KLAI-tis **Definition** inflammation of the iris and ciliary body	irido / cycl / itis iris / ciliary body / inflammation
iridokeratitis EAR-ih-doh-keh-rah-TAI-tis **Definition** inflammation of the iris and cornea	irido / kerat / itis iris / cornea / inflammation
iridopathy EAR-ih-DOP-ah-thee **Definition** disease of the iris	irido / pathy iris / disease
iritis ai-RAI-tis **Definition** inflammation of the iris	ir / itis iris / inflammation
optic neuritis OP-tik nir-AI-tis **Definition** inflammation of the optic nerve	opt / ic — neur / itis eye / pertaining to — nerve / inflammation

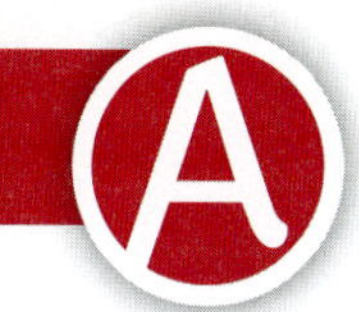

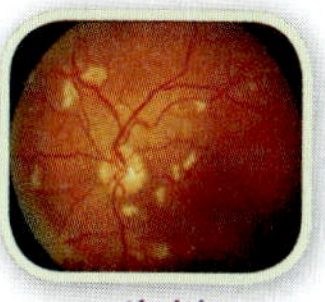

eye *continued*

Term	Word Analysis
phakitis fah-KAI-tis **Definition** inflammation of the lens	**phak / itis** lens / inflammation
Note: *Phak* is written with a *k* instead of a *c*. Although both are acceptable spellings, some people use a *k* to make sure the word is pronounced fah-KAI-tis instead of fah-SAI-tis, which could be confused with other terms.	
retinitis REH-tih-NAI-tis **Definition** inflammation of the retina	**retin / itis** retina / inflammation
retinopathy REH-tih-NOP-ah-thee **Definition** disease of the retina	**retino / pathy** retina / disease
retinosis REH-tih-NOH-sis **Definition** retinal condition	**retin / osis** retina / condition

retinitis

ear

Term	Word Analysis
Outer Ear	
cerumen impaction SEH-roo-men im-PAK-shun **Definition** buildup of ear wax blocking ear canal	**cerumen im / pac / tion** ear wax in / drive / condition
mastoiditis MAS-toi-DAI-tis **Definition** inflammation of the mastoid	**mastoid / itis** mastoid / inflammation
otitis externa oh-TAI-tis eks-TERN-nah **Definition** inflammation of the outer ear	**ot / itis externa** ear / inflammation outside
otomycosis oh-toh-mai-KOH-sis **Definition** fungal ear condition	**oto / myc / osis** ear / fungus / condition
Middle Ear	
aerotitis AIR-oh-TAI-tis **Definition** inflammation of the ear caused by air	**aer / ot / itis** air / ear / inflammation
Note: This one is tricky because, unless you are careful, you will be tempted to miss the *ot* root in the middle. Most people want to divide the word *aero* + *itis*. The problem is the *t* in the middle. That is your clue that a root is hiding in the middle.	
conductive hearing loss con-DUK-tiv **Definition** hearing loss caused by sound not getting to the middle/inner ear (due to blockages)	**con / duct / ive** together / lead / pertaining to

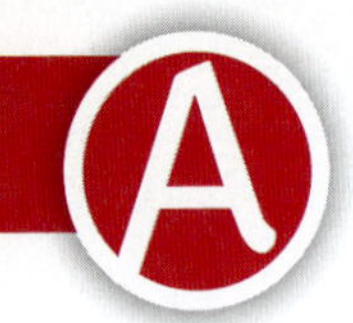

6.4 Diagnosis and Pathology

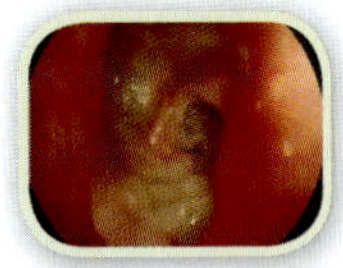
myringitis

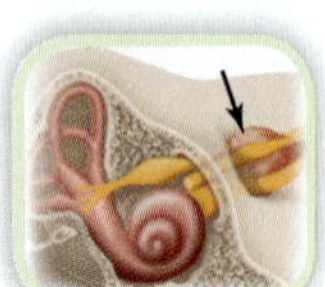
acoustic neuroma

ear *continued*

Term	Word Analysis
myringitis MIR-in-JAI-tis **Definition** inflammation of the eardrum	**myring / itis** eardrum / inflammation
myringodermatitis mir-IN-goh-DER-mah-TAI-tis **Definition** inflammation of the eardrum and surrounding skin	**myringo / dermat / itis** eardrum / skin / inflammation
myringomycosis mir-IN-goh-mai-KOH-sis **Definition** fungal condition of the eardrum	**myringo / myc / osis** eardrum / fungus / condition
otitis media oh-TAI-tis MEH-dee-ah **Definition** inflammation of the middle ear	**ot / itis media** ear / inflammation middle
otosclerosis oh-toh-skleh-ROH-sis **Definition** hearing loss caused by the hardening of the bones of the middle ear	**oto / scler / osis** ear / hardening / condition
rhinosalpingitis RAI-noh-SAL-pin-JAI-tis **Definition** inflammation of the nose and eustachian tubes	**rhino / salping / itis** nose / eustachian / tube inflammation
Inner Ear	
acoustic neuroma ah-KOO-stik nir-OH-mah **Definition** tumor on the acoustic nerve	**acous / tic neur / oma** hearing / pertaining to nerve / tumor
cochleitis KOH-klee-AI-tis **Definition** inflammation of the cochlea	**cochle / itis** cochlea / inflammation
labyrinthitis LAB-uh-rinth-AI-tis **Definition** inflammation of the labyrinth	**labyrinth / itis** labyrinth / inflammation
sensorineural hearing loss SEN-sor-ee-NIR-al **Definition** hearing loss caused by sound not being transmitted from the inner ear to the brain (due to problems with the sensory organs or nerves)	**sensori / neur / al** sense / nerve / pertaining to
vestibular neuritis ves-TIH-byoo-lar nir-AI-tis **Definition** inflammation of the vestibular nerve	**vestibul / ar neur / itis** vestibule / pertaining to nerve / inflammation
vestibulitis ves-TIH-byoo-LAI-tis **Definition** inflammation of the vestibule	**vestibul / itis** vestibule / inflammation

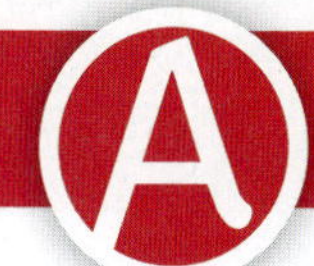

Learning Outcome 6.4 Exercises

PRONUNCIATION

EXERCISE 1 *Break down the following words into syllables.*

EXAMPLE: synesthesia *syn | es | the | sia*

1. retinopathy ______
2. ophthalmopathy ______
3. cochleitis ______
4. mastoiditis ______
5. scleroiritis ______
6. sclerokeratitis ______
7. sclerokeratoiritis ______
8. otosclerosis ______
9. dacryolithiasis ______
10. dacryostenosis ______
11. conjunctivitis ______
12. blepharoconjunctivitis ______
13. ophthalmomyitis ______
14. myringomycosis ______
15. rhinosalpingitis ______

EXERCISE 2 *Indicate which syllable is emphasized when pronounced.*

EXAMPLE: bronchitis bron**chi**tis

1. acoustic ______
2. neuroma ______
3. vestibular ______
4. neuritis ______
5. iritis ______
6. aphakia ______
7. trichiasis ______
8. otomycosis ______

TRANSLATION

EXERCISE 3 *Break down the following words into their component parts.*

EXAMPLE: nasopharyngoscope *naso | pharyngo | scope*

1. iridemia ______
2. retinopathy ______
3. ophthalmopathy ______
4. dacryostenosis ______
5. dacryocystitis ______
6. dacryoadenitis ______
7. otomycosis ______
8. myringomycosis ______
9. ophthalmomycosis ______
10. blepharoconjunctivitis ______
11. sclerokeratoiritis ______

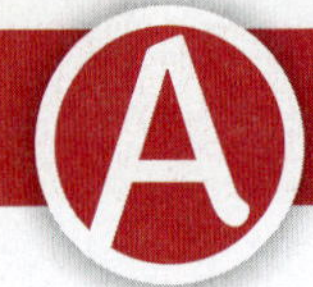

Learning Outcome 6.4 Exercises

EXERCISE 4 *Underline and define the word parts from this chapter in the following terms.*

1. corneal abrasion ____________
2. conjunctivitis ____________
3. mastoiditis ____________
4. cochleitis ____________
5. labyrinthitis ____________
6. vestibulitis ____________
7. myringitis ____________
8. blepharitis ____________
9. retinosis ____________
10. otosclerosis ____________
11. oculopathy ____________
12. keratopathy ____________
13. iridopathy ____________
14. cerumen impaction ____________
15. sclerectasia ____________
16. aniridia ____________
17. aphakia ____________
18. ophthalmomyitis ____________

EXERCISE 5 *Match the term on the left with its definition on the right.*

____ 1. cataract
____ 2. oculomycosis
____ 3. ophthalmatrophy
____ 4. dacryolithiasis
____ 5. dacryohemorrhea
____ 6. trichiasis

a. fungal eye condition
b. atrophy (wasting away) of the eye
c. condition caused by eyelashes growing backward and coming in contact with the eye
d. discharge of blood in the tears
e. opacity (cloudiness) of the lens of the eye
f. presence of hard formations (stones) in the tear system

EXERCISE 6 *Match the term on the left with its definition on the right.*

____ 1. retinitis
____ 2. keratitis
____ 3. iritis
____ 4. ophthalmitis
____ 5. phakitis
____ 6. optic neuritis
____ 7. iridokeratitis
____ 8. iridocyclitis
____ 9. scleroiritis
____ 10. sclerokeratitis
____ 11. cyclokeratitis

a. inflammation of the ciliary body and cornea
b. inflammation of the cornea
c. inflammation of the eye
d. inflammation of the iris
e. inflammation of the iris and ciliary body
f. inflammation of the iris and cornea
g. inflammation of the lens
h. inflammation of the optic nerve
i. inflammation of the retina
j. inflammation of the sclera and cornea
k. inflammation of the sclera and iris

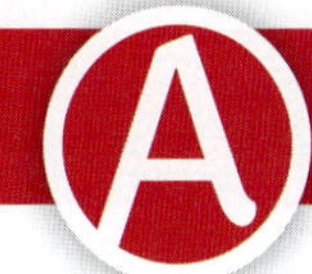

Learning Outcome 6.4 Exercises

EXERCISE 7 *Match the term on the left with its definition on the right.*

e	1. otitis media	a.	inflammation of the outer ear
a	2. otitis externa	b.	inflammation of the ear caused by air
b	3. aerotitis	c.	hearing loss caused by sound not getting to the middle/ inner ear (due to blockages)
c	4. conductive hearing loss	d.	inflammation of the eardrum and surrounding skin
h	5. sensorineural hearing loss	e.	inflammation of the middle ear
i	6. vestibular neuritis	f.	inflammation of the nose and eustachian tubes
g	7. acoustic neuroma	g.	tumor on the acoustic nerve
d	8. myringodermatitis	h.	hearing loss caused by sound not being transmitted from the inner ear to the brain (due to problems with the sense organs or nerves)
f	9. rhinosalpingitis	i.	inflammation of the vestibular nerve

EXERCISE 8 *Translate the following terms as literally as possible.*

EXAMPLE: nasopharyngoscope *an instrument for looking at the nose and throat*

1. oculopathy ______
2. ophthalmopathy ______
3. iridemia ______
4. iridokeratitis ______
5. cyclokeratitis ______
6. sclerectasia ______
7. scleroiritis ______
8. sclerokeratoiritis ______
9. blepharoconjunctivitis ______
10. dacryohemorrhea ______
11. dacryolithiasis ______
12. ophthalmomycosis ______
13. myringomycosis ______
14. trichiasis ______
15. optic neuritis ______
16. acoustic neuroma ______
17. vestibular neuritis ______
18. rhinosalpingitis ______

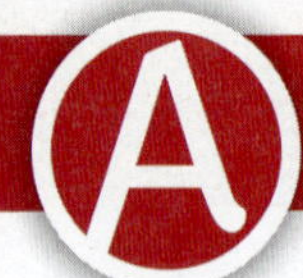

Learning Outcome 6.4 Exercises

GENERATION

EXERCISE 9 *Build a medical term from the information provided.*

EXAMPLE: inflammation of the sinuses *sinusitis*

1. inflammation of the retina ______
2. inflammation of the mastoid ______
3. inflammation of the cochlea ______
4. inflammation of the labyrinth ______
5. inflammation of the vestibule ______
6. inflammation of the lens ______
7. inflammation of the iris ______
8. inflammation of the iris and ciliary body ______
9. inflammation of the cornea (use *kerat/o*) ______
10. inflammation of the sclera and cornea ______
11. inflammation of the eardum (use *myring/o*) ______
12. inflammation of the eardrum and surrounding skin ______
13. inflammation of the eye (use *ophthalm/o*) ______
14. inflammation of the eye muscles ______
15. Inflammation of the eyelid ______
16. Inflammation of the eyelid and conjunctiva ______

EXERCISE 10 *Multiple-choice questions. Select the correct answer(s).*

1. Select the terms that pertain to the eye.
   a. aerotitis
   b. aphakia
   c. cataract
   d. cerumen impaction
   e. corneal abrasion
   f. ophthalmatrophy
   g. otitis media
2. Select the terms that pertain to the ear.
   a. aerotitis
   b. aphakia
   c. cataract
   d. cerumen impaction
   e. corneal abrasion
   f. ophthalmatrophy
   g. otitis media
3. The medical term that refers to the atrophy of the eye is
   a. oculosclerosis
   b. ophthalmatrophy
   c. otomatrophy
   d. otosclerosis

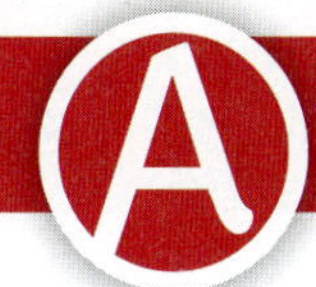

Learning Outcome 6.4 Exercises

4. A cataract affects what part of the eye?
   a. cornea
   b. lens
   c. optic nerve
   d. retina
5. A scratch on the cornea is called a(n)
   a. aphakia
   b. cataract
   c. corneal abrasion
   d. oculitis externa
6. Cerumen impaction is a
   a. buildup of ear wax blocking the ear canal
   b. buildup of ear wax hindering the function of the eardrum
   c. buildup of fluid causing pain in the ear canal
   d. buildup of fluid causing pain in the eardrum
7. Inflammation of the ear caused by air is
   a. aerotitis
   b. otitis externa
   c. otitis media
   d. pneumatic acoustitis

EXERCISE 11 *Briefly describe the difference between each pair of terms.*

1. iridopathy, keratopathy ____________________
2. retinopathy, retinosis ____________________
3. otitis externa, otitis media ____________________
4. dacryocystitis, dacryoadenitis ____________________
5. oculomycosis, otomycosis ____________________
6. dacryostenosis, otosclerosis ____________________
7. aniridia, aphakia ____________________
8. conductive hearing loss, sensorineural hearing loss ____________________

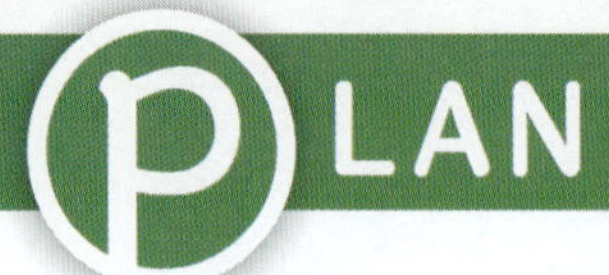

6.5 Treatments and Therapies

The Eye

Many advances have been made in eye surgery in recent years. A skilled surgeon can treat many disorders that could lead to blindness. In the outer layer, the sclera is a common site for making a cut (*sclerotomy*) in order to perform surgery in other parts of the eye.

The cornea is another common site for eye surgery. In a *corneal transplant,* a diseased cornea is removed and replaced with a donor cornea. Another type of corneal surgery, which involves making cuts in the cornea like spokes in a wheel (*radial keratotomy*), corrects myopia.

Many surgeries involve the next layer of the eye. The most common eye surgery is *cataract extraction.* The modern approach involves breaking the original lens up into small pieces, aspirating the pieces out of the eye through a needle (*phacoemulsification*), and then installing a new lens (*intraocular lens implantation*). *Iridotomy* and *iridectomy* are procedures used to treat glaucoma. Retinal detachment requires immediate reattachment (*retinopexy*) in order to prevent blindness.

In the most dire situations, such as aggressive cancer, an eye may need complete removal (*enucleation*). Cosmetic surgeries of the eye usually involve the eyelid (*blepharoplasty*) to remove wrinkles.

There are limited medicines specific to ophthalmology. *Cycloplegics* are used prior to surgery to temporarily paralyze the pupil. *Mydriatics* are used prior to a thorough eye exam to dilate the eyes. *Miotics* were commonly used to treat glaucoma before more effective treatments were discovered.

The Ear

Many treatments of the outer ear first involve a thorough cleaning of the ear canal. This can be done with washing (*ear lavage*) or inserting medicine to clear out the wax (*ceruminolytic*). One outer ear surgery (*otoplasty*) can make a deformed ear appear more normal. Another outer ear intervention is putting in a hearing aid (*auditory prosthesis*). This very common device is used to help people with hearing loss.

Middle ear procedures usually involve just the eardrum. Perhaps the most common surgery children undergo involves making a cut in the eardrum (*myringotomy*) and putting in a *tympanostomy* tube to drain fluid from the ear. Occasionally, when the tube falls out over time, it may leave a hole. In that case, the eardrum will need patching (*tympanoplasty*). In the inner ear, a more advanced electronic device can be placed in the cochlea (*cochlear implant*). Another inner ear surgery, *labryinthectomy,* can be used to treat severe vertigo.

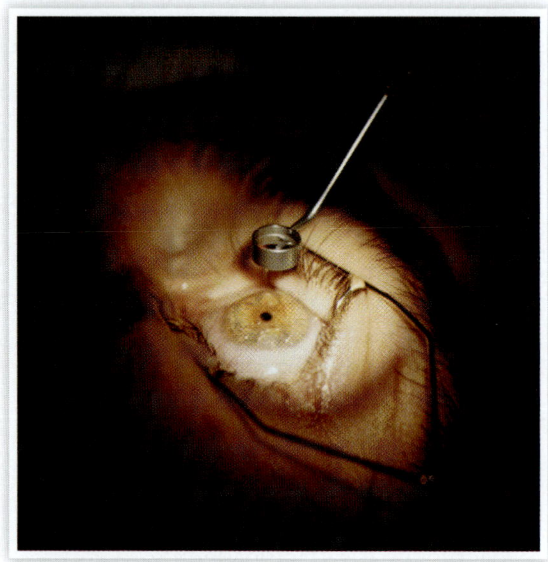

Surgery may be performed to treat a variety of eye disorders.

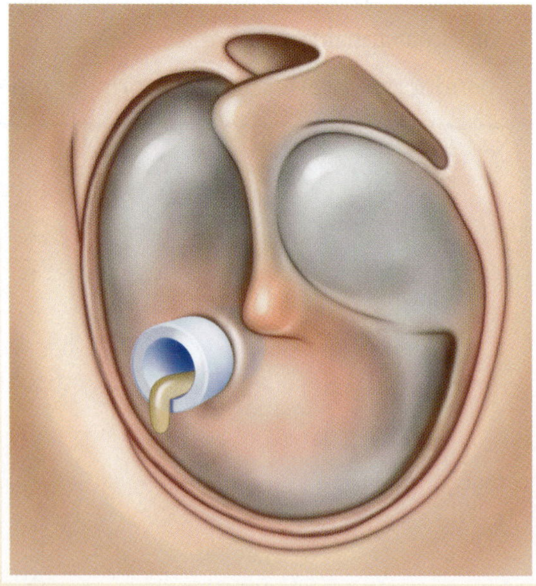

Tubes may be surgically installed in the eardrum to drain fluid from the ear.

6.5 Treatments and Therapies

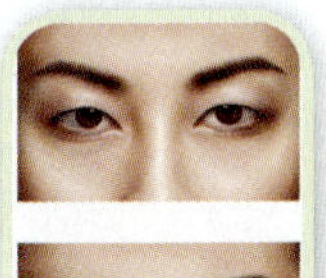

blepharoplasty

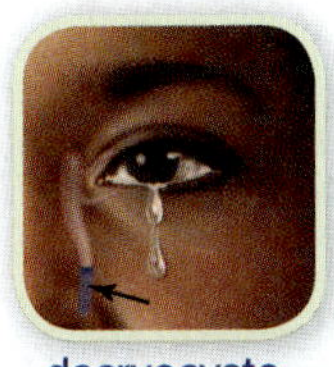

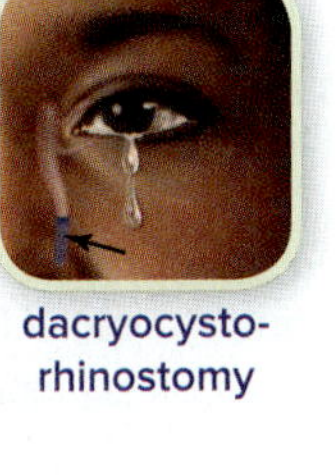

dacryocysto-rhinostomy

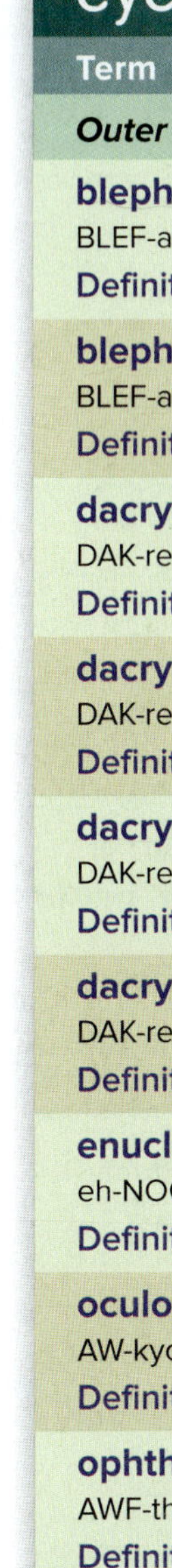

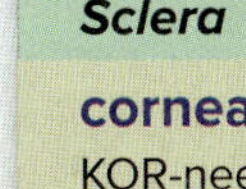

keratoplasty

eye

Term	Word Analysis
Outer Structures and Vision	
blepharoplasty BLEF-ah-roh-PLAS-tee **Definition** surgical reconstruction of the eyelid	blepharo / plasty eyelid / reconstruction
blepharotomy BLEF-ah-RAW-toh-mee **Definition** incision into the eyelid	blepharo / tomy eyelid / cut
dacryoadenectomy DAK-ree-oh-AD-en-EK-toh-mee **Definition** removal of the tear gland	dacryo / aden / ec / tomy tear / gland / out / cut
dacryocystectomy DAK-ree-oh-sis-TEK-toh-mee **Definition** removal of the tear sac	dacryo / cyst / ec / tomy tear / sac / out / cut
dacryocystorhinostomy DAK-ree-oh-SIS-toh-rai-NAWS-toh-mee **Definition** creation of an opening between the tear sac and the nose	dacryo / cysto / rhino / stom / y tear / sac / nose / opening / procedure
dacryocystotomy DAK-ree-oh-sis-TAWT-oh-mee **Definition** incision into the tear sac	dacryo / cysto / tomy tear / sac / cut
enucleation eh-NOO-clee-AY-shun **Definition** removal of an eye	e / nucle / ation out / nucleus / procedure
oculoplasty AW-kyoo-loh-PLAS-tee **Definition** surgical reconstruction of the eye	oculo / plasty eye / reconstruction
ophthalmectomy AWF-thal-MEK-toh-mee **Definition** removal of the eye	ophthalm / ec / tomy eye / out / cut
Sclera	
corneal transplant KOR-nee-al TRANZ-plant **Definition** replacement of damaged cornea with donated tissue	corne / al trans / plant cornea / pertaining to across / place
keratoplasty ker-A-toh-PLAS-tee **Definition** surgical reconstruction of the cornea	kerato / plasty cornea / reconstruction
keratotomy KER-ah-TAW-toh-mee **Definition** incision into the cornea	kerato / tomy cornea / cut
miotic mai-AW-tik **Definition** drug that causes the abnormal contraction of the pupil	miot / ic constriction / pertaining to

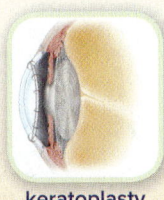

6.5 Treatments and Therapies

eye *continued*

Term	Word Analysis
mydriatic MID-ree-AT-ik	mydriat / ic dilation / pertaining to
Definition drug that causes the abnormal dilation of the pupil	
sclerotomy skler-AW-toh-mee	sclero / tomy sclera / cut
Definition incision into the sclera	
Choroid/Retina	
cycloplegic SAI-kloh-PLEE-jik	cyclo / pleg / ic ciliary body / paralysis / pertaining to
Definition drug that paralyzes the ciliary body	
cyclotomy sai-KLAW-toh-mee	cyclo / tomy ciliary body / cut
Definition incision into the ciliary body	
intraocular lens implant IN-trah-AW-kyoo-lar lenz IM-plant	intra / ocul / ar lens im / plant inside / eye / pertaining to lens in / place
Definition insertion of a new lens inside the eye	
intravitreal antibiotics IN-trah-VEE-tree-al AN-tai-bai-AW-tiks	intra / vitre / al anti / biot / ics inside / vitreous / pertaining to against / life / agent
Definition antibiotics administered directly into the vitreous gel liquid	
iridectomy EAR-id-EK-toh-mee	irid / ec / tomy iris / out / cut
Definition removal of the iris	
iridocyclectomy EAR-ih-doh-sai-KLEK-toh-mee	irido / cycl / ec / tomy iris / ciliary body / out / cut
Definition removal of the iris and ciliary body	
iridotomy EAR-id-AW-toh-mee	irido / tomy iris / cut
Definition incision into the iris	
phacoemulsification FAY-koh-ee-MUL-sih-fih-KAY-shun	phaco / emulsific / ation lens / mix up / condition
Definition fragmentation of an existing lens in order to remove and replace it	
retinopexy reh-TIH-noh-PEK-see	retino / pexy retina / surgical fixation
Definition surgical fixation (reattachment) of a retina	
retinotomy REH-tih-NAW-toh-mee	retino / tomy retina / cut
Definition incision into the retina	
vitrectomy vih-TREK-toh-mee	vitr / ec / tomy vitreous / out / cut
Definition removal of the vitreous liquid from the eye	

intraocular lens implant

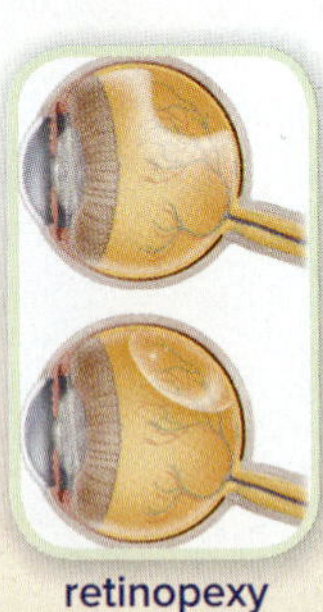

retinopexy

6.5 Treatments and Therapies

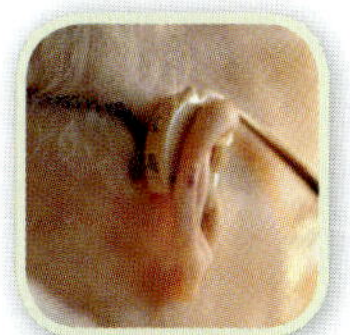

auditory prosthesis

ear

Term	Word Analysis
Outer Ear	
auditory prosthesis AW-dih-TOR-ee praws-THEE-sis **Definition** hearing aid	auditory pros / thesis hearing toward / place
ceruminolysis seh-ROO-min-AW-lih-sis **Definition** breakdown of ear wax	cerumino / lysis ear wax / loose
ceruminolytic seh-ROO-min-oh-LIH-tik **Definition** drug that aids in the breakdown of ear wax	cerumino / lyt / ic ear wax / loose / pertaining to
ear instillation ee-ir in-stil-AY-shun **Definition** ear drops	ear in / still / ation ear in / drop / condition
ear lavage ee-ir lah-VAJ **Definition** rinsing/washing the external ear canal (usually to remove ear wax) NOTE: It's the origin of the English word *lavatory.*	from Latin, for *to wash, bathe*
mastoidectomy MAS-toy-DEK-toh-mee **Definition** removal of the mastoid	mastoid / ec / tomy mastoid / out / cut
mastoidocentesis mas-TOY-doh-sin-TEE-sis **Definition** puncture of the mastoid	mastoido / centesis mastoid / puncture
otoplasty OH-toh-PLAS-tee **Definition** surgical reconstruction of the ear	oto / plasty ear / reconstruction
Middle Ear	
myringectomy MIR-in-JEK-toh-mee **Definition** removal of the eardrum	myring / ec / tomy eardrum / out / cut
myringoplasty mir-IN-goh-PLAS-tee **Definition** surgical reconstruction of the eardrum	myringo / plasty eardrum / reconstruction
myringotomy mir-in-GAW-toh-mee **Definition** incision into the eardrum	myringo / tomy eardrum / cut
tympanocentesis tim-PAN-oh-sin-TEE-sis **Definition** puncture of the eardrum	tympano / centesis eardrum / puncture

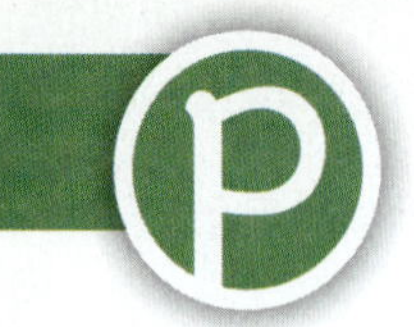

6.5 Treatments and Therapies

ear *continued*

Term	Word Analysis
tympanolabyrinthopexy tim-PAN-oh-lah-buh-RINTH-oh-PEK-see **Definition** surgical fixation of the eardrum to the labyrinth	**tympano / labyrintho / pexy** eardrum / labyrinth / surgical fixation
tympanoplasty tim-PAN-oh-PLAS-tee **Definition** surgical reconstruction of the eardrum	**tympano / plasty** eardrum / reconstruction
tympanostomy TIM-pan-AW-stoh-mee **Definition** creation of an opening in the eardrum	**tympano / stom / y** eardrum / opening / procedure
Inner Ear	
cochlear implant KOH-klee-ar IM-plant **Definition** electronic device that stimulates the cochlea; it can give a sense of sound to those who are profoundly deaf	**cochle / ar im / plant** cochlea / pertaining to in / place
labyrinthectomy LAB-uh-rinth-EK-toh-mee **Definition** removal of the labyrinth	**labyrinth / ec / tomy** labyrinth / out / cut
labyrinthotomy LAB-uh-rinth-AW-toh-mee **Definition** incision into the labyrinth	**labyrintho / tomy** labyrinth / cut
ototoxic OH-toh-TOK-sik **Definition** drug that is damaging to the ear/hearing	**oto / poison / ic** ear / poision / pertaining to
vestibulotomy ves-TIH-byoo-LAW-toh-mee **Definition** incision into the vestibule	**vestibulo / tomy** vestibule / cut

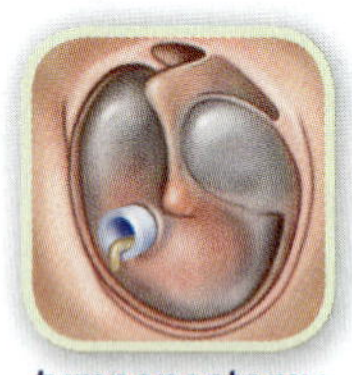
tympanostomy

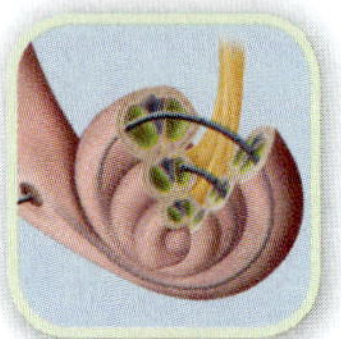
cochlear implant

Learning Outcome 6.5 Exercises

PRONUNCIATION

EXERCISE 1 *Break down the following words into syllables.*

EXAMPLE: synesthesia *syn | es | the | sia*

1. ototoxic ________
2. retinopexy ________
3. retinotomy ________
4. iridectomy ________
5. keratoplasty ________
6. blepharotomy ________
7. myringotomy ________
8. tympanostomy ________
9. labyrinthotomy ________
10. labyrinthectomy ________
11. mastoidectomy ________
12. tympanocentesis ________
13. vestibulotomy ________
14. dacryoadenectomy ________
15. ceruminolytic ________
16. phacoemulsification ________
17. dacryocystorhinostomy ________
18. tympanolabyrinthopexy ________

EXERCISE 2 *Indicate which syllable is emphasized when pronounced.*

EXAMPLE: bronchitis bron**chi**tis

1. cochlear ________
2. lavage ________
3. miotic ________
4. vitrectomy ________

TRANSLATION

EXERCISE 3 *Break down the following words into their component parts.*

EXAMPLE: nasopharyngoscope *naso | pharyngo | scope*

1. keratotomy ________
2. labyrinthotomy ________
3. myringotomy ________
4. cyclotomy ________
5. blepharotomy ________
6. tympanostomy ________
7. labyrinthectomy ________
8. vitrectomy ________
9. myringectomy ________
10. mastoidectomy ________
11. ophthalmectomy ________
12. iridocylcectomy ________
13. dacryoadenectomy ________
14. dacryocystectomy ________
15. dacryocystotomy ________
16. tympanolabyrinthopexy ________

Learning Outcome 6.5 Exercises

EXERCISE 4 *Underline and define the word parts from this chapter in the following terms.*

1. iridectomy ______
2. iridotomy ______
3. retinotomy ______
4. vestibulotomy ______
5. sclerotomy ______
6. oculoplasty ______
7. blepharoplasty ______
8. cycloplegic ______
9. otoplasty ______
10. keratoplasty ______
11. tympanoplasty ______
12. myringoplasty ______
13. ceruminolysis ______
14. mastoidocentesis ______
15. tympanocentesis ______
16. intravitreal antibiotics ______
17. intraocular lens implant ______
18. dacryocystorhinostomy ______

EXERCISE 5 *Match the term on the left with its definition on the right.*

Term	Definition
__i__ 1. corneal transplant	a. drug that is damaging to the ear/hearing
__c__ 2. cochlear implant	b. hearing aid
__a__ 3. ototoxic	c. electronic device that stimulates the cochlea
__b__ 4. auditory prosthesis	d. drug that causes the abnormal contraction of the pupil
__f__ 5. ear instillation	e. drug that causes the abnormal dilation of the pupil
__j__ 6. ear lavage	f. ear drops
__l__ 7. ceruminolytic	g. fragmentation of an existing lens in order to remove and replace it
__k__ 8. retinopexy	h. removal of an eye
__e__ 9. mydriatic	i. replacement of damaged cornea with donated tissue
__d__ 10. miotic	j. rinsing/washing the external ear canal (usually to remove ear wax)
__h__ 11. enucleation	k. surgical fixation (reattachment) of a retina
__g__ 12. phacoemulsification	l. breakdown of ear wax

Learning Outcome 6.5 Exercises

EXERCISE 6 *Translate the following terms as literally as possible.*

EXAMPLE: nasopharyngoscope *an instrument for looking at the nose and throat*

1. ototoxic ______
2. cycloplegic ______
3. tympanostomy ______
4. iridectomy ______
5. vitrectomy ______
6. mastoidectomy ______
7. labyrinthectomy ______
8. myringectomy ______
9. ophthalmectomy ______
10. iridocyclectomy ______
11. phacoemulsification ______
12. dacryocystorhinostomy ______

GENERATION

EXERCISE 7 *Build a medical term from the information provided.*

EXAMPLE: inflammation of the sinuses *sinusitis*

1. incision into the eardrum (use *myringo*) ______
2. incision into the cornea ______
3. incision into the retina ______
4. incision into the iris ______
5. incision into the sclera ______
6. incision into the labyrinth ______
7. incision into the vestibule ______
8. incision into the eyelid ______
9. incision into the ciliary body ______
10. incision into the tear sac ______

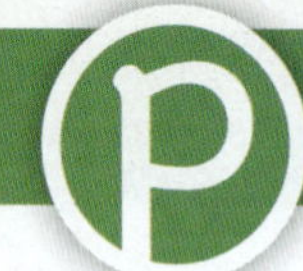

Learning Outcome 6.5 Exercises

EXERCISE 8 *Multiple-choice questions. Select the correct answer(s).*

1. Select the terms that pertain to the ear.
   - a. blepharoplasty
   - b. keratoplasty
   - c. myringoplasty
   - d. oculoplasty
   - e. otoplasty
   - f. tympanoplasty
2. Select the terms that pertain to the eye.
   - a. blepharoplasty
   - b. keratoplasty
   - c. myringoplasty
   - d. oculoplasty
   - e. otoplasty
   - f. tympanoplasty
3. Select the terms that mean *removal of an eye.*
   - a. corneal transplant
   - b. enucleation
   - c. intraocular lens implant
   - d. ophthalmectomy
4. Select the terms than involve surgery of the choroid/retina layer of the eye.
   - a. corneal transplant
   - b. enucleation
   - c. intraocular lens implant
   - d. ophthalmectomy
5. Intravitreal antibiotics are administered to which part of the body?
   - a. blood vessels in the outer eye
   - b. vein
   - c. vitreous liquid of the eye
   - d. vitreous liquid of the inner ear

EXERCISE 9 *Briefly describe the difference between each pair of terms.*

1. ear instillation, ear lavage ______________________
2. mastoidocentesis, tympanocentesis ______________________
3. dacryoadenectomy, dacryocystectomy ______________________
4. retinopexy, tympanolabyrinthopexy ______________________
5. ceruminolysis, ceruminolytic ______________________
6. auditory prosthesis, cochlear implant ______________________
7. mydriatic, miotic ______________________

6.6 Abbreviations

Abbreviations provide a shorthand way of referring to things that either recur often or are too long to write out. When dealing with the eyes and ears, these abbreviations can refer to everything from body parts (OD, OS, AD, AS, TM) to common observations (PERRLA), common diagnoses (ARMD, OM), and common procedures (LASIK).

eye

Abbreviation	Definition
ARMD	age-related macular degeneration
HEENT	head, eyes, ears, nose, and throat
IOL	intraocular lens
IOP	intraocular pressure
LASIK	laser-assisted in situ keratomileusis
OD	right eye (from Latin—*oculus dexter*)
OS	left eye (from Latin—*oculus sinister*)
OU	both eyes (from Latin—*oculus uterque*)
PERRLA	pupils are equal, round, and reactive to light and accommodation
VA	visual acuity
VF	visual field

ear

Abbreviation	Definition
AD	right ear (from Latin—*auris dextra*)
AS	left ear (from Latin—*auris sinistra*)
AU	both ears (from Latin—*auris utraque*)
AOM	acute otitis media
EENT	eye, ear, nose, and throat
ENT	ear, nose, and throat
OM	otitis media
TM	tympanic membrane

Learning Outcome 6.6 Exercises

EXERCISE 1 *Match the abbreviation on the left with its definition on the right.*

__e__	1. AD	a. both ears
__c__	2. AS	b. both eyes
__a__	3. AU	c. left ear
__f__	4. OD	d. left eye
__d__	5. OS	e. right ear
__b__	6. OU	f. right eye

EXERCISE 2 *Define the following abbreviations.*

1. ARMD __________
2. HEENT __________
3. IOL __________
4. OD __________
5. OS __________
6. OU __________
7. PERRLA __________
8. ENT __________
9. AOM __________
10. OM __________
11. TM __________
12. EENT __________

EXERCISE 3 *Give the abbreviations for the following definitions.*

1. intraocular pressure __________
2. laser-assisted in situ keratomileusis __________
3. right eye __________
4. left eye __________
5. both eyes __________
6. visual acuity __________
7. visual field __________
8. right ear __________
9. left ear __________
10. both ears __________

Learning Outcome 6.6 Exercises

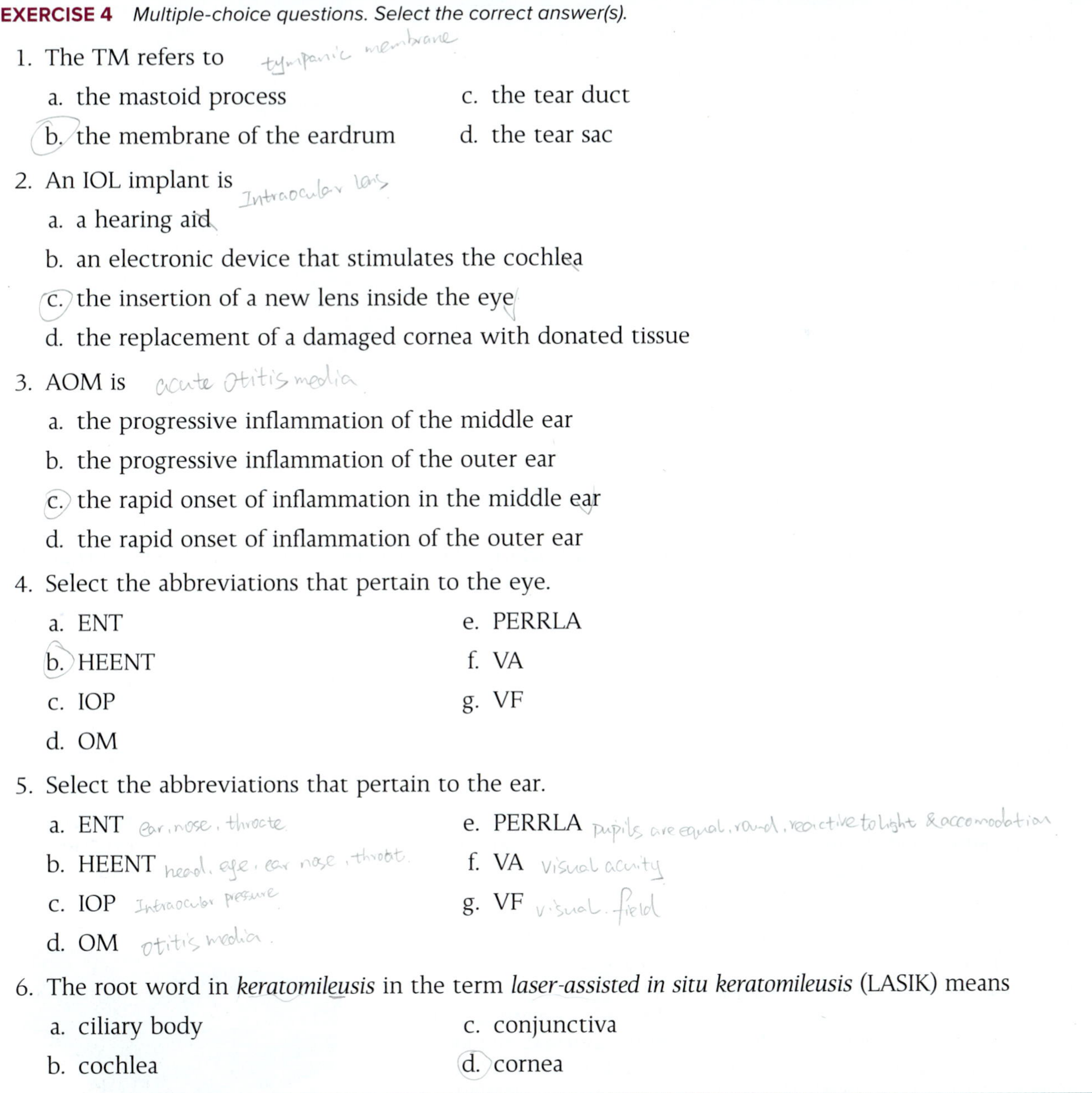

EXERCISE 4 *Multiple-choice questions. Select the correct answer(s).*

1. The TM refers to
   a. the mastoid process
   b. the membrane of the eardrum
   c. the tear duct
   d. the tear sac

2. An IOL implant is
   a. a hearing aid
   b. an electronic device that stimulates the cochlea
   c. the insertion of a new lens inside the eye
   d. the replacement of a damaged cornea with donated tissue

3. AOM is
   a. the progressive inflammation of the middle ear
   b. the progressive inflammation of the outer ear
   c. the rapid onset of inflammation in the middle ear
   d. the rapid onset of inflammation of the outer ear

4. Select the abbreviations that pertain to the eye.
   a. ENT
   b. HEENT
   c. IOP
   d. OM
   e. PERRLA
   f. VA
   g. VF

5. Select the abbreviations that pertain to the ear.
   a. ENT
   b. HEENT
   c. IOP
   d. OM
   e. PERRLA
   f. VA
   g. VF

6. The root word in *keratomileusis* in the term *laser-assisted in situ keratomileusis* (LASIK) means
   a. ciliary body
   b. cochlea
   c. conjunctiva
   d. cornea

6.7 Electronic Health Records

Discharge Summary

Patient Name: Ms. Susan Cloud
Date of Admission: 6/23/15
Date of Discharge: 6/28/15

Admission Diagnosis

1. **Cataract** extraction

Discharge Diagnosis

1. Post-cataract extraction
2. **Endophthalmitis**

Discharge Condition
Stable

Consultations
Infectious disease

Procedures

1. **Extracapsular cataract** extraction with **phacoemulsification** and implantation of a posterior chamber **intraocular lens,** right eye.
2. **Vitrectomy.**

Labs
CBC: WBC 22.4 on 6/24; 18.5 6/25; 15.1 on 6/27; BCx. negative; **vitreous** culture: *Staphylococcus epidermidis*

Imaging
Ocular u/s: **vitreous** inflammation. No **retinal** detachment.

HPI
Ms. Cloud is a 58-year-old woman who first presented to her **ophthalmologist** with c/o **leukocoria.** She was also noted to have **nystagmus** and **strabismus.** She was diagnosed with a **cataract.** She was treated surgically with **cataract** extraction and **lens** implantation. She was admitted to the hospital on 6/23/2015 for postoperative observation.

Hospital Course
On postop day 2, Ms. Cloud began complaining of increasing right **ophthalmalgia.** She was noted to be febrile to 102.2. Exam revealed **conjunctival** infection and edema. She was presumed to have postoperative endophthalmitis. **Vitrectomy** was performed under sterile conditions, and samples were sent to lab for culture. She was given **intravitreal** antibiotics. Over the next couple of days, her fever curve trended down and her WBC count improved. Cultures came back positive for *S. epidermidis.* Infectious disease was consulted; they recommended two weeks of IV therapy. A PICC line was placed and she was discharged with care instructions.

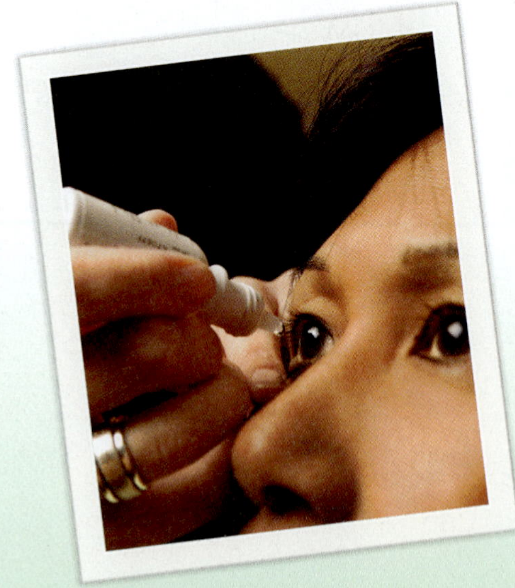

Activity
Eye rest

Diet
No restrictions

Meds
IV vancomycin via PICC

Follow-Up Appointments
Ophthalmology outpatient clinic in 2 days
Infectious disease clinic in 1 week

–Lynn Holmes, MD

Learning Outcome 6.7 Exercises

EXERCISE 1 *Match the term on the left with its definition on the right.*

h	1. conjunctival	a.	condition where the eyes deviate when looking at the same object
j	2. retinal	b.	eye specialist
i	3. ocular	c.	fragmentation of an existing lens in order to remove and replace it
b	4. ophthalmologist	d.	inflammation of the eye
d	5. ophthalmitis	e.	involuntary back-and-forth movement of the eyes
g	6. ophthalmalgia	f.	opacity (cloudiness) of the lens of the eye
f	7. cataract	g.	pain in the eye
e	8. nystagmus	h.	pertaining to the conjunctiva
a	9. strabismus	i.	pertaining to the eye
c	10. phacoemulsification	j.	pertaining to the retina

EXERCISE 2 *Fill in the blanks.*

1. According to the admission diagnosis, Ms. Cloud was admitted for a(n) ________________.
2. The images performed on Ms. Cloud revealed that she had no *retinal detachment*, or that her ________________ was still properly attached.
3. Ms. Cloud was first presented to her ________________ (eye specialist) with c/o leukocoria, and was noted to have *nystagmus* (give definition: ________________) and *strabismus* (give definition: ________________).
4. During her surgery, her ________________ was removed and a(n) ________________ was implanted.
5. On *postop* (give definition: ________________) day, 2 Ms. Cloud began complaining of increasing right eye pain, or ________________.
6. A *vitrectomy* (give definition: ________________) was performed under sterile conditions, and samples were sent to the lab for culture. She was then begun on ________________ (antibiotics administered directly inside the vitreous gel liquid).

EXERCISE 3 *True or false questions. Indicate true answers with a T and false answers with an F.*

1. This health record was created at an ophthalmology clinic. ________
2. Ms. Cloud began complaining that her eye felt inflamed the second day after her operation. ________
3. During her second postop day, Ms. Cloud was noted to have a fever. ________
4. The cultures came back negative for an infection. ________
5. Ms. Cloud will need to follow-up with an optometrist in 2 days. ________

Learning Outcome 6.7 Exercises

EXERCISE 4 *Multiple-choice questions. Select the correct answer(s).*

1. The patient was admitted to the hospital for

   a. a cataract extraction
   b. a lens implantation
   c. ophthalmalgia and a fever
   d. postoperative observation

2. The health record indicates that the patient "was presumed to have post-operative endophthalmitis." The term *endophthalmitis* is created by combining the prefix *endo-* with the term *ophthalmitis,* which means

   a. discharge from the cornea
   b. discharge from the eye
   c. inflammation in the cornea
   d. inflammation in the eye

3. The patient will receive antibiotics via a PICC line, which is a

   a. peripherally inserted central catheter
   b. peripherally inserted corneal control
   c. phacoemulsification inserted corneal control
   d. phacoemulsification iridocyclectal catheter

4. The abbreviation for the term *intraocular lens* is

   a. IL
   b. IOL
   c. ICL
   d. OL

5. *Staph epidermidis* is a staph infection of the *epidermis,* which is the

   a. eye
   b. lens
   c. nerves
   d. skin

Eye Consult

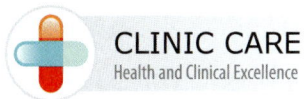

Dr. Strauss,

I saw Mrs. Kelly Robison in my office on 5/7/2015 for routine follow-up. As you know, Mrs. Robison initially presented with nystagmus, strabismus, and noted photophobia. She was diagnosed at the time with aniridia. I have been treating her medically with miotics.

Her resultant refractive errors have been corrected with glasses, and she had strabismus surgery in 2013 to help improve her binocular vision. Last year, she was noted to have significant corneal clouding that was successfully treated with keratoplasty.

As is common with this condition, the medicine alone was not enough to prevent glaucoma. I have been routinely monitoring her IOP, and it has risen in the recent past. It is my recommendation to perform a trabeculotomy to relieve the pressure. I discussed the risks and benefits from the surgery with Mrs. Robison, and she is interested in proceeding. She will contact my staff for scheduling.

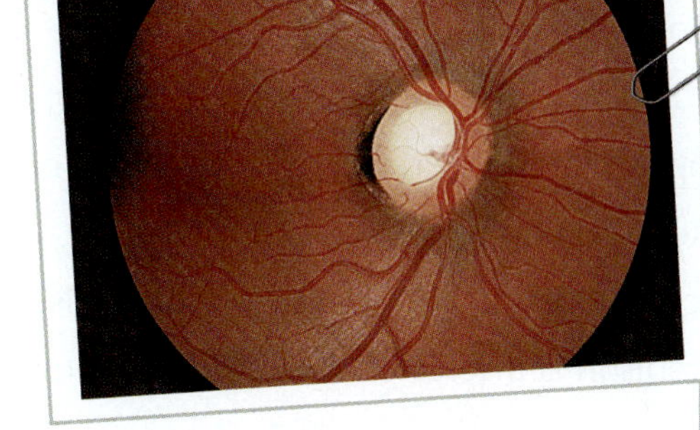

If you have any questions, please call me.

Sincerely,

Theodora McIntosh, MD

Learning Outcome 6.7 Exercises

EXERCISE 5 *Match the term on the left with its definition on the right.*

	Term	Definition
e.	1. binocular	a. condition where the eyes deviate when looking at the same object
b	2. aniridia	b. absence of an iris
f.	3. keratoplasty	c. drug that causes the abnormal contraction of the pupil
a.	4. strabismus	d. involuntary back-and-forth movement of the eyes
d.	5. nystagmus	e. pertaining to both eyes
c.	6. miotic	f. surgical reconstruction of the cornea

EXERCISE 6 *Fill in the blanks.*

1. Mrs. Robison initially presented with ______________ (involuntary back-and-forth movement of the eyes), ______________ (a condition where the eyes deviate when looking at the same object), and ______________ (extreme sensitivity to light).
2. Mrs. Robison was diagnosed with *aniridia* (give definition: ______________) and treated with *miotics* (give definition: ______________).
3. Mrs. Robison's corneal clouding was successfully treated with ______________ (surgical reconstruction of the ______________).

EXERCISE 7 *True or false questions. Indicate true answers with a T and false answers with an F.*

1. Mrs. Robison is having difficulty hearing. ________
2. Mrs. Robison's initial diagnosis included the absence of a lens in her eye. ________
3. A miotic causes the abnormal contraction of the pupil. ________
4. Keratoplasty was successful in treating the clouding that occurred in the patient's cornea. ________
5. Mrs. Robison has developed glaucoma. ________
6. Dr. McIntosh has been monitoring the pressure in the patient's cornea. ________
7. Mrs. Robison is interested in a trabeculotomy. ________

EXERCISE 8 *Multiple-choice questions. Select the correct answer(s).*

1. The abbreviation IOP stands for
   - a. internal ophthalmopathy
   - b. intraocular phacoscopy
   - c. intraocular pressure
   - d. iridopathy
2. Dr. McIntosh recommends a *trabeculotomy*, a medical term formed by combining *trabecula* (part of the anatomy of the eye) and *-otomy*, which means
   - a. creation of an opening
   - b. incision
   - c. removal
   - d. surgical reconstruction
3. A drug that causes the abnormal contraction of the pupil is called a(n)
   - a. ectropion
   - b. miotic
   - c. mydriatic
   - d. ototoxic

Ear Consult

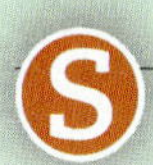

Subjective

Johnny Masur is a 4-year-old boy referred to my clinic for evaluation of chronic otitis media. He began with a 1-week history of nasal congestion, runny nose, and cough. He has had a low-grade temperature up to 100.2. He went to his PCP last week for **otopyorrhea** on the left side and **otalgia** on the right side. He was diagnosed with bilateral acute otitis media and treated with oral antibiotics. He has failed three separate courses of oral antibiotics.

PMHx

Johnny's history is significant for **tympanostomy** tubes placed bilaterally when he was 2 years old. One tube left a persistent perforation in the tympanic membrane, so he had **tympanoplasty** at 3 years of age. He has not had any episodes of **otitis media** in the past 2 years.

Objective

Physical Exam

RR: 24; HR: 88; Temp: 99.9; BP: 98/68.

Gen: Well-developed 4y/o in no acute distress.

HEENT: Normocephalic. PERRLA. No conjunctival erythema; mild clear nasal discharge; right canal blocked with cerumen–after ceruminolytic placed and canal clear, the tympanic membrane was seen. It was erythematous and full. Some mild tympanosclerosis of TM noted; the left ear was erythematous and full. Mild mastoidalgia on the left, but the ear is not displaced forward.

CV: RRR without murmur.

Resp: CTA.

Assessment

Johnny has chronic otitis media failing three courses of oral antibiotics.

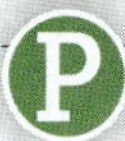

Plan

I have performed **tympanocentesis** in the office and sent the fluid for culture. While awaiting the result, we will treat him with an IM antibiotic. I will also send a fungal culture to rule out otomycosis. While Johnny has mild mastoidalgia, he is afebrile today and in no distress, and his ear is not displaced. Thus, I do not think he has acute **mastoiditis,** but I told Johnny's parents what to look for. Given how long Johnny has had this infection, he will need to see audiology for audiometry when he is better.

–Johanna Long, MD

Learning Outcome 6.7 Exercises

EXERCISE 9 *Match the term on the left with its definition on the right.*

	Term		Definition
____	1. otitis media	a.	drug that aids in the breakdown of ear wax
____	2. audiometry	b.	fungal ear condition
____	3. tympanoplasty	c.	creation of an opening in the eardrum
____	4. otalgia	d.	discharge of pus from the ear
____	5. mastoidalgia	e.	ear pain
____	6. mastoiditis	f.	hardening of the eardrum
____	7. tympanostomy	g.	inflammation of the mastoid
____	8. ceruminolytic	h.	inflammation of the middle ear
____	9. tympanocentesis	i.	pain in the mastoid
____	10. otopyorrhea	j.	procedure for measuring hearing
____	11. otomycosis	k.	puncture of the eardrum
____	12. tympanosclerosis	l.	surgical reconstruction of the eardrum

EXERCISE 10 *Match the abbreviation on the left with its definition on the right.*

____	1. TM	a.	clear to auscultation
____	2. PCP	b.	head, eyes, ears, nose, and throat
____	3. RRR	c.	primary care provider
____	4. CTA	d.	pupils are equal, round, and reactive to light and accommodation
____	5. HEENT	e.	regular rate and rhythm
____	6. PERRLA	f.	tympanic membrane

EXERCISE 11 *Fill in the blanks.*

1. The patient went to his PCP (give definition: ________________________________) for *otopyorrhea* (discharge of ________________ from the ear) and *otalgia* (give definition: ________________________).
2. Johnny had a(n) ________________ (surgical reconstruction of the eardrum) at 3 years of age.
3. Patient's heart rate: ________________; respiratory rate: ________________; blood pressure: ________________________________
4. Johnny's right ear canal was blocked with *cerumen* (give definition: ________________________), and was given a(n) ________________ (a drug that aids in the breakdown of ear wax).

EXERCISE 12 *True or false questions. Indicate true answers with a T and false answers with an F.*

1. The patient was diagnosed by his primary care physician with AOM in both ears. ________
2. Oral antibiotics was an effective treatment for the patient's symptoms in the past. ________
3. Johnny had tubes placed in both of his eardrums when he was 2 years old. ________
4. One tube left a hole in his TM. ________
5. Upon exam, the patient's eardrums were red on both sides. ________
6. Upon exam, the patient had pain in his left ear. ________
7. Part of the physician's plan for care included the puncturing of Johnny's eardrum. ________
8. The patient was diagnosed with otomycosis. ________

Learning Outcome 6.7 Exercises

EXERCISE 13 *Multiple-choice questions. Select the correct answer(s).*

1. The patient visited his physician for *otalgia,* or ear pain. Another medical term for *ear pain* is
   a. mastoidalgia
   b. myringodynia
   c. ophthalmalgia
   d. otodynia
2. *Otitis media* is an inflammation of the middle ear. An inflammation of the outer ear is called
   a. macrotia
   b. osteoacusis
   c. otitis externa
   d. otomycosis
3. The patient was referred to this clinic for *chronic otitis media,* which is
   a. inflammation of the middle ear that has been going on for a while
   b. inflammation of the middle ear that just started recently
   c. inflammation of the outer ear that has been going on for a while
   d. inflammation of the outer ear that just started recently
4. The abbreviation PCP stands for
   a. past care provider
   b. patient care provider
   c. primary care patient
   d. primary care provider
5. The abbreviation for *acute otitis media* is
   a. AO
   b. AOM
   c. AOTM
   d. OM
6. Johnny's history is significant for tubes placed in his
   a. cerumen
   b. cochlea
   c. eardrum
   d. mastoid
7. After clearing the ear canal from ear wax, the tympanic membrane was "*erythematous* and full." The root *erythro* means
   a. black
   b. red
   c. white
   d. yellow
8. Because Johnny's ear infection persisted for so long, Dr. Long recommended that the patient visit with audiology for a(n) ______________________________ when he is better.
   a. antibiotic screening
   b. auditory prosthesis
   c. hearing test
   d. tympanocentesis

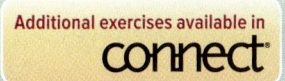

Chapter Review exercises, along with additional practice items, are available in Connect!

Quick Reference

quick reference glossary of roots

Root	Definition	Root	Definition
acous/o	sound	**mastoid/o**	mastoid process
-acusis	hearing condition	**myring/o**	eardrum
audi/o	sound	**ocul/o**	eye
aur/o	ear	**ophthalm/o**	eye
blephar/o	eyelid	**-opia**	vision condition
cerumin/o	ear wax	**-opsia**	vision condition
cochle/o	cochlea	**opt/o**	eye
conjunctiv/o	conjunctiva	**ot/o**	ear
corne/o	cornea	**phac/o**	lens
cycl/o	ciliary body	**phak/o**	lens
dacry/o	tear	**retin/o**	retina
irid/o	iris	**salping/o**	eustachian tube
ir/o	iris	**scler/o**	sclera (the white of the eye)
kerat/o	cornea	**tympan/o**	eardrum
labyrinth/o	labyrinth	**vestibul/o**	vestibule
lacrim/o	tear		

quick reference glossary of terms

Term	Definition
acoustic neuroma	a tumor on the acoustic nerve
aerotitis	inflammation of the ear caused by air
akinetopsia	the inability to see objects in motion
ambiopia	double vision
amblyopia	decreased vision (when it occurs in one eye, it is referred to as *lazy eye*)
aniridia	absence of an iris
aphakia	absence of a lens
asthenopia	weak vision (i.e., eye *strain*)
astigmatism	vision problem caused by the fact that light rays entering the eye aren't focused on a single point in the back of the eye

quick reference glossary of terms *continued*

Term	Definition
audiogram	record produced by an audiometer
audiologist	hearing specialist
audiometer	instrument for measuring hearing
audiometry	procedure for measuring hearing
auditory prosthesis	hearing aid
aural	pertaining to the ear
binocular	pertaining to both eyes
blepharedema	eyelid swelling
blepharitis	eyelid inflammation
blepharoconjunctivitis	inflammation of the eyelid and conjunctiva
blepharoplasty	surgical reconstruction of the eyelid
blepharoplegia	paralysis of the eyelid
blepharoptosis	drooping eyelid
blepharopyorrhea	discharge of pus from the eyelid
blepharospasm	involuntary contraction of an eyelid
blepharotomy	incision into the eyelid
cataract	opacity (cloudiness) of the lens of the eye (from Latin, for *waterfall*)
cerumen impaction	buildup of ear wax blocking the ear canal
ceruminolysis	breakdown of ear wax
ceruminolytic	drug that aids in the breakdown of ear wax
ceruminoma	benign tumor of the cerumen-secreting glands of the ear
ceruminosis	excessive formation of ear wax
cochlear implant	electronic device that stimulates the cochlea; it can give the sense of sound to those who are profoundly deaf
cochleitis	inflammation of the cochlea
conductive hearing loss	sound does not get to the middle/inner ear (due to blockages)
conjunctivitis	inflammation of the conjunctiva (also known as *pink eye*)
corneal abrasion	scratch on the cornea
corneal transplant	replacement of damaged cornea with donated tissue
corneal xerosis	dryness of the cornea
cyclokeratitis	inflammation of the ciliary body and cornea
cycloplegia	paralysis of the ciliary body

quick reference glossary of terms *continued*

Term	Definition
cycloplegic	drug that paralyzes the ciliary body
cyclotomy	incision into the ciliary body
dacrocystitis	inflammation of the tear sac
dacryadenitis	inflammation of the tear gland
dacryoadenalgia	pain in the tear gland
dacryoadenectomy	removal of the tear gland
dacryocystalgia	pain in the tear sac
dacryocystectomy	removal of the tear sac
dacryocystorhinostomy	creation of an opening between the tear sac and the nose
dacryocystotomy	incision into the tear sac
dacryohemorrhea	discharge of blood in the tears
dacryolith	hard formation (stone) in the tear system
dacryolithiasis	presence of hard formations (stones) in the tear system
dacryopyorrhea	discharge of pus in tears
dacryorrhea	excessive tearing
dacryostenosis	narrowing of the tear duct
diplopia	double vision
ear instillation	ear drops
ear lavage	rinsing/washing the external ear canal (usually to remove ear wax); from Latin, for *to wash, bathe*
ectropion	outward turning of the eyelid, away from the eye
entropion	inward turning of the eyelid, toward the eye
enucleation	removal of an eye
esotropia	inward turning of the eye, toward the nose
exophthalmus	protrusion of the eye out of the eye socket
exotropia	outward turning of the eye, away from the nose
hemianopsia	blindness in half the visual field
hyperacusis	excessively sensitive hearing
hyperopia	farsightedness
hypoacusis	excessively insensitive hearing
intraocular lens implant	insertion of a new lens inside the eye
iridalgia	pain in the iris

quick reference glossary of terms *continued*

Term	Definition
iridectomy	removal of the iris
iridemia	bleeding from the iris
iridocyclectomy	removal of the iris and ciliary body
iridocyclitis	inflammation of the iris and ciliary body
iridokeratitis	inflammation of the iris and cornea
iridokinesis	movement of the iris
iridopathy	disease of the iris
iridotomy	incision into the iris
iritis	inflammation of the iris
keratalgia	pain in the cornea
keratitis	inflammation of the cornea
keratomalacia	abnormal softening of the cornea
keratopathy	disease of the cornea
keratoplasty	surgical reconstruction of the cornea
keratotomy	incision into the cornea
labyrinthectomy	removal of the labyrinth
labyrinthitis	inflammation of the labyrinth
labyrinthotomy	incision into the labyrinth
lacrimation	formation of tears (i.e., crying)
macrotia	abnormally large ears
mastoidalgia	pain in the mastoid
mastoidectomy	removal of the mastoid
mastoiditis	inflammation of the mastoid
mastoidocentesis	puncture of the mastoid
microtia	abnormally small ears
miosis	abnormal contraction of the pupil (from Greek, for *to lessen*)
miotic	drug that causes the abnormal contraction of the pupil
mydriasis	abnormal dilation of the pupil
mydriatic	drug that causes the abnormal dilation of the pupil
myopia	nearsightedness
myringectomy	removal of the eardrum

quick reference glossary of terms *continued*

Term	Definition
myringitis	inflammation of the eardrum
myringodermatitis	inflammation of the eardrum and surrounding skin
myringomycosis	fungal condition of the eardrum
myringoplasty	surgical reconstruction of the eardrum
myringotomy	incision into the eardrum
nasolacrimal	pertaining to the nose and tear system
nystagmus	involuntary back-and-forth movement of the eyes (from Greek, for *to nod*)
oculomycosis	a fungal eye condition
oculopathy	disease of the eye
oculoplasty	surgical reconstruction of the eye
ophthalmatrophy	atrophy (wasting away) of the eye
ophthalmectomy	removal of the eye
ophthalmic	pertaining to the eye
ophthalmitis	inflammation of the eye
ophthalmologist	eye specialist
ophthalmomycosis	fungal eye condition
ophthalmomyitis	inflammation of the eye muscles
ophthalmopathy	eye disease
ophthalmoplegia	eye paralysis
ophthalmoscope	instrument for looking at the eye
ophthalmalgia	eye pain
optic	pertaining to the eye
optic neuritis	inflammation of the optic nerve
optokinetic	pertaining to eye movement
optometrist	specialist in measuring the eye
optomyometer	device used to determine the strength of eye muscles
osteoacusis	hearing through bone
otalgia	ear pain
otitis externa	inflammation of the outer ear
otitis media	inflammation of the middle ear
otodynia	ear pain

quick reference glossary of terms *continued*

Term	Definition
otolaryngologist	specialist in the ear and throat
otomycosis	fungal ear condition
otoneurology	specialist in the nerve connections between the ear and brain
otoplasty	surgical reconstruction of the ear
otopyorrhea	discharge of pus from the ears
otorhinolaryngologist	specialist in the ear, nose, and throat
otorrhea	discharge from the ear
otosclerosis	hearing loss caused by the hardening of the bones of the middle ear
otoscope	instrument for looking in the ear
otoscopy	procedure for looking in the ear
otosteal	pertaining to the bones of the ear
ototoxic	drug that is damaging to the ear/hearing
papilledema	swelling of the optic nerve where it enters the retina
phacoemulsification	fragmentation of an existing lens in order to remove and replace it
phacomalacia	abnormal softening of the lens
phacosclerosis	abnormal hardening of the lens
phacoscope	instrument for looking at the lens
phakitis	inflammation of the lens
pneumatic otoscopy	procedure for looking in the ear using air
presbycusis	loss of hearing in old age
presbyopia	decreased vision caused by old age
pterygium	winglike growth of conjunctival tissue extending to the cornea (from Greek, for *wing*)
retinal	pertaining to the retina
retinitis	inflammation of the retina
retinopathy	disease of the retina
retinopexy	surgical fixation (reattachment) of a retina
retinoscope	instrument for looking at the retina
retinoscopy	procedure for looking at the retina
retinosis	retinal condition
retinotomy	incision into the retina
rhinosalpingitis	inflammation of the nose and eustachian tubes

quick reference glossary of terms *continued*

Term	Definition
salpingopharyngeal	pertaining to the eustachian tubes and the throat
salpingoscope	instrument for looking at the eustachian tubes
sclerectasia	overexpansion of the sclera
scleroiritis	inflammation of the sclera and iris
sclerokeratitis	inflammation of the sclera and cornea
sclerokeratoiritis	inflammation of the sclera, cornea, and iris
scleromalacia	abnormal softening of the sclera
sclerotomy	incision into the sclera
scotoma	dark spot in the visual field
scotopia	adjustment of the eye to seeing in darkness
sensorineural hearing loss	sound is not transmitted from the inner ear to the brain (due to problems with the sense organs or nerves)
strabismus	condition where the eyes deviate when looking at the same object (from Latin, for *to squint*)
tinnitus	ringing in the ears (from Latin, for *to ring* or *jingle*)
tonometer	instrument for measuring tension or pressure in the eye (intraocular pressure)
trichiasis	condition caused by eyelashes growing backward and coming in contact with the eye
tympanic perforation	tear or hole in the eardrum
tympanocentesis	puncture of the eardrum
tympanolabyrinthopexy	surgical fixation of the eardrum to the labyrinth
tympanometry	procedure for measuring the eardrum
tympanoplasty	surgical reconstruction of the eardrum
tympanosclerosis	hardening of the eardrum
tympanostomy	creation of an opening in the eardrum
vertigo	sensation of moving through space (while stationary); from Latin, for *to whirl around*
vestibular neuritis	inflammation of the vestibular nerve
vestibulitis	inflammation of the vestibule
vestibulotomy	incision into the vestibule
xerophthalmia	dry eyes

review of terms by roots

Root	Term(s)	
acous/o	acoustic neuroma	
-acusis	hyperacusis hypoacusis	osteoacusis presbycusis
audi/o	audiogram audiologist audiometer	audiometry auditory prosthesis
aur/o	aural	
blephar/o	blepharedema blepharitis blepharoconjunctivitis blepharoplasty blepharoplegia	blepharoptosis blepharopyorrhea blepharospasm blepharotomy
cerumin/o	cerumen impaction ceruminolysis ceruminolytic	ceruminoma ceruminosis
cochle/o	cochlear implant cochleitis	
conjunctiv/o	blepharoconjunctivitis conjunctivitis	
corne/o	corneal abrasion corneal transplant	corneal xerosis
cycl/o	cyclokeratitis cycloplegia cycloplegic	cyclotomy iridocyclectomy iridocyclitis
dacry/o	dacrocystitis dacryadenitis dacryoadenalgia dacryoadenectomy dacryocystalgia dacryocystectomy dacryocystorhinostomy	dacryocystotomy dacryohemorrhea dacryolith dacryolithiasis dacryopyorrhea dacryorrhea dacryostenosis
irid/o	aniridia	
ir/o	iridalgia iridectomy iridemia iridocyclectomy iridocyclitis iridokeratitis	iridokinesis iridopathy iridotomy iritis scleroiritis sclerokeratoiritis
kerat/o	iridokeratitis keratalgia keratitis keratomalacia keratopathy	keratoplasty keratotomy sclerokeratitis sclerokeratoiritis

review of terms by roots *continued*

Root	Term(s)	
labyrinth/o	labyrinthectomy labyrinthitis	labyrinthotomy tympanolabyrinthopexy
lacrim/o	lacrimation nasolacrimal	
mastoid/o	mastoidalgia mastoidectomy	mastoiditis mastoidocentesis
myring/o	myringectomy myringitis myringodermatitis	myringomycosis myringoplasty myringotomy
ocul/o	binocular intraocular lens implant oculomycosis	oculopathy oculoplasty
ophthalm/o	exophthalmus ophthalmalgia ophthalmatrophy ophthalmectomy ophthalmic ophthalmitis ophthalmologist	ophthalmomycosis ophthalmomyitis ophthalmopathy ophthalmoplegia ophthalmoscope xerophthalmia
-opia **-opsia**	akinetopsia ambiopia amblyopia asthenopia diplopia	hemianopsia hyperopia myopia presbyopia scotopia
opt/o	optic optic neuritis optokinetic	optometrist optomyometer
ot/o	aerotitis macrotia microtia otalgia otitis externa otitis media otodynia otolaryngologist otomycosis otoneurology	otoplasty otopyorrhea otorhinolaryngologist otorrhea otosclerosis otoscope otoscopy otosteal ototoxic pneumatic otoscopy
phac/o	phacoemulsification phacomalacia	phacosclerosis phacoscope
phak/o	aphakia	phakitis

review of terms by roots *continued*

Root	Term(s)	
retin/o	retinal retinitis retinopathy retinopexy	retinoscope retinoscopy retinosis retinotomy
salping/o	rhinosalpingitis salpingopharyngeal	salpingoscope
scler/o	sclerectasia scleroiritis sclerokeratitis	sclerokeratoiritis scleromalacia sclerotomy
tympan/o	tympanic perforation tympanocentesis tympanolabyrinthopexy tympanometry	tympanoplasty tympanosclerosis tympanostomy
vestibul/o	vestibular neuritis vestibulitis	vestibulotomy

other terms

astigmatism	mydriasis
cataract	mydriatic
conductive hearing loss	nystagmus
ear instillation	papilledema
ear lavage	pterygium
ectropion	scotoma
entropion	sensorineural hearing loss
enucleation	strabismus
esotropia	tinnitus
exotropia	tonometer
miosis	trichiasis
miotic	vertigo

The Endocrine System–Endocrinology 7

Introduction and Overview of the Endocrine System

Any building with heating or air conditioning also has a thermostat. A thermostat watches for changes in the temperature of a space and then responds to keep it in a desired range. When the building is too warm or too cold, the thermostat sends a signal to the heater or air conditioner to turn on or off. For the human body, the endocrine system serves this function of sending signals to keep all the body's many functions in balance.

The endocrine system can be broken down into signal senders, the signals they send, and the signals' outcomes. The main signal senders are the endocrine glands, which include the hypothalamus, pituitary, thyroid, parathyroid, adrenal, pancreas, and gonads (ovaries and testicles). Endocrine glands specifically send chemical signals to different parts of the body. These chemical signals, which are hormones, generally cause slower, subtler changes than the nervous system, which uses electric signals.

The signals travel through the rest of the body via the bloodstream, but only the intended cells in the body respond to these hormonal signals. These cells are keyed with receptors that fit with the hormone–just like two matching puzzle pieces. The hormone then signals the cell to perform a desired job, such as releasing another hormone, releasing or taking in nutrients, or changing the speed at which the body makes certain proteins.

The end result is that the endocrine system can adjust the levels of nutrients in the blood, excrete excess nutrients, help the body respond to its environment, and direct growth and development. For example, the pancreas secretes hormones that help the body control the level of sugar in the blood. The adrenal glands, thyroid gland, and parathyroid gland keep critical minerals like calcium and sodium in balance. The adrenal glands also make hormones for the fight-or-flight response to danger. Growth hormone helps the body grow to adult height and affects metabolism. The gonads make hormones that help drive sexual development. The endocrine system even stimulates milk production in new mothers.

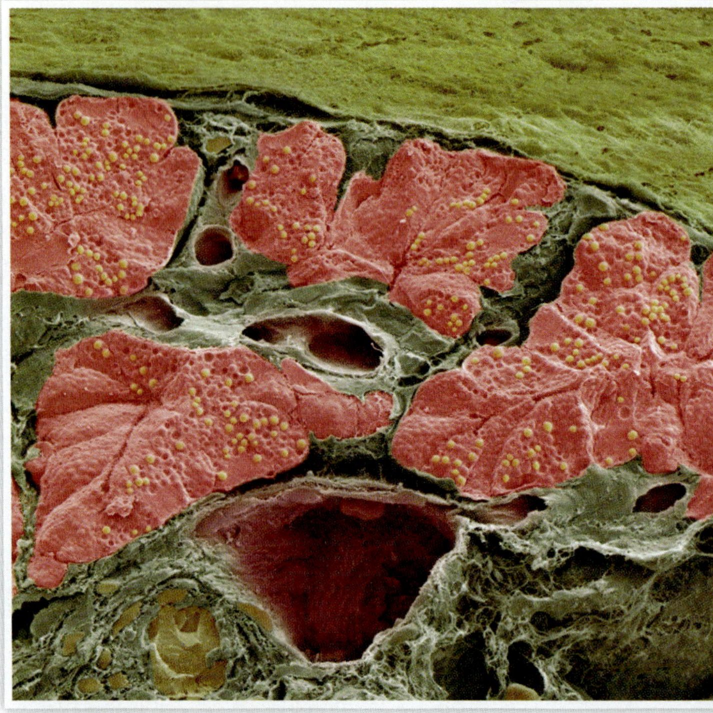

learning outcomes

Upon completion of this chapter, you will be able to:

7.1 Identify the **roots/word parts** associated with the **endocrine system.**

S **7.2** Translate the **Subjective** terms associated with the **endocrine system.**

O **7.3** Translate the **Objective** terms associated with the **endocrine system.**

A **7.4** Translate the **Assessment** terms associated with the **endocrine system.**

P **7.5** Translate the **Plan** terms associated with the **endocrine system.**

7.6 Use **abbreviations** associated with the **endocrine system.**

7.7 Distinguish terms associated with the **endocrine system** in the context of **electronic health records.**

7.1 Word Parts of the Endocrine System

Word Roots for Endocrine Glands

As you recall, the signal makers and senders of the endocrine system are called *glands*. They are located throughout your body, including in your brain, in the area above your kidneys, in your genitals, and in the front part of your neck.

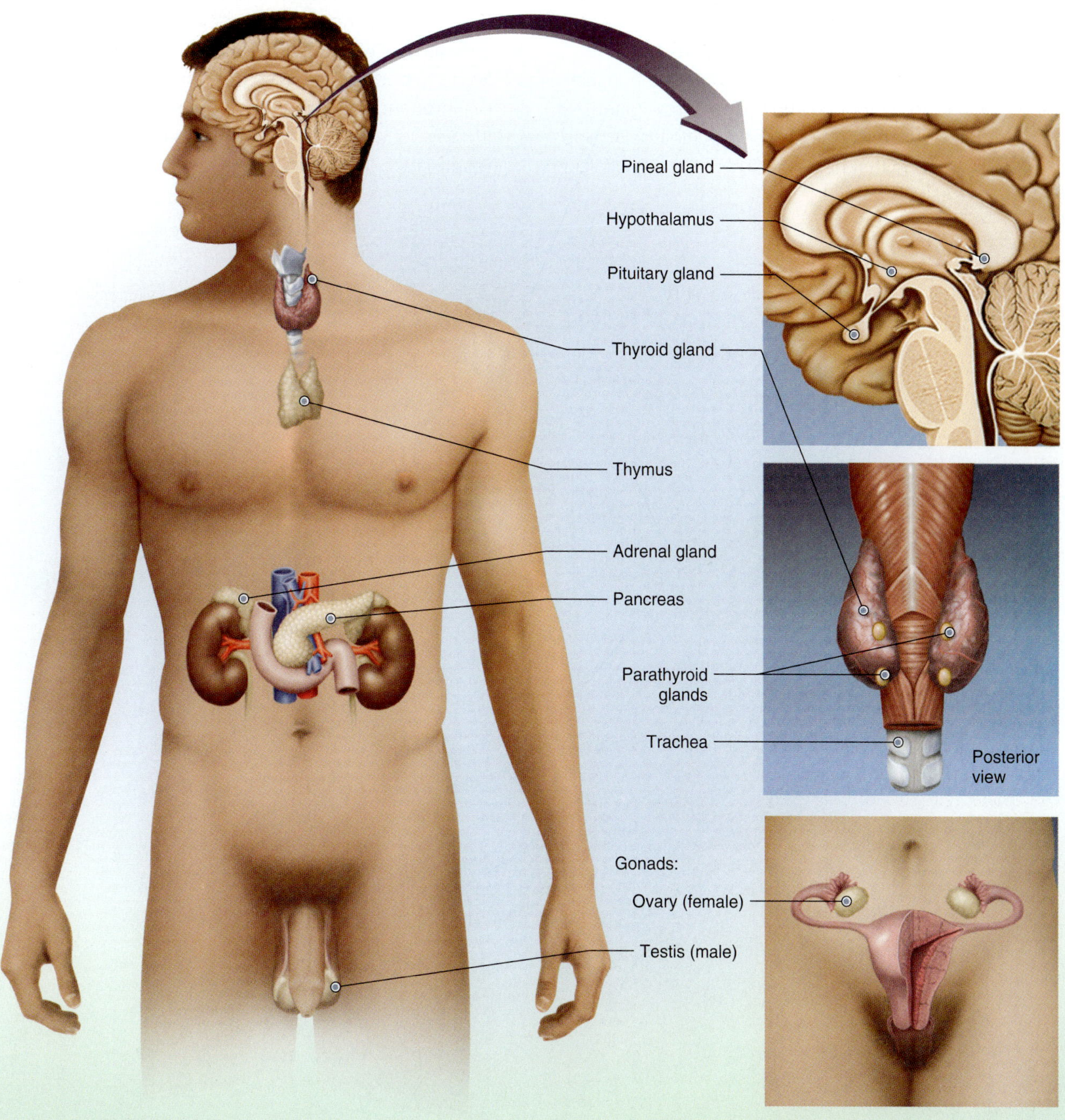

The main gland that affects most of the other glands in your body is named the *hypothalamus*, because it sits just under a part of your brain known as the *thalamus*. The main role of the hypothalamus is to direct the activity of the *pituitary gland*. It can cause the pituitary to make and release its chemical signals via chemicals called *releasing hormones* (example: *gonadotropin-releasing hormone*).

The pituitary gland is made of two parts: the *anterior* (front) and *posterior* (back) pituitary. The anterior pituitary gland is the origin for many very important hormones. These hormones travel by blood and stimulate many other endocrine glands, including your *thyroid* gland, *adrenal* glands, and *gonads*.

Located in the front part of your neck resting just below the Adam's apple is your thyroid gland and just behind it, the *parathyroid* glands. The thyroid gland makes hormones that affect the body's metabolism, as well as a hormone that helps control the level of calcium in the blood. The parathyroid glands also make a hormone that works along with the thyroid hormone to control the blood's calcium level.

The *pancreas*, an interesting gland that sits just under your stomach, is both an endocrine gland and a gastrointestinal organ. As an endocrine gland, it sends hormones directly into the bloodstream that help keep blood sugar level in balance. As a gastrointestinal organ, it secretes enzymes by ducts (*exocrine*) directly into your intestines to help with digestion.

The adrenal gland gets its name from its location in your body, as it lies on top of your kidneys. The adrenal gland has an inner layer that makes the fight-or-flight hormone, *adrenaline*. Its outer layer, or cortex, makes two general types of hormones. One type keeps mineral levels in balance and also maintains the proper volume of water and salt in the blood. The other helps keep blood sugar levels in balance and affects your body's response to inflammation.

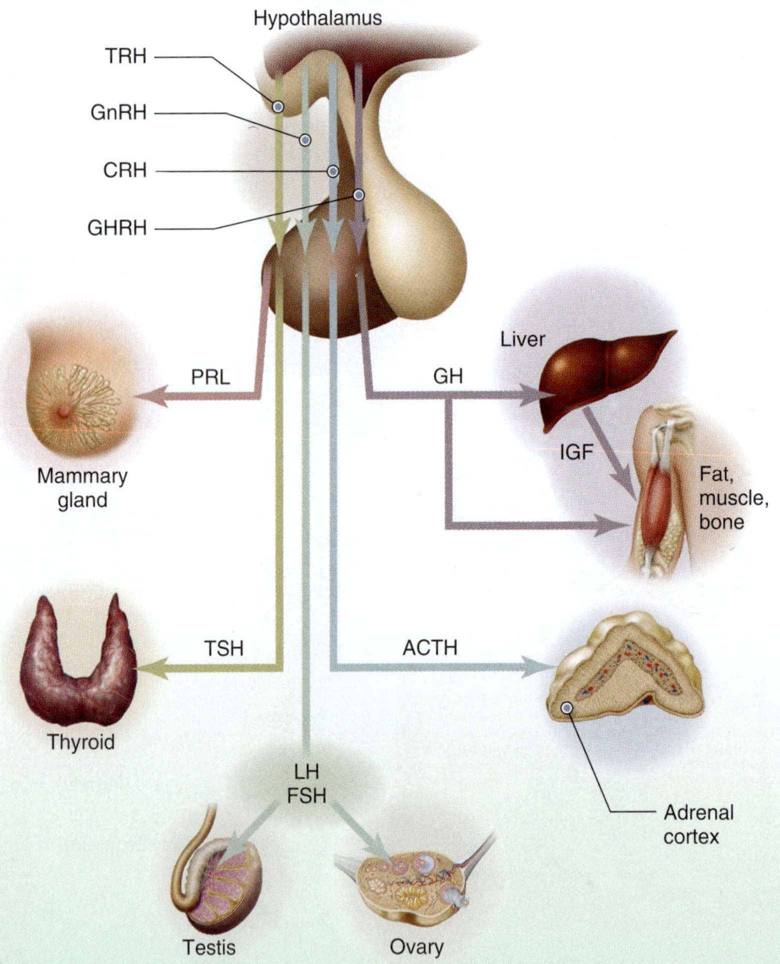

The gonads help with reproduction and with expression of male and female characteristics. The male gonads are the *testes.* They produce the male hormone *testosterone. Ovaries,* the female gonads, secrete *estrogens,* which help the body develop female attributes and help prepare the body for pregnancy.

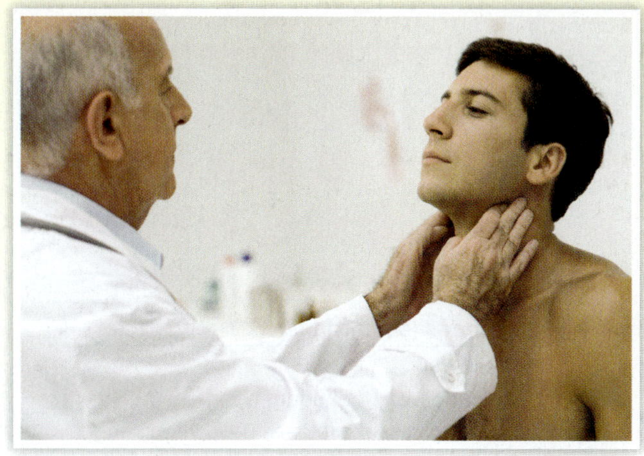

One indicator doctors use in determining health is whether or not the patient has swollen glands.

gland

ROOT: ***aden/o***

EXAMPLES: adenoma, adenopathy

NOTES: This root refers to any gland. Since the endocrine system has a lot of glands, the term comes up often.

adrenal gland

ROOTS: ***adren/o, adrenal/o***

EXAMPLES: adrenarche, adrenalitis

NOTES: The name *adrenal* describes where this gland is located in the body. It literally means *on the kidney—ad* (to, on) + *renal* (kidney).

outer surface

ROOT: ***cortic/o***

EXAMPLES: corticotropic, adrenocorticohyperplasia

NOTES: The root *cortico* and the noun *cortex* both come from a Latin word meaning *bark* or *husk.* It refers to the outer surface of any organ.

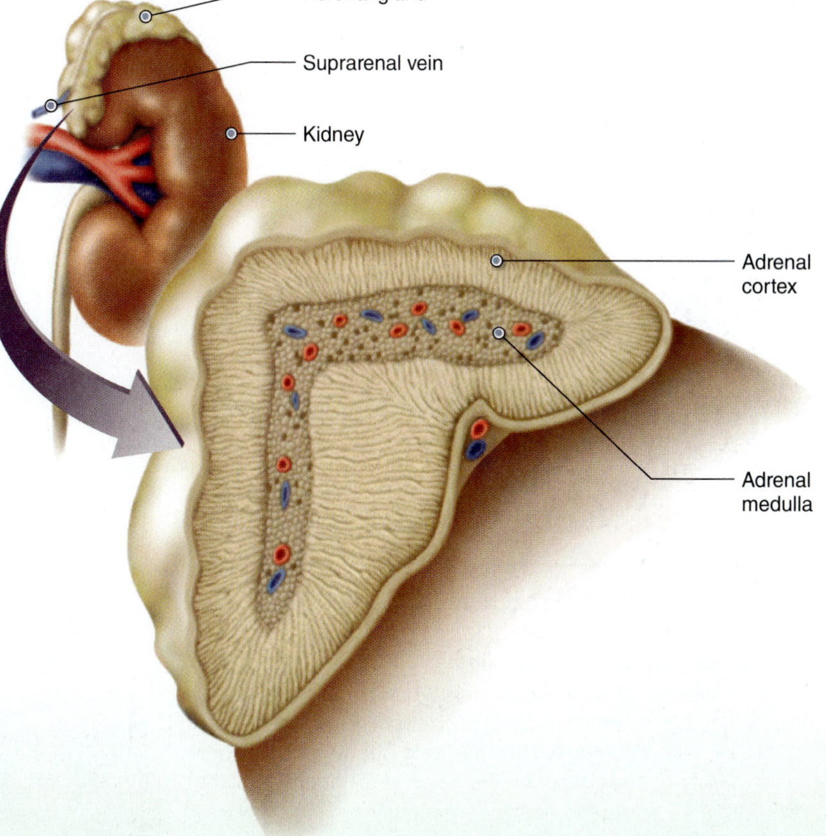

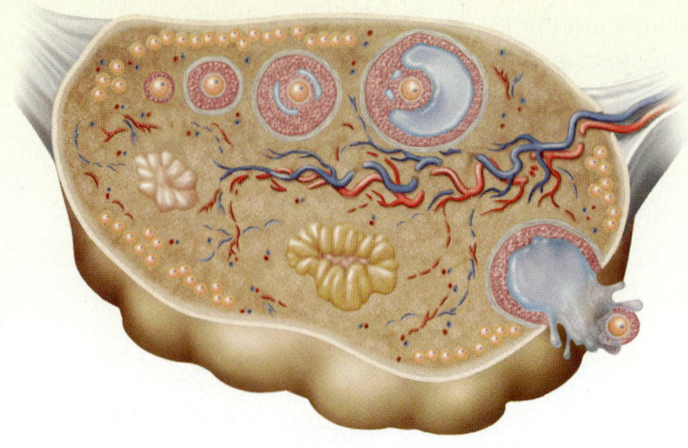

gonads (sex organs)

ROOT: ***gonad/o***

EXAMPLES: gonadopathy, gonadogenesis

NOTES: Although it is sometimes used interchangeably with the term *testicles,* the term *gonad* actually refers to the sex organs of both men and women. In males, of course, the gonads are the testicles, and in females, they are the ovaries.

You can easily recall the term *gonad* by remembering that its first three letters, *gon,* are from the same Greek root that places *gen* in the word *genesis,* which means *to create.* That makes sense, because the gonads are the organs that aid in pro*creation.*

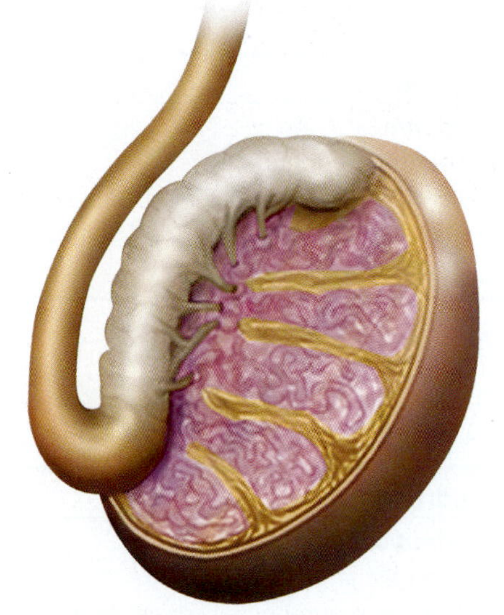

pancreas

ROOT: ***pancreat/o***

EXAMPLES: pancreatitis, pancreatolith

NOTES: The term *pancreas* comes from two Greek words: *pan* (all) and *kreas* (flesh). The reasoning for this has long been debated; some people think the name stuck because of the organ's fleshy consistency.

If you ever find yourself tempted by the word *sweetbreads* on a menu, think carefully before ordering. That's the term used by chefs to mean *cooked pancreas.*

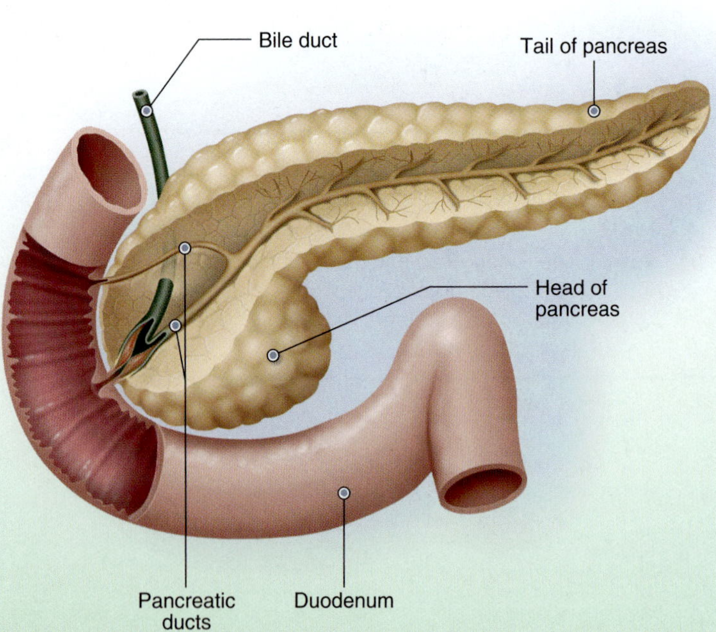

pituitary gland

ROOTS: ***pituitar/o, hypophys/o***

EXAMPLES: hyperpituitarism, hypophysitis

NOTES: The word *pituitary* comes from a Latin word meaning *mucus,* because the Romans believed that the pituitary gland channeled mucus from the brain to the nose. The other root, *hypophyso,* comes from the Greek words *hypo* (under) + *physis* (growth) and refers to the appearance and location of the pituitary gland, a pea-sized gland located under the brain right behind the eyes. It looks a little like an abnormal growth underneath the brain—but it is a critical part of the endocrine system.

thymus

ROOT: ***thym/o***

EXAMPLES: *thymoma, thymectomy*

NOTES: The *thymus* is an organ found in the upper chest, under the sternum and in front of the heart. Its name is derived from the name of the herb *thyme.* To those who first discovered it, the organ looked like a bunch of thyme.

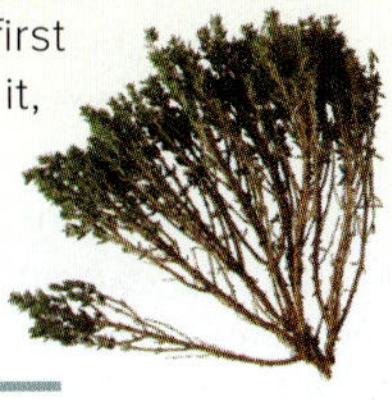

thyroid

ROOTS: ***thyr/o, thyroid/o***

EXAMPLES: thyrotoxin, thyroidectomy

NOTES: The word *thyroid* comes from the Greek word *thyros,* meaning *shield. Thyro* (shield) + *oid* (resembling) = the gland resembling a shield. It really does look like a shield spread out over the throat, doesn't it?

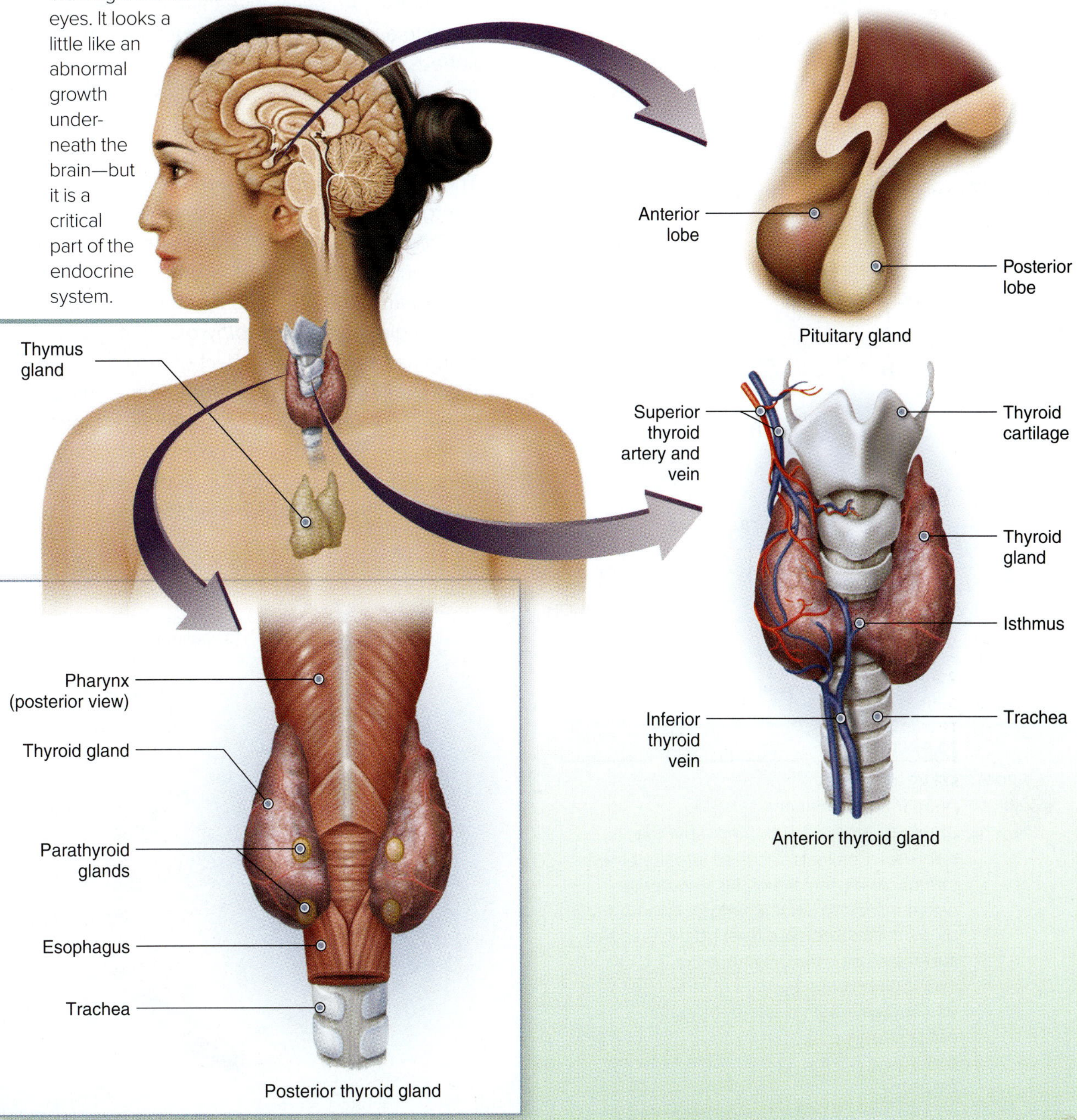

sugar

ROOTS: ***gluc/o, glucos/o, glyc/o***

EXAMPLES: glucocorticoid, glucosuria, hypoglycemia

NOTES: Three common types of sugar are: sucrose, glucose, and fructose. *Sucrose* is a complex molecule made up of glucose and fructose. *Glucose* and *fructose* have the same chemical composition but different molecular structures. For some reason, glucose (which requires insulin to break it down) is the universal fuel of all living things and is also used in brain functions. Neurologists often use glucose consumption as an indicator of brain activity. When the brain lacks glucose, certain mental functions, like self-control and decision making, become more difficult.

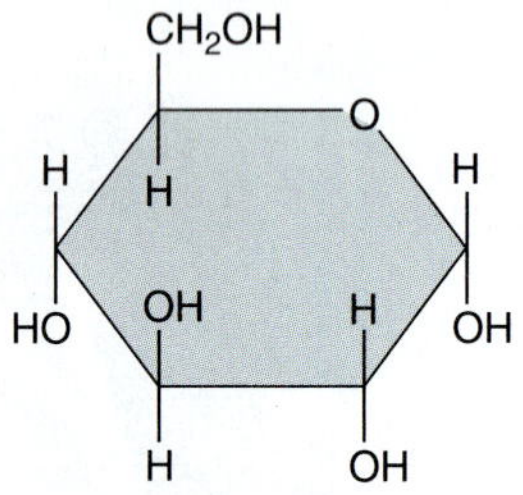

Glucose

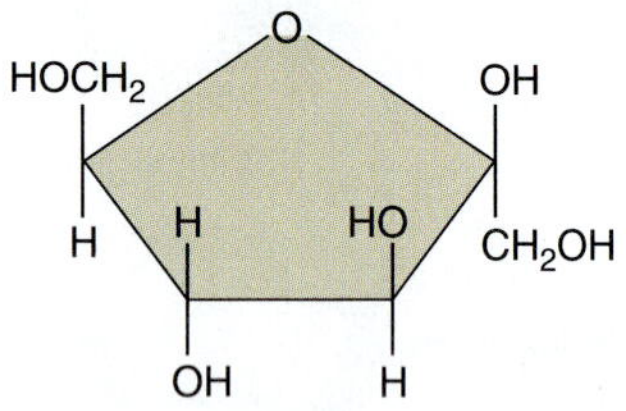

Fructose

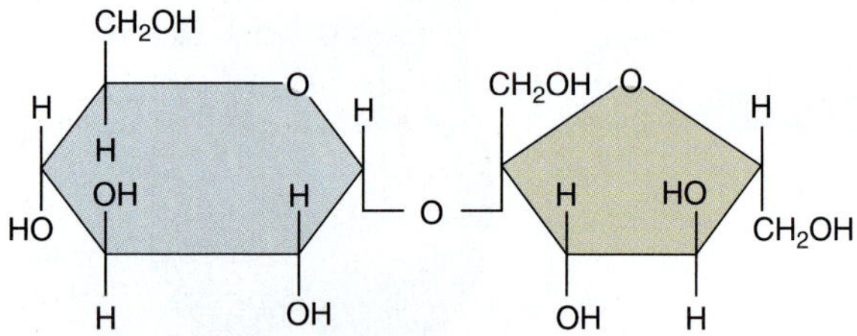

Sucrose

to secrete

ROOT: ***crin/o***

EXAMPLES: endocrine, exocrine

NOTES: *Endocrine* means *to secrete internally;* it refers to chemicals secreted into the bloodstream. The opposite of this is *exocrine,* which means *to secrete externally* and refers to chemicals secreted through ducts to the surface of an organ. Examples of this include sweat glands and salivary glands. Next time you find yourself sweating through a workout or drooling over some food, you can say that you're having an excessive exocrine response.

Word Roots for Secretions, Chemicals, and Blood Work

Once the signals (*hormones*) are made in the endocrine organs, they wait to be secreted (*crino*) to their target body part. Endocrine signals travel via the bloodstream. The *pituitary* gland makes many hormones that encourage other endocrine glands in the body to work. *Adrenocorticotropic hormone (ACTH)* stimulates the outer part of the adrenal gland. *Thyroid-stimulating hormone* (*TSH)* stimulates the thyroid gland. *Luteinizing (LH)* and *follicle-stimulating hormone (FSH)* stimulate the gonads. The pituitary gland also makes growth hormone and prolactin.

The thyroid makes three very important hormones: *T4, T3,* and *calcitonin.* T4 and T3 affect the body's metabolism. An overactive thyroid (*hyperthyroidism*) leads to a higher than normal metabolism—everything speeds up. As a result, a person suffering from hyperthyroidism experiences weight loss, increased hunger, diarrhea, and nervousness. On the opposite end, for people with *hypothyroidism,* everything slows down. They typically experience weight gain, decreased energy and appetite, and constipation.

Calcitonin is a hormone that encourages the uptake of calcium in the blood into bone. This keeps the level of calcium in the blood from getting too high. The parathyroid glands make *parathyroid hormone.* This hormone has the opposite effect of calcitonin. It helps keep the level of calcium in the blood from getting too low.

As you recall, the pancreas is both a digestive organ and an endocrine organ. The endocrine part of the pancreas makes two hormones that work together to keep the level of sugar in the blood in balance. *Insulin*

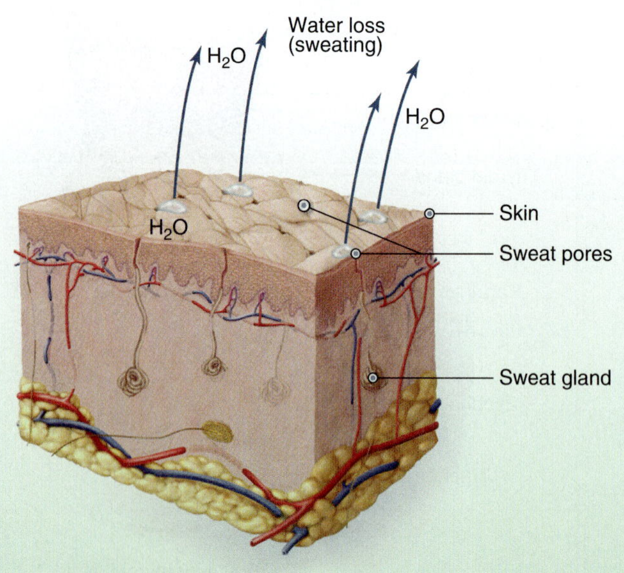

decreases the level of sugar in the blood. It encourages cells to open up to the blood sugar (*glucose*) and take it in. *Glucagon* works against insulin. It tells the liver to make more sugar and thus increases the level of sugar in the blood.

The adrenal gland creates hormones in two parts—the inner part or the outer part. The inner part of the adrenal gland makes *epinephrine,* which was once known as adrenaline. Many people know adrenaline as the chemical that surges in danger and helps mothers lift cars off their babies. While it doesn't truly gift people with super powers, it does play an important role in the fight-or-flight response by increasing your heart rate and opening your airways to get more oxygen. Norepinephrine, also made in the adrenal gland, causes very similar changes.

The outer part of the adrenal gland (*cortex*) also makes very important hormones. ACTH stimulates the cortex to release *corticosteroids,* which are steroid hormones made in the cortex. The two types of corticosteroids are hormones dealing with mineral balance (*mineralcorticoids*) and hormones dealing with sugar balance (*glucocorticoids*).

Last, the adrenal glands are an extra location for secretion of the sex hormones, testosterone and estrogen. The main source of these hormones, however, is the gonads. The gonads of men and women make different hormones. In men, the testes make testosterone. The testes trigger the production of sperm and the development of masculine body characteristics, like increased muscle and facial hair. Ovaries, the female gonads, secrete estrogens, which cause the development and release of eggs as well as the development of feminine attributes, like breasts and wide hips.

Measuring the level of certain hormones and how they affect the patient's blood is one way of checking the function of the endocrine system. The most common example is checking the glucose level in the blood (*glycemia*). These levels may be high (*hyperglycemia*), low (*hypoglycemia*), or normal (*euglycemia*). Another body fluid that is often measured is a patient's *urine.* Substances like sugar (*glucosuria*) or ketones (*ketonuria*) may be found in the urine.

hormone

ROOT: ***hormon/o***

EXAMPLE: hormonopoesis

NOTES: From the Greek word meaning to *rush* or *push, hormones* are chemicals secreted by certain glands for the purpose of stimulating an organ or part of the body to do something.

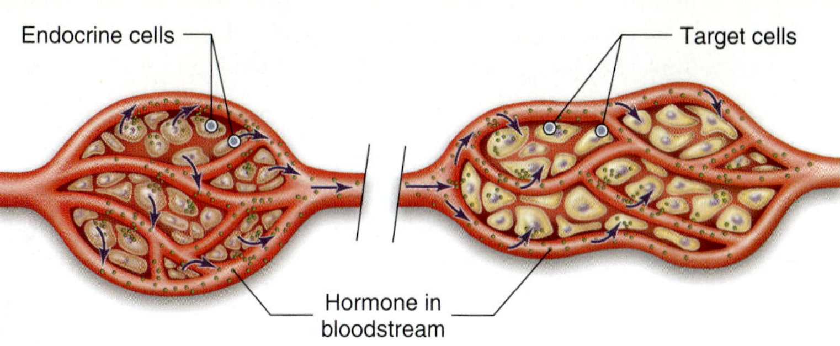

ketone body

ROOT: ***ket/o***

EXAMPLES: ketosis, ketogenic

NOTES: A *ketone body* is a substance that increases in the blood as a result of faulty carbohydrate metabolism. Ketone bodies are toxic chemicals that build up in the blood and are detectable in the urine. When there isn't enough insulin in the blood, the body cannot use sugar for energy, so it breaks down fat instead. The presence of ketone bodies is normally a sign of untreated or poorly controlled diabetes. Oddly enough, although ketones can be secreted in the urine, the primary way the body gets rid of them is through the lungs, giving sufferers fruity-smelling breath.

Suffixes for Secretions, Chemicals, and Blood Work

stimulating hormone

SUFFIX: *-tropin*

EXAMPLES: thyrotropin, gonadotropin

NOTES: If a term has the suffix *-tropin,* it refers to a hormone that has a stimulating effect on a target organ. The suffix comes from a Greek word meaning *to turn*—perhaps because it turns the target organ on and tells it to start working.

-Tropin has the same root as the word *trophy.* In ancient Greece, a *trophy* was a monument built on a battlefield to mark the spot where the battle *turned* in the victor's favor.

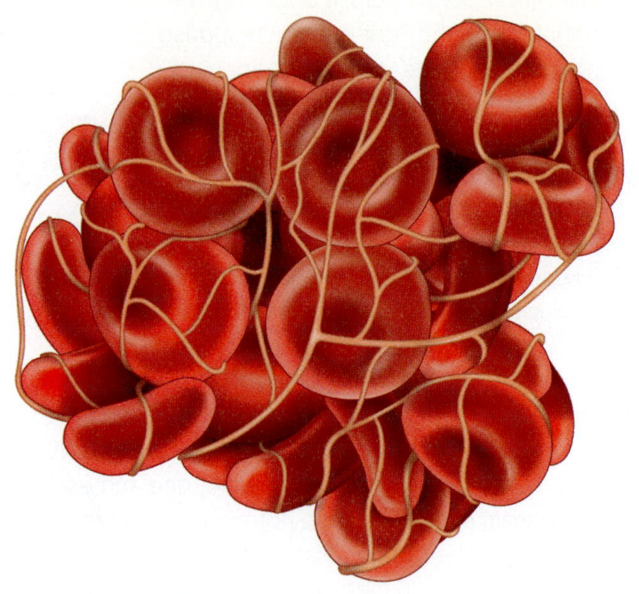

blood condition

SUFFIX: *-emia*

EXAMPLES: glycemia, calcemia

NOTES: Because the endocrine system deals with internal secretions, blood analysis (which is, of course, analysis of a secretion of the body) is usually the best way to detect problems.

urine condition

SUFFIX: *-uria*

EXAMPLE: polyuria

NOTES: Substances in the urine can be useful clues in diagnosing endocrine problems.

For example, in 1889, Oscar Minkowski and Joseph von Mering removed the pancreas of a healthy dog. Several days after the dog's pancreas was removed, the researchers noticed that flies were feeding on the dog's urine—something that was not the case prior to the removal of the pancreas. Analysis of the dog's urine revealed the presence of sugar—a discovery that helped established the relationship between the pancreas and diabetes.

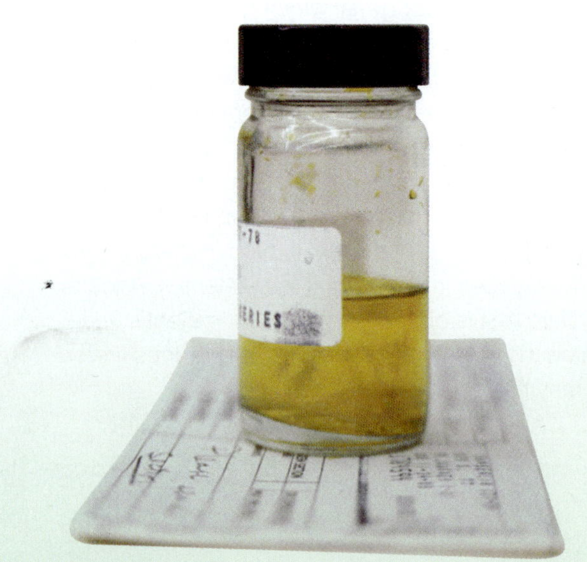

Learning Outcome 7.1 Exercises

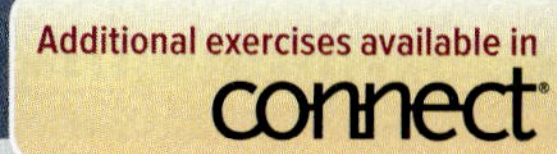
Additional exercises available in
connect

TRANSLATION

EXERCISE 1 *Match the root on the left with its definition on the right.*

e	1. pancreat/o	a. adrenal gland
c	2. gonad/o	b. gland
f	3. pituitar/o	c. gonads (sex organs)
a	4. adren/o	d. outer surface
g	5. thym/o	e. pancreas
h	6. thyr/o	f. pituitary gland
b	7. aden/o	g. thymus
d	8. cortic/o	h. thyroid

EXERCISE 2 *Translate the following roots.*

1. adrenal/o ______
2. gonad/o ______
3. pancreat/o ______
4. thyroid/o ______
5. thym/o ______
6. aden/o ______
7. cortic/o ______
8. hypophys/o ______

EXERCISE 3 *Break down the following words into their component parts and translate.*

EXAMPLE: sinusitis *sinus | itis* *inflammation of the sinuses*

1. thyroidectomy ______
2. thymectomy ______
3. adrenalectomy ______
4. pancreatectomy ______
5. hypophysectomy ______
6. hypopituitarism ______
7. hypogonadism ______
8. adenopathy ______

Learning Outcome 7.1 Exercises

EXERCISE 4 *Match the word part on the left with its definition on the right. Some definitions will be used more than once.*

b	1. hormon/o	a.	blood condition
c	2. ket/o	b.	hormone
e	3. glyc/o	c.	ketone body
e	4. gluc/o	d.	stimulating hormone
a	5. -emia	e.	sugar
g	6. -uria	f.	to secrete
d	7. -tropin	g.	urine condition
f	8. crin/o		

EXERCISE 5 *Translate the following word parts.*

1. hormon/o ______
2. glucos/o ______
3. ket/o ______
4. crin/o ______
5. glyc/o ______
6. -uria ______
7. -emia ______
8. -tropin ______

EXERCISE 6 *Break down the following words into their component parts and translate.*

EXAMPLE: sinusitis *sinus | itis* *inflammation of the sinuses*

1. hyperglycemia ______
2. euglycemia ______
3. ketonuria ______
4. glucosuria ______
5. gonadotropin ______
6. endocrine ______

Learning Outcome 7.1 Exercises

GENERATION

EXERCISE 7 *Identify the word parts from this chapter for the following terms.*

1. adrenomegaly ____________________
2. pancreatalgia ____________________
3. corticotropin ____________________
4. gonadogenesis ____________________
5. hypophysitis ____________________
6. thymoma ____________________
7. polyadenopathy ____________________
8. panhypopituitarism ____________________
9. thyrotoxicosis ____________________
10. hypothyroidism ____________________

EXERCISE 8 *Build a medical term from the information provided.*

1. inflammation of the pancreas ____________________
2. inflammation of the thyroid ____________________
3. inflammation of a gland ____________________
4. good thyroid ____________________

EXERCISE 9 *Identify the word parts from this chapter for the following terms.*

1. polyuria ____________________
2. exocrine ____________________
3. glucogenesis ____________________
4. endocrinologist ____________________
5. hyperphosphatemia ____________________
6. ketogenic diet ____________________
7. adrenocortical insufficiency (2 roots) ____________________
8. euglycemia (2 roots) ____________________
9. adrenocorticotropic hormone (4 roots) ____________________

EXERCISE 10 *Build a medical term from the information provided.*

1. sugar urine condition (use *glucoso*) ____________________
2. ketone urine condition ____________________
3. low blood sugar condition (use *glyco*) ____________________
4. thyroid-stimulating hormone (use *thyro*) ____________________

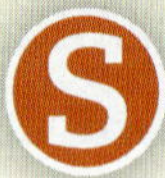

Subjective

Patient History, Problems, Complaints

Adrenal
Gonad
Pancreas
Pituitary
Thyroid

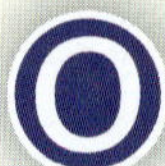

Objective

Observation and Discovery

-Emia/-uria
Hormones
Results
Professional terms, diagnostic procedures

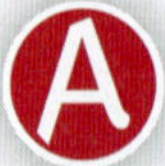

Assessment

Diagnosis and Pathology

General Terms
Adrenal
Pancreas
Pituitary
Thyroid

Plan

Treatments and Therapies

General terms
Adrenal
Pancreas
Pituitary
Thyroid

This section contains medical terms built from the roots presented in the previous section. The purpose of this section is to expose you to words used in the endocrine system that are built from the word roots presented earlier. The focus of this book is to teach you the process of learning roots and translating them in context. Each term is presented with the correct pronunciation, followed by a word analysis that breaks down the word into its component parts, a definition that provides a literal translation of the word, as well as supplemental information if the literal translation deviates from its medical use.

The terms are organized using a health care professional's SOAP note (first introduced in Chapter 2) as a model.

SUBJECTIVE

7.2 Patient History, Problems, Complaints

The symptoms a patient experiences from an endocrine problem all depend on which organ is affected. Patients with pituitary problems may present to a health care provider with growth disturbances. This can be on either extreme, from the abnormally large (*pituitary gigantism*) or small (*pituitary dwarfism*). If the extra growth is disproportionate in the face and long bones of the body, it is known as *acromegaly*.

Patients with an overactive thyroid (*hyperthyroidism*) have higher-than-normal metabolism—everything speeds up. As a result, a person suffering from hyperthyroidism experiences weight loss, increased hunger, diarrhea, and nervousness. Some also have bulging eyes (*exophthalmos*).

On the opposite end, for someone with *hypothyroidism,* everything slows down. Patients with this disease typically experience weight gain, decreased energy, hair loss, decreased appetite, and constipation. They may also experience swelling and puffiness in the hands and face. This grouping of symptoms is called *myxedema*. Both hyperthyroidism and hypothyroidism can present with an enlarged thyroid (*goiter*).

7.2 Patient History, Problems, Complaints

Decreased pancreatic endocrine activity leads to diabetes. Patients with diabetes may complain of excessive thirst (*polydipsia*), excessive urination (*polyuria*), and constant hunger (*polyphagia*), with an unexpected weight loss.

Premature sexual traits may represent a problem with the adrenal gland or the gonads. Males may experience premature puberty from an overactive adrenal gland (*adrenal virilism*). Females with the same problem may report facial hair (*hirsutism*). When a female has a hyperactive gonad (*hypergonadism*) she may present with periods (*menarche*) or breast development (*thelarche*) at a premature age. Females with under-functioning gonads may complain of lack of menstruation (*amenorrhea*). Males may experience breast development (*gynecomastia*). This is very common in puberty.

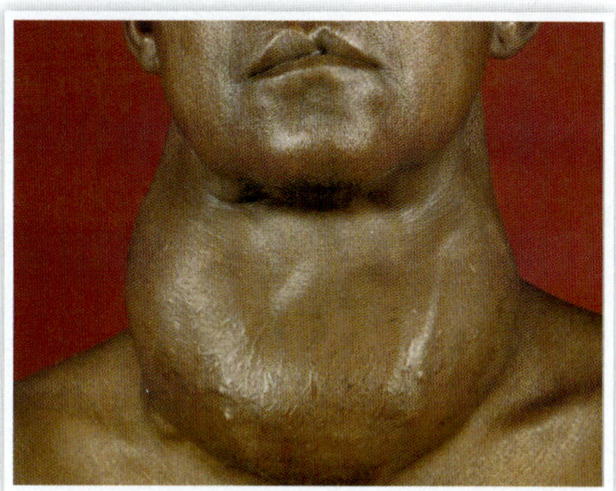

Goiter, or swollen thyroid gland, is most commonly caused by iodine deficiency. The easy solution to this, and to other health problems caused by low iodine, is to add iodine to salt. Check the container of table salt in your home. Chances are good that it's iodized salt.

adrenal

Term	Word Analysis
adenalgia AD-en-AL-jah **Definition** pain in a gland	**aden / algia** gland / pain
adrenal virilism ad-REE-nal VIR-il-izm **Definition** development of male secondary sexual characteristics caused by excessive secretion of the adrenal gland	**adrenal viril / ism** adrenal man / condition
adrenarche AD-ren-AR-kay **Definition** beginning of adrenal secretion (at puberty)	**adren / arche** adrenal / beginning
hirsutism HIR-soo-tizm **Definition** excessive growth of facial and body hair in women	**from Latin, for *shaggy***

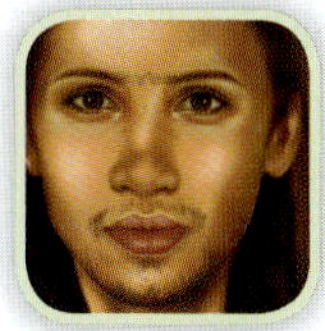

hirsutism

gonad

Term	Word Analysis
amenorrhea ah-MEN-oh-REE-ah **Definition** lack of menstrual flow	**a / meno / rrhea** no / menstrual / flow
gynecomastia GAI-neh-koh-MAS-tee-ah **Definition** development of breast tissue in males	**gyneco / mast / ia** woman / breast / condition
hypergonadism HAI-per-GOH-nad-izm **Definition** excessive secretion of the sex glands	**hyper / gonad / ism** over / gonad / condition

gynecomastia

7.2 Patient History, Problems, Complaints

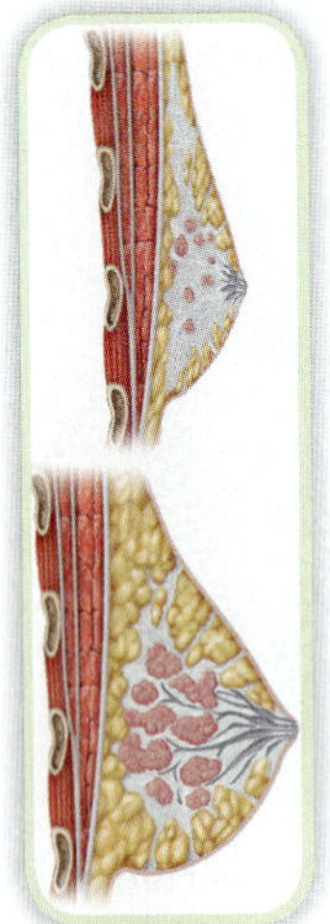
thelarche

gonad *continued*

Term	Word Analysis
hypogonadism HAI-poh-GOH-nad-izm **Definition** undersecretion of the sex glands	hypo / gonad / ism under / gonad / condition
menarche MEN-ar-kee **Definition** beginning or first menstruation	men / arche menstrual / beginning
thelarche thee-LAR-kay **Definition** beginning of breast development	thel / arche breast / beginning

pancreas

Term	Word Analysis
hypoglycemic HAI-poh-glai-SEE-mik **Definition** pertaining to low blood sugar	hypo / glyc / em / ic under / sugar / blood / pertaining to
pancreatalgia PAN-kree-ah-TAL-jah **Definition** pain in the pancreas	pancreat / algia pancreas / pain
polydipsia PAW-lee-DIP-see-ah **Definition** excessive thirst	poly / dips / ia excessive / thirst / condition

Note: You might expect *hyperdipsia*, but the term uses *poly* instead. The reason is because this word is not first a medical word but the ancient Greek term for *excessively thirsty.* In Greek, *poly* can mean *excessive* as well as *many*.

Term	Word Analysis
polyphagia PAW-lee-FAY-jah **Definition** excessive eating	poly / phag / ia excessive / eating / condition
polyuria PAW-lee-YOO-ree-ah **Definition** excessive urination	poly / uria excessive / urine condition

pituitary

Term	Word Analysis
acromegaly AK-roh-MEH-gah-lee **Definition** abnormal enlargement of the extremities	acro / megaly extremities / abnormal enlargement

Note: The term *acro* can mean *top* or *high*, as in *acrophobia*, the fear of heights, or it can mean *the end* or *extremity*, as it does here.

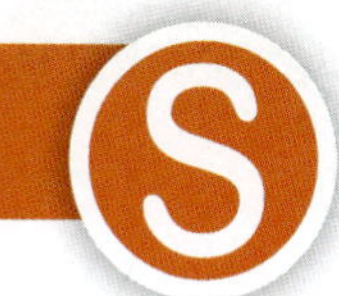

pituitary *continued*

Term	Word Analysis
galactorrhea gah-LAK-toh-REE-ah **Definition** discharge of milk **NOTE:** The word *galaxy* comes from this root. Our galaxy is called the Milky Way because early star-gazers thought it looked like someone sprayed milk in the sky.	galacto / rrhea milk / discharge
pituitary dwarfism pih-TOO-ih-TER-ee DWAR-fizm **Definition** abnormally short height caused by undersecretion of growth hormone from the pituitary gland	pituitary dwarfism
pituitary gigantism pih-TOO-ih-TER-ee jai-GAN-tizm **Definition** abnormally tall height caused by oversecretion of growth hormone from the pituitary gland	pituitary gigantism

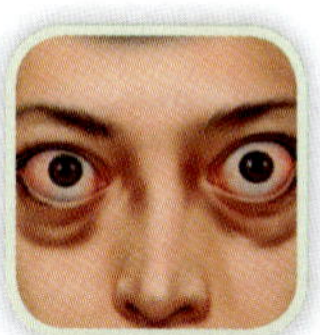

exophthalmos

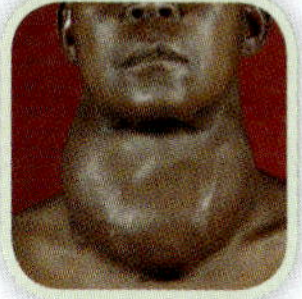

goiter

thyroid

Term	Word Analysis
exophthalmos EKS-of-THAL-mohs **Definition** protrusion of the eyes out of the eye socket	ex / ophthalmos out / eye
goiter GOY-ter **Definition** swollen thyroid gland **NOTE:** The most common cause of goiter is iodine deficiency. The easy solution to this, and to other health problems caused by low iodine, is to add iodine to salt.	from Latin, for *gutter* (meaning *throat*)
myxedema MIX-eh-DEE-mah **Definition** swelling of the skin caused by deposits under the skin **NOTE:** Though the deposits under the skin aren't mucus, they appear to have the consistency of mucus, so that's the root that was used to describe it.	myx / edema mucus / swelling
thyrocele THAI-roh-seel **Definition** another name for goiter	thyro / cele thyroid / tumor
thyromegaly THAI-roh-MEH-gah-lee **Definition** enlargement of the thyroid	thyro / megaly thyroid / enlargement
thyroptosis THAI-rop-TOH-sis **Definition** downward displacement (drooping) of the thryoid	thyro / pt / osis thyroid / drooping / condition

Learning Outcome 7.2 Exercises

PRONUNCIATION

EXERCISE 1 *Break down the following words into syllables.*

EXAMPLE: synesthesia *syn | es | the | sia*

1. adenalgia ______
2. myxedema ______
3. thyroptosis ______
4. adrenal virilism ______
5. hypergonadism ______
6. hypogonadism ______

EXERCISE 2 *Indicate which syllable is emphasized when pronounced.*

EXAMPLE: bronchitis bron**chi**tis

1. menarche ______
2. thelarche ______
3. polydipsia ______

TRANSLATION

EXERCISE 3 *Underline and define the word parts from this chapter in the following terms.*

1. adenalgia ______
2. thyrocele ______
3. thyromegaly ______
4. polyuria ______
5. adrenal virilism ______
6. hypergonadism ______
7. hypogonadism ______
8. pituitary dwarfism ______
9. pituitary gigantism ______
10. thyroptosis ______
11. exophthalmus ______

Learning Outcome 7.2 Exercises

EXERCISE 4 *Match the term on the left with its definition on the right.*

b	1. galactorrhea	a.	abnormal enlargement of the extremities
g	2. amenorrhea	b.	discharge of milk
m	3. gynecomastia	c.	excessive eating
f	4. polyuria	d.	excessive growth of facial and body hair in women
c	5. polyphagia	e.	excessive thirst
e	6. polydipsia	f.	excessive urination
l	7. menarche	g.	lack of menstrual flow
k	8. thelarche	h.	swelling of the skin caused by deposits under the skin
j	9. adrenarche	i.	swollen thyroid gland
i	10. goiter	j.	beginning of adrenal secretion
a	11. acromegaly	k.	beginning of breast development
h	12. myxedema	l.	beginning or first menstruation
d	13. hirsutism	m.	development of breast tissue in males

EXERCISE 5 *Translate the following terms as literally as possible.*

EXAMPLE: nasopharyngoscope *an instrument for looking at the nose and throat*

1. thyroptosis ____________________
2. exophthalmus ____________________
3. galactorrhea ____________________
4. amenorrhea ____________________
5. adrenarche ____________________
6. gynecomastia ____________________

GENERATION

EXERCISE 6 *Build a medical term from the information provided.*

EXAMPLE: inflammation of the sinuses *sinusitis*

1. pain in the pancreas ____________________
2. pain in a gland ____________________
3. thyroid tumor (use *-cele*) ____________________
4. excessive urination ____________________
5. pertaining to low blood sugar ____________________

Learning Outcome 7.2 Exercises

EXERCISE 7 *Multiple-choice questions. Select the correct answer.*

1. In the condition known as *adrenal virilism,* the adrenal gland secretes excess hormones causing the development of
   a. a swollen thyroid gland
   b. abnormal enlargement of the extremities
   c. breast tissue in males
   d. male secondary sexual characteristics
   e. all of these
2. The "bearded lady" at the carnival is displaying which condition?
   a. gynecomastia
   b. hirsutism
   c. myxedema
   d. polydipsia
   e. none of these
3. Another word for *goiter* is
   a. parathyroid
   b. thyrocele
   c. thyromegaly
   d. thyroptosis
   e. none of these
4. A term that describes the swelling of the skin caused by deposits under the skin is called
   a. gynecomastia
   b. hirsutism
   c. myxedema
   d. polydipsia
   e. none of these
5. A person with hyperthyroidism can display which symptoms?
   a. exophthalmos
   b. nervousness
   c. polyphagia
   d. weight loss
   e. all of these
6. Decreased pancreatic endocrine activity leads to diabetes. If a patient has diabetes he or she may complain of
   a. polydipsia
   b. polyuria
   c. polyphagia
   d. unexpected weight loss
   e. all of these
7. When a female has a hyperactive gonad (*hypergonadism*) she may present with premature
   a. periods
   b. menarche
   c. breast development
   d. thelarche
   e. all of these
8. A person who is experiencing weight gain, decreased energy, hair loss, decreased appetite, constipation, or puffy hands and face may be experiencing which of the following conditions?
   a. hyperthyroidism
   b. hypothyroidism
   c. polydipsia
   d. polyphagia
   e. none of these

Learning Outcome 7.2 Exercises

9. Premature sexual traits may represent a problem with the adrenal gland or the gonads. Males may experience
   a. adrenal virilism
   b. hirsutism
   c. premature puberty from an overactive adrenal gland
   d. adrenal virilism and hirsutism
   e. adrenal virilism and premature puberty from an overactive adrenal gland
10. Premature sexual traits may represent a problem with the adrenal gland or the gonads. Females may come to health care providers complaining of
    a. facial hair
    b. gynecomastia
    c. hirsutism
    d. facial hair and gynecomastia
    e. facial hair and hirsutism
11. Females with underfunctioning gonads may complain of
    a. amenorrhea
    b. lack of menstruation
    c. thelarche
    d. amenorrhea and lack of menstruation
    e. lack of menstruation and thelarche
12. Males with underfunctioning gonads may complain of
    a. breast development
    b. gynecomastia
    c. hirsutism
    d. breast development and gynecomastia
    e. breast development and hirsutism

EXERCISE 8 *Briefly describe the difference between each pair of terms.*

1. hypergonadism, hypogonadism ______________________________
2. pituitary dwarfism, pituitary gigantism ______________________________
3. menarche, thelarche ______________________________
4. polydipsia, polyphagia ______________________________
5. acromegaly, thyromegaly ______________________________

OBJECTIVE

7.3 Observation and Discovery

When a patient is examined for endocrine problems, many of the findings are the same things that the patient noticed and reported. The examiner may notice that the patient is much taller or shorter than average, or that he or she is overweight or underweight. Patients may have incorrect sexual traits, like a male with breast development. Patients may have swelling or fat that is more pronounced in certain parts of their bodies.

Much of what is left for data collection relates to laboratory testing. There are numerous tests in endocrinology. The tests check either the level of hormones in the blood or their effect. Many of the hormones take on similar names to the gland that made them. For example, one of the hormones that the parathyroid glands makes is parathyroid hormone. Adrenal glands make adrenaline (also known as *epinephrine*). They may take on the name from the part of the gland in which they are made. Cortisol is made in the cortex of the adrenal gland. Other hormones are named for the organ they "turn on." These types of hormones are known as *-tropins*. For example, adrenocorticotropic hormone stimulates the cortex of the adrenal gland. Other -tropins include gonadotropins (*LH* and *FSH*) and thyrotopin (*TSH*).

There are two general fluids that can be checked to see the results of hormones: blood and urine. Any lab level that represents a substance in the blood ends in *-emia*. For instance, magnesemia is the level of magnesium in the blood. If the level is higher than normal it has the prefix *hyper-*, and if it is lower than normal it has the prefix *hypo-*. For instance, if a patient has a lower than expected level of magnesium in his or her blood, the patient has hypomagnesemia. Any lab level for a substance in the urine ends with *-uria*. If a patient has calcium in his or her urine, the patient has calciuria.

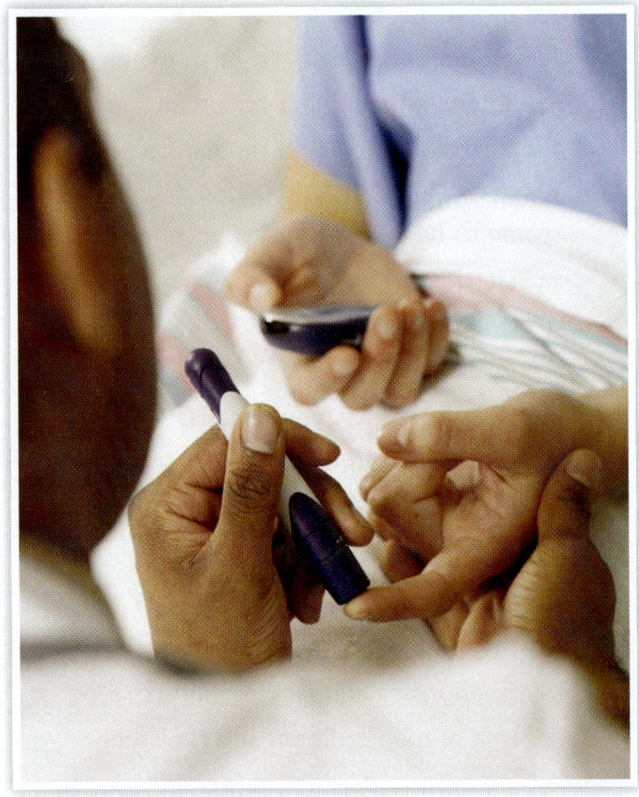

Testing blood is central to gathering data for the endocrine system. A finger prick is the easiest and least invasive path when only a little blood is needed.

One specific nutrient the endocrine system manages is the sugar level in the blood. It controls how fast sugar is being made (*gluconeogenesis*) and how fast it is broken down (*glycolysis*). If someone has low blood sugar (*hypoglycemia*) then the body releases a hormone to increase the production of sugar and slow the breakdown of sugar. Ketones are a by-product of this.

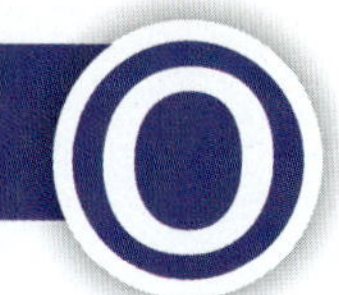

7.3 Observation and Discovery

-emia/-uria

Term	Word Analysis
acidemia A-sih-DEE-mee-ah **Definition** abnormal acidity of the blood	acid / emia acid / blood condition
alkalemia AL-kah-LEE-mee-ah **Definition** abnormal alkalinity (opposite of acidity) of the blood **NOTE:** Alkali is a strong base and is the opposite of an acid. The term *alkali* comes from the Arabic, for *al-qaliy,* which means *the ashes* and is the name of a plant that grows well in alkaline soil.	alkal / emia alkali / blood condition
calciuria CAL-sih-YOO-ree-ah **Definition** calcium in the urine	calci / uria calcium / urine condition
chloremia klor-EE-mee-ah **Definition** increased chloride in the blood	chlor / emia chloride / blood condition
euglycemia YOO-glai-SEE-mee-ah **Definition** good blood sugar	eu / glyc / emia good / sugar / blood condition
glucosuria GLOO-koh-SOO-ree-ah **Definition** sugar in the urine	glucos / uria sugar / urine condition
hypercalcemia HAI-per-kal-SEE-mee-ah **Definition** excessive calcium in the blood	hyper / calc / emia over / calcium / blood condition
hypercholesterolemia HAI-per-koh-LES-ter-aw-LEE-mee-ah **Definition** excessive cholesterol in the blood **NOTE:** The term *cholesterol* breaks down as *chole* (bile) + *stero* (solid) + *ol* (substance) and means a *solid bile substance.* It gets the name because it was first discovered in gallstones.	hyper / cholesterol / emia excessive / cholesterol / blood condition
hyperglycemia HAI-per-glai-SEE-mee-ah **Definition** high blood sugar	hyper / glyc / emia excessive / sugar / blood condition
hyperkalemia HAI-per-kah-LEE-mee-ah **Definition** excessive potassium in the blood **NOTE:** The *kal* root comes from the Latin word *kalium*, which means *pot ash.* The name comes from the fact that potassium is obtained by soaking ashes in water and then evaporating the liquid. This explains why the periodic table's abbreviation for potassium is *K.* The name *potassium* is a Latinization of the words *pot ash.* Potassium really does mean *pot-ash-ium.*	hyper / kal / emia over / potassium / blood condition
hyperlipidemia HAI-per-lih-pih-DEE-mee-ah **Definition** excessive fat in the blood	hyper / lipid / emia excessive / fat / blood condition

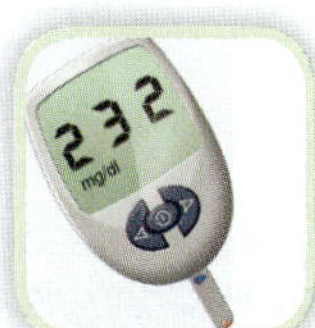

hyperglycemia

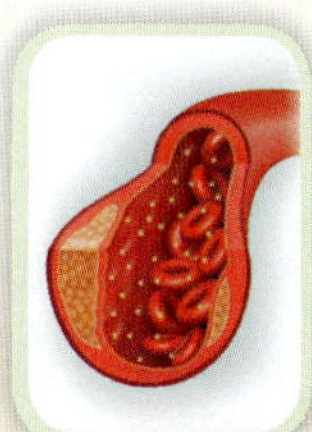
hyperlipidemia

-emia/-uria *continued*

Term	Word Analysis
hypernatremia HAI-per-nah-TREE-mee-ah **Definition** excessive salt in the blood	hyper / natr / emia excessive / salt / blood condition
hyperphosphatemia HAI-per-FAWS-fay-TEE-mee-ah **Definition** excessive phosphate in the blood	hyper / phosphat / emia excessive / phosphate / blood condition
hypoglycemia HAI-poh-glai-SEE-mee-ah **Definition** low blood sugar	hypo / glyc / emia under / sugar / blood condition
ketonuria KEE-toh-NYOO-ree-ah **Definition** ketone bodies in the urine	keton / uria ketone / urine condition
polyuria PAW-lee-YOO-ree-ah **Definition** excessive urination	poly / uria excessive / urine condition
uremia yoo-REE-mee-ah **Definition** presence of urinary waste in the blood	ur / emia urine / blood condition

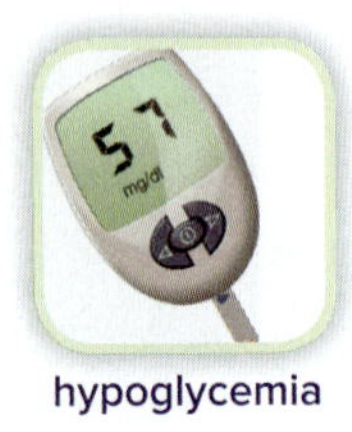

hypoglycemia

hormones

Term	Word Analysis
adrenaline ad-REN-ah-lin **Definition** hormone secreted by the adrenal gland	ad / renal / ine on / kidney / chemical
epinephrine EH-pee-NEF-rin **Definition** hormone secreted by the adrenal gland NOTE: Both *adrenaline* and *epinephrine* mean the same thing and can be used interchangeably. *Adrenaline* comes from Latin and *epinephrine* from Greek. In America, health care professionals prefer *epinephrine*.	epi / nephr / ine upon / kidney / chemical
adrenocorticotropic hormone (ACTH) ah-DREH-noh-KOR-tih-koh-TROH-pik HOR-mohn **Definition** hormone secreted by the pituitary gland that stimulates the cortex of the adrenal gland	adreno / cortico / trop / ic adrenal / cortex / stimulating / pertaining to
corticotropin KOR-tih-koh-TROH-pin **Definition** shorter name for adrenocorticotropic hormone	cortico / tropin cortex / stimulating
glucagon GLOO-kah-gawn **Definition** hormone secreted by the pancreas that stimulates the liver to increase blood sugar levels	gluc / agon sugar / lead

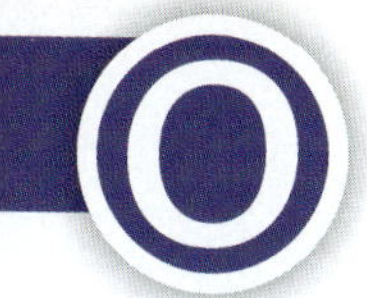

7.3 Observation and Discovery

hormones *continued*

Term	Word Analysis
glucocorticoid GLOO-koh-KOR-tih-koyd **Definition** hormone produced by the adrenal cortex with a role in carbohydrate metabolism	gluco / cortic / oid sugar / cortex / resembling
gonadotropin goh-NAD-oh-TROH-pin **Definition** hormone that stimulates the gonads	gonado / tropin gonad / stimulating
insulin IN-suh-lin **Definition** hormone secreted by the pancreas that controls the metabolism and uptake of sugar and fats **Note:** The root used to name this hormone comes from the fact that insulin is secreted by a cluster or *island* of cells in the pancreas called the *islet of Langerhans*.	insul / in island / chemical
thyrotropin THAI-roh-TROH-pin **Definition** hormone that stimulates the thyroid	thyro / tropin thyroid / stimulating

results

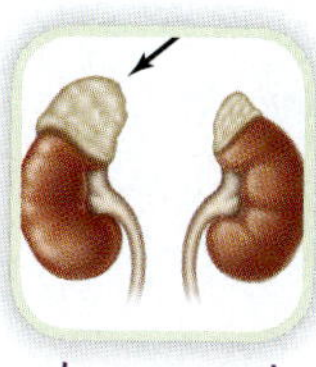

adrenomegaly

Term	Word Analysis
adenomegaly ah-DEN-oh-MEH-gah-lee **Definition** abnormal enlargement of a gland	adeno / megaly gland / enlargement
adrenomegaly ad-REN-oh-MEH-gah-lee **Definition** abnormal enlargement of the adrenal gland	adreno / megaly adrenal / enlargement
euthyroid YOO-thai-royd **Definition** normal functioning thyroid	eu / thyroid good / thyroid
gluconeogenesis GLOO-koh-NEE-oh-JIN-eh-sis **Definition** formation of glucose from noncarbohydrate sources	gluco / neo / genesis sugar / new / formation
glycolysis glai-KAW-lih-sis **Definition** breakdown of sugar **Note:** This is done in cells in order to release energy.	glyco / lysis sugar / loosen
glycopenia GLAI-koh-PEE-nee-ah **Definition** deficiency of sugar	glyco / penia sugar / deficiency

results *continued*

Term	Word Analysis
gonadogenesis goh-NAD-oh-JIN-eh-sis **Definition** creation/development of gonads	gonado / genesis gonad / formation
metabolism meh-TAB-oh-LIZM **Definition** breakdown of matter into energy NOTE: The root *bol* is the source of the English word *ball*.	meta / bol / ism over / throw / condition

professional terms, diagnostic procedures

Term	Word Analysis
endocrine EN-doh-krin **Definition** to secrete internally (i.e., into the bloodstream)	endo / crine inside / secretion
endocrinologist EN-doh-krih-NAW-loh-jist **Definition** specialist in internal secretions	endo / crino / logist inside / secretion / specialist
exocrine EKS-oh-krin **Definition** to secrete externally (through ducts to the surface of an organ, i.e., sweat glands and salivary glands)	exo / crine outside / secretion
glycemic index glai-SEE-mik IN-deks **Definition** ranking of food based on the way it affects sugar levels in the blood	glyc / em / ic sugar / blood / pertaining to

Glycemic Index (GI) and Glycemic Load (GL) for Common Foods

Food	GI	Serving Size (g)	Carbs per Serving (g)	GL
Cornflakes	92	1 cup (28 g)	23	21.1
Grape-Nuts	75	1/2 cup (58 g)	42	31.5
Muesli	66	2/3 cup (55 g)	36	23.8
Bran muffin	59	1 med (113 g)	51	30
Soy milk	44	1 cup (245 g)	9	4
Lentils	29	1 cup (198 g)	24	7

Term	Word Analysis
ketogenesis KEE-toh-JIN-eh-sis **Definition** creation of ketone bodies	keto / genesis ketone / creation

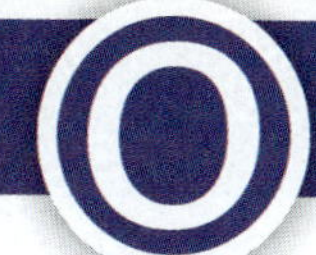

Learning Outcome 7.3 Exercises

PRONUNCIATION

EXERCISE 1 *Break down the following words into syllables.*

EXAMPLE: synesthesia *syn | es | the | sia*

1. glycopenia __________
2. glucosuria __________
3. glucocorticoid __________
4. hypercalcemia __________
5. hyperlipidemia __________
6. hypomagnesemia __________
7. endocrinologist __________
8. adrenocorticotropic hormone __________

EXERCISE 2 *Indicate which syllable is emphasized when pronounced.*

EXAMPLE: bronchitis bron**chi**tis

1. uremia __________
2. chloremia __________
3. hypernatremia __________
4. insulin __________
5. adrenaline __________
6. endocrine __________
7. exocrine __________
8. glycolysis __________
9. euthyroid __________

TRANSLATION

EXERCISE 3 *Break down the following words into their component parts.*

EXAMPLE: synesthesia *syn | es | the | sia*

1. euthyroid __________
2. adrenomegaly __________
3. gonadogenesis __________
4. gluconeogenesis __________
5. endocrinologist __________

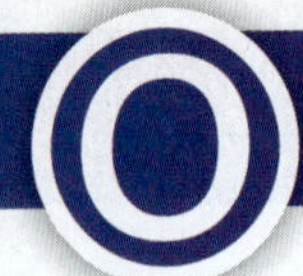

Learning Outcome 7.3 Exercises

6. hyperlipidemia ______________________________
7. hypercholesterolemia ______________________________
8. adrenocorticotropic hormone ______________________________

EXERCISE 4 *Underline and define the word parts from this chapter in the following terms.*

1. glucagon ______________________________
2. glycolysis ______________________________
3. glycopenia ______________________________
4. ketogenesis ______________________________
5. adenomegaly ______________________________
6. endocrine ______________________________
7. exocrine ______________________________
8. adrenaline ______________________________
9. glycemic index ______________________________
10. hyperkalemia ______________________________
11. glucocorticoid (2 roots) ______________________________
12. gonadotropin (2 roots) ______________________________
13. ketonuria (2 roots) ______________________________
14. corticotropin (2 roots) ______________________________
15. thyrotropin (2 roots) ______________________________

EXERCISE 5 *Match the term on the left with its definition on the right.*

______	1. hypoglycemia	a.	abnormal acidity of the blood
______	2. acidemia	b.	abnormal alkalinity (opposite of acidity) of the blood
______	3. chloremia	c.	calcium in the urine
______	4. polyuria	d.	excessive urination
______	5. euglycemia	e.	good blood sugar
______	6. alkalemia	f.	increased chloride in the blood
______	7. calciuria	g.	ketone bodies in the urine
______	8. ketonuria	h.	low blood sugar
______	9. uremia	i.	presence of urinary waste in the blood
______	10. glucosuria	j.	sugar in the urine

EXERCISE 6 *Fill in the blanks.*

1. hypercholesterolemia = excessive ______________ in the blood
2. hypercalcemia = excessive ______________ in the blood

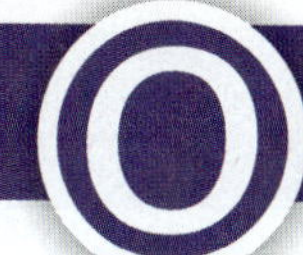

Learning Outcome 7.3 Exercises

3. hyperlipidemia = excessive ______________ in the blood
4. hyperglycemia = excessive ______________ in the blood
5. hyperkalemia = excessive ______________ in the blood
6. hyperphosphatemia = excessive ______________ in the blood
7. hypernatremia = excessive ______________ in the blood

EXERCISE 7 *Translate the following terms as literally as possible.*

EXAMPLE: nasopharyngoscope *an instrument for looking at the nose and throat*

1. euthyroid ______________
2. calciuria ______________
3. glycolysis ______________
4. glycopenia ______________
5. glucocorticoid ______________
6. glucagon ______________
7. endocrinologist ______________
8. hyperlipidemia ______________
9. gluconeogenesis ______________
10. hypernatremia ______________

GENERATION

EXERCISE 8 *Build a medical term from the information provided.*

EXAMPLE: inflammation of the sinuses *sinusitis*

1. sugar in the urine (use *glucos/o*) ______________
2. high blood sugar ______________
3. low blood sugar ______________
4. good blood sugar ______________
5. ketone bodies in the urine ______________
6. presence of urinary waste in the blood ______________
7. a hormone that stimulates the gonads ______________
8. a hormone that stimulates the thyroid ______________
9. abnormal enlargement of a gland ______________
10. abnormal enlargement of the adrenal gland ______________

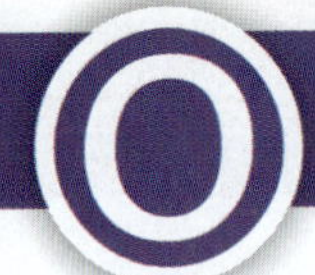

Learning Outcome 7.3 Exercises

EXERCISE 9 *Multiple-choice questions. Select the correct answer(s).*

1. Select all of the terms below that pertain to blood conditions.
   a. chloremia
   b. glucosuria
   c. hypomagnesemia
   d. hypernatremia
   e. hyperphosphatemia
   f. polyuria
   g. uremia

2. Select all of the terms below that pertain to urine conditions.
   a. chloremia
   b. glucosuria
   c. hypomagnesemia
   d. hypernatremia
   e. hyperphosphatemia
   f. polyuria
   g. uremia

3. The breakdown of matter into energy is called
   a. adrenaline
   b. epinephrine
   c. glycolysis
   d. metabolism
   e. none of these

4. The *glycemic index* ranks foods based on
   a. the way they affect sugar levels in the blood
   b. the way they affect sugar levels in the urine
   c. the way the body forms sugar from them
   d. the way the body metabolizes sugar
   e. none of these

5. Select all of the terms below that refer to a hormone secreted by the pituitary gland, which stimulates the cortex of the adrenal gland.
   a. ACTH
   b. adrenaline
   c. adrenocorticotropic hormone
   d. corticotropin
   e. epinephrine

6. Select all of the terms below that refer to a hormone secreted by the adrenal gland.
   a. ACTH
   b. adrenaline
   c. adrenocorticotropic hormone
   d. corticotropin
   e. epinephrine
   f. glucagon
   g. insulin

7. Select all of the terms below that refer to hormones secreted by the pancreas.
   a. ACTH
   b. adrenaline
   c. adrenocorticotropic hormone
   d. corticotropin
   e. epinephrine
   f. glucagon
   g. insulin

EXERCISE 10 *Briefly describe the difference between each pair of terms.*

1. acidemia, alkalemia ______________________
2. hypercalcemia, calciuria ______________________
3. adenomegaly, adrenomegaly ______________________
4. endocrine, exocrine ______________________
5. gonadogenesis, ketogenesis ______________________
6. insulin, glucagon ______________________

ASSESSMENT

7.4 Diagnosis and Pathology

The main types of disorders of the endocrine system result from an organ either making too much of a hormone or not enough of it. When a gland is producing too much hormone, it is labeled with the prefix *hyper-*. An overactive thyroid gland, for example, causes *hyperthyroidism*. A gland that doesn't make enough hormone is labeled with the prefix *hypo-*. When a patient's thyroid gland does not make enough thyroid hormone, the patient develops *hypothyroidism*.

Another way of saying a gland doesn't make enough hormone is to call it *insufficient*. When the cortex of the adrenal gland doesn't make enough cortisol, the condition is called *adrenocortical insufficiency*.

The pancreas is a bit different than many of the other glands in this regard. It produces competing hormones that work against each other: *glucagon* and *insulin*. While problems can occur with either hormone, underproduction of insulin is the most common disorder. This condition leads to *diabetes*.

Many times, overproduction of a hormone is caused by a tumor in the gland that causes it to secrete too much hormone. When a tumor on a gland is benign, it is called an *adenoma;* when a tumor is malignant, it is called an *adenocarcinoma*.

Another cause for the change in the function of a gland is *inflammation*. A patient with *thyroiditis* may initially have high levels of thyroid hormone in his or her blood, followed by hypothyroidism. This initial thyroid hormone is not from overproduction, however. Instead, it originates from the release of already-made hormones. This condition is called *thyrotoxicosis*.

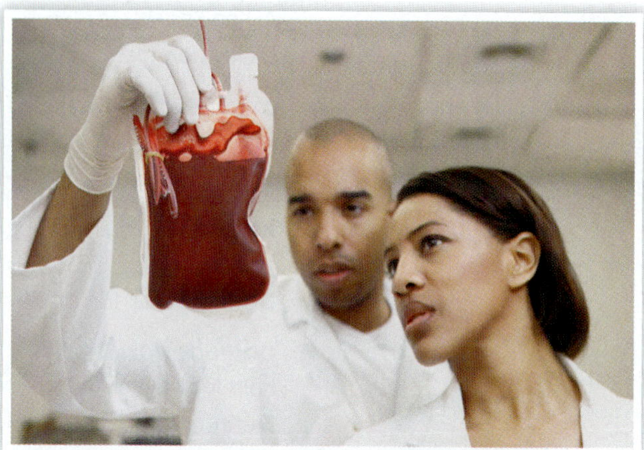

Analyzing blood and urine provides key information about the functioning of the endocrine system.

Bleeding into a gland, which causes cells in the gland to die, can also lead to common gland problems. This happens in the case of *pituitary infarctions*. Bleeding into the pituitary decreases the number of gland cells available to make the hormones, thus causing it to function abnormally.

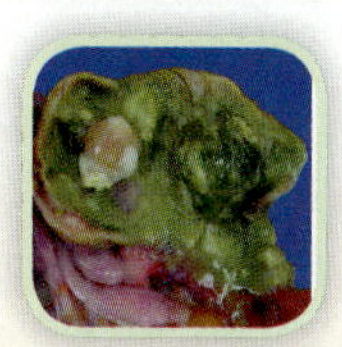

adenocarcinoma

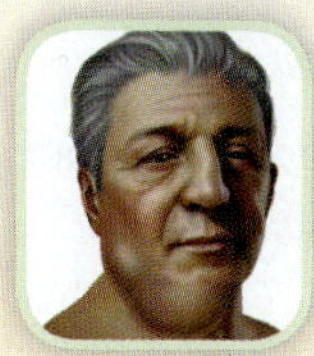

adenoma

general terms

Term	Word Analysis
adenitis AD-en-AI-tis **Definition** inflammation of a gland	**aden / itis** gland / inflammation
adenocarcinoma ad-EN-oh-KAR-sih-NOH-mah **Definition** cancerous tumor of a gland	**adeno / carcin / oma** gland / cancer / tumor
adenoma AD-eh-NOH-mah **Definition** glandular tumor	**aden / oma** gland / tumor
adenopathy AD-en-AW-pah-thee **Definition** gland disease	**adeno / pathy** gland / disease

general terms *continued*

Term	Word Analysis
adenosis AD-en-OH-sis **Definition** gland condition	aden / osis gland / condition
dysmetabolic syndrome DIS-meh-tah-BAW-lik SIN-drohm **Definition** combination of medical disorders associated with faulty metabolism	dys / metabolic syn / drome bad / metabolism together / running
ketosis kee-TOH-sis **Definition** condition characterized by elevated levels of ketone bodies in the blood	ket / osis ketone body / condition
polyadenopathy PAW-lee-AD-en-AW-pah-thee **Definition** disease involving many glands	poly / adeno / pathy many / gland / disease
thymoma thai-MOH-mah **Definition** tumor of the thymus	thym / oma thymus / tumor

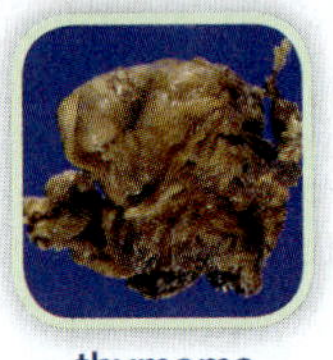
thymoma

adrenal

Term	Word Analysis
adrenal adenoma ad-REE-nal AD-en-OH-mah **Definition** tumor of the adrenal gland	adrenal aden / oma adrenal gland / tumor
adrenal insufficiency ad-REE-nal IN-suh-FIH-shun-see **Definition** condition in which the adrenal glands underproduce necessary hormones	adrenal in / sufficiency adrenal not / adequate
adrenalitis ad-REE-nah-LAI-tis **Definition** inflammation of the adrenal gland	adrenal / itis adrenal / inflammation
adrenocortical carcinoma ad-REE-noh-KOR-tih-kal KAR-sih-NOH-mah **Definition** cancerous tumor originating in the cortex of the adrenal gland	adreno / cortic / al carcin / oma adrenal / cortex / pertaining to cancer / tumor
adrenocortical insufficiency ad-REE-noh-KOR-tih-kal IN-suh-FIH-shun-see **Definition** condition in which the adrenal cortex underproduces necessary hormones	adreno / cortic / al in / sufficiency adrenal / cortex / pertaining to not / adequate
adrenocorticohyperplasia ad-REE-noh-KOR-tih-koh-HAI-per-PLAY-zhah **Definition** overdevelopment of the cortex of the adrenal gland	adreno / cortico / hyper / plasia adrenal / cortex / over / formation
congenital adrenal hyperplasia kon-JEN-ih-tal ad-REE-nal HAI-per-PLAY-zhah **Definition** genetic disease in which the adrenal gland is overdeveloped, resulting in a deficiency of certain hormones and an overproduction of others	con / genit / al adrenal hyper / plasia with / birth / pertaining to adrenal over / formation

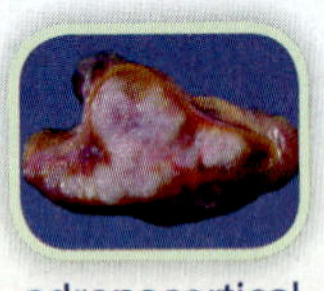
adrenocortical carcinoma

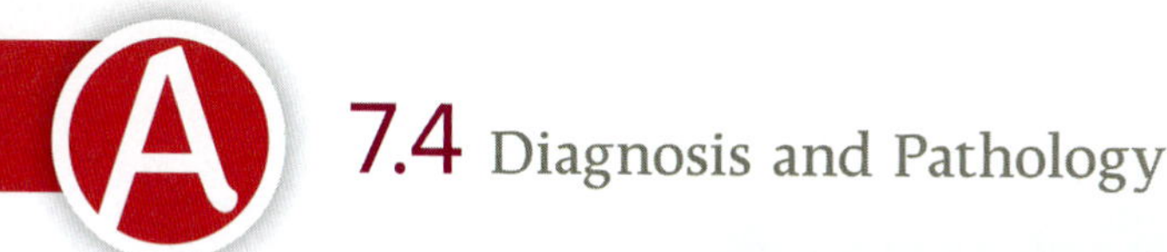

7.4 Diagnosis and Pathology

pancreas

Term	Word Analysis
diabetes mellitus DAI-ah-BEE-teez MEH-lih-tis	diabetes / mellitus pass through / honey
Definition metabolic disease characterized by excessive urination and hyperglycemia NOTE: *Diabetes* is an ancient Greek word that refers to any condition that causes excessive urination. *Mellitus* (which means *honey*) was added to describe a specific kind of diabetes characterized by excessive sugar in the urine.	
diabetic ketoacidosis DAI-ah-BEH-tik KEE-toh-ASS-ih-DOH-sis	diabet / ic keto / acid / osis diabetes / pertaining to ketone / acid / condition
Definition acidity of the blood caused by the presence of ketone bodies produced when the body is unable to burn sugar; thus, it must burn fat for energy	
insulinoma IN-suh-lin-OH-mah	insulin / oma insulin / tumor
Definition tumor that secretes insulin (found in the insulin-producing cells in the pancreas)	
pancreatic pseudocyst PAN-kree-at-ik SOO-doh-sist	pancreat / ic pseudo / cyst pancreas / pertaining to false / cyst
Definition abnormally expanded area in the pancreas resembling a cyst	
pancreatitis PAN-kree-ah-TAI-tis	pancreat / itis pancreas / inflammation
Definition inflammation of the pancreas	
pancreatolith PAN-kree-AT-oh-lith	pancreato / lith pancreas / stone
Definition stone in the pancreas	
pancreatolithiasis PAN-kree-at-oh-lih-THAI-ah-sis	pancreato / lith / iasis pancreas / stone / presence
Definition presence of a stone in the pancreas	

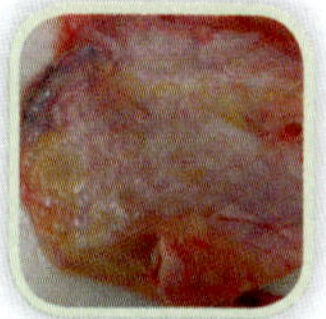
pancreatitis

pituitary

Term	Word Analysis
hyperpituitarism HAI-per-pih-TOO-ih-tar-IZM	hyper / pituitar / ism over / pituitary / condition
Definition overfunctioning of the pituitary gland	
hypophysitis hai-PAWF-ih-SAI-tis	hypophys / itis pituitary / inflammation
Definition inflammation of the pituitary gland	
hypopituitarism HAI-poh-pih-TOO-ih-tar-IZM	hypo / pituitar / ism under / pituitary / condition
Definition condition caused by the undersecretion of the pituitary gland	
panhypopituitarism PAN-HAI-poh-pih-TOO-ih-tar-IZM	pan / hypo / pituitar / ism all / under / pituitary / condition
Definition defective or absent function of the entire pituitary gland	

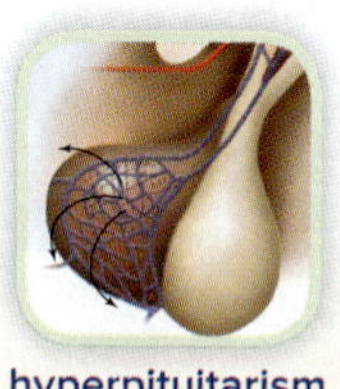
hyperpituitarism

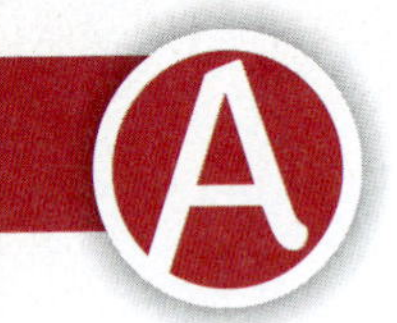

7.4 Diagnosis and Pathology

pituitary *continued*

Term	Word Analysis
pituitary adenoma pih-TOO-ih-TEH-ree AD-en-OH-mah **Definition** tumor on the pituitary gland	pituitary aden / oma pituitary gland / tumor
pituitary infarction pih-TOO-ih-TEH-ree in-FARK-shun **Definition** death of the pituitary gland	pituitary in / farc / tion pituitary in / stuff / condition

Note: The term *infarction* normally refers to a blocked blood vessel, but it can also refer to the death of tissue resulting from the blockage. In fact, it can refer to the death of any tissue—as is the case here—whether or not a blockage is involved.

thyroid

Term	Word Analysis
hyperparathyroidism HAI-per-PAR-ah-THAI-roid-IZM **Definition** overproduction by the parathyroid glands	hyper / para / thyroid / ism over / beside / thyroid / condition
hyperthyroidism HAI-per-THAI-roid-IZM **Definition** overproduction by the thyroid	hyper / thyroid / ism over / thyroid / condition
hypoparathyroidism HAI-poh-PAR-ah-THAI-roid-IZM **Definition** underproduction by the parathyroid	hypo / para / thyroid / ism under / beside / thyroid / condition
hypothyroidism HAI-poh-THAI-roid-IZM **Definition** underproduction by the thyroid	hypo / thyroid / ism under / thyroid / condition
parathyroidoma PAR-ah-THAI-roid-OH-mah **Definition** tumor of the parathyroid	para / thyroid / oma beside / thyroid / tumor
thyroiditis THAI-roid-AI-tis **Definition** inflammation of the thyroid	thyroid / itis thyroid / inflammation
thyrotoxicosis THAI-roh-TOKS-ih-KOH-sis **Definition** condition caused by the exposure of body tissue to excessive levels of thyroid hormone (an extreme version of this is known as "thyroid storm.")	thyro / toxic / osis thyroid / poison / condition

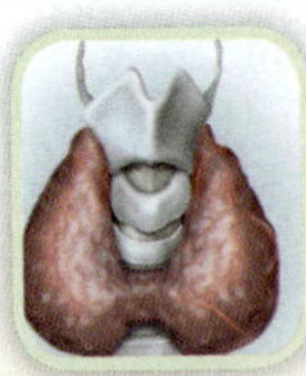
thyroiditis

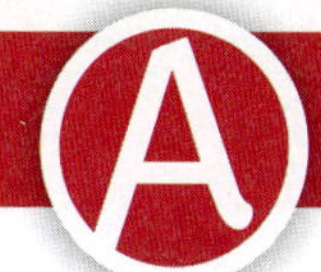

Learning Outcome 7.4 Exercises

PRONUNCIATION

EXERCISE 1 *Break down the following words into syllables.*

EXAMPLE: synesthesia *syn | es | the | sia*

1. adenoma
2. pituitary adenoma
3. diabetes mellitus
4. insulinoma
5. adenopathy
6. polyadenopathy
7. thyrotoxicosis
8. diabetic ketoacidosis
9. pancreatolith
10. pancreatolithiasis
11. parathyroidoma
12. hyperthyroidism
13. hypothyroidism
14. hyperparathyroidism
15. hypoparathyroidism
16. adrenocorticohyperplasia

TRANSLATION

EXERCISE 2 *Break down the following words into their component parts.*

EXAMPLE: nasopharyngoscope *naso | pharyngo | scope*

1. adenosis
2. adrenalitis
3. thyroiditis
4. pancreatitis
5. adenopathy
6. adenoma
7. insulinoma
8. adrenal adenoma
9. parathyroidoma

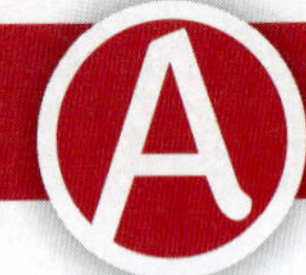

Learning Outcome 7.4 Exercises

10. hypopituitarism ____________
11. panhypopituitarism ____________
12. pancreatolithiasis ____________
13. hyperparathyroidism ____________
14. hypoparathyroidism ____________
15. adrenocortical carcinoma ____________
16. adrenocorticohyperplasia ____________

EXERCISE 3 *Underline and define the word parts from this chapter in the following terms.*

1. ketosis ____________
2. thymoma ____________
3. adenitis ____________
4. pancreatolith ____________
5. pancreatic pseudocyst ____________
6. hyperpituitarism ____________
7. hyperthyroidism ____________
8. hypothyroidism ____________
9. adrenal insufficiency ____________
10. congenital adrenal hyperplasia ____________
11. adenocarcinoma ____________
12. polyadenopathy ____________
13. hypophysitis ____________
14. thyrotoxicosis ____________
15. adrenocortical insufficiency (2 roots) ____________
16. pituitary adenoma (2 roots) ____________

EXERCISE 4 *Multiple-choice questions. Select the correct answer.*

1. *Dysmetabolic syndrome* is a combination of medical disorders associated with faulty
   a. hormone production
   b. metabolism
   c. breakdown of matter into energy
   d. hormone production and metabolism
   e. metabolism and breakdown of matter into energy
2. *Diabetes mellitus* is a metabolic disease characterized by
   a. excessive urination
   b. hyperglycemia
   c. high blood sugar
   d. polyuria
   e. all of these

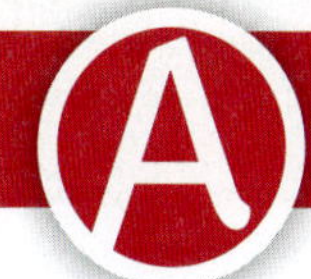

Learning Outcome 7.4 Exercises

3. The name for an acidity of the blood caused by the presence of ketone bodies produced when the body is unable to burn sugar, thus forcing the body to burn fat for energy is
   a. acidemia
   b. diabetes mellitus
   c. diabetic ketoacidosis
   d. hyperlipidemia
   e. ketonuria

4. The death of the pituitary gland is called
   a. pituitary adenoma
   b. pituitary infarction
   c. pituitary dwarfism
   d. pituitary gigantism
   e. none of these

EXERCISE 5 *Translate the following terms as literally as possible.*

EXAMPLE: nasopharyngoscope *an instrument for looking at the nose and throat*

1. adenopathy ____________________
2. polyadenopathy ____________________
3. adenosis ____________________
4. ketosis ____________________
5. pancreatolith ____________________
6. pancreatolithiasis ____________________
7. hyperthyroidism ____________________
8. hypothyroidism ____________________
9. hyperpituitarism ____________________
10. hypopituitarism ____________________
11. panhypopituitarism ____________________
12. hyperparathyroidism ____________________
13. hypoparathyroidism ____________________
14. pancreatic pseudocyst ____________________
15. thyrotoxicosis ____________________

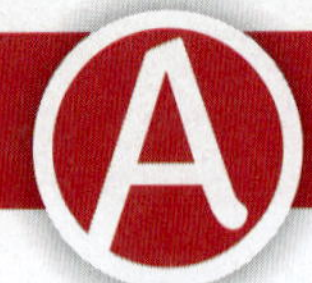

Learning Outcome 7.4 Exercises

GENERATION

EXERCISE 6 *Build a medical term from the information provided.*

EXAMPLE: inflammation of the sinuses *sinusitis*

1. inflammation of the pituitary gland (use *hypophyso*) _______________
2. inflammation of the thyroid _______________
3. inflammation of the pancreas _______________
4. inflammation of the adrenal gland _______________
5. inflammation of a gland _______________
6. a tumor of the thymus _______________
7. a tumor of the adrenal gland (2 words) _______________
8. a tumor of the parathyroid _______________
9. a tumor on the pituitary gland (2 words) _______________
10. a cancerous tumor of a gland _______________
11. a glandular tumor _______________
12. a tumor that secretes insulin _______________

EXERCISE 7 *Match the term on the left with its definition on the right.*

_____ 1. dysmetabolic syndrome

_____ 2. diabetes mellitus

_____ 3. pituitary infarction

_____ 4. adrenocortical insufficiency

_____ 5. adrenal insufficiency

_____ 6. adrenocortical carcinoma

_____ 7. congenital adrenal hyperplasia

_____ 8. adrenocorticohyperplasia

_____ 9. diabetic ketoacidosis

a. cancerous tumor originating in the cortex of the adrenal gland

b. combination of medical disorders associated with faulty metabolism

c. condition in which the adrenal cortex underproduces necessary hormones

d. condition in which the adrenal glands underproduce necessary hormones

e. genetic disease in which the adrenal gland is overdeveloped

f. metabolic disease characterized by excessive urination and hyperglycemia

g. acidity of the blood caused by the presence of ketone bodies produced when the body is unable to burn sugar, thus it must burn fat for energy

h. death of the pituitary gland

i. overdevelopment of the cortex of the adrenal gland

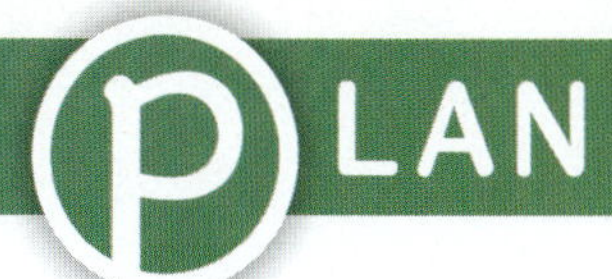

7.5 Treatments and Therapies

Most treatments of endocrine problems involve correcting abnormal hormone levels. If the level of a particular hormone, such as insulin, is too low, the proper treatment involves giving the patient supplemental hormones to bring the levels to normal (*hormone replacement therapy*). There are many routes for delivering the supplemental hormones, including injection, oral, and topical. An even more advanced method is continuous subcutaneous insulin infusion, which is an insulin pump that injects insulin under the skin as needed.

When the hormone level disorder is caused by a tumor or an overactive organ, more aggressive measures may be needed. This can involve taking a medicine that destroys all or part of the problematic gland or undergoing surgery to partially or completely remove the gland (i.e., *adenectomy*).

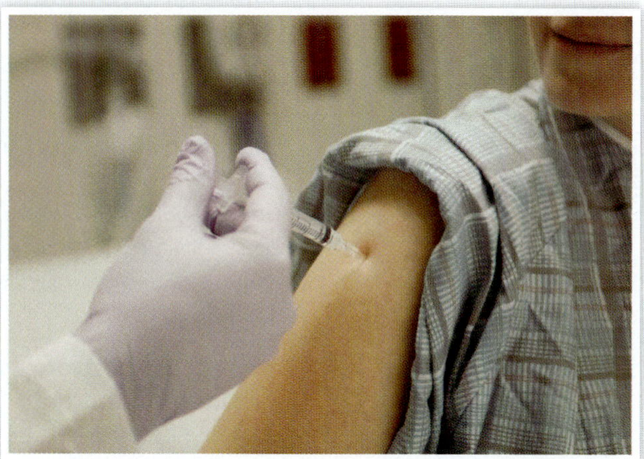

Once an endocrine imbalance has been diagnosed, sometimes the treatment is as easy as supplying the needed hormone.

general terms

Term	Word Analysis
adenectomy AD-en-EK-toh-mee **Definition** removal of a gland	aden / ec / tomy gland / out / cut
ketogenic diet KEE-toh-JIN-ik DAI-et **Definition** diet that aids in the production of ketones in the body	keto / genic diet ketone body / creating
thymectomy thai-MEK-toh-mee **Definition** removal of the thymus	thym / ec / tomy thymus / out / cut

adrenal

Term	Word Analysis
adrenalectomy ad-REE-nal-EK-toh-mee **Definition** removal of the adrenal gland	adrenal / ec / tomy adrenal / out / cut
laparascopic adrenalectomy LAP-rah-SKAW-pik ad-REE-nal-EK-toh-mee **Definition** removal of an adrenal gland by means of a laparascope (instrument inserted into the abdomen for viewing)	lapara / scop / ic adrenal / ec / tomy abdomen / looking / pertaining to adrenal / out / cut

laparascopic adrenalectomy

7.5 Treatments and Therapies

pancreas

Term	Word Analysis
cholangiopancreatography KOHL-AN-jee-oh-PAN-kree-ah-TAW-grah-fee	chol / angio / pancreato / graph / y bile / vessel / pancreas / writing / procedure
Definition procedure used to examine the bile ducts and pancreas	
continuous subcutaneous insulin infusion kun-TIN-yoo-us SUB-koo-TAY-nee-us IN-suh-lin in-FYOO-zhun	continuous sub / cutaneous insulin in / fus / ion continuous beneath / skin insulin in / pour / process
Definition continuous injection of insulin into the blood from a pump inserted under the skin	
endoscopic retrograde cholangiopancreatography EN-doh-SKAW-pik REH-troh-GRAYD KOHL-AN-jee-oh-PAN-kree-ah-TAW-grah-fee	endo / scop / ic retro / grade inside / looking / pertaining to backward / step chol / angio / pancreato / graphy bile / vessel / pancreas / writing procedure
Definition procedure used to examine the bile ducts and pancreas in which an endoscope is passed backward from the digestive tract into the bile duct	
pancreatectomy PAN-kree-ah-TEK-toh-mee	pancreat / ec / tomy pancreas / out / cut
Definition removal of the pancreas	
pancreatolithectomy PAN-kree-ah-toh-lith-EK-toh-mee	pancreato / lith / ec / tomy pancreas / stone / out / cut
Definition removal of a stone in the pancreas	

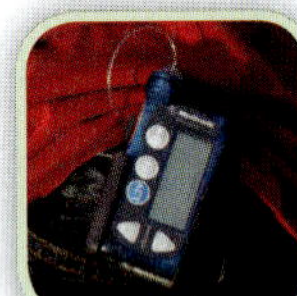
continuous subcutaneous insulin infusion

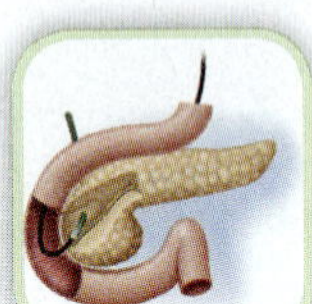
endoscopic retrograde cholangiopancreatography

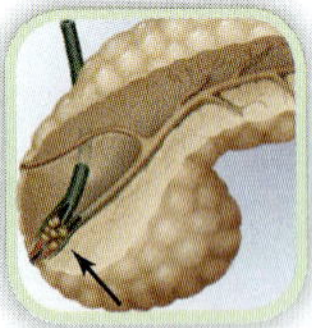
pancreatolithectomy

pituitary

Term	Word Analysis
hypophysectomy hai-POF-is-EK-toh-mee	hypophys / ec / tomy pituitary / out / cut
Definition removal of the pituitary gland	

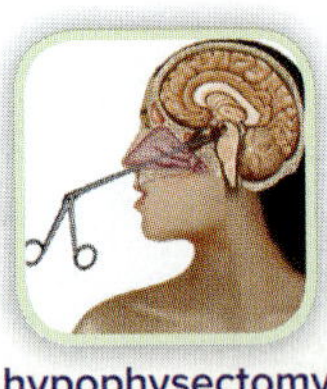
hypophysectomy

thyroid

Term	Word Analysis
parathyroidectomy PAR-ah-THAI-roid-EK-toh-mee	para / thyroid / ec / tomy beside / thyroid / out / cut
Definition removal of the parathyroid	

7.5 Treatments and Therapies

thyroid *continued*

Term	Word Analysis
thyroid function tests THAI-roid FUNK-shun TESTS **Definition** tests performed to evaluate the function of the thyroid	thyroid function tests
thyroidectomy THAI-roid-EK-toh-mee **Definition** removal of the thyroid	thyroid / ec / tomy thyroid / out / cut
thyroidotomy THAI-roid-AW-toh-mee **Definition** incision into the thyroid	thyroido / tomy thyroid / cut
thyroidotoxin thai-ROI-doh-TOK-sin **Definition** substance poisonous to the thyroid gland	thyroido / toxin thyroid / poison
thyroparathyroidectomy THAI-roh-PAR-ah-THAI-roid-EK-toh-me **Definition** removal of the thyroid and parathyroid glands	thyro / para / thyroid / ec / tomy thyroid / beside / thyroid / out / cut

Learning Outcome 7.5 Exercises

PRONUNCIATION

EXERCISE 1 *Break down the following words into syllables.*

EXAMPLE: synesthesia *syn | es | the | sia*

1. thyroidectomy ______
2. thyroidotomy ______
3. thyroidotoxin ______
4. adenectomy ______
5. thymectomy ______
6. adrenalectomy ______
7. laparascopic adrenalectomy ______
8. pancreatectomy ______
9. pancreatolithectomy ______
10. parathyroidectomy ______

TRANSLATION

EXERCISE 2 *Break down the following words into their component parts.*

EXAMPLE: nasopharyngoscope *naso | pharyngo | scope*

1. thymectomy ______
2. adenectomy ______
3. adrenalectomy ______
4. pancreatolithectomy ______
5. thyroidectomy ______
6. parathyroidectomy ______
7. thyroparathyroidectomy ______

EXERCISE 3 *Underline and define the word parts from this chapter in the following terms.*

1. thyroid function tests ______
2. thyroidotomy ______
3. ketogenic diet ______
4. thyroidotoxin ______
5. pancreatectomy ______
6. hypophysectomy ______

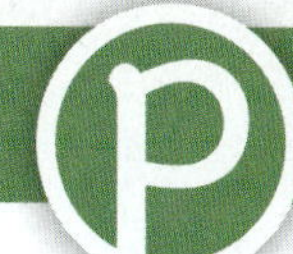

Learning Outcome 7.5 Exercises

7. laparascopic adrenalectomy ______________________
8. cholangiopancreatography ______________________
9. endoscopic retrograde cholangiopancreatography ______________________

EXERCISE 4 *Match the term on the left with its definition on the right.*

__e__ 1. thyroid function tests
__a__ 2. continuous subcutaneous insulin infusion
__d__ 3. laparascopic adrenalectomy
__b__ 4. cholangiopancreatography
__c__ 5. endoscopic retrograde cholangiopancreatography

a. continuous injection of insulin into the blood from a pump inserted under the skin
b. procedure used to examine the bile ducts and pancreas
c. procedure used to examine the bile ducts and pancreas in which an endoscope is passed backward from the digestive tract into the bile duct
d. removal of an adrenal gland by means of a laparascope (an instrument inserted into the abdomen for viewing)
e. tests performed to evaluate the function of the thyroid

EXERCISE 5 *Translate the following terms as literally as possible.*

EXAMPLE: nasopharyngoscope *an instrument for looking at the nose and throat*

1. thyroidotomy ______________________
2. thyroidotoxin ______________________
3. ketogenic diet ______________________
4. pancreatolithectomy ______________________
5. laparascopic adrenalectomy ______________________

GENERATION

EXERCISE 6 *Build a medical term from the information provided.*

EXAMPLE: inflammation of the sinuses *sinusitis*

1. removal of the pituitary gland (use *hypophys/o*) ______________________
2. removal of the pancreas ______________________
3. removal of the thymus ______________________
4. removal of the adrenal gland ______________________
5. removal of a gland ______________________
6. removal of the thyroid ______________________
7. removal of the parathyroid ______________________
8. removal of the thyroid and parathyroid glands ______________________

7.6 Abbreviations

Abbreviations provide a shorthand way of referring to things that either recur often or are too long to write out. When dealing with the endocrine system, these can refer to common tests (TFT), hormones (GH), diagnoses (DM), or treatments (CSII).

endocrine system abbreviations

Abbreviation	Definition
ACTH	adrenocorticotropic hormone
BS	blood sugar
CSII	continuous subcutaneous insulin infusion
CGM	continuous glucose monitor
DI	diabetes insipidus
DM	diabetes mellitus
GDM	gestational diabetes mellitus
ERCP	endoscopic retrograde cholangiopancreatography
FBS	fasting blood sugar
GH	growth hormone
GTT	glucose tolerance test
HgA1C	hemoglobin A1C test (used by diabetes patients to monitor blood sugar levels)
HRT	hormone replacement therapy
IDDM	insulin-dependent diabetes mellitus (type 1)
NIDDM	noninsulin-dependent diabetes mellitus (type 2)
TFT	thyroid function test
TSH	thyroid stimulating hormone (also known as thyrotropin)
T3	triiodothyronine (one of two primary hormones produced by the thyroid)
T4	thyroxine (one of two primary hormones produced by the thyroid)

Learning Outcome 7.6 Exercises

EXERCISE 1 *Define the following abbreviations.*

1. BS ____________________
2. FBS ____________________
3. TFT ____________________
4. DM ____________________
5. DI ____________________
6. IDDM ____________________
7. CSII ____________________
8. NIDDM ____________________
9. T4 ____________________
10. GH ____________________
11. GTT ____________________
12. CGM ____________________
13. HRT ____________________
14. ERCP ____________________
15. GDM ____________________

EXERCISE 2 *Give the abbreviations for the following definitions.*

1. blood sugar ____________________
2. thyroid function test ____________________
3. continuous subcutaneous insulin infusion ____________________
4. diabetes insipidus ____________________
5. diabetes mellitus ____________________
6. fasting blood sugar ____________________
7. growth hormone ____________________
8. glucose tolerance test ____________________
9. continuous glucose monitor ____________________
10. hormone replacement therapy ____________________
11. insulin-dependent diabetes mellitus ____________________
12. noninsulin-dependent diabetes mellitus ____________________
13. endoscopic retrograde cholangiopancreatography ____________________
14. thyroxin levels ____________________
15. thyroid stimulating hormone ____________________

Learning Outcome 7.6 Exercises

EXERCISE 3 *Multiple-choice questions. Select the correct answer(s).*

1. Select all the abbreviations below that pertain to diabetes.
   a. BS
   b. CGM
   c. DI
   d. DM
   e. FBS
   f. GH
   g. HRT
   h. IDDM

2. Select all the abbreviations below that pertain to hormones.
   a. BS
   b. CGM
   c. DI
   d. DM
   e. FBS
   f. GH
   g. HRT
   h. IDDM

3. Select all the abbreviations below that pertain to blood sugar.
   a. BS
   b. CGM
   c. DI
   d. DM
   e. FBS
   f. GH
   g. HRT
   h. IDDM

4. Which of the following types of diabetes is dependent on insulin?
   a. CSII
   b. ERCP
   c. IDDM
   d. NIDDM

5. GTT is a test that determines how a patient's body tolerates
   a. calcium
   b. excess water
   c. fat
   d. sugar

6. A test to evaluate the function of the thyroid is a(n)
   a. CGM
   b. GTT
   c. HRT
   d. TFT

7. Continuous injection of insulin into the blood from a pump inserted under the skin is abbreviated as
   a. CGM
   b. CSII
   c. ERCP
   d. IDDM

7.7 Electronic Health Records

Endocrinology Clinic Note

S Subjective

Mrs. Moon returned to the clinic today to discuss her blood tests. She first came to the office with a chief complaint of **amenorrhea.** She had also noticed a hump developing on the back of her neck, recent weight gain, and **hirsutism.**

O Objective

Temp: 98.6; HR: 70; RR: 16; BP: 150/94.

Gen: WDWN, NAD. AOx3.

HEENT: NCAT. PERRLA. White sclera. No conjunctival injection. Mucous membranes moist and pink. Normal dentition.

Neck: Supple. No LAD. Enlarged fat pad over extensor surface of neck.

Resp: CTA without wheezes, rales, or rhonchi.

CV: RRR without murmurs, gallops, or rubs; radial pulse 2+.

Abd: Soft, nontender, nondistended. No masses. Striae over abdomen.

Neuro: CN II-XII grossly intact. No focal neurologic deficit.

Ext: Feet pink and warm. No cyanosis, clubbing, or edema.

Skin: Mild increase in hair growth over lip and chin.

Tests revealed low **ACTH,** increased cortisol, **hyperlipidemia,** and **hyperglycemia.**

A Assessment

Mrs. Moon has **glucocorticoid** excess (specifically cortisol). The differential diagnosis at this point includes adrenal cortical nodular hyperplasia and an adrenal adenoma.

P Plan

We will schedule Mrs. Moon for abdominal CT to help clarify the diagnosis. I discussed the case with Dr. Glenz, who is in agreement.

–Mary Masterson, NP

Learning Outcome 7.7 Exercises

EXERCISE 1 *Match the term on the left with its definition on the right.*

f	1. hyperglycemia	a.	hormone produced by the adrenal cortex with a role in carbohydrate metabolism
g	2. amenorrhea	b.	hormone secreted by the pituitary gland, which stimulates the cortex of the adrenal gland
d	3. hyperlipidemia	c.	tumor of the adrenal gland
a	4. glucocorticoid	d.	excessive fat in the blood
c	5. adrenal adenoma	e.	excessive growth of facial and body hair in women
e	6. hirsutism	f.	high blood sugar
b	7. ACTH	g.	lack of menstrual flow

EXERCISE 2 *Fill in the blanks.*

1. Using the data recorded at the patient's discharge physical examination, fill in the following blanks.
   a. The patient's temperature: ______________________________
   b. The patient's heart rate: ______________________________
   c. The patient's respiratory rate: ______________________________
   d. The patient's blood pressure: ______________________________
   e. HEENT (______________________________):
   NCAT. ______________________________
   (pupils equal, round, and reactive to light and accommodation).
2. Her tests revealed low ACTH (give definition: ____________________), increased cortisol, ____________________ (excessive fat in the blood), and *hyperglycemia* (give definition: ______________________________).
3. The patient will be scheduled for an abdominal ____________________ (computed axial tomography) to help clarify the diagnosis.

EXERCISE 3 *True or false questions. Indicate true answers with a T and false answers with an F.*

1. The patient's tests showed too much fat in the blood and high blood sugar. ________
2. One possible diagnosis is an adrenal tumor. ________
3. The patient has a mild increase in hair growth over the lip and chin, which could indicate she has hirsutism. ________

Emergency Department Visit

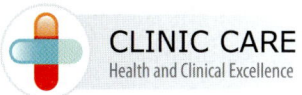

Patient Name: Olivia Sweet
Chief Complaint: Vomiting, lethargy.
History of Present Illness:

Miss Sweet is a 13-year-old female who presented to the ER with a several-hour history of vomiting. She awoke this morning with abdominal pain, which progressed to vomiting. She has not had any fever. She has not been able to keep any food or liquid down, and when she began to look tired, Miss Sweet's parents brought her to the Emergency Department.
Per Miss Sweet's parents, she has had a two-month history of **polydipsia**, **polyuria**, and **polyphagia**. Despite a recent increase in appetite, they have noticed that she has lost weight.

Past Medical History: Normal. She has not had **menarche**.
Medications: None.
Allergies: NKDA.
Social History: Lives with her parents and two siblings. A/B student on the honor roll.
Surgical History: None.
Family History: Mother: Rheumatoid arthritis; maternal aunt: **IDDM**.

Physical Exam:

Temperature: 98.6; Heart Rate: 100; Respiratory Rate: 32; BP: 84/60.
General: Thin. Lethargic.
Head: Normocephalic atraumatic, very dry mucous membranes. **Ketotic** breath. Pupils equal, round, and reactive to light. TMs normal.
Neck: Supple.
Cardiovascular: Mild tachycardia. No murmur, gallop, or rub.
Respiratory: Deep, rapid breathing. Clear to auscultation. No retractions.
Abdomen: Soft, nontender, nondistended. Spleen and liver edge not palpable.
Neurologic: DTRs: patellar and brachial present and equal.
Skin: Dry. Cap refill > 3 seconds.
Extremities: No cyanosis, clubbing, or edema.

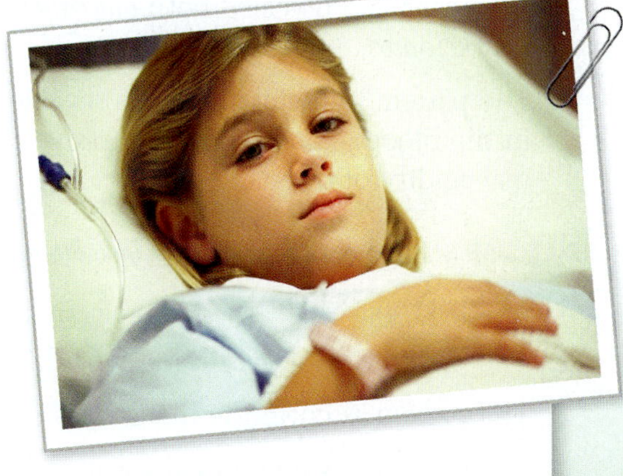

Emergency Department Course:

Miss Sweet arrived in the ED lethargic, but responsive. Given her history and vomiting, we were concerned about **diabetic ketoacidosis**. The patient's finger stick blood sugar test result of 320 confirmed **hyperglycemia**, and a urinalysis revealed both **glucosuria** and **ketonuria**. An IV was started and labs were sent. Chemistry profile showed **hypernatremia**, **hypokalemia**, and **acidemia**. The pediatric intensive care team was contacted for transfer to the PICU.

Disposition: Transfer to PICU.

—Ed Rhume, MD

Learning Outcome 7.7 Exercises

EXERCISE 4 *Match the term on the left with its definition on the right.*

_____ 1. hyperglycemia
_____ 2. ketonuria
_____ 3. acidemia
_____ 4. polyuria
_____ 5. glucosuria
_____ 6. menarche
_____ 7. diabetic ketoacidosis
_____ 8. polydipsia
_____ 9. polyphagia
_____ 10. hypernatremia

a. abnormal acidity of the blood
b. acidity of the blood caused by the presence of ketone bodies produced when the body is unable to burn sugar; thus, it must burn fat for energy
c. excessive eating
d. excessive salt in the blood
e. excessive thirst
f. excessive urination
g. high blood sugar
h. ketone bodies in the urine
i. sugar in the urine
j. beginning or first menstruation

EXERCISE 5 *Fill in the blanks.*

1. Using the data recorded at the patient's discharge physical examination, fill in the following blanks.
   a. T:_____
   b. HR:_____
   c. RR:_____
   d. BP:_____
   e. The patient has a two-month history of _____ (excessive thirst), _____ (excessive hunger), and _____ (excessive urination).
2. The urinalysis revealed both *glucosuria* (give definition: _____) and *ketonuria* (give definition: _____).
3. The patient's chemistry profile revealed *hypernatremia* (excessive _____ in the blood), *hypokalemia* (excessive _____ in the blood), and *acidemia* (abnormal acidity of the _____).

EXERCISE 6 *True or false questions. Indicate true answers with a T and false answers with an F.*

1. The patient is afebrile. _____
2. The patient is not very hungry or thirsty. _____
3. The patient is currently menstruating. _____
4. The patient has high blood sugar. _____
5. The patient has sugar and ketone bodies in her urine. _____

Learning Outcome 7.7 Exercises

EXERCISE 7 *Multiple-choice questions. Select the correct answer.*

1. *Hypernatremia* is a condition of the
   a. adrenal gland
   b. blood
   c. thyroid
   d. urine
2. A person with excessive potassium in the blood has
   a. acidemia
   b. glucosuria
   c. hyperkalemia
   d. hypernatremia
3. PICU stands for
   a. pediatric intensive care unit
   b. postoperative intensive care unit
   c. preoperative intensive care unit
   d. none of these
4. When a person has faulty carbohydrate metabolism, the result is increased ketone bodies. The body gets rid of them through the lungs, giving sufferers fruity-smelling breath.
   a. Miss Sweet has ketotic breath.
   b. Miss Sweet is experiencing normal carbohydrate metabolism.
   c. Miss Sweet is suffering from faulty carbohydrate metabolism.
   d. Miss Sweet has ketotic breath and is experiencing normal carbohydrate metabolism.
   e. Miss Sweet has ketotic breath and is suffering from faulty carbohydrate metabolism.

Surgery Follow-Up Note

Subjective

Mr. Shield presented to our office today for follow-up from his **thyroidectomy.** He initially presented to his primary care physician with concerns over a **goiter.** His PCP noticed mild **exophthlamos** and an enlarged thyroid with palpable nodules. He had **thyroid scintigraphy** and **TFTs** that both revealed active nodules. After discussion with Dr. Sharp during a consultation, Mr. Shield elected for surgical correction. Dr. Sharp performed a thyroidectomy 2 weeks ago. Mr. Shield had postoperative **hypocalcemia** but otherwise had an unremarkable hospital stay. Since discharge, Mr. Shield has done very well.

Objective

Temp: 98.6; HR 60; RR: 16; BP 102/62; Wt: 176.
General: No acute distress. Alert and oriented.
HEENT: PERRLA. No conjunctival injection. Mucous membranes moist and pink. TMs normal.
Neck: Postop incision site is clean, dry and intact. No erythema induration or discharge. No goiter.
Resp: CTA. w/o wheezes, rales, or rhonchi.
CV: RRR without murmur.
Gen: Soft, nontender, nondistended.
Ext: No c/c/e. Labs: Mildly elevated **TSH** and low T4.
Calcium—normal.

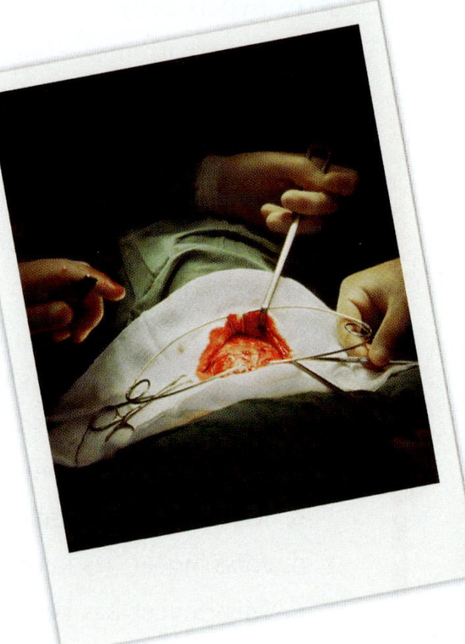

Impression/Plan

Mr. Shield's thyroid labs are still not where I want them to be. We will increase his medicine to help get him **euthyroid.**
No lasting **hypoparathyroidism** from the surgery.
Return for follow-up visit including labs in 1 month.

—Sue Stenson, NP

Learning Outcome 7.7 Exercises

EXERCISE 8 *Match the term on the left with its definition on the right.*

	Term		Definition
c	1. hypocalcemia	a.	"good thyroid"
d	2. thyroidectomy	b.	swollen thyroid gland
a	3. euthyroid	c.	low calcium levels in the blood
e	4. exophthalmos	d.	removal of the thyroid
f	5. hypoparathyroidism	e.	protrusion of the eyes out of the eye socket
b	6. goiter	f.	underproduction by the parathyroid

EXERCISE 9 *Fill in the blanks.*

1. Mr. Shield is at the office today to follow up from his *thyroidectomy* (give definition: ______________________________).

2. Using the data recorded at the patient's discharge physical examination, fill in the following blanks.
   a. The patient's temperature: ______________
   b. The patient's heart rate: ______________
   c. The patient's respiratory rate: ______________
   d. The patient's blood pressure: ______________
   e. HEENT (______________________________): ______________ (pupils equal, round, and reactive to light and accommodation).
   f. Resp: CTA (______________ to ______________).
   g. CV: ______________ (regular rate and rhythm).

EXERCISE 10 *True or false questions. Indicate true answers with a T and false answers with an F.*

1. The patient recently had his thyroid removed. ________
2. He initially presented to his PCP with concerns over a swollen thyroid gland. ________
3. His thyroid function tests revealed active nodules. ________
4. After Mr. Shield's operation, he had normal blood sugar. ________
5. According to the patient's labs, he has low thyroxin levels. ________

EXERCISE 11 *Multiple-choice questions. Select the correct answer.*

1. The patient suffered from postoperative *hypocalcemia.* Which of the following is a correct breakdown of the term?
   a. *hypo* (over) + *calc* (calcium) + *-emia* (blood condition)
   b. *hypo* (over) + *calc* (calcium) + *-emia* (urine condition)
   c. *hypo* (under) + *calc* (calcium) + *-emia* (blood condition)
   d. *hypo* (under) + *calc* (calcium) + *-emia* (urine condition)

2. The patient has no lasting *hypoparathyroidism.* Which of the following is a correct breakdown of the term?
   a. *hypo* (over) + *para* (in addition to) + *thyroid* (the thyroid organ) + *-ism* (condition)
   b. *hypo* (over) + *parathyroid* (the parathyroid organ) + *-ism* (condition)
   c. *hypo* (under) + *parathyroid* (the parathyroid organ) + *-ism* (condition)
   d. *hypo* (under) + *para* (in addition to) + *thyroid* (the thyroid organ) + *-ism* (condition)

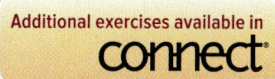

Chapter Review exercises, along with additional practice items, are available in Connect!

Quick Reference

quick reference glossary of roots

Root	Definition	Root	Definition
aden/o	gland	**hypophys/o**	pituitary gland
adren/o, adrenal/o	adrenal gland	**ket/o**	ketone body
cortic/o	outer surface	**pancreat/o**	pancreas
crin/o	secrete	**pituitar/o**	pituitary gland
-emia	blood condition	**thym/o**	thymus
gluc/o, glucos/o, glyc/o	sugar	**thyr/o, thyroid/o**	thyroid
gonad/o	gonads (sex organs)	**-tropin**	stimulating hormone
hormon/o	hormone	**-uria**	urine condition

quick reference glossary of terms

Term	Definition
acidemia	abnormal acidity of the blood
acromegaly	abnormal enlargement of the extremities
adenalgia	pain in a gland
adenectomy	removal of a gland
adenitis	inflammation of a gland
adenocarcinoma	cancerous tumor of a gland
adenoma	glandular tumor
adenomegaly	abnormal enlargement of a gland
adenopathy	gland disease
adenosis	gland condition
adrenal adenoma	tumor of the adrenal gland
adrenal insufficiency	condition in which the adrenal glands underproduce necessary hormones
adrenal virilism	development of male secondary sexual characteristics caused by excessive secretion of the adrenal gland
adrenalectomy	removal of the adrenal gland
adrenaline	hormone secreted by the adrenal gland (from Latin; see also *epinephrine*)
adrenalitis	inflammation of the adrenal gland

quick reference glossary of terms *continued*

Term	Definition
adrenarche	beginning of adrenal secretion (at puberty)
adrenocortical carcinoma	cancerous tumor originating in the cortex of the adrenal gland
adrenocortical insufficiency	condition in which the adrenal cortex underproduces necessary hormones
adrenocorticohyperplasia	overdevelopment of the cortex of the adrenal gland
adrenocorticotropic hormone (ACTH)	hormone secreted by the pituitary gland, which stimulates the cortex of the adrenal gland
adrenomegaly	abnormal enlargement of the adrenal gland
alkalemia	abnormal alkalinity (opposite of acidity) of the blood
amenorrhea	lack of menstrual flow
calciuria	calcium in the urine
chloremia	increased chloride in the blood
cholangiopancreatography	procedure used to examine the bile ducts and pancreas
congenital adrenal hyperplasia	genetic disease in which the adrenal gland is overdeveloped, resulting in a deficiency of certain hormones and an overproduction of others
continuous subcutaneous insulin infusion	continuous injection of insulin into the blood from a pump inserted under the skin
corticotropin	shorter name for adrenocorticotropic hormone
diabetes mellitus	metabolic disease characterized by excessive urination and hyperglycemia
diabetic ketoacidosis	acidity of the blood caused by the presence of ketone bodies produced when the body is unable to burn sugar; thus, it must burn fat for energy
dysmetabolic syndrome	combination of medical disorders associated with faulty metabolism
endocrine	secrete internally (i.e., into the bloodstream)
endocrinologist	specialist in internal secretions
endoscopic retrograde cholangiopancreatography	procedure used to examine the bile ducts and pancreas in which an endoscope is passed backward from the digestive tract into the bile duct
epinephrine	hormone secreted by the adrenal gland (from Greek; see also *adrenaline*)
euglycemia	good blood sugar
euthyroid	a normal functioning thyroid
exocrine	secrete externally through ducts to the surface of an organ (i.e., sweat glands and salivary glands)
exophthalmus	protrusion of the eyes out of the eye socket

quick reference glossary of terms *continued*

Term	Definition
galactorrhea	discharge of milk
glucagon	hormone secreted by the pancreas that stimulates the liver to increase blood sugar levels
glucocorticoid	a hormone produced by the adrenal cortex with a role in carbohydrate metabolism
gluconeogenesis	the formation of glucose from noncarbohydrate sources
glucosuria	sugar in the urine
glycemic index	ranking of food based on the way it affects sugar levels in the blood
glycolysis	breakdown of sugar
glycopenia	deficiency of sugar
goiter	swollen thyroid gland
gonadogenesis	creation/development of gonads
gonadotropin	hormone that stimulates the gonads
gynecomastia	development of breast tissue in males
hirsutism	excessive growth of facial and body hair in women
hypercalcemia	excessive calcium in the blood
hypercholesterolemia	excessive cholesterol in the blood
hyperglycemia	high blood sugar
hypergonadism	excessive secretion of the sex glands
hyperkalemia	excessive potassium in the blood
hyperlipidemia	excessive fat in the blood
hyperparathyroidism	overproduction by the parathyroid glands
hyperpituitarism	overfunctioning of the pituitary gland
hyperthyroidism	overproduction by the thyroid
hypoglycemia	low blood sugar
hypoglycemic	pertaining to low blood sugar
hypogonadism	undersecretion of the sex glands
hypomagnesemia	deficient magnesium in the blood
hypernatremia	excessive salt in the blood
hypoparathyroidism	underproduction by the parathyroid
hyperphosphatemia	excessive phosphate in the blood
hypophysectomy	removal of the pituitary gland

quick reference glossary of terms *continued*

Term	Definition
hypophysitis	inflammation of the pituitary gland
hypopituitarism	condition caused by the undersecretion of the pituitary gland
hypothyroidism	underproduction by the thyroid
insulin	hormone secreted by the pancreas that controls the metabolism and uptake of sugar and fats
insulinoma	tumor that secretes insulin (found in the insulin-producing cells in the pancreas)
ketogenesis	creation of ketone bodies
ketogenic diet	diet that aids in the production of ketones in the body
ketonuria	ketone bodies in the urine
ketosis	condition characterized by elevated levels of ketone bodies in the blood
laparascopic adrenalectomy	removal of an adrenal gland by means of a laparascope (an instrument inserted into the abdomen for viewing)
menarche	beginning or first menstruation
metabolism	breakdown of matter into energy
myxedema	swelling of the skin caused by deposits under the skin
pancreatalgia	pain in the pancreas
pancreatectomy	removal of the pancreas
pancreatic pseudocyst	abnormally expanded area in the pancreas resembling a cyst
pancreatitis	inflammation of the pancreas
pancreatolith	stone in the pancreas
pancreatolithectomy	removal of a stone in the pancreas
pancreatolithiasis	presence of a stone in the pancreas
panhypopituitarism	defective or absent function of the entire pituitary gland
parathyroid	removal of the parathyroid
parathyroidoma	tumor of the parathyroid
pituitary adenoma	tumor on the pituitary gland
pituitary dwarfism	abnormally short height caused by undersecretions of growth hormone from the pituitary gland

quick reference glossary of terms *continued*

Term	Definition
pituitary gigantism	abnormally tall height caused by oversecretion of growth hormone from the pituitary gland
pituitary infarction	death of the pituitary gland
polyadenopathy	disease involving many glands
polydipsia	excessive thirst
polyphagia	excessive eating
polyuria	excessive urination
thelarche	beginning of breast development
thymectomy	removal of the thymus
thymoma	tumor of the thymus
thyrocele	see *goiter*
thyroid function tests	tests performed to evaluate the function of the thyroid
thyroidectomy	removal of the thyroid
thyroiditis	inflammation of the thyroid
thyroidotomy	incision into the thyroid
thyroidotoxin	substance poisonous to the thyroid gland
thyromegaly	enlargement of the thyroid
thyroparathyroidectomy	removal of the thyroid and parathyroid glands
thyroptosis	downward displacement (drooping) of the thyroid
thyrotoxicosis	condition caused by the exposure of body tissue to excessive levels of thyroid hormone
thyrotropin	hormone that stimulates the thyroid
uremia	presence of urinary waste in the blood

review of terms by roots

Root	Term(s)	
aden/o	adenalgia adenectomy adenitis adenocarcinoma adenoma adenomegaly	adenopathy adenosis adrenal adenoma pituitary adenoma polyadenopathy
adren/o	adrenal adenoma adrenal insufficiency adrenal virilism adrenalectomy adrenaline adrenalitis adrenarche	adrenocortical carcinoma adrenocortical insufficiency adrenocorticohyperplasia adrenocorticotropic hormone (ACTH) adrenomegaly congenital adrenal hyperplasia laparascopic adrenalectomy
cortic/o	adrenocortical carcinoma adrenocortical insufficiency	adrenocorticohyperplasia adrenocorticotropic hormone (ACTH) corticotropin glucocorticoid
crin/o	endocrine endocrinologist	exocrine
-emia	acidemia alkalemia chloremia euglycemia hypercalcemia hypercholesterolemia hyperglycemia hyperkalemia	hyperlipidemia hypernatremia hyperphosphatemia hypoglycemia hypoglycemic hypomagnesemia uremia
gluc/o	glucagon	
glucos/o	glucocorticoid glucogenesis glucosuria	
glyc/o	euglycemia glycemic index glycolysis glycopenia	hyperglycemia hypoglycemia hypoglycemic
gonad/o	gonadogenesis gonadotropin	hypergonadism hypogonadism
hormon/o	adrenocorticotropic hormone (ACTH)	
hypophys/o	hypophysectomy hypophysitis	
ket/o	diabetic ketoacidosis ketogenesis ketogenic diet	ketonuria ketosis

review of terms by roots *continued*

Root	Term(s)	
pancreat/o	cholangiopancreatography endoscopic retrograde pancreatalgia pancreatectomy pancreatic pseudocyst	pancreatitis pancreatolith pancreatolithectomy pancreatolithiasis
pituitar/o	hyperpituitarism hypopituitarism panhypopituitarism pituitary adenoma	pituitary dwarfism pituitary gigantism pituitary infarction
thym/o	thymectomy thymoma	
thyr/o	euthyroid	
thyroid/o	hyperparathyroidism hyperthyroidism hypoparathyroidism hypothyroidism parathyroidectomy parathyroidoma thyrocele thyroid function tests thyroidectomy	thyroiditis thyroidotomy thyroidotoxin thyromegaly thyroparathyroidectomy thyroptosis thyrotoxicosis thyrotropin
-tropin	adrenocorticotropic hormone (ACTH) corticotropin gonadotropin	thyrotropin
-uria	calciuria glucosuria ketonuria	polyuria uremia

other terms

acromegaly	hirsutism
amenorrhea	insulin
continuous subcutaneous insulin infusion	insulinoma
diabetes mellitus	menarche
dysmetabolic syndrome	metabolism
epinephrine	myxedema
exophthalmos	polydipsia
galactorrhea	polyphagia
goiter	thelarche
gynecomastia	

The Blood and Lymphatic Systems—Hematology and Immunology

8

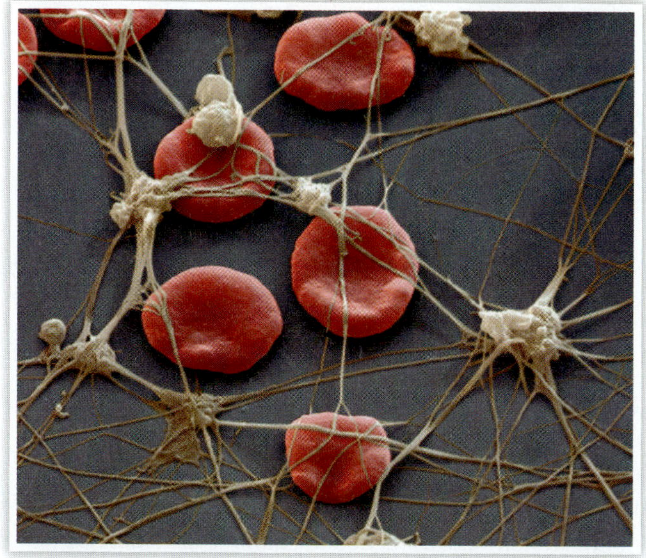

learning outcomes

Upon completion of this chapter, you will be able to:

8.1 Identify the **roots/word parts** associated with the **hematological/immunological systems.**

S **8.2** Translate the **Subjective** terms associated with the **hematological/immunological systems.**

O **8.3** Translate the **Objective** terms associated with the **hematological/immunological systems.**

A **8.4** Translate the **Assessment** terms associated with the **hematological/immunological systems.**

P **8.5** Translate the **Plan** terms associated with the **hematological/immunological systems.**

8.6 Use **abbreviations** associated with the **hematological/immunological systems.**

8.7 Distinguish terms associated with the **hematological/immunological systems** in the context of **electronic health records.**

Introduction and Overview of Hematology and Immunology

People who live together in a community, like an apartment complex or neighborhood, all need certain services. A community needs energy, such as electricity, to provide power for all its lights and appliances. A community needs ways to communicate, like phones or mail service. A community needs recycling and garbage removal systems. Finally, a community needs protection, such as the services rendered by police officers and firefighters.

In many ways, the body is a collection of many communities. The blood and lymphatic systems provide many of these valuable services and resources to the body's communities. These services are absolutely critical to life. If blood flow stops even for a few minutes, hazardous waste will accumulate, and cells will starve. For example, the blood provides energy by delivering sugar and oxygen. The blood carries signals from other parts of the body, allowing for communication. The blood also takes away the waste made by the body's cells.

The lymphatic system provides constant protection by repairing injuries and fighting infections.

8.1 Word Parts Associated with the Hematological/Immunological Systems

Word Roots of the Hematological System

Blood has three main types of cells (*cytes*). Red blood cells (*erythrocytes*) are the transport trucks that bring oxygen to all the cells of the body and take away the waste. White blood cells (*leukocytes*) fight infection. Platelets (*thrombocytes*) are the small scab-makers of the body. They patch things up.

Red blood cells (*hemo/hemato*) are the most common cells in the blood. They contain a substance called *hemoglobin.* Hemoglobin grabs on to oxygen when the surrounding oxygen levels are high and releases it when the ambient oxygen levels are low. In this way, it helps carry fresh oxygen from the lungs to all the parts of the body that need it.

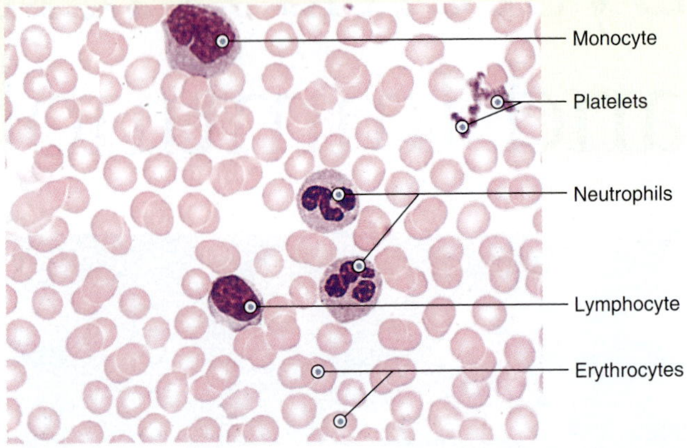

White blood cells protect the body from invasion. The blood contains different types of white blood cells that fight different types of infections (*neutrophils, lymphocytes, basophils,* and *eosinophils*). Each carries out a different job.

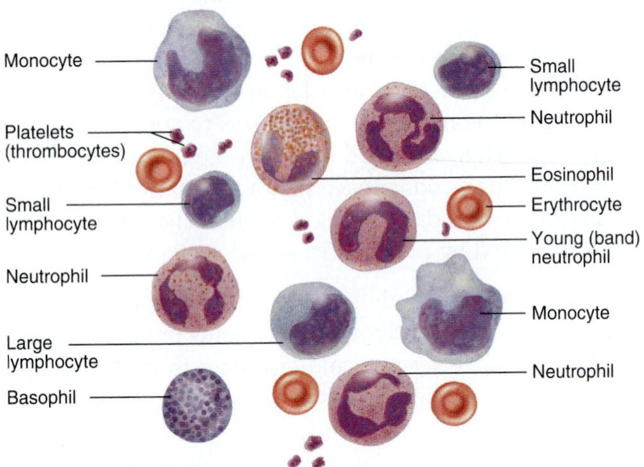

These white blood cells aren't the body's only defense, though. The body also makes special protective proteins as well. These proteins are called *immunoglobulins.* Just like the white blood cells, different types of immunoglobulins are designed for specific tasks. In fact, immunizations are means of forcing the body to make immunoglobulins against dangerous illnesses.

Platelets are the smallest of the cells in the blood. Their job is to patch up any broken blood vessels. Blood vessels constantly develop small leaks. They need a patch system to keep them functioning properly. When a vessel is injured, it attracts platelets that clump together to form a sticky patch. They also send signals that help further form a permanent clot.

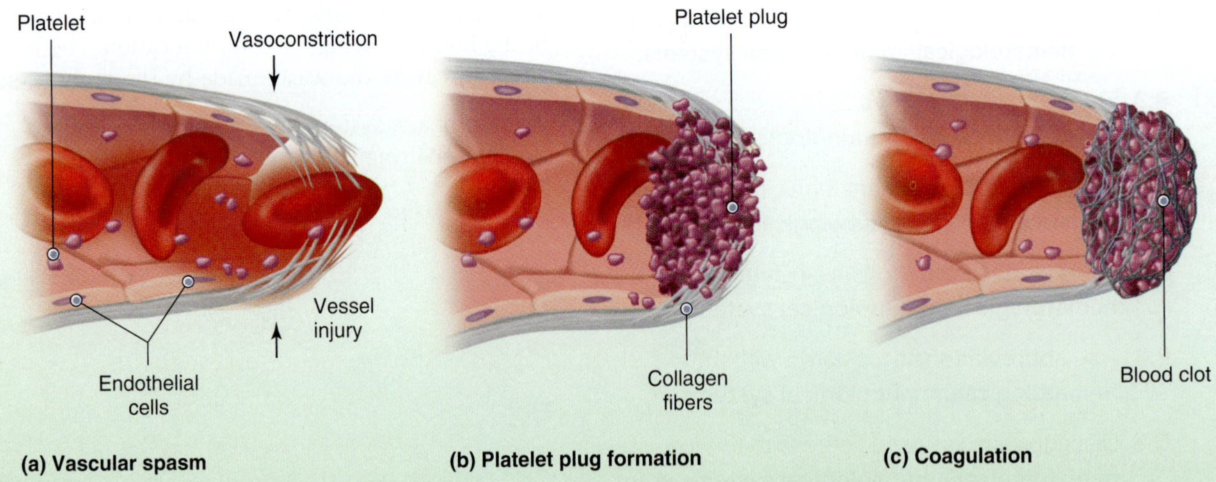

This shows the process of coagulation and the formation of a clot.

BLOOD

coagulation

ROOT: ***coagul/o***

EXAMPLES: anticoagulant, coagulopathy

NOTES: *Coagulo* refers to the blood's ability to form clots. It comes from a Latin word, *coagulum,* which comes from the world of cheese making. *Coagulum* is added to milk to make it curdle and begin the process of turning milk into cheese.

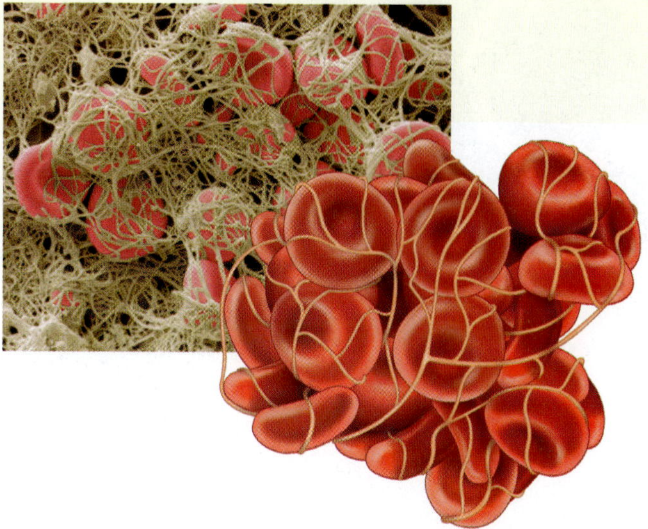

clot

ROOT: ***thromb/o***

EXAMPLES: thrombocyte, thrombosis

NOTES: The blood's ability to clot can be both life saving and life threatening. When the body is wounded, clotting enables the body to stop the bleeding and begin the healing process. *Hemophilia* is a disease in which the blood doesn't clot well, potentially causing minor cuts to become life-threatening injuries. Clots become life threatening when they form in the bloodstream in places where they aren't needed, which could block blood flow to vital organs.

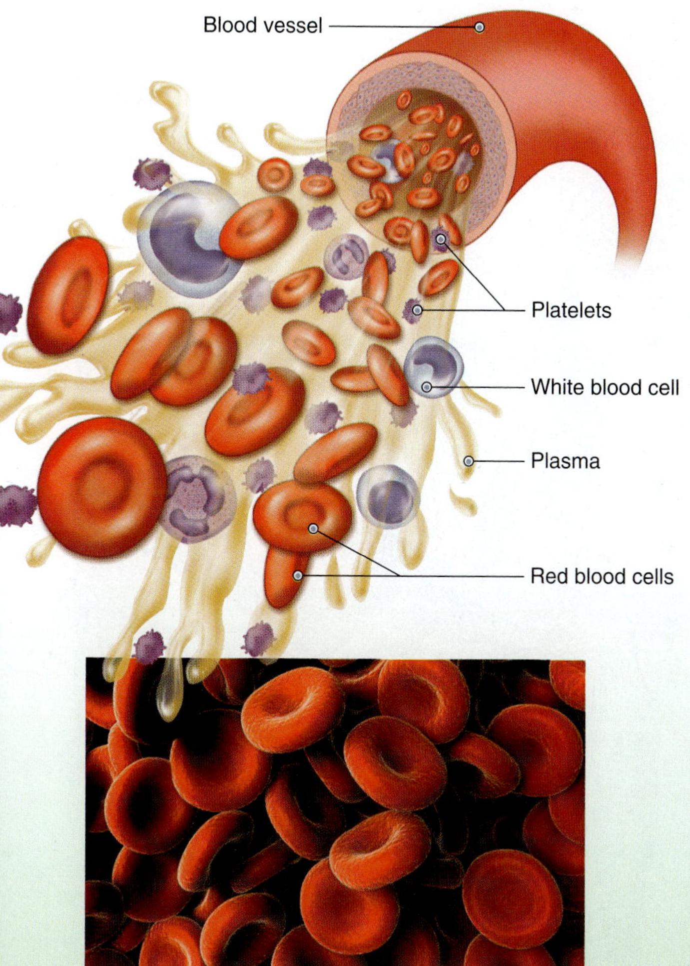

blood

ROOTS: ***hem/o, hemat/o***

EXAMPLES: hemolysis, hematology

NOTES: The average-sized man has almost 6 quarts of blood in his body. The average-sized woman has almost 4 quarts.

cell

ROOT: ***cyt/o***

EXAMPLES: erythrocyte, thrombocytosis

NOTES: *Cyto* comes from a Greek word meaning *jar* or *basket.* The word in Greek can also refer to the individual units of a beehive, which is probably where the connection with human cells comes from.

white

ROOT: ***leuk/o***

EXAMPLES: leukocytes, leukemia

NOTES: Leukocytes, which are white blood cells, act as the bloodstream's police force and garbage collectors. They are the primary responders to infection and tissue damage. They also remove debris from the bloodstream through a process called *phagocytosis* (remember: *phago* means *to eat)* and begin the process of cell repair.

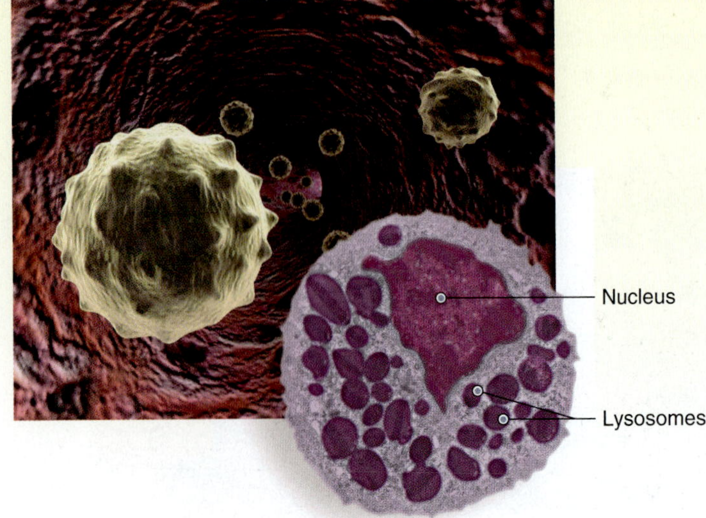

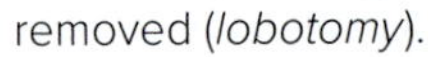

vein

ROOTS: ***phleb/o, ven/o***

EXAMPLES: phlebotomy, venospasm

NOTES: The term *phlebotomy* comes from *phlebo* (vein) and *tomy* (incision). It is the term used for drawing blood. But make sure you pronounce the word carefully: You don't want to get some blood drawn (*phlebotomy*) and end up having a portion of your brain removed (*lobotomy*).

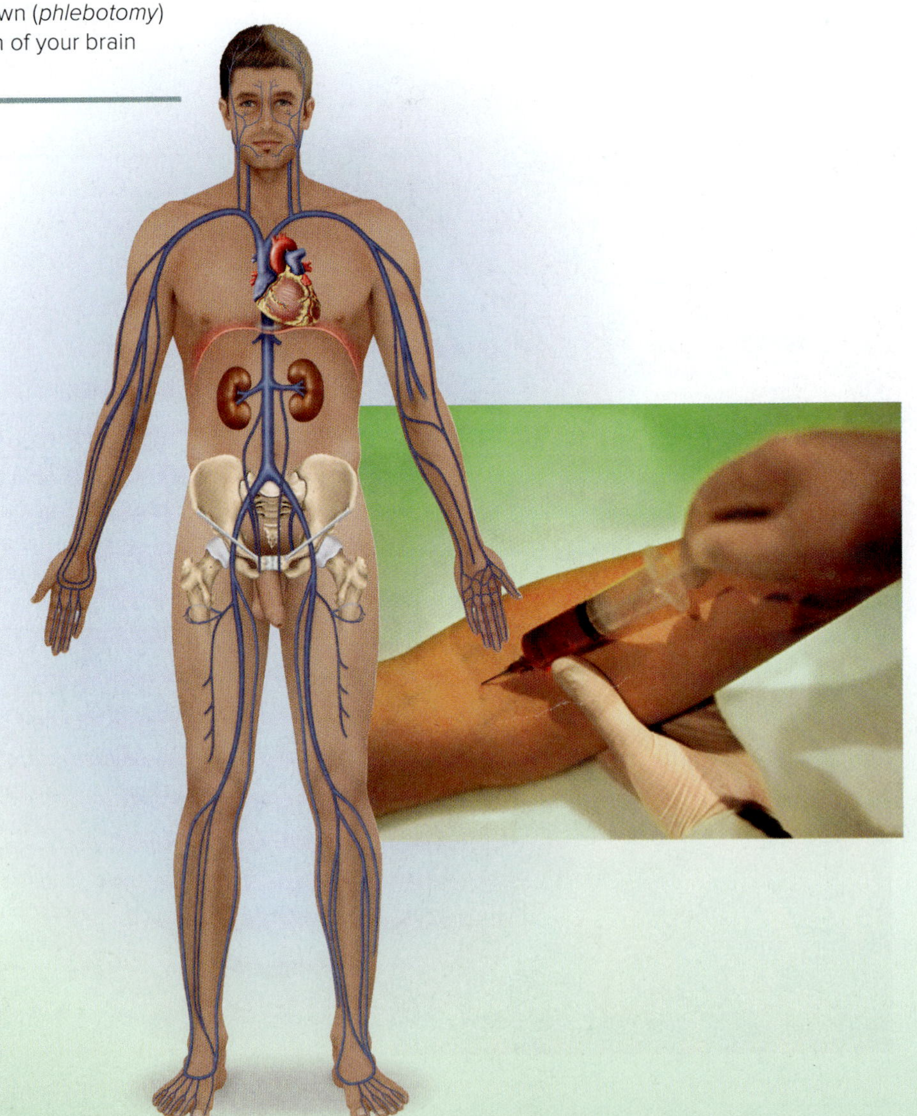

Word Roots of the Immunological System

LYMPHATIC SYSTEM

Runoff water from mountains collects into small tributaries that collect into larger streams, then into rivers, and eventually into the ocean.

The lymphatic system works in a similar way. Excess fluid from body tissues collects into lymph vessels that pour into larger vessels. This fluid then eventually pours back into the "ocean" of the body's blood supply. Along with lymphatic vessels, the lymph system includes lymph nodes, tonsils, a spleen, and a thymus.

Together, the lymphatic system plays a large role in the body's immune system. Lymph vessels carry immune proteins to all parts of the body. Lymph nodes and the spleen act as filters in the body, filtering out dangerous things like infectious agents and cancerous cells.

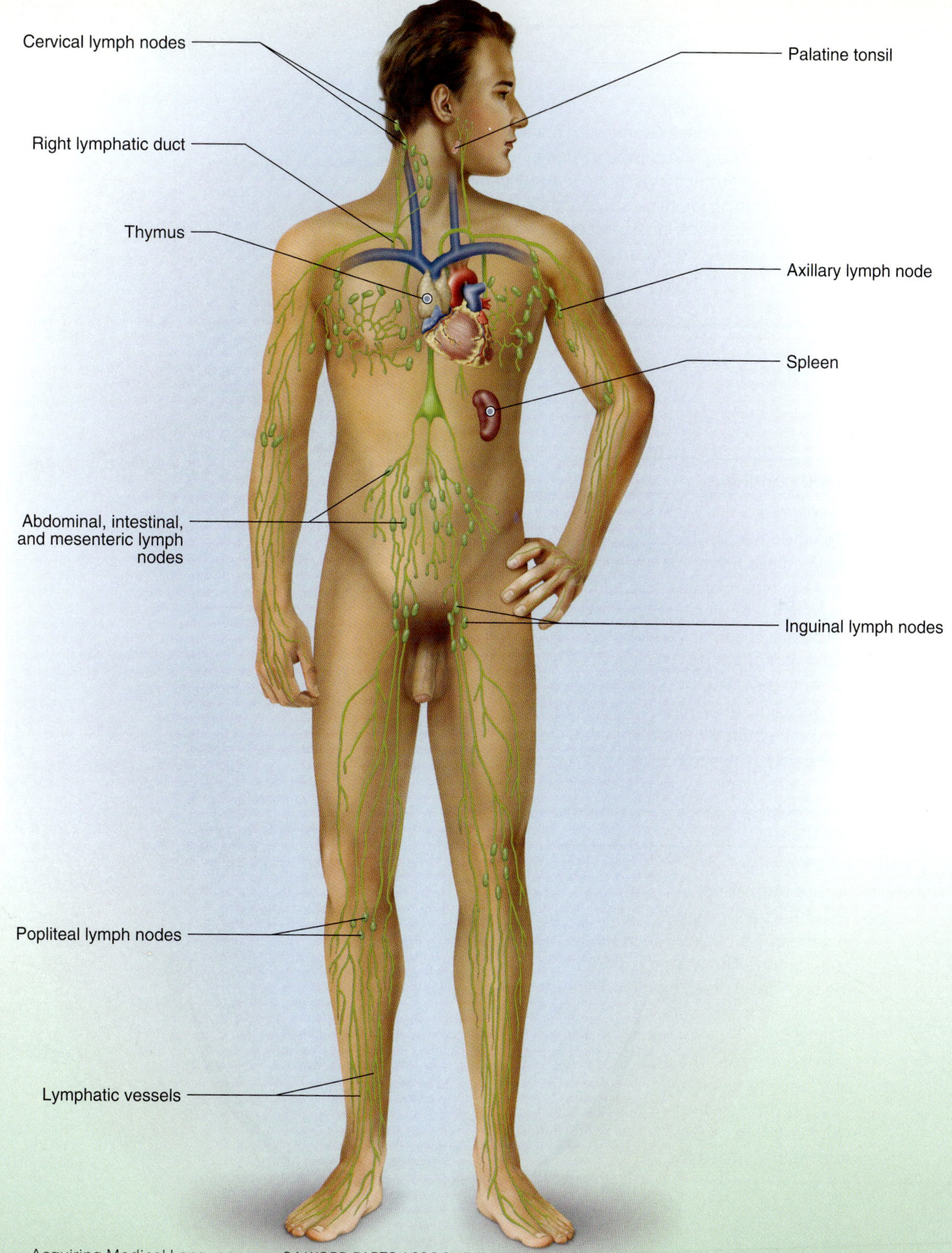

lymph

ROOT: ***lymph/o***

EXAMPLES: lymphadenitis, lymphoma

NOTES: *Lymph* comes from a Latin word meaning *water* or *spring* and refers to a clear liquid that circulates in the body, providing nutrients to cells and removing waste from them.

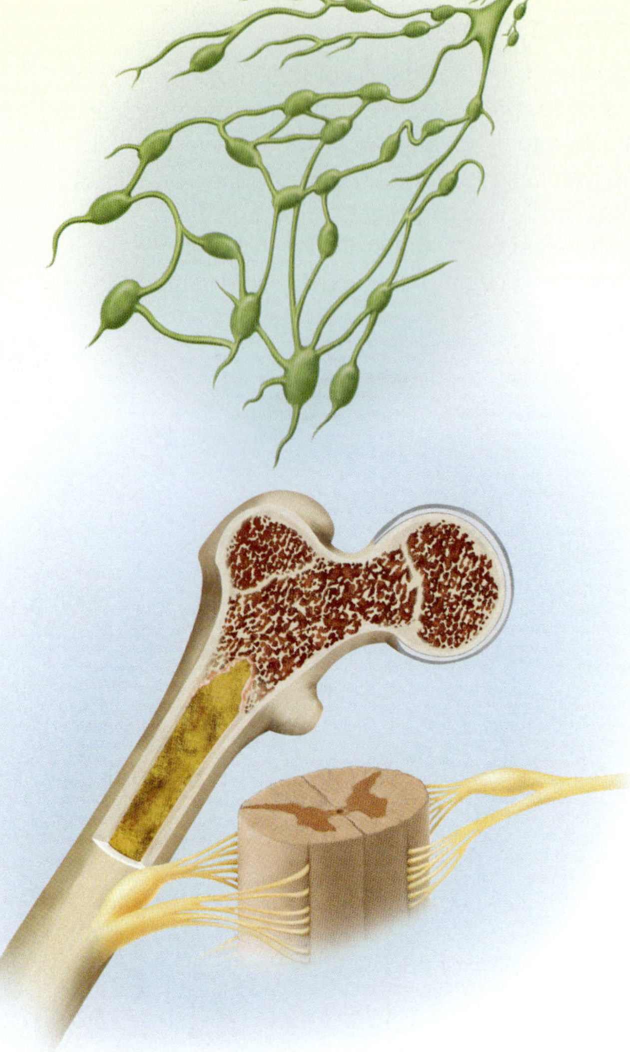

bone marrow, spine

ROOT: ***myel/o***

EXAMPLES: myelitis, myelodysplasia

NOTES: This root comes from a Greek word meaning *the innermost part* and is used in medicine to refer to two different things: bone marrow and the spinal cord. If you think about, it makes sense: Both are in the innermost part of something else. Bone marrow is in the center of bones. The spinal cord is in the center of the spine.

blood condition

SUFFIX: ***-emia***

EXAMPLES: anemia, leukemia

NOTES: *-Emia* comes from a combination of *hemo,* meaning *blood,* and *-ia,* meaning *condition.* The *h* at the beginning of *hemo* got dropped because it is hard to pronounce when added to the end of a word. Think about it. Which is easier to say: *anemia* or *anhemia?*

On occasion, the *h* makes a comeback, in words like *polycythemia.* So watch out.

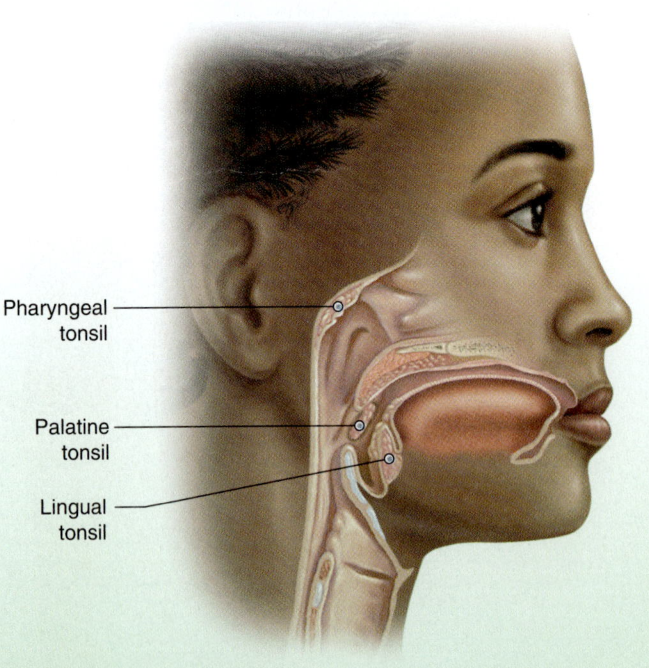

tonsils

ROOT: ***tonsill/o***

EXAMPLES: tonsillitis, tonsillectomy

NOTES: The *tonsils* are masses of lymphoid tissue located in the back of the mouth at the top of the throat. The word *tonsil* comes from the Latin word meaning *almond,* no doubt because of its appearance. The fact that the root has two, and not one, letter *l* is not a spelling mistake. The English word tonsil has one l, but its root form has two. That's why the words *tonsillitis* and *tonsillectomy* have two.

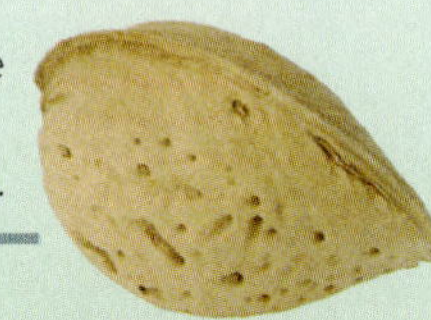

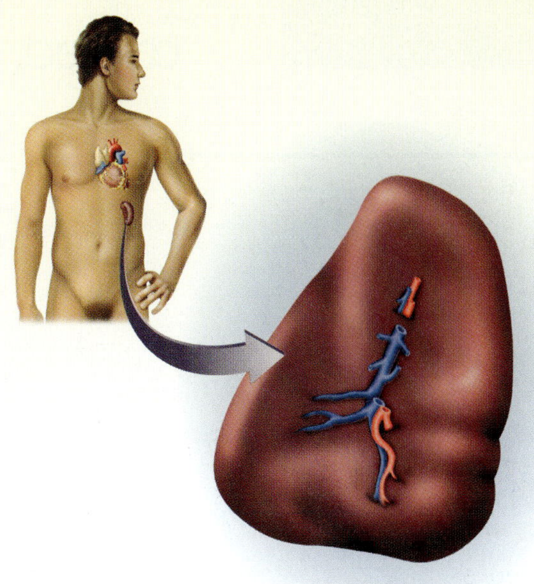

spleen

ROOT: ***splen/o***

EXAMPLES: splenomegaly, splenectomy

NOTES: The spleen is an organ in the upper left portion of your abdomen. One of its jobs is to filter old red blood cells out of your blood. A human can live without a spleen with no adverse effects, which is good news for motocross and BMX bikers, who have a high rate of spleen injury and removal. Why? Because when they have accidents, their abdomens often crash into the handlebars of their bikes.

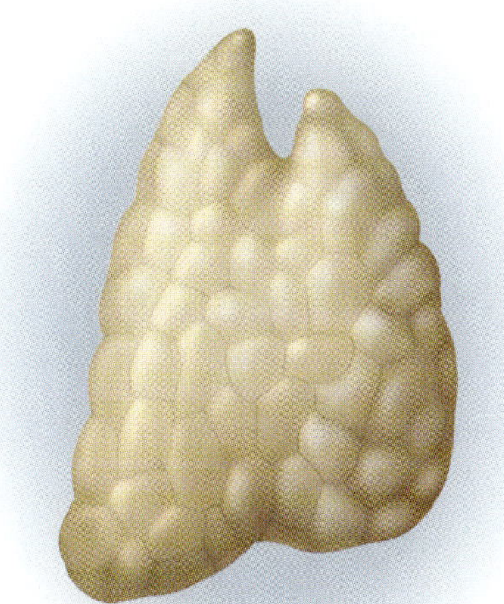

thymus

ROOT: ***thym/o***

EXAMPLES: thymoma, thymectomy

NOTES: The *thymus* is an organ found at the base of the neck. Its name is derived from the herb *thyme*. Evidently, the organ looked like a bunch of thyme to the folks who first discovered it.

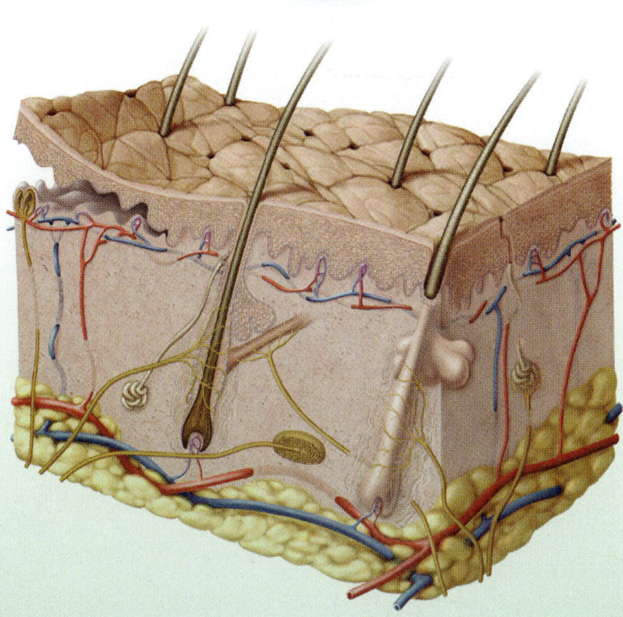

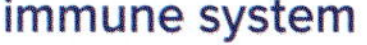

immune system

ROOT: ***immun/o***

EXAMPLES: immunology, immunoglobulin

NOTES: The immune system is the body's defensive system against foreign invaders. Most people don't realize that the skin is a layer of the immune system. It functions as a physical barrier between your vital organs and a world of organisms intent on causing harm to them.

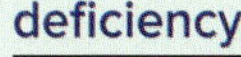

deficiency

SUFFIX: ***-penia***

EXAMPLE: cytopenia

NOTES: -*Penia* comes from a Greek word meaning *poverty* or *famine*. It is related to the English word *penury*, which means *poverty*. But that's a word that doesn't get used much these days.

Learning Outcome 8.1 Exercises

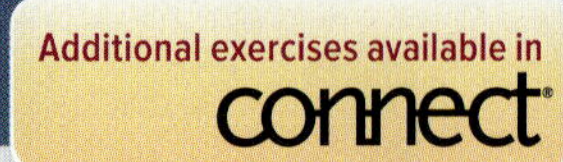
Additional exercises available in
connect

TRANSLATION

EXERCISE 1 *Match the root on the left with its definition on the right. Some definitions will be used more than once.*

f	1. leuk/o	a.	blood
b	2. cyt/o	b.	cell
e	3. ven/o	c.	clot
a	4. hem/o	d.	coagulation
a	5. hemat/o	e.	vein
d	6. coagul/o	f.	white
c	7. thromb/o		
e	8. phleb/o		

EXERCISE 2 *Translate the following roots.*

1. leuk/o ______
2. cyt/o ______
3. ven/o ______
4. hem/o ______
5. hemat/o ______
6. coagul/o ______
7. thromb/o ______
8. phleb/o ______

EXERCISE 3 *Underline and define the word parts from this chapter for the following terms.*

1. leukemia ______
2. hematopoiesis ______
3. hemoglobinopathy ______
4. thromboembolism ______
5. hypercoagulability ______
6. phlebarteriectasia ______
7. phagocytosis ______
8. thrombophlebitis (2 roots) ______

EXERCISE 4 *Break down the following words into their component parts and translate.*

EXAMPLE: sinusitis *sinus | itis* *inflammation of the sinuses*

1. anticoagulant ______
2. leukocyte ______
3. thrombocyte ______
4. phlebotomy ______
5. hematoma ______
6. hemolysis ______

Learning Outcome 8.1 Exercises

EXERCISE 5 *Match the word part on the left with its definition on the right.*

__h__	1. tonsill/o	a. blood condition
____	2. immun/o	b. bone marrow
____	3. lymph/o	c. deficiency
____	4. splen/o	d. immune system
____	5. thym/o	e. lymph
____	6. -emia	f. spleen
____	7. myel/o	g. thymus
____	8. -penia	h. tonsil

EXERCISE 6 *Translate the following word parts.*

1. tonsill/o ____________________
2. immun/o ____________________
3. lymph/o ____________________
4. splen/o ____________________
5. thym/o ____________________
6. myel/o ____________________
7. -emia ____________________
8. -penia ____________________

EXERCISE 7 *Underline and define the word parts from this chapter for the following terms.*

1. tonsillectomy ____________________
2. thymic hyperplasia ____________________
3. autoimmune disease ____________________
4. hypervolemia ____________________
5. myelodysplasia ____________________
6. lymphangiectasia ____________________
7. laparosplenectomy ____________________
8. pancytopenia (2 roots) ____________________

EXERCISE 8 *Break down the following words into their component parts and translate.*

> EXAMPLE: sinusitis *sinus | itis* *inflammation of the sinuses*

1. tonsillectomy ____________________
2. thymectomy ____________________
3. immunologist ____________________
4. lymphedema ____________________
5. splenalgia ____________________
6. myeloma ____________________
7. lymphocyte ____________________
8. leukopenia ____________________
9. hypercholesterolemia ____________________

Learning Outcome 8.1 Exercises

GENERATION

EXERCISE 9 *Identify the word parts for the following terms.*

1. white ______
2. cell ______
3. coagulation ______
4. clot ______
5. blood (2 roots) ______
6. vein (2 roots) ______

EXERCISE 10 *Build a medical term from the information provided.*

1. normal-sized cell (use the prefix *normo-*) ______
2. the study of the blood ______
3. the study of veins ______
4. coagulation disease ______
5. white cell ______
6. clot cell ______

EXERCISE 11 *Multiple-choice questions. Select the correct answer.*

1. What are the names of the body's three different types of blood cells?
   a. leukocytes, red blood cells, white blood cells
   b. leukocytes, thrombocytes, white blood cells
   c. leukocytes, platelets, thrombocytes
   d. platelets, red blood cells, white blood cells
   e. platelets, red blood cells, thrombocytes
2. The function of a red blood cell is to
   a. bring oxygen to cells and remove waste
   b. fight infection
   c. patch up broken blood vessels
   d. all of these
   e. none of these
3. The function of a white blood cell is to
   a. bring oxygen to cells and remove waste
   b. fight infection
   c. patch up broken blood vessels
   d. all of these
   e. none of these
4. The function of a platelet is to
   a. bring oxygen to cells and remove waste
   b. fight infection
   c. patch up broken blood vessels
   d. all of these
   e. none of these
5. A scab is formed by which type of blood cell?
   a. erythrocyte
   b. leukocyte
   c. platelet
   d. red blood cell
   e. white blood cell

Learning Outcome 8.1 Exercises

6. Neutrophils, lymphocytes, basophils, and eosinophils are all types of
   a. erythrocytes
   b. platelets
   c. red blood cells
   d. thrombocytes
   e. white blood cells
7. The type of blood cell that contains *hemoglobin* is a
   a. leukocyte
   b. platelet
   c. red blood cell
   d. thrombocyte
   e. white blood cell
8. Another name for *red blood cell* is
   a. erythrocyte
   b. leukocyte
   c. platelet
   d. thrombocyte
   e. white blood cell
9. Another name for *white blood cell* is
   a. erythrocyte
   b. leukocyte
   c. platelet
   d. red blood cell
   e. thrombocyte
10. Another name for *platelet* is
    a. erythrocyte
    b. leukocyte
    c. red blood cell
    d. thrombocyte
    e. white blood cell
11. Which of the following substances assists a cell in grabbing oxygen where levels are low and then releasing them when the levels are high?
    a. hemoglobin
    b. immunoglobulin
    c. leukocyte
    d. thrombocyte
    e. none of these
12. Which of the following substances is a protein that assists white blood cells in fighting infection?
    a. hemoglobin
    b. immunoglobulin
    c. leukocyte
    d. thrombocyte
    e. none of these

Learning Outcome 8.1 Exercises

EXERCISE 12 *Identify the word parts for the following terms.*

1. immune system ____________________
2. tonsil ____________________
3. lymph ____________________
4. thymus ____________________
5. spleen ____________________
6. bone marrow ____________________
7. blood condition ____________________
8. deficiency ____________________

EXERCISE 13 *Build a medical term from the information provided.*

1. study of the immune system ____________________
2. inflammation of the tonsil ____________________
3. inflammation of the spleen ____________________
4. disease of the thymus ____________________
5. bone marrow tumor ____________________
6. lymph cell ____________________
7. lymph deficiency ____________________
8. white blood condition ____________________

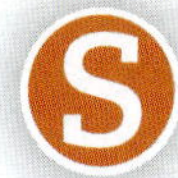

Subjective
Patient History, Problems, Complaints
Blood
Lymph

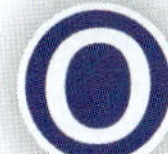

Objective
Observation and Discovery
Blood
Lymph
Professional terms

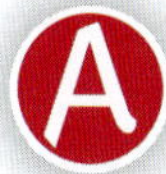

Assessment
Diagnosis and Pathology
Blood
Blood Conditions
Lymph

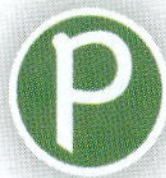

Plan
Treatments and Therapies
Drugs
Surgery
Transfusions

This section contains medical terms built from the roots presented in the previous section. The purpose of this section is to expose you to words used in hematology and immunology that are built from the word roots presented earlier. The focus of this book is to teach you the process of learning roots and translating them in context. Each term is presented with the correct pronunciation, followed by a word analysis that breaks down the word into its component parts, a definition that provides a literal translation of the word, as well as supplemental information if the literal translation deviates from its medical use.

The terms are organized using a health care professional's SOAP note (first introduced in Chapter 2) as a model.

SUBJECTIVE

8.2 Patient History, Problems, Complaints

Patients with blood disorders normally present with the same general symptoms. They usually seek medical care because they suffer from secondary effects of having a low amount of a specific blood cell type.

A patient with anemia may feel weak and run down, and may look paler than normal. If patients' *platelet* levels are too low, they may notice they bruise easily (*ecchymosis*) or that they develop small, flat, red spots on their body (*petechiae*). They may also complain that they tend to bleed (*hemorrhage*) more easily than most people. This can also result from *hemophilia*.

A patient who has a low white blood cell count is more vulnerable to infection; thus, he or she will suffer from more infections than normal. A patient may even present with the chief concern of possible immune deficiency.

Disorders of the lymphatic system also have few symptoms. Most commonly, a patient will present with swollen lymph nodes (*lymphadenopathy*). This can be a sign of many different types of illnesses, which range from mild to serious. Another concern may be swelling in their extremities (*lymphedema*), which can also have serious or harmless causes.

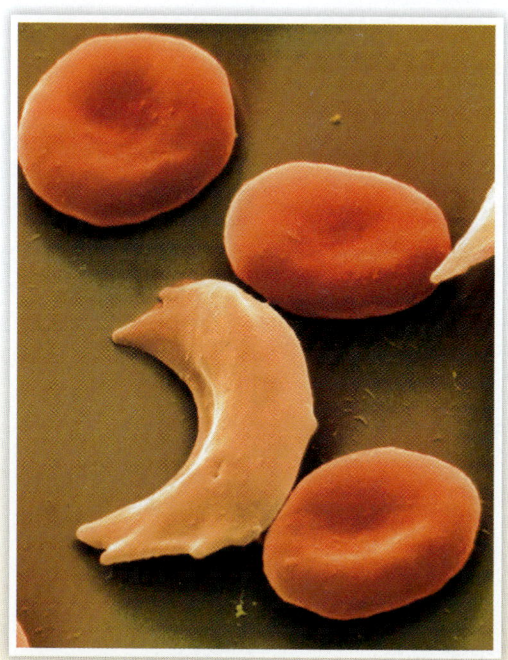

A common type of anemia is sickle-cell anemia, called that because affected red blood cells develop a hard, rigid "sickle" shape that can cause frequent clots in the sufferer.

8.2 Patient History, Problems, Complaints

blood

Term	Word Analysis
anemia ah-NEE-mee-ah **Definition** reduction of red blood cells noticed by the patient by weakness and fatigue.	an / emia no / blood condition
ecchymosis eh-kih-MOH-sis **Definition** large bruise	from Greek, for *to pour out*
hematoma HEE-mah-TOH-mah **Definition** mass of blood within an organ, cavity, or tissue	hemat / oma blood / tumor
hemophilia HEE-moh-FEE-lee-ah **Definition** condition in which the blood doesn't clot, thus causing excessive bleeding	hemo / phil / ia blood / love / condition
hemorrhage HIM-or-rij **Definition** excessive blood loss	hemo / rrhage blood / burst forth
petechia puh-TEE-kee-yah **Definition** small bruise	from Latin, for *freckle* or *spot*
reperfusion injury REE-pir-FYOO-zhun IN-jir-ee **Definition** injury to tissue that occurs after blood flow is restored	re / per / fusion injury again / through / pour

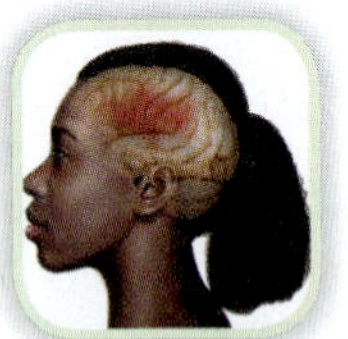

hematoma

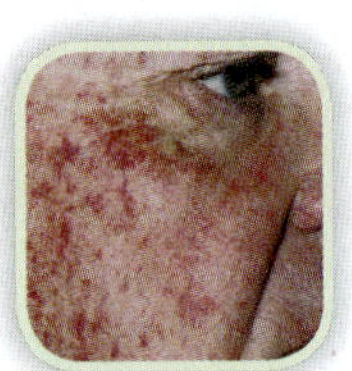

petechia

lymph

Term	Word Analysis
lymphadenopathy lim-FAD-eh-NAW-pah-thee **Definition** any disease of a lymph gland (node); used to refer to noticeably swollen lymph nodes, especially in the neck	lymph / adeno / pathy lymph / gland / disease
lymphedema LIMF-ah-DEE-mah **Definition** swelling caused by abnormal accumulation of lymph, usually in the extremities	lymph / edema lymph / swelling
splenalgia splee-NAL-jah **Definition** pain in the spleen	splen / algia spleen / pain
splenodynia SPLEE-noh-DAI-nee-ah **Definition** pain in the spleen	spleno / dynia spleen / pain

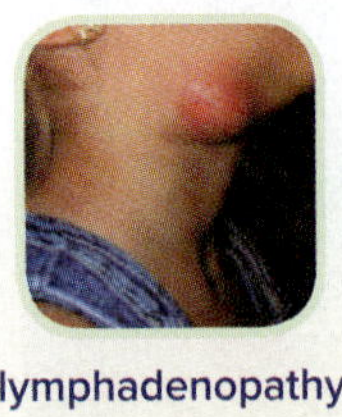

lymphadenopathy

Learning Outcome 8.2 Exercises

PRONUNCIATION

EXERCISE 1 *Break down the following words into syllables.*

EXAMPLE: synesthesia *syn | es | the | sia*

1. anemia ______
2. hemophilia ______
3. hemorrhage ______
4. hematoma ______
5. splenodynia ______
6. splenalgia ______
7. lymphedema ______
8. reperfusion injury ______

TRANSLATION

EXERCISE 2 *Break down the following words into their component parts.*

EXAMPLE: nasopharyngoscope *naso | pharyngo | scope*

1. hematoma ______
2. hemorrhage ______
3. splenodynia ______
4. splenalgia ______
5. lymphedema ______
6. hemophilia ______
7. anemia ______
8. lymphadenopathy ______

EXERCISE 3 *Underline and define the word parts from this chapter in the following terms.*

1. hemophilia ______
2. hemorrhage ______
3. hematoma ______
4. splenodynia ______
5. splenalgia ______
6. lymphedema ______
7. anemia ______

Learning Outcome 8.2 Exercises

EXERCISE 4 *Match the term on the left with its definition on the right. Some definitions may be used more than once.*

___	1. anemia	a.	a condition in which the blood doesn't clot, thus causing excessive bleeding
___	2. hemophilia	b.	a mass of blood within an organ, cavity, or tissue
___	3. hemorrhage	c.	excessive blood loss
___	4. hematoma	d.	injury to tissue that occurs after blood flow is restored
___	5. splenalgia	e.	large bruise
___	6. splenodynia	f.	pain in the spleen
___	7. lymphedema	g.	reduction of red blood cells noticed by the patient as weakness and fatigue
___	8. reperfusion injury	h.	small bruise
___	9. ecchymosis	i.	swelling caused by abnormal accumulation of lymph
___	10. petechia		

EXERCISE 5 *Translate the following terms as literally as possible.*

EXAMPLE: nasopharyngoscope *an instrument for looking at the nose and throat*

1. splenodynia ___
2. splenalgia ___
3. hematoma ___
4. hemorrhage ___
5. anemia ___
6. lymphedema ___

GENERATION

EXERCISE 6 *Build a medical term from the information provided.*

EXAMPLE: inflammation of the sinuses *sinusitis*

1. spleen pain (use *-dynia*) ___
2. spleen pain (use *-algia*) ___
3. blood tumor ___
4. lymph swelling ___
5. no blood condition ___
6. any disease of a lymph gland (node) ___

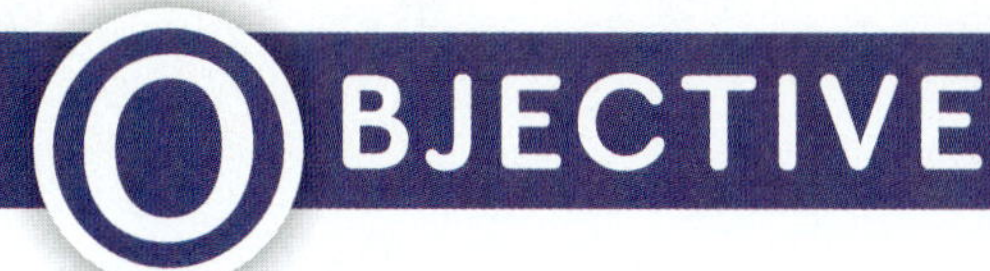

8.3 Observation and Discovery

There are two ways of looking at blood cells. The first is to count them. A *complete blood count (CBC)* is one of the most common tests in medicine. A machine counts the number of each type of cells in the blood.

A lower-than-normal number of red blood cells is known as *anemia.* It is the most common blood problem and has a variety of causes. A higher-than-normal number of red blood cells (*erythrocytosis* or *polycythemia*) is much less common. When it is severe, it can be dangerous because the blood becomes too thick to flow well.

A low number of white blood cells (*leukopenia*) can be caused by an infection. If the number is too low, however, it may mean the patient has a weakened immune system (*immunodeficiency*). In general, people are more at risk if they are low in a specific type of white blood cell, neutrophils (*neutropenia*). Having a high number of white blood cells in the blood (*leukocytosis*) is a common marker for infection. Less commonly, it can indicate cancer.

Low platelet numbers (*thrombocytopenia*) can lead to easy bleeding and bruising. Having too many platelets in the blood (*thrombocytosis*) indicates inflammation. If platelet levels are too high, the patient runs the risk of experiencing abnormal blood clotting and forming a floating clot (*thromboembolism*).

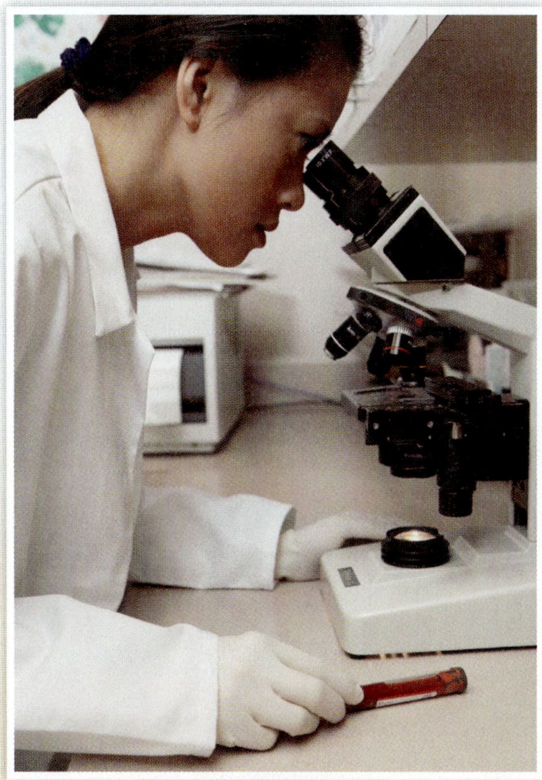

In hematology, a great deal of information is gathered through microscopic analysis of blood samples.

Another way of evaluating blood cells is by looking at their size and shape. The size of red blood cells helps distinguish among different causes for anemia. In fact, it is generally the first step in diagnosing the cause.

Causes for anemia with small red blood cells (*microcytosis*) include iron deficiency and lead poisoning. Anemias with enlarged blood cells (*macrocytosis*) can be a result of folate deficiency or B_{12} deficiency. Normal-sized blood cell (*normocytic*) anemias include bleeding and anemia from chronic disease. Some problems with the makeup of a red blood cell can cause it to assume abnormal shapes. *Spherocytes* and *elliptocytes* are two types of blood cells with abnormal shapes.

The physical exam of the lymphatic system focuses mainly on the few organs of the system, including the lymph nodes and the spleen. The lymph nodes may be swollen and painful (*lymphadenopathy*). The spleen may also be enlarged (*splenomegaly*). When lymph vessels become swollen, they can cause swelling in arms and legs (*lymphedema*).

There are no lab tests specific to the lymphatic system, but there is a special type of image that examines the lymph vessels (*lymphangiogram*). Most other lymphatic system issues, such as the absence of a spleen (*asplenia*), can be seen on a CT scan.

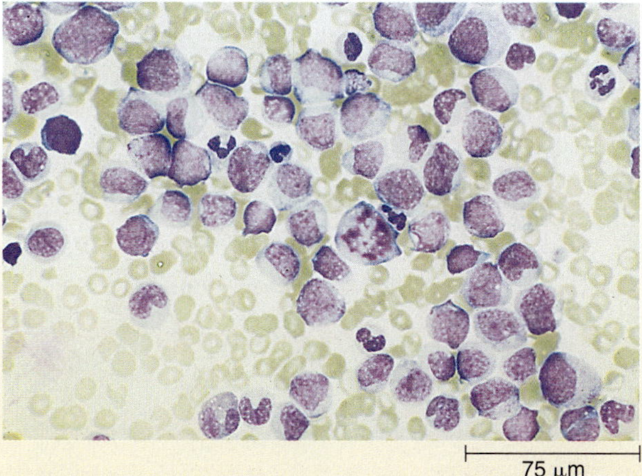

Blood from a patient with acute monocytic leukemia. Note the abnormally high number of white blood cells, especially monocytes.

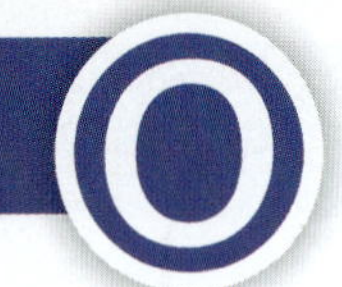

8.3 Observation and Discovery

blood

Term	Word Analysis
anisocytosis AN-ai-soh-SAI-toh-sis	an / iso / cyt / osis not / equal / cell / condition
Definition condition characterized by a great inequality in the size of red blood cells	
elliptocyte ee-LIP-toh-SAIT	ellipto / cyte oval-shaped / cell
Definition oval red blood cells	
elliptocytosis ee-LIP-toh-SAI-toh-sis	ellipto / cyt / osis oval-shaped / cell / condition
Definition condition characterized by an increase in the number of oval-shaped red blood cells	
embolism EM-boh-LIZ-um	embol / ism embolus / condition
Definition blockage in a blood vessel caused by an embolus	
embolus EM-boh-lus	em / bolus in / throw
Definition mass of matter present in the blood Note: In Greek, this word means stopper, as in a cap for a bottle.	
erythrocyte eh-RIH-throh-SAIT	erythro / cyte red / cell
Definition red blood cell	
erythrocytosis eh-RIH-throh-sai-TOH-sis	erythro / cyt / osis red / cell / condition
Definition abnormal increase in the number of red blood cells	
hematopoiesis heh-MAH-toh-poh-EE-sis	hemato / poiesis blood / formation
Definition formation of blood cells	
hemolysis hee-MAW-lih-sis	hemo / lysis blood / breakdown
Definition breakdown of blood cells	
leukocyte LOO-koh-sait	leuko / cyte white / cell
Definition white blood cell	
leukocytosis LOO-koh-sai-TOH-sis	leuko / cyt / osis white / cell / condition
Definition increase in the number of white blood cells	
leukopenia LOO-koh-PEE-nee-ah	leuko / penia white / deficiency
Definition deficiency in white blood cells	

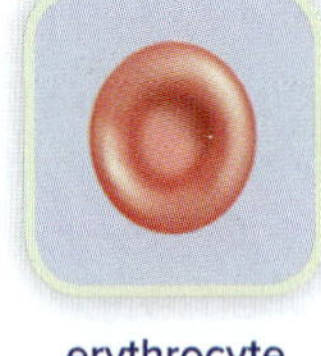

erythrocyte

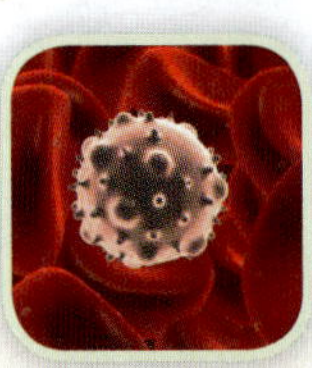

leukocyte

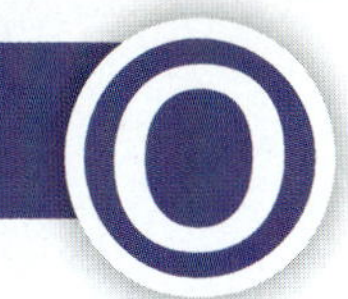

8.3 Observation and Discovery

myelopoiesis

blood *continued*

Term	Word Analysis
macrocytosis MAH-kroh-sai-TOH-sis **Definition** condition characterized by large red blood cells	macro / cyt / osis large / cell / condition
microcytosis MAI-kroh-sai-TOH-sis **Definition** condition characterized by small red blood cells	micro / cyt / osis small / cell / condition
myelopoiesis MAI-eh-loh-poh-EE-sis **Definition** formation of bone marrow	myelo / poiesis bone marrow / formation
neutropenia NOO-troh-PEE-nee-ah **Definition** deficiency in neutrophil NOTE: A neutrophil is a type of white blood cell.	neutro / penia neutrophil / deficiency
normocyte NOR-moh-sait **Definition** normal-sized red blood cell	normo / cyte normal / cell
oligocythemia AW-lih-goh-sih-THEE-mee-ah **Definition** deficiency in the number of red blood cells	oligo / cyt / hemia few / cell / blood condition
pancytopenia PAN-SAI-toh-PEE-nee-ah **Definition** deficiency in all cellular components of the blood	pan / cyto / penia all / cell / deficiency
phagocytosis FAG-oh-sai-TOH-sis **Definition** process in which phagocytes (a type of white blood cell) destroy (or eat) foreign microorganisms or cell debris	phago / cyt / osis eat / cell / condition
poikilocytosis POI-kih-loh-sai-TOH-sis **Definition** condition characterized by red blood cells in a variety of shapes	poikilo / cyt / osis various / cell / condition
polycythemia PAW-lee-sih-THEE-mee-ah **Definition** excess of red blood cells	poly / cyt / hemia many / cell / blood condition
reticulocyte reh-TIK-yoo-loh-SAIT **Definition** immature red blood cell; the root comes from its netlike appearance	reticulo / cyte net / cell
spherocyte SFEE-roh-SAIT **Definition** red blood cell that assumes a spherical shape	sphero / cyte sphere / cell

blood *continued*

Term	Word Analysis
thrombocyte THROM-boh-sait **Definition** cell that helps blood clot; also known as a platelet	**thrombo / cyte** clot / cell
thrombocytopenia THROM-boh-SAI-toh-PEE-nee-ah **Definition** deficiency in the number of platelets (clot cells)	**thrombo / cyto / penia** clot / cell / deficiency
thrombocytosis THROM-boh-sai-TOH-sis **Definition** increase in the number of platelets (clot cells)	**thrombo / cyt / osis** clot / cell / condition
thromboembolism THROM-boh-EM-boh-LIZ-um **Definition** blockage of a vessel (embolism) caused by a clot that has broken off from where it formed	**thrombo / embol / ism** clot / embolus / condition
thrombogenic THROM-boh-JIN-ik **Definition** capable of producing a blood clot	**thrombo / gen / ic** clot / formation / pertaining to
thrombosis throm-BOH-sis **Definition** the formation of a blood clot	**thromb / osis** clot / condition
thrombus THROM-bus **Definition** blood clot NOTE: The difference between a thrombus and an embolus is twofold. A thrombus is a clot of blood and is stationary. An embolus is foreign material and is in motion. When a thrombus breaks off, it becomes a *thromboembolus.*	from Greek, for *lump, clot,* or even *curd of milk*

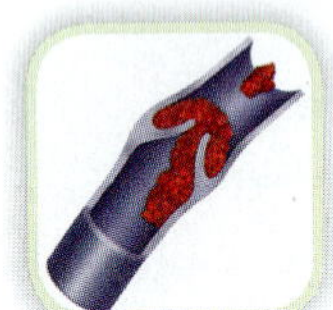
thromboembolism

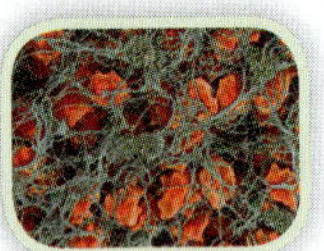
thrombosis

lymph

Term	Word Analysis
asplenia ah-SPLEE-nee-ah **Definition** absence of a spleen or of spleen function	**a / splen / ia** no / spleen / condition
hepatosplenomegaly heh-PAT-oh-SPLEE-noh-MEH-gah-lee **Definition** enlargement of the liver and spleen	**hepato / spleno / megaly** liver / spleen / enlargement
lymphocyte LIM-foh-SAIT **Definition** lymph cell	**lympho / cyte** lymph / cell

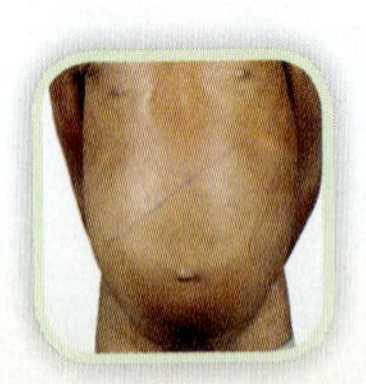
hepatosplenomegaly

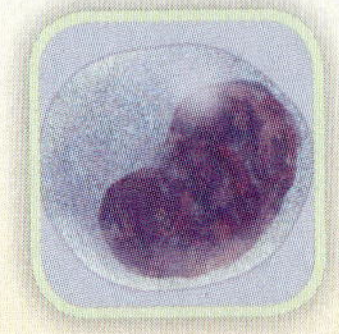
lymphocyte

lymph *continued*

Term	Word Analysis
lymphopenia LIM-foh-PEE-nee-ah **Definition** abnormal deficiency in lymph	lympho / penia lymph / deficiency
splenectopy splee-NEK-toh-pee **Definition** displacement of the spleen; sometimes called floating spleen	splen / ec / top / y spleen / out / place / condition
splenolysis splee-NAW-lih-sis **Definition** breakdown (destruction) of spleen tissue	spleno / lysis spleen / breakdown
splenomalacia SPLEE-noh-mah-LAY-shah **Definition** softening of the spleen	spleno / malacia spleen / softening
splenomegaly SPLEE-noh-MEH-gah-lee **Definition** enlargement of the spleen	spleno / megaly spleen / enlargement
splenoptosis SPLEE-nawp-TOH-sis **Definition** downward displacement (drooping) of the spleen	spleno / pt / osis spleen / drooping / condition
thymic hyperplasia THAI-mik HAI-per-PLAY-zhah **Definition** overdevelopment of the thymus	thym / ic hyper / plasia thymus / pertaining to over / formation

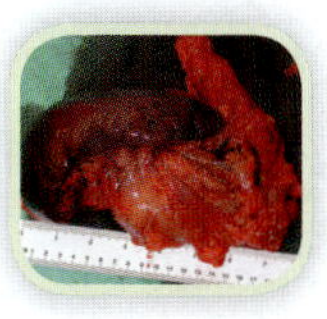

splenomegaly

professional terms

Term	Word Analysis
antibody AN-tih-BAW-dee **Definition** substance produced by the body in response to an antigen **Note:** If you think the word *antibody* seems incomplete and keep asking yourself "an anti-*what* body," you're right. Something *is* missing. This word is a shortened form of *antitoxic body*—that means *against poison*, which makes more sense.	anti / body against / body
antigen AN-th-JIN **Definition** substance that causes the body to produce antibodies	anti / gen against / creator

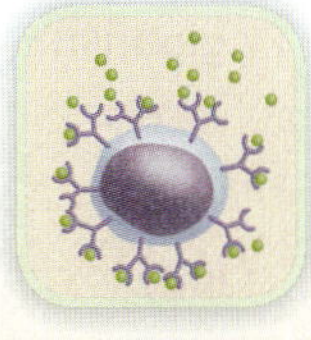

antigen

professional terms *continued*

Term	Word Analysis

hematocrit
hee-MAT-oh-krit

hemato / crit
blood / judge (separate)

Definition test to judge or separate the blood; it is used to determine the ratio of red blood cells to total blood volume

Note: The root *crit* comes from the Greek word that is the basis of the English word *critic.*

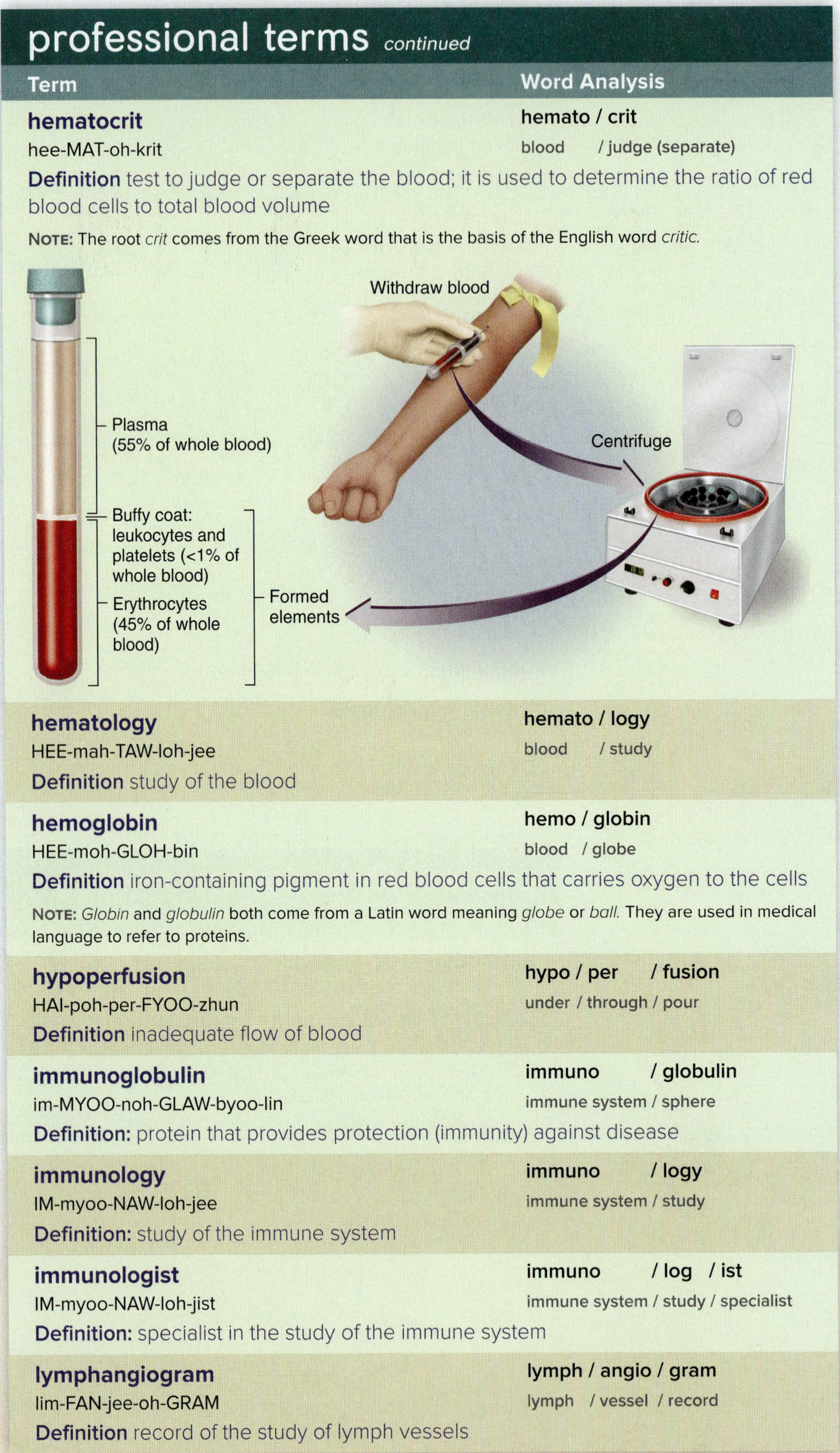

hematology
HEE-mah-TAW-loh-jee

hemato / logy
blood / study

Definition study of the blood

hemoglobin
HEE-moh-GLOH-bin

hemo / globin
blood / globe

Definition iron-containing pigment in red blood cells that carries oxygen to the cells

Note: *Globin* and *globulin* both come from a Latin word meaning *globe* or *ball.* They are used in medical language to refer to proteins.

hypoperfusion
HAI-poh-per-FYOO-zhun

hypo / per / fusion
under / through / pour

Definition inadequate flow of blood

immunoglobulin
im-MYOO-noh-GLAW-byoo-lin

immuno / globulin
immune system / sphere

Definition: protein that provides protection (immunity) against disease

immunology
IM-myoo-NAW-loh-jee

immuno / logy
immune system / study

Definition: study of the immune system

immunologist
IM-myoo-NAW-loh-jist

immuno / log / ist
immune system / study / specialist

Definition: specialist in the study of the immune system

lymphangiogram
lim-FAN-jee-oh-GRAM

lymph / angio / gram
lymph / vessel / record

Definition record of the study of lymph vessels

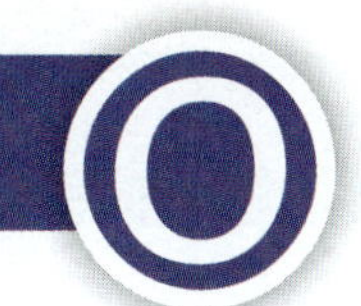

professional terms *continued*

Term	Word Analysis
lymphangiography lim-FAN-jee-AW-grah-fee **Definition** procedure to study the lymph vessels	lymph / angio / graphy lymph / vessel / writing procedure
perfusion per-FYOO-zhun **Definition** circulation of blood through tissue	per / fusion through / pour
phlebology fleh-BAW-loh-jee **Definition** study of veins	phlebo / logy vein / study of
phlebotomist fleh-BAW-toh-mist **Definition** specialist in drawing blood	phlebo / tom / ist vein / cut / specialist
phlebotomy fleh-BAW-toh-mee **Definition** incision into a vein; another name for drawing blood	phlebo / tom / y vein / cut / procedure
sphygmomanometer SFIG-moh-mah-NAW-meh-ter **Definition** fancy name for the device used to measure blood pressure	sphygmo / mano / meter strangle / thin / instrument for measuring

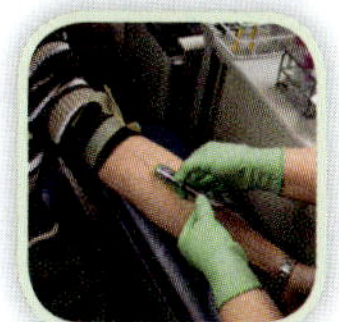

phlebotomy

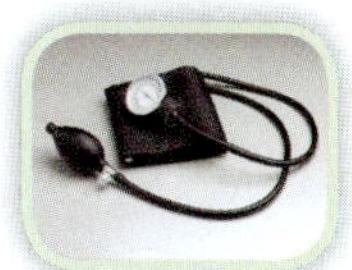

sphygmomanometer

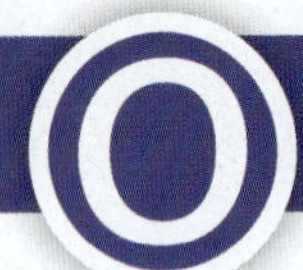

Learning Outcome 8.3 Exercises

PRONUNCIATION

EXERCISE 1 *Break down the following words into syllables.*

EXAMPLE: synesthesia *syn | es | the | sia*

1. splenomegaly __________
2. macrocytosis __________
3. microcytosis __________
4. leukocytosis __________
5. thrombocytosis __________
6. elliptocytosis __________
7. erythrocytosis __________
8. poikilocytosis __________
9. splenoptosis __________
10. neutropenia __________
11. pancytopenia __________
12. thrombocytopenia __________
13. pyelopoiesis __________
14. lymphangiogram __________
15. hepatosplenomegaly __________
16. sphygmomanometer __________

EXERCISE 2 *Indicate which syllable is emphasized when pronounced.*

EXAMPLE: bronchitis bron**chi**tis

1. splenectopy __________
2. perfusion __________
3. embolus __________
4. thrombus __________
5. thrombosis __________
6. leukocyte __________
7. normocyte __________
8. thrombocyte __________
9. phlebotomy __________
10. phlebotomist __________
11. asplenia __________
12. hemolysis __________
13. splenolysis __________

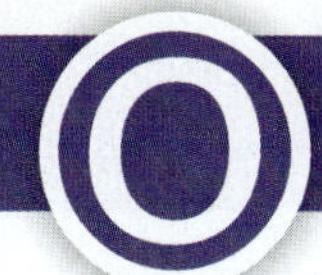

Learning Outcome 8.3 Exercises

TRANSLATION

EXERCISE 3 *Break down the following words into their component parts.*

EXAMPLE: nasopharyngoscope *naso | pharyngo | scope*

1. hemolysis ______
2. hematocrit ______
3. thrombosis ______
4. immunoglobulin ______
5. hepatosplenomegaly ______
6. splenolysis ______
7. splenomalacia ______
8. splenomegaly ______
9. antibody ______
10. antigen ______
11. hemoglobin ______
12. hypoperfusion ______
13. immunologist ______
14. lymphangiography ______
15. perfusion ______
16. phlebotomist ______
17. sphygmomanometer ______

EXERCISE 4 *Underline and define the word parts from this chapter in the following terms.*

1. immunology ______
2. hematology ______
3. phlebology ______
4. thymic hyperplasia ______
5. splenectopy ______
6. phlebotomy ______
7. splenoptosis ______
8. hematopoiesis ______
9. myelopoiesis ______
10. neutropenia ______
11. asplenia ______
12. lymphangiography ______
13. leukopenia (2 roots) ______
14. lymphopenia (2 roots) ______
15. pancytopenia (2 roots) ______
16. oligocythemia (2 roots) ______
17. polycythemia (2 roots) ______
18. thrombocytopenia (3 roots) ______

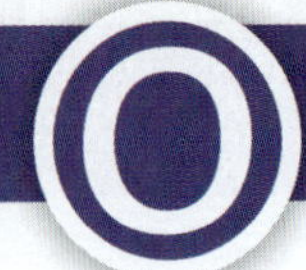

Learning Outcome 8.3 Exercises

EXERCISE 5 *Match the term on the left with its definition on the right.*

______	1. normocyte	a.	cell that helps blood clot (platelet)
______	2. lymphocyte	b.	immature red blood cell (net-like appearance)
______	3. spherocyte	c.	lymph cell
______	4. leukocyte	d.	normal-sized red blood cell
______	5. thrombocyte	e.	oval-shaped red blood cell
______	6. erythrocyte	f.	red blood cell
______	7. elliptocyte	g.	spherical red blood cell
______	8. reticulocyte	h.	white blood cell

EXERCISE 6 *Match the term on the left with its definition on the right.*

______	1. thrombogenic	a.	blockage in a blood vessel caused by an embolus
______	2. thrombus	b.	blockage of a vessel (embolism) caused by a blood clot (thrombus) that has broken off from where it formed
______	3. embolism	c.	a mass of matter present in the blood; from the Greek word for *stopper,* as in the cap on a bottle
______	4. embolus	d.	stationary blood clot
______	5. thromboembolism	e.	capable of producing a blood clot

EXERCISE 7 *Fill in the blanks.*

1. macrocytosis = ______________________ cell condition
2. microcytosis = ______________________ cell condition
3. leukocytosis = ______________________ cell condition
4. thrombocytosis = ______________________ cell condition
5. elliptocytosis = ______________________ cell condition
6. erythrocytosis = ______________________ cell condition
7. phagocytosis = ______________________ cell condition
8. poikilocytosis = ______________________ cell condition
9. anisocytosis = ______________________ cell condition

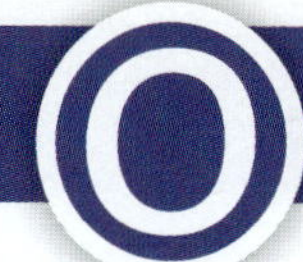

Learning Outcome 8.3 Exercises

EXERCISE 8 *Translate the following terms as literally as possible.*

EXAMPLE: nasopharyngoscope *an instrument for looking at the nose and throat*

1. immunologist ______
2. immunoglobulin ______
3. thrombogenic ______
4. lymphopenia ______
5. neutropenia ______
6. pancytopenia ______
7. splenolysis ______
8. splenoptosis ______
9. hematocrit ______
10. erythrocytosis ______
11. phagocytosis ______
12. anisocytosis ______
13. poikilocytosis ______
14. thymic hyperplasia ______
15. hepatosplenomegaly ______

GENERATION

EXERCISE 9 *Build a medical term from the information provided.*

EXAMPLE: inflammation of the sinuses *sinusitis*

1. study of the immune system ______
2. study of blood ______
3. study of veins ______
4. lymph cell ______
5. white blood cell ______
6. clot cell ______
7. red blood cell ______
8. sphere cell ______
9. normal cell ______
10. softening of the spleen ______
11. enlargement of the spleen ______
12. no spleen condition ______
13. formation of bone marrow ______

Learning Outcome 8.3 Exercises

EXERCISE 10 *Multiple-choice questions. Select the correct answer(s).*

1. A *sphygmomanometer* measures
   a. blood pressure
   b. red blood cells
   c. white blood cells
   d. none of these
2. A *floating spleen* is called a
   a. splenectopy
   b. splenolysis
   c. splenomalacia
   d. splenomegaly
   e. splenoptosis
3. An immature red blood cell that has a netlike appearance is called a(n)
   a. elliptocyte
   b. erythrocyte
   c. reticulocyte
   d. spherocyte
   e. thrombocyte
4. *Hemoglobin* (select all that apply)
   a. carries oxygen to cells
   b. contains antibodies
   c. contains iron
   d. helps the body fight infection
   e. is found in red blood cells
   f. is found in white blood cells
5. The circulation of blood through tissue is called
   a. hyperplasia
   b. hypoperfusion
   c. perfusion
   d. none of these
6. An inadequate flow of blood is called
   a. hyperplasia
   b. hypoperfusion
   c. perfusion
   d. none of these
7. An *embolism* is
   a. a blockage in a blood vessel caused by a foreign material in motion
   b. a cell capable of producing a blood clot
   c. the formation of a blood clot
   d. none of these
8. A blockage of a vessel caused by a clot that has broken off from where it formed is a(n)
   a. embolism
   b. thromboembolism
   c. thrombosis
   d. thrombus
9. The formation of a blood clot is a(n)
   a. embolism
   b. thromboembolism
   c. thrombosis
   d. thrombus

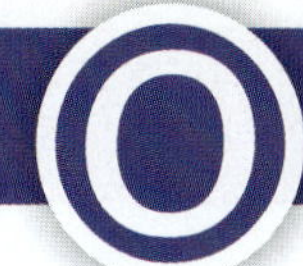

Learning Outcome 8.3 Exercises

EXERCISE 11 *Briefly describe the difference between each pair of terms.*

1. macrocytosis, microcytosis ______________________________
2. elliptocyte, elliptocytosis ______________________________
3. phlebotomist, phlebotomy ______________________________
4. hematopoiesis, hemolysis ______________________________
5. lymphangiogram, lymphangiography ______________________________
6. leukocytosis, leukopenia ______________________________
7. thrombocytopenia, thrombocytosis ______________________________
8. oligocythemia, polycythemia ______________________________
9. antibody, antigen ______________________________
10. embolus, thrombus ______________________________

ASSESSMENT

8.4 Diagnosis and Pathology

Diseases affecting the blood often affect one specific blood cell type. The most common type of red blood cell problem is not having enough of them to do their job (*anemia*), which results from the body not being able to make enough of them. Iron is a necessary mineral for generating blood cells. As a result, a low level of iron can cause a decreased production of red blood cells *(iron deficiency anemia).* The available red blood cells may also be low because they break too easily (*hemolytic anemia*).

Even if there are enough red blood cells, there may be a problem with the blood's *hemoglobin,* the protein that actually carries oxygen. In less common situations, a patient may have too many red blood cells (*polycythemia*). This condition can make the blood thicker, making the flow of blood more difficult.

As with red blood cells, an insufficient number of white blood cells in the body can cause serious problems. A deficiency of white blood cells may cause the patient to be more vulnerable to infections (*immune deficiency*). Sometimes this can be caused by an outside force (*immunosuppression*) like a medication or illness. When the body has a problem with making white blood cells, it may make way too many of them. This is what happens in people who have *leukemia.*

Not having enough platelets in the blood (*thrombocytopenia*) can cause problems with bleeding. It can be mild, causing bruising and bloody noses, or it can be more severe, creating risk for bleeding into major organs like the brain.

On the other hand, if the blood has too many platelets, spontaneous clots (*thrombosis*) may occur. Problems also arise when other parts of the body's clotting team are not working well—whether the blood is not clotting enough (*coagulopathy*) or clotting too easily (*hypercoagulability*).

Finally, blood diseases can be caused by things that are carried in the blood along with blood cells. Infection can spread to the bloodstream (*septicemia*), which can be very dangerous. Fat floats in the blood as well. Too much fat (*hyperlipidemia*) in the blood can eventually lead to heart problems. Another thing that may be seen in the blood is the recycled blood product *bilirubin.* Too much bilirubin in the blood may cause the skin to appear yellow.

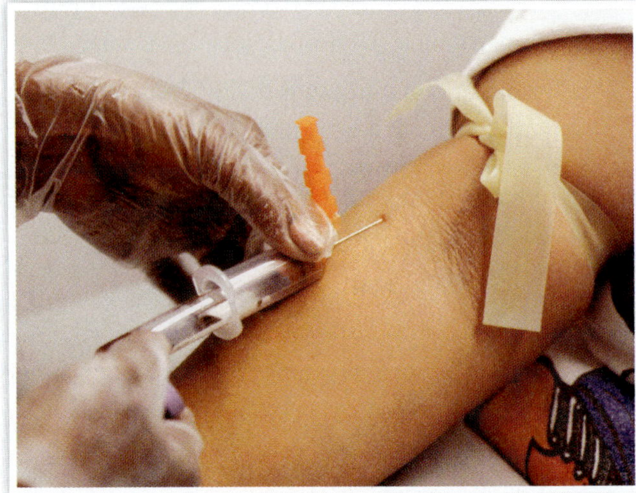

Often, a phlebotomy is the first step in diagnosing blood conditions.

Problems in the lymphatic system are mainly seen in lymph nodes. Lymph nodes can become sore (*lymphadenopathy*) when overworked or infected (*lymphadenitis*). They are also a common site for cancer (*lymphoma*). The main spleen condition patients encounter is an enlarged spleen (*splenomegaly*), which can happen when it is overactive (*hypersplenism*) or, more commonly, as a result of an infection. The most common infection that affects the spleen is *mononucleosis.*

Bone marrow can become infected (*osteomyelitis*) from the bloodstream or from an injury to the bone. These infections are hard to treat and require a long course of antibiotics.

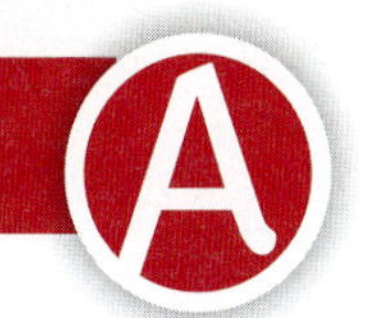

8.4 Diagnosis and Pathology

blood

Term	Word Analysis
autoimmune disease AW-toh-ih-MYOON dih-ZEEZ	auto / immune self / immune
Definition disease caused by the body's immune system attacking the body's own healthy tissue	
coagulopathy coh-AG-yoo-LAW-pah-thee	coagulo / pathy coagulation / disease
Definition any disease that deals with problems in blood coagulation	
deep vein thrombosis DEEP VAYN throm-BOH-sis	deep vein thromb / osis deep vein clot / condition
Definition formation of a blood clot in a vein deep in the body, most commonly the leg	
hemoglobinopathy HEE-maw-GLOH-bin-AW-pah-thee	hemo / globino / pathy blood / globe / disease
Definition disease of the hemoglobin	
hypercoagulability HAI-per-koh-AG-yoo-lah-BIL-ih-tee	hyper / coagul / ability over / coagulation / ability
Definition increased ability of the blood to coagulate	
immunocompromised ih-MYOO-noh-COM-proh-MAIZD	immuno / compromised immune / compromised
Definition having an immune system incapable of responding normally and completely to a pathogen or disease	
immunodeficiency ih-MYOO-noh-deh-FIH-shin-see	immuno / deficiency immune / deficiency
Definition immune system with decreased or compromised response to disease-causing organisms	
immunosuppresion ih-MYOO-noh-suh-PREH-shun	immuno / suppression immune / suppression
Definition reduction in the activity of the body's immune system	
ischemia ih-SKEE-mee-ah	isch / emia hold back / blood condition
Definition blockage of blood flow to an organ	
phlebarteriectasia FLEB-ar-TER-ee-ek-TAY-zhah	phleb / arteri / ectasia vein / artery / dilation
Definition dilation of blood vessels	
spherocytosis SFEER-oh-sai-TOH-sis	sphero / cyt / osis sphere / cell / condition
Definition condition in which red blood cells assume a spherical shape	
thrombophlebitis THROM-boh-fleh-BAI-tis	thrombo / phleb / itis clot / vein / inflammation
Definition inflammation of vein caused by a clot	

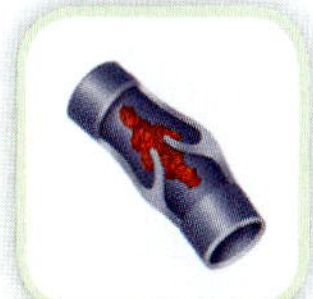
deep vein thrombosis

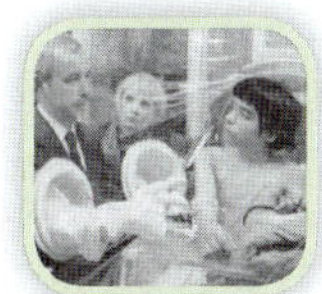
immunodeficiency

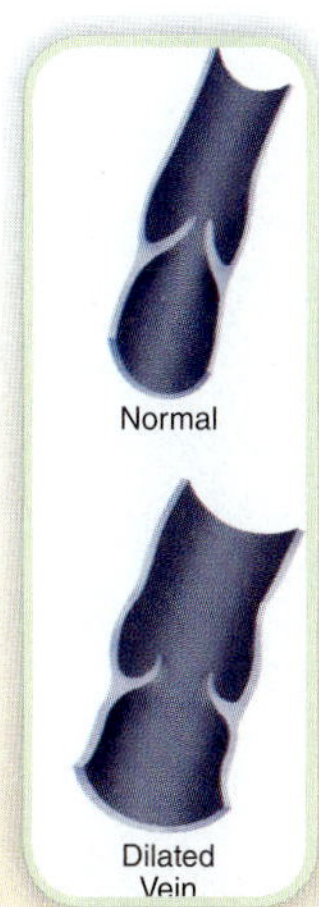

phlebarteriectasia

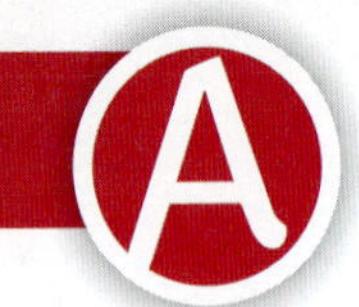

8.4 Diagnosis and Pathology

blood conditions

Term	Word Analysis
anemia ah-NEE-mee-ah **Definition** reduced red blood cells	an / emia no / blood condition
aplastic anemia AY-plas-tik ah-NEE-mee-ah **Definition** anemia caused by red blood cells not being formed in sufficient quantities	a / plast / ic an / emia no / formation / pertaining to no / blood condition
hemolytic anemia HEE-moh-LIH-tiok ah-NEE-mee-ah **Definition** anemia caused by the destruction of red blood cells	hemo / lytic an / emia blood / breakdown no / blood condition
iron deficiency anemia AI-ern deh-FIH-shin-see ah-NEE-mee-ah **Definition** anemia caused by inadequate iron intake	iron deficiency an / emia iron deficiency no / blood condition
bilirubinemia BIH-lee-ROO-bin-EE-mee-ah **Definition** presence of bilirubin in the blood **NOTE:** *Bilirubin* (red bile) is a substance derived from red blood cells that have completed their life span. Bilirubin is secreted by the liver into the digestive tract.	bili / rubin / emia bile / red / blood condition
hyperbilirubinemia HAI-per-BIH-lee-ROO-bin-EE-mee-ah **Definition** excessive bilirubin in the blood	hyper / bili / rubin / emia over / bile / red / blood condition
hypercholesterolemia HAI-per-koh-LES-ter-ol-EE-mee-ah **Definition** excessive cholesterol in the blood	hyper / cholesterol / emia over / cholesterol / blood condition
hyperlipidemia HAI-per-LIH-pid-EE-mee-ah **Definition** excessive fat in the blood	hyper / lipid / emia over / fat / blood condition
hypervolemia HAI-per-voh-LEE-mee-ah **Definition** increased blood volume	hyper / vol / emia over / volume / blood condition
hypovolemia HAI-poh-voh-LEE-mee-ah **Definition** decreased blood volume	hypo / vol / emia under / volume / blood condition
leukemia loo-KEE-mee-ah **Definition** cancer of the blood or bone marrow characterized by the abnormal increase in white blood cells	leuk / emia white / blood condition

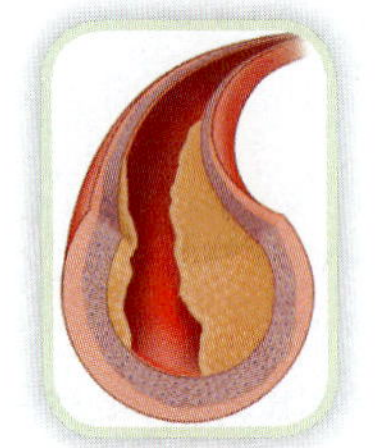

hypercholesterolemia

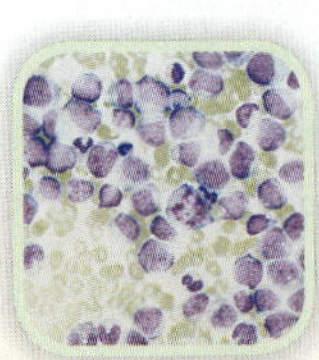

leukemia

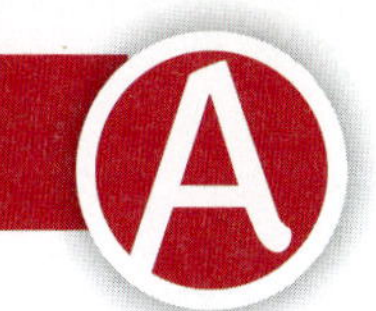

blood conditions *continued*

Term	Word Analysis
septicemia SEP-tih-SEE-mee-ah	septic / emia rotting / blood condition
Definition presence of disease-causing microorganisms in the blood	
uremia yoo-REE-mee-ah	ur / emia urine / blood condition
Definition presence of urine in the blood	

lymph

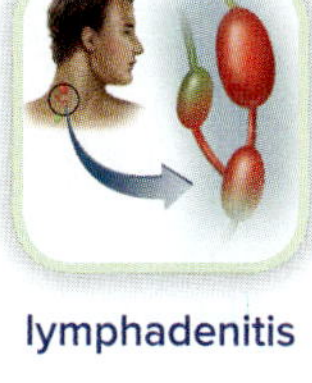

lymphadenitis

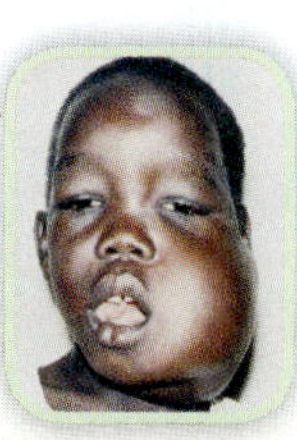

lymphoma

Term	Word Analysis
hepatosplenitis hih-PAT-oh-SPLEEN-ai-tis	hepato / splen / itis liver / spleen / inflammation
Definition inflammation of the liver and spleen	
hypersplenism HAI-per-SPLEE-niz-um	hyper / splen / ism over / spleen / condition
Definition increased spleen activity	
lymphadenitis LIM-fad-eh-NAI-tis	lymph / aden / itis lymph / gland / inflammation
Definition inflammation of a lymph gland (node)	
lymphangiesctasia lim-FAN-jee-ek-TAY-zhah	lymph / angi / ectasia lymph / vessel / dilation
Definition dilation of a lymph vessel, normally noticed by swelling in the extremities	
lymphangitis LIM-fan-JAI-tis	lymph / ang / itis lymph / vessel / inflammation
Definition inflammation of lymph vessels	
lymphoma lim-FOH-mah	lymph / oma lymph / tumor
Definition tumor originating in lymphocytes	
mononucleosis MAW-noh-NOO-klee-OH-sis	mono / nucle / osis one / nucleus / condition
Definition condition characterized by an abnormally large number of mononuclear leukocytes	
myelodysplasia MAI-el-oh-dis-PLAY-zhah	myelo / dys / plas / ia bone marrow / bad / formation / condition
Definition disease characterized by poor production of blood cells by the bone marrow	

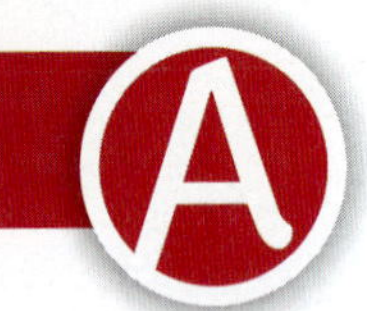

8.4 Diagnosis and Pathology

lymph *continued*

Term	Word Analysis
myeloma MAI-eh-LOH-mah **Definition** cancerous tumor of the bone marrow; when the tumors are present in several bones, it is called multiple myeloma	myel / oma bone marrow / tumor
osteomyelitis AW-stee-oh-MAI-eh-LAI-tis **Definition** inflammation of bone and bone marrow	osteo / myel / itis bone / bone marrow / inflammation
splenitis splee-NAI-tis **Definition** inflammation of the spleen	splen / itis spleen / inflammation
splenopathy splee-NAW-pah-thee **Definition** any disease of the spleen	spleno / pathy spleen / disease
splenorrhexis SPLEE-noh-REK-sis **Definition** rupture of the spleen	spleno / rrhexis spleen / rupture
thymoma thai-MOH-mah **Definition** tumor of the thymus	thym / oma thymus / tumor
thymopathy thai-MAW-pah-thee **Definition** disease of the thymus	thymo / pathy thymus / disease
tonsillitis TON-sil-AI-tis **Definition** inflammation of a tonsil	tonsill / itis tonsil / inflammation

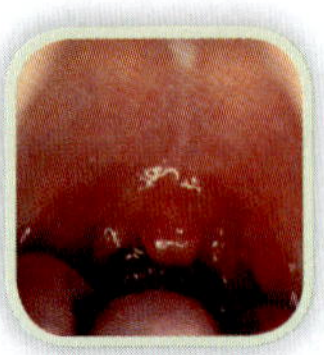

tonsillitis

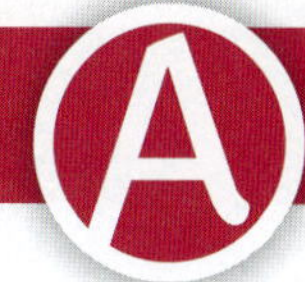

Learning Outcome 8.4 Exercises

PRONUNCIATION

EXERCISE 1 *Break down the following words into syllables.*

EXAMPLE: synesthesia *syn | es | the | sia*

1. coagulopathy __________
2. hemoglobinopathy __________
3. hypercoagulability __________
4. thrombophlebitis __________
5. bilirubinemia __________
6. hyperbilirubinemia __________
7. hypervolemia __________
8. hypovolemia __________
9. hepatosplenitis __________
10. hypersplenism __________
11. osteomyelitis __________

EXERCISE 2 *Indicate which syllable is emphasized when pronounced.*

EXAMPLE: bronchitis bron**chi**tis

1. anemia __________
2. leukemia __________
3. uremia __________
4. lymphoma __________
5. splenitis __________
6. splenopathy __________
7. thymoma __________
8. thymopathy __________

TRANSLATION

EXERCISE 3 *Break down the following words into their component parts.*

EXAMPLE: nasopharyngoscope *naso | pharyngo | scope*

1. autoimmune __________
2. splenitis __________
3. splenopathy __________
4. thymopathy __________
5. hemoglobinopathy __________
6. immunocompromised __________
7. immunosuppression __________
8. hypersplenism __________

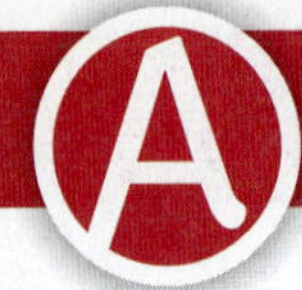

Learning Outcome 8.4 Exercises

9. hyperbilirubinemia ______________________________
10. lymphangitis ______________________________
11. osteomyelitis ______________________________
12. hypercoagulability ______________________________

EXERCISE 4 *Underline and define the word parts from this chapter in the following terms.*

1. tonsillitis ______________________________
2. immunodeficiency ______________________________
3. lymphoma ______________________________
4. thymoma ______________________________
5. myeloma ______________________________
6. coagulopathy ______________________________
7. lymphadenitis ______________________________
8. anemia ______________________________
9. deep vein thrombosis ______________________________
10. phlebarteriectasia ______________________________
11. spherocytosis ______________________________
12. lymphangiectasia ______________________________
13. myelodysplasia ______________________________
14. splenorrhexis ______________________________
15. hepatosplenitis ______________________________
16. leukemia (2 roots) ______________________________
17. thrombophlebitis (2 roots) ______________________________

EXERCISE 5 *Match the term on the left with its definition on the right.*

____	1. hypercholesterolemia	a. anemia caused by inadequate iron intake
____	2. iron deficiency anemia	b. anemia caused by red blood cells not being formed in sufficient quantities
____	3. bilirubinemia	c. anemia caused by the destruction of red blood cells
____	4. hemolytic anemia	d. blockage of blood flow to an organ
____	5. aplastic anemia	e. decreased blood volume
____	6. hyperlipidemia	f. excessive cholesterol in the blood
____	7. hypervolemia	g. excessive fat in the blood
____	8. hypovolemia	h. increased blood volume
____	9. septicemia	i. the presence of bilirubin in the blood
____	10. ischemia	j. the presence of disease-causing microorganisms in the blood
____	11. uremia	k. the presence of urine in the blood

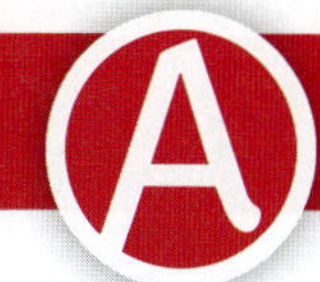

Learning Outcome 8.4 Exercises

EXERCISE 6 *Translate the following terms as literally as possible.*

EXAMPLE: nasopharyngoscope *an instrument for looking at the nose and throat*

1. hypercoagulability ______
2. phlebarteriectasia ______
3. spherocytosis ______
4. thrombophlebitis ______
5. anemia ______
6. hyperbilirubinism ______
7. septicemia ______
8. hepatosplenitis ______
9. hypersplenism ______
10. lymphadenitis ______
11. lymphangiectasia ______
12. lymphangitis ______
13. osteomyelitis ______
14. splenitis ______
15. splenorrhexis ______
16. tonsillitis ______

GENERATION

EXERCISE 7 *Build a medical term from the information provided.*

EXAMPLE: inflammation of the sinuses *sinusitis*

1. lymph tumor ______
2. spleen disease ______
3. thymus disease ______
4. coagulation disease ______
5. a disease of the hemoglobin ______
6. *white blood condition* ______
7. presence of bilirubin in the blood ______
8. presence of urine in the blood ______
9. excessive cholesterol in the blood ______
10. excessive fat in the blood ______

Learning Outcome 8.4 Exercises

EXERCISE 8 *Multiple-choice questions. Select the correct answer.*

1. The root word in *immunocompromised* is
   a. *compromo*–the lymph system
   b. *compromo*–to protect
   c. *immuno*–the immune system
   d. *immuno*–the platelets and white cells of the body
   e. none of these
2. An immune system with decreased or compromised response to disease-causing organisms is called
   a. autoimmune
   b. immunodeficiency
   c. immunogenic
   d. immunosuppression
   e. none of these
3. Anemia caused by inadequate iron intake is known as
   a. aplastic anemia
   b. hematopenia
   c. hemolytic anemia
   d. iron deficiency anemia
   e. none of these
4. The term *ischemia* means
   a. blockage of blood flow to an organ
   b. decreased blood volume
   c. dilation of blood vessels
   d. inflammation of a vein caused by a clot
   e. none of these
5. The formation of a blood clot deep in the body, most commonly in the leg, is called
   a. deep vein thrombosis
   b. hyperthrombopathy
   c. phlebarteriectasia
   d. thrombophlebitis
   e. none of these
6. *Bilirubin* is
   a. red bile
   b. a substance derived from red blood cells
   c. secreted by the liver into the digestive tract
   d. a substance that has completed its life span
   e. all of these
7. A cancer of the blood or bone marrow characterized by the abnormal increase in white blood cells is known as
   a. leukemia
   b. myeloma
   c. lymphoma
   d. osteomyelitis
   e. none of these

Learning Outcome 8.4 Exercises

8. A disease characterized by poor production of blood cells by the bone marrow is called
   a. myelodysplasia
   b. osteomyelitis
   c. myeloma
   d. hematomyelogenopathy
   e. none of these

EXERCISE 9 *Briefly describe the difference between each pair of terms.*

1. myeloma, thymoma ______________________________
2. hypervolemia, hypovolemia ______________________________
3. autoimmune disease, immunosuppression ______________________________
4. aplastic anemia, hemolytic anemia ______________________________

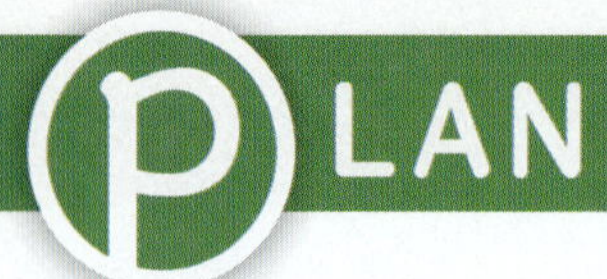

8.5 Treatments and Therapies

Treatment for blood problems generally involves both medicine and transfusions. With red blood cell problems, the treatment often involves blood transfusions (for severe problems), and then fixing the cause. Many times, iron supplements can also be helpful.

White blood cell problems—in particular, severely low white blood cell counts—can be treated with transfusions too. A patient with leukemia is treated with chemotherapy.

When the problem is significant enough, patients with very low platelet levels often are treated with transfusions as well. Other medicines that can help with platelet problems include medicines to break clots (*thrombolytics*) and those that prevent clots (*anticoagulants*).

Treating diseases of the lymphatic system generally involves surgery. Organs of the lymphatic system may be removed, such as the spleen (*splenectomy*) or the thymus (*thymectomy*). Lymph nodes may need removal (*lymphadenectomy*) as well, usually for the purpose of a biopsy.

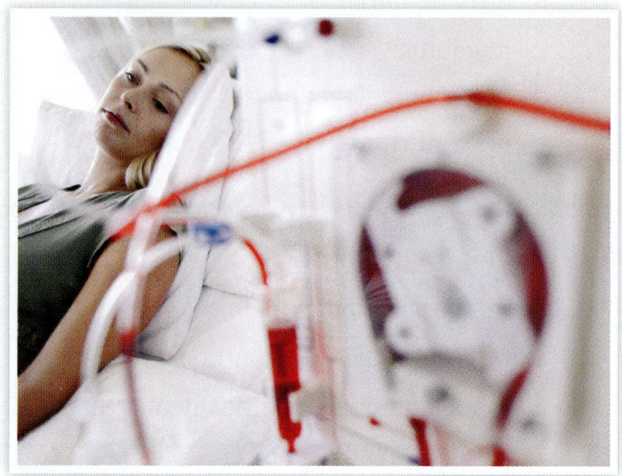

Transfusions and apheresis are important components of treating blood problems.

drugs

Term	Word Analysis
anticoagulant AN-tee-coh-AG-yoo-lant **Definition** drug that prevents the coagulation of blood	anti / coagul / ant against / coagulation / agent
hemostatic HEE-moh-STAT-ik **Definition** drug that stops the flow of blood	hemo / static blood / standing
thrombolytic THROM-boh-LIH-tik **Definition** drug that breaks down blood clots	thrombo / lyt / ic clot / breakdown / agent

surgery

Term	Word Analysis
laparosplenectomy LAP-ah-roh-splee-NEK-toh-mee **Definition** surgical removal of the spleen through the abdomen	laparo / splen / ec / tomy abdomen / spleen / out / cut
lymphadenectomy lim-FAD-eh-NEK-toh-mee **Definition** surgical removal of a lymph gland (node)	lymph / aden / ec / tomy lymph / gland / out / cut

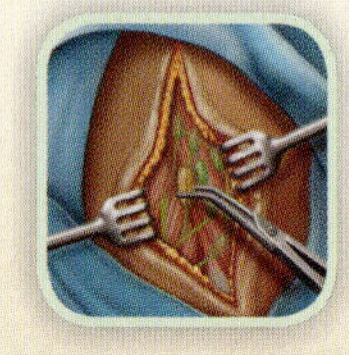

lymphadenectomy

Learning Outcome 8.5 Exercises

surgery *continued*

Term	Word Analysis
lymphadenotomy lim-FAD-eh-NAW-toh-mee **Definition** incision into a lymph gland (node)	lymph / adeno / tomy lymph / gland / cut
nephrosplenopexy NEF-roh-SPLEE-noh-PEK-see **Definition** surgical fixation of the spleen and a kidney	nephro / spleno / pexy kidney / spleen / fixation
splenectomy spleh-NEK-toh-mee **Definition** surgical removal of the spleen	splen / ec / tomy spleen / out / cut
thymectomy thai-MEK-toh-mee **Definition** surgical removal of the thymus	thym / ec / tomy thymus / out / cut
tonsillectomy TON-sil-EK-toh-mee **Definition** surgical removal of a tonsil	tonsill / ec / tomy tonsil / out / cut

transfusions

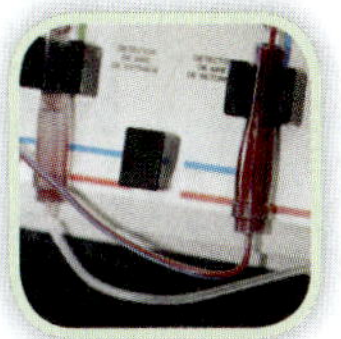

apheresis

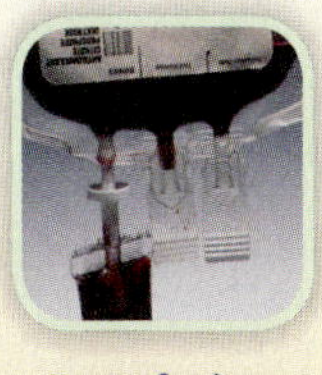

transfusion

Term	Word Analysis
apheresis AH-fer-EE-sis **Definition** general term for a process, similar to dialysis, that draws out a patient's blood, removes something from it, then returns the rest of the blood to the patient's body **NOTE:** *Apheresis* can also refer to the use of this process to remove unwanted or disease-causing components from the blood.	from Greek, for *separation* **NOTE:** This is the same word that was the origin of the word *heretic,* meaning one who has separated from the traditional teachings of a group.
cytapheresis SAI-tah-fer-EE-sis **Definition** apheresis to remove cellular material	cyt / apheresis cell / separation
plasmapheresis PLAZ-mah-fer-EE-sis **Definition** apheresis to remove plasma	plasm / apheresis plasma / separation
plateletpheresis PLAYT-let-fer-EE-sis **Definition** apheresis to remove platelets (for the purpose of donating them to patients in need of platelets) **NOTE:** Where did the *a* in *apheresis* go? Probably, this term was developed from the term *plasmapheresis.* But because the first root in that word is *plasma,* someone thought that the *a* in *apheresis* went with it, so when they made this new word, they left the *a* out. Either that, or *platelet-AH-pheresis* didn't sound as good.	platelet / pheresis platelet / separation
transfusion tranz-FYOO-zhun **Definition** infusion into a patient of blood from another source	trans / fusion across / pour

Learning Outcome 8.5 Exercises

PRONUNCIATION

EXERCISE 1 *Break down the following words into syllables.*

EXAMPLE: synesthesia *syn | es | the | sia*

1. hemostatic ______
2. tonsillectomy ______
3. anticoagulant ______
4. plasmapheresis ______
5. plateletpheresis ______
6. laparosplenectomy ______

EXERCISE 2 *Indicate which syllable is emphasized when pronounced.*

EXAMPLE: bronchitis bron**chi**tis

1. transfusion ______
2. thymectomy ______
3. splenectomy ______

TRANSLATION

EXERCISE 3 *Break down the following words into their component parts.*

EXAMPLE: nasopharyngoscope *naso | pharyngo | scope*

1. thymectomy ______
2. laparosplenectomy ______
3. transfusion ______
4. plasmapheresis ______
5. plateletpheresis ______
6. lymphadenotomy ______

EXERCISE 4 *Underline and define the word parts from this chapter in the following terms.*

1. tonsillectomy ______
2. thymectomy ______
3. splenectomy ______
4. thrombolytic ______
5. anticoagulant ______
6. hemostatic ______

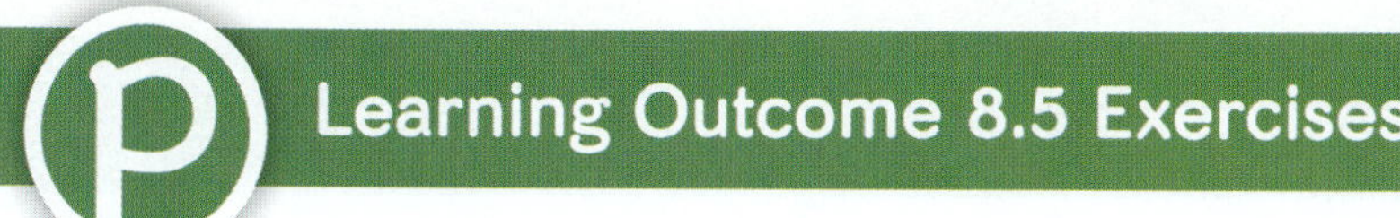

Learning Outcome 8.5 Exercises

7. cytapheresis ____________________
8. lymphadenectomy ____________________
9. laparosplenectomy ____________________
10. nephrosplenopexy ____________________

EXERCISE 5 *Match the term on the left with its definition on the right.*

__d__	1. transfusion	a. apheresis to remove cellular material
__c__	2. apheresis	b. apheresis to remove platelets
__b__	3. plasmapheresis	c. general term for a process, similar to dialysis, that draws blood, removes something from it, then returns the rest of the blood to the patient
__a__	4. cytapheresis	d. infusion into a patient of blood from another source

EXERCISE 6 *Translate the following terms as literally as possible.*

> EXAMPLE: nasopharyngoscope *an instrument for looking at the nose and throat*

1. thrombolytic ____________________
2. hemostatic ____________________
3. cytapheresis ____________________
4. plateletpheresis ____________________
5. plasmapheresis ____________________
6. laparosplenectomy ____________________
7. nephrosplenopexy ____________________

GENERATION

EXERCISE 7 *Build a medical term from the information provided.*

> EXAMPLE: inflammation of the sinuses *sinusitis*

1. surgical removal of the spleen ____________________
2. surgical removal of the thymus ____________________
3. surgical removal of the tonsil ____________________
4. surgical removal of a lymph gland (node) ____________________
5. incision into a lymph gland (node) ____________________
6. a drug that prevents the coagulation of blood ____________________

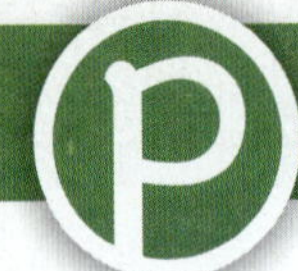

Learning Outcome 8.5 Exercises

EXERCISE 8 *Multiple-choice questions. Select the correct answer(s).*

1. A *laparosplenectomy* is
   a. an incision into the spleen through the abdomen
   b. an incision into the spleen with a laser
   c. the surgical removal of the spleen through the abdomen
   d. the surgical removal of the spleen with a laser
   e. none of these
2. Select all of the below statements that apply to the term *apheresis*.
   a. a process similar to dialysis
   b. can refer to the removal of unwanted or disease-causing components from the blood
   c. from the Greek word meaning *separation*
   d. requires a transfusion
   e. the blood is not returned to the patient once removed
3. After a patient has undergone *plateletpheresis*,
   a. the patient receives a transfusion to replace lost blood
   b. the plasma is cleaned and then returned to the patient
   c. the platelets are often donated to another person in need
   d. the platelets are then returned to the patient
   e. none of these

8.6 Abbreviations

Abbreviations provide a shorthand way of referring to things that either recur often or are too long to write out. When dealing with the the blood and lymph systems, these can refer to common examination findings (NCAT), common lab work (PLT, RBC, WBC), diseases (ALL, AIDS), or treatments (BMT).

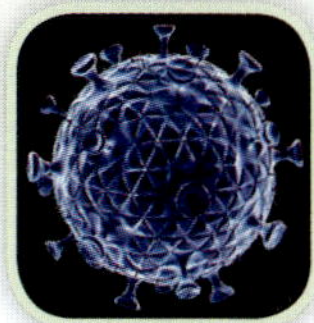
AIDS

blood and lymph abbreviations

Abbreviation	Definition
AIDS	acquired immunodeficiency syndrome
ALL	acute lymphoblastic leukemia
AML	acute myeloid leukemia
BMT	bone marrow transplant
CBC	complete blood count
CML	chronic myeloid leukemia
DIC	disseminated intravascular coagulopathy
EBV	Epstein-Barr virus
ESR	erythrocyte sedimentation rate
Hct	hematocrit
Hgb	hemoglobin
HIV	human immunodeficiency virus
HSM	hepatosplenomegaly
HUS	hemolytic uremic syndrome
INR	international normalized ratio
ITP	idiopathic thrombocytopenic purpura
IV	intravenous
IVIG	intravenous immunoglobulin
LAD	lymphadenopathy
NCAT	no cervical adenopathy or tenderness
PLT	platelet count
PT	prothrombin time
PTT	partial thromboplastin time
RBC	red blood count
TTP	thrombotic thrombocytopenic purpura
WBC	white blood count

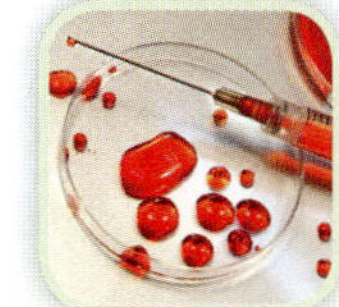
RBC (red blood count)

Learning Outcome 8.6 Exercises

EXERCISE 1 *Define the following abbreviations.*

1. HIV ______
2. AIDS ______
3. CBC ______
4. WBC ______
5. RBC ______
6. Hgb ______
7. PLT ______
8. INR ______
9. AML ______
10. BMT ______
11. CML ______
12. LAD ______
13. IV ______

EXERCISE 2 *Give the abbreviations for the following definitions.*

1. no cervical adenopathy or tenderness ______
2. acute lymphoblastic leukemia ______
3. disseminated intravascular coagulopathy ______
4. erythrocyte sedimentation rate ______
5. hemolytic uremic syndrome ______
6. prothrombin time ______
7. partial thromboplastin time ______
8. idiopathic thrombocytopenic purpura ______
9. thrombotic thrombocytopenic purpura ______
10. intravenous immunoglobulin ______
11. hepatosplenomegaly ______
12. hematocrit ______
13. Epstein-Barr virus ______

EXERCISE 3 *Multiple-choice questions. Select the correct answer(s).*

1. Both AIDS and HIV have to do with the
   a. blood count
   b. bone marrow
   c. immune system
   d. leukemia
   e. none of these
2. BMT is
   a. blood microcytosis time
   b. blood microcytosis transplant
   c. bone marrow time
   d. bone marrow transplant
   e. none of these

Learning Outcome 8.6 Exercises

3. PLT is

    a. partial leukocyte time
    b. platelet count
    c. prothrombin time
    d. thrombocytopenic purpura
    e. none of these

4. HUS, *hemolytic uremic syndrome,* comes from the roots

    a. *hemo:* blood + *lytic:* breakdown agent + *ur:* urine + *emia:* blood condition
    b. *hemo:* blood + *lytic:* clotting agent + *ur:* urine + *emia:* blood deficiency
    c. *hemo:* liver + *lytic:* breakdown agent + *ur:* urine + *emia:* blood condition
    d. *hemo:* liver + *lytic:* clotting agent + *ur:* urine + *emia:* blood deficiency
    e. *hemo:* spleen + *lytic:* clotting agent + *ur:* urine + *emia:* blood deficiency

5. A person with HSM has

    a. a hardened and enlarged spleen
    b. a hardened liver and spleen
    c. a small and hardened spleen
    d. a small liver and spleen
    e. an enlarged liver and spleen

6. A person with LAD has

    a. any disease of a lymph gland (node)
    b. lymphadenopathy
    c. noticeably swollen lymph nodes, especially in the neck
    d. all of these
    e. none of these

7. Select the abbreviations below that pertain to leukemia.

    a. ALL
    b. ALT
    c. AML
    d. CML
    e. ITP
    f. PT
    g. PTT
    h. TTP

8. Select the abbreviations below that pertain to blood counts.

    a. BMT
    b. CBC
    c. ESR
    d. Hct
    e. Hgb
    f. RBC
    g. WBC

9. Select the abbreviations below that pertain to red blood cells.

    a. BMT
    b. CBC
    c. ESR
    d. Hct
    e. Hgb
    f. RBC
    g. WBC

8.7 Electronic Health Records

Heme/Onc Clinic

Subjective

Jerry is a 4-year-old male sent to our clinic for evaluation of ostealgia. He has had a 1-month history of intermittent pain in his distal left femur. He also been febrile on and off for the past month and had night sweats. He denies weight loss, weakness, or limping. No other extremities are hurting him.

ROS: No shortness of breath, no chest pain; no headaches; no arthralgias; no new rashes; no gastrointestinal complaints.

Objective

Physical Exam

RR: 20; HR: 88; Temp: 100; BP: 80/60.

Gen: WDWN, active, playful 4-year-old boy in NAD. AOx3.

HEENT: NCAT. PERRLA. White sclera. No conjunctival injection. Mucous membranes moist and pink. Normal dentition.

Neck: Supple. No LAD.

Resp: CTAB without wheezes, rales, or rhonchi; no retractions. Good air exchange.

CV: RRR without murmurs.

Abd: Soft, nontender, nondistended. Mild hepatosplenomegaly. No masses.

Neuro: CN II-XII grossly intact. No focal neurologic deficit.

Ext: Distal left femur has mild edema and is tender to palpation. No erythema, warmth, or induration. Multiple palpable inguinal lymph nodes on the left.

Skin: Scattered **petechiae** generalized over body, both above and below the midchest.

Genitalia: SMR I male testes descended bilaterally.

Laboratory Data: WBC: 6,200 (20 neutrophils, 2 bands, 10 lymphocytes, 1 mono, 67 lymphoblasts); hemoglobin 10.1, hematocrit 30.6, platelet count 54,000.

Assessment

4-year-old male with anemia, leukopenia, and thrombocytopenia. The lymphoblasts on the peripheral blood smear indicate an acute lymphoblastic leukemia.

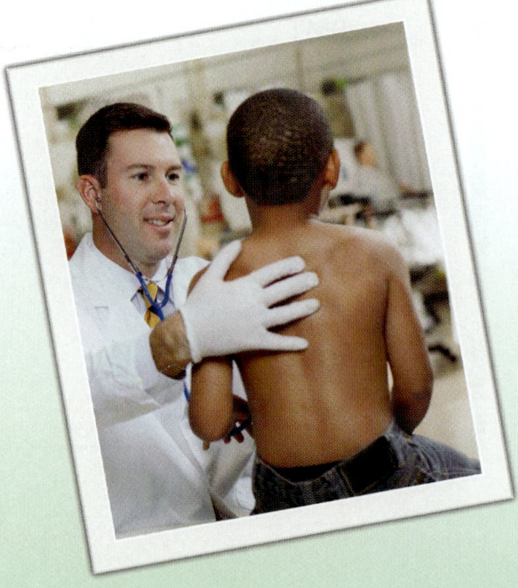

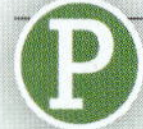

Plan

1. We will schedule him for a diagnostic bone marrow aspirate and biopsy.
2. Lumbar puncture to rule out CNS involvement.
3. Ab CT to evaluate for nodes.

–Rodger Dodger, PA

Learning Outcome 8.7 Exercises

EXERCISE 1 *Match the term on the left with its definition on the right.*

_____	1. anemia	a.	deficiency in the number of platelets (clot cells)
_____	2. hemoglobin	b.	deficiency in white blood cells
_____	3. leukopenia	c.	enlargement of the liver and spleen
_____	4. thrombocytopenia	d.	reduction of red blood cells noticed by the patient by weakness and fatigue
_____	5. hepatosplenomegaly	e.	the iron-containing pigment in red blood cells that carries oxygen to the cells

EXERCISE 2 *Fill in the blanks.*

1. Using the data recorded at the patient's physical examination, fill in the following blanks.
   a. The patient's temperature: ______________________________
   b. The patient's heart rate: ______________________________
   c. The patient's respiratory rate: ______________________________
   d. The patient's blood pressure: ______________________________
   e. WDWN (____________________) active playful 4-year-old boy in NAD (____________________).
   f. HEENT: NCAT (______________________________).
   g. Neck: no LAD (define abbreviation: ______________________________).
   h. CV: ______________________________ (regular rate and rhythm).
2. Using the patient's laboratory data, fill in the following blanks.
   a. WBC (____________________): 6,200
   b. 10 *lymphocytes* (give definition:______________________________)
   c. *hemoglobin* (give definition: ____________________) 10.1
   d. Hct (define abbreviation: ____________________) 30.6
   e. Platelet count (give abbreviation: ____________________) 54,000

EXERCISE 3 *True or false questions. Indicate true answers with a T and false answers with an F.*

1. The patient has had intermittent pain in his *distal* (farther away from the center) left femur. _____
2. The patient has not had a fever. _____
3. The patient has lymphadenopathy in his neck. _____
4. Several of the patient's left lymph nodes are *palpable* (large enough to feel). _____
5. A neutrophil is a type of white blood cell. _____
6. The patient's blood smear indicated an ALL. _____
7. The patient does not need to have a Bx. _____

Learning Outcome 8.7 Exercises

EXERCISE 4 *Multiple-choice questions. Select the correct answer.*

1. The health care professional noticed the patient had *hepatosplenomegaly*, which is a(n)
   a. enlarged spleen and liver
   b. small spleen and liver
   c. displaced spleen and liver
   d. none of these
2. Which of the following is *not* included in the patient's assessment?
   a. reduction of red blood cells
   b. deficiency in white blood cells
   c. deficiency in clotting cells
   d. decreased blood volume
3. The patient's blood smear indicated an *acute lymphoblastic leukemia*, which is
   a. a cancer of the blood or bone marrow characterized by the abnormal increase in white blood cells, specifically lymphoblasts, that started recently
   b. a cancer of the blood or bone marrow characterized by the abnormal increase in white blood cells, specifically lymphoblasts, that has been going on for a while now
   c. a cancer of the blood or bone marrow characterized by the abnormal increase in red blood cells, specifically lymphoblasts, that started recently
   d. a cancer of the blood or bone marrow characterized by the abnormal increase in red blood cells, specifically lymphoblasts, that has been going on for a while now
4. Which of the following is *not* part of the patient's plan for treatment?
   a. abdominal computer axial tomography
   b. Bx
   c. LP to rule out central nervous system involvement
   d. PTT to determine if there is an additional bleeding disorder

Hospital Progress Note

Subjective

Mrs. Campos was admitted last night for fever and elevated WBC. Initial blood culture is coming back positive from gram-positive cocci. She has been on antibiotics for 10 hours now. Last night, the nurses noted hemorrhages. She had **hematuria, hemoptysis,** and **epistaxis.** In addition, she developed painful swelling in her right calf. She remains febrile, but the fever is improving since admission. She is still very tired. She denies vomiting.

Objective

RR: 18; HR: 70; Temp 101.2; BP: 102/74.

General: Sleeping. Tired but responsive to questions.

HEENT: NCAT, dried bloody crusts in nostrils, Mucous membranes moist and pink; PERRLA, EOMI, conjunctivae clear.

Neck: Supple, no **adenopathy,** no JVD.

Resp: No increased effort, clear breath sounds.

CV: Regular, S1, S2, no murmur/rub; pedal pulses 2+ .

Abd: Soft, nontender, nondistended, normoactive bowel sounds, no **HSM.**

Lymph: No enlarged cervical, axillary, or inguinal lymph nodes.

Skin: Scattered **petechiae,** CR 2 seconds.

Ext: Right swelling with tender subcutaneous nodule.

Neuro: Alert and oriented, CN II-XII grossly intact, normal and symmetric strength in UEs and LEs, DTRs 2+ and symmetric.

Labs

Total bilirubin: 6.2

Hgb: 9.2; **WBC:** 20.2; **PLT:** 24.

PT and **PTT** both elevated.

Microangiopathic hemolysis seen on peripheral smear.

Assessment/Plan

1. **Septicemia:** Fever down slightly and WBC decreased from 25.4 to 20.2. Continue current IV antibiotics.
2. **Anemia/Coagulopathy/Thrombocytopenia:** Clinically consistent with **DIC.** We will transfuse a unit of platelets and follow labs in 6 hours.
3. Calf swelling: Suspect superficial **thromboembolism.** We will consult hematology/oncology in regard to their opinion on beginning **anticoagulant** medicine.
4. **Hyperbilrubinemia:** I suspect the etiology is liver dysfunction from DIC. Follow labs in the AM.

–Linda Lovegood, MD

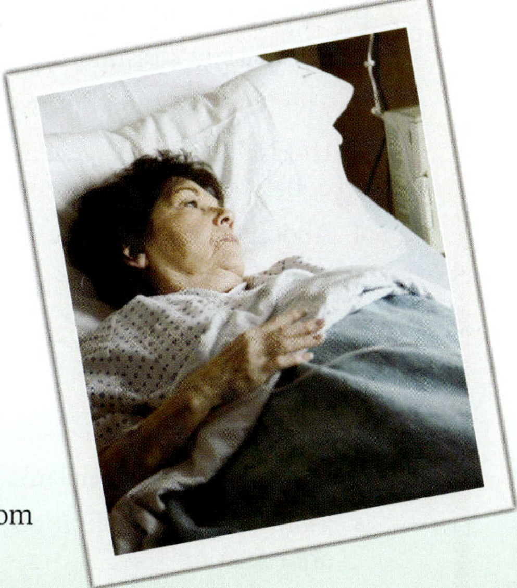

Learning Outcome 8.7 Exercises

EXERCISE 5 *Match the term on the left with its definition on the right.*

______	1. anemia	a.	a blockage of a vessel (embolism) caused by a clot that has broken off from where it formed
______	2. transfusion	b.	a drug that prevents the coagulation of blood
______	3. hematology	c.	any disease that deals with problems in blood coagulation
______	4. hemorrhage	d.	breakdown of blood cells
______	5. hemolysis	e.	deficiency in the number of platelets (clot cells)
______	6. anticoagulant	f.	enlargement of the spleen and liver
______	7. coagulopathy	g.	excessive bilirubin in the blood
______	8. hyperbilirubinemia	h.	excessive blood loss
______	9. septicemia	i.	reduction of red blood cells noticed by the patient by weakness and fatigue
______	10. thrombocytopenia	j.	the infusion into a patient of blood from another source
______	11. hepatosplenomegaly	k.	the presence of disease-causing microorganisms in the blood
______	12. thromboembolism	l.	the study of the blood

EXERCISE 6 *Fill in the blanks.*

1. Using the data recorded at the patient's physical examination, fill in the following blanks.
   a. The patient's temperature: ______________________________
   b. The patient's heart rate: ______________________________
   c. The patient's respiratory rate: ______________________________
   d. The patient's blood pressure: ______________________________
   e. HEENT (______________________): NCAT. ______________________ (pupils equal, round, and reactive to light and accommodation).
   f. Abdomen: no HSM (give definition for abbreviation: ______________________)
2. Using the patient's laboratory data, fill in the following blanks.
   a. Hemoglobin: ______________________________
   b. White blood count: ______________________________
   c. Platelet count: ______________________________
3. According to the physician's assessment/plan,
   a. *septicemia* (give definition: ______________________); WBC (give definition for abbreviation: ______________________) decreased from 25.4 to 20.2.
   b. ______________________ (decreased red blood cells)/ ______________________ (any disease that deals with problems in blood coagulation)/ ______________________ (deficiency in the number of platelets): clinically consistent with DIC (give definition for abbreviation: ______________________________).
   c. For suspected ______________________ (a blockage of a vessel [embolism] caused by a clot that has broken off from where it formed), the hematology/oncology department will be consulted before beginning *anticoagulants* (give definition: ______________________).

Learning Outcome 8.7 Exercises

EXERCISE 7 *True or false questions. Indicate true answers with a T and false answers with an F.*

1. The patient was admitted for an elevated red blood count. ________
2. Upon admission, the patient was afebrile. ________
3. The patient's spleen and liver are enlarged. ________
4. The patient's prothrombin time and partial thromboplastin time are elevated. ________
5. The patient will receive blood and/or blood components from another source. ________
6. The patient has increased bilirubin in the blood. ________

EXERCISE 8 *Multiple-choice questions. Select the correct answer.*

1. The patient has *hematuria,* which is
   a. blood in the urine
   b. a condition of the liver and blood
   c. decreased blood volume
   d. none of these
2. The patient had *hemoptysis,* which comes from the root *ptysis,* which means cough, and *hemo,* which means
   a. blood
   b. bone marrow
   c. liver
   d. lymph system
3. The patient's peripheral blood smear revealed *microangiopathic hemolysis.* The term *microangiopathic* refers to a disease of the small blood vessels. The term *hemolysis* refers to
   a. breakdown of blood cells
   b. breakdown of clotting cells
   c. creation of blood cells
   d. creation of clotting cells
4. The patient has *hyperbilirubinemia,* which is
   a. excessive bilirubin in the blood
   b. excessive red bile in the blood
   c. excessive bilirubin in the blood and excessive red bile in the blood
   d. none of these

Hospital Consult

Subjective

Reason for Consult: I was asked to see this 8-year-old boy to evaluate his **anemia.**

History of Present Illness: Billy Caspar presented initially to his primary care provider with decreased energy and **pallor.** He had recently had rash on his hands and a fever, both of which have improved over the past few days. A **hematocrit** was performed in the office and it was critically low. In addition, the patient had a flow murmur and appeared lethargic. He was sent to the hospital for admission. He was **transfused** with 2 units of **prbcs** and **hematology** was consulted.

Past Medical History: Term delivery. Normal newborn screen. Specifically, no **hemoglobinopathy** on screen. Normal development.

Past Surgical History: None.

Family History: Father with **hereditary spherocytosis.**

Medications: Daily vitamin.

Objective

Exam

Temp: 99.4; Heart Rate: 100; Respiratory Rate: 22; Blood Pressure: 88/64; Pulse Ox 98%.

General: Tired, pale young man in no acute distress.

HEENT: PERRLA. Pale palpebral conjunctiva. Pale, dry mucous membranes. Normal dentition.

Neck: Supple. No **LAD.**

CV: Mild tachycardia and soft systolic flow murmur. No gallop or rub.

Resp: CTA.

Abd: Soft, nontender, nondistended. **Splenomegaly:** spleen tip palpates 3 finger breadths below ribs. No hepatomegaly.

Ext: Cool to touch. No cyanosis, clubbing, or edema. Delayed capillary refill.

Laboratory Data

CBC: **Normocytic anemia. Reticulocytosis.**

BMP: **Hyperbilirubinemia.**

Smear: **Poikilocytosis.**

Assessment

Billy clearly has a **hemolytic anemia** that is consistent with hereditary spherocytosis. I believe that, given his sudden and severe presentation along with his recent illness, he has **aplastic** crisis. This is likely brought on from infection from the parvo B19 virus. His flow murmur and slow cap refill are concerning for continued **hypovolemia.**

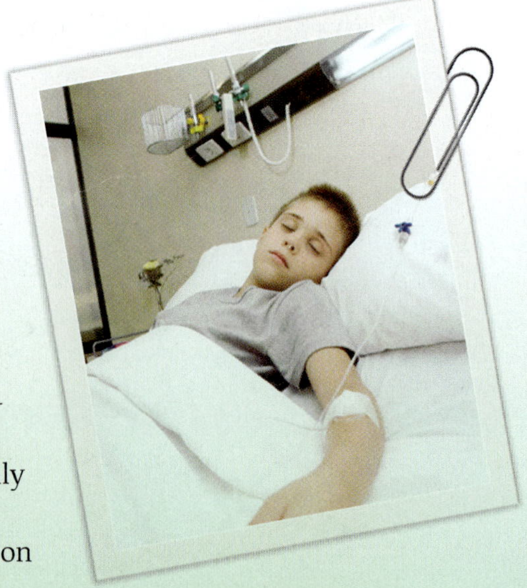

Recommendation

Billy needs another transfusion immediately. I have already ordered this. Once his anemia is stabilized, I think he should be seen by surgery to assess for a **splenectomy.** If he does get a splenectomy, he will, of course, need a pneumococcus **vaccine,** as he will be partially **immunocompromised** due to **asplenia.**

Thank you for this interesting consult. I will continue to follow up on a daily basis.

–Red Barnes, MD

Learning Outcome 8.7 Exercises

EXERCISE 9 *Match the term on the left with its definition on the right.*

_____	1. hematology	a.	a condition characterized by red blood cells in a variety of shapes
_____	2. anemia	b.	a disease of the hemoglobin
_____	3. immunocompromised	c.	a normal-sized red blood cell
_____	4. transfusion	d.	condition in which red blood cells assume a spherical shape
_____	5. normocyte	e.	absence of a spleen or of spleen function
_____	6. hypovolemia	f.	an immature red blood cell (net-like appearance)
_____	7. hyperbilirubinemia	g.	anemia caused by the destruction of red blood cells
_____	8. hemolytic anemia	h.	decreased blood volume
_____	9. splenomegaly	i.	enlargement of the spleen
_____	10. splenectomy	j.	excessive bilirubin in the blood
_____	11. hemoglobinopathy	k.	having an immune system incapable of responding normally and completely to a pathogen or disease
_____	12. spherocytosis	l.	reduction of red blood cells noticed by the patient by weakness and fatigue
_____	13. asplenia	m.	study of the blood
_____	14. reticulocyte	o.	surgical removal of the spleen
_____	15. poikilocytosis	p.	the infusion into a patient of blood from another source

EXERCISE 10 *Fill in the blanks.*

1. The reason for the consult was to evaluate Billy's *anemia* (give definition: _______________).
2. According to Billy's past medical history, he did not have _______________ (disease of the hemoglobin).
3. Billy's family has a history of *spherocytosis* (give definition: _______________).
4. Using the data recorded at Billy's physical examination, fill in the following blanks.
   a. Temp: _______________
   b. HR: _______________
   c. RR: _______________
   d. BP: _______________
   e. Neck: no _______________ (lymphadenopathy)
   f. Abdomen: _______________ (enlarged spleen)
5. Using Billy's laboratory data, fill in the following blanks.
   a. CBC (define abbreviation: _______________): *normocytic anemia, reticulocytosis* (condition of the _______________ red blood cells).
   b. BMP: *hyperbilirubinemia* (give definition: _______________).
   c. Smear: *poikilocytosis* (condition characterized by _______________ blood cells in a variety of _______________).

Learning Outcome 8.7 Exercises

EXERCISE 11 *True or false questions. Indicate true answers with a T and false answers with an F.*

1. An Hct was performed in the office. ________
2. Billy needs to be given more blood from an outside source. ________
3. Billy's spleen does not need to be removed. ________
4. Without a spleen, Billy's immune system will not be compromised. ________

EXERCISE 12 *Multiple-choice questions. Select the correct answer(s).*

1. Billy has been assessed with *hemolytic anemia,* which is
   a. anemia caused by red blood cells not being formed in sufficient quantities
   b. anemia caused by the destruction of red blood cells
   c. anemia caused by the destruction of white blood cells
   d. anemia caused by white blood cells not being formed in sufficient quantities
2. The term *normocytic anemia* refers to an anemia of the *normocytes,* which are
   a. clotting cells
   b. red blood cells
   c. white blood cells
   d. none of these
3. Bilirubin is (select all that apply)
   a. a substance derived from red blood cells that have completed their life span
   b. a substance derived from white blood cells that have completed their life span
   c. also known as red bile
   d. also known as white bile
   e. normally found in the blood
   f. normally found in the digestive tract
   g. secreted by the liver
   h. secreted by the spleen

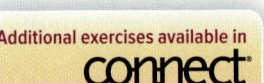

Chapter Review exercises, along with additional practice items, are available in Connect!

Quick Reference

quick reference glossary of roots

Root	Definition	Root	Definition
coagul/o	coagulation	**-penia**	deficiency
cyt/o	cell	**phleb/o**	vein
-emia	blood condition	**splen/o**	spleen
hem/o, hemat/o	blood	**thromb/o**	clot
immun/o	immune system	**thym/o**	thymus
leuk/o	white	**tonsill/o**	tonsils
lymph/o	lymph	**ven/o**	vein
myel/o	bone marrow		

quick reference glossary of terms

Term	Definition
anemia	reduction of red blood cells noticed by the patient by weakness and fatigue
anisocytosis	condition characterized by a great inequality in the size of red blood cells
antibody	substance produced by the body in response to an antigen
anticoagulant	drug that prevents the coagulation of blood
antigen	substance that causes the body to produce antibodies
apheresis	general term for a process, similar to dialysis, that draws blood, removes something from it, then returns the rest of the blood to the patient
aplastic anemia	anemia caused by red blood cells not being formed in sufficient quantities
asplenia	absence of a spleen or of spleen function
autoimmune disease	a disease caused by the body's immune system attacking the body's own healthy tissue
bilirubinemia	the presence of bilirubin (red bile; a substance derived from red blood cells that have completed their life span) in the blood
coagulopathy	any disease that deals with problems in blood coagulation
cytapheresis	apheresis to remove cellular material
deep vein thrombosis	the formation of a blood clot in a vein deep in the body, most commonly the leg

quick reference glossary of terms *continued*

Term	Definition
ecchymosis	large bruise
elliptocyte	oval-shaped red blood cell
elliptocytosis	condition characterized by an increase in the number of oval-shaped red blood cells
embolism	blockage in a blood vessel caused by an embolus
embolus	mass of matter present in the blood
erythrocyte	red blood cell
erythrocytosis	abnormal increase in the number of red blood cells
hematocrit	test to judge or separate the blood; used to determine the ratio of red blood cells to total blood volume
hematology	study of the blood
hematoma	mass of blood within an organ, cavity, or tissue
hematopoiesis	formation of blood cells
hemoglobin	iron-containing pigment in red blood cells that carries oxygen to the cells
hemoglobinopathy	disease of the hemoglobin
hemolysis	breakdown of blood cells
hemolytic anemia	anemia caused by the destruction of red blood cells
hemophilia	condition in which the blood doesn't clot, thus causing excessive bleeding
hemorrhage	excessive blood loss
hemostatic	drug that stops the flow of blood
hepatosplenitis	inflammation of the liver and spleen
hepatosplenomegaly	enlargement of the liver and spleen
hyperbilirubinemia	excessive bilirubin in the blood
hypercholesterolemia	excessive cholesterol in the blood
hypercoagulability	increased ability of the blood to coagulate
hyperlipidemia	excessive fat in the blood
hypersplenism	increased spleen activity
hypervolemia	increased blood volume
hypoperfusion	inadequate flow of blood
hypovolemia	decreased blood volume

quick reference glossary of terms *continued*

Term	Definition
immunocompromised	having an immune system incapable of responding normally and completely to a pathogen or disease
immunodeficiency	immune system with decreased or compromised response to disease-causing organisms
immunoglobulin	protein that provides protection (immunity) against disease
immunologist	specialist in the immune system
immunology	study of the immune system
immunosuppression	reduction in the activity of the body's immune system
iron deficiency anemia	anemia caused by inadequate iron intake
ischemia	blockage of blood flow to an organ
laparosplenectomy	surgical removal of the spleen through the abdomen
leukemia	cancer of the blood or bone marrow characterized by the abnormal increase in white blood cells
leukocyte	white blood cell
leukocytosis	increase in the number of white blood cells
leukopenia	deficiency in white blood cells
lymphadenectomy	surgical removal of a lymph gland (node)
lymphadenitis	inflammation of a lymph gland (node)
lymphadenopathy	any disease of a lymph gland (node); used to refer to noticeably swollen lymph nodes, especially in the neck
lymphadenotomy	incision into a lymph gland (node)
lymphangiectasia	dilation of a lymph vessel, normally noticed by swelling in the extremities
lymphangiogram	record of the study of lymph vessels
lymphangiography	procedure to study the lymph vessels
lymphangitis	inflammation of the lymph vessels
lymphedema	swelling caused by abnormal accumulation of lymph
lymphocyte	lymph cell
lymphoma	tumor originating in lymphocytes
lymphopenia	abnormal deficiency in lymph
macrocytosis	condition characterized by large red blood cells

quick reference glossary of terms *continued*

Term	Definition
microcytosis	condition characterized by small red blood cells
myelodysplasia	disease characterized by poor production of blood cells by the bone marrow
myeloma	cancerous tumor of the bone marrow
myelopoiesis	formation of bone marrow
nephrosplenopexy	surgical fixation of the spleen and a kidney
neutropenia	deficiency in neutrophil
normocyte	normal-sized red blood cell
oligocythemia	deficiency in the number of red blood cells
osteomyelitis	inflammation of bone and bone marrow
pancytopenia	deficiency in all cellular components of the blood
perfusion	circulation of blood through tissue
petechia	small bruise
phagocytosis	process in which phagocytes (a type of white blood cell) destroy (or eat) foreign microorganisms or cell debris
phlebarteriectasia	dilation of blood vessels
phlebology	study of veins
phlebotomist	specialist in drawing blood
phlebotomy	incision into a vein (another name for drawing blood)
plasmapheresis	apheresis to remove plasma
plateletpheresis	apheresis to remove platelets (for the purpose of donating them to patients in need of platelets)
poikilocytosis	condition characterized by red blood cells in a variety of shapes
polycythemia	excess of red blood cells
reperfusion injury	injury to tissue that occurs after blood flow is restored
reticulocyte	immature red blood cell
septicemia	presence of disease-causing microorganisms in the blood
spherocyte	red blood cell that assumes a spherical shape
spherocytosis	condition in which red blood cells assume a spherical shape
sphygmomanometer	fancy name for the device used to measure blood pressure
splenalgia	pain in the spleen

quick reference glossary of terms *continued*

Term	Definition
splenectomy	surgical removal of the spleen
splenectopy	displacement of the spleen, sometimes called *floating spleen*
splenitis	inflammation of the spleen
splenodynia	pain in the spleen
splenolysis	breakdown (destruction) of spleen tissue
splenomalacia	softening of the spleen
splenomegaly	enlargement of the spleen
splenopathy	any disease of the spleen
splenoptosis	downward displacement (drooping) of the spleen
splenorrhexis	rupture of the spleen
thrombocyte	cell that helps blood clot (also known as a platelet)
thrombocytopenia	deficiency in the number of platelets (clot cells)
thrombocytosis	increase in the number of platelets (clot cells)
thromboembolism	blockage of a vessel (embolism) caused by a clot that has broken off from where it formed
thrombogenic	capable of producing a blood clot
thrombolytic	drug that breaks down blood clots
thrombophlebitis	inflammation of a vein caused by a clot
thrombosis	formation of a blood clot
thrombus	blood clot
thymectomy	surgical removal of the thymus
thymic hyperplasia	overdevelopment of the thymus
thymoma	tumor of the thymus
thymopathy	disease of the thymus
tonsillectomy	surgical removal of a tonsil
tonsillitis	inflammation of a tonsil
transfusion	infusion into a patient of blood from another source
uremia	presence of urine in the blood

review of terms by roots

Root	Term(s)	
coagul/o	anticoagulant coagulopathy	hypercoagulability
cyt/o	anisocytosis cytapheresis elliptocyte elliptocytosis erythrocyte erythrocytosis leukocyte leukocytosis lymphocyte macrocytosis microcytosis normocyte	oligocythemia pancytopenia phagocytosis poikilocytosis polycythemia reticulocyte spherocyte spherocytosis thrombocyte thrombocytopenia thrombocytosis
-emia	anemia aplastic anemia bilirubinemia hemolytic anemia hyperbilirubinemia hypercholesterolemia hyperlipidemia hypervolemia	hypovolemia iron deficiency anemia ischemia leukemia oligocythemia polycythemia septicemia uremia
hem/o, hemat/o	hematocrit hematology hematoma hematopoiesis hemoglobin hemoglobinopathy	hemolysis hemolytic anemia hemophilia hemorrhage hemostatic
immun/o	autoimmune disease immunocompromised immunodeficiency immunoglobulin	immunologist immunology immunosuppression
leuk/o	leukemia leukocyte	leukocytosis leukopenia
lymph/o	lymphadenectomy lymphadenitis lymphadenopathy lymphadenotomy lymphangiectasia lymphangiogram	lymphangiography lymphangitis lymphedema lymphocyte lymphoma lymphopenia

review of terms by roots *continued*

Root	Term(s)	
myel/o	myelodysplasia myeloma	myelopoiesis osteomyelitis
-penia	leukopenia lymphopenia neutropenia	pancytopenia thrombocytopenia
phleb/o	phlebarteriectasia phlebology phlebotomist	phlebotomy thrombophlebitis
splen/o	asplenia hepatosplenitis hepatosplenomegaly hypersplenism laparosplenectomy nephrosplenopexy splenalgia splenectomy splenectopy	splenitis splenodynia splenolysis splenomalacia splenomegaly splenopathy splenoptosis splenorrhexis
thromb/o	deep vein thrombosis thrombocyte thrombocytopenia thrombocytosis thromboembolism	thrombogenic thrombolytic thrombophlebitis thrombosis thrombus
thym/o	thymectomy thymic hyperplasia	thymoma thymopathy
tonsill/o	tonsillectomy tonsillitis	

other terms

antibody	perfusion
antigen	petechia
apheresis	plasmapheresis
ecchymosis	plateletpheresis
embolism	reperfusion injury
embolus	sphygmomanometer
hypoperfusion	transfusion

The Cardiovascular System—Cardiology 9

Introduction and Overview of the Cardiovascular System

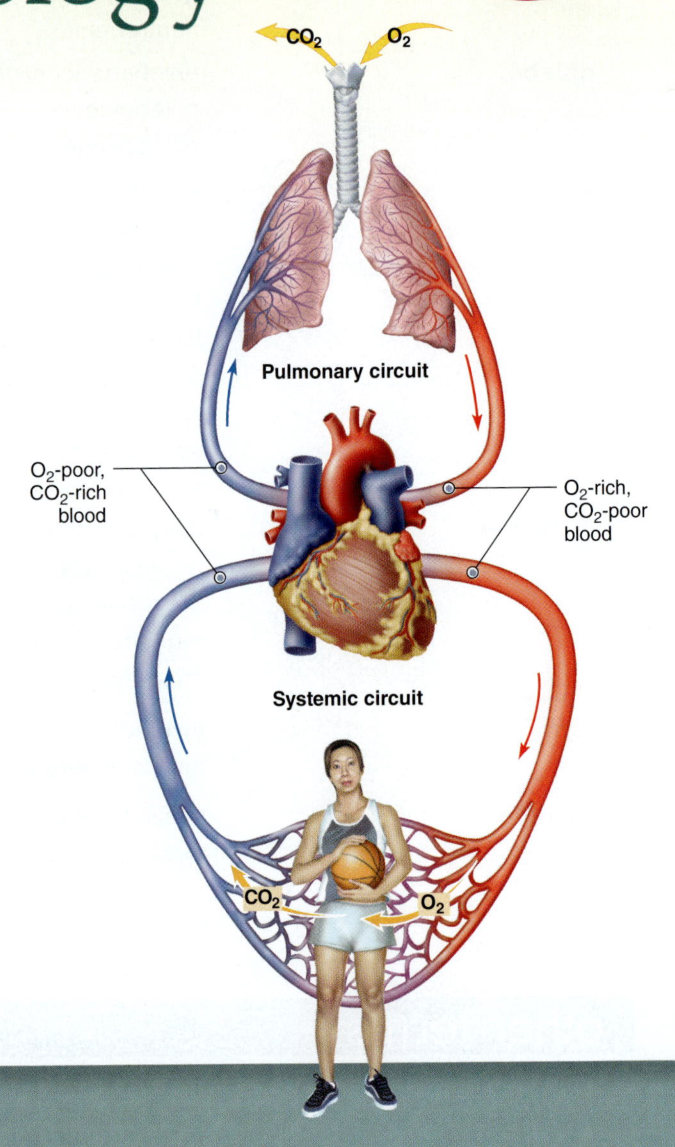

Imagine a large city without roads or transportation of any type. There would be no way for food to get to stores, no access for emergency services to get to people in need of rescue, and no means for trash to be collected. It wouldn't take long for the city to fall into chaos.

The body is much the same. It needs a system to continually deliver fresh supplies to the cells of the body and remove waste. The body also needs a means to deliver chemical messages from one part of the body to another. The cardiovascular system is the body's transport system that provides nourishment, cleanup services, and communication.

There are two parts to the cardiovascular system: the *cardio* (heart) and the *vascular* (blood vessels). The heart is a big pump that squeezes blood out to the body, and the vessels are the tubes that carry the blood. Together, they transport all manner of essential nutrients, blood cells, and chemical signals. They also work together to help rid the body of waste.

learning outcomes

Upon completion of this chapter, you will be able to:

9.1 Identify the **roots/word parts** associated with the **cardiovascular system.**

S **9.2** Translate the **Subjective** terms associated with the **cardiovascular system.**

O **9.3** Translate the **Objective** terms associated with the **cardiovascular system.**

A **9.4** Translate the **Assessment** terms associated with the **cardiovascular system.**

P **9.5** Translate the **Plan** terms associated with the **cardiovascular system.**

9.6 Use **abbreviations** associated with the **cardiovascular system.**

9.7 Distinguish terms associated with the **cardiovascular system** in the context of **electronic health records.**

9.1 Word Parts of the Cardiovascular System

Heart

The heart is the workhorse of this critical transport system. It constantly pumps, getting blood moving to where it needs to go. The heart is divided into four "rooms" or chambers: the left and right receiving rooms (*atria*) and the left and right sending rooms (*ventricles*).

The left side of the heart handles oxygen-rich blood, and the right side handles the oxygen-poor blood. A thick wall of muscle, the *septum,* divides the left and right sides.

Blood constantly cycles between the body and the heart, and it collects in the atria. Blood that has nourished the body and is ready to go to the lungs for more oxygen collects in the right atrium. After getting a fresh supply of oxygen, blood returns to the heart via the left atrium. From the atria, blood—on both sides—passes through the one-way doors of the valves into the ventricles.

In a normal heart, there is no blood flow between the left and right side. There are connections between the atria and ventricles, and between the ventricles and the blood vessels. The connection between each atrium and ventricle is a valve that allows blood to flow in one direction. On the left side, the *mitral valve* connects the left atrium and ventricle. Then the *aortic valve* connects the left ventricle to the outgoing blood vessel, the *aorta.*

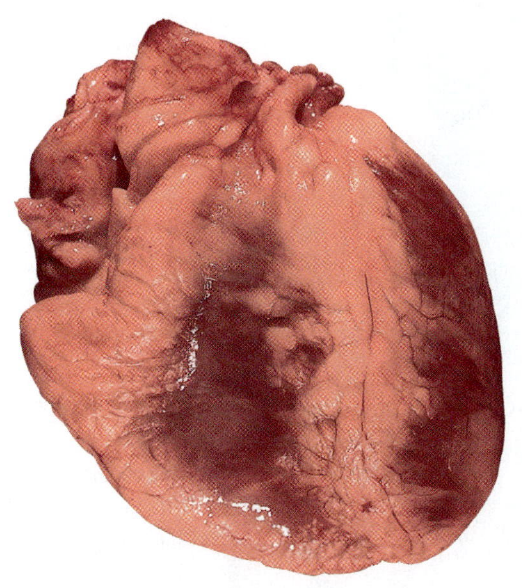

valve

ROOT: ***valvul/o***

EXAMPLES: valvulotomy, valvulitis

NOTES: The heart has four valves: two atrioventricular valves and two valves between the ventricles and arteries. The purpose of heart valves is to prevent blood from flowing backward.

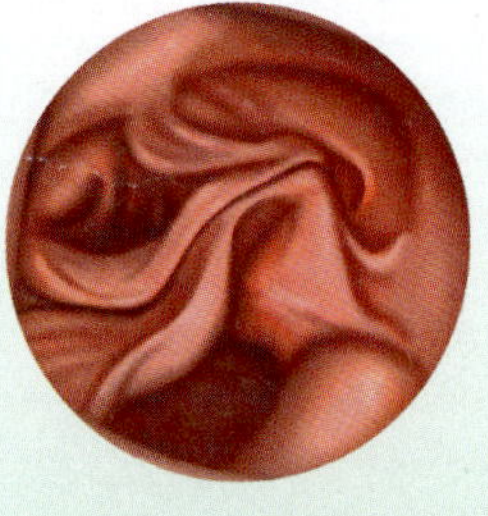

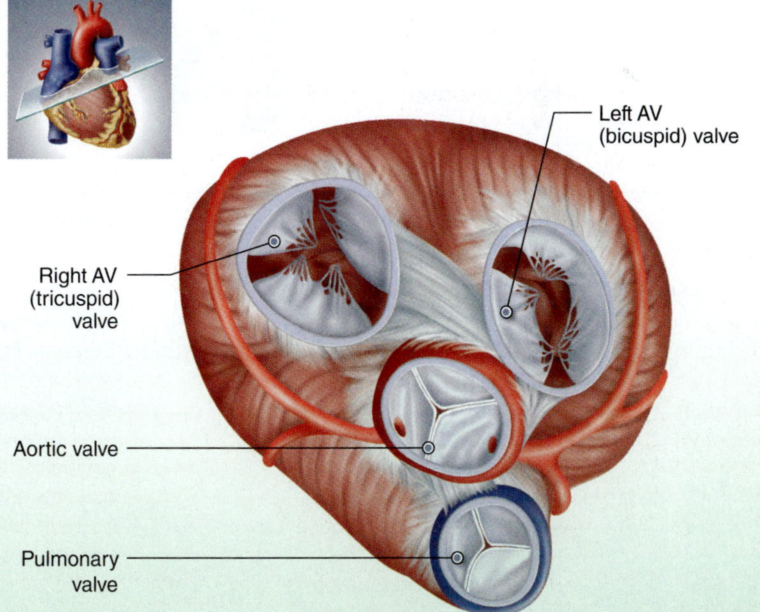

On the right side, the connector between the atrium and ventricle is the *tricuspid valve.* The *pulmonic valve* connects the right ventricle and the outgoing blood vessel, the *pulmonary artery.*

Ventricles are strong and muscular. When the heart compresses, the ventricles force the blood out into the outgoing blood vessels (*arteries*). The right ventricle sends blood to the lungs to get fresh oxygen and to discard excess carbon dioxide. The fresh blood is sent out from the heart by the left ventricle to the rest of the body to provide oxygen and collect the body's carbon dioxide waste.

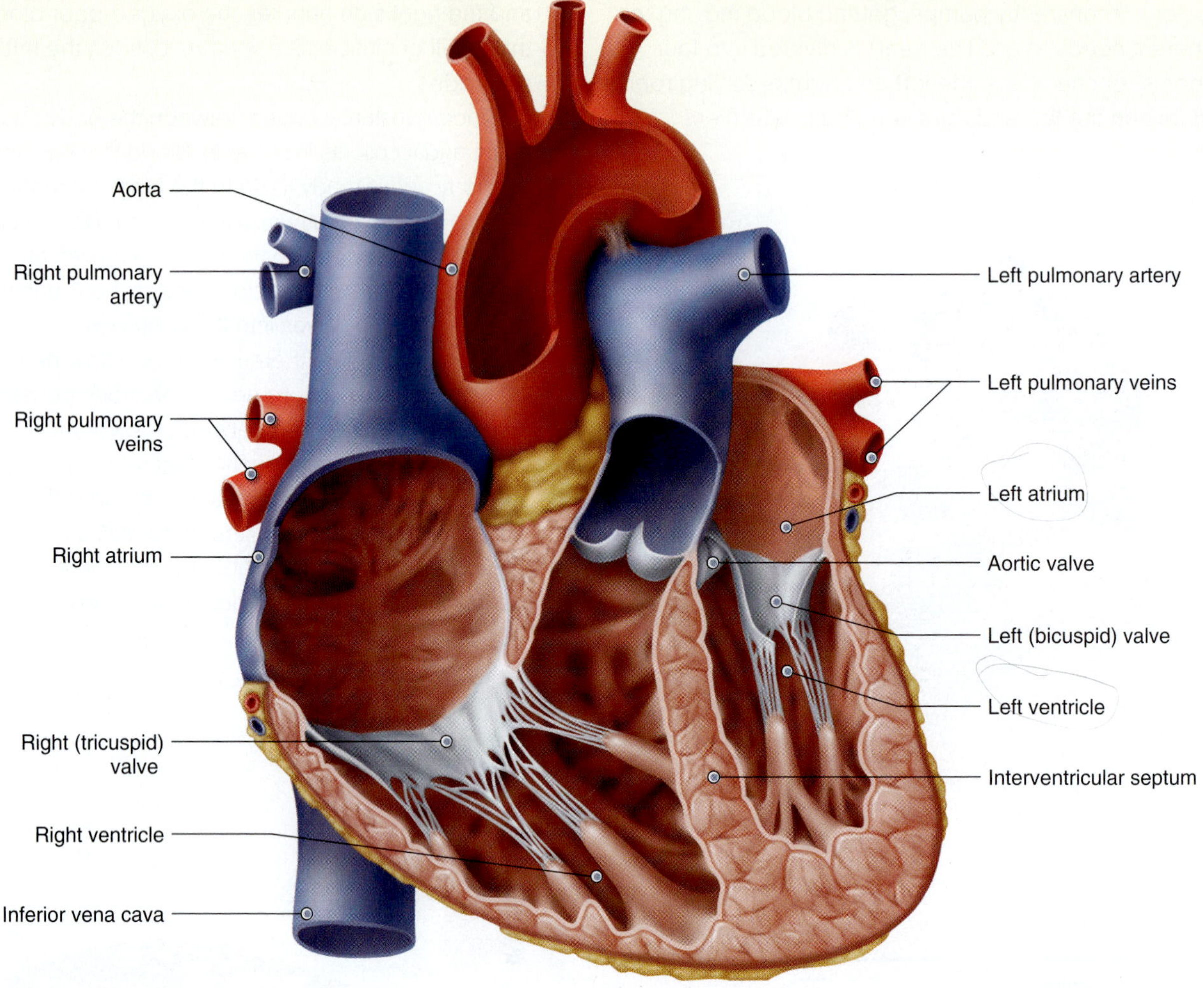

atrium (upper chamber)

ROOT: ***atri/o***

EXAMPLES: atrium, atrial fibrillation

NOTES: The *atrium* is the upper portion of each side of the heart. The term comes from Roman architecture, where it referred to the large open area that was characteristic of most Roman houses; typically, all the other rooms of the house would branch off from this center space. Even today, a large central area in building is often called its *atrium.*

septum (plural: septa)

ROOT: ***sept/o***

EXAMPLES: atrial septal defect, septoplasty

NOTES: *Septum* comes from a Latin word meaning *partition* or *dividing structure* and can refer to any wall dividing two cavities. There are numerous septa throughout the body, including between the two sides of the heart. The easiest to find is the nasal septum. If you place an index finger in each nostril and try to make them touch, what you are feeling is the nasal septum. If you find that your nasal septum leans to one side, you have a deviated septum.

ventricle (lower chamber)

ROOT: ***ventricul/o***

EXAMPLE: ventriculotomy

NOTES: The ventricle is the lower portion of each side of the heart. The word is a combination of *venter* (stomach) plus the diminutive suffix-*icle,* and means *little stomach.*

heart

ROOT: ***cardi/o***

EXAMPLES: cardiology, cardiac arrest, myocarditis

NOTES: The root *cardio* can be tricky because it ends in the double vowel *io*. You expect the *o* to go away sometimes, but when a suffix beginning with an *i* is added to this root, not just the *o*, but also an *i* disappears as well. For example: *myo* (muscle) + *cardio* (heart) + *itis* (inflammation) = myocard-*I*-tis.

heart

ROOT: ***coron/o***

EXAMPLES: coronary artery, coronary thrombosis

NOTES: The term *corona* literally means crown and refers to the way the blood vessels that supply the heart descend and support the heart like a crown. The term *coronary* is in medical language to refer specifically to the heart's blood supply.

Circulation

There are miles of blood vessels in the body. From vessels the size of a garden hose down to tiny capillaries much thinner than a human hair, blood vessels make up a large transportation network that acts like a road system. This system is a closed loop.

The left ventricle forces blood into the main outgoing vessel (*aorta*). The aorta branches into smaller arteries, just as highways have exits to smaller roads. These branches break off further still. Eventually, they reach their destinations: the brain, stomach, muscles, and so on.

By this point, the blood is flowing in tiny vessels known as *capillaries*. The oxygen and other nutrients pass out into the tissues that need it, and they give back their waste.

Once the blood has made the delivery and picked up the waste, it begins its journey back to the heart through veins. Smaller veins collect into larger veins, which collect into the upper (*superior*) and lower (*inferior*) *vena cava*. These main veins return blood to the right atrium.

At the same time that the left ventricle pumps blood into the aorta, the right ventricle pumps blood into the

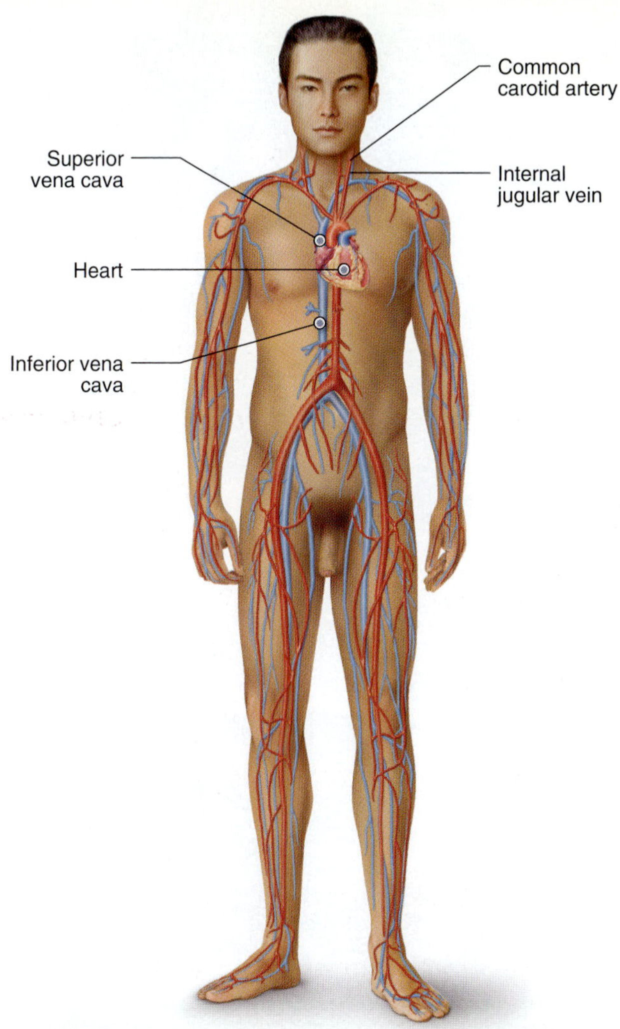

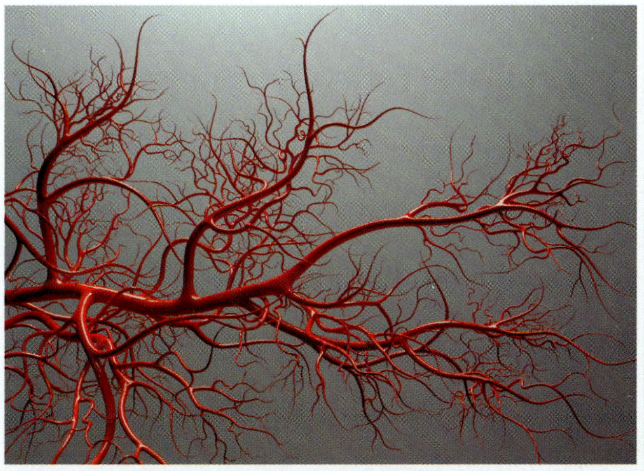

vessel

ROOTS: ***angi/o, vas/o, vascul/o***

EXAMPLES: angioplasty, angiogram, vasodilator, vasculitis

NOTES: All these roots come from words meaning *jar* or *pitcher*. *Angio* comes from Greek, and *vaso* and *vasculo* come from Latin. Although blood vessels don't look like jars, they do hold a lot of liquid—almost 6 quarts in the average man and almost 4 quarts in the average woman.

pulmonary artery. The pulmonary artery carries blood to the lungs to attain oxygen and discard carbon dioxide. Once these gases are traded, the blood returns to the heart through a system of veins that lead to the main *pulmonary vein.* The pulmonary vein dumps the oxygen-rich blood into the left atrium. When the valve opens between the left atrium and left ventricle, the blood fills the ventricle and the cycle continues.

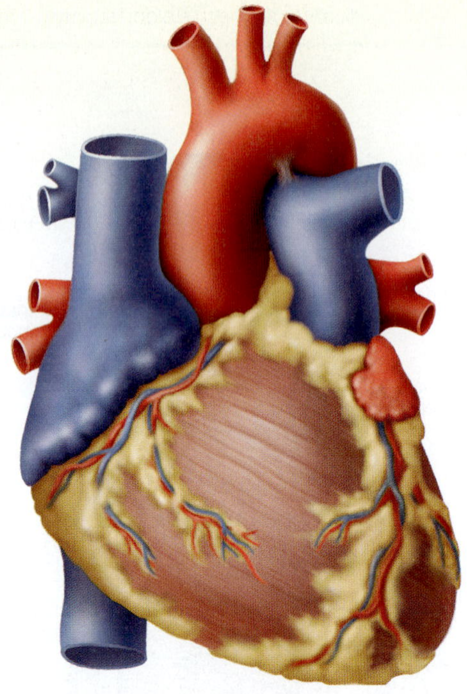

aorta

ROOT: ***aort/o***

EXAMPLES: aortitis, aortolith

NOTES: The *aorta* is the main artery leaving the heart and distributing oxygenated blood throughout the body. Its name means *to rise up* and refers to the fact that as the aorta leaves the heart, it rises up briefly and branches off into the arteries that supply the upper body before making what is called the *arch of the aorta* and descending into the lower body.

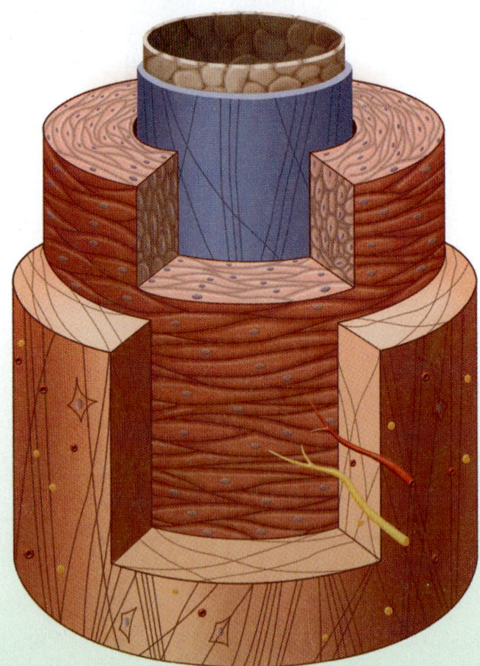

artery

ROOT: ***arteri/o***

EXAMPLES: arteriosclerosis, endarterectomy

NOTES: Arteries are the large blood vessels that carry oxygenated blood from heart to body tissue. It's funny that the word *artery* is actually a Greek word for *trachea* or *windpipe,* a reference to the fact that some of the body's arteries are so large that early students of anatomy thought they carried air.

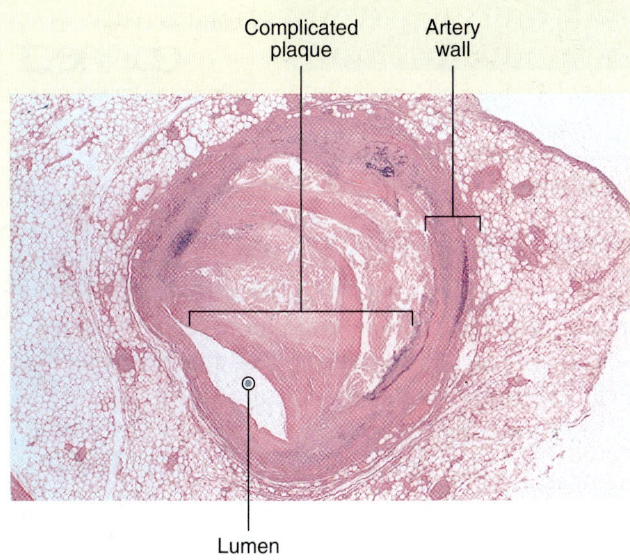

fatty plaque

ROOT: ***ather/o***

EXAMPLE: atherosclerosis

NOTES: This root comes from Greek, for *gruel* or *porridge.* Be careful: This root is easily confused with *arterio,* especially in the words *arteriosclerosis* and *atherosclerosis.* There's another reason for the confusion: atherosclerosis is actually a form of arteriosclerosis. Arteriosclerosis means *hardening of an artery* and atherosclerosis means *hardening of an artery due specifically to build-up of fatty plaque.*

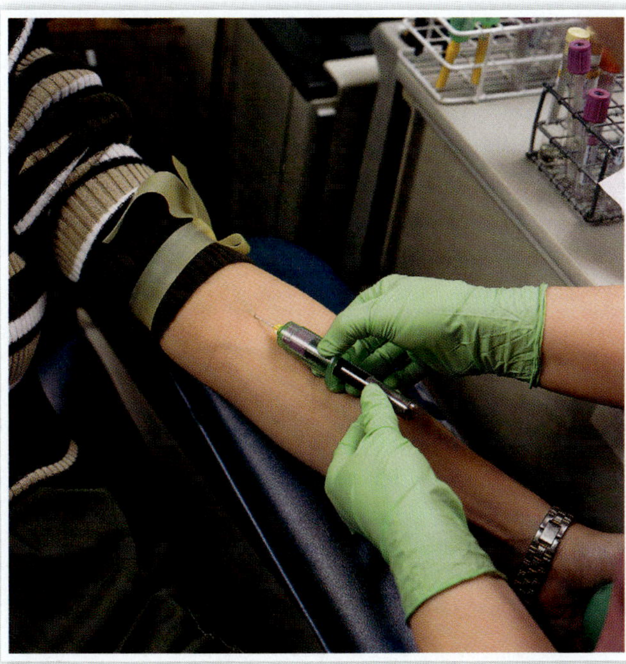

vein

ROOTS: ***phleb/o, ven/o***

EXAMPLES: phlebotomy, venospasm

NOTES: The term *phlebotomy* comes from *phlebo* (vein) and *tomy* (incision). It's the term used for drawing blood. But always make sure you pronounce the word carefully. You don't want to go to the hospital to get some blood drawn (*phlebotomy*) and end up having a portion of your brain removed (*lobotomy*).

Learning Outcome 9.1 Exercises

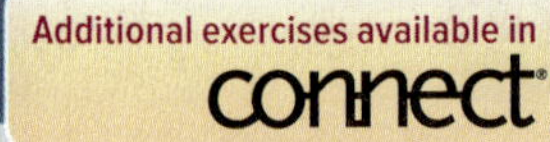
Additional exercises available in
connect

TRANSLATION

EXERCISE 1 *Match the word part on the left with its definition on the right.*

_____ 1. valvul/o

_____ 2. atri/o

_____ 3. ventricul/o

_____ 4. sept/o

_____ 5. coron/o

a. from Latin, for *partition* or *dividing structure;* can refer to any wall dividing two cavities

b. literally means *crown* and refers to the way the blood vessels that supply the heart descend and support the heart like a crown; the term is used in medical language to refer specifically to the heart's blood supply

c. lower chamber of the heart

d. upper chamber of the heart

e. valve

EXERCISE 2 *Translate the following word parts.*

1. cardi/o _____
2. atri/o _____
3. valvul/o _____
4. ventricul/o _____
5. sept/o _____
6. coron/o _____

EXERCISE 3 *Underline and define the word parts from this chapter in the following terms.*

1. cardiac arrest _____
2. endocarditis _____
3. valvuloplasty _____
4. coronary thrombosis _____
5. ventricular septal defect (2 roots) _____
6. atrial septal defect (2 roots) _____

EXERCISE 4 *Break down the following words into their component parts and translate.*

EXAMPLE: sinusitis *sinus | itis inflammation of the sinuses*

1. cardiology _____
2. valvulotomy _____
3. cardiomegaly _____
4. coronary circulation _____
5. atrial septal defect _____
6. ventricular septal defect _____

Learning Outcome 9.1 Exercises

EXERCISE 5 *Match the word part on the left with its definition on the right. Some definitions will be used more than once.*

______ 1. ven/o		a. blood vessel
______ 2. aort/o		b. fatty plaque
______ 3. phleb/o		c. large blood vessels that carry oxygenated blood from heart to body tissue
______ 4. vas/o		d. main artery leaving the heart and distributing oxygenated blood throughout the body
______ 5. vascul/o		e. vein
______ 6. arteri/o		
______ 7. angi/o		
______ 8. ather/o		

EXERCISE 6 *Translate the following word parts.*

1. arteri/o ______________________________
2. aort/o ______________________________
3. ven/o ______________________________
4. vas/o ______________________________
5. vascul/o ______________________________
6. angi/o ______________________________
7. phleb/o ______________________________
8. ather/o ______________________________

EXERCISE 7 *Underline and define the word parts from this chapter in the following terms.*

1. angiosclerosis ______________________________
2. venosclerosis ______________________________
3. atherosclerosis ______________________________
4. phlebosclerosis ______________________________
5. arteriectomy ______________________________
6. aortolith ______________________________
7. vasoconstrictor ______________________________
8. vascular endoscopy ______________________________
9. aortic stenosis ______________________________
10. thrombophlebitis ______________________________
11. superior vena cava ______________________________
12. cardiovascular (2 roots) ______________________________
13. angiocarditis (2 roots) ______________________________
14. coronary artery bypass surgery (2 roots) ______________________________

Learning Outcome 9.1 Exercises

EXERCISE 8 *Break down the following words into their component parts and translate.*

EXAMPLE: sinusitis *sinus | itis inflammation of the sinuses*

1. angioplasty ______
2. aortotomy ______
3. arterioplasty ______
4. atherectomy ______
5. coronary arterectomy ______
6. phlebotomy ______
7. vasculitis ______
8. vasodilator ______
9. venectomy ______

GENERATION

EXERCISE 9 *Identify the roots for the following definitions.*

1. septum ______
2. valve ______
3. ventricle ______
4. atrium ______
5. upper chamber of the heart ______
6. lower chamber of the heart ______
7. heart (2 roots) ______

EXERCISE 10 *Build a medical term from the information provided.*

1. inflammation of the heart (use *cardi/o*) ______
2. inflammation of a heart valve ______
3. heart specialist (use *cardi/o*) ______
4. inflammation of the tissue around the heart (use *cardi/o*) ______

EXERCISE 11 *Identify the roots for the following definitions.*

1. aorta ______
2. artery ______
3. fatty plaque ______
4. vein (2 roots) ______
5. vessel (3 roots) ______

EXERCISE 12 *Build a medical term from the information provided.*

1. record of a vessel (use *angi/o*) ______
2. record of a vein (use ven/o) ______
3. record of the aorta ______
4. record of an artery ______
5. inflammation of a vein ______
6. involuntary contraction of a vessel (use *vas/o*) ______
7. the formation of a fatty plaque (use *-genesis*) ______

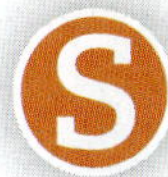

Subjective

Patient History, Problems, Complaints

Heart

Circulation

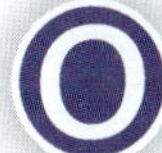

Objective

Observation and Discovery

Heart—structure

Heart

Circulation—structure

Circulation

Diagnostic procedures

Professional terms

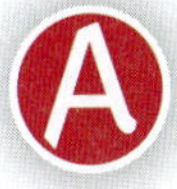

Assessment

Diagnosis and Pathology

Heart

Circulation

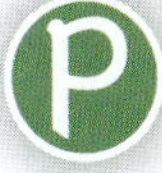

Plan

Treatments and Therapies

Drugs

Heart procedures

Circulation procedures

This section contains medical terms built from the roots presented in the previous section. The purpose of this section is to expose you to words used in cardiology that are built from the word roots presented earlier. The focus of this book is to teach you the process of learning roots and translating them in context. Each term is presented with the correct pronunciation, followed by a word analysis that breaks down the word into its component parts, a definition that provides a literal translation of the word, as well as supplemental information if the literal translation deviates from its medical use.

The terms are organized using a health care professional's SOAP note (first introduced in Chapter 2) as a model.

SUBJECTIVE

9.2 Patient History, Problems, Complaints

The most common heart problem patients report is chest pain (*pectoralgia*). The causes can range from minor issues, like muscle soreness, to the pain associated with a heart attack (*angina pectoris*). Patients can occasionally feel pain in their blood vessels. This is most common with enlarged surface veins (*phlebalgia*).

While the heart never stops beating, we are rarely aware of its rhythm. When the heart beats out of pace, a patient might feel a jumping sensation (*palpitation*). If the heart continues to beat in an odd rhythm (*arrhythmia, dysrhythmia*), a patient may notice this as well.

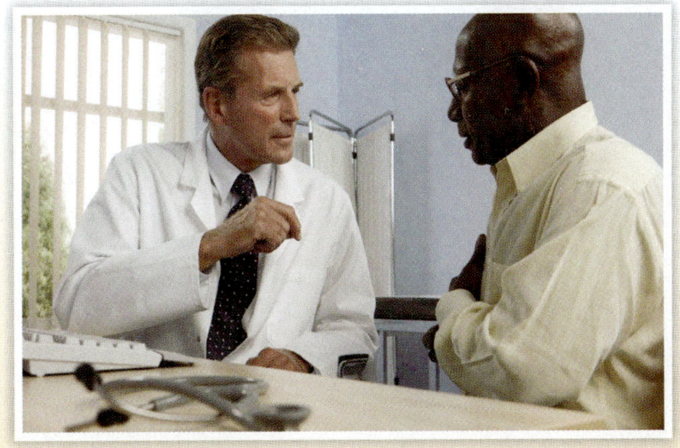

9.2 Patient History, Problems, Complaints

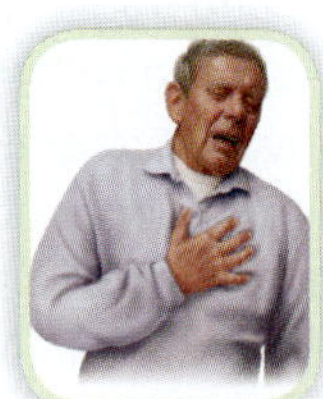
angina pectoris

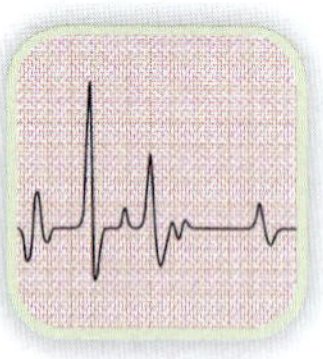
arrhythmia

heart

Term	Word Analysis
angina pectoris an-JAI-nah PEK-tor-is **Definition** oppressive pain in the chest caused by irregular blood flow to the heart	angina pectoris to choke chest
arrhythmia ay-RITH-mee-ah **Definition** irregular heartbeat	a / rrhythm / ia no / rhythm / condition
dysrhythmia dis-RITH-mee-ah **Definition** irregular heartbeat (*arrhythmia* is more common)	dys / rhythm / ia bad / rhythm / condition
palpitation PAL-pih-TAY-shun **Definition** rapid or irregular beating of the heart	from Latin, for *to flutter*
pectoralgia PEK-tor-AL-jah **Definition** chest pain	pector / algia chest / pain

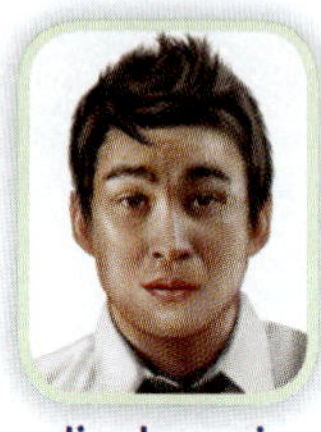
diaphoresis

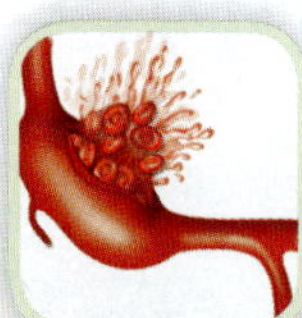
hemorrhage

circulation

Term	Word Analysis
aortalgia AY-or-TAL-jah **Definition** pain in the aorta	aort / algia aorta / pain
diaphoresis DAI-ah-for-EE-sis **Definition** profuse sweating	dia / phoresis through / carry
hemorrhage HEM-oh-RIJ **Definition** loss of blood	hemo / rrhage blood / burst forth
phlebalgia fleh-BAL-jah **Definition** pain in a vein	phleb / algia vein / pain

Learning Outcome 9.2 Exercises

PRONUNCIATION

EXERCISE 1 *Break down the following words into syllables.*

EXAMPLE: synesthesia *syn | es | the | sia*

1. palpitation ______
2. pectoralgia ______
3. hemorrhage ______
4. aortalgia ______
5. diaphoresis ______

EXERCISE 2 *Indicate which syllable is emphasized when pronounced.*

EXAMPLE: bronchitis bron**chi**tis

1. phlebalgia ______
2. dysrhythmia ______
3. arrhythmia ______
4. angina pectoris ______

TRANSLATION

EXERCISE 3 *Break down the following words into their component parts.*

EXAMPLE: nasopharyngoscope *naso | pharyngo | scope*

1. pectoralgia ______
2. aortalgia ______
3. phlebalgia ______
4. arrhythmia ______
5. dysrhythmia ______
6. hemorrhage ______

EXERCISE 4 *Underline and define the word parts from this chapter in the following terms.*

1. aortalgia ______
2. phlebalgia ______
3. hemorrhage ______

Learning Outcome 9.2 Exercises

EXERCISE 5 *Match the term on the left with its definition on the right. Some definitions may be used more than once.*

____ 1. aortalgia	a. oppressive pain in the chest caused by irregular blood flow to the heart
____ 2. phlebalgia	b. chest pain
____ 3. pectoralgia	c. irregular heartbeat
____ 4. arrhythmia	d. loss of blood
____ 5. dysrhythmia	e. pain in a vein
____ 6. palpitation	f. pain in the aorta
____ 7. hemorrhage	g. profuse sweating
____ 8. angina pectoris	h. rapid or irregular beating of the heart
____ 9. diaphoresis	

EXERCISE 6 *Translate the following terms as literally as possible.*

EXAMPLE: nasopharyngoscope *an instrument for looking at the nose and throat*

1. aortalgia ____________________
2. phlebalgia ____________________
3. pectoralgia ____________________
4. arrhythmia ____________________
5. dysrhythmia ____________________
6. angina pectoris ____________________

GENERATION

EXERCISE 7 *Build a medical term from the information provided.*

EXAMPLE: inflammation of the sinuses *sinusitis*

1. pain in a vein (use *phleb/o*) ____________________
2. chest pain ____________________
3. pain in the aorta ____________________
4. no rhythm condition ____________________
5. bad rhythm condition ____________________

S Learning Outcome 9.2 Exercises

EXERCISE 8 *Multiple-choice questions. Select the correct answer(s).*

1. Select the terms that pertain to heartbeat (select all that apply).
   a. angina pectoris
   b. aortalgia
   c. arrhythmia
   d. diaphoresis
   e. hemorrhage
   f. palpitation
   g. pectoralgia
   h. phlebalgia
2. Select the terms that pertain to pain in the heart or chest (select all that apply).
   a. angina pectoris
   b. aortalgia
   c. arrhythmia
   d. diaphoresis
   e. hemorrhage
   f. palpitation
   g. pectoralgia
   h. phlebalgia
3. Which of the following types of pain in the chest is caused by irregular blood flow to the heart?
   a. angina pectoris
   b. diaphoresis
   c. hemorrhage
   d. palpitation
   e. phlebalgia
4. Which of the following terms is from Latin, for *to flutter*?
   a. angina pectoris
   b. diaphoresis
   c. hemorrhage
   d. palpitation
   e. phlebalgia
5. Which of the following terms means *profuse sweating*?
   a. angina pectoris
   b. diaphoresis
   c. hemorrhage
   d. palpitation
   e. phlebalgia
6. Which of the following terms literally means *blood burst forth*?
   a. angina pectoris
   b. diaphoresis
   c. hemorrhage
   d. palpitation
   e. phlebalgia

OBJECTIVE

9.3 Observation and Discovery

During a patient consultation about a heart or circulation problem, the first thing the examiner might notice is a change in the color of the patient's skin. Patients with very poor circulation or low oxygen in their blood may appear a bit blue (*cyanosis*). Generally, cyanosis is seen in emergency situations; it signals the need for immediate action.

While skin color change may not be noted in most cardiac patients, hearts will almost always be examined by measuring patients' vital signs. The two vital signs most closely related to the heart are pulse and blood pressure. As a patient's heart squeezes, it is possible to feel throbbing when placing a finger over certain blood vessels.

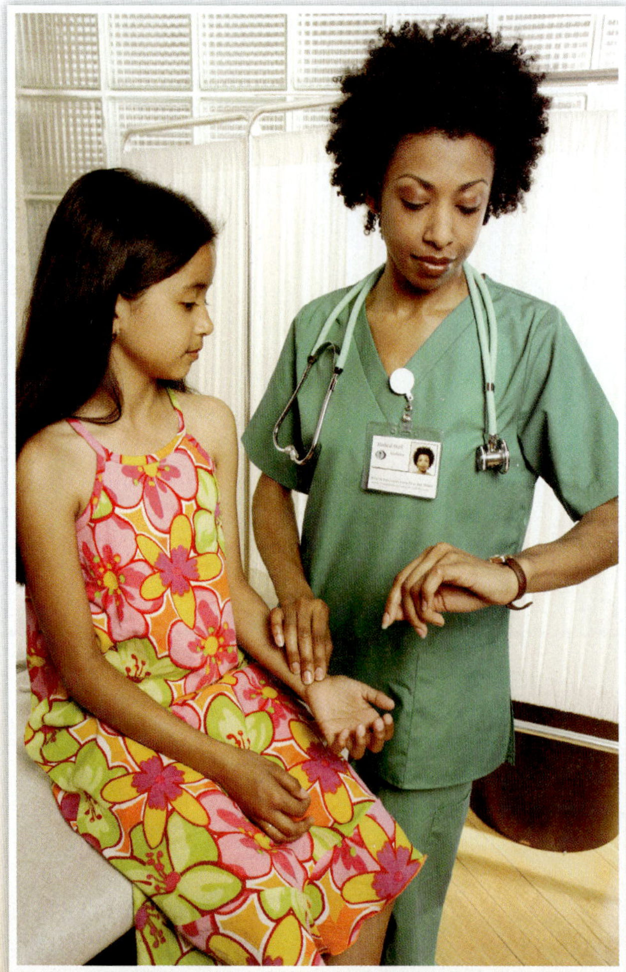

The most basic piece of observable data about the heart is the heart rate, discovered easiest through taking the patient's pulse at the wrist.

This is the *pulse*. A pulse is described as either strong or weak and can be a very helpful indicator in heart health. When a pulse is very weak, it may be an indication of dangerously low blood pressure (*hypotension*).

A pulse reading can also indicate how fast the patient's heart is beating (*heart rate*). If the patient's heart is beating too fast (*tachycardia*) or too slow (*bradycardia*), this may be an indication of disease. The rate at which a heart beats is controlled by electrical signals. The signals travel throughout the heart muscle fibers to get them to work together.

Have you ever noticed that in some houses the water comes out of the shower faster and harder than in others? This is due to differences in water pressure. Blood pressure works in the same way—it measures how strong the flow of blood is in the body. When a patient's heart muscle fibers are contracting and sending blood out of the ventricles, the pressure in the arteries is at its highest. This arterial pressure, the *systole,* is the first number of a blood pressure reading.

The second number of a blood pressure reading is called the *diastole*. It refers to the pressure on the vessels when the heart is relaxed and filling with blood. When a patient's blood vessels are caked with hard deposits, higher pressure is needed to force blood through them. This is the most common cause of high blood pressure (*hypertension*). The blood pressure is another vital sign and is measured by listening to changes in the sound of blood flow through an artery as a special cuff is constricted.

Chief among the means of evaluating the heart is listening directly to the heartbeat. There are two heart sounds that are caused by the closing of valves in the heart. The first heart sound (S1) is due to the closing of the valves between the atria and ventricles. This represents the beginning of heart contraction *(systole)*. Systole ends with closing of the pulmonary and aortic valves, which creates the second heart sound (S2). When listening to the heart, the examiner listens for abnormal sounds *(murmurs)* or a disturbance in the rhythm.

Two very common tests are used to observe the heart: *electrocardiograms* and *echocardiograms*. An electrocardiogram measures the electrical signals in the heart. During the test, electrodes are placed on different parts of a patient's body and measure electrical signals from the heart. One important reason for this test is to

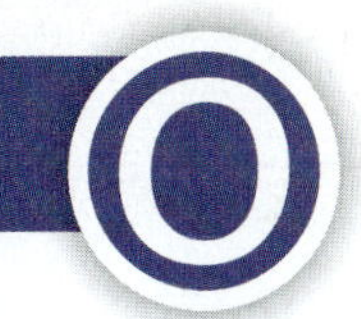

9.3 Observation and Discovery

check for signs of decreased blood flow to the heart (*ischemia*). Sometimes a patient must exercise in order to exhibit these signs (*stress electrocardiogram*).

An echocardiogram uses ultrahigh sound frequencies (*ultrasound*) to watch the heart as it works. With an echocardiogram it is possible to view the layers of the heart (*pericardium, myocardium,* and *endocardium*), the *valves,* and the wall of the heart (*septum*). An examiner can also visualize the flow of blood through the heart. The flow through the valves may be tight (*stenosis*) or may flow back the wrong direction (*regurgitation*).

The most common way to examine blood vessels is to inject dye into the blood and view the results using an x-ray (*angiogram*). This type of study can show all sorts of problems, including deposits of fat (*atherosclerosis*), a floating object that blocks blood flow (*embolus*), a cutoff in blood flow (*occlusion*), or the dilation of a vessel (*ectasia*).

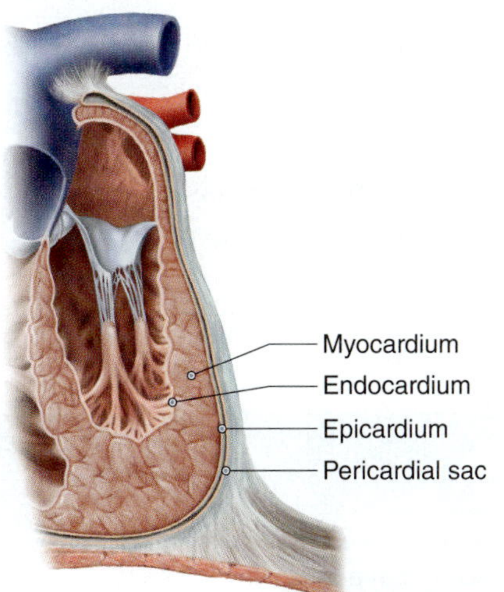

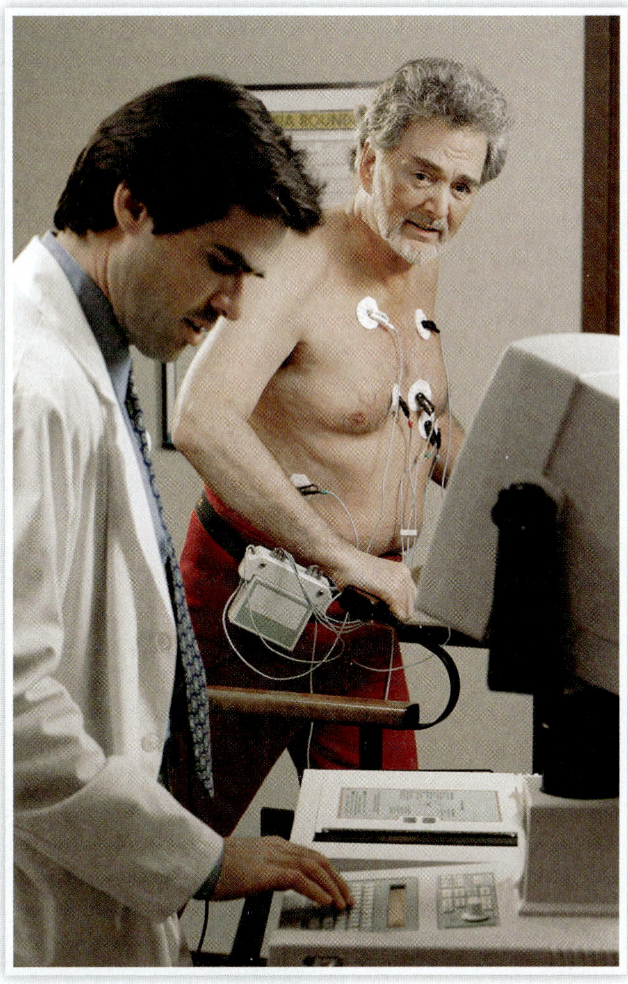

A stress echocardiogram observes the patient's heart while the patient exercises.

heart—structure

Term	Word Analysis
endocardium EN-doh-KAR-dee-um **Definition** tissue lining the inside of the heart	endo / card / ium inside / heart / tissue
epicardium EH-pee- KAR-dee-um **Definition** tissue lining the outside of the heart	epi / card / ium upon / heart / tissue
myocardium MAI-oh-KAR-dee-um **Definition** heart muscle tissue	myo / card / ium muscle / heart / tissue
pericardium PER-ee- KAR-dee-um **Definition** tissue around the heart	peri / card / ium around / heart / tissue

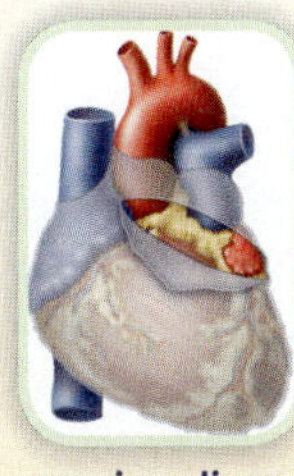

pericardium

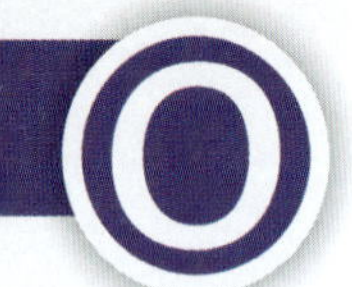

9.3 Observation and Discovery

heart

Term	Word Analysis
bradycardia BRAY-dih- KAR-dee-ah **Definition** slow heartbeat	brady / card / ia slow / heart / condition
cardiomegaly KAR-dee-oh-MEH-gah-lee **Definition** enlarged heart	cardio / megaly heart / enlargement
cardiotoxic KAR-dee-oh-TOK-sik **Definition** poisonous to the heart	cardio / toxic heart / poison
cyanosis SAI-ah-NOH-sis **Definition** bluish appearance to the skin—a sign that the tissue isn't receiving enough oxygen	cyan / osis blue / condition
murmur MIR-mir **Definition** abnormal heart sound	from Latin, for *to grumble or hum*
tachycardia TAK-ih- KAR-dee-ah **Definition** rapid heartbeat	tachy / card / ia fast / heart / condition

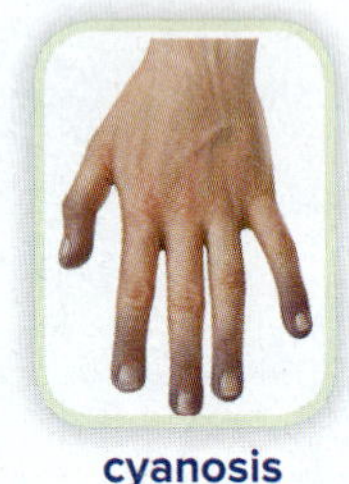

cyanosis

circulation—structure

Term	Word Analysis
vena cava VEE-nah CAY-vah **Definition** large-diameter vein that gathers blood from the body and returns it to the heart	vena cava vein hollow
inferior vena cava in-FEER-ee-or VEE-nah CAY-vah **Definition** portion of the vena cava that gathers blood from the lower portion of the body	inferior vena cava lower vein hollow

circulation—structure *continued*

Term	Word Analysis		
superior vena cava soo-PEER-ee-or VEE-nah CAY-vah	superior upper	vena vein	cava hollow

Definition portion of the vena cava that gathers blood from the upper portion of the body (head and arms)

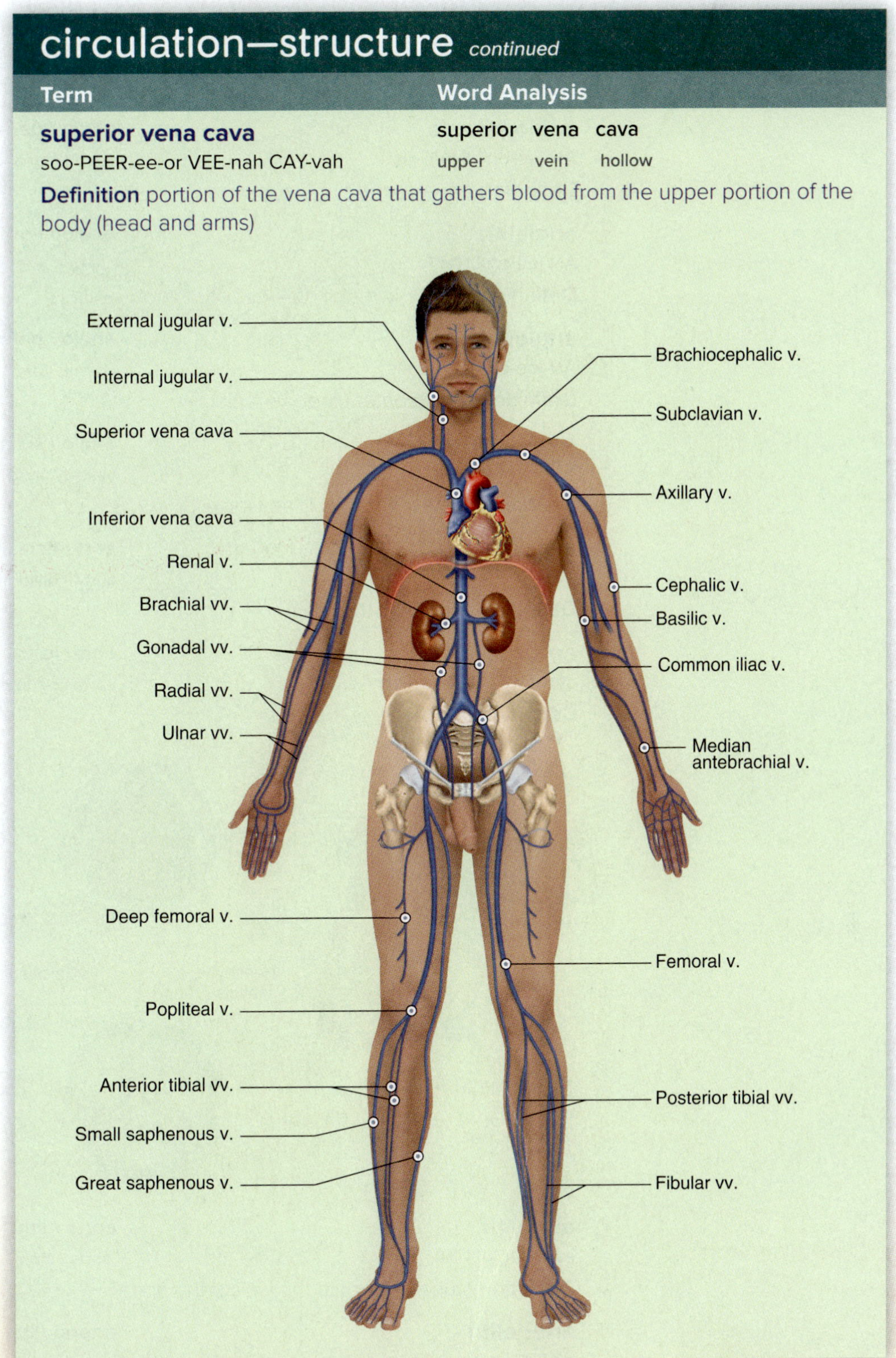

9.3 Observation and Discovery

circulation

Term	Word Analysis
angiogenesis AN-jee-oh-JIN-eh-sis **Definition** development of blood vessels	angio / genesis vessel / creation
angiolith AN-jee-oh-LITH **Definition** stone forming in the wall of a blood vessel	angio / lith vessel / stone
angiopoiesis AN-jee-oh-poh-EE-sis **Definition** formation of blood vessels	angio / poiesis vessel / formation
angiosclerosis AN-jee-oh-skleh-ROH-sis **Definition** hardening of a blood vessel	angio / scler / osis vessel / hard / condition
aortectasia ay-OR-tek-TAY-zhah **Definition** dilation of the aorta	aort / ectasia aorta / dilation
aortic stenosis ay-OR-tik stih-NOH-sis **Definition** narrowing of the aorta	aort / ic sten / osis aorta / pertaining to narrow / condition
aortolith ay-OR-toh-LITH **Definition** stone deposit in the wall of the aorta	aorto / lith aorta / stone
arteriolith ar-TER-ee-oh-LITH **Definition** stone in the artery	arterio / lith artery / stone

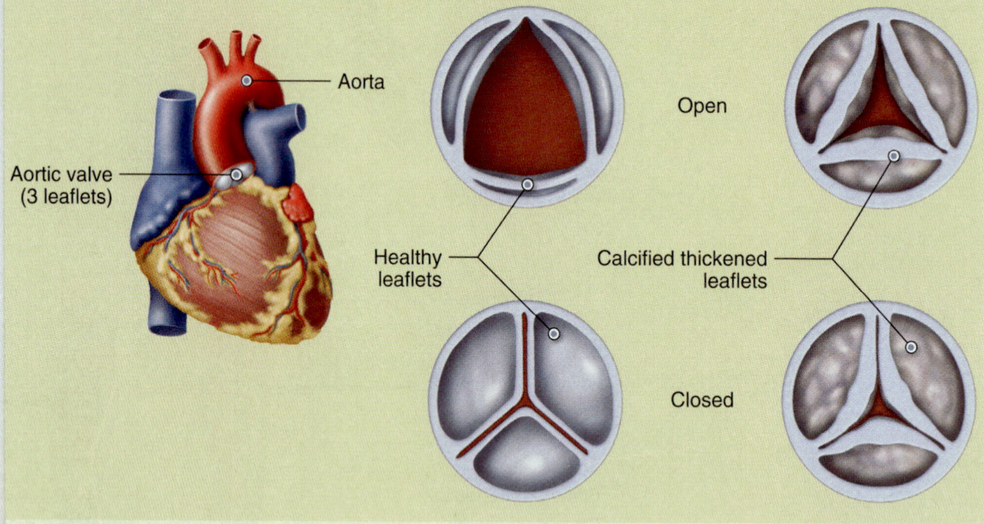

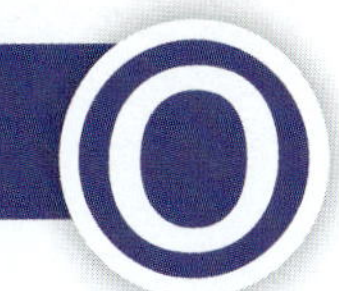

9.3 Observation and Discovery

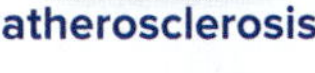

atherosclerosis

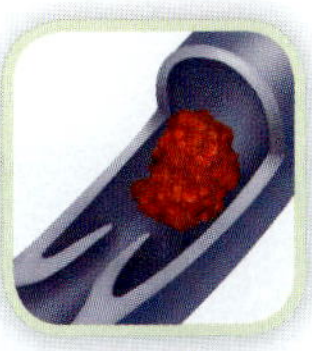
embolism

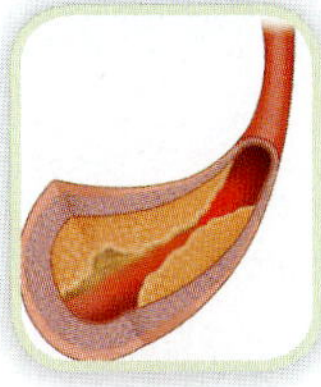
occlusion

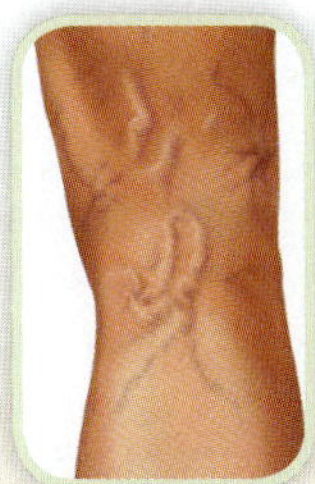
varicose veins

circulation *continued*

Term	Word Analysis
arteriorrhexis ar-TER-ee-oh-REK-sis **Definition** rupture of an artery	arterio / rrhexis artery / rupture
arteriosclerosis ar-TER-ee-oh-skleh-ROH-sis **Definition** hardening of an artery	arterio / scler / osis artery / hard / condition
atherogenesis A-ther-oh-JIN-eh-sis **Definition** formation of fatty plaque on the wall of an artery	athero / genesis fatty plaque / creation
atherosclerosis A-ther-oh-skleh-ROH-sis **Definition** hardening of an artery due to build-up of fatty plaque	athero / scler / osis fatty plaque / hard / condition
embolus EM-boh-lus **Definition** mass of matter present in the blood **Note:** In Greek, this word was used to mean *stopper*, as in the opening of a bottle.	em / bolus in / throw
embolism EM-boh-LIZ-um **Definition** blockage in a blood vessel caused by an embolus	embol / ism embolus / condition
ischemia ih-SKEE-mee-ah **Definition** blockage of blood flow to an organ	isch / emia hold back / blood condition
occlusion oh-KLOO-zhun **Definition** closing or blockage of a passage	from Latin, for *to close off*
phlebosclerosis FLEB-oh-skleh-ROH-sis **Definition** hardening of a vein	phlebo / scler / osis vein / hard / condition
thrombus THROM-bus **Definition** blood clot **Note:** The difference between a thrombus and an embolus is twofold. A *thrombus* is a clot of blood and is stationary. An *embolus* is foreign material and is in motion. When a thrombus breaks off, it becomes a *thromboembolus*.	from Greek, for *lump, clot,* or even *curd of milk*
varicose veins VAR-ih-kohs VAYNS **Definition** an enlarged, dilated vein toward the surface of the skin	varicose veins swollen / twisted veins

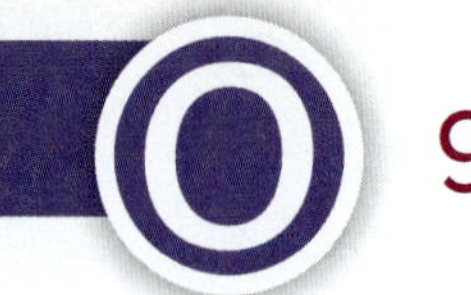

9.3 Observation and Discovery

circulation *continued*

Term	Word Analysis
vasospasm VAS-oh-SPAZ-um **Definition** involuntary contraction of a blood vessel	**vaso / spasm** vessel / involuntary contraction
venosclerosis VEE-noh-skleh-ROH-sis **Definition** hardening of a vein	**veno / scler / osis** vein / hard / condition
venospasm VEE-noh-SPAZ-um **Definition** involuntary contraction of a vein	**veno / spasm** vein / involuntary contraction
venostasis VEE-noh-STA-sis **Definition** trapping of blood in an extremity due to compression **NOTE:** This name refers not to the fact that the blood is trapped but, instead, to the fact that the blood is standing still and not moving.	**veno / stasis** vein / standing

diagnostic procedures

Term	Word Analysis
angiogram AN-jee-oh-GRAM **Definition** record of the blood vessels	**angio / gram** vessel / record
angiography AN-jee-AW-grah-fee **Definition** procedure to describe the blood vessels	**angio / graph / y** vessel / writing / procedure
angioscope AN-jee-oh-SKOWP **Definition** device for looking into a blood vessel	**angio / scope** vessel / device for looking
aortogram ay-OR-tah-GRAM **Definition** record of the aorta	**aorto / gram** aorta / record
arteriogram ar-TER-ee-oh-GRAM **Definition** record of an artery	**arterio / gram** artery / record

diagnostic procedures *continued*

Term	Word Analysis
cardiac catheterization KAR-dee-ak KATH-eh-ter-ih-ZAY-shun	cardi / ac — catheter / ization heart / pertaining to — catheter / procedure
Definition process of inserting a tube (catheter) into the heart NOTE: The word *catheter* comes from Greek words meaning *to go inside*. By passing a tube through arteries, doctors are able to diagnose and treat heart problems without performing major surgery.	
echocardiogram EK-oh-KAR-dee-oh-GRAM	echo / cardio / gram echo / heart / record
Definition image of the heart produced using sound waves; the same procedure as an ultrasound performed on pregnant women, but instead it is performed on a heart	
echocardiography EK-oh-KAR-dee-AW-grah-fee	echo / cardio / graph / y echo / heart / writing / procedure
Definition use of sound waves to produce an image of the heart; the same procedure as an ultrasound performed on pregnant women, but instead it is performed on a heart	
electrocardiogram eh-LEK-troh-KAR-dee-oh-GRAM	electro / cardio / gram electricity / heart / record
Definition record of the electrical currents of the heart	
electrocardiography eh-LEK-troh-KAR-dee- AW-grah-fee	electro / cardio / graph / y electricity / heart / writing / procedure
Definition procedure for recording the electrical currents of the heart	
sonography saw-NAW-grah-fee	sono / graph / y sound / writing / procedure
Definition use of sound waves to produce diagnostic images; also called ultrasound	
stress electrocardiogram stres eh-LEK-troh-KAR-dee-oh-GRAM	stress electro / cardio / gram stress electricity / heart / record
Definition image of the heart produced using sound waves while the patient experiences increases of exercise stress	
transesophageal echocardiogram TRANZ-eh-SOF-ah-JEE-al EK-oh-KAR-dee-oh-GRAM	trans / esophag / eal through / esophagus / pertaining to echo / cardio / gram echo / heart / record
Definition record of the heart using sound waves performed by inserting the sonograph into the esophagus	
vascular endoscopy VAS-kyoo-lar en-DAW-skoh-pee	vascul / ar — endo / scop / y vessel / pertaining to — inside / looking / procedure
Definition procedure to look inside a blood vessel	
venogram VEE-noh-gram	veno / gram vein / record
Definition record of a vein	

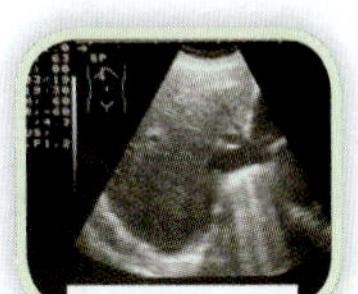
echocardiogram

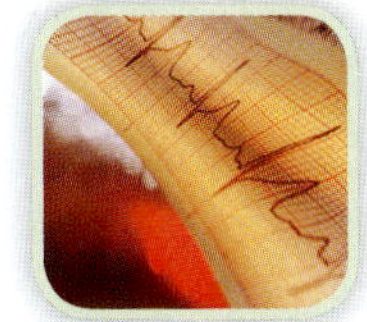
electrocardiogram

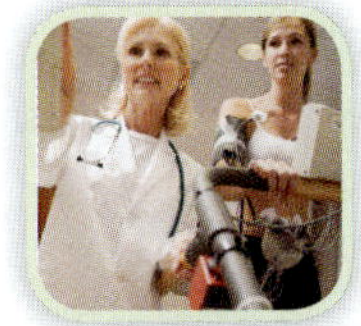
stress electrocardiogram

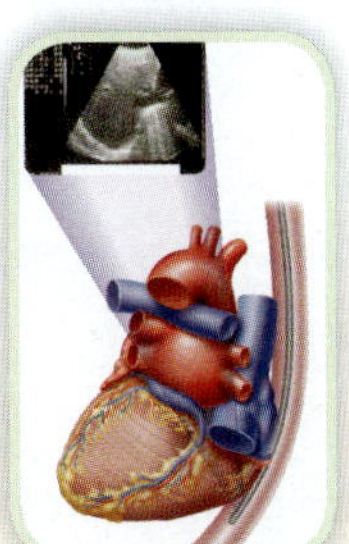
transesophageal echocardiogram

9.3 Observation and Discovery

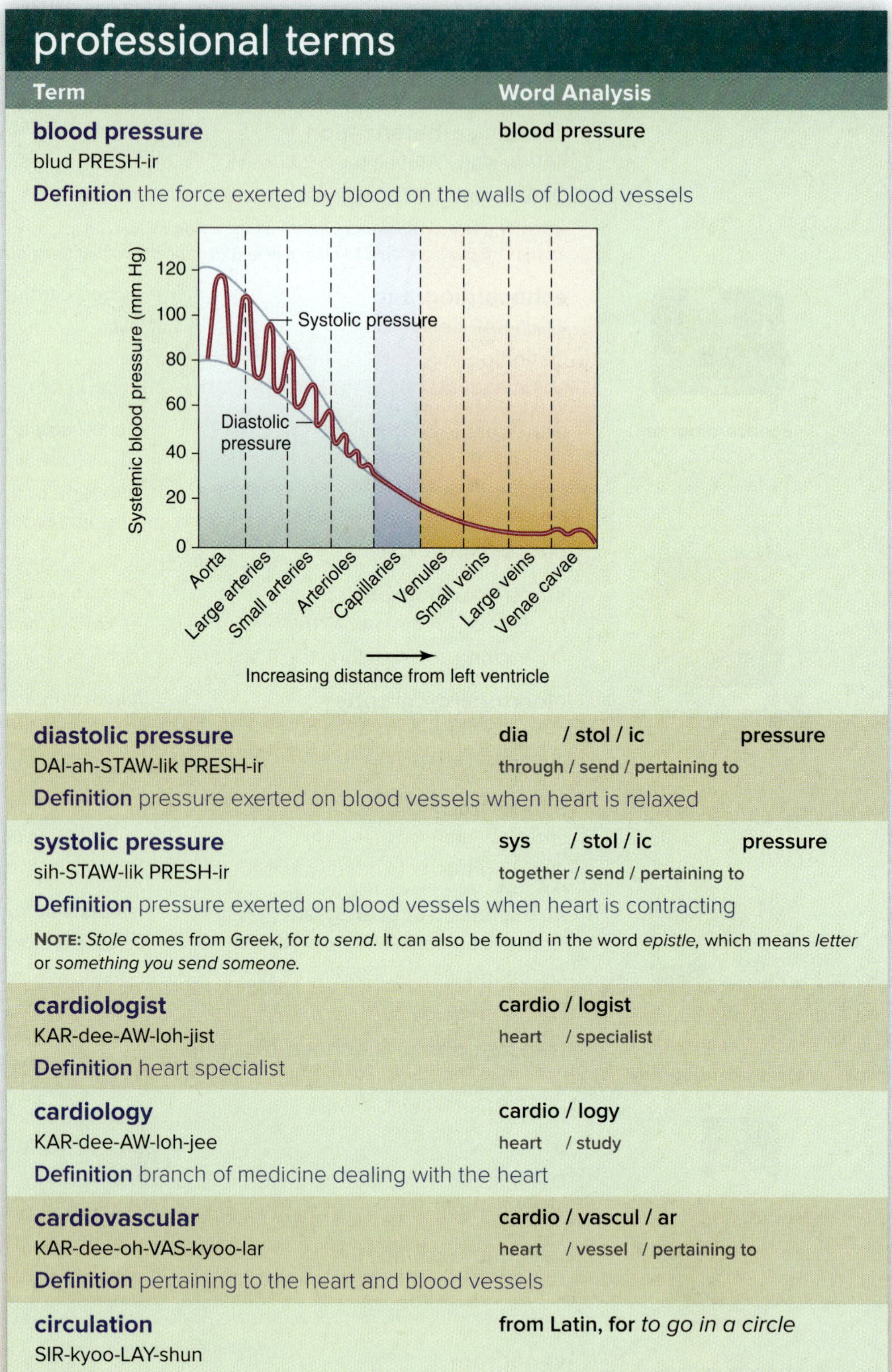

professional terms

Term	Word Analysis
blood pressure blud PRESH-ir **Definition** the force exerted by blood on the walls of blood vessels	blood pressure

Term	Word Analysis
diastolic pressure DAI-ah-STAW-lik PRESH-ir **Definition** pressure exerted on blood vessels when heart is relaxed	**dia / stol / ic pressure** through / send / pertaining to
systolic pressure sih-STAW-lik PRESH-ir **Definition** pressure exerted on blood vessels when heart is contracting **NOTE:** *Stole* comes from Greek, for *to send.* It can also be found in the word *epistle,* which means *letter* or *something you send someone.*	**sys / stol / ic pressure** together / send / pertaining to
cardiologist KAR-dee-AW-loh-jist **Definition** heart specialist	**cardio / logist** heart / specialist
cardiology KAR-dee-AW-loh-jee **Definition** branch of medicine dealing with the heart	**cardio / logy** heart / study
cardiovascular KAR-dee-oh-VAS-kyoo-lar **Definition** pertaining to the heart and blood vessels	**cardio / vascul / ar** heart / vessel / pertaining to
circulation SIR-kyoo-LAY-shun **Definition** moving of blood from the heart through the vessels and back to the heart	**from Latin, for** ***to go in a circle***

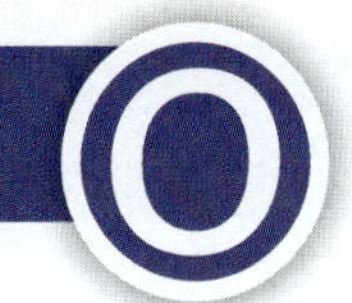

professional terms *continued*

Term	Word Analysis
coronary circulation KOR-ah-NAR-ee SIR-kyoo-LAY-shun **Definition** circulation of blood from the heart to the heart muscle (the heart always feeds itself first)	coron / ary circulation heart / pertaining to
pulmonary circulation PUL-mon-AR-ee SIR-kyoo-LAY-shun **Definition** circulation of blood from the heart to the lungs (to oxygenate it)	pulmon / ary circulation lung / pertaining to
systemic circulation sih-STEM-ik SIR-kyoo-LAY-shun **Definition** circulation of blood from the heart to the rest of the body	sys / stem / ic circulation together / stand / pertaining to
phlebologist fleb-AW-loh-jist **Definition** specialist in veins	phlebo / logist vein / specialist
phlebology fleb-AW-loh-jee **Definition** study of veins	phlebo / logy vein / study
phlebotomist fleh-BAW-toh-mist **Definition** one who draws blood	phlebo / tom / ist vein / incision / specialist
phlebotomy fleh-BAW-toh-mee **Definition** incision into a vein—the technical term for drawing blood	phlebo / tom / y vein / incision / procedure

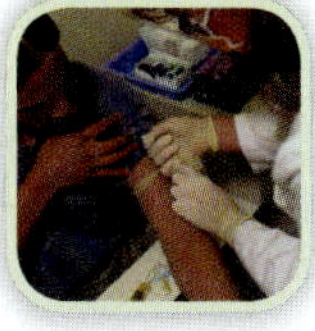

phlebotomist

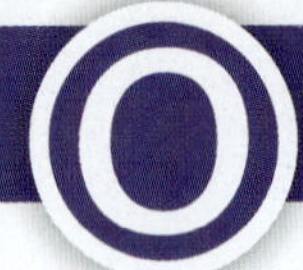

Learning Outcome 9.3 Exercises

PRONUNCIATION

EXERCISE 1 *Break down the following words into syllables.*

EXAMPLE: synesthesia *syn | es | the | sia*

1. circulation ______
2. embolism ______
3. cardiology ______
4. cardiovascular ______
5. angiolith ______
6. aortolith ______
7. arteriolith ______
8. angiogram ______
9. aortogram ______
10. arteriogram ______
11. angioscope ______
12. aortectasia ______
13. superior vena cava ______
14. venostasis ______
15. atherogenesis ______
16. venosclerosis ______
17. atherosclerosis ______
18. phlebosclerosis ______
19. arteriosclerosis ______
20. diastolic pressure ______
21. systolic pressure ______
22. pulmonary circulation ______
23. cardiac catheterization ______
24. echocardiogram ______
25. electrocardiogram ______

EXERCISE 2 *Indicate which syllable is emphasized when pronounced.*

EXAMPLE: bronchitis bron**chi**tis

1. murmur ______
2. thrombus ______
3. embolus ______

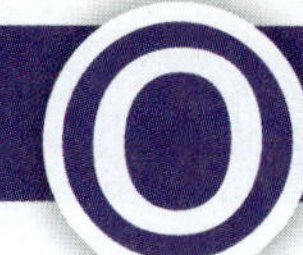

Learning Outcome 9.3 Exercises

4. venogram ______
5. phlebology ______
6. ischemia ______
7. occlusion ______
8. phlebotomist ______
9. phlebotomy ______
10. varicose veins ______
11. aortic stenosis ______
12. vascular endoscopy ______

TRANSLATION

EXERCISE 3 *Break down the following words into their component parts.*

EXAMPLE: synesthesia *syn | es | the | sia*

1. cardiology ______
2. phlebology ______
3. angiography ______
4. sonography ______
5. cardiotoxic ______
6. cyanosis ______
7. phlebotomist ______
8. angiogenesis ______
9. atherogenesis ______
10. aortic stenosis ______
11. echocardiography ______
12. electrocardiography ______

EXERCISE 4 *Underline and define the word parts from this chapter in the following terms.*

1. cardiologist ______
2. phlebologist ______
3. cardiomegaly ______
4. angiogram ______
5. aortogram ______
6. arteriogram ______
7. venogram ______
8. angiopoiesis ______

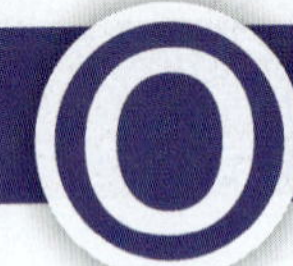

9. aortectasia ______
10. venostasis ______
11. phlebotomy ______
12. arteriorrhexis ______
13. atherosclerosis ______
14. vena cava ______
15. echocardiogram ______
16. electrocardiogram ______
17. stress electrocardiogram ______
18. transesophageal echocardiogram ______
19. vascular endoscopy ______
20. cardiovascular (2 roots) ______
21. coronary circulation ______

EXERCISE 5 *Select the correct option for each given translation.*

EXAMPLE: hypoglycemia *hypo over | under glyc salt | sugar -emia blood | urine condition*

1. *tachycardia* = fast/slow (*tachy*) + heart condition (*cardia*)
2. *bradycardia* = fast/slow (*brady*) + heart condition (*cardia*)
3. *venospasm* = artery/blood vessel/vein (*veno*) + involuntary contraction (*spasm*)
4. *vasospasm* = artery/blood vessel/vein (*vaso*) + involuntary contraction (*spasm*)
5. *arteriosclerosis* = artery/blood vessel/vein (*arterio*) + hard condition (*sclerosis*)
6. *venosclerosis* = artery/blood vessel/vein (*veno*) + hard condition (*sclerosis*)
7. *phlebosclerosis* = artery/blood vessel/vein (*phlebo*) + hard condition (*sclerosis*)
8. *angiosclerosis* = artery/blood vessel/vein (*angio*) + hard condition (*sclerosis*)

EXERCISE 6 *Fill in the blanks.*

1. *angioscope* = device for looking into a(n) ______
2. *aortolith* = stone forming in the wall of the ______
3. *arteriolith* = stone forming in a(n) ______
4. *angiolith* = stone forming in the wall of a(n) ______
5. *myocardium* = heart ______ tissue
6. *pericardium* = tissue ______ the heart
7. *endocardium* = tissue lining the ______ of the heart
8. *epicardium* = tissue lining the ______ of the heart

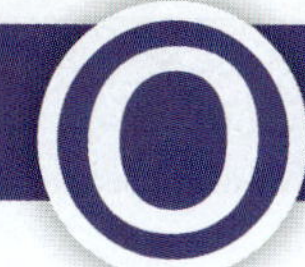

Learning Outcome 9.3 Exercises

EXERCISE 7 *Match the term on the left with its definition on the right.*

h	1. blood pressure	a.	abnormal heart sound
i	2. circulation	b.	blood clot; from Greek, for *lump, clot,* or even *curd of milk*
a	3. murmur	c.	bluish appearance to the skin; a sign that the tissue isn't receiving enough oxygen
c	4. cyanosis	d.	mass of matter present in the blood; from Greek, for *stopper,* as in the opening of a bottle
e	5. varicose veins	e.	enlarged, dilated vein toward the surface of the skin
g	6. occlusion	f.	blockage of blood flow to an organ
f	7. ischemia	g.	closing or blockage of a passage; from Latin, for *to close off*
j	8. cardiac catheterization	h.	force exerted by blood on the walls of blood vessels
d	9. embolus	i.	moving of blood from the heart through the vessels and back to the heart
b	10. thrombus	j.	process of inserting a tube into the heart

EXERCISE 8 *Translate the following terms as literally as possible.*

EXAMPLE: nasopharyngoscope *an instrument for looking at the nose and throat*

1. cardiovascular ______
2. cardiotoxic ______
3. angiogenesis ______
4. endocardium ______
5. epicardium ______
6. myocardium ______
7. pericardium ______
8. bradycardia ______
9. tachycardia ______
10. angiography ______
11. sonography ______
12. atherosclerosis ______
13. angiopoiesis ______
14. arteriorrhexis ______
15. cyanosis ______
16. inferior vena cava ______
17. superior vena cava ______
18. vascular endoscopy ______

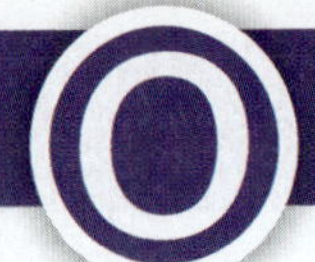

Learning Outcome 9.3 Exercises

GENERATION

EXERCISE 9 *Build a medical term from the information provided.*

EXAMPLE: inflammation of the sinuses *sinusitis*

1. study of veins (use *phleb/o*) ______
2. study of the heart ______
3. record of a vein (use *ven/o*) ______
4. record of the blood vessels (use *angi/o*) ______
5. record of the aorta ______
6. record of an artery ______
7. hardening of a blood vessel (use *angi/o*) ______
8. hardening of a vein (use *phleb/o*) ______
9. hardening of a vein (use *ven/o*) ______
10. hardening of an artery ______
11. involuntary contraction of a blood vessel (use *vas/o*) ______
12. involuntary contraction of a vein (use *ven/o*) ______
13. device for looking into a blood vessel (use *angi/o*) ______
14. vessel stone (use *angi/o*) ______
15. enlarged heart ______
16. fatty plaque creation ______
17. record of the electrical currents of the heart ______

EXERCISE 10 *Multiple-choice questions. Select the correct answer(s).*

1. A *stress electrocardiogram* is
   a. a record of the heart using sound waves performed by inserting the sonograph into the esophagus
   b. an image of the heart produced using sound waves while the patient experiences increases of exercise stress
   c. a procedure to look inside blood vessels that are currently undergoing stress
   d. none of these

2. A *transesophageal echocardiogram* is
   a. a record of the heart using sound waves performed by inserting the sonograph into the esophagus
   b. an image of the heart produced using sound waves while the patient experiences increases of exercise stress
   c. a procedure to look inside blood vessels that are currently undergoing stress
   d. none of these

3. Which of the following statements about the term *echocardiogram* is true? (select all that apply)
   a. image of heart produced using sound waves
   b. image of the heart produced using electrical currents
   c. procedure to look inside blood vessels
   d. ultrasound of the heart

Learning Outcome 9.3 Exercises

4. *Circulation* is (select all that apply)
   a. from Latin, for *to go in a circle*
   b. the force exerted by blood on the walls of vessels
   c. the moving of blood from the heart through the vessels and back to the heart
   d. none of these
5. *Systemic circulation* is
   a. circulation of blood from the heart to the heart muscle
   b. circulation of blood from the heart to the lungs
   c. circulation of blood from the heart to the rest of the body
   d. all of these
6. *Pulmonary circulation* is
   a. circulation of blood from the heart to the heart muscle
   b. circulation of blood from the heart to the lungs
   c. circulation of blood from the heart to the rest of the body
   d. all of these
7. *Coronary circulation* is
   a. circulation of blood from the heart to the heart muscle
   b. circulation of blood from the heart to the lungs
   c. circulation of blood from the heart to the rest of the body
   d. all of these
8. *Blood pressure* is (select all that apply)
   a. from Latin, for *to go in a circle*
   b. the force exerted by blood on the walls of vessels
   c. the moving of blood from the heart through the vessels and back to the heart
   d. none of these
9. *Diastolic pressure* is
   a. the force exerted on blood vessels when the heart is contracting
   b. the pressure exerted on blood vessels when the heart is relaxed
   c. both the force exerted on blood vessels when the heart is contracting and the pressure exerted on blood vessels when the heart is relaxed
   d. none of these
10. *Systolic pressure* is
   a. the force exerted on blood vessels when the heart is contracting
   b. the pressure exerted on blood vessels when the heart is relaxed
   c. both the force exerted on blood vessels when the heart is contracting and the pressure exerted on blood vessels when the heart is relaxed
   d. none of these

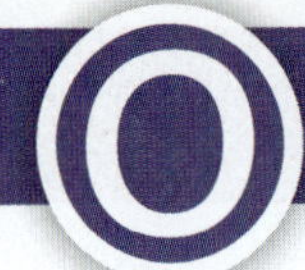

Learning Outcome 9.3 Exercises

11. The *inferior vena cava* is the (select all that apply)
    a. portion of the vena cava that gathers blood from the lower portion of the body
    b. portion of the vena cava that gathers blood from the upper portion of the body (head and arms)
    c. large-diameter vein that gathers blood from the body and returns it to the heart
    d. none of these
12. The *superior vena cava* is the (select all that apply)
    a. portion of the vena cava that gathers blood from the lower portion of the body
    b. portion of the vena cava that gathers blood from the upper portion of the body (head and arms)
    c. large-diameter vein that gathers blood from the body and returns it to the heart
    d. none of these
13. A blockage in a blood vessel caused by a mass of matter present in the blood is known as a(n)
    a. atherosclerosis
    b. embolism
    c. thrombus
    d. venostasis
14. The trapping of blood in an extremity due to compression is known as
    a. atherosclerosis
    b. embolism
    c. thrombus
    d. venostasis
15. An abnormal heart sound is a
    a. cardiac anomaly
    b. cardiophony
    c. coronary anomaly
    d. murmur
16. Which of the following statements about the term *cardiac catheterization* is true? (select all that apply)
    a. It is the process of inserting a tube into the heart.
    b. Doctors are able to diagnose and treat heart problems without performing major surgery by performing this process.
    c. It comes from the root *cardio*, meaning heart, and Greek words meaning *to go inside*.
    d. None of these.

EXERCISE 11 *Briefly describe the difference between each pair of terms.*

1. cardiologist, phlebologist ____________________
2. phlebotomist, phlebotomy ____________________
3. aortolith, arteriolith ____________________
4. echocardiography, electrocardiography ____________________
5. pulmonary circulation, systemic circulation ____________________
6. diastolic pressure, systolic pressure ____________________
7. aortectasia, aortic stenosis ____________________
8. embolus, embolism ____________________
9. embolus, thrombus ____________________
10. ischemia, occlusion ____________________

9.4 Diagnosis and Pathology

Problems with the heart can begin as early as birth. Patients may be born with flaws in the structure of their heart (*congenital heart defect*). Among the most common flaws are holes in the wall of the heart (*atrial septal defect* and *ventricular septal defect*).

Another type of flaw the heart can have is in its electrical system. A problem with electrical signals can cause an abnormal rhythm in the heartbeat (*arrhythmia, dysrhythmia*). Some rhythm problems are very minor and don't even require treatment. Others, like *ventricular fibrillation,* are medical emergencies. Ventricular fibrillation occurs when the main squeezing muscle fibers of the heart do not coordinate. As a result, no blood flow occurs. Unless treated, a patient will likely die of the condition.

When the muscle fibers of the heart do not work as well as they are supposed to (*cardiomyopathy*), the heart may cease to function properly (*cardiac insufficiency*). These problems usually develop over time. Cardiomyopathies can involve muscle that is too floppy (*dilated*), too tight (*restrictive*), or too weak (*congestive*). One type involves muscle that is too thick (*hypertrophic*) and can cause sudden death while a person is playing sports. This is a major reason for physical exams prior to playing sports.

The heart is not a common site for infection, but when it does become infected, the condition is usually very serious. Infection can be inside the muscle (*myocarditis*) or along the lining of the heart and vessels (*endocarditis*).

The heart can be inflamed as a result of other illnesses as well. One site for inflammation is the thin lining on the outside of the heart (*pericarditis*), which can cause fluid to collect around the heart (*pericardial effusion*) and make it more difficult for the heart to work well.

The most common heart problem involves the blood supply to the muscle fibers of the heart. Just as the rest of the body needs blood to take in nutrients and remove harmful waste, the heart needs it too. Coronary arteries serve this purpose. Floating fat in the blood (*cholesterol*) can accumulate and harden in the arteries of the heart. This process is called *atherosclerosis.* When the coronary arteries get blocked enough that it prevents sufficient blood flow, the heart muscle fibers do not get the oxygen they need. As a result, the muscle dies—a heart attack (*myocardial infarction*).

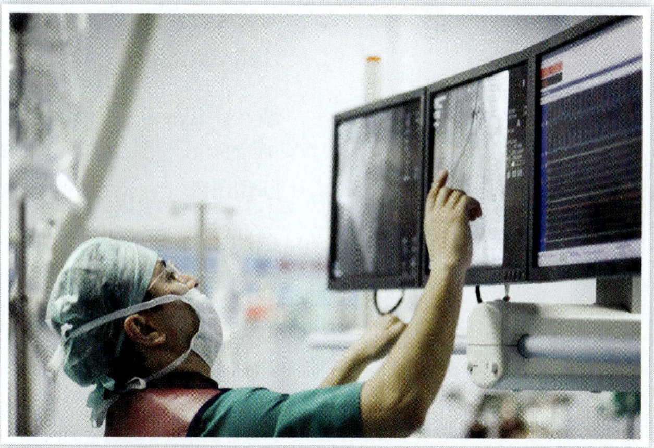

Imaging procedures are the most frequently used tools doctors use to diagnose heart issues.

Common to all heart problems is the possibility of the heart failing to adequately pump the blood to the rest of the body *(congestive heart failure).* The heart's inability to pump all the blood that reaches it creates a bottleneck effect, which leads to fluid accumulation in the lungs or body. The symptoms of heart failure depend on which side of the heart is affected.

Other blood vessel problems include a blockage (*deep vein thrombosis*) or bulge (*aneurysm*) in the vessel. Vessels can also become inflamed. An inflamed vein (*phlebitis*) is usually a problem involving just one part of a single vein. Inflammation of several blood vessels (*vasculitis*) can present in many different ways, depending on the type of vessels affected.

9.4 Diagnosis and Pathology

heart

Term	Word Analysis
angiocarditis AN-jee-oh-kar-DAI-tis	angio / card / itis vessel / heart / inflammation
Definition inflammation of the heart vessels	
atrial fibrillation AY-tree-al FIB-rih-LAY-shun	atri / al fibrill / ation atrium / pertaining to little fibers / process
Definition quivering or spontaneous contraction of muscle fibers in the heart's atrium	
atrial septal defect AY-tree-al SEP-tal DEE-fekt	atri / al sept / al de / fect atrium / pertaining to septum / pertaining to bad / made
Definition flaw in the septum that divides the two atria of the heart	
cardiac arrest KAR-dee-ak ah-REST	cardi / ac arrest heart / pertaining to stop
Definition cessation of functional circulation	
cardiomyopathy KAR-dee-oh-mai-AW-pah-thee	cardio / myo / pathy heart / muscle / disease
Definition disease of the heart muscle	
congestive cardiomyopathy con-JES-tiv KAR-dee-oh-mai-AW-pah-thee	con / gestive cardiomyopathy together / bring
Definition heart cavity is unable to pump all the blood out of itself (*congestive*) and becomes stretched (*dilated*), which causes weak/slow pumping of blood	
dilated cardiomyopathy DAI-lay-ted KAR-dee-oh-mai-AW-pah-thee	dilated cardiomyopathy expanded
Definition another term for congestive cardiomyopathy	

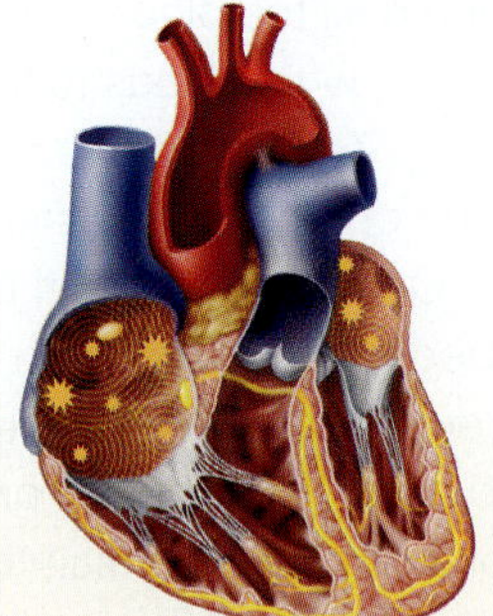

atrial fibrillation

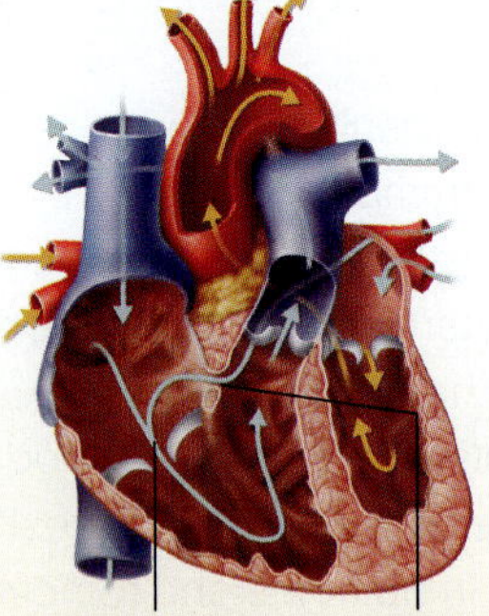

atrial septal defect

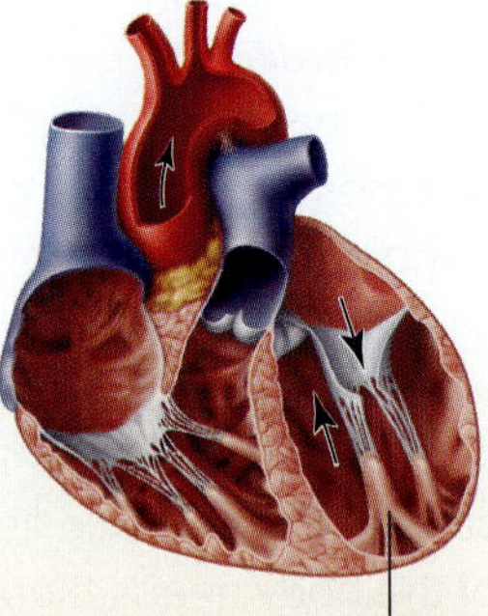

congestive cardiomyopathy

heart *continued*

Term	Word Analysis
hypertrophic cardiomyopathy HAI-per-TROH-fik KAR-dee-oh-mai-AW-pah-thee	hyper / troph / ic — over / developed / pertaining to; cardiomyopathy
Definition heart muscle becomes enlarged and blocks blood flow	
restrictive cardiomyopathy ree-STRIK-tiv KAR-dee-oh-mai-AW-pah-thee	re / strict / ive — back / tied / pertaining to; cardiomyopathy
Definition heart muscle hardens, restricting the expansion of the heart, thus limiting the amount of blood it can pump to the rest of the body	
carditis kar-DAI-tis	card / itis — heart / inflammation
Definition inflammation of the heart	
congenital heart defect con-JEN-ih-tal HART DEE-fekt	con / genit / al — together / birth / pertaining to; heart — heart; de / fect — bad / made
Definition flaw in the structure of the heart present at birth	
congestive heart failure con-JES-tiv HART FAYL-yir	con / gest / ive — together / bring / pertaining to; heart failure
Definition heart failure characterized by the heart cavity being unable to pump all the blood out of itself (*congestive*)	
coronary thrombosis KOR-ah-NAR-ee throm-BOH-sis	coron / ary — heart / pertaining to; thromb / osis — clot / condition
Definition obstruction of a coronary artery by a clot	
endocarditis EN-doh-kar-DAI-tis	endo / card / itis — inside / heart / inflammation
Definition inflammation of the tissue lining the inside of the heart	
myocardial infarction MAI-oh-KAR-dee-al in-FARK-shun	myo / cardi / al — muscle / heart / pertaining to; in / farc / tion — in / stuff / condition
Definition death of heart muscle tissue **NOTE:** The term *infarction* originally referred to a blocked blood vessel, but it came to refer to the death of tissue resulting from the blockage.	
myocardial ischemia MAI-oh-KAR-dee-al ih-SKEE-mee-ah	myo / cardi / al — muscle / heart / pertaining to; isch / emia — hold back / blood condition
Definition blockage of blood to the heart muscle	
myocarditis MAI-oh-kar-DAI-tis	myo / card / itis — muscle / heart / inflammation
Definition inflammation of the heart muscle	
pericardial effusion PER-ee-KAR-dee-al ee-FYOO-zhun	peri / cardi / al — around / heart / pertaining to; ef / fusion — out / pour
Definition fluid pouring out into the tissue around the heart	

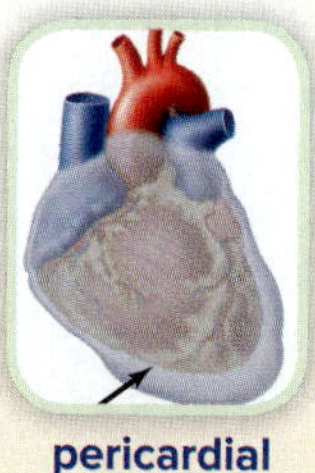

pericardial effusion

9.4 Diagnosis and Pathology

heart *continued*

Term	Word Analysis
pericarditis PER-ee-kar-DAI-tis	peri / card / itis around / heart / inflammation
Definition inflammation of the tissue around the heart	
valvulitis VAL-vyoo-LAI-tis	valvul / itis valve / inflammation
Definition inflammation of a heart valve	
ventricular septal defect (VSD) ven-TRIK-yoo-lar SEP-tal DEE-fekt	ventricul / ar sept / al de / fect ventricle / pertaining to septum / pertaining to bad / made
Definition flaw in the septum that divides the two ventricles of the heart	

circulation

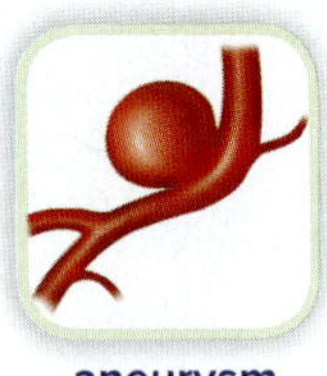
aneurysm

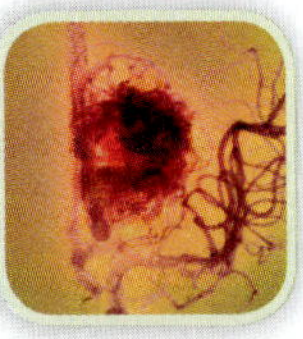
angioma

Term	Word Analysis
aneurysm AN-yir-IZ-um	an / eury / sm up / wide / condition
Definition bulge in a blood vessel	
Note: The *an-* prefix here doesn't meet *not;* rather, it is short for *ana* and means *up* or *out*. The *not* meaning is much more common, but there are also a few important examples of the *up/out* meaning, such as *anabolic*.	
angioedema AN-jee-oh-eh-DEE-mah	angio / edema vessel / swelling
Definition swelling of the blood vessels	
angioma AN-jee-OH-mah	angi / oma vessel / tumor
Definition blood vessel tumor	
aortic aneurysm ay-OR-tik AN-yir-IZ-um	aort / ic an / eury / sm aorta / pertaining to up / wide / condition
Definition bulging or swelling of the aorta	
aortic regurgitation ay-OR-tik ree-GIR-jih-TAY-shun	aort / ic re / gurgit / ation aorta / pertaining to back / bubble / condition
Definition flow of blood backward from the aorta into the heart; caused by a weak heart valve	
aortitis ay-or-TAI-tis	aort / itis aorta / inflammation
Definition inflammation of the aorta	

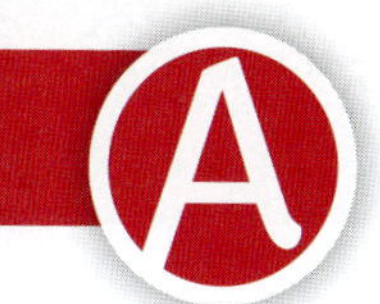

circulation *continued*

Term	Word Analysis
arteriopathy ar-TER-ee-AW-pah-thee **Definition** disease of the arteries	arterio / pathy artery / disease
arteritis AR-ter-AI-tis **Definition** inflammation of the arteries	arter / itis artery / inflammation
deep vein thrombosis DEEP VAYN throm-BOH-sis **Definition** formation of a blood clot in a vein deep in the body, most commonly the leg	deep vein thromb / osis deep vein clot / condition
hypertension HAI-per-TEN-shun **Definition** high blood pressure	hyper / tens / ion over / stretch / condition
hypotension HAI-poh-TEN-shun **Definition** low blood pressure	hypo / tens / ion under / stretch / condition
normotension NOR-moh-TEN-shun **Definition** normal blood pressure	normo / tens / ion normal / stretch / condition
phlebitis fleh-BAI-tis **Definition** inflammation of the veins	phleb / itis vein / inflammation
phlebostenosis FLEB-oh-sten-OH-sis **Definition** narrowing of the veins	phlebo / sten / osis vein / narrow / condition
thrombophlebitis THROM-boh-fleh-BAI-tis **Definition** inflammation of vein caused by a clot	thrombo / phleb / itis clot / vein / inflammation
vasculitis VAS-kyoo-LAI-tis **Definition** inflammation of blood vessels	vascul / itis vessel / inflammation

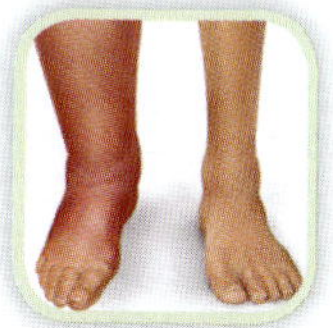

deep vein thrombosis

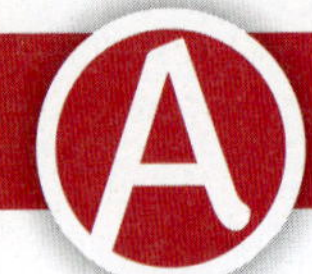

Learning Outcome 9.4 Exercises

PRONUNCIATION

EXERCISE 1 *Break down the following words into syllables.*

EXAMPLE: synesthesia *syn | es | the | sia*

1. vasculitis ____________
2. pericarditis ____________
3. myocarditis ____________
4. endocarditis ____________
5. valvulitis ____________
6. normotension ____________
7. coronary thrombosis ____________
8. pericardial effusion ____________
9. angioedema ____________
10. arteriopathy ____________
11. aortic regurgitation ____________
12. thrombophlebitis ____________

EXERCISE 2 *Indicate which syllable is emphasized when pronounced.*

EXAMPLE: bronchitis bron**chi**tis

1. cardiac arrest ____________
2. aortitis ____________
3. phlebitis ____________
4. atrial septal defect ____________
5. ventricular septal defect ____________

TRANSLATION

EXERCISE 3 *Break down the following words into their component parts.*

EXAMPLE: nasopharyngoscope *naso | pharyngo | scope*

1. angioma ____________
2. aortitis ____________
3. arteritis ____________
4. phlebitis ____________
5. endocarditis ____________
6. myocarditis ____________
7. pericarditis ____________
8. cardiomyopathy ____________
9. dilated cardiomyopathy ____________
10. myocardial ischemia ____________

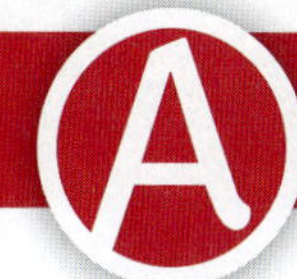

Learning Outcome 9.4 Exercises

EXERCISE 4 *Underline and define the word parts from this chapter in the following terms.*

1. carditis ________________
2. valvulitis ________________
3. vasculitis ________________
4. cardiac arrest ________________
5. angioedema ________________
6. arteriopathy ________________
7. aortic aneurysm ________________
8. phlebostenosis ________________
9. thrombophlebitis ________________
10. coronary thrombosis ________________
11. pericardial effusion ________________
12. angiocarditis (2 roots) ________________
13. myocardial infarction (2 roots) ________________
14. atrial septal defect (2 roots) ________________
15. ventricular septal defect (2 roots) ________________

EXERCISE 5 *Match the term on the left with its definition on the right.*

Term	Definition
____ 1. normotension	a. bulge in a blood vessel
____ 2. hypertension	b. flaw in the structure of the heart, present at birth
____ 3. hypotension	c. heart failure characterized by the heart cavity being unable to pump all the blood out of itself
____ 4. deep vein thrombosis	d. high blood pressure
____ 5. atrial fibrillation	e. low blood pressure
____ 6. congestive heart failure	f. normal blood pressure
____ 7. congenital heart defect	g. quivering or spontaneous contraction of muscle fibers in the heart's atrium
____ 8. aortic regurgitation	h. flow of blood backward from the aorta into the heart; caused by a weak heart valve
____ 9. aneurysm	i. formation of a blood clot in a vein deep in the body, most commonly the leg
____ 10. restrictive cardiomyopathy	j. heart is unable to pump all the blood out of itself and becomes stretched, which causes weak/slow blood pumping
____ 11. congestive cardiomyopathy	k. heart muscle fibers become enlarged and block blood flow
____ 12. hypertropic cardiomyopathy	l. heart muscle fibers harden, restricting the expansion of the heart and thus limiting the amount of blood it can pump to the rest of the body

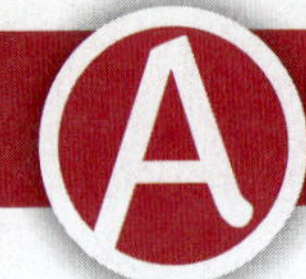

Learning Outcome 9.4 Exercises

EXERCISE 6 *Translate the following terms as literally as possible.*

EXAMPLE: nasopharyngoscope *an instrument for looking at the nose and throat*

1. arteriopathy ______
2. angioedema ______
3. phlebostenosis ______
4. coronary thrombosis ______
5. normotension ______
6. atrial septal defect ______
7. ventricular septal defect ______
8. dilated cardiomyopathy ______
9. hypertrophic cardiomyopathy ______

GENERATION

EXERCISE 7 *Build a medical term from the information provided.*

EXAMPLE: inflammation of the sinuses *sinusitis*

1. inflammation of the veins (use *phleb/o*) ______
2. inflammation of blood vessels (use *vascul/o*) ______
3. blood vessel tumor (use *angi/o*) ______
4. inflammation of the heart ______
5. inflammation of a heart valve ______
6. inflammation of the aorta ______
7. inflammation of the arteries ______
8. inflammation of the heart vessels ______
9. inflammation of the heart muscle ______
10. disease of the heart muscle ______
11. inflammation of the tissue lining the inside of the heart ______
12. inflammation of the tissue around the heart ______
13. inflammation of a vein caused by a clot ______

EXERCISE 8 *Multiple-choice questions. Select the correct answer.*

1. *Cardiac arrest* is
   a. bulge in a blood vessel
   b. cessation of functional circulation
   c. death of heart muscle tissue
   d. fluid pouring out into the tissue around the heart
   e. flow of blood backward from the aorta back into the heart

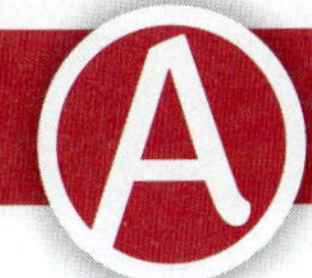

Learning Outcome 9.4 Exercises

2. *Pericardial effusion* is
   a. bulge in a blood vessel
   b. cessation of functional circulation
   c. death of heart muscle tissue
   d. fluid pouring out into the tissue around the heart
   e. flow of blood backward from the aorta back into the heart
3. An *aneurysm* is
   a. bulge in a blood vessel
   b. cessation of functional circulation
   c. death of heart muscle tissue
   d. fluid pouring out into the tissue around the heart
   e. flow of blood backward from the aorta back into the heart
4. The formation of a blood clot in a vein deep in the body, most commonly the leg, is known as
   a. aneurysm
   b. angioedema
   c. angioma
   d. deep vein thrombosis
   e. thrombophlebitis
5. Quivering or spontaneous contraction of muscle fibers in the heart's upper chamber is known as
   a. atrial fibrillation
   b. atriospasm
   c. ventricular fibrillation
   d. ventriculospasm
   e. none of these

EXERCISE 9 *Briefly describe the difference between each pair of terms.*

1. hypertension, hypotension ____________________
2. congestive cardiomyopathy, restrictive cardiomyopathy ____________________
3. congenital heart defect, congestive heart failure ____________________
4. myocardial infarction, myocardial ischemia ____________________
5. aortic aneurysm, aortic regurgitation ____________________

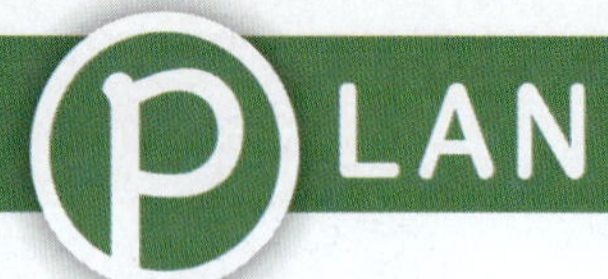

9.5 Treatments and Therapies

Medications for treating the heart deal with helping the pain associated with low oxygen to the heart (*antianginal*) and medicines that correct the heart's electrical signals (*cardioversion, antiarrhythmics*). Medicine can also work on blood vessels. They can cause the vessels to squeeze down (*vasoconstrictor, vasopressor*), which causes blood pressure to increase, or they can cause them to dilate (*vasodilator*), which lowers the blood pressure. *Thrombolytics* can work on both the heart and blood vessels. They work by breaking down dangerous accumulations that can develop in the heart or blood vessels.

In the past, the vast majority of procedures to physically correct heart problems used to include cutting open the patient's chest (*cardiothoracic surgery*) for direct access to the heart. While these more invasive means are now less common, they are still necessary for some types of surgeries like making an alternate blood vessel route (*anastomosis*) for congenital heart defects. A similar procedure is a very common treatment for blocked heart vessels. In a procedure known as coronary artery bypass graft, a blood vessel from another part of the body is used to make an alternate route for blood to get to the heart around an area of blockage. This is the most common type of heart surgery. Now, less invasive techniques are often preferred. One such treatment for coronary artery disease involves passing instruments up a patient's blood vessels into the heart (*percutaneous coronary intervention*). Once the instrument is inside the coronary artery, there are several options for treatment. A balloon can be inflated to crush the build-up (*balloon angioplasty*), a mesh tube can be inserted (*stent*), or the build-up can be destroyed (*atherectomy*).

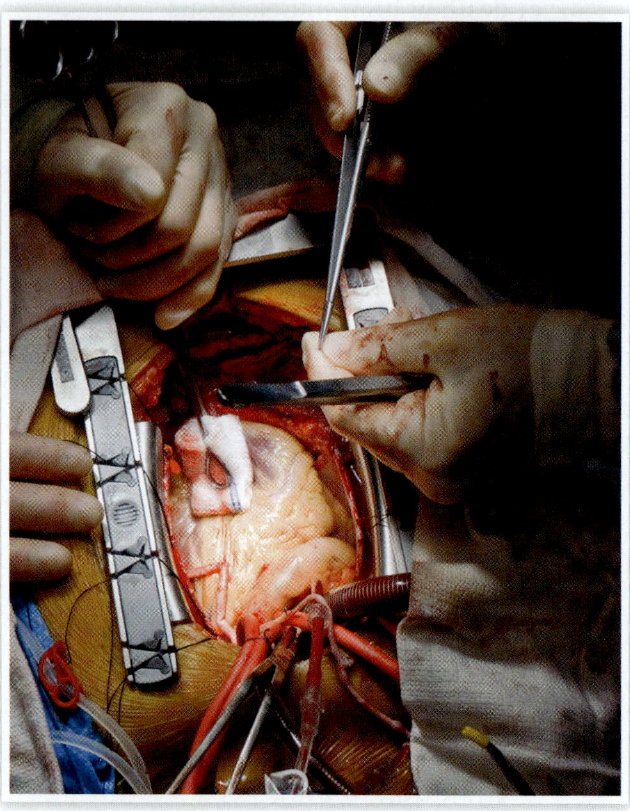

Though less-invasive techniques have been developed in recent years for a variety of heart procedures, for certain procedures—such as coronary artery bypass surgery—doctors still must employ cardiothoracic surgery.

drugs

Term	Word Analysis
antianginal AN-tee-AN-jih-nal	anti / angin / al against / *angina* (choke) / agent
Definition drug that prevents or relieves the symptoms of angina pectoris	
antiarrhythmic AN-tee-a-RITH-mik	anti / a / rrhythm / ic against / no / rhythm / agent
Definition drug that opposes an irregular heartbeat	
anticoagulant AN-tee-koh-AG-yoo-lant	anti / coagul / ant against / coagulation / agent
Definition drug that opposes the coagulation of the blood	

drugs *continued*

thrombolytic

Term	Word Analysis
antihypertensive	anti / hyper / tens / ive
AN-tee-HAI-per-TEN-siv	against / over / stretch / agent
Definition drug that opposes high blood pressure	
cardiotonic	cardio / ton / ic
KAR-dee-oh-TAW-nik	heart / tone / agent
Definition drug that increases the strength of the heart contractions	
thrombolytic	thrombo / lyt / ic
THROM-boh-LIH-tik	clot / loose / agent
Definition drug that breaks down clots	
vasoconstrictor	vaso / constrict / or
VAS-oh-kin-STRIK-tor	vessel / narrowing / agent
Definition drug that constricts or narrows the diameter of a blood vessel	
vasodilator	vaso / dilat / or
VAS-oh-DAI-lay-tor	vessel / expanding / agent
Definition drug that causes the relaxation or expansion of a blood vessel	
vasopressor	vaso / press / or
VAS-oh-PRES-or	vessel / press / agent
Definition drug that constricts or narrows the diameter of a blood vessel	

heart procedures

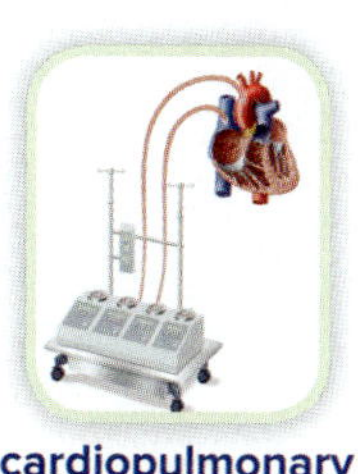
cardiopulmonary bypass

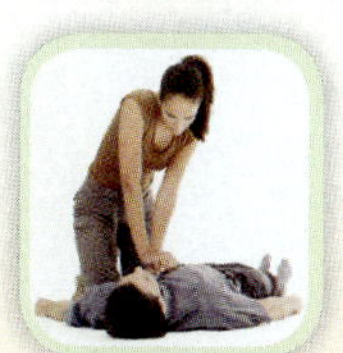
cardiopulmonary resuscitation (CPR)

Term	Word Analysis
cardiomyotomy	cardio / myo / tomy
KAR-dee-oh-mai-AW-toh-mee	heart / muscle / cut
Definition incision into the heart muscle	
cardiopulmonary bypass	cardio / pulmon / ary bypass
KAR-dee-oh-PUL-mon-AR-ee BAI-pas	heart / lung / pertaining to
Definition procedure that temporarily circulates and oxygenates a patient's blood during the portion of heart surgery where the heart is stopped	
cardiopulmonary resuscitation (CPR)	cardio / pulmon / ary re / suscit / ation
KAR-dee-oh-PUL-mon-AR-ee re-SIS-ih-TAY-shun	heart / lung / pertaining to again / stir up / procedure
Definition basic life support	
NOTE: Despite its name, CPR does not actually *resuscitate* an unconscious patient. Rather, through artificial breathing and chest compression, an unresponsive patient's blood circulates and is kept oxygenated until further steps can be taken.	
cardiothoracic surgery	cardio / thorac / ic surgery
KAR-dee-oh-thoh-RA-sik SIR-jir-ee	heart / chest / pertaining to
Definition surgery that involves cutting through the patient's chest to get to the heart	
NOTE: Remember, a *c* before an *a*, *o*, or *u* makes a *k* sound (*KAR-dee-oh*) but before an *i* or *e*, it makes an *s* sound (*thoh-RA-sik*).	

heart procedures *continued*

Term	Word Analysis
cardioversion KAR-dee-oh-VER-zhun	cardio / vers / ion heart / turn / procedure
Definition returning a heart to normal rhythm	
coronary arterectomy KOR-ah-NAR-ee AR-ter-EK-toh-mee	coron / ary arter / ec / tomy heart / pertaining to artery / out / cut
Definition surgical removal of a coronary artery	
coronary artery bypass graft (CABG) KOR-ah-NAR-ee AR-ter-ee BAI-pas GRAFT	coronary artery bypass graft
Definition borrowed piece of blood vessel used to bypass a blocked artery in the heart	
coronary artery bypass surgery KOR-ah-NAR-ee AR-ter-ee BAI-pas SIR-jir-ee	coronary artery bypass surgery
Definition surgery to bypass a blocked artery in the heart	
percutaneous coronary intervention PER-koo-TAY-nee-us KOR-ah-NAR-ee IN-ter-VEN-shun	per / cutaneo / us coron / ary through / skin / pertaining to heart / pertaining to
Definition alternate treatment for a coronary artery that passes instruments up a patient's blood vessels into the heart	
pericardiocentesis PER-ee-KAR-dee-oh-sin-TEE-sis	peri / cardio / centesis around / heart / puncture
Definition puncture of the tissue around the heart	
pericardiotomy PER-ee-KAR-dee-AW-toh-mee	peri / cardio / tomy around / heart / cut
Definition incision into the tissue around the heart	
valvectomy val-VEK-toh-mee	valv / ec / tomy valve / out / cut
Definition surgical removal of a heart valve	
valvotomy val-VAW-toh-mee	valvo / tomy valve / cut
Definition incision into a heart valve	
valvuloplasty VAL-voo-loh-PLAS-tee	valvulo / plasty valve / reconstruction
Definition surgical reconstruction of a heart valve	
ventriculotomy ven-TRIK-yoo-LAW-toh-mee	ventriculo / tomy ventricle / cut
Definition incision into a ventricle	

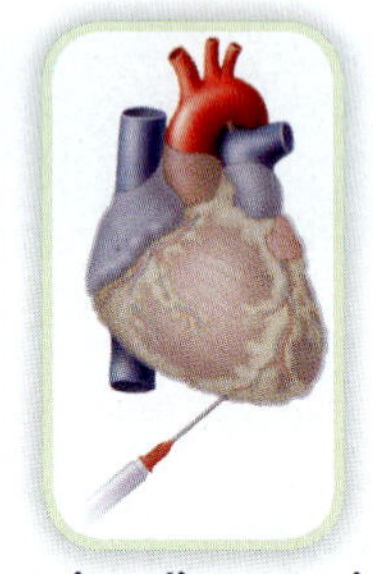
pericardiocentesis

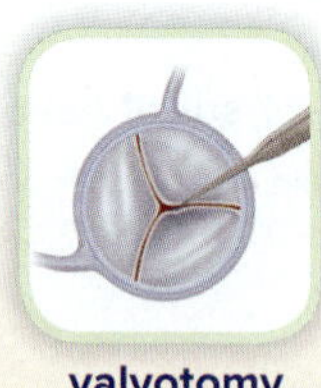
valvotomy

circulation procedures

Term	Word Analysis
anastomosis ah-NAS-tah-moh-sis	ana / stom / osis up / mouth / condition
Definition creation of an opening between two normally separate structures	
Note: The *an-* prefix here doesn't mean *not;* rather, it is short for *ana* and means *up* or *out*. The *not* meaning is much more common, but there are also a few important examples of the *up/out* meaning, such as *anabolic*.	
aneurysmectomy AN-yir-IZ-um-EK-toh-mee	an / eury / sm / ec / tomy up / wide / condition / out / cut
Definition surgical removal of an aneurysm	
angioplasty AN-jee-oh-PLAS-tee	angio / plasty vessel / reconstruction
Definition surgical reconstruction of a vessel	
angiorrhaphy AN-jee-OR-ah-fee	angio / rrhaphy vessel / suture
Definition suture of a vessel	
aortorrhaphy ay-or-TOR-ah-fee	aorto / rrhaphy aorta / suture
Definition suture of the aorta	
aortotomy ay-or-TAW-toh-mee	aorto / tomy aorta / cut
Definition incision into the aorta	
arteriectomy ar-TER-ee-EK-toh-mee	arteri / ec / tomy artery / out / cut
Definition surgical removal of an artery	
arterioplasty ar-TER-ee-oh-PLAS-tee	arterio / plasty artery / reconstruction
Definition surgical reconstruction of an artery	
arteriorrhaphy ar-TER-ee-OR-ah-fee	arterio / rrhaphy artery / suture
Definition suture of an artery	
atherectomy A-ther-EK-toh-mee	ather / ec / tomy fatty plaque / out / cut
Definition surgical removal of fatty plaque within an artery	
embolectomy EM-boh-LEK-toh-mee	embol / ec / tomy embolus / out / cut
Definition surgical removal of an embolus	

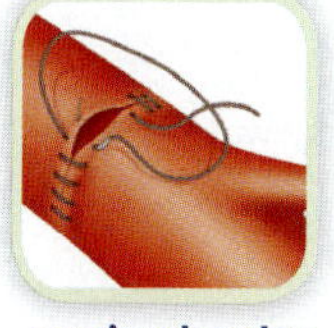
angiorrhaphy

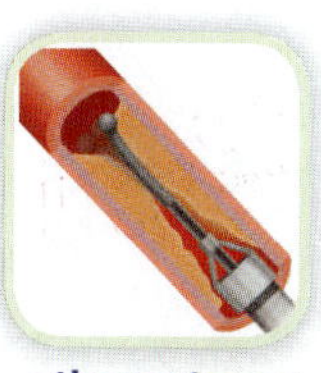
atherectomy

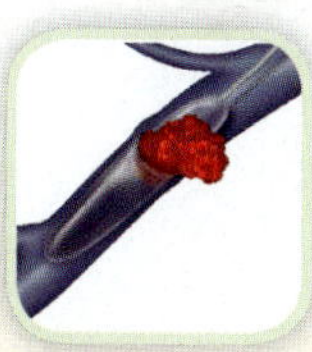
embolectomy

circulation procedures *continued*

Term	Word Analysis
endarterectomy END-ar-ter-EK-toh-me	end / arter / ec / tomy inside / artery / out / cut
Definition surgical removal of the inside of an artery	
phlebectomy fleb- EK-toh-mee	phleb / ec / tomy vein / out / cut
Definition surgical removal of a vein	
phlebophlebostomy FLEB-oh-fleb-AW-stoh-mee	phlebo / phlebo / stom / y vein / vein / mouth / procedure
Definition procedure to create an opening between two veins	
varicotomy VAR-ih-KAW-toh-mee	varico / tomy swollen / cut
Definition surgical removal of a varicose vein **NOTE:** Normally, you would expect *-ectomy* to mean *removal*, but *varicectomy* was probably too much of a mouthful.	
venectomy vee-NEK-toh-mee	ven / ec / tomy vein / out / cut
Definition surgical removal of a vein	

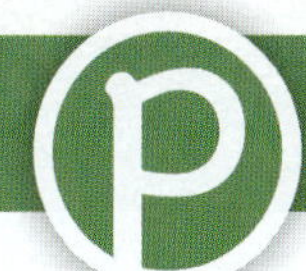

Learning Outcome 9.5 Exercises

PRONUNCIATION

EXERCISE 1 *Break down the following words into syllables.*

EXAMPLE: synesthesia *syn | es | the | sia*

1. vasopressor ____________
2. cardioversion ____________
3. valvuloplasty ____________
4. atherectomy ____________
5. embolectomy ____________
6. arteriectomy ____________
7. arterioplasty ____________
8. ventriculotomy ____________
9. angiorrhaphy ____________
10. aortorrhaphy ____________
11. arteriorrhaphy ____________
12. endarterectomy ____________
13. anastomosis ____________
14. pericardiotomy ____________
15. antiarrhythmic ____________
16. pericardiocentesis ____________

EXERCISE 2 *Indicate which syllable is emphasized when pronounced.*

EXAMPLE: bronchitis bron**chi**tis

1. valvectomy ____________
2. valvotomy ____________
3. varicotomy ____________
4. venectomy ____________
5. phlebectomy ____________
6. aortotomy ____________
7. anastomosis ____________

TRANSLATION

EXERCISE 3 *Break down the following words into their component parts.*

EXAMPLE: nasopharyngoscope *naso | pharyngo | scope*

1. vasodilator ____________
2. arterioplasty ____________
3. angioplasty ____________
4. antihypertensive ____________
5. anticoagulant ____________
6. thrombolytic ____________
7. valvectomy ____________
8. embolectomy ____________
9. aortotomy ____________
10. cardiomyotomy ____________
11. cardioversion ____________
12. pericardiotomy ____________
13. phlebophlebostomy ____________
14. cardiothoracic surgery ____________

Learning Outcome 9.5 Exercises

EXERCISE 4 *Underline and define the word parts from this chapter in the following terms.*

1. valvectomy ______________________
2. venectomy ______________________
3. atherectomy ______________________
4. phlebectomy ______________________
5. arteriectomy ______________________
6. endarterectomy ______________________
7. valvotomy ______________________
8. ventriculotomy ______________________
9. valvuloplasty ______________________
10. angiorrhaphy ______________________
11. aortorrhaphy ______________________
12. arteriorrhaphy ______________________
13. cardiotonic ______________________
14. vasoconstrictor ______________________
15. percutaneous coronary intervention ______________________
16. vasopressor ______________________
17. pericardiocentesis ______________________
18. cardiopulmonary bypass ______________________
19. coronary arterectomy (2 roots) ______________________

EXERCISE 5 *Match the term on the left with its definition on the right.*

f	1. coronary artery bypass surgery	a.	borrowed piece of blood vessel used to bypass a blocked artery in the heart
a	2. coronary artery bypass graft	b.	drug that opposes an irregular heartbeat
b	3. antiarrhythmic	c.	drug that prevents or relieves the symptoms of angina pectoris
e	4. cardiopulmonary resuscitation	d.	alternate treatment for the coronary artery that passes instruments up a patient's blood vessels into the heart
d	5. percutaneous coronary intervention	e.	basic life support: artificial breathing and chest compression
c	6. antianginal	f.	surgery to bypass a blocked artery in the heart
h	7. aneurysmectomy	g.	surgical removal of a varicose vein
g	8. varicotomy	h.	surgical removal of an aneurysm
i	9. anastomosis	i.	creation of an opening between two normally separate structures

Learning Outcome 9.5 Exercises

EXERCISE 6 *Translate the following terms as literally as possible.*

EXAMPLE: *nasopharyngoscope* *an instrument for looking at the nose and throat*

1. arterioplasty ______
2. valvuloplasty ______
3. angioplasty ______
4. angiorrhaphy ______
5. aortorrhaphy ______
6. arteriorrhaphy ______
7. vasoconstrictor ______
8. vasodilator ______
9. vasopressor ______
10. cardioversion ______
11. pericardiocentesis ______

EXERCISE 7 *Fill in the blanks.*

1. *antihypertensive* = drug that opposes ______
2. *anticoagulant* = drug that opposes ______
3. *thrombolytic* = drug that ______
4. *antiarrhythmic* = drug that opposes a(n) ______
5. *antianginal* = drug that prevents or relieves the symptoms of ______

GENERATION

EXERCISE 8 *Build a medical term from the information provided.*

EXAMPLE: inflammation of the sinuses *sinusitis*

1. surgical removal of a vein (use *phleb/o*) ______
2. surgical removal of a vein (use *ven/o*) ______
3. surgical removal of an aneurysm ______
4. surgical removal of a heart valve ______
5. incision into a heart valve ______
6. incision into a ventricle ______
7. incision into the aorta ______
8. incision into the heart muscle ______
9. incision into the tissue around the heart ______
10. surgical removal of an artery ______

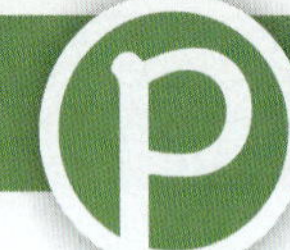

Learning Outcome 9.5 Exercises

11. surgical removal of a coronary artery ____________________
12. surgical removal of the inside of an artery ____________________
13. surgical removal of fatty plaque (within an artery) ____________________
14. surgical removal of an aneurysm ____________________
15. surgical removal of an embolus ____________________

EXERCISE 9 *Multiple-choice questions. Select the correct answer.*

1. A *cardiotonic*
   a. breaks down clots
   b. causes the relaxation of expansion of a blood vessel
   c. increases the strength of heart contractions
   d. opposes an irregular heartbeat
   e. prevents or relieves the symptoms of angina pectoris
2. A procedure that temporarily circulates and oxygenates a patient's blood during the portion of heart surgery where the heart is stopped is known as
   a. anastomosis
   b. cardiopulmonary bypass
   c. cardiopulmonary resuscitation
   d. percutaneous coronary intervention
   e. none of these
3. Which of the following statements about the abbreviation *CPR* is *not* true?
   a. It is basic life support.
   b. It keeps a patient's blood circulating and oxygenated.
   c. It is a process of artificial breathing and chest compression.
   d. It resuscitates an unconscious patient.
   e. It stands for cardiopulmonary resuscitation.
4. The surgical removal of a varicose vein is known as
   a. varicectomy
   b. varicotomy
   c. vasectomy
   d. venectomy
   e. none of these
5. Surgery that involves cutting through the patient's chest to get to the heart is known as
   a. cardiopulmonary bypass surgery
   b. cardiopulmonary resuscitation
   c. cardiothoracic surgery
   d. percutaneous coronary intervention
   e. none of these

EXERCISE 10 *Briefly describe the difference between each pair of terms.*

1. vasoconstrictor, vasodilator ____________________
2. coronary artery bypass graft, coronary artery bypass surgery ____________________
3. anastomosis, phlebophlebostomy ____________________

9.6 Abbreviations

Abbreviations provide a shorthand way of referring to things that either recur often or are too long to write out. When dealing with the heart and circulatory system, these can refer to diseases (CAD), test data (CO, SV), test procedures (EKG, MRA), diagnoses (CHF, HTN, SCA), and treatments (CABG, PCI).

cardiovascular system abbreviations

Abbreviation	Definition
AA	abdominal aortic aneurysm
A-fib	atrial fibrillation
ASD	atrial septal defect
BP	blood pressure
CABG	coronary artery bypass graft
CAD	coronary artery disease
CHF	congestive heart failure
CO	cardiac output
CTA	computed tomographic angiography
DVT	deep vein thrombosis
ECHO	echocardiogram
EKG	electrocardiogram
HTN	hypertension
MI	myocardial infarction
MRA	magnetic resonance angiography
MVP	mitral valve prolapse
NSR	normal sinus rhythm
PCI	percutaneous coronary intervention
SCA	sudden cardiac arrest
SV	stroke volume
TEE	transesophageal echocardiogram
VSD	ventricular septal defect

Learning Outcome 9.6 Exercises

EXERCISE 1 *Define the following abbreviations.*

1. BP ____________________
2. CABG ____________________
3. ECHO ____________________
4. EKG ____________________
5. DVT ____________________
6. TEE ____________________
7. MRA ____________________
8. NSR ____________________
9. CAD ____________________
10. CHF ____________________
11. CO ____________________
12. SCA ____________________

13 A-fib ____________________

EXERCISE 2 *Give the abbreviations for the following terms.*

1. atrial septal defect ____________________
2. computed tomography angiography ____________________
3. hypertension ____________________
4. myocardial infarction ____________________
5. mitral valve prolapse ____________________
6. percutaneous coronary intervention ____________________
7. stroke volume ____________________
8. ventricular septal defect ____________________
9. coronary artery disease ____________________
10. cardiac output ____________________
11. normal sinus rhythm ____________________
12. abdominal aortic aneurysm ____________________

EXERCISE 3 *Match the abbreviation on the left with its full definition on the right.*

______ 1. BP	a.	borrowed piece of blood vessel used to bypass a blocked artery in the heart
______ 2. PCI	b.	alternate treatment for the coronary artery that passes instruments up a patient's blood vessels into the heart
______ 3. CABG	c.	death of heart muscle tissue
______ 4. CHF	d.	heart failure characterized by the heart cavity being unable to pump all the blood out of itself (*congestive*)
______ 5. MI	e.	high blood pressure
______ 6. DVT	f.	force exerted by blood on the walls of blood vessels
______ 7. HTN	g.	formation of a blood clot deep in the body, most commonly in the leg

Learning Outcome 9.6 Exercises

EXERCISE 4 *Multiple-choice questions. Select the correct answer(s).*

1. *Stroke volume* is the volume of blood pumped from one ventricle of the heart with each beat. The abbreviation for this is

   a. BP
   b. NSR
   c. SV
   d. Svol
   e. vol

2. *Cardiac output* is the volume of blood being pumped by the heart, in particular by a left or right ventricle, in the time interval of one minute. The abbreviation for this is

   a. CAD
   b. CO
   c. CTA
   d. SCA
   e. SV

3. *MRA* is

   a. a procedure to describe blood vessels using magnetic resonance
   b. a procedure to describe heart muscle fibers using magnetic resonance
   c. a procedure to treat blood vessels using multiple radiations
   d. a procedure to treat heart muscle fibers using multiple radiations
   e. none of these

4. *MVP* stands for

   a. mitral valve prolapse
   b. mitral ventricle procedure
   c. mitral ventricle prolapse
   d. myocardial valve procedure
   e. myocardial valve prolapse

5. Which of the following abbreviations refer to a diagnostic procedure (select all that apply)?

   a. ASD arterial septal defect
   b. ECHO
   c. EKG
   d. TEE transesphageal echocardiogram
   e. VSD ventricular septal defect

6. Which of the following abbreviations refer to defects in the septa of the heart (select all that apply)?

   a. ASD
   b. ECHO
   c. EKG
   d. TEE
   e. VSD

7. *Sinus rhythm* is a term used in medicine to describe the normal beating of the heart. A person with *NSR* has

   normal

   a. a fast heartbeat
   b. a normal heartbeat
   c. a slow heartbeat
   d. a stopped heartbeat
   e. an irregular heartbeat

9.7 Electronic Health Records

Cardiology Admission Note

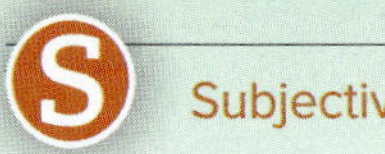

Subjective

Chief Complaint: VSD, postop.

History of Present Illness:

Sharon Jackson is a 12-month-old female with a history of **VSD** first discovered on **echocardiogram** shortly after birth. She has been followed by cardiology. She had been **hemodynamically** stable until the past month, when her parents noticed that she had increased difficulty eating. She would sweat after eating and become **cyanotic** with exertion. Her mother followed up with Sharon's **cardiologist,** who sent her to our office for consult.

Sharon's symptoms were consistent with congestive heart failure. It was decided to surgically correct her VSD. She underwent a sternotomy and atriotomy for patch placement in the ventricular septum to correct her VSD. This was performed with cardiopulmonary bypass under the guidance of a perfusionist. Sharon tolerated the procedure well and is now being admitted for postoperative observation and care.

Review of Systems: No fever, cough, congestion, vomiting, diarrhea.

Medications: IV antibiotics.

Allergies: No known drug allergies.

Past Medical History: No contributory.

Past Surgical History: None.

Social History: Stays at home with mother.

Two school-aged siblings.

Family History: Noncontributory.

Objective

Vital Signs: Temp: 99.2; Heart rate: 94;
Respiratory rate: 26; Blood pressure: 94/64.

Physical Exam

General: Sedated and intubated.

Head: NCAT. Mucous membranes moist. PERRLA.

Cardiovascular: RRR with soft systolic murmur.

Respiratory: CTA.

Abdomen: Soft, nontender, nondistended.

Neurologic: Sedated.

Skin: No cyanosis, clubbing, edema.

Labs: CBC normal.

Imaging: CXR–No cardiomegaly.

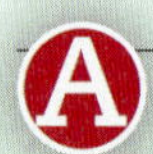

Assessment

1. Postop for VSD repair–routine postop orders and care.
2. When patient switches to PO, we will d/c IV ABx, and at discharge, she will continue antibiotics as needed for endocarditis prophylaxis.

–Miles O'Keefe, PA

Learning Outcome 9.7 Exercises

EXERCISE 1 *Match the term on the left with its definition on the right.*

_____ 1. cardiology

_____ 2. cardiologist

_____ 3. cardiomegaly

_____ 4. echocardiogram

_____ 5. endocarditis

_____ 6. ventricular septal defect

_____ 7. congestive heart failure

_____ 8. cardiopulmonary bypass

a. procedure that temporarily circulates and oxygenates a patient's blood during a portion of heart surgery where the heart is stopped

b. image of the heart produced using sound waves; the same procedure as an ultrasound performed on pregnant women, but instead is performed on the heart

c. branch of medicine dealing with the heart

d. enlarged heart

e. flaw in the septum that divides the two ventricles of the heart

f. heart failure characterized by the heart cavity being unable to pump all the blood out of itself

g. heart specialist

h. inflammation of the tissue lining the inside of the heart

EXERCISE 2 *Fill in the blanks.*

1. Using the data recorded at the patient's physical examination, fill in the following blanks.
   a. T: ______________________________
   b. HR: ______________________________
   c. RR: ______________________________
   d. Cardiovascular (*give definition:* ______________________________)
   RRR (define abbreviation: ______________________________)
2. According to the history of present illness, Sharon's symptoms were consistent with *congestive heart failure* (give abbreviation: ______________________________).
3. Sharon's sternotomy (*sterno* = sternum + *tomy* = ____________________) and atriotomy were performed with ____________________ (a procedure that temporarily circulates and oxygenates a patient's blood during a portion of heart surgery where the heart is stopped).

EXERCISE 3 *True or false questions. Indicate true answers with a T and false answers with an F.*

1. The patient is 12 years old. _________
2. The patient has a Hx of ventricular septal defect. _________
3. The patient's VSD was first discovered on EKG shortly after birth. _________
4. The patient has CHF. _________
5. The patient has an enlarged heart. _________
6. The patient will not need to continue her antibiotics once she is discharged. _________

Learning Outcome 9.7 Exercises

EXERCISE 4 *Multiple-choice questions. Select the correct answer(s).*

1. Sharon underwent an *atriotomy*. Which of the following is an accurate breakdown of the term?
   a. *atrio* (aorta) + *tomy* (cut) = incision into the upper chamber of the heart
   b. *atrio* (aorta) + *tomy* (removal) = incision into the lower chamber of the heart
   c. *atrio* (atrium) + *tomy* (cut) = incision into the lower chamber of the heart
   d. *atrio* (atrium) + *tomy* (cut) = incision into the upper chamber of the heart
   e. *atrio* (atrium) + *tomy* (removal) = incision into the upper chamber of the heart
2. To correct her VSD, a patch was placed on Sharon's *ventricular septum*. Select all that apply to the term *ventricular septum:*
   a. Septum comes from a Latin word meaning *partition or dividing structure* and can refer to any wall dividing two cavities.
   b. The term comes from Roman architecture where it referred to the large open area in the center of every Roman house off of which all the other rooms of the house branched out.
   c. The ventricle is the lower portion of each side of the heart.
   d. The ventricle is the upper portion of each side of the heart.
   e. The word *ventricle* is a combination of *venter* (stomach) plus the diminutive suffix *-icle,* and means *little stomach.*
3. Sharon was "*hemodynamically* stable until the past month." The root *hemo* means
   a. artery
   b. blood
   c. heart
   d. vein
   e. vessel
4. Sharon will be given antibiotic as needed for *endocarditis prophylaxis*. Which of the following is an accurate breakdown of the term?
   a. *endo* (inside) + *card* (heart) + *itis* (inflammation) + *prophylaxis* (preventative treatment)
   b. *endo* (inside) + *card* (heart) + *itis* (inflammation) + *prophylaxis* (treatment of symptoms)
   c. *endo* (outside) + *card* (heart) + *itis* (inflammation) + *prophylaxis* (treatment of symptoms)
   d. *endo* (outside) + *card* (heart) + *itis* (inflammation) + *prophylaxis* (preventative treatment)
   e. none of these
5. During Sharon's physical examination, the physician noted a "soft systolic murmur," which indicates that she has
   a. abnormal heart rate when the heart is contracting
   b. abnormal heart rate when the heart is relaxed
   c. abnormal heart sound when the heart is contracting
   d. abnormal heart sound when the heart is relaxed
   e. none of these

Cardiology Consult Note

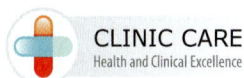

Reason for Consult: 65-year-old male with chest pain consistent with **myocardial ischemia**.

History of Present Illness: Chester Payne is a 65-year-old white male who presented to the emergency department with a one-day history of worsening **cardiodynia**. The pain began as a dull pressure sensation 6/10 in severity. He had taken sublingual nitroglycerin at home. Despite taking two pills, Mr. Payne reported that the pain worsened to 8/10 and radiated up his neck and down his left arm. At this point, his wife insisted he seek medical attention. Upon arrival at the ED, Mr. Payne was treated according to routine cardiac protocol and the **cardiology** service was consulted.

Past Medical History:
CAD with **PTCA** in 20xx. **Hypertension.** Hypertriglyceridemia.
Medications: Beta blocker, nitroglycerin prn, **ASA,** antilipidemic agent.
Allergies: Penicillin.
Family History: Brother deceased from an **MI** at 69 years of age.
Social: Patient does not smoke. He drinks 1–2 beers per week. Denies illicit drug use. He is married with two grown children and three grandchildren.

Review of Systems: Mr. Payne denies any new neurologic problems. Other than mild gastroesophageal reflux, which responds to OTC antacid medication, there is no GI disease. He denies asthma or any other respiratory issues.

Physical Exam:
Temp: 98.6; HR: 72; RR: 24; BP: 90/60. Pulse Ox: 99% on 3L per nasal cannula.
General: Diaphoretic, mildly uncomfortable but responsive to questions. Alert and oriented.
HEENT: Pupils equal round and reactive to light bilaterally; mucous membranes moist and pink, nares patent, no flaring.
Neck: Supple. No goiter. No **JVD** or **bruits.**
Resp: Clear to auscultation.
CV: Regular rate and rhythm. Soft **systolic** ejection **murmur**, no gallop or rub. No thrills.
Abdomen: Soft, nontender, nondistended. No abdominal bruits.
Skin: No tenting of skin. Cap refill 2 seconds.
Ext: No cyanosis, clubbing, or edema.

EKG: Ischemic changes.
Lab: Cardiac enzymes elevated.
CXR: No **cardiomegaly.**

Impression: **Acute myocardial infarction.**

Plan: Patient has already had an emergent **coronary arteriography,** which showed three **stenotic** vessels. I have recommended **CABG** over **percutaneous catheterization** due to three-vessel involvement, and the patient agrees.

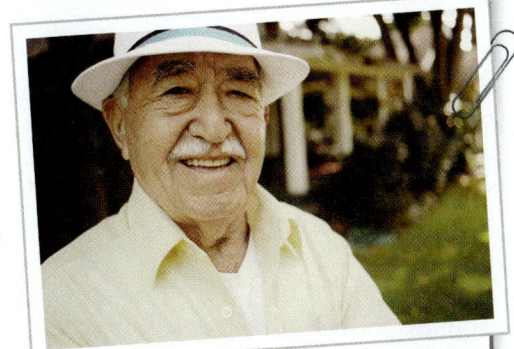

—Ramon Sinclar, MD

Learning Outcome 9.7 Exercises

EXERCISE 5 *Match the term on the left with its definition on the right.*

	Term		Definition
______	1. cardiology	a.	borrowed piece of blood vessel used to bypass a blocked artery in the heart
______	2. cardiomegaly	b.	abnormal heart sound
______	3. murmur	c.	blockage of blood flow to an organ
______	4. electrocardiogram	d.	blockage of blood to the heart muscle
______	5. coronary artery bypass graft	e.	branch of medicine dealing with the heart
______	6. ischemia	f.	death of heart muscle tissue
______	7. myocardial ischemia	g.	enlarged heart
______	8. myocardial infarction	h.	record of the electrical currents of the heart

EXERCISE 6 *Fill in the blanks.*

1. Using the data recorded at Mr. Payne's physical examination, fill in the following blanks.
   a. The patient's temperature: ______________________________
   b. The patient's heart rate: ______________________________
   c. The patient's respiratory rate: ______________________________
   d. The patient's blood pressure: ______________________________
   e. CV (give definition for abbreviation: ______________________________)
2. Past medical history: *hypertension* (give definition: ______________________________).
3. Past medical history: ______________________________ (coronary artery disease).
4. EKG (give definition for abbreviation: ______________________________): ischemic changes.
5. CXR (chest x-ray): no *cardiomegaly* (give definition: ______________________________).

EXERCISE 7 *True or false questions. Indicate true answers with a T and false answers with an F.*

1. Mr. Payne presented to the ED with cardiodynia. ______
2. Mr. Payne has high blood pressure. ______
3. Mr. Payne's heart sounds normal. ______
4. Mr. Payne has HTN. ______
5. Mr. Payne's brother died of a myocardial ischemia. ______
6. Dr. Sinclar recommends a coronary artery bypass graft. ______

EXERCISE 8 *Multiple-choice questions. Select the correct answer.*

1. The patient's past medical history shows *coronary artery disease,* which is
   a. a disease of the arteries
   b. a disease of the arteries of the heart
   c. a disease of the heart
   d. none of these

Learning Outcome 9.7 Exercises

2. The patient has already had a *coronary arteriography*. Which of the following is an accurate breakdown of the term *coronary arteriography*?
   a. *coronary* (heart) + *arterio* (artery) + *graphy* (record)
   b. *coronary* (heart) + *arterio* (artery) + *graphy* (writing procedure)
   c. *coronary* (heart) + *arterio* (vein) + *graphy* (record)
   d. *coronary* (heart) + *arterio* (vein) + *graphy* (writing procedure)
3. The patient presented to the emergency department with *cardiodynia*. Which of the following is an accurate breakdown of the term *cardiodynia*?
   a. *cardio* (blood vessel) + *dynia* (dilation)
   b. *cardio* (blood vessel) + *dynia* (pain)
   c. *cardio* (heart) + *dynia* (dilation)
   d. *cardio* (heart) + *dynia* (pain)
4. The patient has a past medical history of *hypertriglyceridemia*. Which of the following is an accurate breakdown of the term *hypertriglyceridemia*?
   a. *hyper* (over) + *triglyceride* (fatty molecule) + *-emia* (blood condition)
   b. *hyper* (over) + *triglyceride* (fatty molecule) + *-emia* (urine condition)
   c. *hyper* (under) + *triglyceride* (fatty molecule) + *-emia* (blood condition)
   d. *hyper* (under) + *triglyceride* (fatty molecule) + *-emia* (urine condition)
5. The patient took *sublingual nitroglycerin*. Nitroglycerin is used medically as a vasodilator to treat heart conditions. A *vasodilator* is a
   a. drug that causes the relaxation or expansion of a blood vessel
   b. drug that causes the relaxation or expansion of the heart
   c. drug that constricts or narrows the diameter of a blood vessel
   d. drug that constricts or narrows the diameter of the heart
6. The physician's impression is that the patient has *acute myocardial infarction*, which is
   a. a blockage of blood to the heart muscle that has been going on for a while
   b. a blockage of blood to the heart muscle that just started recently
   c. a death of heart muscle tissue that has been going on for a while
   d. a death of heart muscle tissue that just started recently
7. The *percutaneous* approach is commonly used in vascular procedures. This involves a needle catheter getting access to a blood vessel, followed by the introduction of a wire through the pathway of the needle. It is over this wire that other catheters can be placed into the blood vessel. According to this medical consult
   a. the consulting physician recommended a coronary artery bypass graft instead of a *percutaneous catheterization*
   b. the patient already had a *percutaneous catheterization*
   c. the patient refused *percutaneous catheterization*
   d. the patient will undergo a *percutaneous catheterization*

Cardiothoracic Surgery Clinic Note

Subjective

Mrs. Short presents to my office for her routine postoperative follow-up following **aortic valvuloplasty.** She has been followed by her cardiologist for known **bicuspid aortic valve** related to her Turner syndrome. She has recently had difficulty breathing with exercise and episodes of syncope. An **echocardiogram** revealed **left ventricular hypertrophy.** Since she was becoming symptomatic, she was referred to my office for surgical correction. She underwent aortic valvuloplasty 5 days previously and discharged 2 days ago.

Since her surgery, she has had a few episodes of **tachycardia** and a funny feeling in her chest. She denies pain or fever.

Objective

Temp: 99.0. HR: 60. RR: 20. BP: 112/70.

General: Pleasant, responsive. No acute distress.

HEENT: Pupils equal, round, and reactive to light. Mucous membranes moist and pink.

Resp: Clear to auscultation. No wheezes, rales, rhonchi or crackles. Good air exchange. No increased work of breathing.

Chest: **Sternotomy** incision healing well without warmth, erythema, or induration. Dressing clean and dry.

CV: Regular in rate and rhythm no murmur. No jugulovenous distention. CR brisk. Radial pulses 2+, dorsal pedal pulses 2+.

Abd: Soft, nontender, nondistended. No hepatosplenomegaly.

Ext: No cyanosis, clubbing, or edema.

CXR: Unremarkable. No **cardiomegaly.**

EKG: Normal.

Labs: No elevated cardiac enzymes. Normal CBC.

Assessment

Given that her chest x-ray is normal, I do not believe that Mrs. Short has postoperative **pericardial effusion.** Since she is afebrile, I do not believe she has **endocarditis.** Her shortness of breath and tachycardic episodes are most likely postoperative **atrial flutter.**

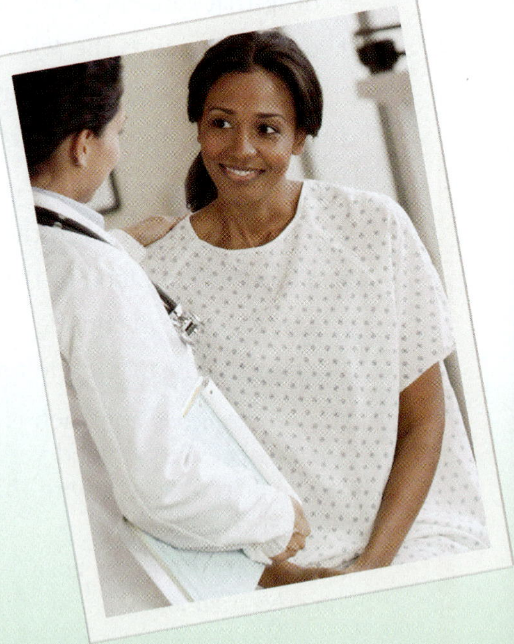

Plan

I will admit her overnight for observation under **telemetry** and **cardioversion,** if needed.

—Anton Valentine, MD

Learning Outcome 9.7 Exercises

EXERCISE 9 *Match the term on the left with its definition on the right.*

	Term		Definition
______	1. cardiomegaly	a.	an image of the heart produced using sound waves; the same procedure as an ultrasound performed on pregnant women, but instead performed on the heart
______	2. echocardiogram	b.	enlarged heart
______	3. endocarditis	c.	fluid pouring out into the tissue around the heart
______	4. tachycardia	d.	inflammation of the tissue lining the inside of the heart
______	5. valvuloplasty	e.	rapid heartbeat
______	6. pericardial effusion	f.	returning a heart to normal rhythm
______	7. cardioversion	g.	surgical reconstruction of a heart valve

EXERCISE 10 *Fill in the blanks.*

1. Using the data recorded at Mrs. Short's physical examination, fill in the following blanks.
   a. Mrs. Short's temperature: ______________________________
   b. Mrs. Short's heart rate: ______________________________
   c. Mrs. Short's respiratory rate: ______________________________
   d. Mrs. Short's blood pressure: ______________________________
   e. CV (*cardiovascular,* give definition: ______________________________):
   regular rate and rhythm (give abbreviation: ______________________________)
2. An *echocardiogram* (give abbreviation: ______________________________)
   revealed left ventricular hypertrophy (enlargement of the ______________________________,
   the lower chamber of the heart).
3. Labs: no elevated cardiac enzymes. Normal ______________________________ (complete blood count).
4. Mrs. Short will be admitted overnight for observation and *cardioversion* (give definition:
   ______________________________) if needed.

EXERCISE 11 *True or false questions. Indicate true answers with a T and false answers with an F.*

1. Since her surgery, Mrs. Short has had a few episodes of her heart beating rapidly. ________
2. Mrs. Short has experienced cardiodynia. ________
3. Mrs. Short has a normal-sized heart. ________
4. Mrs. Short has a fever. ________
5. Mrs. Short has pericardial effusion and endocarditis. ________

EXERCISE 12 *Multiple-choice questions. Select the correct answer(s).*

1. The patient's labs revealed no *cardiac enzymes.* The root *cardio* means
   a. blood vessel
   b. circulation
   c. heart
   d. vein

Learning Outcome 9.7 Exercises

2. Mrs. Short came into the office for a follow-up after her *aortic valvuloplasty*. The aortic valve is one of the valves of the heart. It lies between the left ventricle and the aorta. Which of the following is an accurate breakdown of the term *aortic valvuloplasty*?
   a. *aortic* (pertaining to the largest artery of the body) + *valvulo* (valve) + *plasty* (reconstruction)
   b. *aortic* (pertaining to the largest artery of the body) + *valvulo* (valve) + *plasty* (incision)
   c. *aortic* (pertaining to the largest vein of the body) + *valvulo* (valve) + *plasty* (reconstruction)
   d. *aortic* (pertaining to the largest vein of the body) + *valvulo* (valve) + *plasty* (incision)
3. Mrs. Short's echocardiogram revealed *left ventricular hypertrophy*. Which of the following is an accurate breakdown of the term *ventricular hypertrophy*?
   a. *ventricular* (pertaining to the lower chamber of the heart) + *hyper* (over) + *trophy* (development)
   b. *ventricular* (pertaining to the lower chamber of the heart) + *hyper* (under) + *trophy* (development)
   c. *ventricular* (pertaining to the upper chamber of the heart) + *hyper* (over) + *trophy* (development)
   d. *ventricular* (pertaining to the upper chamber of the heart) + *hyper* (under) + *trophy* (development)
4. Atrial flutter (AFL) is an abnormal heart rhythm that occurs in the atria of the heart. According to this clinic note (select all that apply)
   a. AFL can possibly be treated with an antianginal medication
   b. AFL is a type of arrhythmia
   c. AFL pertains to the lower chamber of the heart
   d. AFL pertains to the upper chamber of the heart
   e. the physician believes AFL is the cause of her episodes of tachycardia
   f. the physician believes AFL is the caused by the patient's endocarditis

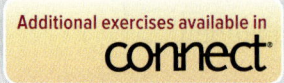

Chapter Review exercises, along with additional practice items, are available in Connect!

Quick Reference

quick reference glossary of roots

Root	Definition	Root	Definition
angi/o	vessel	**phleb/o**	vein
aort/o	aorta	**sept/o**	septum (plural, septa)
arteri/o	artery	**valvul/o**	valve
ather/o	fatty plaque	**vas/o, vascul/o**	vessel
atri/o	atrium (upper chamber)	**ven/o**	vein
cardi/o	heart	**ventricul/o**	ventricle (lower chamber)
coron/o	heart		

quick reference glossary of terms

Term	Definition
anastomosis	creation of an opening between two normally separate structures
aneurysm	bulge in a blood vessel
aneurysmectomy	surgical removal of an aneurysm
angina pectoris	oppressive pain in the chest caused by irregular blood flow to the heart
angiocarditis	inflammation of the heart vessels
angioedema	swelling of the blood vessels
angiogenesis	development of blood vessels
angiogram	record of the blood vessels
angiography	procedure to describe the blood vessels
angiolith	stone forming in the wall of a blood vessel
angioma	blood vessel tumor
angioplasty	surgical reconstruction of a vessel
angiopoiesis	formation of blood vessels
angiorrhaphy	suture of a vessel
angiosclerosis	hardening of a blood vessel
angioscope	device for looking into a blood vessel
antianginal	drug that prevents or relieves the symptoms of angina pectoris

quick reference glossary of terms *continued*

Term	Definition
antiarrhythmic	drug that opposes an irregular heartbeat
anticoagulant	drug that opposes the coagulation of blood
antihypertensive	drug that opposes high blood pressure
aortalgia	pain in the aorta
aortectasia	dilation of the aorta
aortic aneurysm	bulging or swelling of the aorta
aortic regurgitation	flow of blood backward from the aorta into the heart; caused by a weak heart valve
aortic stenosis	narrowing of the aorta
aortitis	inflammation of the aorta
aortogram	record of the aorta
aortolith	stone deposit in the wall of the aorta
aortorrhaphy	suture of the aorta
aortotomy	incision into the aorta
arrhythmia	irregular heartbeat
arteriectomy	surgical removal of an artery
arteriogram	record of an artery
arteriolith	stone in an artery
arteriopathy	disease of the arteries
arterioplasty	surgical reconstruction of an artery
arteriorrhaphy	suture of an artery
arteriorrhexis	rupture of an artery
arteriosclerosis	hardening of an artery
arteritis	inflammation of the arteries
atherectomy	surgical removal of fatty plaque within an artery
atherogenesis	formation of fatty plaque on the wall of an artery
atherosclerosis	hardening of an artery due to build-up of fatty plaque
atrial fibrillation	quivering or spontaneous contraction of muscle fibers in the heart's atrium
atrial septal defect	flaw in the septum that divides the two atria of the heart
blood pressure	force exerted by blood on the walls of blood vessels
bradycardia	slow heartbeat
cardiac arrest	cessation of functional circulation

quick reference glossary of terms *continued*

Term	Definition
cardiac catheterization	the process of inserting a tube (catheter) into the heart
cardiologist	heart specialist
cardiology	branch of medicine dealing with the heart
cardiomegaly	enlarged heart
cardiomyopathy	disease of the heart muscle
cardiomyotomy	incision into the heart muscle
cardiopulmonary bypass	procedure that temporarily circulates and oxygenates a patient's blood during a portion of heart surgery where the heart is stopped
cardiopulmonary resuscitation	basic life support
cardiothoracic surgery	surgery that involves cutting through the patient's chest to get to the heart
cardiotonic	a drug that increases the strength of heart contractions
cardiotoxic	poisonous to the heart
cardiovascular	pertaining to the heart and blood vessels
cardioversion	returning a heart to normal rhythm
carditis	inflammation of the heart
congenital heart defect	flaw in the structure of the heart, present at birth
congestive cardiomyopathy	heart cavity is unable to pump all the blood out of it (congestive) and becomes stretched (dilated), which causes weak/slow pumping of blood
congestive heart failure	heart failure characterized by the heart cavity being unable to pump all the blood out of it (congestive)
coronary arterectomy	surgical removal of a coronary artery
coronary artery bypass graft (CABG)	borrowed piece of blood vessel used to bypass a blocked artery in the heart
coronary artery bypass surgery	surgery to bypass a blocked artery in the heart
coronary circulation	circulation of blood from the heart to the heart muscle
coronary thrombosis	obstruction of a coronary artery by a clot
cyanosis	a bluish appearance to the skin; a sign that the tissue isn't receiving enough oxygen
deep vein thrombosis	the formation of a blood clot deep in the body, most commonly in the leg

quick reference glossary of terms *continued*

Term	Definition
diaphoresis	profuse sweating
diastolic pressure	pressure exerted on blood vessels when the heart is relaxed
dilated cardiomyopathy	see *congestive cardiomyopathy*
dysrhythmia	irregular heartbeat
echocardiogram	image of the heart produced using sound waves; it is the same procedure as an ultrasound performed on pregnant women, but done on the heart
echocardiography	use of sound waves to produce an image of the heart
electrocardiogram	record of the electrical currents of the heart
electrocardiography	procedure for recording the electrical currents of the heart
embolectomy	surgical removal of an embolus
embolism	blockage in a blood vessel caused by an embolus
embolus	mass of matter present in the blood
endarterectomy	surgical removal of the inside of an artery
endocarditis	inflammation of the tissue lining the inside of the heart
endocardium	tissue lining the inside of the heart
epicardium	tissue lining the outside of the heart
hemorrhage	loss of blood
hypertension	high blood pressure
hypertropic cardiomyopathy	heart muscle becomes enlarged and blocks blood flow
hypotension	low blood pressure
ischemia	blockage of blood flow to an organ
murmur	abnormal heart sound
myocardial infarction	death of heart muscle tissue
myocardial ischemia	blockage of blood to the heart muscle
myocarditis	inflammation of the heart muscle
myocardium	heart muscle tissue
normotension	normal blood pressure
occlusion	closing or blockage of a passage
palpitation	rapid or irregular beating of the heart
pectoralgia	chest pain

quick reference glossary of terms *continued*

Term	Definition
percutaneous coronary intervention	alternate treatment for the coronary artery that passes instruments up a patient's blood vessels into the heart
pericardial effusion	fluid pouring out into the tissue around the heart
pericardiocentesis	puncture of the tissue around the heart
pericardiotomy	incision into the tissue around the heart
pericarditis	inflammation of the tissue around the heart
pericardium	tissue around the heart
phlebalgia	pain in a vein
phlebectomy	surgical removal of a vein
phlebitis	inflammation of the veins
phlebologist	specialist in veins
phlebology	study of veins
phlebophlebostomy	procedure to create an opening between two veins
phlebosclerosis	hardening of a vein
phlebostenosis	narrowing of the veins
phlebotomist	one who draws blood
phlebotomy	incision into a vein (the technical term for drawing blood)
pulmonary circulation	circulation of blood from the heart to the lungs
restrictive cardiomyopathy	heart muscle hardens, restricting the expansion of the heart and thus limiting the amount of blood it can pump to the rest of the body
sonography	use of sound waves to produce diagnostic images; also called an ultrasound
stress electrocardiogram	image of the heart produced using sound waves while the patient experiences increases of exercise stress
superior vena cava	portion of the vena cava that gathers blood from the upper portion of the body (head and arms)
systemic circulation	circulation of blood from the heart to the rest of the body
systolic pressure	pressure exerted on blood vessels when the heart is contracting
tachycardia	rapid heartbeat
thrombolytic	drug that breaks down clots
thrombophlebitis	inflammation of a vein caused by a clot
thrombus	blood clot (from Greek, for *lump, clot,* or *curd of milk*)

quick reference glossary of terms *continued*

Term	Definition
transesophageal electrocardiogram	recording of the heart using sound waves performed by inserting the sonograph into the esophagus
valvectomy	surgical removal of a heart valve
valvotomy	incision into a heart valve
valvulitis	inflammation of a heart valve
valvuloplasty	surgical reconstruction of a heart valve
varicose veins	enlarged, dilated vein toward the surface of the skin
varicotomy	surgical removal of a varicose vein
vascular endoscopy	procedure to look inside a blood vessel
vasculitis	inflammation of blood vessels
vasoconstrictor	drug that constricts or narrows the diameter of a blood vessel
vasodilator	drug that causes the relaxation or expansion of a blood vessel
vasopressor	drug that constricts or narrows the diameter of a blood vessel
vasospasm	involuntary contraction of a blood vessel
vena cava	large-diameter vein that gathers blood from the body and returns it to the heart
vena cava inferior	portion of the vena cava that gathers blood from the lower portion of the body
venectomy	surgical removal of a vein
venogram	record of a vein
venosclerosis	hardening of a vein
venospasm	involuntary contraction of a vein
venostasis	trapping of blood in an extremity due to compression
ventricular septal defect	flaw in the septum that divides the two ventricles of the heart
ventriculotomy	incision into a ventricle

review of terms by roots

Root	Term(s)	
angi/o	angiocarditis	angioma
	angioedema	angioplasty
	angiogenesis	angiopoiesis
	angiogram	angiorrhaphy
	angiography	angiosclerosis
	angiolith	angioscope
aort/o	aortalgia	aortitis
	aortectasia	aortogram
	aortic aneurysm	aortolith
	aortic regurgitation	aortorrhaphy
	aortic stenosis	aortotomy
arteri/o	arteriectomy	arteriosclerosis
	arteriogram	arteritis
	arteriolith	coronary arterectomy
	arteriopathy	coronary artery bypass graft
	arterioplasty	coronary artery bypass surgery
	arteriorrhaphy	endarterectomy
	arteriorrhexis	
ather/o	atherectomy	atherosclerosis
	atherogenesis	
atri/o	atrial fibrillation	
	atrial septal defect	
cardi/o	angiocarditis	cardiopulmonary resuscitation
	bradycardia	cardiothoracic surgery
	cardiac arrest	cardiotonic
	cardiac catheterization	cardiotoxic
	cardiologist	cardiovascular
	cardiology	cardioversion
	cardiomegaly	carditis
	cardiomyopathy	congestive cardiomyopathy
	cardiomyotomy	dilated cardiomyopathy
	cardiopulmonary bypass	echocardiogram

review of terms by roots *continued*

Root	Term(s)	
cardi/o (continued)	echocardiography	myocardium
	electrocardiogram	pericardial effusion
	electrocardiography	pericardiocentesis
	endocarditis	pericardiotomy
	endocardium	pericarditis
	epicardium	pericardium
	hypertropic cardiomyopathy	restrictive cardiomyopathy
	myocardial ischemia	stress electrocardiogram
	myocardial infarction	tachycardia
	myocarditis	transesophageal echocardiogram
coron/o	coronary arterectomy	coronary circulation
	coronary artery bypass graft (CABG)	coronary thrombosis
	coronary artery bypass surgery	percutaneous coronary intervention
phleb/o	phlebalgia	phlebosclerosis
	phlebectomy	phlebostenosis
	phlebitis	phlebotomist
	phlebologist	phlebotomy
	phlebology	thrombophlebitis
	phlebophlebostomy	
sept/o	atrial septal defect	
	ventricular septal defect	
valvul/o	valvectomy	valvulitis
	valvotomy	valvuloplasty
varic/o	varicose veins	
	varicotomy	
vas/o, vascul/o	cardiovascular	vasodilator
	vascular endoscopy	vasopressor
	vasculitis	vasospasm
	vasoconstrictor	

review of terms by roots *continued*

Root	Term(s)	
ven/o	superior vena cava	venogram
	vena cava	venosclerosis
	vena cava inferior	venospasm
	venectomy	venostasis
ventricul/o	ventricular septal defect	
	ventriculotomy	

other terms

anastomosis	embolism
aneurysm	embolus
aneurysmectomy	hemorrhage
angina pectoris	hypertension
antianginal	hypotension
antiarrhythmic	ischemia
anticoagulant	murmur
antihypertensive	normotension
arrhythmia	occlusion
blood pressure	palpitation
congenital heart defect	pectoralgia
congestive heart failure	pulmonary circulation
cyanosis	sonography
deep vein thrombosis	systemic circulation
diaphoresis	systolic pressure
diastolic pressure	thrombolytic
dysrhythmia	thrombus
embolectomy	

The Respiratory System—Pulmonology 10

Introduction and Overview of the Respiratory System

Spiro is the root of the word *spirit*. A person with spirit is full of enthusiasm. While we cannot actually visualize enthusiasm, we can certainly see its effect; for example, it's "team spirit" that drives sports fans to go to games shirtless in the middle of winter! In the same way, we can't see the air we breathe, but we know it gives life.

Simply put, the main job of the respiratory system is to deliver oxygen to the blood and carry carbon dioxide away from it. As we breathe in (*inhale*), we are taking in oxygen-rich air. As air passes through the respiratory tract, it is cleaned, warmed, and moistened. The air reaches its end point in the lungs, where it comes in contact with the blood. There, oxygen is exchanged for carbon dioxide. Finally, the waste air passes back out through the nose and mouth (*exhale*).

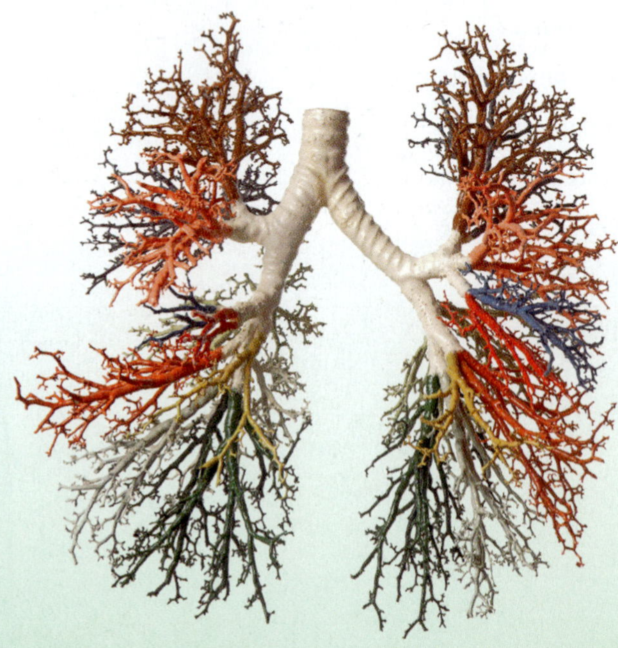

This image of the lungs shows the branching of the airways from the trachea to the bronchi, bronchioles, and down to the alveoli.

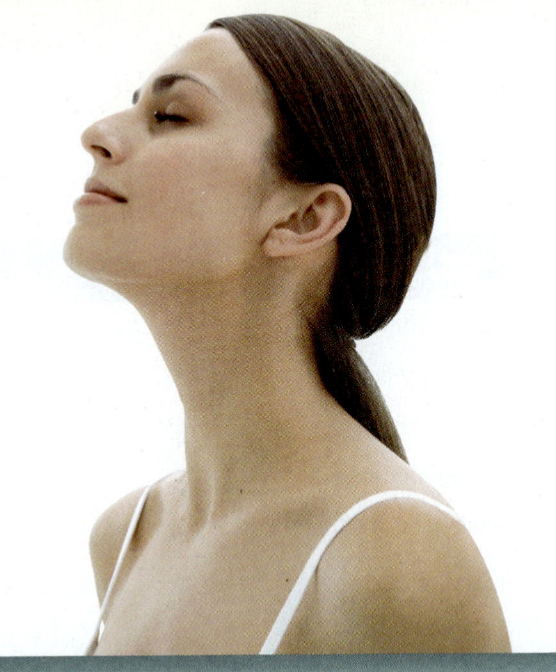

learning outcomes

Upon completion of this chapter, you will be able to:

10.1 Identify the **roots/word parts** associated with the **respiratory system.**

S **10.2** Translate the **Subjective** terms associated with the **respiratory system.**

O **10.3** Translate the **Objective** terms associated with the **respiratory system.**

A **10.4** Translate the **Assessment** terms associated with the **respiratory system.**

P **10.5** Translate the **Plan** terms associated with the **respiratory system.**

10.6 Use **abbreviations** associated with the **respiratory system.**

10.7 Distinguish terms associated with the **respiratory system** in the context of **electronic health records**.

It helps to view the anatomy of the respiratory system as a tree. The mouth, nose, and throat form the tree's roots. The trachea is the tree's trunk; it leads to large branches (*bronchi*). Each branch splits into more branches (other bronchi) that further lead to twigs (*bronchioles*) and leaves (*alveoli*).

10.1 Word Parts of the Respiratory System

Upper Respiratory System

adenoid

ROOT: ***adenoid/o***

EXAMPLES: adenoidectomy, adenoiditis

NOTES: The word *adenoid* is formed by adding a suffix to the root *adeno,* which means *gland: aden/o + oid* = resembling a gland.

tonsil

ROOT: ***tonsill/o***

EXAMPLES: tonsillectomy, tonsillitis

NOTES: The word *tonsil* comes from a Latin word meaning *almond*. The Latin word has two *l*s, but in English, one disappears.

nose

ROOTS: ***nas/o (Latin for* nose*), rhin/o (Greek for* nose*)***

EXAMPLES: nasogastric tube, nasendoscope, rhinorrhea, rhinoplasty

NOTES: Rhinoceros is the combination of *rhino* and *ceros* (horn), which means *horn nose*.

A poet named Publius Ovidius Naso (43 BC–17 AD) lived in ancient Rome. Perhaps you know him by the much shorter name Ovid. Apparently, he or one of his ancestors had quite a prominent nose—hence the root *naso*.

palate

ROOT: ***palat/o***

EXAMPLES: palatoplasty, palatoschisis

NOTES: This term means *the roof of the mouth.*

mouth

ROOT: ***or/o***

EXAMPLES: orofacial, oronasal

NOTES: This comes from the Latin for *mouth*.

larynx (voice box)

ROOT: ***laryng/o***

EXAMPLES: laryngospasm, laryngitis

NOTES: Remember: the letter *g* is soft when followed by an *i* and hard when followed by an *o* (e.g., laryn**GO**-spasm vs. laryn**JI**tis).

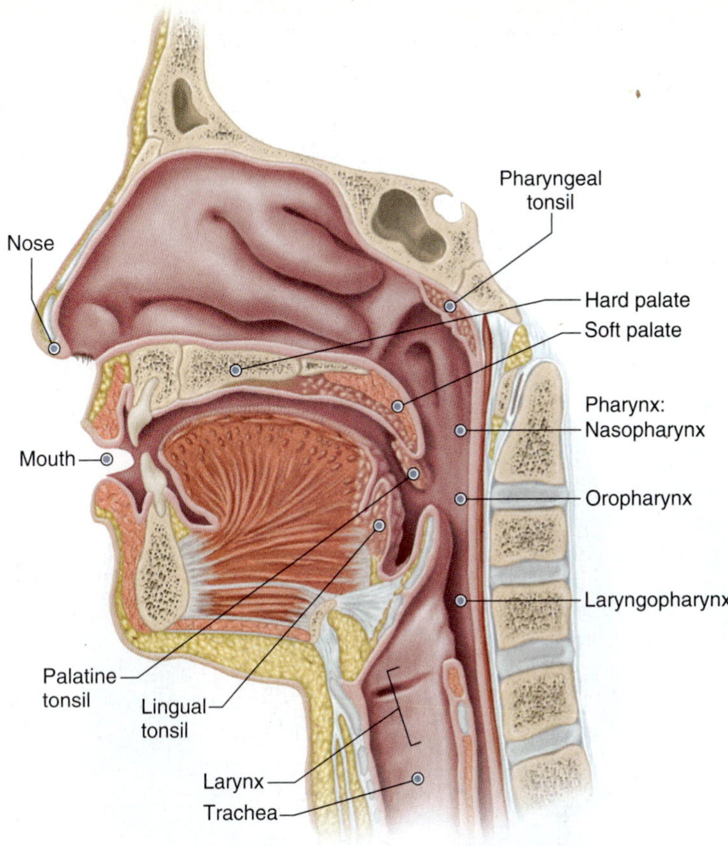

pharynx (throat)

ROOT: ***pharyng/o***

EXAMPLES: pharyngitis, pharyngostenosis

NOTES: The pharynx is the pathway used by both food and air.

trachea (windpipe)

ROOT: ***trache/o***

EXAMPLES: tracheotomy, tracheostomy

NOTES: From the Greek word for *rough*, because of the bumpy ridges that line the outside of the trachea.

The entry point for air into the body is primarily through the nose, with some air entering through the mouth. The nose serves to warm, clean, and moisten the air. The nose consists of two nostrils (*nares*), a septum (*septum*), and tube-shaped cartilage inside the nose (*turbinates*). The nose is very vascular, which means that it contains many blood vessels, which is why the nose bleeds easily. The blood in these vessels warms the air as it enters the rest of the respiratory tract. In addition, multiple hairs line the nose and filter out dust and other particles. Finally, the nose produces mucus, which helps clean and moisten the air.

The air passes through the nose or mouth and proceeds into the throat (*pharynx*). There are three parts to the pharynx: the nasopharynx, the oropharynx, and the laryngopharynx. The laryngopharynx contains the vocal cords (*larynx*). When air passes across these cords upon exhalation, the cords vibrate at certain speeds—just like a harmonica or saxophone. These vibrations make sounds, which we use to form speech. The air continues down the windpipe (*trachea*). The trachea is surrounded by bumpy rings of cartilage that prevent it from caving in.

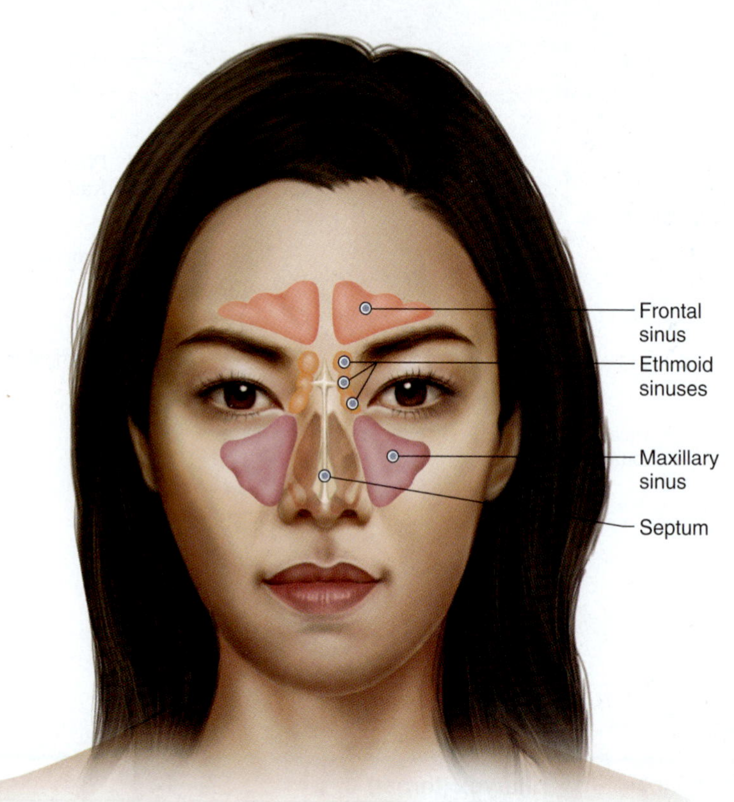

septum (plural: septa)

ROOT: ***sept/o***

EXAMPLES: septectomy, septoplasty

NOTES: *Septum* comes from a Latin word meaning *partition or dividing structure* and can refer to any wall dividing two cavities. Of the numerous septa throughout the body, the easiest to find is the nasal septum. If you place your index fingers in each nostril and press them together, you will feel the nasal septum. If your nasal septum leans to one side, you have a deviated septum.

sinus

ROOTS: ***sin/o, sinus/o***

EXAMPLES: sinusitis, sinusotomy

NOTES: From a Latin word meaning *hollow or cavity, sinus* refers generally to any hollow area—specifically, those in bones.

air or lungs

ROOTS: ***pneum/o, pneumat/o, pneumon/o***

EXAMPLES: pneumomelanosis, pneumatology, pneumonia

NOTES: These roots can mean either *lung* or *air.* Context and familiarity will help in determining which to use. For instance, it makes more sense to translate *pneumothorax* as *air in the chest* rather than *lung in the chest.*

The term *pneumatic* can also be found in the construction world. It refers to any tool that moves by forcing air into it (i.e., a pneumatic drill), as opposed to hydraulic tools, which involve the use of water instead of air (i.e., a hydraulic lift).

lungs

ROOT: ***pulmon/o***

EXAMPLES: pulmonologist, pulmonary

NOTES: *Pulmon/o* is listed by itself instead of with the various forms of *pneum/o* because while *pulmon/o* means only lung, *pneum/o* can mean both lung (as in *pneumonia*) and air (as in *pneumothorax*).

lobe

ROOT: ***lob/o***

EXAMPLES: lobectomy, lobotomy

NOTES: A *lobe* is a well-defined portion of any organ. The main organs that have lobes are the lungs, brain, and liver.

What is the difference between a *lobectomy* and a *lobotomy?*

bronchus

ROOTS: ***bronch/o, bronchi/o***

EXAMPLES: bronchoscope, bronchiostenosis

NOTES: The main branches from the trachea into each lung.

bronchiole

ROOT: ***bronchiol/o***

EXAMPLES: bronchiolitis, bronchiolectasis

NOTES: The root *bronchiole* is actually formed by adding a diminutive suffix to another root: *bronch/o* + *iole* = *little bronchus,* which is a smaller subdivision of the bronchial tubes.

alveolus (air sac)

ROOT: ***alveol/o***

EXAMPLES: alveolitis, alveolar

NOTES: *Alveolus* comes from a Latin word meaning *hollow* or *cavity.* The two main types are *pulmonary alveoli,* the air sacs in the lungs, and *dental alveoli,* the sockets in the jaw from which teeth emerge.

If you place your tongue on the roof of your mouth and move it forward, you will feel a bump called the *alveolar ridge* right before you get to your teeth.

Lower Respiratory System

After passing the *trachea,* the air finally makes its way to the lungs via two main *bronchi* (right and left). Like the trachea, rings of cartilage surround the bronchi for support. The bronchi further branch into five *lobar bronchi*—three on the right and two on the left. These branches define the five *lobes* of the lung. Each lobar

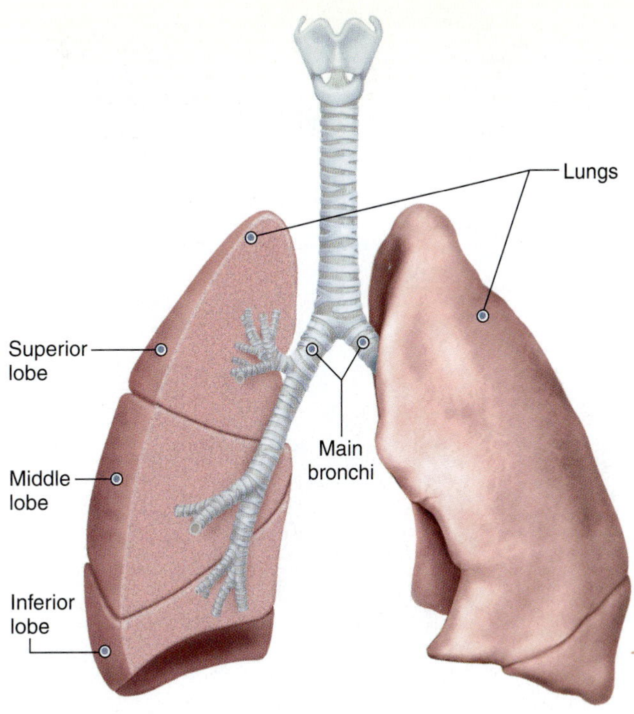

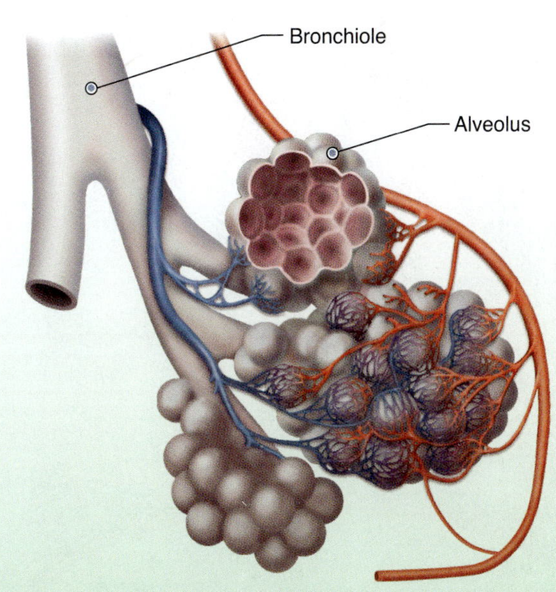

bronchus breaks into smaller segments (*segmental bronchi*) that further branch into smaller airways known as *bronchioles*. The bronchioles end in clusters of *alveoli,* tiny balloon-like structures surrounded by small blood vessels. At this point, oxygen passes into the blood, and carbon dioxide passes out of the blood.

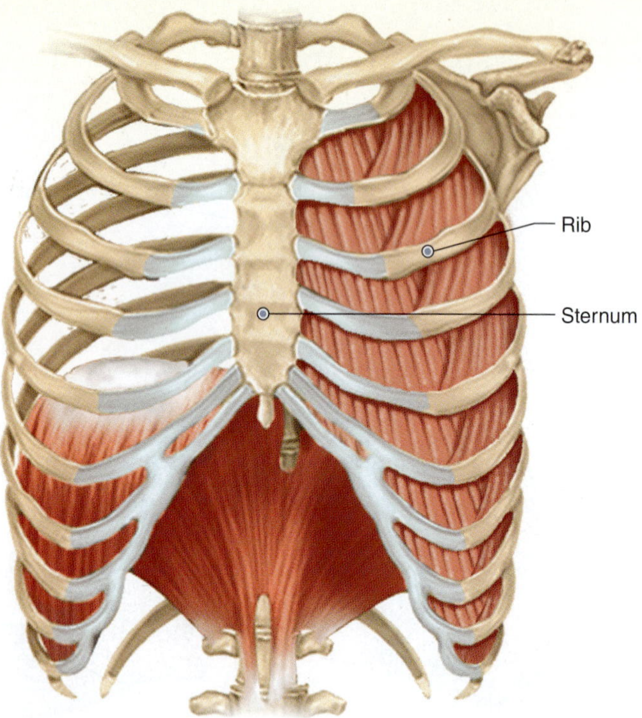

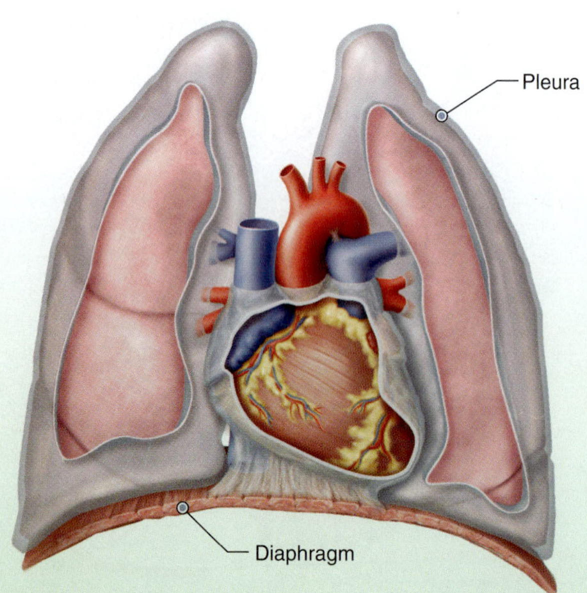

sternum

ROOT: ***stern/o***

EXAMPLES: sternocostal, sternotomy

NOTES: The *sternum* (also known as the breastbone) comes to a point at the bottom called the *xiphoid* (ZAI-foid) *process.* The term comes from the Greek word *xiphos,* meaning *sword.* Therefore, *xiphoid* means *resembling a sword.*

rib

ROOT: ***cost/o***

EXAMPLES: costectomy, costophrenic

NOTES: *Ribs* are sometimes grouped into three categories: true, false, and floating. The top seven ribs are called "true" ribs because they attach to both the spine and the sternum. The next three ribs are called "false" ribs because they connect to the spine and to the lowest true rib instead of the sternum. The lowest two ribs are called "floating" ribs because they attach only to the spine.

chest

ROOTS: ***thorac/o, pector/o (also pectus), steth/o***

EXAMPLES: thoracic, pectoralgia, pectus excavatum, stethoscope

NOTES: The root *pector/o* can also stand as a word by itself. When it does, however, the ending changes slightly, from *pectoro* to *pectus.* Hence, pectus excavatum.

The term *stethoscope* literally means *an instrument for looking at the chest,* but of course, you do not look with a stethoscope—you listen.

pleura

ROOT: ***pleur/o***

EXAMPLES: pleuritis, pleurectomy

NOTES: The *pleura* is a membrane surrounding the lungs.

diaphragm

ROOT: ***phren/o***

EXAMPLES: phrenospasm, phrenoplegia

NOTES: In addition to the diaphragm, *phren/o* can also refer to the brain (as in the term *schizophrenia*). The rationale comes from the ancient Greek view of the mind. The Greeks believed that the chest was the seat of emotion and reason. As that view changed and the location of the mind moved from the chest to the brain, the word for mind became applied to both regions of the body.

Process of Respiration

Although air begins its journey in the nose and mouth, the work of breathing actually starts with two sets of muscles: the muscles between the ribs (*intercostal*) and a horizontal muscle (*diaphragm*) that lies between the chest and the abdomen. When these muscles shorten (*contract*), they cause the chest to enlarge, which decreases chest (*thoracic*) pressure. As a result, air is literally sucked into the lungs.

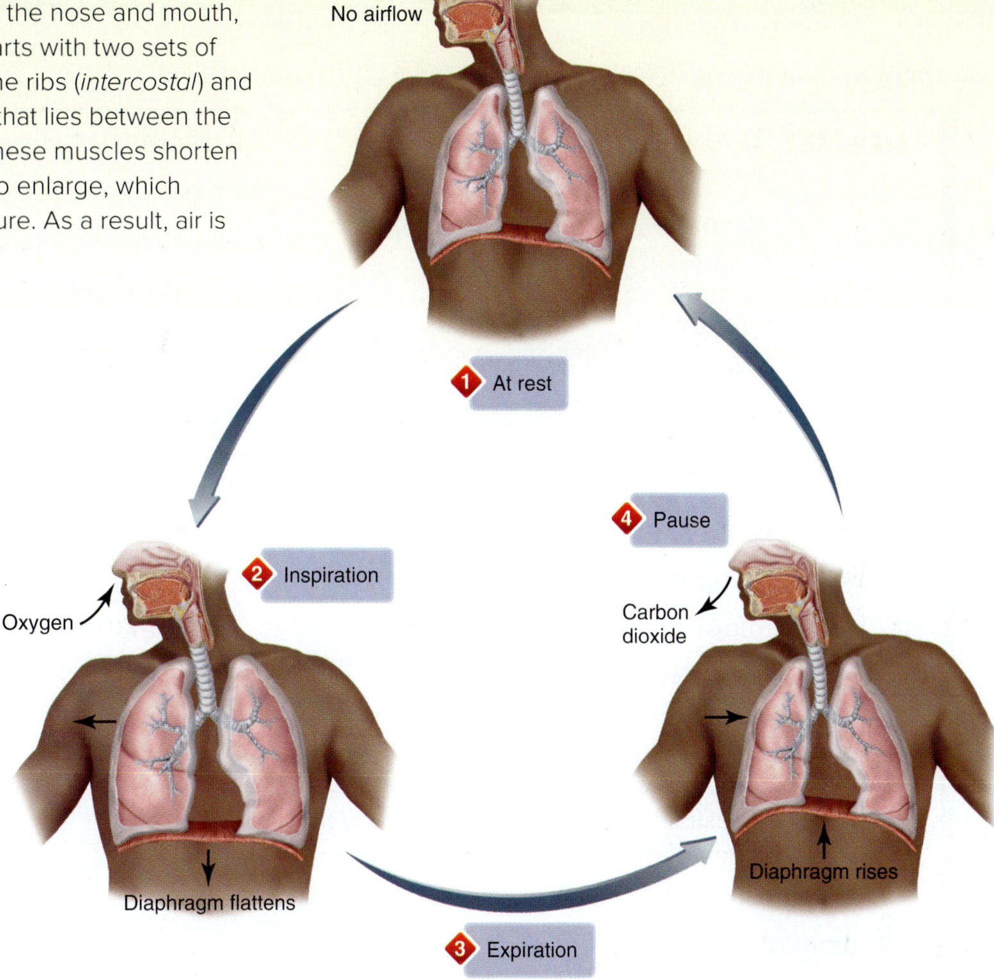

oxygen

ROOT: ***ox/o***

EXAMPLES: hypoxia, hypoxemia

NOTES: *Hypoxia* refers to a lack of oxygen in tissue cells. *Hypoxemia* refers to lack of oxygen in the blood. If a hypoxic patient is also hypoxemic, then oxygen is not getting into the blood. If the person is not hypoxemic, then the problem lies in the transfer of oxygen from blood to tissue. Diagnosing this problem is similar to tracking a package: If a customer does not receive a package, the delivery chain could have broken down in any number of places along the way. The package might never have been sent, might not have made it on the delivery truck, or might not have been delivered to the right door.

breathing

WORD PARTS: ***spir/o, -pnea***

EXAMPLES: spirometry, sleep apnea

NOTES: *Spir/o* also occurs in other words:

- *Perspire* translates as *to breathe through*.
- *Conspire* translates as *to breathe together*—no doubt coming from the idea that people who are *conspiring* can be thought of as being huddled together and breathing the same air.
- *Expire* also contains the *spir/o* root and means *to breathe out*. It was originally written as *exspire,* but the letter *s* was dropped because *x* is made up of two *k* sounds. To test this, say *expire* and *exspire*. They are rarely pronounced differently.

carbon dioxide

ROOTS: ***capn/o (Greek for* smoke*), carb/o (Latin for* coal*)***

EXAMPLES: hypercapnia, hypocarbia

NOTES: One of the treatments for hyperventilation is to have the person breathe into a paper bag. A person who is hyperventilating has *hypocarbia* and thus needs to increase the carbon dioxide in his or her respiratory system.

Learning Outcome 10.1 Exercises

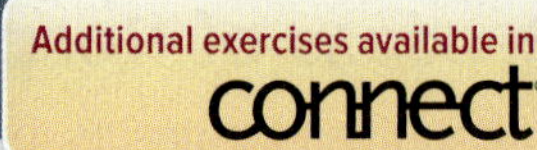

TRANSLATION

EXERCISE 1 *Match the word part on the left with its definition on the right.*

____	1. adenoid/o		a. windpipe
____	2. sin/o		b. tonsil
____	3. tonsill/o		c. sinus
____	4. sept/o		d. mouth
____	5. pharyng/o		e. nose
____	6. palat/o		f. adenoids
____	7. or/o		g. septum
____	8. laryng/o		h. voice box
____	9. rhin/o		i. pharynx
____	10. trache/o		j. palate

EXERCISE 2 *Translate the following word parts.*

1. sinus/o ____________________
2. adenoid/o ____________________
3. pharyng/o ____________________
4. tonsill/o ____________________
5. palat/o ____________________
6. nas/o ____________________
7. or/o ____________________
8. sept/o ____________________
9. trache/o ____________________
10. laryng/o ____________________

EXERCISE 3 *Break down the following words into their component parts and define.*

> **EXAMPLE:** sinusitis *sinus | itis* *inflammation of the sinuses*

1. laryngitis ____________________
2. oronasal ____________________
3. tonsillitis ____________________
4. septectomy ____________________
5. nasendoscope ____________________
6. palatoplasty ____________________
7. pharyngostenosis ____________________

EXERCISE 4 *Match the word part on the left with its definition on the right.*

____	1. bronch/o		a. air
____	2. pleur/o		b. lung
____	3. lob/o		c. lobe
____	4. alveol/o		d. sternum
____	5. stern/o		e. alveolus
____	6. pneum/o		f. chest
____	7. phren/o		g. bronchus
____	8. pulmon/o		h. pleura
____	9. thorac/o		i. rib
____	10. cost/o		j. diaphragm

Learning Outcome 10.1 Exercises

EXERCISE 5 *Translate the following word parts.*

1. lob/o ______
2. stern/o ______
3. pleur/o ______
4. bronchiol/o ______
5. steth/o ______
6. pneumat/o ______
7. alveol/o ______
8. pneumon/o ______
9. pector/o ______
10. pulmon/o ______
11. phren/o ______
12. cost/o ______

EXERCISE 6 *Break down the following words into their component parts and define.*

EXAMPLE: sinusitis *sinus | itis* *inflammation of the sinuses*

1. pneumonia ______
2. bronchitis ______
3. pleuritis ______
4. lobectomy ______
5. alveolitis ______
6. stethoscope ______
7. phrenoplegia ______
8. bronchiostenosis ______

EXERCISE 7 *Match the word part on the left with its definition on the right.*

__a__	1. ox/o	a. oxygen
__c__	2. capn/o	b. breathing
__b__	3. spir/o	c. carbon dioxide

EXERCISE 8 *Translate the following word parts.*

1. ox/o ______
2. carb/o ______
3. capn/o ______
4. spir/o ______
5. -pnea ______

Learning Outcome 10.1 Exercises

GENERATION

EXERCISE 9 *Identify the roots for the following definitions.*

1. tonsil ______
2. adenoid ______
3. pharynx ______
4. mouth ______
5. trachea ______
6. nose ______
7. palate ______
8. throat ______
9. voice box ______

EXERCISE 10 *Build a medical term from the information provided.*

1. inflammation of the throat ______
2. inflammation of the sinus ______
3. incision into the trachea ______
4. discharge from the nose ______
5. surgical removal of the tonsils ______
6. creation of an opening in the trachea ______
7. surgical reconstruction of the septum ______

EXERCISE 11 *Identify the roots for the following definitions.*

1. bronchus ______
2. sternum ______
3. pleura ______
4. lobe ______
5. bronchiole ______
6. alveolus ______
7. diaphragm ______
8. lungs ______
9. chest ______
10. air or lungs ______
11. rib ______
12. air sac ______

Learning Outcome 10.1 Exercises

EXERCISE 12 *Build a medical term from the information provided.*

1. chest pain ________________
2. the study of the lungs ________________
3. instrument to look into the bronchus ________________
4. surgical removal of a rib ________________
5. involuntary contraction of the diaphragm ________________
6. inflammation of the smaller subdivisions of the bronchus ________________
7. pertaining to the sternum and ribs ________________
8. a black lung condition ________________

EXERCISE 13 *Break down the following words into their component parts and define.*

EXAMPLE: sinusitis *sinus | itis* *inflammation of the sinuses*

1. hypercapnia ________________
2. hypoxemia ________________
3. apnea ________________

EXERCISE 14 *Identify the roots for the following definitions.*

1. breathing ________________
2. oxygen ________________
3. carbon dioxide ________________

EXERCISE 15 *Build a medical term from the information provided.*

1. deficient oxygen ________________
2. excessive carbon dioxide ________________
3. instrument for measuring breathing ________________

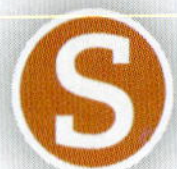

Subjective

Patient History, Problems, Complaints

Breathing processes

Upper respiratory

Lower respiratory

Discharges and secretions

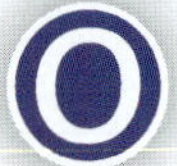

Objective

Observation and Discovery

Physical findings and examination methods

Pathological findings

Laboratory data

Diagnostic procedures

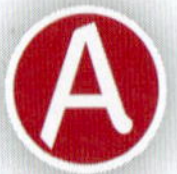

Assessment

Diagnosis and pathology

Upper respiratory

Lower respiratory

Plan

Treatments and Therapies

Upper respiratory

Lower respiratory

Drugs

The focus of this book is to teach you the process of learning roots and translating them in context. This section contains medical terms built from the roots presented in the previous section. The purpose of this section is to expose you to words used in pulmonology that are built from the word roots presented earlier in the chapter. In this section, each term is presented with the correct pronunciation. This is followed by a word analysis that breaks down the word into its component parts, a definition that provides a literal translation of the word, and supplemental information if the word's literal translation deviates from its medical use.

The terms are organized using a health care professional's SOAP note (first introduced in Chapter 2) as a model.

SUBJECTIVE

10.2 Patient History, Problems, Complaints

The most common patient respiratory complaint is coughing. Depending on whether *sputum* is present, a cough can be described as either *productive* or *nonproductive.* A productive cough is also known as *expectoration.* Coughing blood (*hemoptysis*) is generally a more worrisome symptom.

Other respiratory symptoms include changes in the breathing patterns and pain. Descriptions of the breathing pattern reflect the speed of breathing (*tachypnea, bradypnea*), the depth of breathing (*hyperventilation, hypoventilation*), or the work involved in breathing (*orthopnea, dyspnea*). While pain is a less frequent symptom in the respiratory system than in other systems, it should never be overlooked. When chest pain happens during *inspiration* or with a cough, it is known as *pleuritic chest pain.* If pain occurs at these intervals, the pain may be distinguished as respiratory in nature.

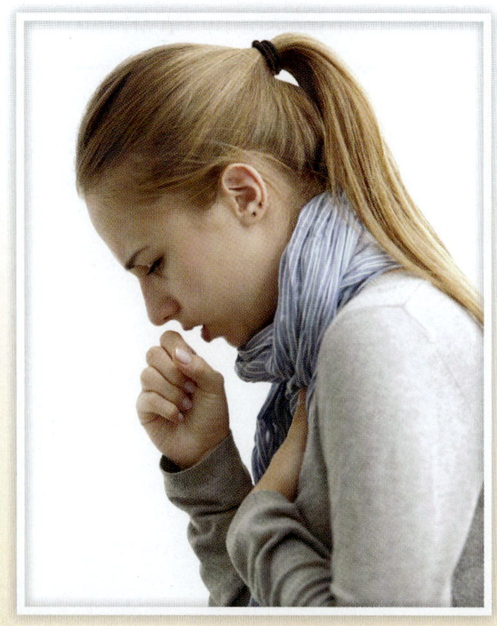

10.2 Patient History, Problems, Complaints

breathing processes

Term	Word Analysis
apnea AP-nee-ah **Definition** cessation of breathing	a / pnea not / breathing
eupnea YOOP-nee-ah **Definition** good/normal breathing	eu / pnea good / breathing
tachypnea ta-KIP-nee-ah **Definition** rapid breathing	tachy / pnea fast / breathing
bradypnea brad-ip-NEE-ah **Definition** slow breathing	brady / pnea slow / breathing
hypopnea hai-POP-nee-ah **Definition** shallow breathing	hypo / pnea under / breathing
hyperpnea hai-perp-NEE-ah **Definition** heavy breathing	hyper / pnea over / breathing
dyspnea disp-NEE-ah **Definition** difficulty breathing	dys / pnea bad / breathing
orthopnea or-thop-NEE-ah **Definition** able to breathe only in an upright position	ortho / pnea straight / breathing
hyperventilation hai-per-ven-ti-LAY-shun **Definition** overbreathing; the condition of having too much air flowing into and out of the lungs; leads to hypocapnia	hyper / ventilation over / breathing
hypoventilation hai-po-ven-ti-LAY-shun **Definition** underbreathing; the condition of having too little air flowing into and out of the lungs; leads to hypercapnia	hypo / ventilation under / breathing

upper respiratory

Term	Word Analysis
dysphonia dis-FON-ia **Definition** bad voice condition (also known as hoarseness)	dys / phonia bad / sound / voice

10.2 Patient History, Problems, Complaints

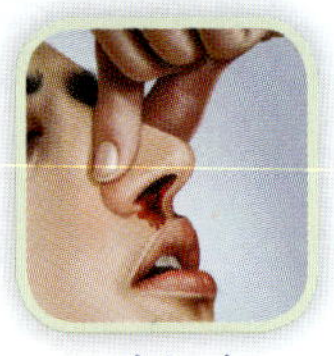
epistaxis

upper respiratory *continued*

Term	Word Analysis
epistaxis ep-ee-STAKS-is **Definition** a nosebleed	from the Greek word *epistazo*, meaning *to drip out or upon*
rhinorrhagia rai-no-RAY-jah **Definition** excessive blood flow from the nose (another term for a nosebleed)	rhino / rrhagia nose / excessive bleeding
rhinorrhea rai-no-REE-yah **Definition** runny nose	rhino / rrhea nose / discharge

lower respiratory

Term	Word Analysis
bronchospasm BRON-ko-spaz-um **Definition** involuntary contraction of the bronchus	broncho / spasm bronchus / involuntary contraction
phrenospasm fre-no-SPAZ-um **Definition** involuntary contraction of the diaphragm (also known as the hiccups)	phreno / spasm diaphragm / involuntary contraction
pleuralgia plur-AL-jah **Definition** pain in the pleura	pleur / algia pleura / pain
pleurodynia plur-oh-DAI-nee-ah **Definition** pain in the pleura	pleuro / dynia pleura / pain
thoracalgia thor-a-KAL-jah **Definition** chest pain	thorac / algia chest / pain

discharges and secretions

Term	Word Analysis
bronchorrhea bron-koh-REE-ah **Definition** discharge from the bronchi	broncho / rrhea bronchus / discharge
expectoration eks-pec-tor-A-shun **Definition** coughing or spitting material out of the lungs	ex / pector / ation out / chest / process
hemoptysis heem-op-TIS-is **Definition** coughing up blood	hemo / ptysis blood / cough
sputum SPYOO-tum **Definition** mucus discharged from the lungs by coughing	Latin for *spit*

S Learning Outcome 10.2 Exercises

PRONUNCIATION

EXERCISE 1 *Indicate which syllable is emphasized when pronounced.*

EXAMPLE: bronchitis bron**chi**tis

1. eupnea ____________________
2. hypopnea ____________________
3. dyspnea ____________________
4. hypoventilation ____________________
5. rhinorrhagia ____________________
6. phrenospasm ____________________
7. bronchospasm ____________________
8. hemoptysis ____________________

TRANSLATION

EXERCISE 2 *Underline and define the word parts from this chapter in the following terms.*

1. tachypnea ____________________
2. hypopnea ____________________
3. rhinorrhagia ____________________
4. bronchospasm ____________________
5. phrenospasm ____________________
6. bronchorrhea ____________________
7. pleuralgia ____________________
8. thoracalgia ____________________
9. hyperventilation ____________________
10. expectoration ____________________

EXERCISE 3 *Match the term on the left with its definition on the right.*

b	1. apnea	a.	hoarseness
d	2. eupnea	b.	cessation of breathing
k	3. dyspnea	c.	pain in the pleura
g	4. orthopnea	d.	normal breathing
i	5. hyperventilation	e.	runny nose
h	6. epistaxis	f.	coughing up blood
a	7. dysphonia	g.	able to breathe only in an upright position
e	8. rhinorrhea	h.	nosebleed
c	9. pleurodynia	i.	overbreathing, or too much air flowing into and out of the lungs
f	10. hemoptysis	j.	mucus discharged from the lungs by coughing
j	11. sputum	k.	difficulty breathing

Learning Outcome 10.2 Exercises

EXERCISE 4 *Break down the following words into their component parts.*

EXAMPLE: nasopharyngoscope *naso | pharyngo | scope*

1. bradypnea ______
2. hyperpnea ______
3. rhinorrhea ______
4. phrenospasm ______
5. pleurodynia ______
6. thoracalgia ______
7. hypoventilation ______
8. hemoptysis ______

EXERCISE 5 *Translate the following terms as literally as possible.*

EXAMPLE: nasopharyngoscope *an instrument for looking at the nose and throat*

1. orthopnea ______
2. hyperpnea ______
3. hypopnea ______
4. rhinorrhagia ______
5. bronchospasm ______
6. pleuralgia ______
7. thoracalgia ______
8. dysphonia ______
9. bronchorrhea ______
10. hyperventilation ______
11. hypoventilation ______

Learning Outcome 10.2 Exercises

GENERATION

EXERCISE 6 *Build a medical term from the information provided.*

EXAMPLE: inflammation of the sinuses *sinusitis*

1. not breathing ______________________
2. good breathing ______________________
3. difficulty breathing ______________________
4. slow breathing ______________________
5. fast breathing ______________________
6. pain in the pleura ______________________
7. runny nose ______________________
8. involuntary contraction of the diaphragm ______________________
9. coughing up blood ______________________

EXERCISE 7 *Multiple-choice questions. Select the correct answer.*

1. *Epistaxis* comes from the Greek word meaning *to drip out or upon* and is used to indicate
   a. a nosebleed
   b. a runny nose
   c. mucus on the lungs
   d. a wet cough
2. The Latin word for *spit,* which indicates mucus discharged by the lungs, is
   a. spasm
   b. sputum
   c. mucus
   d. wet cough
3. Which of the following is NOT a term related to describing a breathing process?
   a. hyperventilation
   b. hypopnea
   c. bradypnea
   d. hemoptysis
4. Which of the following is NOT a term to describe pain in the lower respiratory system?
   a. pleuralgia
   b. rhinorrhagia
   c. pleurodynia
   d. thoracalgia
5. Which term describes a patient who is coughing up blood?
   a. rhinorrhagia
   b. epistaxis
   c. hemoptysis
   d. dyspnea

OBJECTIVE

10.3 Observation and Discovery

When gathering clues about the status of a patient's respiration, a health care professional may use physical findings, labs, and specialized tests or imaging. Sights and sounds are valuable tools in the physical exam of a patient with a respiratory problem. Inspection may reveal an abnormal chest shape, a patient working harder to breathe, or a change in skin color. When listening to the patient's chest (*auscultation*), an examiner may notice changes in breathing sounds.

Lab data mainly deal with the levels of carbon dioxide and oxygen in the blood. *Capnography* and *oximetry* are fast tests that provide this information, but more specialized tests examine how well the lungs work.

Spirometry measures the strength of breathing, while a *ventilation–perfusion scan* measures how effectively oxygen and blood reach different parts of the lungs. Finally, it may be necessary to get a closer look to get to the root of the problem (e.g., *bronchoscopy* and *thorascopy*).

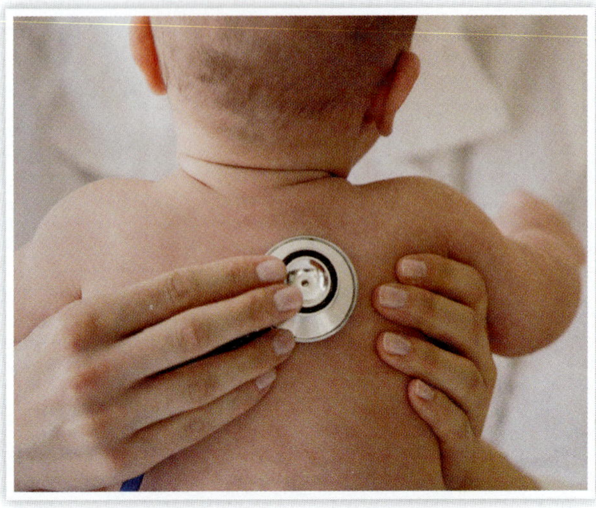

A doctor's first step in gathering data for a diagnosis is to listen to lung function using a stethoscope.

physical findings and examination methods

Term	Word Analysis
auscultation ah-skul-TAY-shun	from the Latin word *ausculto,* meaning *to listen*
Definition a health care professional using a stethoscope	
cyanosis sai-an-O-sis	cyan / osis blue / condition
Definition a bluish color in the skin caused by insufficient oxygen	
pectoriloquy pek-tor-IH-low-kwee	pectori / loquy chest / speak
Definition speaking from the chest; used as a means of finding masses in the lung. A health professional listening to a patient's chest asks the patient to whisper a word. The word will be audible in areas where fluid or a mass is present. Hence the chest "speaks" in those places. **NOTE:** A common related word is *ventriloquist,* a person who makes a puppet appear to talk. *Venter* means *stomach;* thus *ventriloquist* translates as *one who speaks from his stomach.*	
pectus carinatum PEK-tus car-ee-NAH-tum	pectus carinatum chest keel
Definition a chest that protrudes like the keel of a ship	
pectus excavatum PEK-tus eks-cuh-VAH-tum	pectus ex / cavatum chest out / hollowed
Definition a chest that is hollowed out	
percussion per-KUH-shun	from the Latin word *percussio,* meaning *to strike*
Definition striking the body surface (in this context, to cause vibrations that can help locate fluid build-up in the chest)	

pectus carinatum

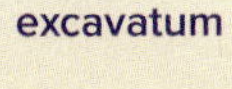

pectus excavatum

pathological findings

Term	Word Analysis
atelectasis ah-tel-EK-ta-sis **Definition** incomplete expansion	a / tel / ectasis not / complete / expansion
bronchiectasis bron-key-EK-ta-sis **Definition** expansion of the bronchi	bronchi / ectasis bronchus / expansion
caseous necrosis KAYZ-ee-us ne-CROW-sis **Definition** the death of tissue with a cheeselike appearance	caseous necr / osis cheeselike death / condition
chylothorax kai-low-THOR-aks **Definition** chyle in the chest **NOTE:** Chyle is a milky bodily fluid formed in the small intestine during digestion of fatty foods and carried through the body via lymph vessels.	chylo / thorax chyle / chest
empyema em-pie-EE-mah **Definition** pus inside the chest	em / py / ema in / pus / condition
hemothorax heem-o-THOR-aks **Definition** blood in the chest	hemo / thorax blood / chest
phrenoplegia fre-no-PLEE-jah **Definition** paralysis of the diaphragm	phreno / plegia diaphragm / paralysis
phrenoptosis fre-nop-TOE-sis **Definition** drooping of the diaphragm	phreno / pt / osis diaphragm / drooping / condition
pleural effusion PLUR-al ef-YOO-zhun **Definition** fluid pouring out into the pleura **NOTE:** The prefix in *effusion* is actually *ex*. The *x* turns to an *f* when followed by an *f*. Why? Say *exfusion* 10 times. Most people slur *exfusion* into *effusion* because it is easier to say.	pleur / al ex / fusion pleura / pertaining to out / pour
pneumohemothorax new-moh-hee-moh-THOR-aks **Definition** air and blood in the chest	pneumo / hemo / thorax air / blood / chest
pneumothorax new-moh-THOR-aks **Definition** air in the chest	pneumo / thorax air / chest
pulmonary edema pul-mon-AIR-ee ah-DEE-ma **Definition** swelling in the lungs	pulmon / ary edema lung / pertaining to swelling

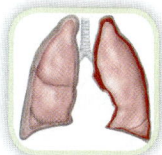

hemothorax

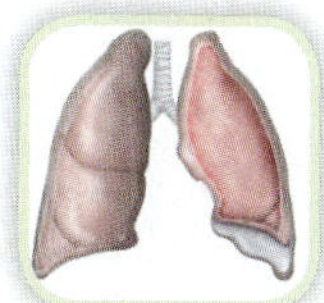
pleural effusion

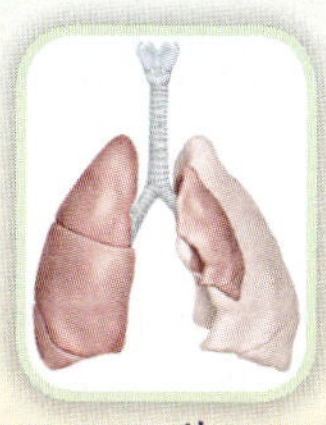
pneumothorax

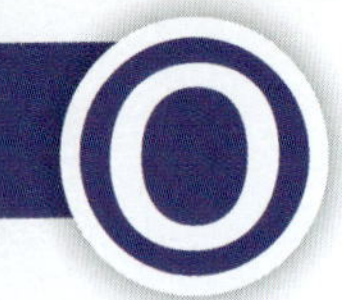

10.3 Observation and Discovery

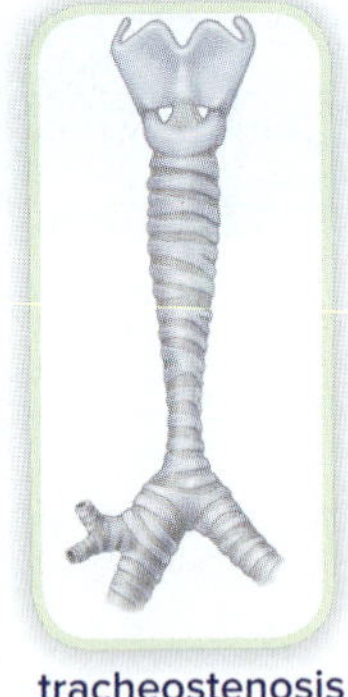

tracheostenosis

pathological finding *continued*

Term	Word Analysis
pyothorax pie-oh-THOR-aks **Definition** pus in the chest	pyo / thorax pus / chest
tracheostenosis tray-kee-oh-sten-OH-sis **Definition** narrowing of the trachea	tracheo / stenosis trachea / narrowing

laboratory data

Term	Word Analysis
hypercapnia hai-per-CAP-nee-yah **Definition** excessive carbon dioxide	hyper / capn / ia over / carbon dioxide / condition
hypercarbia hai-per-CAR-bee-yah **Definition** excessive carbon dioxide	hyper / carb / ia over / carbon dioxide / condition
hypocapnia hai-po-CAP-nee-yah **Definition** insufficient carbon dioxide	hypo / capn / ia under / carbon dioxide / condition
hypocarbia hai-po-CAR-bee-yah **Definition** insufficient carbon dioxide	hypo / carb / ia under / carbon dioxide / condition
hypoxemia hai-poks-EEM-ee-yah **Definition** insufficient oxygen in the blood	hypo / ox / em / ia under / oxygen / blood / condition
hypoxia hai-POKS-ee-yah **Definition** insufficient oxygen	hypo / ox / ia under / oxygen / condition

diagnostic procedures

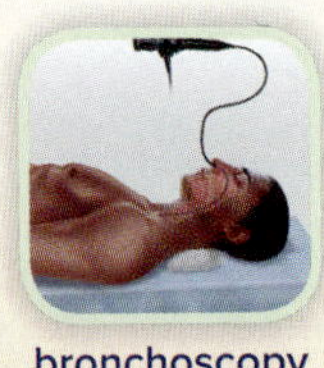

bronchoscopy

Term	Word Analysis
bronchoscopy bron-KOS-koh-pee **Definition** procedure to look inside the bronchi	broncho / scop / y bronchus / look / procedure
capnography cap-NAH-gra-fee **Definition** procedure to record carbon dioxide levels	capno / graph / y carbon dioxide / recording / process

diagnostic procedures *continued*

Term	Word Analysis	Definition
capnometer cap-NOM-eh-ter	capno / meter carbon dioxide / instrument to measure	instrument to measure carbon dioxide levels
computed tomography com-PYOO-ted tom-O-grah-fee	computed tomo / graph / y cut / writing / procedure	an imaging procedure using a computer to cut **NOTE:** *Cut* in this context does not mean incision but rather using a computer to view “slices” of a patient’s organs.
endoscope EN-doh-SKOHP	endo / scope inside / instrument to look	instrument to look inside
nasopharyngoscope nay-zoh-fa-RIN-go-skope	naso / pharyngo / scope nose / throat / instrument to look	an instrument to look at the nose and throat
oximetry ok-SIM-ah-tree	oxi / metr / y oxygen / measure / procedure	procedure to measure oxygen levels
polysomnography po-lee-som-NAH-gra-fee	poly / somno / graph / y multiple / sleep / recording / procedure	recording multiple aspects of sleep
pulmonary angiography pul-mon-AIR-ee an-jee-O-grah-fee	pulmon / ary lung / pertaining to angio / graph / y blood vessel / recording / procedure	an imaging procedure for recording pulmonary blood vessel activity
pulmonary function testing pul-mon-AIR-ee funk-shun TES-ting	pulmon / ary function testing lung / pertaining to	a group of tests used to evaluate the condition and operation of the lungs
spirometry speer-O-me-tree	spiro / metr / y breathing / measure / procedure	procedure to measure breathing
thoracoscopy thor-a-KOS-koh-pee	thoraco / scopy chest / procedure to look	examination of the chest **NOTE:** This word is sometimes shortened to *thorascopy* to make it easier to say.
ventilation–perfusion scan ven-ti-LAY-shun–per-FYOO-shun skan	ventil / ation – per / fusion breathing / process – through / pour	a scan that tests whether a problem in the lungs is caused by airflow (ventilation) or blood flow (perfusion)

endoscope

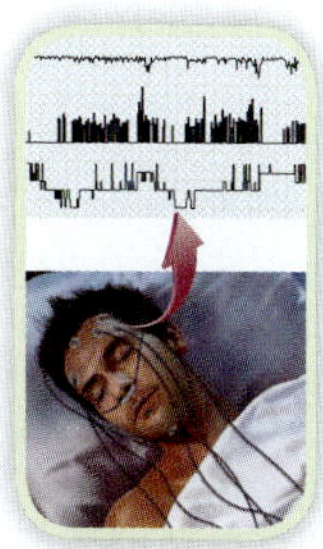

polysomnography

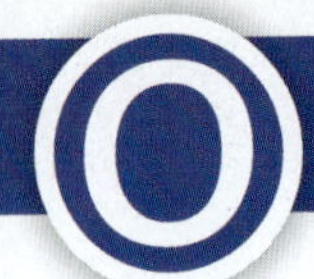

Learning Outcome 10.3 Exercises

PRONUNCIATION

EXERCISE 1 *Indicate which syllable is emphasized when pronounced.*

EXAMPLE: bronchitis bron**chi**tis

1. capnometer ____________
2. hemothorax ____________
3. hypoxia ____________
4. empyema ____________
5. phrenoptosis ____________
6. pyothorax ____________
7. pneumohemothorax ____________
8. atelectasis ____________
9. hypocarbia ____________
10. pectoriloquy ____________
11. endoscopy ____________
12. polysomnography ____________
13. thoracoscopy ____________

TRANSLATION

EXERCISE 2 *Underline and define the word parts from this chapter in the following terms.*

1. pectoriloquy ____________
2. pulmonary ____________
3. chylothorax ____________
4. hypercarbia ____________
5. hypocapnia ____________
6. hypoxia ____________
7. capnography ____________
8. bronchoscopy ____________
9. spirometry ____________
10. thoracoscopy ____________

EXERCISE 3 *Match the term on the left with its definition on the right.*

____	1. percussion	a.	a scan that tests whether a problem in the lungs is caused by airflow or blood flow
____	2. cyanosis	b.	death of tissue with a cheeselike appearance
____	3. pectus excavatum	c.	an instrument to look at the nose and throat
____	4. pectus carinatum	d.	chest that is hollowed out
____	5. auscultation	e.	a bluish color in the skin
____	6. caseous necrosis	f.	instrument to look inside
____	7. atelectasis	g.	a recording procedure using a computer to view "cuts" of a patient's organs
____	8. pleural effusion	h.	fluid pouring out into the pleura
____	9. hypoxemia	i.	deficient oxygen in the blood
____	10. endoscope	j.	using a stethoscope to listen to the chest
____	11. nasopharyngoscope	k.	a group of tests used to evaluate the condition and operation of the lungs
____	12. ventilation-perfusion scan	l.	incomplete expansion
____	13. computed tomography	m.	striking the body surface to help locate fluid build-up in the chest
____	14. pulmonary function testing	n.	a chest that protrudes

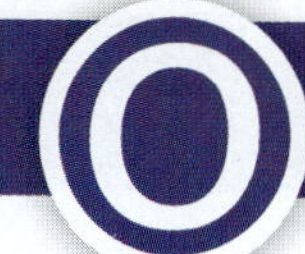

Learning Outcome 10.3 Exercises

EXERCISE 4 *Break down the following words into their component parts.*

EXAMPLE: nasopharyngoscope *naso | pharyngo | scope*

1. hemothorax ______
2. phrenoplegia ______
3. capnometer ______
4. oximetry ______
5. hypercapnia ______
6. hypocarbia ______
7. pyothorax ______
8. pneumothorax ______
9. pneumohemothorax ______
10. empyema ______
11. tracheostenosis ______
12. bronchiectasis ______
13. polysomnography ______
14. phrenoptosis ______
15. pulmonary angiography ______

EXERCISE 5 *Translate the following terms as literally as possible.*

EXAMPLE: nasopharyngoscope *an instrument for looking at the nose and throat*

1. oximetry ______
2. hypercapnia ______
3. hypocarbia ______
4. hypercarbia ______
5. hypocapnia ______
6. hypoxia ______
7. thoracoscopy ______
8. capnography ______
9. hemothorax ______
10. pneumohemothorax ______
11. bronchiectasis ______
12. polysomnography ______
13. pulmonary angiography ______
14. phrenoptosis ______
15. pectus excavatum ______
16. pectoriloquy ______

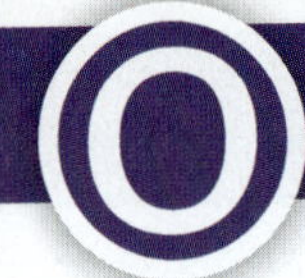

Learning Outcome 10.3 Exercises

GENERATION

EXERCISE 6 *Build a medical term from the information provided.*

EXAMPLE: inflammation of the sinuses *sinusitis*

1. swelling in the lungs ______
2. air in the chest ______
3. pus inside the chest ______
4. pus in the chest ______
5. chyle in the chest ______
6. paralysis of the diaphragm ______
7. narrowing of the trachea ______
8. instrument to measure carbon dioxide levels ______
9. procedure to look inside the bronchi ______
10. procedure to measure breathing ______

EXERCISE 7 *Multiple-choice questions. Select the correct answer.*

1. A health care professional uses a stethoscope as part of the following procedure:
   a. auscultation
   b. polysomnography
   c. endoscopy
   d. capnography
2. Which of the following terms pertains to the diaphragm?
   a. pleural effusion
   b. pulmonary edema
   c. phrenoplegia
   d. pneumothorax
3. Which procedure measures oxygen levels?
   a. spirometry
   b. capnography
   c. bronchoscopy
   d. oximetry
4. The term *hemothorax* means that there is which of the following in the chest?
   a. blood
   b. pus
   c. chyle
   d. air

ASSESSMENT

10.4 Diagnosis and Pathology

Since the upper respiratory tract is the first line of defense, infections in this area are very common. While inflammation in these areas (*rhinitis, sinusitis, pharyngitis, laryngitis,* etc.) is not *always* caused by infection, infection is certainly the most common cause. The lower respiratory tract has its share of infections as well, with the most common being *bronchitis* and *pneumonia*. *Asthma* and *chronic obstructive pulmonary disorder* are long-term, noninfectious causes of illness that can be serious.

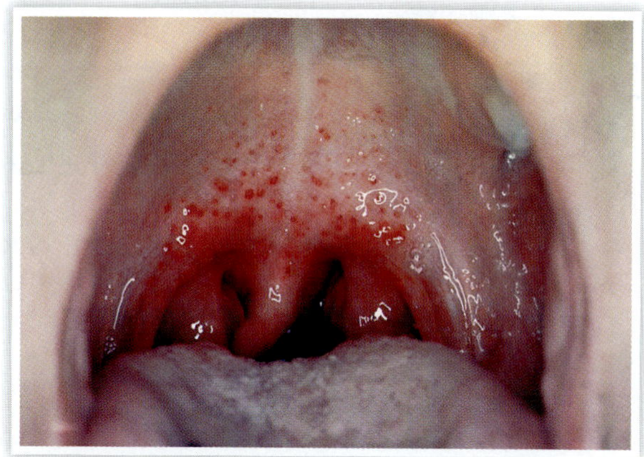

"Open up and say 'Ah'" is the way many examinations involving the respiratory system begin.

upper respiratory

Term	Word Analysis
laryngitis la-rin-JAI-tis	laryng / itis larynx / inflammation
Definition inflammation of the larynx	
laryngotracheobronchitis la-rin-go-tray-key-o-bron-KAI-tis	laryngo / tracheo / bronch / itis larynx / trachea / bronchus / inflammation
Definition inflammation of the larynx, trachea, and bronchi	
rhinitis rai-NAI-tis	rhin / itis nose / inflammation
Definition inflammation of the nasal passages	
sinusitis sai-nus-AI-tis	sinus / itis sinus / inflammation
Definition inflammation of the sinus	
pansinusitis pan-sai-nus-AI-tis	pan / sinus / itis all / sinus / inflammation
Definition inflammation of all sinuses	
sleep apnea sleep AP-nee-ah	a / pnea not / breathing
Definition a condition where the patient ceases to breathe while asleep	
tonsillitis ton-sil-AI-tis	tonsill / itis tonsil / inflammation
Definition inflammation of the tonsils	
tracheitis tray-kee-AI-tis	trache / itis trachea / inflammation
Definition inflammation of the trachea	
tracheomalacia tray-kee-oh-ma-LAY-shah	tracheo / malac / ia trachea / softening / condition
Definition softening of the trachea	

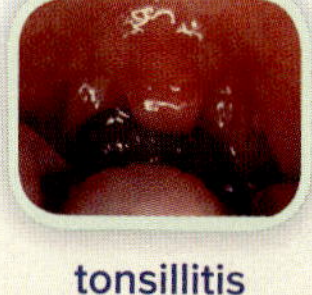

tonsillitis

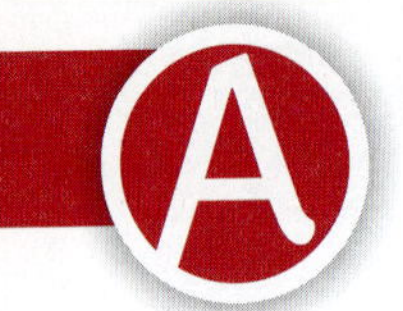

10.4 Diagnosis and Pathology

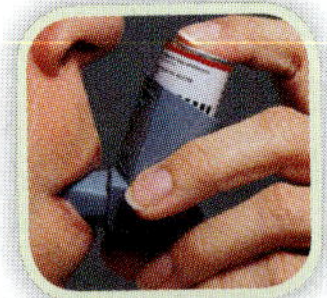

asthma

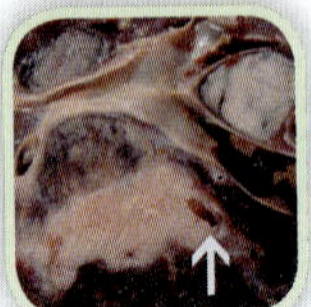

bronchiogenic carcinoma

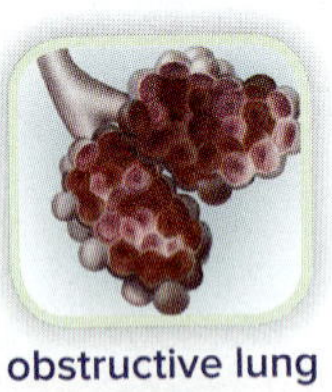

obstructive lung disorder

lower respiratory

Term	Word Analysis
asthma AZ-ma	from the Greek word for *panting* or *gasping*
Definition a disease causing episodic narrowing and inflammation of the airway **NOTE:** The name describes the wheezing and shortness of breath that accompanies an attack.	
bronchiogenic carcinoma bron-kee-oh-JEN-ic car-si-NO-ma	bronchio / genic — bronchus / beginning in carcin / oma — cancer / tumor
Definition a cancerous tumor originating in the bronchi	
bronchiolitis bron-kee-yo-LAI-tis	bronchiol / itis — bronchiole / inflammation
Definition inflammation of a bronchiole	
bronchitis bron-KAI-tis	bronch / itis — bronchus / inflammation
Definition inflammation of the bronchi	
chronic obstructive pulmonary disease (COPD) KRON-ik ob-STRUKT-iv pul-mon-AIR-ee diz-EEZ	chron / ic — time / pertaining to ob / struct / ive — in the way / build / pertaining to pulmon / ary — lung / pertaining to
Definition a group of lung diseases characterized by the continual blockage of lung passages	
diaphragmatocele dai-a-frag-MAT-o-seel	diaphragmato / cele — diaphragm / pouch / tumor / hernia
Definition hernia of the diaphragm	
emphysema im-fi-ZEE-ma	from the Greek word *emphysan*, meaning *to inflate*
Definition a disease that causes the alveoli to lose elasticity; emphysema patients can inhale but have difficulty exhaling	
obstructive lung disorder ob-STRUKT-iv	ob / struct / ive — in the way / build / pertaining to lung disorder
Definition a lung disorder caused by a blockage	
pleuritis plur-AI-tis	pleur / itis — pleura / inflammation
Definition inflammation of the pleura	
pleurisy PLUR-ih-see	pleur / isy — pleura / inflammation
Definition another word for pleuritis	
pneumatocele new-MAT-o-seel	pneumato / cele — lung / pouch / tumor / hernia
Definition hernia of the lung	

10.4 Diagnosis and Pathology

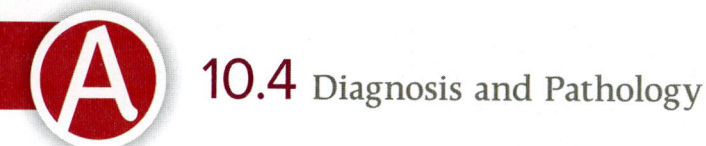

lower respiratory *continued*

Term	Word Analysis
pneumoconiosis new-moh-con-i-O-sis **Definition** a lung condition caused by dust	pneumo / coni / osis lung / dust / condition
pneumonia new-MOH-nee-yah **Definition** a lung condition	pneumon / ia lung / condition
pneumonitis new-moh-NAI-tis **Definition** inflammation of the lung	pneumon / itis lung / inflammation
pulmonary embolism pul-mon-AIR-ee em-bol-IZ-um **Definition** blockage in the pulmonary blood supply	pulmon / ary em / bol / ism lung / pertaining to in / throw / condition
pulmonary neoplasm pul-mon-AIR-ee nee-oh-PLAZ-sum **Definition** new growth (tumor) in the lung	pulmon / ary neo / plasm lung / pertaining to new / formation
restrictive lung disorder re-STRIKT-iv **Definition** a lung disorder caused by the limiting of air into the lungs	re / strict / ive lung disorder back / bind / tie / pertaining to

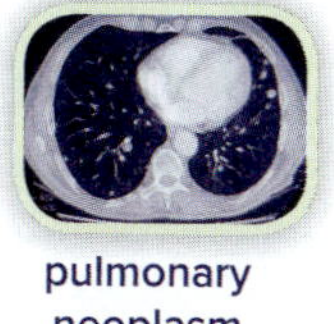

pulmonary neoplasm

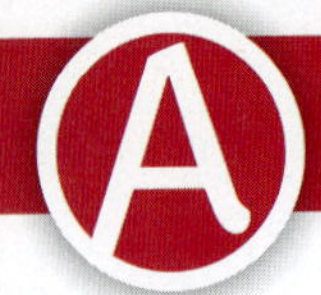

Learning Outcome 10.4 Exercises

PRONUNCIATION

EXERCISE 1 *Indicate which syllable is emphasized when pronounced.*

EXAMPLE: bronchitis bron**chi**tis

1. rhinitis ____________
2. pleuritis ____________
3. pleurisy ____________
4. asthma ____________
5. pneumonia ____________
6. sinusitis ____________
7. emphysema ____________

TRANSLATION

EXERCISE 2 *Break down the following words into their component parts.*

EXAMPLE: nasopharyngoscope *naso | pharyngo | scope*

1. bronchiolitis ____________
2. pansinusitis ____________
3. tracheomalacia ____________
4. pneumoconiosis ____________
5. pulmonary embolism ____________
6. laryngotracheobronchitis ____________
7. bronchiogenic carcinoma ____________

EXERCISE 3 *Underline and define the word parts from this chapter in the following terms.*

1. laryngitis ____________
2. rhinitis ____________
3. sinusitis ____________
4. tonsillitis ____________
5. bronchitis ____________
6. pulmonary ____________
7. tracheitis ____________
8. pleuritis ____________

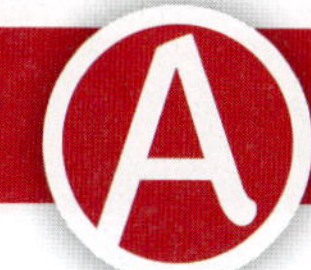

Learning Outcome 10.4 Exercises

EXERCISE 4 *Match the term on the left with its definition on the right.*

__d__ 1. sleep apnea
__f__ 2. obstructive lung disorder
__h__ 3. restrictive lung disorder
__g__ 4. asthma
__a__ 5. emphysema
__c__ 6. chronic obstructive pulmonary disease (COPD)
_____ 7. pleurisy
__b__ 8. pulmonary embolism

a. a disease that causes the alveoli to lose their elasticity
b. blockage in the pulmonary blood supply
c. a lung disease caused by the continual blocking of lung passages
d. a condition where the patient ceases to breathe while asleep
e. inflammation of the pleura
f. a lung disorder caused by a blockage
g. a disease causing episodic narrowing and inflammation of the airway
h. a lung disorder caused by the limiting of air into the lungs

EXERCISE 5 *Translate the following terms as literally as possible.*

EXAMPLE: nasopharyngoscope *an instrument for looking at the nose and throat*

1. pneumonia __________
2. pleuritis __________
3. rhinitis __________
4. pansinusitis __________
5. tracheomalacia __________
6. pneumatocele __________
7. diaphragmatocele __________
8. pulmonary neoplasm __________
9. laryngotracheobronchitis __________
10. bronchiogenic carcinoma __________

GENERATION

EXERCISE 6 *Build a medical term from the information provided.*

EXAMPLE: inflammation of the sinuses *sinusitis*

1. inflammation of the larynx __________
2. inflammation of all sinuses __________
3. inflammation of the tonsils __________
4. inflammation of the lung __________
5. inflammation of the trachea __________
6. inflammation of the bronchi __________
7. a lung condition caused by dust __________

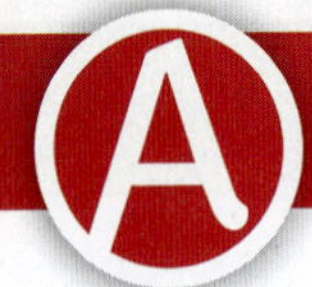

Learning Outcome 10.4 Exercises

EXERCISE 7 *Multiple-choice questions. Select the correct answer(s).*

1. The Greek word for *panting* or *gasping* is

   a. emphysema
   b. asthma
   c. pleurisy
   d. embolism

2. *Emphysema* comes from the Greek word meaning ________________ and describes a disease that causes the alveoli to lose their elasticity.

   a. to deflate
   b. to stretch
   c. to inflate
   d. to loosen

3. Select the terms that pertain to the upper respiratory system.

   a. bronchitis
   b. laryngitis
   c. laryngotracheobronchitis
   d. pansinusitis
   e. pleuritis
   f. pneumonitis
   g. rhinitis
   h. sinusitis
   i. tonsillitis
   j. tracheitis

4. Select the terms that pertain to the lower respiratory system.

   a. bronchitis
   b. laryngitis
   c. laryngotracheobronchitis
   d. pansinusitis
   e. pleuritis
   f. pneumonitis
   g. rhinitis
   h. sinusitis
   i. tonsillitis
   j. tracheitis

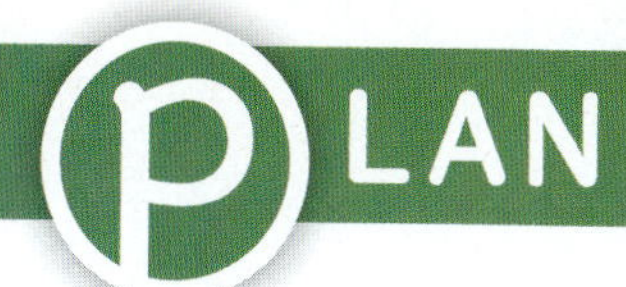

10.5 Treatments and Therapies

Most respiratory illnesses respond to medicines. Bronchi-opening medicines (*bronchodilators*) given through an *inhaler device* or a machine (*nebulizer*) help people with asthma or chronic obstructive pulmonary disorder. Cough-stopping (*antitussive*) medicines are popular, but not necessarily very helpful.

With some illnesses, more aggressive intervention is needed. Surgeries of the upper airway are among the most common procedures. Lower airway surgeries, such as cutting out part of the lung (*lobectomy*), are less common. Very ill patients or patients who are undergoing surgery may need to have a tube placed in the mouth and into the windpipe (*endotracheal tube*). The tube is then attached to a breathing machine.

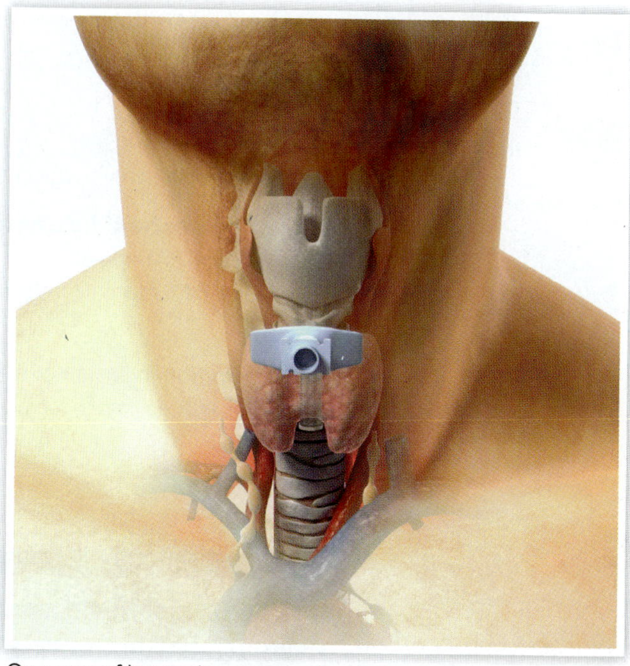

One way of bypassing a patient's obstructed airway is through a tracheostomy, creating an artificial opening in the trachea to allow air to enter the lungs easier.

upper respiratory

Term	Word Analysis
adenoidectomy a-din-oid-EK-toe-mee **Definition** removal of the adenoids	adenoid / ec / tomy adenoid / out / cut
laryngectomy la-rin-JEK-toe-mee **Definition** removal of the larynx	laryng / ec / tomy larynx / out / cut
laryngoplasty la-rin-GO-plas-stee **Definition** reconstruction of the larynx	laryngo / plasty larynx / reconstruction
palatoplasty pal-e-toe-PLAS-tee **Definition** reconstruction of a palate	palato / plasty palate / reconstruction
septoplasty sep-toe-PLAS-tee **Definition** reconstruction of a septum	septo / plasty septum / reconstruction
tonsillectomy ton-sil-EK-toe-mee **Definition** removal of the tonsils	tonsill / ec / tomy tonsil / out / cut

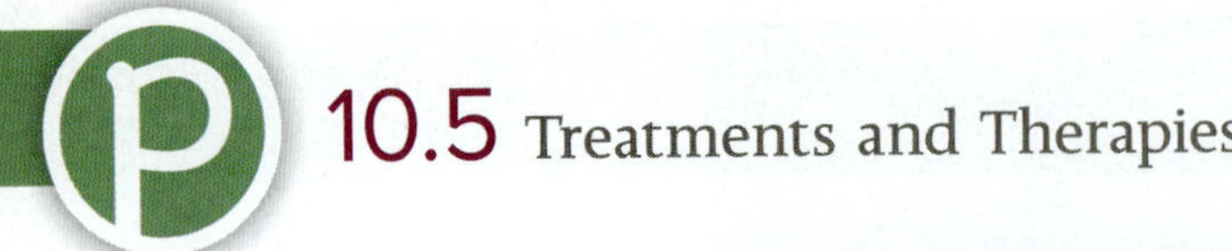

10.5 Treatments and Therapies

upper respiratory *continued*

Term	Word Analysis
tracheostomy tray-kee-AH-stoh-mee **Definition** creation of an opening in the trachea	tracheo / stomy trachea / creation of an opening
tracheotomy tray-kee-AH-toe-mee **Definition** incision into the trachea	tracheo / tomy trachea / cut
endotracheal intubation en-doh-TRAY-kee-al in-too-BAY-shun **Definition** insertion of a tube inside the trachea	endo / trache / al inside / trachea / pertaining to in / tub / ation in / tube / process

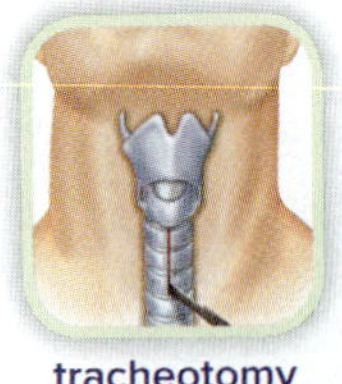
tracheotomy

lower respiratory

Term	Word Analysis
bronchoplasty bron-koh-PLAS-tee **Definition** reconstruction of a bronchus	broncho / plasty bronchus / reconstruction
cardiopulmonary resuscitation (CPR) kar-dee-oh-pul-mon-AIR-ee ree-sus-i-TAY-shun **Definition** method of artificially maintaining blood flow and airflow when breathing and pulse have stopped NOTE: *Suscit* is formed by adding the prefix *sub-* to the Latin word *cito*, which means *to move*. *Suscit* = *sub* + *cito* = *to move from beneath*, and thus *to raise* or *awaken*. The *cito* root is found in other words like *excite*, *incite*, and *recite*.	cardio / pulmon / ary heart / lung / pertaining to re / suscit / ation again / awaken / process
lobectomy loh-BEK-toe-mee **Definition** removal of a lobe	lob / ec / tomy lobe / out / cut
pleuropexy ploo-rah-PEK-see **Definition** reattachment of the pleura	pleuro / pexy pleura / fixation
pneumonectomy new-mon-EK-toe-mee **Definition** removal of a lung	pneumon / ec / tomy lung / out / cut

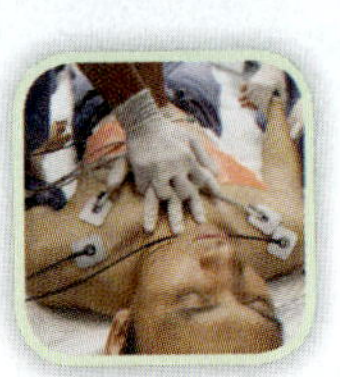
cardiopulmonary resuscitation

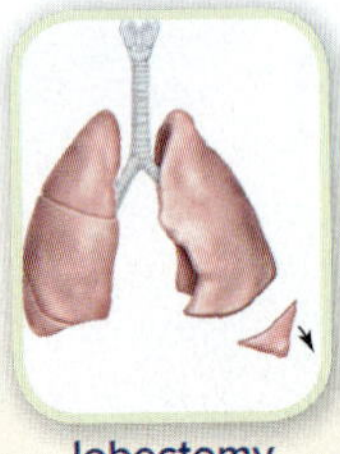
lobectomy

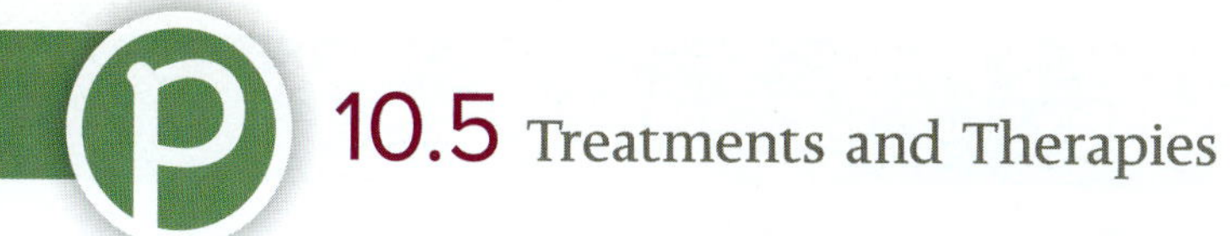

10.5 Treatments and Therapies

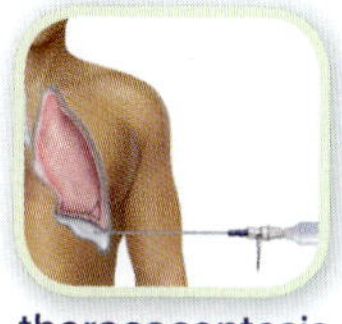
thoracocentesis

lower respiratory *continued*

Term	Word Analysis
thoracocentesis thor-a-koh-sin-TEE-sis **Definition** puncture of the chest	thoraco / centesis chest / puncture
thoracentesis thor-a-sin-TEE-sis **Definition** puncture of the chest **NOTE:** This word drops a syllable from *thoracocentesis* to make it easier to say.	thora [co] / centesis chest / puncture
thoracoplasty thor-a-koh-PLAS-tee **Definition** reconstruction of the chest	thoraco / plasty chest / reconstruction
thoracostomy thor-a-KOS-toe-mee **Definition** creation of an opening in the chest	thoraco / stomy chest / creation of an opening
thoracotomy thor-a-KAH-toe-mee **Definition** incision into the chest	thoraco / tomy chest / cut

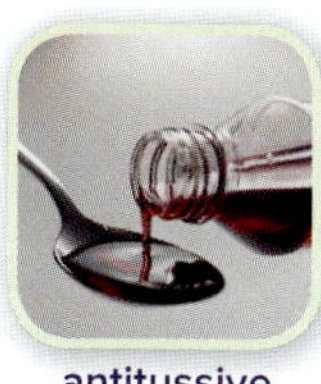
antitussive

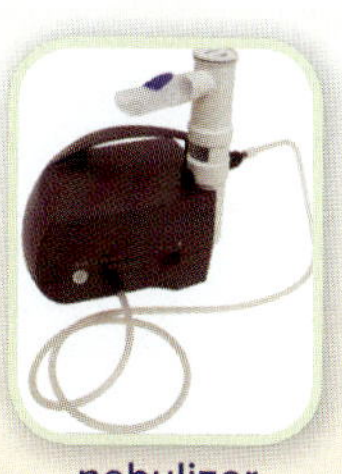
nebulizer

drugs

Term	Word Analysis
antitussive an-tee-TUSS-iv **Definition** a drug that prevents coughing	anti / tuss / ive against / cough / agent
bronchodilator bron-koh-DAI-lay-tor **Definition** a drug that expands the walls of the bronchi	broncho / dilator bronchus / expander
expectorant eks-PEK-tor-ant **Definition** a drug that encourages the expulsion of material from the lungs	ex / pector / ant out / chest / agent
mucolytic myoo-koh-LIT-ik **Definition** a drug that aids in the breakdown of mucus	muco / lytic mucus / break down
nebulizer neh-byoo-LAI-zir **Definition** a machine that administers respiratory medication by creating a "cloud" or mist that is inhaled by the patient	from the Latin word *nebula*, meaning *cloud*

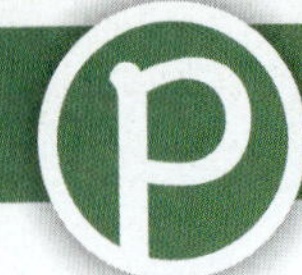

Learning Outcome 10.5 Exercises

PRONUNCIATION

EXERCISE 1 *Indicate which syllable is emphasized when pronounced.*

EXAMPLE: bronchitis bron**chi**tis

1. lobectomy ______
2. antitussive ______
3. adenoidectomy ______
4. palatoplasty ______
5. tracheostomy ______
6. thoracentesis ______
7. thoracostomy ______

TRANSLATION

EXERCISE 2 *Break down the following words into their component parts.*

EXAMPLE: nasopharyngoscope *naso | pharyngo | scope*

1. septoplasty ______
2. laryngoplasty ______
3. tracheotomy ______
4. adenoidectomy ______
5. pneumonectomy ______
6. thoracostomy ______
7. tracheostomy ______
8. pleuropexy ______
9. thoracocentesis ______
10. antitussive ______
11. expectorant ______
12. mucolytic ______

EXERCISE 3 *Underline and define the word parts from this chapter in the following terms.*

1. laryngectomy ______
2. bronchoplasty ______
3. thoracocentesis ______
4. expectorant ______
5. endotracheal ______

Learning Outcome 10.5 Exercises

EXERCISE 4 *Match the term on the left with its definition on the right.*

e	1. thoracotomy	a.	insertion of a tube inside the trachea
b	2. nebulizer	b.	a machine that administers respiratory medication by creating a "cloud" or mist that is inhaled by the patient
c	3. thoracentesis (puncture)	c.	a puncture of the chest
a	4. endotracheal intubation	d.	a method of artificially maintaining blood flow and airflow when breathing and pulse have stopped
d	5. cardiopulmonary resuscitation	e.	incision into the chest

EXERCISE 5 *Translate the following terms as literally as possible.*

EXAMPLE: nasopharyngoscope *an instrument for looking at the nose and throat*

1. antitussive ______
2. expectorant ______
3. laryngoplasty ______
4. septoplasty ______
5. adenoidectomy ______
6. pneumonectomy ______
7. tracheotomy ______
8. tracheostomy ______
9. thoracostomy ______
10. pleuropexy ______
11. thoracocentesis ______
12. mucolytic ______

GENERATION

EXERCISE 6 *Build a medical term from the information provided.*

EXAMPLE: inflammation of the sinuses *sinusitis*

1. removal of the larynx ______
2. removal of the tonsils ______
3. removal of a lobe ______
4. reconstruction of a palate ______
5. reconstruction of a bronchus ______
6. reconstruction of the chest ______
7. a drug that expands the walls of the bronchi ______

Learning Outcome 10.5 Exercises

EXERCISE 7 *Multiple-choice questions. Select the correct answer(s).*

1. A *nebulizer* administers medication by creating a mist to be inhaled by a patient. It comes from the Latin word *nebula,* meaning
   a. mist
   b. smoke
   c. cloud
   d. medication

2. Select the terms that pertain to the upper respiratory system.
   a. adenoidectomy
   b. bronchoplasty
   c. laryngectomy
   d. laryngoplasty
   e. lobectomy
   f. palatoplasty
   g. pneumonectomy
   h. septoplasty
   i. thoracoplasty
   j. tonsillectomy

3. Select the terms that pertain to the lower respiratory system.
   a. adenoidectomy
   b. bronchoplasty
   c. laryngectomy
   d. laryngoplasty
   e. lobectomy
   f. palatoplasty
   g. pneumonectomy
   h. septoplasty
   i. thoracoplasty
   j. tonsillectomy

4. Select the terms that involve removal of a part of the respiratory system.
   a. adenoidectomy
   b. bronchoplasty
   c. laryngectomy
   d. laryngoplasty
   e. lobectomy
   f. palatoplasty
   g. pneumonectomy
   h. septoplasty
   i. thoracoplasty
   j. tonsillectomy

5. Select the terms that involve reconstruction of a part of the respiratory system.
   a. adenoidectomy
   b. bronchoplasty
   c. laryngectomy
   d. laryngoplasty
   e. lobectomy
   f. palatoplasty
   g. pneumonectomy
   h. septoplasty
   i. thoracoplasty
   j. tonsillectomy

6. Which drug is used to break down mucus?
   a. antitussive
   b. bronchodilator
   c. expectorant
   d. mucolytic

10.6 Abbreviations

Abbreviations provide a shorthand way of referring to things that either recur often or are too long to write out. When dealing with the respiratory system, those terms include clinical observations (CTA), diagnostic tests (CXR, V/Q), diagnoses (LTB, COPD, URI), and treatments (T&A, CPAP).

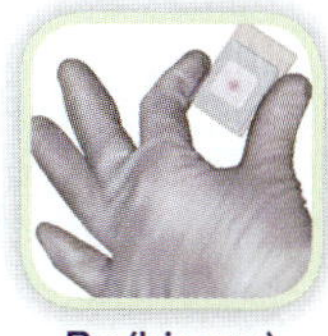

Bx (biopsy)

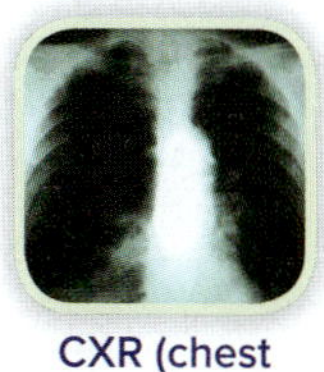

CXR (chest x-ray)

respiratory system abbreviations

Abbreviation	Definition
ABG	arterial blood gas analysis of the gases in the blood; used to determine the effectiveness of the lungs in exchanging gases
Bx	biopsy
COPD	chronic obstructive pulmonary disease
CPAP	continuous positive airway pressure a treatment for apnea involving keeping a patient's airways open using air pressure delivered via a face mask
CPR	cardiopulmonary resuscitation
CT	computed tomography
CTA	clear to auscultation when an examination reveals nothing abnormal about a patient's lung
CXR	chest x-ray
ET	endotracheal
IRDS	infant respiratory distress syndrome
LTB	laryngotracheobronchitis
MRI	magnetic resonance imaging
OSA	obstructive sleep apnea
PE	pulmonary embolism
PET	positron emission tomography
PFT	pulmonary function test
PSG	polysomnography
SOB	shortness of breath
T&A	tonsillectomy and adenoidectomy
TB	tuberculosis
URI	upper respiratory infection
V/Q	ventilation–perfusion scan

Learning Outcome 10.6 Exercises

TRANSLATION

EXERCISE 1 *Define the following abbreviations.*

1. CPR ________________
2. MRI ________________
3. PET ________________
4. CT ________________
5. CTA ________________
6. URI ________________
7. T&A ________________
8. ABG ________________
9. CXR ________________
10. CPAP ________________
11. SOB ________________
12. IRDS ________________

EXERCISE 2 *Give the abbreviations for the following terms.*

1. biopsy ________________
2. pulmonary embolism ________________
3. clear to auscultation ________________
4. ventilation-perfusion scan ________________
5. chronic obstructive pulmonary disease ________________
6. laryngotracheobronchitis ________________
7. polysomnography ________________
8. obstructive sleep apnea ________________
9. pulmonary function test ________________
10. endotracheal ________________
11. tuberculosis ________________

EXERCISE 3 *Multiple-choice questions. Select the correct answer.*

1. CPAP is a treatment for
   a. bronchitis
   b. thoracalgia
   c. apnea
   d. hyperventilation
2. A patient with an infection in the upper respiratory system has a(n)
   a. CTA
   b. URI
   c. PSG
   d. ABG
3. A patient with a blockage in the blood supply to the lungs has a(n)
   a. URI
   b. PE
   c. LTB
   d. T&A

Learning Outcome 10.6 Exercises

4. A T&A involves the removal of

   a. tonsils and adenoids
   c. tonsils and alveolus
   b. trachea and adenoids
   d. trachea and alveolus

5. LTB is an inflammation of the

   a. larynx, trachea, and bronchi
   c. lung, trachea, and breathing
   b. lobe, trachea, and bronchi
   d. larynx, tonsil, and bronchi

6. A patient with OSA

   a. has difficulty sleeping due to obstructive sputum
   b. has overactive sinuses when awake
   c. has obstructive adenoids when asleep
   d. stops breathing when asleep

7. An analysis of gases in the blood to determine the effectiveness of the lungs in exchanging gases is

   a. ABG
   c. LGE
   b. AGB
   d. GBLE

8. Which of the following is NOT a diagnostic procedure?

   a. V/S
   c. PFT
   b. CT
   d. LTB

10.7 Electronic Health Records

Primary Care Visit

S Subjective

The patient is a 4 month old with a 4-day history of **nasal** congestion, **rhinorrhea,** and a dry cough. He also has been **wheezing** for the past 2 days. His congestion is getting worse. He has had a fever up to 103.4°F. His parents say he has not had any **apnea, cyanosis,** or trouble breathing. No one in his family has **asthma.** His mother was recently diagnosed with **bronchitis.**

O Objective

Objective: Temp: 101.1°F; HR: 110; **RR:** 32; BP: 84/60; **Pulse ox:** 93%

Gen: He is alert and in no apparent distress.

HEENT: His ear canals are clear. There is no evidence of an ear infection. There is congestion in his **nares.** His lips and mouth are moist. He does not have any **pharnygeal exudate.**

Resp: He is wheezing **bilaterally** on **auscultation.**

CV: His heart is beating with a regular rate and rhythm and without a murmur.

Skin: His skin is warm, dry, and pink.

CXR: There is **peribronchial** fluid with mild **hyperinflation** of his lungs. An **opacity** is seen on one x-ray view but not the other. This is likely from **atelectasis.**

A Assessment

Since he is wheezing, his cough is probably **bronchospastic.** He did not improve after using a bronchodilator in the office. Therefore, I believe the patient has a URI and **bronchiolitis.**

P Plan

Use a humidifier in his room at night and clean his nose with a suction bulb.

Learning Outcome 10.7 Exercises

EXERCISE 1 *Fill in the blanks.*

1. The patient has a history of *rhinorrhea* (define rhinorrhea: ____________________).
2. The parents deny ____________ (that the patient is not breathing) or *cyanosis* (define cyanosis: ____________________).
3. Respiratory observation revealed bilateral wheezing on auscultation (define auscultation: ____________________).
4. The cough is most likely caused by ____________________ (involuntary contraction of the bronchus).
5. The patient did not respond to ____________________ (drug that expands the walls of the bronchi).
6. The patient has URI (____________________) and ____________________ (inflammation of the bronchioles).

EXERCISE 2 *True or false questions. Indicate true answers with a T and false answers with an F.*

1. The doctor noticed the patient had cyanosis. ________
2. The parents claim the patient had stopped breathing. ________
3. The doctor attempted to open the patient's bronchial tubes using medication. ________

EXERCISE 3 *Multiple-choice questions. Select the correct answer.*

1. What test indicated incomplete expansion of the bronchial tubes?
   a. chest x-ray
   b. CT scan
   c. ABG
   d. auscultation
2. The patient's cough is probably caused by
   a. overexpansion of the bronchial tubes
   b. incomplete expansion of the bronchial tubes
   c. involuntary contraction of the bronchial tubes
   d. blockage of the bronchial tubes

Emergency Department Visit

Chief Complaint: **Hemoptysis**

History of Present Illness: The patient has been brought to the emergency department by her mother. She is a 22-year-old female with **cystic fibrosis.** She has had a 1-day history of **hemoptysis.** She has been feeling tired for 5 days. Her mother says that the patient has had mild **dyspnea** and cough. The patient's last **PFTs** were much worse than normal for her. She has not had any **epistaxis,** bleeding from her gums, bloody stool, or easy bruising.

Past Medical History: Cystic fibrosis; bronchiectasis.

Medications: **Inhaled** antibiotic (tobramycin inhaled); **mucolytic** agent (pulmozyme); vitamins ADEK; **bronchodilator** (albuterol).

Allergies: NKDA.

Social: She is a nonsmoker. She is a sophomore in college and lives with her parents.

Surgical History: None.

Physical Exam: RR: 30; HR: 92; Temp: 102.1°F; BP: 90/57; **Pulse ox:** 89%

Gen: Mildly **cyanotic.** In mild **respiratory distress.**
Her nose and mouth are a little dry.

HEENT: Her ear drums and ear canals are normal.

CV: Mildly **tachycardic.** No murmur. Her pulses are a little weak.

Resp: **Tachypneic,** shallow breaths, breath sounds are weaker than normal **bilaterally.**

GI: Normal. Her liver and spleen are not large.

Emergency Department Course: When she came to the **ED,** the patient was in **acute respiratory distress.** She was **intubated** with an **endotracheal tube** and placed on **SIMV.** A **CXR** verified correct placement in her trachea. She had poor circulation, so she was given **IVF** and transfused with 2 units of blood **(prbcs).** An **ABG** showed **hypoxemia** and **hypercapnia,** both of which improved on follow-up **ABG** after she was intubated. The **pulmonology** team was contacted; the team decided **bronchoscopy** would be best. The team found that she was bleeding in her **bronchi** and treated her with **endobronchial electrocautery.** Afterward, she was transferred to the **ICU** for further care.

Learning Outcome 10.7 Exercises

EXERCISE 4 *Fill in the blanks.*

1. The patient has cystic fibrosis and a 1-day history of ______________ (coughing up blood).
2. The patient has had *dyspnea* (give definition: ______________).
3. Her recent PFTs (give definition: ______________) were significantly worse than previously.
4. Her medical history includes cystic fibrosis as well as ______________ (expansion of the bronchi).
5. Among her medications is albuterol, a *bronchodilator* (give definition: ______________).
6. Her physical exam revealed that she has mild cyanosis (give definition: ______________) and her breathing was rapid or ______________.
7. The patient was then intubated with a tube in her ______________. They used a bedside CXR (give definition: ______________) to confirm correct placement.
8. ABG (give definition: ______________) revealed *hypoxemia* (give definition: ______________) and ______________ (excessive carbon dioxide).
9. The pulmonologist performed a bronchoscopy (give definition: ______________).
10. A(n) ______________ (inside the bronchi) electrocautery was used for hemostasis.

EXERCISE 5 *Multiple-choice questions. Select the correct answer.*

1. Which is a symptom mentioned by the patient?
   a. coughing up blood
   b. runny nose
   c. sleeplessness
   d. sore throat
2. How was the patient breathing when examined in the ED?
   a. rapidly
   b. slowly
   c. not at all
   d. heavily
3. The chart says the patient was taking shallow breaths. What is another term for that?
   a. hyperpnea
   b. hypopnea
   c. orthopnea
   d. apnea
4. Where was a tube placed in the patient?
   a. nowhere
   b. into the nose
   c. into the trachea
   d. into the nose and throat
5. What did the analysis of the patient's arterial blood gases reveal?
   a. deficient oxygen levels
   b. excessive carbon dioxide
   c. both
   d. neither

EXERCISE 6 *True or false questions. Indicate true answers with a T and false answers with an F.*

1. The patient has had a recent nosebleed. _____
2. The patient takes medication for constricted bronchial tubes. _____
3. The patient takes medication for insufficient mucus secretion. _____
4. The doctor noted the patient's skin had a slight blue color. _____
5. An examination of the patient's bronchial tubes was performed. _____

Pulmonology Consult

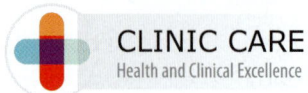

Reason for Consult: Cough and dyspnea.

The patient is a 64-year-old male who has had a cough for 2 months. His cough has had a lot of **sputum** in it. Now he also has **dyspnea**. He has been sweating at night and has lost 5 pounds in the past 2 months. He does not have any **hemoptysis, dysphonia,** or fever. He is a 2-pack-per-day smoker.

On physical exam, the patient is alert. He takes occasional pauses when he says long sentences, but otherwise, he is not in any distress. He has an occasional cough during his exam. His skin is pink and dry, and his lips are moist. His heartbeat is regular in rate and rhythm, without a murmur. On lung examination, he has **whispered pectoriloquy** on the right side with decreased breath sounds. He does not have any **retractions** or **nasal flaring** noted. His liver and spleen are not large.

A **CT** of his lungs revealed **opacities** and **air bronchograms** in his right upper lobe, with a small area of **pleural effusion** on the right. There are also two large **lymph nodes** in his **mediastinum.**

An **ABG** shows mild **hypoxemia**. I believe this is from the large amount of **bronchorrhea.**

Thoracoscopy with **biopsy** was then done under sedation in the surgical suite. The biopsy sample was sent to the pathology lab. The results showed **bronchioloalveolar carcinoma.**

I have discussed the results with the patient, including his treatment options. I explained he would need a partial **lobectomy.** He is scheduled for a surgical consultation later this week. After surgical resection of the tumor and lobectomy, he will need to begin chemotherapy.

Learning Outcome 10.7 Exercises

EXERCISE 7 *Fill in the blanks.*

1. The patient's cough has clear ________________ and progressed to *dyspnea* (give definition: ________________).
2. He denies ________________ (coughing up blood), dysphonia, and fever.
3. The CT, or ________________, of his lungs revealed a small area of fluid pouring into the pleura, or a(n) ________________.
4. Arterial blood gases, or ________________, revealed *hypoxemia* (give definition: ________________).
5. The chest examination, or ________________, with biopsy revealed a *bronchioloalveolar* (give definition: ________________) carcinoma.
6. Treatment will include partial removal of a lobe of the lung, or ________________.

EXERCISE 8 *True or false questions. Indicate true answers with a T and false answers with an F.*

1. *Thorascopy* is a shortening of the word *thoracoscopy*. ________
2. The patient was diagnosed with cancer. ________
3. The patient had a lung removed. ________
4. The patient has sufficient oxygen in his blood. ________
5. The patient's lung was CTA. ________
6. The patient has been coughing up blood. ________
7. The patient complains of hoarseness. ________
8. The lining of the patient's lungs has excess fluid in it. ________

Quick Reference

quick reference glossary of roots

Root	Definition	Root	Definition
adenoid/o	adenoid	**phren/o**	diaphragm
bronch/o, bronchi/o	bronchus	**pleur/o**	pleura
bronchiol/o	bronchiole	**-pnea**	breathing
capn/o	carbon dioxide	**pneum/o, pneumat/o, pneumon/o**	air or lungs
carb/o	carbon dioxide	**pulmon/o**	lungs
laryng/o	larynx (voice box)	**rhin/o**	nose
lob/o	lobe	**sept/o**	septum
nas/o	nose	**sin/o, sinus/o**	sinus
ox/o	oxygen	**spir/o**	breathing
palat/o	palate	**thorac/o**	chest
pector/o	chest	**tonsill/o**	tonsil
pharyng/o	pharynx (throat)	**trache/o**	trachea (windpipe)

quick reference glossary of terms

Terms	Definition
adenoidectomy	removal of the adenoids
antitussive	a drug that prevents coughing
apnea	cessation of breathing
asthma	a disease caused by episodic narrowing and inflammation of the airway
atelectasis	incomplete expansion
auscultation	from the Latin word *ausculto,* meaning *to listen;* a doctor using a stethoscope is performing an auscultation
bradypnea	slow breathing
bronchiectasis	expansion of the bronchi
bronchiogenic carcinoma	a cancerous tumor originating in the bronchi
bronchiolitis	inflammation of the bronchiole

quick reference glossary of terms *continued*

Terms	Definition
bronchioplasty	reconstruction of a bronchus
bronchitis	inflammation of the bronchi
bronchodilator	a drug that expands the walls of the bronchi
bronchorrhea	discharge from the bronchi
bronchoscopy	a procedure to look inside the bronchi
bronchospasm	involuntary contraction of the bronchia
capnography	a procedure to record carbon dioxide levels
capnometer	instrument to measure carbon dioxide levels
cardiopulmonary resuscitation (CPR)	a method of artificially maintaining blood flow and airflow when breathing and pulse have stopped
caseous necrosis	the death of tissue with a cheeselike appearance
chronic obstructive pulmonary disease (COPD)	a lung disease caused by the continual blockage of lung passages
chylothorax	chyle in the chest
computed tomography	a recording procedure using a computer to "cut" or view "slices" of a patient's organs
cyanosis	a bluish color in the skin caused by insufficient oxygen
diaphragmatocele	hernia of the diaphragm
dysphonia	"bad voice condition"; hoarseness
dyspnea	difficulty breathing
emphysema	a disease that causes the alveoli to lose their elasticity; patients can inhale but have difficulty exhaling
empyema	pus inside (the chest)
endoscopy	instrument to look inside
endotracheal intubation	insertion of a tube inside the trachea
epistaxis	nosebleed
eupnea	good/normal breathing
expectorant	a drug that encourages that explusion of material from the lungs
expectoration	coughing or spitting material out of the lungs
hemoptysis	coughing up blood

quick reference glossary of terms *continued*

Terms	Definition
hemothorax	blood in the chest
hypercapnia	condition of having excessive carbon dioxide in the blood
hypercarbia	excessive carbon dioxide
hyperpnea	heavy breathing
hyperventilation	overbreathing; condition of having too much air flowing into and out of the lungs; leads to hypocapnia
hypocapnia	insufficient carbon dioxide
hypocarbia	insufficient carbon dioxide
hypopnea	shallow breathing
hypoventilation	underbreathing; condition of having too little air flowing into and out of the lungs; leads to hypercapnia
hypoxemia	insufficient oxygen in the blood
hypoxia	insufficient oxygen
laryngectomy	removal of the larynx
laryngitis	inflammation of the larynx
laryngoplasty	reconstruction of the larynx
laryngotracheobronchitis	inflammation of the larynx, trachea, and bronchi
lobectomy	removal of a lobe
mucolytic	a drug that aids in the breakdown of mucus
nasopharyngoscope	an instrument to look at the nose and throat
nebulizer	a machine that administers respiratory medication by creating a "cloud" or mist that is inhaled by the patient
obstructive lung disorder	a lung disorder caused by a blockage
orthopnea	able to breathe only in an upright position
oximetry	a procedure to measure oxygen levels
palatoplasty	reconstruction of the palate
pansinusitis	inflammation of all sinuses
pectoriloquy	*speaking from the chest;* used as a means of finding masses in the lung
pectus carinatum	a chest that protrudes like the keel of a ship
pectus excavatum	a chest that is hollowed out

quick reference glossary of terms *continued*

Terms	Definition
percussion	the body surface; in this context, to cause vibrations that can help locate fluid build-up in the chest
phrenoplegia	paralysis of the diaphragm
phrenoptosis	drooping of the diaphragm
phrenospasm	involuntary contraction of the diaphragm
pleuradynia	pain in the pleura
pleural effusion	fluid pouring out into the pleura
pleuralgia	pain in the pleura
pleurisy	inflammation of the pleura; another word for pleuritis
pleuritis	inflammation of the pleura
pleuropexy	reattachment of the pleura
pneumatocele	hernia of the lung
pneumoconiosis	a lung condition caused by dust
pneumohemothorax	air and blood in the chest
pneumonectomy	removal of a lung
pneumonia	a lung condition
pneumonitis	inflammation of the lung
pneumothorax	air in the chest
polysomnography	recording multiple aspects of sleep
pulmonary angiography	a procedure for recording pulmonary blood vessel activity
pulmonary edema	swelling in the lungs
pulmonary embolism	blockage in the pulmonary blood supply
pulmonary function testing	a group of tests used to evaluate the condition of the lungs
pulmonary neoplasm	new growth (tumor) in the lung
pyothorax	pus in the chest
restrictive lung disorder	a lung disorder caused by the limiting of air into the lungs
rhinitis	inflammation of the nasal passages
rhinorrhagia	excessive blood flow from the nose (another term for nosebleed)
rhinorrhea	runny nose

quick reference glossary of terms *continued*

Terms	Definition
septoplasty	reconstruction of a septum
sinusitis	inflammation of the sinus
sleep apnea	a condition where the patient ceases to breathe while asleep
spirometry	a procedure to measure breathing
sputum	mucus discharged from the lungs by coughing
tachypnea	rapid breathing
thoracalgia	chest pain
thoracentesis	puncture of the chest
thoracocentesis	puncture of the chest
thoracoplasty	reconstruction of the chest
thoracoscopy	examination of the chest
thoracostomy	creation of an opening in the chest
thoracotomy	incision into the chest
tonsillectomy	removal of the tonsils
tonsillitis	inflammation of the tonsils
tracheitis	inflammation of the trachea
tracheomalacia	softening of the trachea
tracheostenosis	narrowing of the trachea
tracheostomy	creation of an opening in the trachea
tracheotomy	incision into the trachea
ventilation–perfusion scan	a scan that tests whether a problem in the lungs is caused by airflow (ventilation) or blood flow (perfusion)

review of terms by roots

Root	Term(s)	
adenoid/o	adenoidectomy	
bronch/o, bronchi/o	bronchiectasis bronchiogenic carcinoma bronchioplasty bronchitis bronchodilator	bronchorrhea bronchoscopy bronchospasm laryngotracheobronchitis
bronchiol/o	bronchiolitis	
capn/o	capnography capnometer	hypercapnia hypocapnia
carb/o	hypercarbia hypocarbia	
laryng/o	laryngectomy laryngitis	laryngoplasty laryngotracheobronchitis
lob/o	lobectomy	
nas/o	nasopharyngoscope	
ox/o	hypoxemia hypoxia	oximetry
palat/o	palatoplasty	
pector/o	expectorant expectoration pectoriloquy	pectus carinatum pectus excavatum
pharyng/o	nasopharyngoscope	
phren/o	phrenoplegia phrenoptosis	phrenospasm
pleur/o	pleural effusion pleuralgia pleuritis	pleurodynia pleuropexy
-pnea	apnea bradypnea dyspnea eupnea hyperpnea	hypopnea orthopnea sleep apnea tachypnea

review of terms by roots *continued*

Root	Term(s)	
pneum/o, pneumat/o, pneumon/o	pneumatocele pneumoconiosis pneumohemothorax pneumonectomy	pneumonia pneumonitis pneumothorax
pulmon/o	cardiopulmonary resuscitation chronic obstructive pulmonary disease pulmonary angiography pulmonary edema	pulmonary embolism pulmonary function testing pulmonary neoplasm
rhin/o	rhinitis rhinorrhagia	rhinorrhea
sept/o	septoplasty	
sin/o, sinus/o	pansinusitis sinusitis	
spir/o	spirometry	
thorac/o	chylothorax hemothorax laryngotracheobronchitis pneumohemothorax pneumothorax pyrothorax thoracalgia	thoracentesis thoracocentesis thoracoplasty thoracoscopy thoracostomy thoracotomy
tonsill/o	tonsillectomy tonsillitis	
trache/o	endotracheal intubation tracheitis tracheomalacia	tracheostenosis tracheostomy tracheotomy

The Gastrointestinal System—Gastroenterology

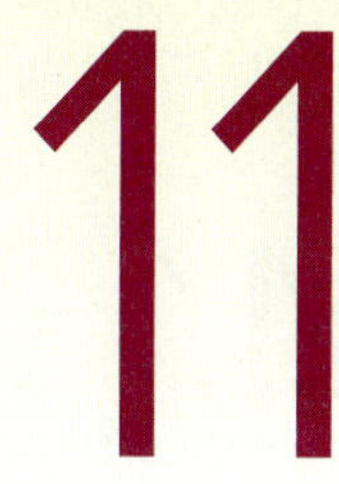

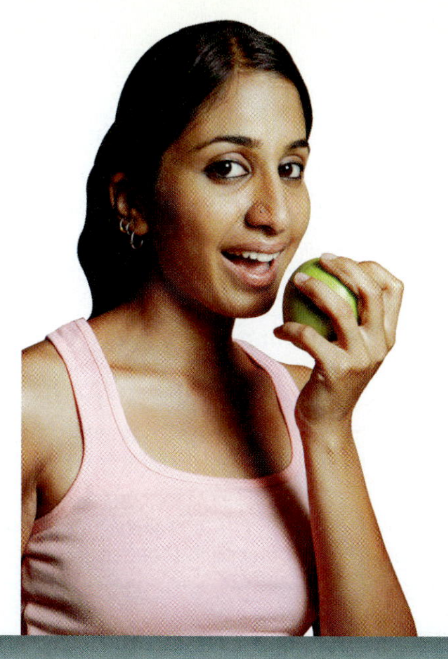

Introduction and Overview of the Gastrointestinal System

Energy is necessary to make machines work, whether it comes from gasoline, batteries, or electricity. The body is the same way–it constantly needs energy. The gastrointestinal (GI) system is responsible for turning food into energy. As a first step, it digests the food. *Digest* comes from *di* (short for dia), meaning *through*, and *gest*, meaning *to carry*. *Digestion* is the process of carrying food through the body and breaking it apart into usable and unusable parts. There are three main types of usable food fuel: *protein, fat,* and *carbohydrates.* As food passes through the digestive system, the body breaks down and absorbs the usable parts and discards any unusable parts.

learning outcomes

Upon completion of this chapter, you will be able to:

11.1 Identify the **roots/word parts** associated with the **gastrointestinal system.**

S **11.2** Translate the **Subjective** terms associated with the **gastrointestinal system.**

O **11.3** Translate the **Objective** terms associated with the **gastrointestinal system.**

A **11.4** Translate the **Assessment** terms associated with the **gastrointestinal system.**

P **11.5** Translate the **Plan** terms associated with the **gastrointestinal system.**

11.6 Use **abbreviations** associated with the **gastrointestinal system.**

11.7 Distinguish terms associated with the **gastrointestinal system** in the context of **electronic health records.**

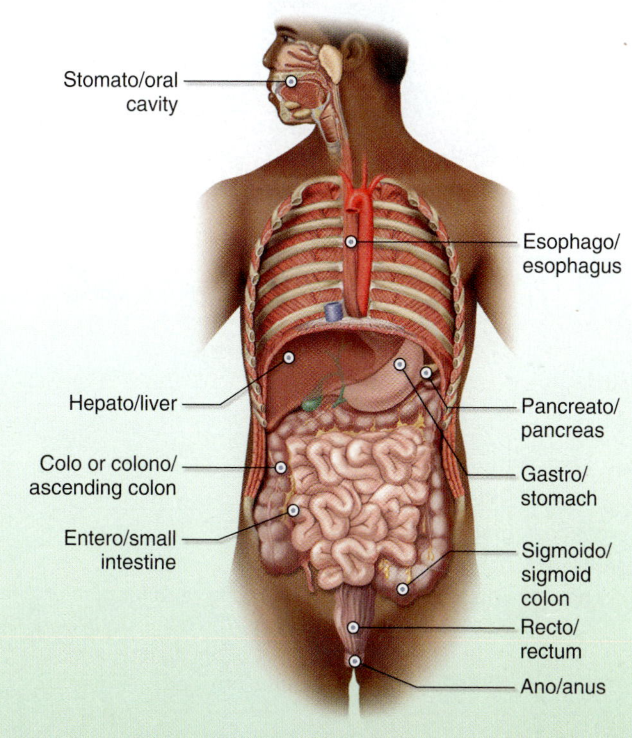

The gastrointestinal system is mainly one long tube. Health care providers often talk about the system's two parts: the *upper* and *lower gastrointestinal (GI) tracts.* The upper GI tract includes the mouth, esophagus, and stomach. The lower GI tract is made up of the small and large intestines. In addition to the stomach and intestines, there are other organs that help in dealing with our nutrition. These organs are the liver, pancreas, and gallbladder.

11.1 Word Parts of the Gastrointestinal System

Upper Gastrointestinal Tract

The process of digestion begins in the mouth. When people eat, they start with chewing their food. When chewing, teeth (*dento*) tear food into smaller parts. At the same time, the salivary glands make saliva (*sialo*). The saliva helps to moisten the food to help it pass down the throat. Saliva also has chemicals that help to break the food apart.

mouth

ROOTS: ***or/o, stomat/o***
EXAMPLES: oral, stomatosis
NOTES: Most people tend to chew on the side of the mouth that corresponds to the hand with which they write. Right-handed folks use the right side of their mouth, and left-handed folks—well, you get the idea.

tooth

ROOTS: ***dent/o, odont/o***
EXAMPLES: dentist, odontalgia
NOTES: The enamel on the outside of the *tooth* is the hardest thing in the human body. Adult humans have 32 teeth (or they're supposed to, anyway). An opossum has 50 teeth, a mosquito has 47 teeth, and sharks have as many as 40 sets of teeth in their lifetime.

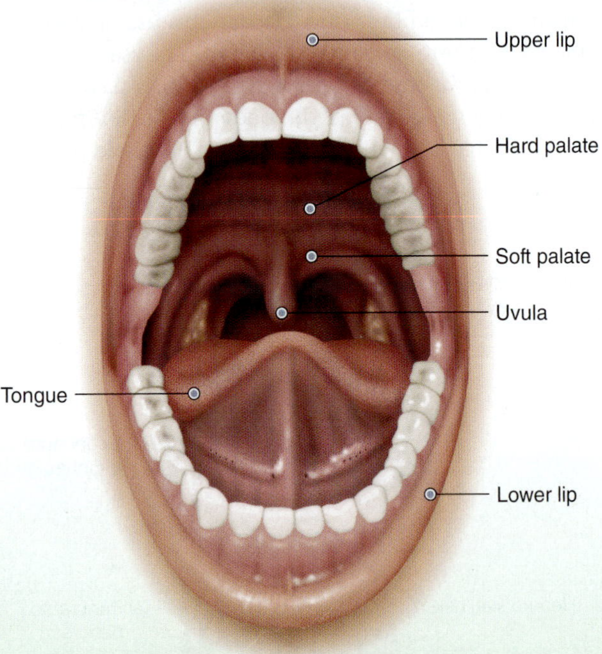

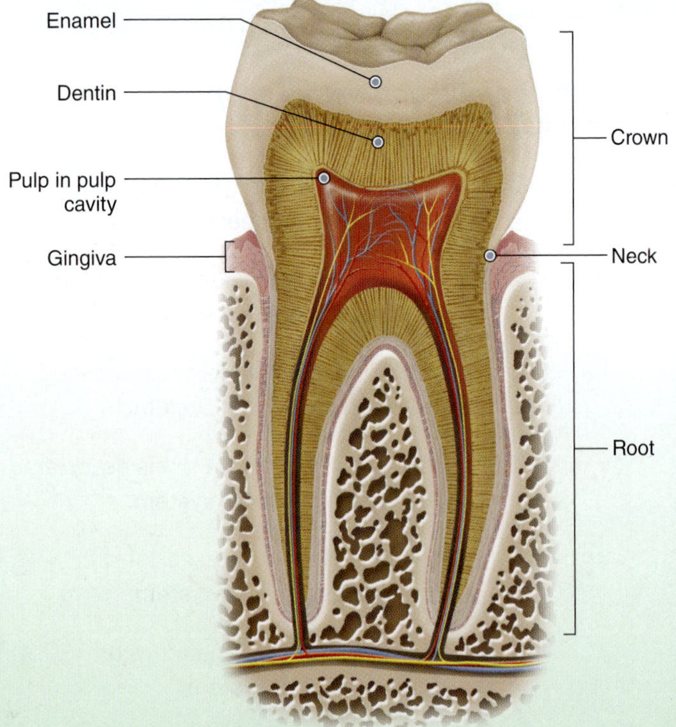

gums

ROOT: ***gingiv/o***
EXAMPLES: gingivitis, gingivostomatitis
NOTES: This root comes from the Latin word for *gums.* Healthy gums are a pinkish-red color, but the color can vary depending on the lightness or darkness of the patient's skin.

The food is passed from the mouth down a tube (*esophagus*) that leads to the stomach (*gastro*). The esophagus has two gates that keep the food moving the right way. The first gate keeps out air from the stomach and the second gate keeps food from leaving the stomach in the wrong direction.

As we eat, food collects in the stomach. The stomach makes acid, which breaks down protein. The stomach acts almost like a blender. Through muscle contractions, the stomach mixes the food with stomach juices, including acid. This mixing process physically and chemically softens the food into a paste-like substance known as *chyme*. Food then passes through a muscle at the end of the stomach, the *pylorus,* and into the small intestine.

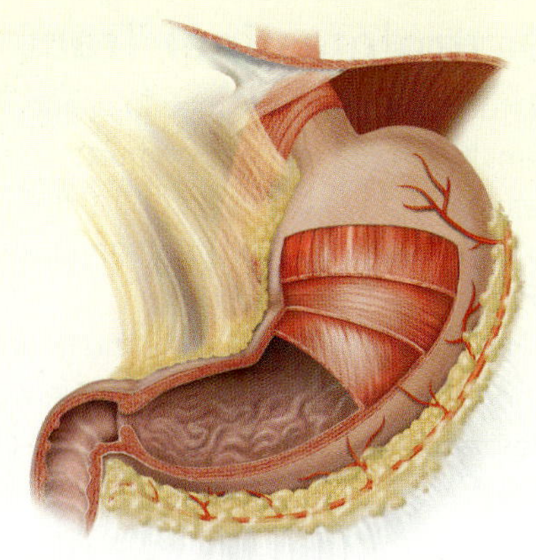

stomach

ROOT: ***gastr/o***

EXAMPLES: gastritis, gastropexy

NOTES: Here are two things you probably don't know about the *stomach:* It must produce a new layer of mucus every 2 weeks or it will digest itself, and when you blush, your stomach changes colors, too.

tongue

ROOTS: ***gloss/o, lingu/o***

EXAMPLES: glossopathy, hypoglossal, sublingual

NOTES: The strongest muscle in the human body, relative to its size, is the *tongue*. It is also the only muscle in the human body that is attached at only one end. Here's an interesting fact: Whether or not you can roll your tongue into a tube or other shapes is predetermined by your genetics.

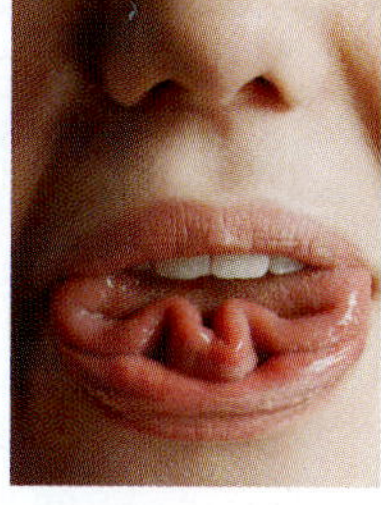

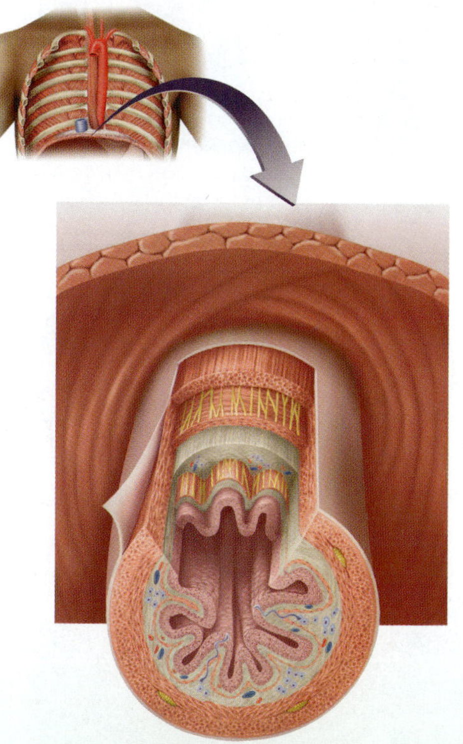

Cross section of the esophagus

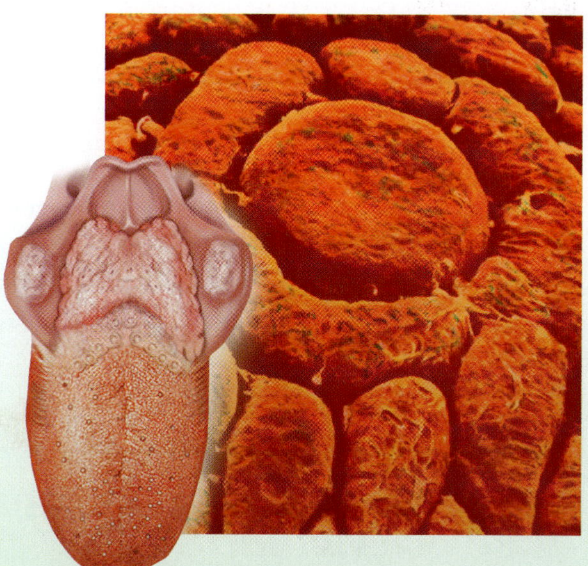

esophagus

ROOT: ***esophag/o***

EXAMPLES: esophageal, esophagitis

NOTES: The *esophagus* is a tube that is about the diameter of a quarter; it connects your mouth to your stomach. The name breaks down into *eso* (carry) and *phagus* (eat) and literally means *the thing that carries what you eat,* presumably to the stomach.

Lower Gastrointestinal Tract

The lower GI tract is made up of the small and large intestines. The small intestine is the longest part of the gastrointestinal system. It is made up of three parts: the *duodenum, jejunum,* and *ileum.* Most of the chemical breakdown in the small intestine happens in its first part, the duodenum. In the duodenum, chemicals from the liver (*bile*) and the pancreas mix with the food. The food continues digestion throughout the rest of the long path of the jejunum and ileum.

From here, the food then passes into the large intestine. By this point, most of the nutrients have been absorbed. The main role of the large intestine is to absorb the water from the remaining food. The stool passes through the *ascending, transverse, descending,* and *sigmoid colon* into the *rectum,* where it waits to be excreted.

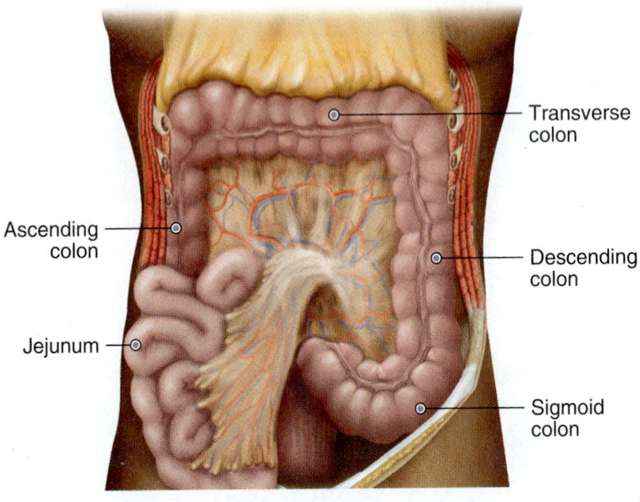

intestines

ROOT: ***enter/o***

EXAMPLES: gastroenterology, dysentery

NOTES: This combining form refers to the intestines in general. It comes from a Greek word meaning *inside.* It's appropriate, because your intestines take up a great deal of space inside you. The average adult has over 20 feet of intestines.

duodenum

ROOT: ***duoden/o***

EXAMPLES: gastroduodenoscope, duodenectomy

NOTES: The small intestine is divided into three sections: the *duodenum, jejunum,* and *ileum.* The duodenum is the first of the three sections. Its name means *twelve* and refers to the fact that its length is about the same as the width of 12 fingers.

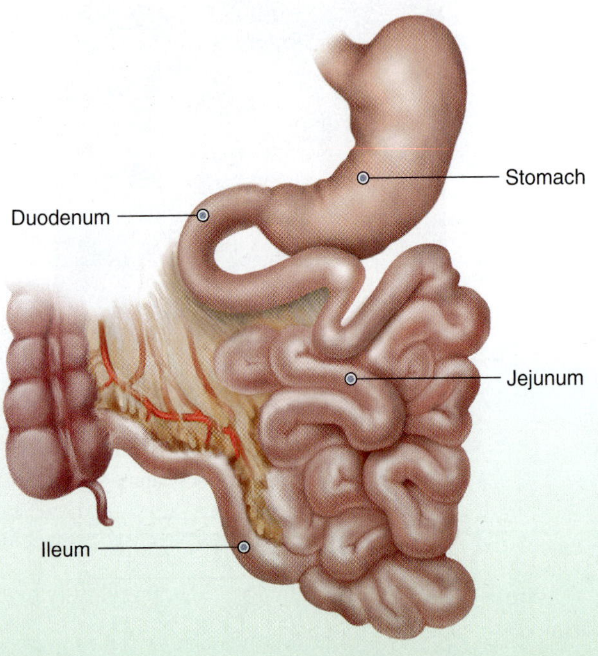

jejunum

ROOT: ***jejun/o***

EXAMPLES: jejunotomy, jejunitis

NOTES: The jejunum is the second of the small intestine's three sections. Its name means *empty* and refers to the fact that it is found empty during dissections.

ileum

ROOT: ***ile/o***

EXAMPLES: ileotomy, ileitis

NOTES: The ileum is the third of the small intestine's three sections. Its name means *groin* and refers to the fact that it is located in the lower abdomen.

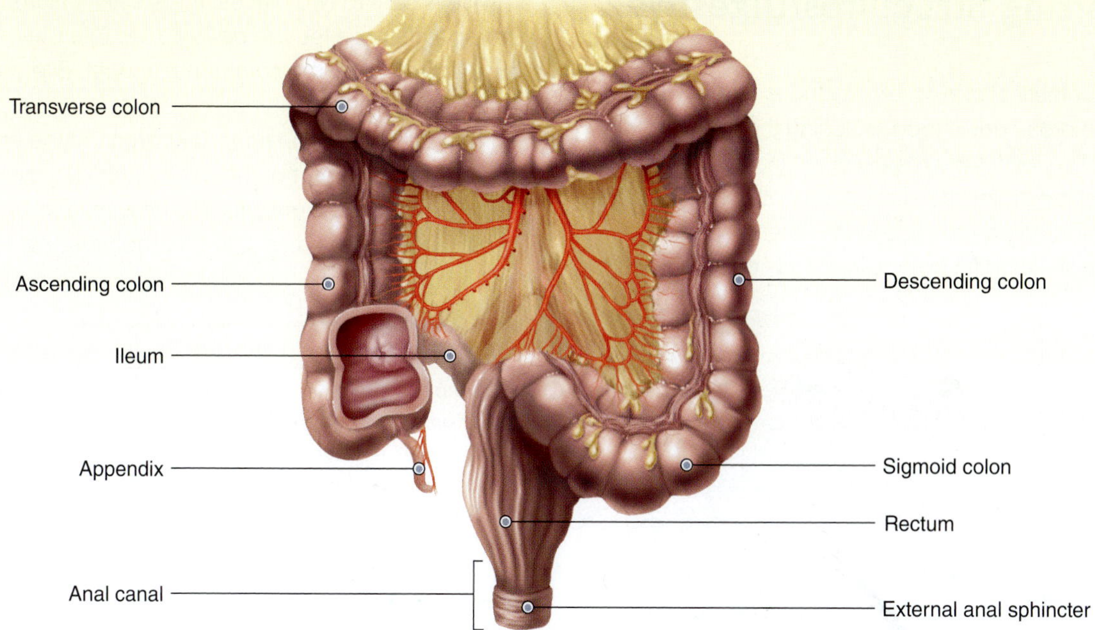

colon (large intestine)

ROOTS: ***col/o, colon/o***

EXAMPLES: colorectal carcinoma, colitis, colonoscopy, colonectomy

NOTES: The colon starts at the bottom of the abdomen (remember, that's where the ileum ends) and is divided into three main sections: the ascending (*going up*) colon, the transverse (*going across*) colon, and the descending (*going down*) colon.

sigmoid colon

ROOT: ***sigmoid/o***

EXAMPLE: sigmoidoscope

NOTES: The sigmoid colon is at the end of the colon, before the rectum begins. Its name is derived from the Greek letter *sigma* (Σ, related to the letter *s*) + *oid* (resembling). It refers to the fact it has an *s*-shaped curve.

rectum

ROOT: ***rect/o***

EXAMPLES: rectoplasty, rectitis

NOTES: *Rectum* is Latin for *straight* and refers to the final portion of the colon before it arrives at the anus. Although it is straight in comparison to the rest of the intestines, the human rectum really isn't straight. It got its name from an ancient doctor named Galen, who dissected animals that really did have straight rectums.

anus

ROOT: ***an/o***

EXAMPLES: anoplasty, anal fistula

NOTES: The *anus* is the sphincter or muscle at the end of the intestines that allows for the passage of feces. Its name comes from the Latin word for *ring*.

anus and rectum

ROOT: ***proct/o***

EXAMPLES: proctology, proctitis

NOTES: The root *ano* refers specifically to the anus and the root *recto* refers specifically to the rectum, but *procto* refers to both the anus and rectum.

Supporting Structures/Digestive Organs

The gastrointestinal system also includes other organs that help to break down food, including the liver and pancreas. The *liver* is the largest gland in the body. It has many roles in nutrition. It helps get rid of dangerous toxins, plays a role in energy storage, and makes a substance used to break down fat in the GI tract, called *bile*.

Bile is sent to two places: the small intestine and a storage gland called the *gallbladder*. Bile enters the small intestine by the common bile duct. Bile breaks big pieces of fat into smaller pieces of fat.

The *pancreas* is an important organ in the endocrine system. It also is part of the gastrointestinal system. The pancreas makes chemicals known as enzymes that break apart proteins, fats, and carbohydrates.

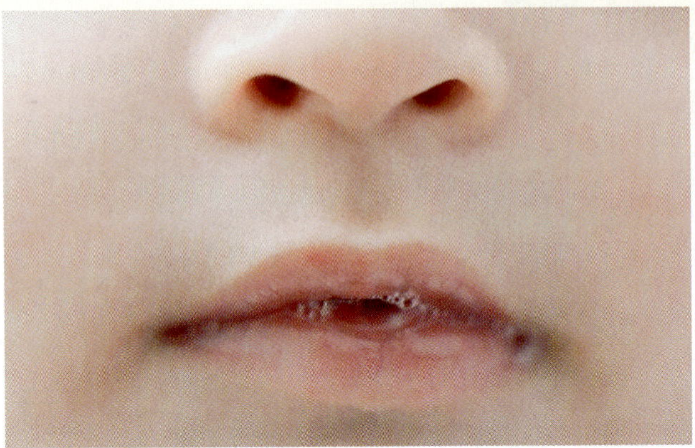

saliva

ROOT: ***sial/o***
EXAMPLE: sialoadenitis
NOTES: The average human produces between 1 and 3 pints of saliva a day. In addition to beginning the process of digestion, saliva is necessary to taste food. You cannot taste food until it is mixed with saliva.

bile (gall)

ROOTS: ***bil/i, chol/e***
EXAMPLES: biligenesis, cholelith
NOTES: *Bile,* which is sometimes called *gall,* is a substance produced in the liver that is required for the body to digest food.

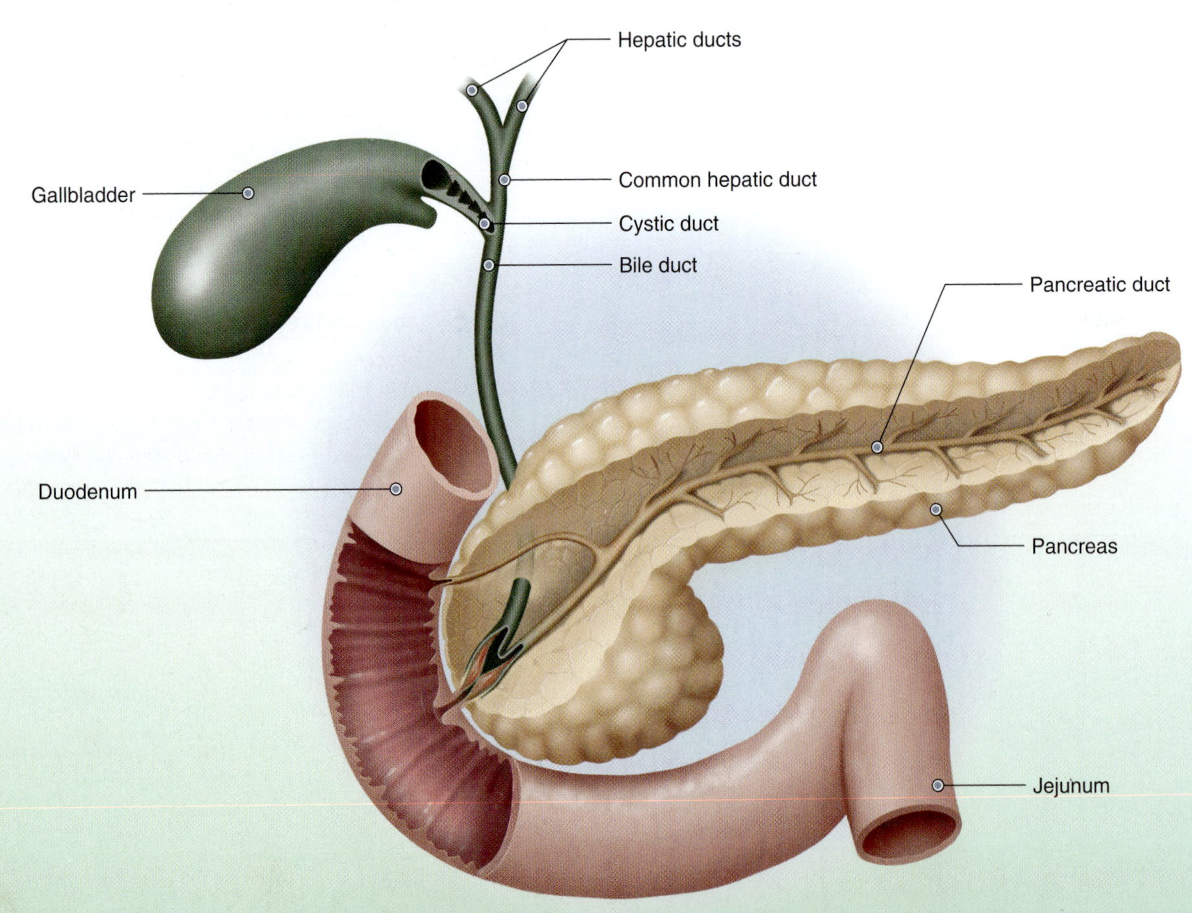

The gastrointestinal organs are located in the part of the body known as the *abdomen* and are surrounded by a membrane that keeps everything in place. This membrane is called the *peritoneum.* It has more specific nerve fibers than the organs it surrounds. If infection or inflammation spreads to the peritoneum, the pain is usually more specific in its nature. This is very helpful when examining a patient with gastrointestinal pain.

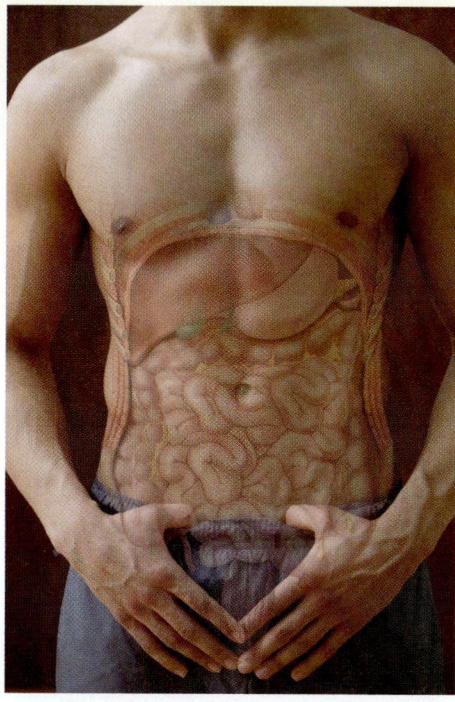

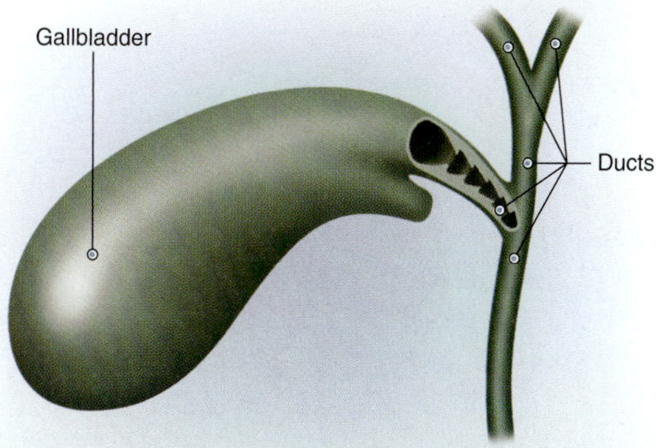

abdomen

ROOTS: ***abdomin/o, celi/o, lapar/o***

EXAMPLES: abdominocentesis, celiopathy, laparoscope

NOTES: Laparoscopic surgery is a way to perform surgery on the *abdomen* without making lengthy incisions. In fact, it is so minimally invasive that it is sometimes referred to as *Band-Aid* or *keyhole* surgery because the incisions are so small. One unique aspect of this procedure, though, is that in order to have enough room to work, surgeons must fill the abdomen with air, or blow it up like a balloon.

bladder

ROOT: ***cyst/o***

EXAMPLES: cholecystogram, cholecystectomy

NOTES: Once bile is produced in the liver, some of it is stored in the *gallbladder,* a small organ about the size of a pear that's located under the liver. While it is being stored, the bile becomes more concentrated in order to increase its potency. It is stored until the body needs it to help digest fatty foods.

duct

ROOT: ***doch/o***

EXAMPLE: choledocholithiasis

NOTES: Okay, this is tricky. Bile leaves the liver through numerous bile *ducts.* The name for these, though, uses the root *choleangio,* for *bile vessels.* All of these little ducts eventually unite to form the *common bile duct,* a single tube that empties into the small intestine. The root *choledocho* means *bile duct* but refers to only this main duct.

liver

ROOTS: ***hepat/o, hepatic/o***

EXAMPLES: hepatitis, hepaticotomy

NOTES: The *liver,* which is located on the right side of your abdomen just below your rib cage, is the largest organ in the human body (except the skin); it can filter more than a liter of blood every minute.

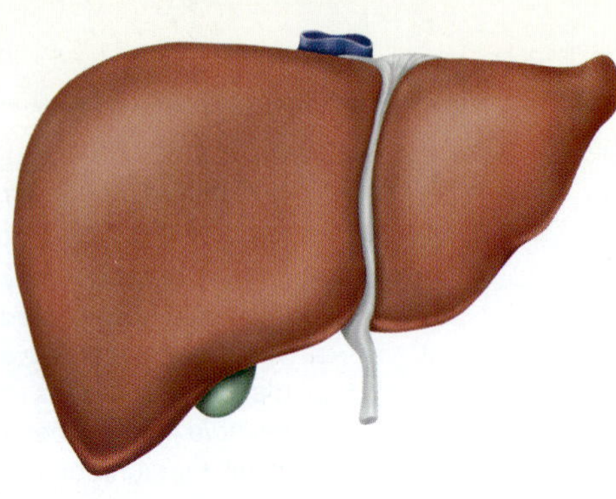

Anterior view

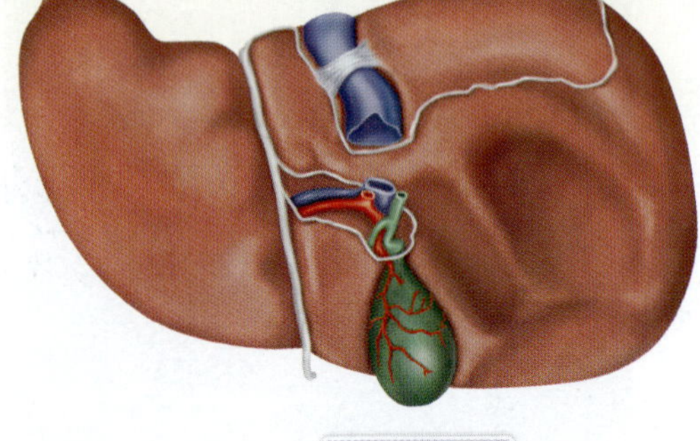

Inferior view

pancreas

ROOT: ***pancreat/o***

EXAMPLES: pancreatitis, pancreatolith

NOTES: The term *pancreas* comes from two Greek words: *pan* (*all*) and *kreas* (*flesh*). People debate the reason why, but some think it is because of the organ's fleshy consistency. If you are in a restaurant and are tempted to order *sweetbreads,* be careful. It's a term used by chefs to mean *cooked pancreas.*

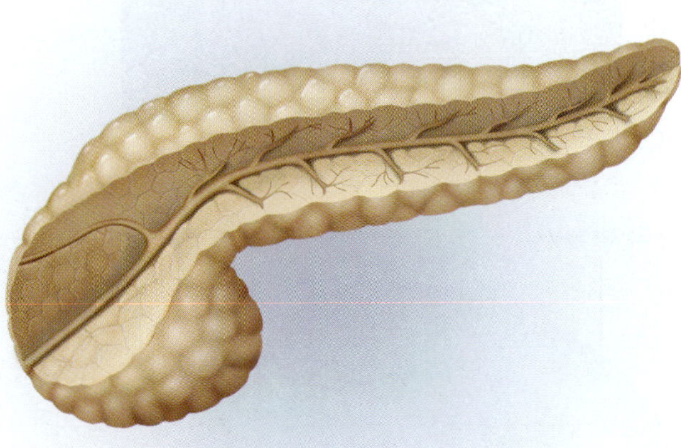

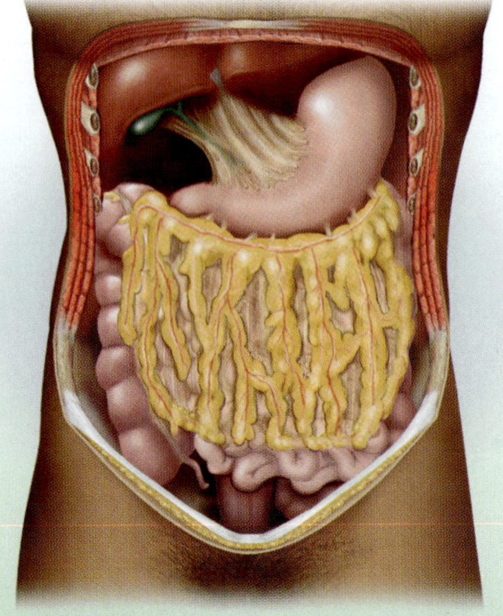

peritoneum

ROOT: ***peritone/o***

EXAMPLE: peritoneotomy

NOTES: The peritoneum is a membrane that lines the abdominal cavity and covers most of the abdominal organs. The name comes from *peri* (*around*) and *teneo* (*stretch*) and refers to the fact that it appears to be *stretched around* the abdominal organs.

Learning Outcome 11.1 Exercises

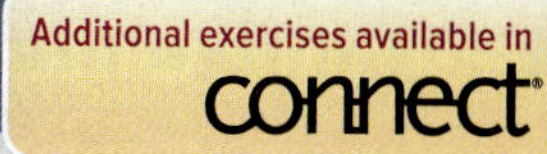

TRANSLATION

EXERCISE 1 *Match the root on the left with its definition on the right. Some definitions will be used more than once.*

__f__	1. dent/o	a. esophagus
__a__	2. esophag/o	b. gums
__b__	3. gingiv/o	c. mouth
__e__	4. lingu/o	d. stomach
__c__	5. or/o	e. tongue
__d__	6. gastr/o	f. tooth
__f__	7. odont/o	
__e__	8. gloss/o	
__c__	9. stomat/o	

EXERCISE 2 *Translate the following roots.*

1. dent/o ______________________
2. esophag/o ______________________
3. gingiv/o ______________________
4. lingu/o ______________________
5. or/o ______________________
6. gastr/o ______________________
7. odont/o ______________________
8. gloss/o ______________________
9. stomat/o ______________________

EXERCISE 3 *Underline and define the roots from this chapter in the following terms.*

1. dentistry ______________________
2. orthodontics ______________________
3. esophageal carcinoma ______________________
4. gingival hyperplasia ______________________
5. nasogastric tube ______________________
6. glossorrhaphy ______________________
7. stomatomycosis ______________________
8. stomatogastric (2 roots) ______________________
9. esophagogastroplasty (2 roots) ______________________

Learning Outcome 11.1 Exercises

EXERCISE 4 *Break down the following words into their component parts and translate.*

EXAMPLE: sinusitis *sinus | itis* *inflammation of the sinuses*

1. dentalgia ______________________
2. odontalgia ______________________
3. stomatoplasty ______________________
4. esophagalgia ______________________
5. gastralgia ______________________
6. gastroplasty ______________________
7. gingivoplasty ______________________
8. glossoplasty ______________________

EXERCISE 5 *Match the root on the left with its definition on the right.*

____ 1. proct/o
____ 2. enter/o
____ 3. an/o
____ 4. rect/o
____ 5. ile/o
____ 6. jejun/o
____ 7. duoden/o
____ 8. col/o
____ 9. sigmoid/o

a. sphincter or muscle at the end of the intestines that allows for the passage of feces; its name comes from the Latin word for *ring*
b. anus and rectum
c. end of the colon before it enters the rectum; its name is derived from the Greek letter *sigma* (Σ, related to the letter *s*) + *oid* (resembling), and it refers to the fact it has an *s*-shaped curve
d. first of three sections of the small intestine; the name means *twelve* and refers to the fact that its length is about the same as the width of 12 fingers
e. intestines
f. Latin for *straight* and refers to the final portion of the colon, before it arrives at the anus
g. starts at the bottom of the abdomen and is divided into three main sections: the ascending, the transverse, and the descending
h. the second of three sections of the small intestine, its name means *empty*, a reference to the fact that it is found empty during dissections
i. the third of three sections of the small intestine, its name means *groin*, a reference to the fact that it is located in the lower abdomen

EXERCISE 6 *Translate the following roots.*

1. proct/o ______________________
2. an/o ______________________
3. rect/o ______________________
4. colon/o ______________________
5. enter/o ______________________
6. col/o ______________________
7. jejun/o ______________________
8. duoden/o ______________________
9. ile/o ______________________
10. sigmoid/o ______________________

Learning Outcome 11.1 Exercises

EXERCISE 7 *Underline and define the roots from this chapter in the following terms.*

1. anal fistula ______
2. colovaginal fistula ______
3. colostomy ______
4. jejunostomy ______
5. sigmoidoscopy ______
6. rectopexy ______
7. enterorrhaphy ______
8. proctoptosis ______
9. colorectal carcinoma (2 roots) ______
10. anosigmoidoscopy (2 roots) ______
11. gastroduodenostomy (2 roots) ______
12. gastroenterostomy (2 roots) ______

EXERCISE 8 *Break down the following words into their component parts and translate.*

EXAMPLE: sinusitis *sinus | itis* *inflammation of the sinuses*

1. rectalgia ______
2. anoplasty ______
3. proctology ______
4. colectomy ______
5. duodenectomy ______
6. enterectomy ______
7. ileotomy ______
8. jejunotomy ______
9. sigmoidoscope ______

Learning Outcome 11.1 Exercises

EXERCISE 9 *Match the root on the left with its definition on the right. Some definitions will be used more than once.*

____ 1. pancreat/o
____ 2. abdomin/o
____ 3. lapar/o
____ 4. sial/o
____ 5. bil/i
____ 6. chol/e
____ 7. hepat/o
____ 8. cyst/o
____ 9. choledoch/o
____ 10. cholangi/o
____ 11. peritone/o
____ 12. celi/o

a. membrane that lines the abdominal cavity and covers most of the abdominal organs; the name comes from *peri* (*around*) and *teneo* (*stretch*) and refers to the fact that it appears to be *stretched around* the abdominal organs
b. a substance produced in the liver and required for the body to digest food
c. abdomen
d. begins the process of digestion; required to taste food
e. bladder
f. located on the right side of your abdomen just below your rib cage, this, the largest organ in the human body (except the skin), can filter over a liter of blood every minute
g. main bile duct
h. pancreas
i. bile vessels through which bile leaves the liver

EXERCISE 10 *Translate the following roots.*

1. abdomin/o ____
2. pancreat/o ____
3. bil/i ____
4. peritone/o ____
5. celi/o ____
6. chol/e ____
7. hepatic/o ____
8. hepat/o ____
9. lapar/o ____
10. doch/o ____
11. cyst/o ____
12. sial/o ____

EXERCISE 11 *Underline and define the roots from this chapter in the following terms.*

1. abdominocentesis ____
2. biligenesis ____
3. celiomyositis ____
4. cholelithotripsy ____
5. peritoneoscopy ____
6. laparoscopic surgery ____
7. sialolithiasis ____
8. hepatomalacia ____
9. pancreatolithiasis ____
10. cholecystectomy (2 roots) ____

Learning Outcome 11.1 Exercises

11. choledocholithiasis (2 roots) ______
12. hepaticogastrostomy (2 roots) ______
13. laparoenterostomy (2 roots) ______
14. cholangiopancreatography (2 roots) ______

EXERCISE 12 *Break down the following words into their component parts and translate.*

EXAMPLE: sinusitis *sinus | itis* *inflammation of the sinuses*

1. cholelith ______
2. celiotomy ______
3. cholelithotomy ______
4. cholecystalgia ______
5. choledochotomy ______
6. sialolith ______
7. abdominoplasty ______
8. hepaticotomy ______
9. laparotomy ______
10. pancreatolith ______
11. peritonitis ______
12. sialolithotomy ______

GENERATION

EXERCISE 13 *Identify the roots for the following definitions.*

1. esophagus ______
2. gums ______
3. stomach ______
4. tooth (2 roots) ______
5. tongue (2 roots) ______
6. mouth (2 roots) ______

EXERCISE 14 *Build a medical term from the information provided.*

EXAMPLE: inflammation of the sinuses *sinusitis*

1. inflammation of the mouth (use *stomat/o*) ______
2. inflammation of the esophagus ______
3. inflammation of the stomach ______
4. inflammation of the gums ______

Learning Outcome 11.1 Exercises

5. tooth specialist (use *dent/o*) __________
6. straight teeth specialist (use *odont/o*) __________
7. inflammation of the gums and tongue (use *gloss/o*) __________
8. around tooth inflammation (use *odont/o*) __________

EXERCISE 15 *Identify the roots for the following definitions.*

1. anus __________
2. rectum __________
3. anus and rectum __________
4. ileum __________
5. jejunum __________
6. duodenum __________
7. intestines __________
8. colon (2 roots) __________
9. sigmoid colon __________

EXERCISE 16 *Build a medical term from the information provided.*

EXAMPLE: inflammation of the sinuses *sinusitis*

1. inflammation of the colon (use *col/o*) __________
2. inflammation of the duodenum __________
3. inflammation of the ileum __________
4. inflammation of the jejunum __________
5. inflammation of the rectum __________
6. surgical reconstruction of the anus __________
7. instrument to look into the sigmoid colon __________
8. inflammation of the anus and rectum (use *proct/o*) __________
9. inflammation of the ileum and colon (use *col/o*) __________
10. inflammation of the jejunum and ileum __________
11. inflammation of the stomach, intestines, and colon (use *col/o*) __________

EXERCISE 17 *Identify the roots for the following definitions.*

1. peritoneum __________
2. pancreas __________
3. bladder __________
4. duct __________
5. saliva __________
6. liver (2 roots) __________
7. bile (2 roots) __________
8. abdomen (3 roots) __________

Learning Outcome 11.1 Exercises

EXERCISE 18 *Build a medical term from the information provided.*

EXAMPLE: inflammation of the sinuses *sinusitis*

1. inflammation of the liver (use *hepat/o*) __________
2. inflammation of the pancreas __________
3. inflammation of the peritoneum __________
4. inflammation of the bile bladder (use *chol/e*) __________
5. incision into the bile duct (use *chol/e*) __________
6. incision into the abdomen (use *lapar/o*) __________
7. surgical reconstruction of the abdomen (use *abdomin/o*) __________
8. disease of the abdomen (use *celi/o*) __________

EXERCISE 19 *Multiple-choice questions. Select the correct answer(s).*

1. Select all of the roots below that pertain to the supporting structures/digestive organs.

a. abdomin/o	g. gingiv/o
b. chol/e	h. hepatic/o
c. colon/o	i. pancreat/o
d. enter/o	j. proct/o
e. esophag/o	k. sial/o
f. gastr/o	l. stomat/o

2. Select all of the roots below that pertain to the lower GI tract.

a. abdomin/o	g. gingiv/o
b. chol/e	h. hepatic/o
c. colon/o	i. pancreat/o
d. enter/o	j. proct/o
e. esophag/o	k. sial/o
f. gastr/o	l. stomat/o

3. Select all of the roots below that pertain to the upper GI tract.

a. abdomin/o	g. gingiv/o
b. chol/e	h. hepatic/o
c. colon/o	i. pancreat/o
d. enter/o	j. proct/o
e. esophag/o	k. sial/o
f. gastr/o	l. stomat/o

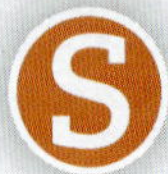

Subjective

Patient History, Problems, Complaints

Upper gastro tract

Lower gastro tract

Supporting organs

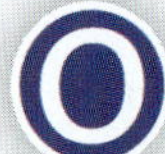

Objective

Observation and Discovery

Upper gastro tract

Lower gastro tract

Supporting organs

Diagnostic procedures

Professional terms

Anatomical regions

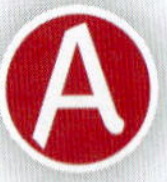

Assessment

Diagnosis and Pathology

Upper gastro tract

Lower gastro tract

Supporting organs

Plan

Treatments and Therapies

Drugs

Upper gastro tract

Lower gastro tract

Supporting organs

This section contains medical terms built from the roots presented in the previous section. The purpose of this section is to expose you to words used in gastroenterology that are built from the word roots presented earlier. The focus of this book is to teach you the process of learning roots and translating them in context. Each term is presented with the correct pronunciation, followed by a word analysis that breaks down the word into its component parts, a definition that provides a literal translation of the word, as well as supplemental information if the literal translation deviates from its medical use.

The terms are organized using a health care professional's SOAP note (first introduced in Chapter 2) as a model.

S UBJECTIVE

11.2 Patient History, Problems, Complaints

Gastrointestinal complaints are a very common reason for patient visits to a health care provider. Problems of the upper gastrointestinal tract differ a bit from problems of the lower gastrointestinal tract. Pain in the upper GI tract is much more common than in the lower GI tract.

A patient may have pain in his or her mouth (*stomatodynia*). This is common with inflammation of the mouth (*stomatitis*), which may include ulcers. Esophageal pain (*esophalgia*) is very common in patients who have acid reflux disease, where stomach acid comes up the wrong way from the stomach. Stomach pain (*gastralgia*) can be from a hole in the lining of the stomach or from inflammation.

The other common type of upper GI complaint is change in function. A patient may have discomfort with

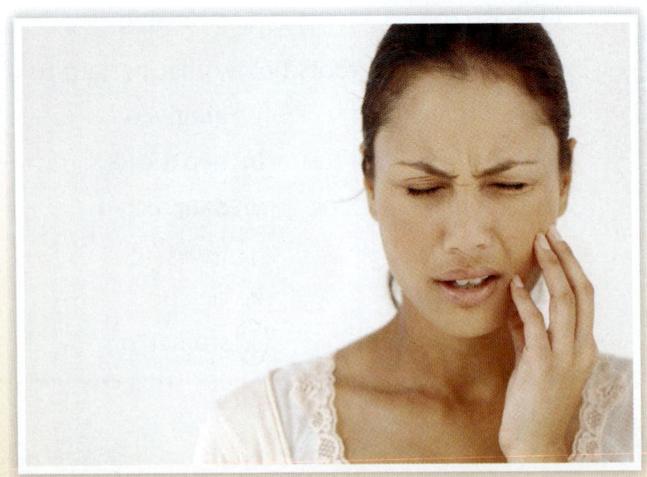

It might not seem like it, but dentalgia, or tooth pain, can be a sign of a gastroenterology problem as well as a dentistry problem.

11.2 Patient History, Problems, Complaints

eating (*dyspepsia*); this may either be pain or general nausea. If nausea becomes severe, the body may vomit (*emesis*) the stomach's contents.

Symptoms of the lower GI tract generally relate to problems with how food moves through the tract. If food moves too fast, less of the water in it is absorbed into the body, and stools may become very watery (*diarrhea*). If food moves too slowly, the stool may become hard, causing constipation. If food doesn't move at all, there may be a blockage (*obstruction*). If the obstruction blocks even gas from passing, it's known as *obstipation*.

The supporting organs of the digestive system can cause pain as well. Gallbladder pain (*cholecystalgia*) is among the more common GI complaints in adult patients. It can be caused by blockage, infection, or both. Pancreatic pain is usually very severe and often requires strong pain medicine for relief. While diseases of the liver can also cause pain, they more often first present as yellow discoloration of the eyes and skin (*jaundice*). This is due to an accumulation of *bilirubin*.

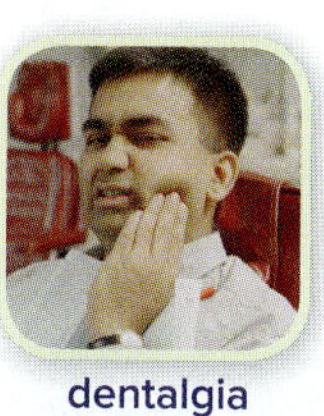
dentalgia

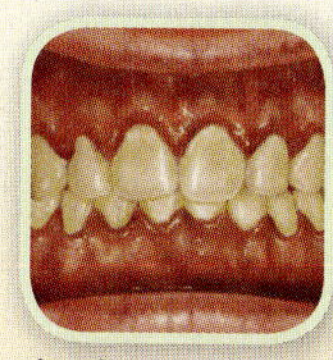
gingivostomatitis

upper gastro tract

Term	Word Analysis
aerodontalgia ER-oh-dawn-TAL-jah **Definition** tooth pain caused by exposure to air	**aer / odont / algia** air / tooth / pain
aphagia a-FAY-jah **Definition** inability to eat	**a / phag / ia** no / eat / condition
dentalgia den-TAL-jah **Definition** tooth pain	**dent / algia** tooth / pain
dyspepsia dis-PEP-see-ah **Definition** bad digestion	**dys / peps / ia** bad / digestion / condition
esophagalgia eh-SAWF-ah-GAL-jah **Definition** pain in the esophagus	**esophag / algia** esophagus / pain
eupepsia yoo-PEP-see-ah **Definition** good digestion	**eu / peps / ia** good / digestion / condition
gastralgia gas-TRAL-jah **Definition** stomach pain	**gastr / algia** stomach / pain
gastrodynia GAS-troh-DAI-nee-ah **Definition** stomach pain	**gastro / dynia** stomach / pain
gingivalgia JIN-jih-VAL-jah **Definition** gum pain	**gingiv / algia** gum / pain
gingivostomatitis JIN-jih-voh-STOH-mah-TAI-tis **Definition** inflammation of the mouth and gums	**gingivo / stomat / itis** gum / mouth / inflammation

11.2 Patient History, Problems, Complaints

upper gastro tract *continued*

Term	Word Analysis
hematemesis HEM-at-EM-eh-sis **Definition** vomiting blood	hemat / emesis blood / vomiting
hyperemesis HAI-per-EM-eh-sis **Definition** excessive vomiting	hyper / emesis over / vomiting
odontalgia OH-dawn-TAL-jah **Definition** tooth pain	odont / algia tooth / pain
odontodynia oh-DAWN-toh-DAI-nee-ah **Definition** tooth pain	odonto / dynia tooth / pain
stomatitis STOH-mah-TAI-tis **Definition** inflammation of the mouth	stomat / itis mouth / inflammation
stomatodynia stoh-MAT-oh-DAI-nee-ah **Definition** mouth pain	stomato / dynia mouth / pain

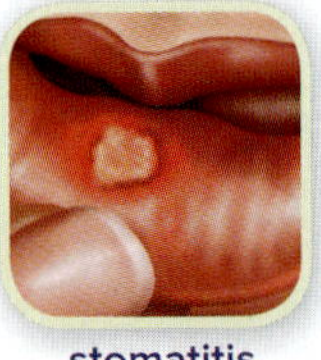
stomatitis

lower gastro tract

Term	Word Analysis
constipation KAWN-stih-PAY-shun **Definition** difficulty passing feces	from Latin, for *to crowd together*
diarrhea DAI-ah-REE-ah **Definition** passing of fluid or unformed feces	dia / rrhea through / excessive discharge
dysentery DIS-en-TER-ee **Definition** another name for diarrhea	dys / enter / y bad / intestine / condition
enterodynia EN-ter-oh-DAI-nee-ah **Definition** pain in the intestines	entero / dynia intestine / pain
hemorrhoid HEM-oh-ROID **Definition** inflammation of the veins surrounding the anus	from a Greek word referring to veins likely to discharge blood
rectalgia rek-TAL-jah **Definition** rectal pain	rect / algia rectum / pain

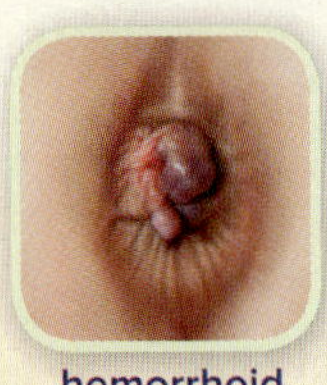
hemorrhoid

11.2 Patient History, Problems, Complaints

supporting organs

Term	Word Analysis
cholecystalgia KOH-lay-sis-TAL-jah **Definition** pain in the gallbladder	chole / cyst / algia bile / bladder / pain
cholemesis koh-LEM-eh-sis **Definition** vomiting bile	chol / emesis bile / vomiting
jaundice JAWN-dis **Definition** yellowing of skin, tissue, and fluids caused by increased levels of bilirubin in the blood	from French, meaning *yellow*
icterus IK-ter-us **Definition** another name for jaundice NOTE: This word has its origins in the name of a bird with a yellow breast; it was once believed that seeing the bird would cure jaundice.	from Greek, for *jaundice*
sialorrhea SAI-ah-loh-REE-ah **Definition** excessive salivation	sialo / rrhea saliva / excessive discharge

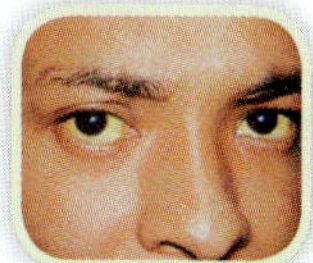

icterus

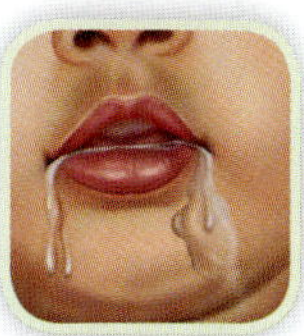

sialorrhea

Learning Outcome 11.2 Exercises

PRONUNCIATION

EXERCISE 1 *Break down the following words into syllables.*

EXAMPLE: synesthesia *syn | es | the | sia*

1. jaundice ____
2. hemorrhoid ____
3. stomatitis ____
4. diarrhea ____
5. gastralgia ____
6. enterodynia ____
7. sialorrhea ____
8. gingivalgia ____
9. hematemesis ____
10. odontodynia ____

EXERCISE 2 *Indicate which syllable is emphasized when pronounced.*

EXAMPLE: bronchitis bron**chi**tis

1. aphagia ____
2. jaundice ____
3. icterus ____
4. dentalgia ____
5. rectalgia ____
6. gastralgia ____
7. eupepsia ____
8. dyspepsia ____
9. cholemesis ____

TRANSLATION

EXERCISE 3 *Break down the following words into their component parts.*

EXAMPLE: nasopharyngoscope *naso | pharyngo | scope*

1. stomatitis ____
2. gastrodynia ____
3. odontodynia ____
4. enterodynia ____

5. hematemesis ______
6. hyperemesis ______
7. gingivalgia ______
8. dyspepsia ______
9. eupepsia ______
10. aerodontalgia ______
11. cholecystalgia ______
12. gingivostomatitis ______

EXERCISE 4 *Underline and define the roots from this chapter in the following terms.*

1. dentalgia ______
2. odontalgia ______
3. gastralgia ______
4. esophagalgia ______
5. rectalgia ______
6. stomatodynia ______
7. enterodynia ______
8. cholemesis ______
9. sialorrhea ______
10. aerodontalgia ______
11. dysentery ______
12. gingivostomatitis (2 roots) ______
13. cholecystalgia (2 roots) ______

EXERCISE 5 *Match the term on the left with its definition on the right.*

d	1. constipation	a.	inability to eat
e	2. diarrhea	b.	bad digestion
f	3. hemorrhoid	c.	good digestion
b	4. dyspepsia	d.	difficulty passing feces
c	5. eupepsia	e.	passing of fluid or unformed feces
g	6. jaundice	f.	inflammation of the veins surrounding the anus
a	7. aphagia	g.	yellowing of the skin, tissue, and fluids caused by increased levels of bilirubin in the blood

EXERCISE 6 *Fill in the blanks.*

1. *rectalgia* = pain in the ______
2. *esophagalgia* = pain in the ______
3. *gastralgia* = pain in the ______

Learning Outcome 11.2 Exercises

4. *gingivalgia* = pain in the ______
5. *dentalgia* = pain in the ______
6. *odontalgia* = pain in the ______

EXERCISE 7 *Translate the following terms as literally as possible.*

EXAMPLE: nasopharyngoscope *an instrument for looking at the nose and throat*

1. odontodynia ______
2. stomatodynia ______
3. enterodynia ______
4. aerodontalgia ______
5. dyspepsia ______
6. eupepsia ______
7. cholemesis ______
8. hematemesis ______
9. hyperemesis ______
10. aphagia ______

GENERATION

EXERCISE 8 *Build a medical term from the information provided.*

EXAMPLE: inflammation of the sinuses *sinusitis*

1. inflammation of the mouth (use *stomat/o*) ______
2. inflammation of the mouth and gums (use *stomat/o*) ______
3. stomach pain (use *-dynia*) ______
4. bad intestine condition ______
5. excessive salivation ______

EXERCISE 9 *Multiple-choice questions. Select the correct answer(s).*

1. Select all of the terms below that pertain to the lower GI tract.
   a. constipation
   b. dentalgia
   c. diarrhea
   d. hematemesis
   e. hemorrhoid
   f. rectalgia
   g. stomatitis

Learning Outcome 11.2 Exercises

2. Select all of the terms below that pertain to the upper GI tract.
   a. constipation
   b. dentalgia
   c. diarrhea
   d. hematemesis
   e. hemorrhoid
   f. rectalgia
   g. stomatitis
3. Which of the terms below literally means *through excessive discharge* and is the passing of fluid or unformed feces?
   a. constipation
   b. diarrhea
   c. dysentery
   d. hemorrhoid
   e. icterus
4. Which of the terms below is generally considered the OPPOSITE of *diarrhea?*
   a. constipation
   b. diarrhea
   c. dysentery
   d. hemorrhoid
   e. icterus
5. Which of the definitions below is the correct definition of the term *hemorrhoid?*
   a. inflammation of the skin surrounding the anus
   b. inflammation of the skin surrounding the rectum
   c. inflammation of the veins surrounding the anus
   d. inflammation of the veins surrounding the rectum
   e. none of these
6. Which of the terms below means *pain in the gallbladder?*
   a. bilemesis
   b. bilidynia
   c. cholecystalgia
   d. choledynia
   e. cholemesis

OBJECTIVE

11.3 Observation and Discovery

The first component to examining a patient with gastrointestinal complaints is visual inspection. Color changes, like jaundice, can indicate problems with the GI system. Another visual finding could be a very large, fluid-filled abdomen (*ascites*). This is usually associated with serious liver problems.

After visually inspecting the patient, the next step is to touch, or *palpate,* the abdomen. During abdominal palpation, an examiner may notice masses, pain, or tensing of the abdominal muscles in response to pain, which is known as *guarding.*

It is important to know where a patient has tenderness during the exam. The abdomen is divided into different regions to help distinguish the types of problems a patient may have. One specific goal of palpation is locating the liver's edge. An enlarged liver (*hepatomegaly*) can be a sign of disease.

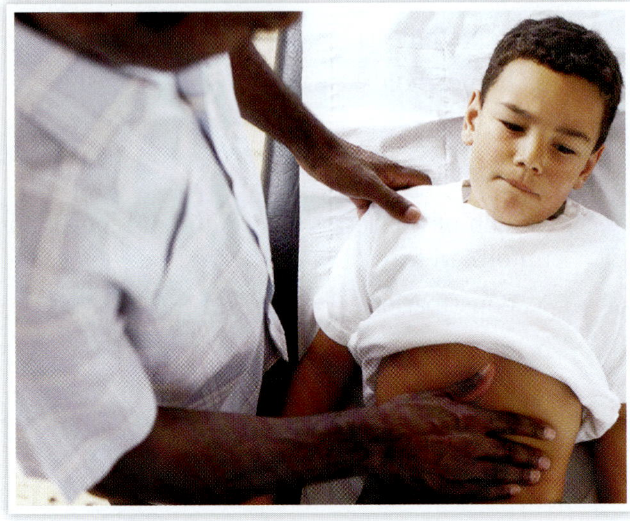

A doctor pressing on a patient's abdomen during a physical exam is checking for hepatomegaly.

Many laboratory tests for the digestive system involve examining the waste product of the digestion—that is, the stool. Some tests look for nutrients that have not been broken down or absorbed correctly. For example, fat in the stool (*steatorrhea*) indicates disease. Other tests look for blood (*fecal occult blood test*) or pus in the stool, and still others look for bacteria (*stool culture*) in the stool.

A few blood tests specifically relate to the GI system. These tests involve the chemicals that organs make to break down food (*enzymes*) and include liver enzymes and pancreatic enzymes.

As with all parts of the body, images can be very helpful in diagnosing disease. X-rays, CT scans, and ultrasounds are all very common ways of assessing the abdomen and GI structures. Because the GI system is one long tube, visual inspection with a camera is also possible (*endoscopy*). Common examples include camera inspection of the entire colon (*colonoscopy*) or just the end part (*sigmoidoscopy*), as well as inspection of the esophagus, stomach, and duodenum (*esophagogastroduodenoscopy*). There are also more specialized tests that examine vessels and ducts. One common example studies the release of bile from the gallbladder (*cholangiogram*).

11.3 Observation and Discovery

gingivitis

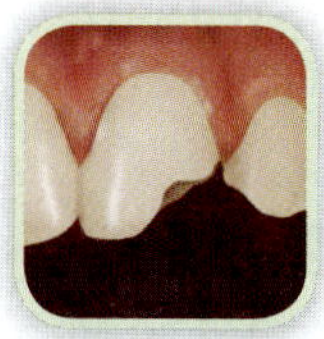

odontoclasis

upper gastro tract

Term	Word Analysis
gastromalacia GAS-troh-mah-LAY-shah **Definition** softening of the stomach	gastro / malacia stomach / softening
gastroparesis GAS-troh-par-EE-sis **Definition** partial paralysis of the stomach	gastro / paresis stomach / partial paralysis
gingivitis JIN-jih-VAI-tis **Definition** inflammation of the gums	gingiv / itis gum / inflammation
gingivoglossitis JIN-jih-voh-glaw-SAI-tis **Definition** inflammation of the gums and tongue	gingivo / gloss / itis gum / tongue / inflammation
glossoplegia GLAW-soh-PLEE-jah **Definition** paralysis of the tongue	glosso / plegia tongue / paralysis
odontoclasis OH-dawn-TAWK-lah-sis **Definition** breaking of a tooth	odonto / clasis tooth / break
stomatogastric stoh-MAT-oh-GAS-trik **Definition** pertaining to the mouth and stomach	stomato / gastr / ic mouth / stomach / pertaining to
stomatosis STOH-mah-TOH-sis **Definition** mouth condition	stomat / osis mouth / condition

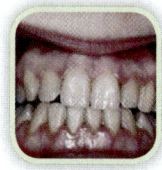

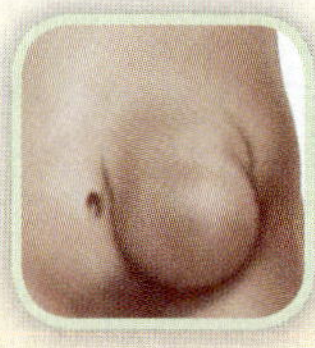

hernia

lower gastro tract

Term	Word Analysis
anophony an-AW-foh-nee **Definition** sound from the anus	ano / phony anus / sound
flatus FLAH-tus **Definition** medical term for passing gas	from Latin, for *to blow*
hernia HER-nee-ah **Definition** rupture or protusion of an organ through the wall that normally contains it	from Latin, for *rupture*
steatorrhea STAY-at-oh-REE-ah **Definition** excessive fat discharged in the feces	steato / rrhea fat / discharge

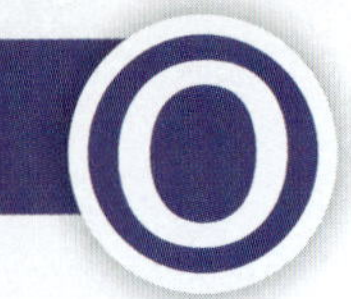

11.3 Observation and Discovery

supporting organs

Term	Word Analysis
ascites ah-SAI-teez	from the Greek word *askos*, referring to a bag made from the skin of a goat that was used to hold wine
Definition retention of fluid in the peritoneum NOTE: The name comes from the patient's resemblence to an askos.	
biligenesis bih-lih-JIN-eh-sis	bili / genesis bile / creation
Definition formation of bile	
cholelith KOH-lay-lith	chole / lith bile / stone
Definition gallstone; literally, *a stone in the bile*	
hepatomalacia heh-PAT-oh-mah-LAY-shah	hepato / malacia liver / softening
Definition softening of the liver	
hepatomegaly heh-PAT-oh-MEG-ah-lee	hepato / megaly liver / enlargement
Definition enlargement of the liver	
hepatoptosis heh-PAT-op-TOH-sis	hepato / pt / osis liver / drooping / condition
Definition downward displacement of the liver	
pancreatolith pan-kree-AT-oh-lith	pancreato / lith pancreas / stone
Definition stone in the pancreas	
sialoangiectasis SAI-ah-loh-AN-jee-EK-tah-sis	sialo / angi / ectasis saliva / vessel / expansion
Definition overexpansion of the salivary vessels	
sialolith sai-AL-oh-lith	sialo / lith saliva / stone
Definition stone in the saliva	
sialostenosis SAI-ah-loh-steh-NOH-sis	sialo / sten / osis saliva / narrowing / condition
Definition narrowing of the salivary glands	

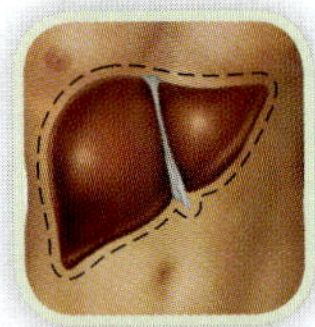

hepatomegaly

diagnostic procedures

Term	Word Analysis
anosigmoidoscopy AN-oh-SIG-moid-AW-skoh-pee	ano / sigmoido / scop / y anus / sigmoid / look / procedure
Definition procedure for looking at the anus and sigmoid colon	
cholangiogram koh-LAN-jee-oh-gram	chol / angio / gram bile / vessel / record
Definition record of the bile vessels (ducts)	
cholangiography koh-LAN-jee-AW-grah-fee	chol / angio / graph / y bile / vessel / writing / procedure
Definition procedure for mapping the bile vessels (ducts)	
cholangiopancreatography koh-LAN-jee-oh-PAN-kree-ah-TAW-grah-fee	chol / angio / pancreato / graph / y bile / vessel / pancreas / writing / procedure
Definition procedure for mapping the bile vessels (ducts) and pancreas	
cholecystogram KOH-lay-SIS-toh-gram	chole / cysto / gram bile / bladder / record
Definition record of the bile (gall) bladder	
colonoscopy COH-lon-AW-skoh-pee	colono / scop / y colon / look / procedure
Definition procedure for looking at the colon	
endoscope EN-doh-SKOHP	endo / scope inside / instrument to look
Definition instrument used to look inside	
endoscopy en-DAW-skoh-pee	endo / scop / y inside / look / procedure
Definition procedure of looking inside	
esophagoscopy eh-SAW-fah-GAW-skoh-pee	esophago / scop / y esophagus / look / procedure
Definition procedure for looking inside the esophagus	
esophagogastroduodenoscopy eh-SAW-fah-goh-GAS-stroh-DOO-aw-den-AW-skoh-pee	esophago / gastro / duodeno / scop / y esophagus / stomach / duodenum / look / procedure
Definition procedure for looking inside the esophagus, stomach, and duodenum	
fecal occult blood test (FOBT) FEE-kal ah-KULT blud test	fec / al occult blood test feces / pertaining to hidden
Definition test of feces to discover blood not visibly apparent	

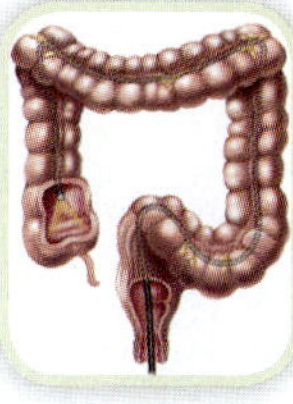
colonoscopy

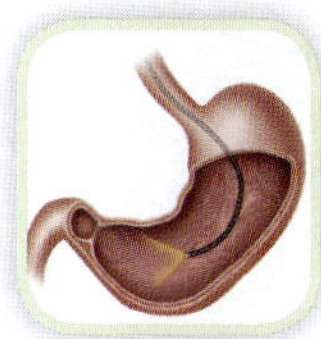
endoscopy

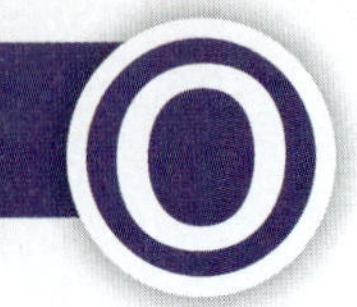

11.3 Observation and Discovery

diagnostic procedures *continued*

Term	Word Analysis
gastroscope GAS-troh-SKOHP	gastro / scope stomach / instrument to look
Definition instrument for looking at the stomach	
gastroscopy gas-STRAW-skoh-pee	gastro / scop / y stomach / look / procedure
Definition procedure for looking at the stomach	
laparoscope LAP-ar-oh-skohp	laparo / scope abdomen / instrument to look
Definition instrument for looking inside the abdomen	
laparoscopy LAP-ar-AW-skoh-pee	laparo / scop / y abdomen / look / procedure
Definition procedure for looking inside the abdomen	
nasogastric tube NAY-soh-GAS-trik TOOB	naso / gastr / ic tube nose / stomach / pertaining to
Definition tube inserted through the nose into the stomach	
pancreatography PAN-kree-ah-TAW-graw-FEE	pancreato / graph / y pancreas / writing / procedure
Definition procedure for mapping the pancreas	
peritoneoscopy PER-ih-TOH-nee-AW-skoh-pee	peritoneo / scop / y peritoneum / look / procedure
Definition procedure for looking at the peritoneum	
proctoscope PRAWK-toh-skohp	procto / scope anus/rectum / instrument to look
Definition instrument for looking at the anus and rectum	
proctoscopy prawk-TAW-skoh-pee	procto / scop / y anus/rectum / look / procedure
Definition procedure for looking at the anus and rectum	
sigmoidoscope sig-MOY-doh-skohp	sigmoido / scope sigmoid / instrument to look
Definition instrument for looking at the sigmoid colon	
sigmoidoscopy sig-moy-DAW-skoh-pee	sigmoido / scop / y sigmoid / look / procedure
Definition procedure for looking at the sigmoid colon	

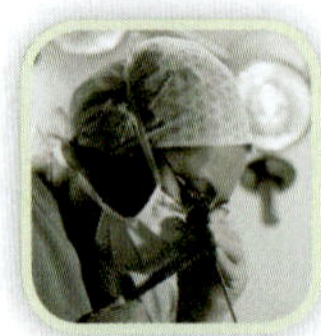

laparoscope

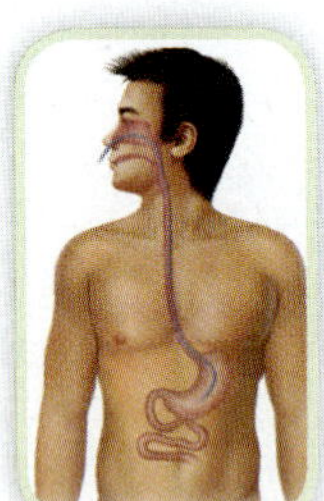

nasogastric tube

professional terms

Term	Word Analysis
bariatrics BAR-ee-ah-triks **Definition** branch of medicine dealing with weight issues NOTE: In weather forecasts, the atmospheric pressure is called *barometric pressure.*	bar / iatr / ics heavy / doctor / pertaining to
dentist DEN-tist **Definition** specialist in teeth	dent / ist tooth / specialist
dentistry DEN-tis-tree **Definition** branch of medicine dealing with teeth	dent / istry tooth / specialty
dentifrice DEN-ti-fris **Definition** toothpaste NOTE: The suffix *-frice* also gives us the word *friction.*	denti / frice tooth / rub
gastroenterologist GAS-troh-EN-ter-AW-loh-jist **Definition** specialist in the stomach and intestines	gastro / entero / logist stomach / intestines / specialist
gastroenterology GAS-troh-EN-ter-AW-loh-jee **Definition** study of the stomach and intestines	gastro / entero / logy stomach / intestines / study
orthodontics or-thoh-DAWN-tiks **Definition** branch of medicine dealing with the straightening of teeth	ortho / dont / ics straight / teeth / pertaining to
orthodontist or-thoh-DAWN-tist **Definition** specialist in straightening teeth	ortho / dont / ist straight / teeth / specialist
proctologist prok-TAW-loh-jist **Definition** specialist in the anus, rectum, and colon	procto / logist anus/rectum / specialist
proctology prok-TAW-loh-jee **Definition** branch of medicine dealing with the anus, rectum, and colon	procto / logy anus/rectum / study

dentistry

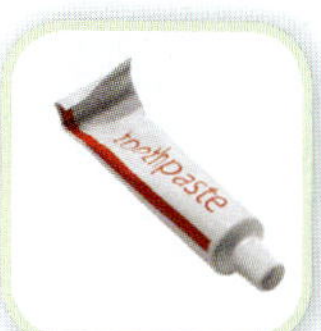

dentifrice

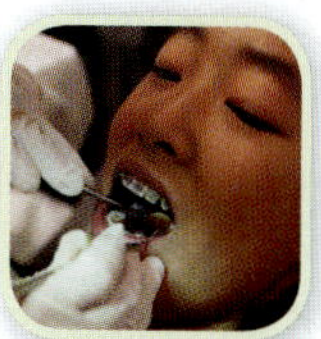
orthodontics

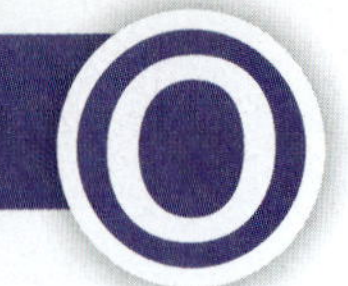

11.3 Observation and Discovery

anatomical regions

Term	Word Analysis
epigastric eh-pee-GAS-trik **Definition** upper center portion of the abdomen	epi / gastr / ic upon / stomach / pertaining to
hypochondriac hai-poh-KON-dree-ak **Definition** upper side portions of the abdomen	hypo / chondr / iac beneath / cartilage / pertaining to
hypogastric hai-poh-GAS-trik **Definition** lower center portion of the abdomen	hypo / gastr / ic beneath / stomach / pertaining to
inguinal IN-gwin-al **Definition** lower side portions of the abdomen	inguin / al groin / pertaining to
lumbar LUM-bar **Definition** middle side portions of the abdomen	lumb / ar loin / pertaining to
umbilical um-BIL-ih-kal **Definition** middle center portion of the abdomen	umbilic / al belly button / pertaining to

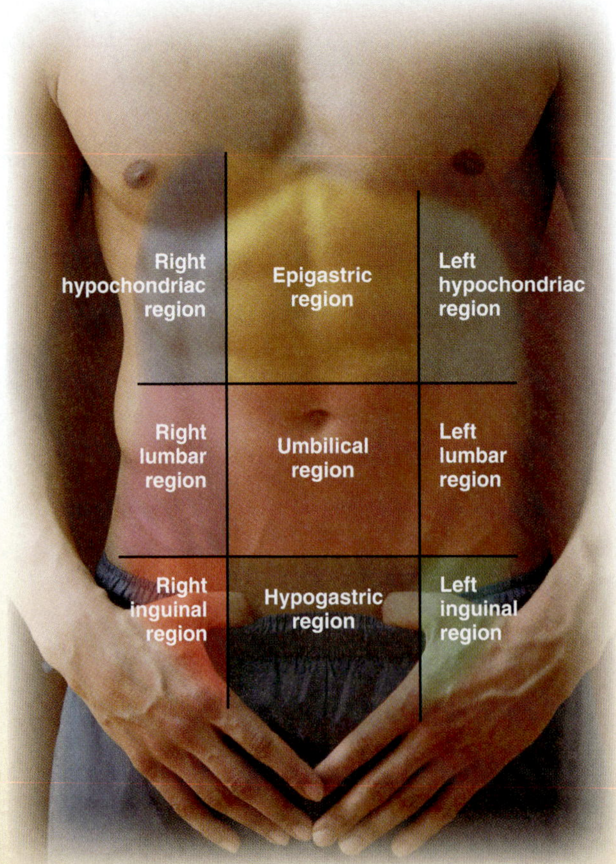

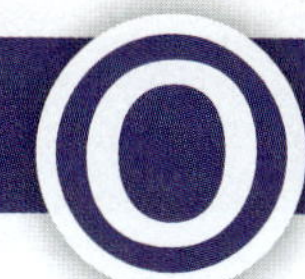

Learning Outcome 11.3 Exercises

PRONUNCIATION

EXERCISE 1 *Break down the following words into syllables.*

EXAMPLE: synesthesia *syn | es | the | sia*

1. hepatomegaly ______
2. endoscope ______
3. gastroscope ______
4. nasogastric tube ______
5. stomatosis ______
6. hepatomalacia ______
7. gastroparesis ______
8. glossoplegia ______
9. odontoclasis ______
10. laparoscopy ______
11. cholangiogram ______
12. sigmoidoscope ______
13. stomatogastric ______
14. pancreatography ______
15. ascites ______
16. hepatoptosis ______
17. sialostenosis ______
18. cholangiography ______
19. peritoneoscopy ______

EXERCISE 2 *Indicate which syllable is emphasized when pronounced.*

EXAMPLE: bronchitis bron**chi**tis

1. lumbar ______
2. hernia ______
3. dentist ______
4. dentistry ______
5. orthodontics ______
6. orthodontist ______
7. proctologist ______
8. proctology ______
9. umbilical ______
10. anophony ______
11. endoscopy ______
12. gastroscopy ______
13. proctoscopy ______
14. flatus ______
15. ascites ______
16. cholelith ______

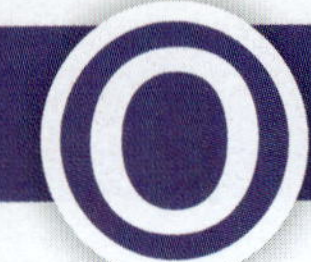

Learning Outcome 11.3 Exercises

17. pancreatolith ______
18. sialolith ______
19. laparoscope ______
20. proctoscope ______
21. sigmoidoscope ______
22. sigmoidoscopy ______
23. bariatrics ______
24. dentifrice ______
25. epigastric ______
26. hypochondriac ______
27. hypogastric ______
28. inguinal ______

TRANSLATION

EXERCISE 3 *Break down the following words into their component parts.*

EXAMPLE: nasopharyngoscope *naso | pharyngo | scope*

1. gastroscope ______
2. laparoscope ______
3. proctoscope ______
4. sigmoidoscope ______
5. endoscope ______
6. endoscopy ______
7. proctology ______
8. dentist ______
9. dentifrice ______
10. gastromalacia ______
11. pancreatolith ______
12. sialostenosis ______
13. hepatomegaly ______
14. anophony ______
15. steatorrhea ______
16. nasogastric tube ______
17. gastroenterology ______
18. orthodontics ______
19. hypochondriac ______
20. cholangiogram ______
21. cholangiography ______
22. hepatoptosis ______
23. sialoangiectasis ______
24. cholangiopancreatography ______

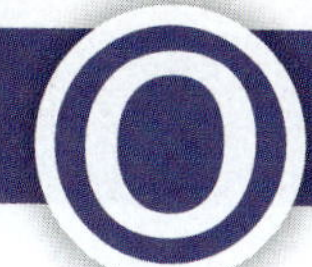

Learning Outcome 11.3 Exercises

EXERCISE 4 *Underline and define the roots from this chapter in the following terms.*

1. dentistry ______________________
2. orthodontist ______________________
3. proctologist ______________________
4. gingivitis ______________________
5. epigastric ______________________
6. hypogastric ______________________
7. gastroparesis ______________________
8. biligenesis ______________________
9. glossoplegia ______________________
10. odontoclasis ______________________
11. stomatosis ______________________
12. anophony ______________________
13. cholelith ______________________
14. hepatomalacia ______________________
15. sialolith ______________________
16. cholecystogram ______________________
17. pancreatography ______________________
18. colonoscopy ______________________
19. esophagoscopy ______________________
20. gastroscopy ______________________
21. laparoscopy ______________________
22. peritoneoscopy ______________________
23. proctoscopy ______________________
24. sigmoidoscopy ______________________
25. stomatogastric (2 roots) ______________________
26. gastroenterologist (2 roots) ______________________
27. gingivoglossitis (2 roots) ______________________
28. anosigmoidoscopy (2 roots) ______________________
29. esophagogastroduodenoscopy (3 roots) ______________________

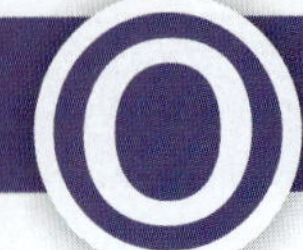

Learning Outcome 11.3 Exercises

EXERCISE 5 *Match the term on the left with its definition on the right.*

g	1. hernia	a.	branch of medicine dealing with weight issues
h	2. fecal occult blood test	b.	lower side portions of the abdomen
a	3. bariatrics	c.	medical term for passing gas; from the Latin word meaning *to blow*
c	4. flatus	d.	middle center portion of the abdomen
e	5. lumbar	e.	middle side portions of the abdomen
d	6. umbilical	f.	retention of fluid in the peritoneum
b	7. inguinal	g.	rupture or protrusion of an organ through the wall that normally contains it
f	8. ascites	h.	test of feces to discover blood not visibly apparent

EXERCISE 6 *Fill in the blanks.*

1. *dentist* = specialist in ______________________
2. *proctologist* = specialist in ______________________
3. *orthodontist* = specialist in ______________________
4. *gastroenterologist* = specialist in ______________________
5. *colonoscopy* = procedure for looking at the ______________________
6. *gastroscopy* = procedure for looking at the ______________________
7. *esophagoscopy* = procedure for looking at the ______________________
8. *peritoneoscopy* = procedure for looking at the ______________________
9. *proctoscopy* = procedure for looking at the ______________________
10. *laparoscopy* = procedure for looking at the ______________________
11. *sigmoidoscopy* = procedure for looking at the ______________________
12. *anosigmoidoscopy* = procedure for looking at the ______________________
13. *esophagogastroduodenoscopy* = procedure for looking at the ______________________

EXERCISE 7 *Translate the following terms as literally as possible.*

EXAMPLE: nasopharyngoscope *an instrument for looking at the nose and throat*

1. biligenesis ______________________
2. pancreatography ______________________
3. stomatosis ______________________
4. gastroparesis ______________________
5. glossoplegia ______________________
6. odontoclasis ______________________
7. stomatogastric ______________________
8. anophony ______________________
9. sialostenosis ______________________

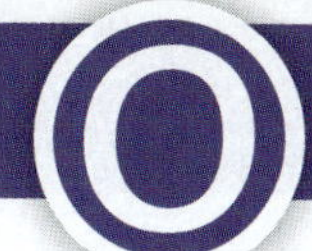

Learning Outcome 11.3 Exercises

10. hepatoptosis ____________
11. nasogastric tube ____________
12. dentistry ____________
13. orthodontics ____________
14. steatorrhea ____________
15. sialoangiectasis ____________
16. cholangiopancreatography ____________

GENERATION

EXERCISE 8 *Build a medical term from the information provided.*

EXAMPLE: inflammation of the sinuses *sinusitis*

1. enlargement of the liver ____________
2. softening of the liver ____________
3. softening of the stomach ____________
4. inflammation of the gums ____________
5. stone in the pancreas ____________
6. stone in the saliva ____________
7. gall (bile) stone ____________
8. record of the bile (gall) bladder ____________
9. instrument for looking at the sigmoid colon ____________
10. instrument for looking at the stomach ____________
11. instrument for looking inside the abdomen ____________
12. instrument for looking at the anus and rectum ____________
13. inflammation of the gums and tongue ____________
14. study of the stomach and intestines ____________
15. study of the anus, rectum, and colon ____________

EXERCISE 9 *Multiple-choice questions. Select the correct answer(s).*

1. Which of the terms below is the technical term for *toothpaste?*
   a. bariatric
   b. dentifrice
   c. inguinal
   d. odontoclasis
   e. none of these
2. A person with *ascites* has fluid retention in which part of the GI system?
   a. esophagus
   b. ileum
   c. mouth
   d. peritoneum
   e. sigmoid colon

Learning Outcome 11.3 Exercises

Fecal. Occult Blood Test.

3. An FOBT tests the feces for what?
   a. allergies
   b. bile
   c. blood
   d. sugar
   e. undigested materials
4. *Bariatrics* is a
   a. branch of medicine dealing with the anus, rectum, and colon
   b. branch of medicine dealing with digestive disorders
   c. branch of medicine dealing with intestinal issues
   d. branch of medicine dealing with weight issues
   e. none of these
5. Which of the terms below comes from the Latin word meaning *to blow*?
   a. anophony
   b. ascites
   c. dentifrice
   d. flatus
   e. hernia
6. Which of the terms below comes from the Latin word meaning *to rupture*?
   a. anophony
   b. ascites
   c. dentifrice
   d. flatus
   e. hernia

EXERCISE 10 *Briefly describe the difference between each pair of terms.*

1. cholangiogram, cholangiography ______
2. endoscope, endoscopy ______
3. gingivitis, gingivoglossitis ______
4. sialoangiectasis, sialostenosis ______
5. gastroparesis, glossoplegia ______
6. epigastric, hypochondriac ______
7. epigastric, hypogastric ______
8. hypochondriac, inguinal ______
9. lumbar, umbilical ______

ASSESSMENT

11.4 Diagnosis and Pathology

GI problems include infection or inflammation, change in function, and problems in the GI tract's structure. Infection of the GI tract is perhaps the most common GI problem seen in the office setting. *Acute gastroenteritis* is infection of the entire tract; it presents with vomiting and/or diarrhea. Most cases are caused by a virus and require no treatment. However, food poisoning can possibly lead to life-threatening illness.

Less-common infections include infection of the liver (*hepatitis*) or pancreas (*pancreatitis*). Infectious hepatitis is generally caused by a virus and presents with pain, jaundice, and/or vomiting. The chief symptom of pancreatitis is intense pain. Inflammation of GI organs can also be caused by inherited disorders like *ulcerative colitis* or acquired due to stress or reaction to a medication, such as stomach inflammation (*gastritis*).

When the GI tract isn't working the way it should, food might travel in the wrong direction. For instance, when food passes from the stomach back up the esophagus (*gastroesophageal reflux*), the result can be a painful burning sensation. While medicine often helps, this problem can become severe enough to require surgery.

When the intestines do not work properly (*enteropathy*), food will often pass through without being completely digested or absorbed. Another functional GI problem occurs when a blockage exists in the tract. This can be caused by an overgrown structure in the body, such as the muscle valve at the end of the stomach (*pyloric stenosis*), or it can be caused by development of stones over time like with gallstones (*cholelithiasis*). This blockage frequently leads to infection of the gallbladder (*cholecystitis*).

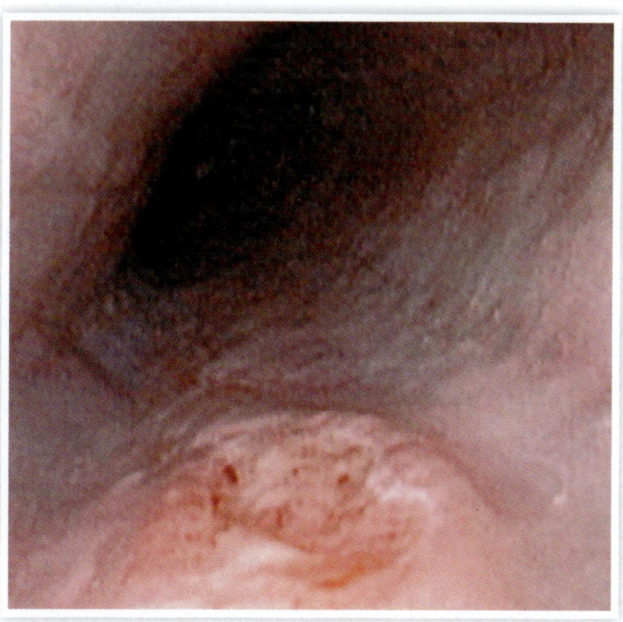

Endoscopes are invaluable tools in diagnosing problems in the digestive tract.

upper gastro tract

Term	Word Analysis
esophagitis eh-SAWF-ah-JAI-tis **Definition** inflammation of the esophagus	esophag / itis esophagus / inflammation
esophageal carcinoma eh-SAWF-ah-JEE-al KAR-sih-NOH-mah **Definition** cancerous tumor of the esophagus	esophag / eal carcin / oma esophagus / pertaining to cancer / tumor
gastritis gas-TRAI-tis **Definition** inflammation of the stomach	gastr / itis stomach / inflammation

11.4 Diagnosis and Pathology

upper gastro tract *continued*

Term	Word Analysis
gastroenteritis GAS-troh-EN-ter-AI-tis **Definition** inflammation of the stomach and intestines	gastro / enter / itis stomach / intestine / inflammation
gastroenterocolitis GAS-troh-EN-ter-oh-coh-LAI-tis **Definition** inflammation of the stomach, intestine, and colon	gastro / entero / col / itis stomach / intestine / colon / inflammation
gastroesophageal reflux disease (GERD) GAS-troh-eh-SOF-ah-JEE-al REE-fluks dih-ZEEZ **Definition** disease in which acid comes up from the stomach and damages the esophagus	gastro / esophag / eal re / flux stomach / esophagus / pertaining to back / flow
gingival hyperplasia JIN-jih-val HAI-per-PLAY-zhah **Definition** overformation of gum tissue	gingiv / al hyper / plasia gum / pertaining to over / formation
glossopathy glaws-AW-pah-thee **Definition** disease of the tongue	glosso / pathy tongue / disease
glossotrichia GLAWS-oh-TRIK-ee-ah **Definition** overdevelopment of bumps on the tongue, making the tongue appear to be hairy	glosso / trich / ia tongue / hair / condition
periodontitis PER-ee-OH-don-TAI-tis **Definition** inflammation of region around the teeth	peri / odont / itis around / tooth / inflammation
pyloric stenosis PAI-lor-ik steh-NOH-sis **Definition** narrowing of the sphincter at the base of the stomach **NOTE:** The body has three muscles called *sphincters* that open and close to allow the passage of fluid and solids—the esophageal (between the esophagus and the stomach), the pyloric (between the stomach and the intestines), and the anus. *Pyloric* comes from Greek, for *gatekeeper.*	pylor / ic sten / osis gatekeeper / pertaining to narrowing / condition
stomatomycosis stoh-MAT-oh-mai-KOH-sis **Definition** fungus condition of the mouth	stomato / myc / osis mouth / fungus / condition
stomatosis STOH-mah-TOH-sis **Definition** mouth condition	stomat / osis mouth / condition

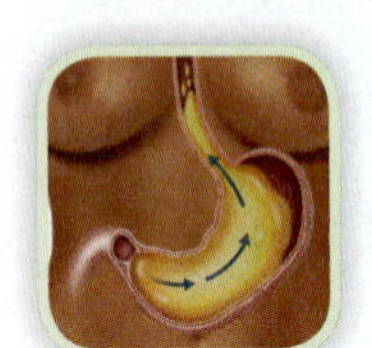

gastroesophageal reflux disease (GERD)

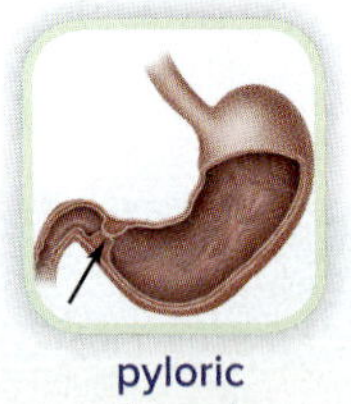

pyloric stenosis

11.4 Diagnosis and Pathology

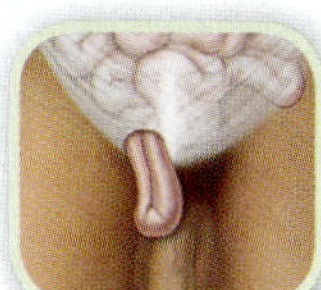
enterocele

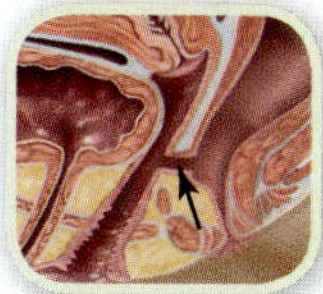
fistula

lower gastro tract

Term	Word Analysis
colitis coh-LAI-tis **Definition** inflammation of the colon	col / itis colon / inflammation
colorectal carcinoma COH-loh-REK-tal KAR-sih-NOH-mah **Definition** cancerous tumor of the colon or rectum	colo / rect / al — carcin / oma colon / rectum / pertaining to — cancer / tumor
duodenitis doo-AH-den-AI-tis **Definition** inflammation of the duodenum	duoden / itis duodenum / inflammation
enterocele EN-ter-oh-seel **Definition** hernia of the intestines	entero / cele intestine / tumor
enteropathy EN-ter-AW-pah-thee **Definition** disease of the intestines	entero / pathy intestine / disease
fistula FIS-tyoo-la **Definition** any abnormal passageway in the body that shouldn't be there	from Latin, for *pipe*
anal fistula AY-nal FIS-tyoo-la **Definition** abnormal opening between the rectum and the exterior perianal skin	an / al — fistula anus / pertaining to — pipe
colovaginal fistula COH-loh-VAJ-in-al FIS-tyoo-la **Definition** abnormal opening between the colon and vagina	colo / vagin / al — fistula colon / vagina / pertaining to — pipe
ileitis IH-lee-AI-tis **Definition** inflammation of the ileum	ile / itis ileum / inflammation
ileocolitis IH-lee-oh-koh-LAI-tis **Definition** inflammation of the ileum and colon	ileocol / itis ileum / inflammation
jejunitis JE-joo-NAI-tis **Definition** inflammation of the jejunum	jejun / itis jejunum / inflammation
jejunoileitis je-JOO-noh-IH-lee-AI-tis **Definition** inflammation of the jejunum and ileum	jejuno / ile / itis jejunum / ileum / inflammation
proctitis prok-TAI-tis **Definition** inflammation of the anus and rectum	proct / itis anus/rectum / inflammation

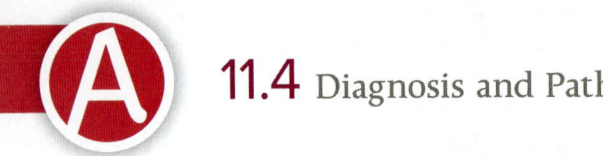

11.4 Diagnosis and Pathology

lower gastro tract *continued*

Term	Word Analysis
proctoptosis prok-TOP-toh-sis **Definition** downward displacement of the rectum and anus	procto / pt / osis anus/rectum / drooping / condition
rectitis rek-TAI-tis **Definition** inflammation of the rectum	rect / itis rectum / inflammation

supporting organs

Term	Word Analysis
celiomyositis SEE-lee-oh-MAI-oh-sai-TOH-sis **Definition** inflammation of the abdominal muscle	celio / myos / itis abdomen / muscle / inflammation
celiopathy see-lee-AW-pah-thee **Definition** disease of the abdomen	celio / pathy abdomen / disease
cholangioma koh-lan-jee-OH-mah **Definition** tumor of the bile vessels (ducts)	chol / angi / oma bile / vessel / tumor
cholangitis KOH-lan-JAI-tis **Definition** inflammation of the bile vessels (ducts)	chol / ang / itis bile / vessel / inflammation
cholecystitis KOH-lay-sis-TAI-tis **Definition** inflammation of the bile (gall) bladder	chole / cyst / itis bile / bladder / inflammation
choledochocele koh-lay-DOH-koh-seel **Definition** hernia of the (common) bile duct	chole / docho / cele bile / duct / tumor
choledocholithiasis koh-lay-DOH-koh-lith-AI-ah-sis **Definition** presence of a stone in the (common) bile duct	chole / docho / lith / iasis bile / duct / stone / presence
cholelithiasis KOH-lay-lih-THAI-ah-sis **Definition** presence of a gallstone	chole / lith / iasis bile / stone / presence
cirrhosis sir-OH-sis **Definition** liver disease named for the change of color in the liver **NOTE:** The standard Greek root for yellow is *xantho*. This word uses a much rarer root for *yellow*.	from the Greek word *cirrho*, for *yellow*

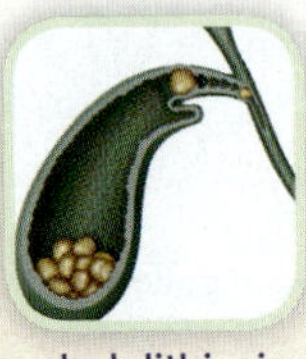

cholelithiasis

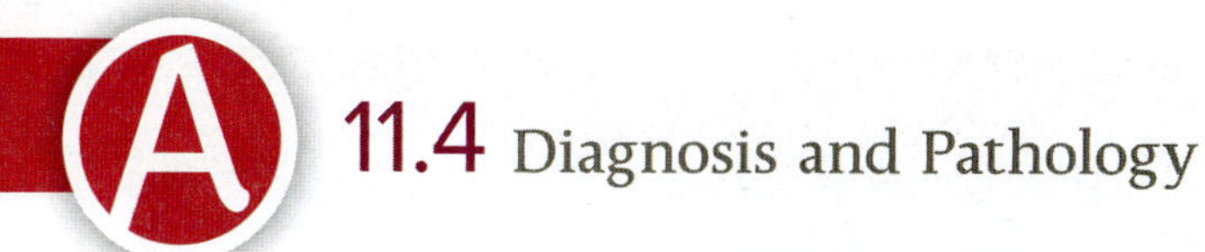

11.4 Diagnosis and Pathology

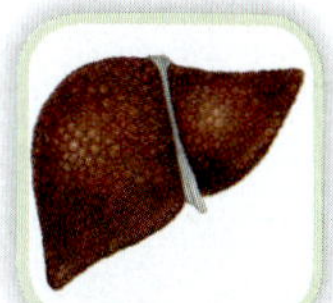

hepatitis

laparocele

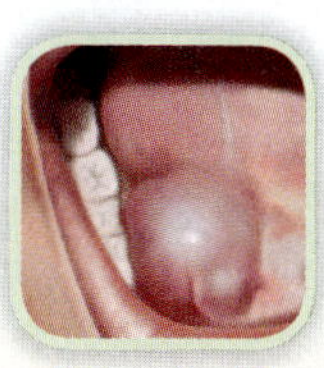

sialoadenitis

supporting organs *continued*

Term	Word Analysis
hepatitis HEH-pah-TAI-tis **Definition** inflammation of the liver	hepat / itis liver / inflammation
hepatocarcinoma heh-PAT-oh-KAR-sih-NOH-mah **Definition** cancerous tumor of the liver	hepato / carcin / oma liver / cancer / tumor
hepatoma HEH-pah-TOH-mah **Definition** tumor of the liver	hepat / oma liver / tumor
hepatosclerosis heh-PAT-oh-skleh-ROH-sis **Definition** hardening of the liver	hepato / scler / osis liver / hardening / condition
laparocele LAP-ar-oh-seel **Definition** abdominal hernia	laparo / cele abdomen / tumor
pancreatitis PAN-kree-ah-TAI-tis **Definition** inflammation of the pancreas	pancreat / itis pancreas / inflammation
pancreatolithiasis PAN-kree-AH-toh-lih-THAI-ah-sis **Definition** presence of a stone in the pancreas	pancreato / lith / iasis pancreas / stone / presence
peritonitis PER-ih-toh-NAI-tis **Definition** inflammation of the peritoneum	periton / itis peritoneum / inflammation
sclerosing cholangitis skleh-ROH-sing KOH-lan-JAI-tis **Definition** inflammation and hardening of the bile vessels (ducts)	scleros / ing chol / ang / itis harden / ing bile / vessel / inflammation
sialoadenitis sai-AL-oh-AD-en-AI-tis **Definition** inflammation of the salivary glands	sialo / aden / itis saliva / gland / inflammation
sialoadenosis sai-AL-oh-AD-en-OH-sis **Definition** a condition of the salivary glands	sialo / aden / osis saliva / gland / condition
sialolithiasis sai-AL-oh-lih-THAI-ah-sis **Definition** presence of salivary stones	sialo / lith / iasis saliva / stone / presence

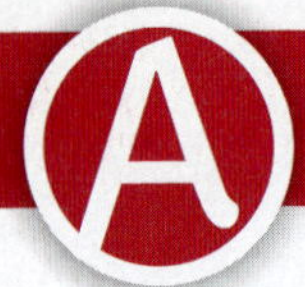

Learning Outcome 11.4 Exercises

PRONUNCIATION

EXERCISE 1 *Break down the following words into syllables.*

EXAMPLE: synesthesia *syn | es | the | sia*

1. hepatitis ______
2. hepatoma ______
3. enteropathy ______
4. stomatosis ______
5. peritonitis ______
6. pancreatitis ______
7. colorectal carcinoma ______
8. ileitis ______
9. gastroenteritis ______
10. periodontitis ______
11. duodenitis ______
12. ileocolitis ______
13. jejunoileitis ______
14. sialoadenitis ______
15. gastroenterocolitis ______
16. proctoptosis ______
17. cholelithiasis ______
18. pancreatolithiasis ______

EXERCISE 2 *Indicate which syllable is emphasized when pronounced.*

EXAMPLE: bronchitis bron**chi**tis

1. celiopathy ______
2. glossopathy ______
3. gastritis ______
4. colitis ______
5. rectitis ______
6. proctitis ______
7. fistula ______
8. anal fistula ______
9. cirrhosis ______
10. laparocele ______
11. enterocele ______
12. pyloric stenosis ______
13. proctoptosis ______
14. cholangioma ______

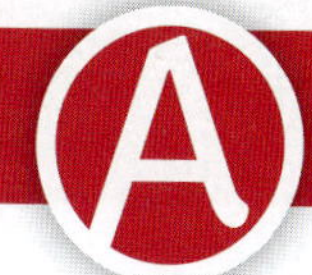

Learning Outcome 11.4 Exercises

TRANSLATION

EXERCISE 3 *Break down the following words into their component parts.*

EXAMPLE: nasopharyngoscope *naso | pharyngo | scope*

1. gastritis ______
2. colitis ______
3. esophagitis ______
4. cholangitis ______
5. hepatoma ______
6. enteropathy ______
7. stomatosis ______
8. glossotrichia ______
9. ileocolitis ______
10. jejunoileitis ______
11. celiomyositis ______
12. hepatosclerosis ______
13. proctoptosis ______
14. sialoadenitis ______
15. sialolithiasis ______
16. cholelithiasis ______
17. pancreatolithiasis ______
18. choledocholithiasis ______

EXERCISE 4 *Underline and define the roots from this chapter in the following terms.*

1. pancreatitis ______
2. rectitis ______
3. peritonitis ______
4. ileitis ______
5. jejunitis ______
6. duodenitis ______
7. hepatitis ______
8. proctitis ______
9. cholangitis ______
10. periodontitis ______
11. gingival hyperplasia ______
12. esophageal carcinoma ______
13. hepatocarcinoma ______
14. enterocele ______

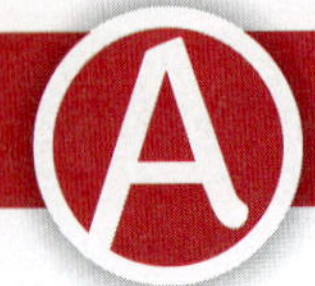

Learning Outcome 11.4 Exercises

15. laparocele ______
16. celiopathy ______
17. glossopathy ______
18. stomatomycosis ______
19. sclerosing cholangitis ______
20. sialoadenosis ______
21. gastroesophageal reflux disease (2 roots) ______
22. gastroenteritis (2 roots) ______
23. colorectal carcinoma (2 roots) ______
24. cholecystitis (2 roots) ______
25. choledochocele (2 roots) ______
26. gastroenterocolitis (3 roots) ______

EXERCISE 5 *Match the term on the left with its definition on the right.*

d	1. cirrhosis	a.	abnormal opening between the colon and vagina
a	2. colovaginal fistula	b.	abnormal opening between the rectum and the exterior perianal skin
b	3. anal fistula	c.	any abnormal passageway in the body that shouldn't be there
c.	4. fistula	d.	liver disease named for the change in color in the liver
e.	5. pyloric stenosis	e.	narrowing of the sphincter at the base of the stomach

EXERCISE 6 *Translate the following terms as literally as possible.*

EXAMPLE: nasopharyngoscope *an instrument for looking at the nose and throat*

1. laparocele ______
2. glossopathy ______
3. stomatosis ______
4. cholangitis ______
5. celiopathy ______
6. hepatosclerosis ______
7. esophageal carcinoma ______
8. colorectal carcinoma ______
9. gingival hyperplasia ______
10. stomatomycosis ______
11. celiomyositis ______
12. proctoptosis ______
13. choledocholithiasis ______
14. sclerosing cholangitis ______

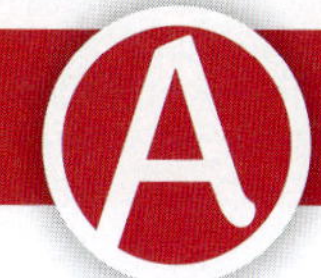

Learning Outcome 11.4 Exercises

GENERATION

EXERCISE 7 *Build a medical term from the information provided.*

EXAMPLE: inflammation of the sinuses *sinusitis*

1. inflammation of the esophagus ____________
2. inflammation of the pancreas ____________
3. inflammation of the rectum ____________
4. inflammation of the colon ____________
5. inflammation of the duodenum ____________
6. inflammation of the jejunum ____________
7. inflammation of the ileum ____________
8. inflammation of the peritoneum ____________
9. inflammation of the stomach ____________
10. inflammation of the liver ____________
11. inflammation of the anus and rectum ____________
12. inflammation of the stomach and intestines ____________
13. inflammation of the ileum and colon ____________
14. inflammation of the jejunum and ileum ____________
15. inflammation of the region around the teeth ____________
16. inflammation of the bile (gall) bladder ____________
17. inflammation of the salivary glands ____________
18. inflammation of the stomach, intestine, and colon ____________

EXERCISE 8 *Multiple-choice questions. Select the correct answer(s).*

1. A person suffering from *cirrhosis* has (select all that apply)
   a. a liver disease
   b. a purple liver
   c. a yellow liver
   d. liver cancer
   e. liver inflammation
2. The pyloric sphincter is located between the stomach and the intestines. A patient with *pyloric stenosis* has
   a. hardening of the sphincter at the base of the stomach
   b. narrowing of the sphincter at the base of the stomach
   c. softening of the sphincter at the base of the stomach
   d. widening of the sphincter at the base of the stomach
   e. none of these

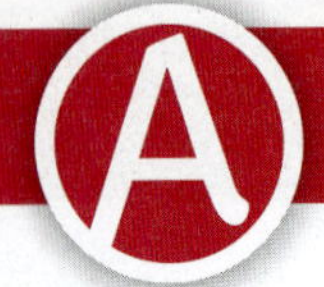

Learning Outcome 11.4 Exercises

3. GERD is
   a. a disease in which acid comes up from the intestines and damages the esophagus
   b. a disease in which acid comes up from the intestines and damages the stomach
   c. a disease in which acid comes up from the stomach and damages the esophagus
   d. a disease in which acid comes up from the stomach and damages the intestines
   e. none of these
4. A person with *glossotrichia* has
   a. abnormal hair growth in the mouth
   b. hair growing on the tongue
   c. overdevelopment of bumps on the tongue, making the tongue appear to be hairy
   d. hair from the nose long enough to touch the tongue
   e. none of these
5. An abnormal passageway (one that shouldn't be there) in the body is called a
   a. carcinoma
   b. cirrhosis
   c. fistula
   d. laparocele
   e. stenosis

EXERCISE 9 *Briefly describe the difference between each pair of terms.*

1. cholelithiasis, pancreatolithiasis ______
2. enterocele, enteropathy ______
3. anal fistula, colovaginal fistula ______
4. cholangioma, choledochocele ______
5. sialoadenosis, sialolithiasis ______
6. hepatocarcinoma, hepatoma ______

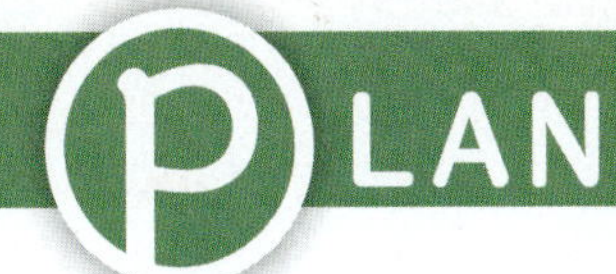

11.5 Treatments and Therapies

Medicines that are utilized to help patients with GI problems generally treat issues with stomach acid and the movement of food through their GI tracts. Patients with gastroesophageal reflux and ulcers may need medicine to decrease levels of stomach acid (*antacids*). Medicines also help with food movement, including medicine to stop vomiting (*antiemetics*) or medicine to help accelerate the movement of food or aid with constipation (*cathartics*).

Nonmedication methods are also commonly used to treat GI problems. Among the most common treatments is keeping the patient from eating or drinking anything (*NPO*), which helps the GI tract rest. Another form of assistance includes inserting a tube into part of the GI tract. The most common tube is the nasogastric tube (*NGT*). This tube can either send food into the stomach, bypassing the throat, or it can be used to suck out (*aspirate*) the contents of the stomach. A tube can also be passed through the anus into the colon to administer fluid (*enema*) to help flush out stool that is stuck there.

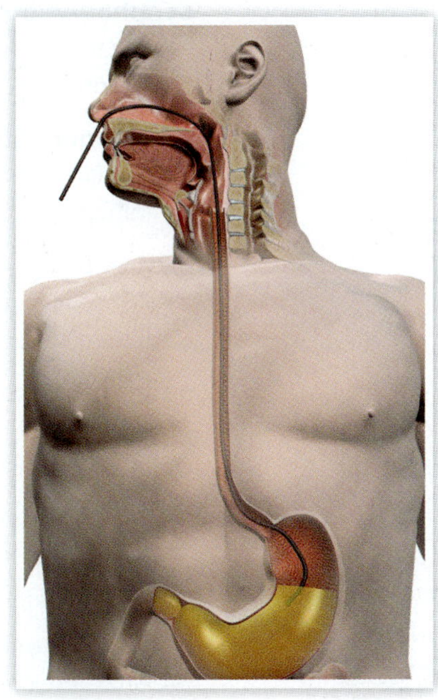

A nasograstric tube can either send food into the stomach, bypassing the throat, or can suck out (aspirate) the contents of the stomach.

There are two types of surgical approaches when operating on the gastrointestinal system: cutting a patient open (*laparotomy*) and inserting a camera and instruments through small holes (*laparoscopic*). The most common type of surgery involves removing part of the GI tract. When a section of the GI tract is removed, the remaining ends need to be reconnected (*anastamosis*). Occasionally, one end is attached to an opening to the outside of the body (*ostomy*), and the part past this is left disconnected. Usually, this is a temporary procedure to give time for the GI tract to heal. The most common of all gastrointestinal surgeries is removal of the appendix (*appendectomy*). The appendix is a small extension off the large intestine with little to no function. If blocked, it can become infected and possibly rupture.

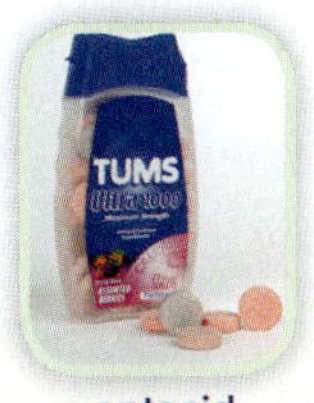

antacid

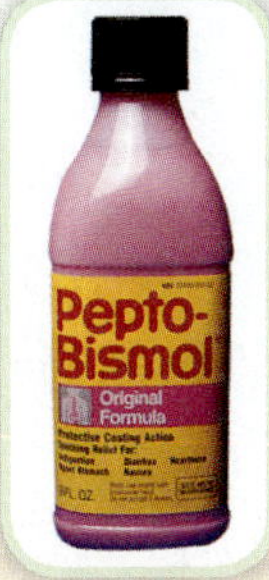

antiemetic

drugs

Term	Word Analysis
antacid ant-AS-id **Definition** agent that neutralizes acid	ant / acid against / acid
antiemetic AN-tih-EE-met-ik **Definition** agent that prevents or relieves nausea or vomiting	anti / emet / ic against / vomiting / pertaining to
cathartic kah-THAR-tik **Definition** agent that produces bowel movels	cathart / ic cleansing / pertaining to
sialagogic sai-AL-ah-GAW-jik **Definition** agent that causes salivation	sial / agog / ic saliva / leading / pertaining to

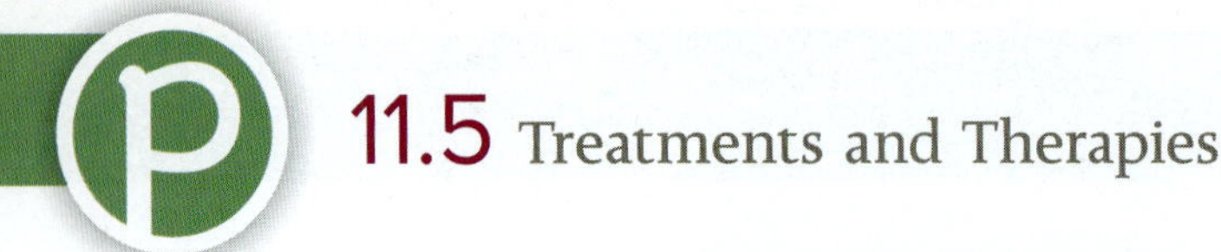

11.5 Treatments and Therapies

upper gastro tract

Term	Word Analysis
esophagectomy eh-SAW-fah-JEK-toh-mee **Definition** surgical removal of the esophagus	esophag / ec / tomy esophagus / out / cut
esophagogastroplasty eh-SAW-fah-goh-GAS-troh-PLAS-tee **Definition** surgical reconstruction of the esophagus and stomach	esophago / gastro / plasty esophagus / stomach / reconstruction
gastrectomy gas-TREK-toh-mee **Definition** surgical removal of the stomach	gastr / ec / tomy stomach / out / cut
gastroduodenostomy GAS-troh-doo-AH-den-AW-stoh-mee **Definition** creation of an opening between the stomach and the duodenum	gastro / duodeno / stom / y stomach / duodenum / mouth / procedure
gastroenterostomy GAS-troh-EN-ter-AW-stoh-mee **Definition** creation of an opening between the stomach and the intestines	gastro / entero / stom / y stomach / intestine / mouth / procedure
gastrojejunostomy GAS-troh-JEH-joo-NAW-stoh-mee **Definition** creation of an opening between the stomach and the jejunum	gastro / jejuno / stom / y stomach / jejunum / mouth / procedure
gastropexy GAS-troh-PEK-see **Definition** surgical fixation of the stomach	gastro / pexy stomach / fixation
gastroplasty GAS-troh-PLAS-tee **Definition** surgical reconstruction of the stomach	gastro / plasty stomach / reconstruction
gingivectomy JIN-jiv-EK-toh-mee **Definition** surgical removal of gum tissue	gingiv / ec / tomy gum / out / cut
gingivoplasty JIN-jiv-oh-PLAS-tee **Definition** surgical reconstruction of gum tissue	gingivo / plasty gum / reconstruction
glossoplasty GLAWS-oh-PLAS-tee **Definition** surgical reconstruction of the tongue	glosso / plasty tongue / reconstruction
glossorrhaphy glaws-OR-ah-fee **Definition** suture of the tongue	glosso / rrhaphy tongue / suture

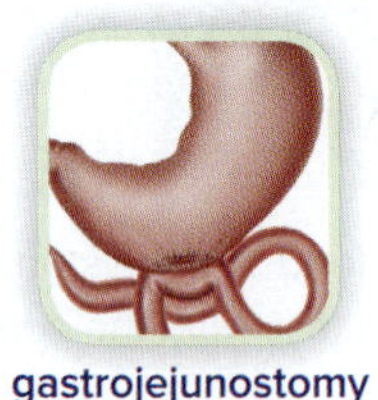

gastrojejunostomy

upper gastro tract *continued*

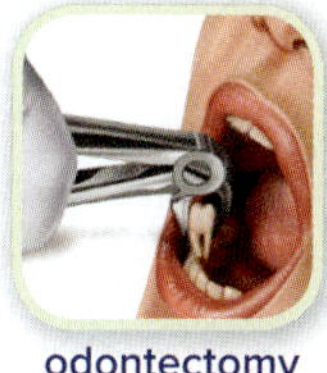
odontectomy

Term	Word Analysis
glossotomy glaws-AW-toh-mee **Definition** incision into the tongue	glosso / tomy tongue / cut
odontectomy oh-dawn-TEK-toh-mee **Definition** surgical removal of a tooth	odont / ec / tomy tooth / out / cut

lower gastro tract

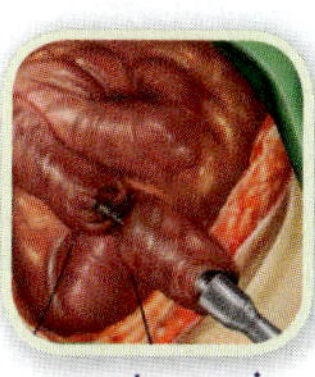
anastomosis

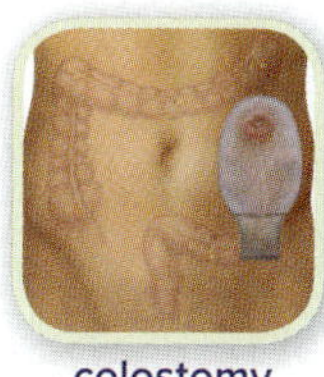
colostomy

Term	Word Analysis
anastomosis ah-NAS-toh-MOH-sis **Definition** creation of an opening; a surgical procedure connecting two previously unconnected hollow tubes **Note:** The prefix *ana-* here means *out* or *up* instead of *no* or *not*. This is the same type of usage as in the word *aneurysm*.	ana / stom / osis up / out / mouth / condition
anoplasty AN-noh-PLAS-tee **Definition** surgical reconstruction of the anus	ano / plasty anus / recontruction
colectomy koh-LEK-toh-mee **Definition** surgical removal of the colon	col / ec / tomy colon / out / cut
colostomy koh-LAW-stoh-mee **Definition** creation of an opening in the colon	colo / stom / y colon / mouth / procedure
duodenectomy doo-AW-den-EK-toh-mee **Definition** surgical removal of the duodenum	dudoden / ec / tomy duodenum / out / cut
enterectomy en-ter-EK-toh-mee **Definition** surgical removal of the intestines	enter / ec / tomy intestine / out / cut
enterorrhaphy en-ter-OR-ah-fee **Definition** suture of the intestines	entero / rrhaphy intestine / suture
enterotomy en-ter-AW-toh-mee **Definition** incision into the intestines	entero / tomy intestine / cut

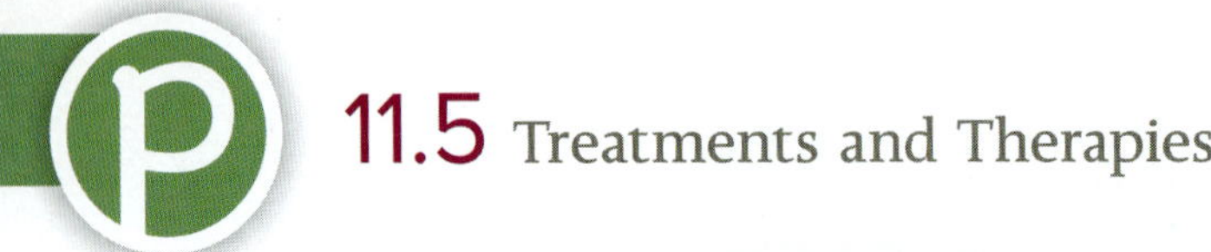

lower gastro tract *continued*

Term	Word Analysis
hemicolectomy HEH-mee-koh-LEK-toh-mee **Definition** surgical removal of half (a portion) of the colon	hemi / col / ec / tomy half / colon / out / cut
hemorrhoidectomy HEM-oh-roi-DEK-toh-mee **Definition** surgical removal of hemorrhoids	hemorrhoid / ec / tomy hemorrhoid / out / cut
herniorrhaphy her-nee-OR-ah-fee **Definition** suture of a hernia	hernio / rrhaphy hernia / suture
ileocolostomy IH-lee-oh-koh-LAW-stoh-mee **Definition** creation of an opening between the ileum and colon	ileo / colo / stom / y ileum / colon / mouth / procedure
ileorrhaphy IH-lee-OR-ah-fee **Definition** suture of the ileum	ileo / rrhaphy ileum / suture
ileostomy IH-lee-AW-stoh-mee **Definition** creation of an opening in the ileum	ileo / stom / y ileum / mouth / procedure
ileotomy IH-lee-AW-toh-mee **Definition** incision into the ileum	ileo / tomy ileum / cut
jejunorrhaphy JE-joo-NOR-ah-fee **Definition** suture of the jejunum	jejuno / rrhaphy jejunum / suture
jejunostomy JE-joo-NAW-stoh-mee **Definition** creation of an opening in the jejunum	jejuno / stom / y jejunum / mouth / procedure
jejunotomy JE-joo-NAW-toh-mee **Definition** incision into the jejunum	jejuno / tomy jejunum / cut
proctoplasty PROK-toh-PLAS-tee **Definition** surgical reconstruction of the anus and rectum	procto / plasty anus/rectum / reconstruction
rectopexy REK-toh-PEK-see **Definition** surgical fixation of the rectum	recto / pexy rectum / fixation

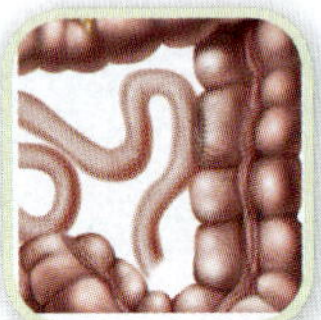
ileocolostomy

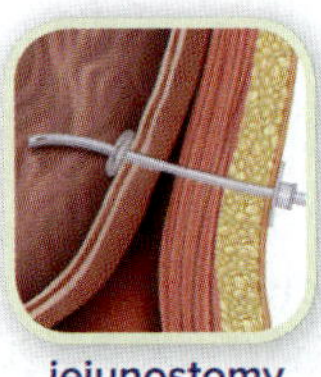
jejunostomy

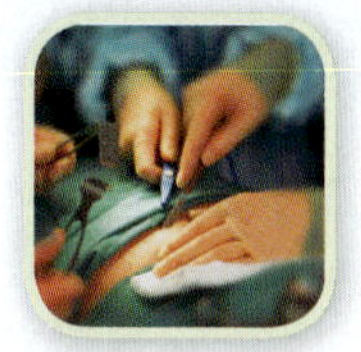
abdominocentesis

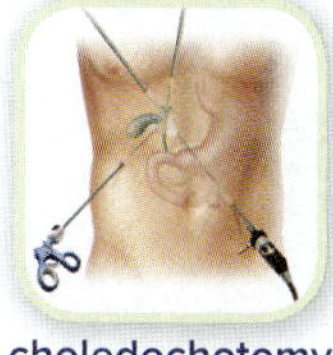
choledochotomy

supporting organs

Term	Word Analysis
abdominocentesis ab-DAW-min-oh-sin-TEE-sis **Definition** puncture of the abdomen (usually for the purpose of withdrawing fluid)	abdomino / centesis abdomen / puncture
abdominoplasty ab-DAW-min-oh-PLAS-tee **Definition** surgical reconstruction of the abdomen	abdomino / plasty abdomen / reconstruction
celiotomy SEE-lee-AW-toh-mee **Definition** incision into the abdomen	celio / tomy abdomen / cut
cholangiogastrostomy koh-LAN-jee-oh-gas-TRAWS-toh-mee **Definition** creation of an opening between the bile vessel (ducts) and the stomach	chol / angio / gastro / stom / y bile / vessel / stomach / mouth / procedure
cholecystectomy KOH-lay-sis-TEK-toh-me **Definition** surgical removal of the bile (gall) bladder	chole / cyst / ec / tomy bile / bladder / out / cut
choledochoenterostomy KOH-leh-DOH-koh-EN-ter-AW-stoh-mee **Definition** creation of an opening between (common) bile duct and the intestines	chole / docho / entero / stom / y bile / duct / intestine / mouth / procedure
choledocholithectomy KOH-leh-DOH-koh-lih-THEK-toh-mee **Definition** surgical removal of a stone from the (common) bile duct	chole / docho / lith / ec / tomy bile / duct / stone / out / cut
choledochotomy KOH-leh-doh-KAW-toh-mee **Definition** incision into the (common) bile duct	chole / docho / tomy bile / duct / cut
cholelithotomy KOH-lay-lih-THAW-toh-mee **Definition** incision to remove bile (gall) stones	chole / litho / tomy bile / stone / cut
cholelithotripsy KOH-lay-lih-THOH-trip-see **Definition** crushing of bile (gall) stones	chole / litho / trips / y bile / stone / rub / procedure
hepatectomy HEP-ah-TEK-toh-me **Definition** surgical removal of the liver	hepat / ec / tomy liver / out / cut
hepaticogastrostomy heh-PAT-ih-koh-gas-TRAW-stoh-me **Definition** creation of an opening between the liver and the stomach	hepatico / gastro / stom / y liver / stomach / mouth / procedure

supporting organs *continued*

Term	Word Analysis
hepaticotomy heh-PAT-ih-KAW-toh-me **Definition** incision into the liver	**hepatico / tomy** liver / cut
hepatopexy heh-PAT-oh-PEK-see **Definition** surgical fixation of the liver	**hepato / pexy** liver / fixation
laparoenterostomy LAP-ar-oh-EN-ter-AW-stoh-me **Definition** creation of an opening between the abdomen and the intestines	**laparo / entero / stom / y** abdomen / intestine / mouth / procedure
laparoscopic surgery LAP-ar-oh-SKAW-pik SIR-jir-ee **Definition** the use of a laparscope to perform minimally invasive surgery	**laparo / scop / ic surgery** abdomen / device to look / pertaining to
laparotomy LAP-ar-AW-toh-mee **Definition** incision into the abdomen	**laparo / tomy** abdomen / cut
pancreatectomy PAN-kree-ah-TEK-toh-mee **Definition** surgical removal of the panceas	**pancreat / ec / tomy** pancreas / out / cut
pancreatoduodenectomy PAN-kree-at-oh-DOO-aw-den-EK-toh-mee **Definition** surgical removal of the pancreas and duodenum	**pancreato / duoden / ec / tomy** pancreas / duodenum / out / cut
pancreatolithectomy PAN-kree-at-oh-lih-THECK-toh-mee **Definition** surgical removal of stones in the pancreas	**pancreato / lith / ec / tomy** pancreas / stone / out / cut
sialoadenectomy sai-AL-oh-AD-en-EK-toh-mee **Definition** surgical removal of a salivary gland	**sialo / aden / ec / tomy** saliva / gland / out / cut
sialolithotomy sai-AL-oh-lih-THAW-toh-mee **Definition** incision to remove salivary stones	**sialo / litho / tomy** saliva / stone / cut
stomatoplasty stoh-MAT-oh-PLAS-tee **Definition** surgical reconstruction of the mouth	**stomato / plasty** mouth / reconstruction

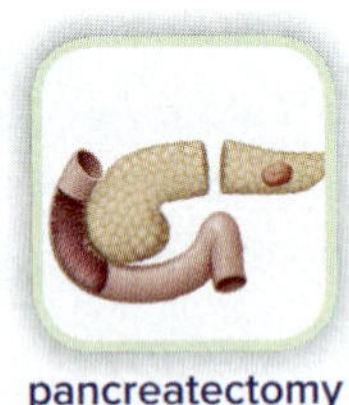
pancreatectomy

Learning Outcome 11.5 Exercises

PRONUNCIATION

EXERCISE 1 *Break down the following words into syllables.*

EXAMPLE: synesthesia *syn | es | the | sia*

1. gastroplasty ______
2. glossoplasty ______
3. anoplasty ______
4. gastropexy ______
5. rectopexy ______
6. antiemetic ______
7. ileostomy ______
8. hepatopexy ______
9. laparotomy ______
10. hepatectomy ______
11. jejunostomy ______
12. gingivoplasty ______
13. ileorrhaphy ______
14. anastomosis ______
15. duodenectomy ______
16. abdominoplasty ______
17. choledochotomy ______
18. cholelithotomy ______
19. cholelithotripsy ______
20. sialolithotomy ______
21. stomatoplasty ______
22. pancreatectomy ______
23. sialoadenectomy ______
24. laparoenterostomy ______
25. pancreatolithectomy ______

EXERCISE 2 *Indicate which syllable is emphasized when pronounced.*

EXAMPLE: bronchitis bron**chi**tis

1. antacid ______
2. cathartic ______
3. glossotomy ______
4. colectomy ______
5. colostomy ______
6. enterotomy ______
7. gastrectomy ______
8. odontectomy ______
9. enterectomy ______
10. glossorrhaphy ______
11. enterorrhaphy ______
12. herniorrhaphy ______

TRANSLATION

EXERCISE 3 *Break down the following words into their component parts.*

EXAMPLE: nasopharyngoscope *naso | pharyngo | scope*

1. hepatopexy ______
2. laparotomy ______
3. ileostomy ______
4. colostomy ______

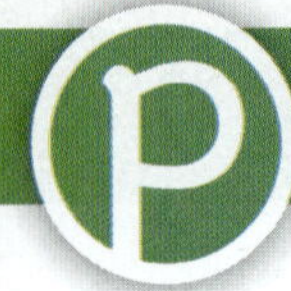

Learning Outcome 11.5 Exercises

5. gastropexy ______
6. jejunostomy ______
7. gingivoplasty ______
8. abdominoplasty ______
9. glossorrhaphy ______
10. herniorrhaphy ______
11. enterorrhaphy ______
12. hemorrhoidectomy ______
13. ileocolostomy ______
14. sialolithotomy ______
15. pancreatolithectomy ______
16. laparoenterostomy ______
17. gastroduodenostomy ______
18. gastroenterostomy ______
19. gastrojejunostomy ______
20. hepaticogastrostomy ______
21. choledochotomy ______
22. cholelithotripsy ______
23. anastomosis ______
24. cholangiogastrostomy ______
25. choledochoenterostomy ______

EXERCISE 4 *Underline and define the roots from this chapter in the following terms.*

1. glossoplasty ______
2. proctoplasty ______
3. stomatoplasty ______
4. gastroplasty ______
5. anoplasty ______
6. glossotomy ______
7. enterotomy ______
8. ileotomy ______
9. jejunotomy ______
10. celiotomy ______
11. hepaticotomy ______
12. cholelithotomy ______
13. ileorrhaphy ______

Learning Outcome 11.5 Exercises

14. jejunorrhaphy ______________________________
15. rectopexy ______________________________
16. esophagectomy ______________________________
17. gastrectomy ______________________________
18. gingivectomy ______________________________
19. odontectomy ______________________________
20. colectomy ______________________________
21. duodenectomy ______________________________
22. enterectomy ______________________________
23. hemicolectomy ______________________________
24. hepatectomy ______________________________
25. pancreatectomy ______________________________
26. sialoadenectomy ______________________________
27. abdominocentesis ______________________________
28. laparoscopic surgery ______________________________
29. esophagogastroplasty (2 roots) ______________________________
30. cholecystectomy (2 roots) ______________________________
31. choledocholithectomy (2 roots) ______________________________
32. pancreatoduodenectomy (2 roots) ______________________________

EXERCISE 5 *Match the term on the left with its definition on the right.*

	Term	Definition
____	1. antacid	a. agent that causes salivation
____	2. sialagogic	b. agent that neutralizes acid
____	3. antiemetic	c. agent that prevents/relieves nausea or vomiting
____	4. cathartic	d. agent that produces bowel movements

EXERCISE 6 *Translate the following terms as literally as possible.*

EXAMPLE: nasopharyngoscope *an instrument for looking at the nose and throat*

1. enterotomy ______________________________
2. jejunotomy ______________________________
3. laparotomy ______________________________
4. celiotomy ______________________________
5. esophagectomy ______________________________
6. herniorrhaphy ______________________________
7. glossorrhaphy ______________________________
8. enterorrhaphy ______________________________

Learning Outcome 11.5 Exercises

9. ileorrhaphy ______
10. jejunorrhaphy ______
11. gastropexy ______
12. duodenectomy ______
13. hemorrhoidectomy ______
14. abdominocentesis ______
15. laparoscopic surgery ______

EXERCISE 7 *Fill in the blanks.*

1. *colostomy* = creation of an opening in the ______
2. *ileostomy* = creation of an opening in the ______
3. *jejunostomy* = creation of an opening in the ______
4. *ileocolostomy* = creation of an opening between ______ and ______
5. *gastroduodenostomy* = creation of an opening between ______ and ______
6. *gastroenterostomy* = creation of an opening between ______ and ______
7. *gastrojejunostomy* = creation of an opening between ______ and ______
8. *hepaticogastrostomy* = creation of an opening between ______ and ______
9. *laparoenterostomy* = creation of an opening between ______ and ______
10. *cholangiogastrostomy* = creation of an opening between ______ and ______
11. *choledochoenterostomy* = creation of an opening between ______ and ______

GENERATION

EXERCISE 8 *Build a medical term from the information provided.*

EXAMPLE: inflammation of the sinuses *sinusitis*

1. surgical reconstruction of the stomach ______
2. surgical reconstruction of gum tissue ______
3. surgical reconstruction of the tongue ______
4. surgical reconstruction of the anus ______
5. surgical reconstruction of the abdomen ______
6. surgical reconstruction of the mouth ______
7. surgical reconstrution of the anus and rectum ______
8. surgical reconstruction of the esophagus and stomach ______
9. incision into the ileum ______
10. incision into the tongue ______
11. incision into the (common) bile duct ______

Learning Outcome 11.5 Exercises

12. surgical removal of the stomach ________________
13. surgical removal of the duodenum ________________
14. surgical fixation of the rectum ________________
15. surgical fixation of the liver ________________

EXERCISE 9 *Multiple-choice questions. Select the correct answer(s).*

1. Select all of the terms below that pertain to the upper GI tract.
   - a. cholecystectomy
   - b. choledocholithectomy
   - c. colectomy
   - d. duodenectomy
   - e. enterectomy
   - f. esophagectomy
   - g. gastrectomy
   - h. gingivectomy
   - i. hepatectomy
   - j. odontectomy
2. Select all of the terms below that pertain to the lower GI tract.
   - a. cholecystectomy
   - b. choledocholithectomy
   - c. colectomy
   - d. duodenectomy
   - e. enterectomy
   - f. esophagectomy
   - g. gastrectomy
   - h. gingivectomy
   - i. hepatectomy
   - j. odontectomy
3. Select all of the terms below that pertain to the supporting organs for the GI system.
   - a. cholecystectomy
   - b. choledocholithectomy
   - c. colectomy
   - d. duodenectomy
   - e. enterectomy
   - f. esophagectomy
   - g. gastrectomy
   - h. gingivectomy
   - i. hepatectomy
   - j. odontectomy

EXERCISE 10 *Briefly describe the difference between each pair of terms.*

1. gingivectomy, odontectomy ________________
2. colectomy, hemicolectomy ________________
3. hepatectomy, hepaticotomy ________________
4. pancreatectomy, pancreatolithectomy ________________
5. cholelithotomy, cholelithotripsy ________________
6. cholecystectomy, choledocholithectomy ________________
7. sialoadenectomy, sialolithotomy ________________
8. antacid, antiemetic ________________
9. cathartic, sialagogic ________________

11.6 Abbreviations

Abbreviations provide a shorthand way of referring to things that either recur often or are too long to write out. When dealing with the digestive system, these abbreviations can refer to regions of the abdomen (RLQ, LUQ), organs (GB), systems (N&V), diseases (PUD), and procedures (PEG, FOBT).

gastrointestinal system abbreviations

Abbreviations	Definition
BE	barium enema
BM	bowel movement
EGD	esophagogastroduodenoscopy
ERCP	endoscopic retrograde cholangiopancreatography
EUS	endoscopic ultrasound
FOBT	fecal occult blood test
GB	gallbladder
GERD	gastroesophageal reflux disease
GI	gastrointestinal
LFT	liver function test
NGT	nasogastric tube
NPO	nothing by mouth (nihil per os)
N&V	nausea and vomiting
PEG	percutaneous endoscopic gastrostomy
PEJ	percutaneous endoscopic jejunostomy
PUD	peptic ulcer disease
RLQ	right lower quadrant
RUQ	right upper quadrant
LLQ	left lower quadrant
LUQ	left upper quadrant
UGI	upper gastrointestinal

Learning Outcome 11.6 Exercises

EXERCISE 1 *Define the following abbreviations.*

1. GERD ____________
2. BM ____________
3. N&V ____________
4. BE ____________
5. FOBT ____________
6. NPO ____________
7. GB ____________
8. PUD ____________
9. EUS ____________
10. RUQ ____________
11. LFT ____________

EXERCISE 2 *Give the abbreviations for the following definitions.*

1. right lower quadrant ____________
2. left upper quadrant ____________
3. left lower quadrant ____________
4. nasogastric tube ____________
5. gastrointestinal ____________
6. esophagogastroduodenoscopy ____________
7. percutaneous endoscopic gastrostomy ____________
8. endoscopic retrograde cholangiopancreatography ____________
9. percutaneous endoscopic jejunostomy ____________
10. upper gastrointestinal ____________

EXERCISE 3 *Multiple-choice questions. Select the correct answer.*

1. The abbreviation *EUS* stands for *endoscopic ultrasound.* Which of the descriptions below is an accurate breakdown of the term *endoscopic*?
   a. *endo* (inside) + *scopic* (pertaining to looking)
   b. *endo* (outside) + *scopic* (pertaining to looking)
   c. *endo* (around) + *scopic* (pertaining to looking)
   d. *endo* (beneath) + *scopic* (pertaining to looking)
   e. *endo* (above) + *scopic* (pertaining to looking)

2. Which of the terms below pertains to the GB?
   a. cholangitis
   b. cholecystalgia
   c. choledochocele
   d. cholelithiasis
   e. cholemesis

Learning Outcome 11.6 Exercises

3. *PEJ* stands for *percutaneous endoscopic jejunostomy*. Which of the definitions below is correct for *jejunostomy*?
   a. creation of an opening in the jejunum
   b. incision into the jejunum
   c. narrowing of the jejunum
   d. removal of the jejunum
   e. suture of the jejunum

EXERCISE 4 *Match the abbreviation on the left with its full definition on the right.*

______	1. RLQ	a. tube inserted through the nose into the stomach
______	2. LUQ	b. disease in which acid comes up from the stomach and damages the esophagus
______	3. LLQ	c. nothing by mouth
______	4. RUQ	d. procedure for looking inside the esophagus, stomach, and duodenum
______	5. GERD	e. test of feces to discover blood not visibly apparent
______	6. FOBT	f.
______	7. NG	g.
______	8. EGD	h.
______	9. NPO	i.

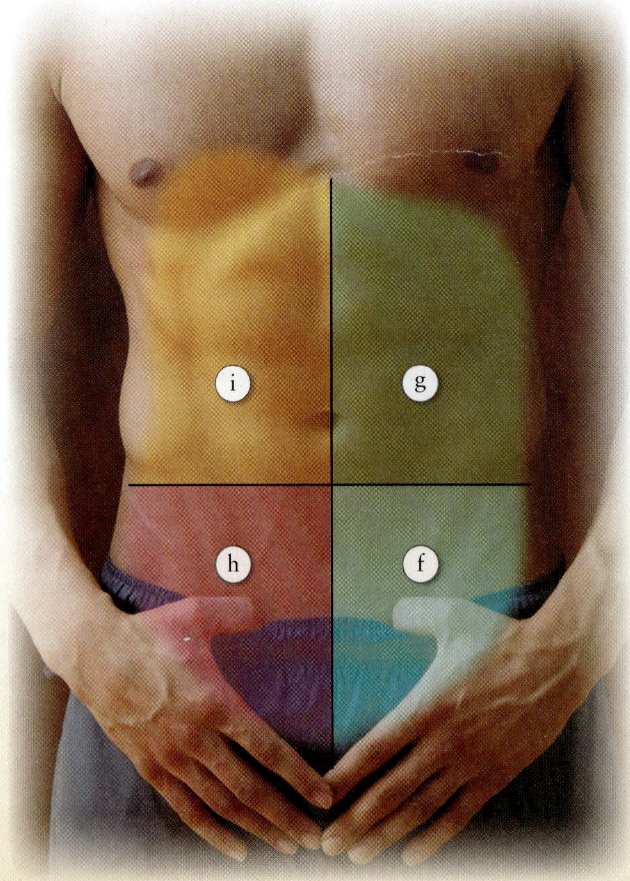

11.7 Electronic Health Records

Clinic Note

S Subjective

Mr. Robert Luno presents to our clinic with a 2-month history of intermittent post-prandial gastralgia and dyspepsia. It has become more and more frequent. He also reports occasional emesis as well, but denies hematemesis and cholemesis. He denies diarrhea and constipation.

O Objective

Temp: 98.6; HR: 64; RR: 16; BP: 120/80.
General: Overweight, middle-aged man in no apparent distress.
HEENT: PERRLA. No conjunctival injection.
No scleral icterus. Mucous membranes moist and pink. TMs normal.
CV: RRR without murmur.
Resp: CTA. Good air entry.
Abd: Soft, nontender, nondistended.
No HSM. Normative bowel sounds.

A Assessment

I suspect Mr. Luno is suffering from gastroesophageal reflux. Other possibilities include gastritis, cholelithiasis, and PUD.

P Plan

I will begin a trial of antacid therapy along with recommended dietary adjustments.
If he does not respond to treatment in 1 month, I will schedule him for an EGD.

–Constance Stiles, NP

Learning Outcome 11.7 Exercises

EXERCISE 1 *Match the term on the left with its definition on the right.*

______	1. constipation	a.	agent that neutralizes acid
______	2. antacid	b.	bad digestion
______	3. diarrhea	c.	difficulty passing feces
______	4. gastritis	d.	disease in which acid comes up from the stomach and damages the esophagus
______	5. dypepsia	e.	inflammation of the stomach
______	6. hematemesis	f.	passing of fluid or unformed feces
______	7. cholemesis	g.	procedure for looking inside the esophagus, stomach, and duodenum
______	8. emesis	h.	presence of a gallstone
______	9. cholelithiasis	i.	vomiting
______	10. gastroesophageal reflux	j.	vomiting bile
______	11. esophagogastroduodenoscopy	k.	vomiting blood

EXERCISE 2 *Fill in the blanks.*

1. Using the data recorded in the patient's clinic note, fill in the following blanks.
   a. The patient's temperature: ______________________________
   b. The patient's heart rate: ______________________________
   c. The patient's respiratory rate: ______________________________
   d. The patient's blood pressure: ______________________________
   e. Abd: No ______________________________ (hepatosplenomegaly)
2. Mr. Luno presents to the clinic with a 2-month history of intermittent *gastralgia* (give definition: ______________________________) and *dyspepsia* (give definition: ______________________________).
3. He occasionally vomits, but has not vomited ______________________________ (*hematemesis*) or vomited ______________________________ (*cholemesis*).

EXERCISE 3 *True or false questions. Indicate true answers with a T and false answers with an F.*

1. The medical professional suspects the patient has GERD. ________
2. The patient has stomach pain and poor digestion. ________
3. The patient has vomited both blood and bile. ________
4. The patient has difficulty passing feces. ________
5. The patient may have a gallstone. ________
6. The patient may have peptic ulcer disease. ________

Learning Outcome 11.7 Exercises

EXERCISE 4 *Multiple-choice questions. Select the correct answer.*

1. Which of the following symptoms did Mr. Luno report to the medical professional?
   a. cholemesis
   b. constipation
   c. diarrhea
   d. gastralgia
   e. hematemesis
2. Which of the following is NOT a possible diagnosis?
   a. cholelithiasis
   b. gastritis
   c. gastroesophageal reflux disease
   d. hepatosplenomegaly
   e. peptic ulcer disease
3. Which is the correct definition for the abbreviation *EGD*?
   a. epigastricduodenectomy
   b. epigastrodynia
   c. esophagogastroduodenoscopy
   d. esophagogastrodynia
   e. none of these

GI Consult

Subjective

Reason for Consult: Jaundice, RUQ pain.

History of Present Illness: Ms. Renata Mendel is a 22-year-old woman well known to the **gastroenterology** service. She was initially diagnosed with **ulcerative colitis** 2 years previously. She had presented to her primary care provider at the time with a history of recurring bloody stools and **constipation.** The symptoms progressed to include fatigue and purulent **rectal** discharge, and she was referred to our clinic.

Colonoscopy confirmed the diagnosis of ulcerative colitis. One year ago, she developed **toxic megacolon**, which eventually led to surgical intervention. She had been doing well until 3 months ago, when she started reporting fatigue, general pruritis, and pain in her **RUQ.** Her primary provider referred her again for evaluation. She reports some history of **steatorrhea,** but denies bright red blood.

Objective

Past Medical History: Ulcerative colitis. **Toxic megacolon.**
Past Surgical History: **Total colectomy with ilieorectal anastomosis.**
Family History: Mother with ulcerative colitis.
Medications: Daily vitamin.

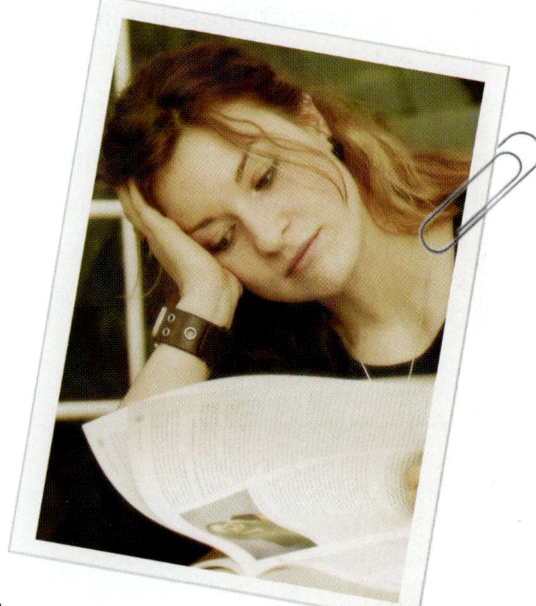

Physical Exam:
Temp: 98.6; Heart Rate: 76; Respiratory Rate: 22;
Blood Pressure: 108/72; Pulse Ox: 98%.

General: **Jaundiced, cachetic**-appearing young woman in no apparent distress. Alert and oriented x3.
HEENT: PERRLA. Scleral **icterus.** Moist mucous membranes. Normal dentition.

Neck: Supple. No LAD.
CV: RRR without murmur, gallop or rub.

Resp: CTA.
Abd: Soft, nontender, nondistended. **Hepatomegaly** two-finger breadths below ribs. No **splenomegaly.**
Ext: No cyanosis, clubbing, or edema. Capillary refill brisk.

Laboratory Data:
Significant for increased **LFTs, hypoalbuminemia,** and **hyperbilirubinemia.**

Assessment

Ms. Mendel's symptoms are concerning for primary sclerosing cholangitis. Other possibilities include hepatitis, cholelithiasis, and biliary obstruction.

Plan

Recommendation:
We need to perform an **endoscopic retrograde cholangiopancreatogram** (**ERCP**) or **magnetic resonance cholangiopancreatogram (MRCP).** Given the less invasive nature, I recommended Ms. Mendel have an MR cholangiogram, which is scheduled for later this week. If the results confirm primary sclerosing cholangitis, we will begin medical treatment and then schedule a **percutaneous hepatic biopsy.**

Thank you for your help with our mutual patient. I will keep your office up to date with further findings.

—Susan Marsden, MD

Learning Outcome 11.7 Exercises

EXERCISE 5 *Match the term on the left with its definition on the right.*

______	1. constipation	a.	creation of an opening; a surgical procedure connecting two previously unconnected hollow tubes
______	2. hepatitis	b.	difficulty passing feces
______	3. jaundice	c.	excessive fat discharged in the feces
______	4. colonoscopy	d.	inflammation and hardening of the bile vessels (ducts)
______	5. colitis	e.	inflammation of the colon
______	6. colectomy	f.	inflammation of the liver
______	7. cholangiogram	g.	procedure for looking at the colon
______	8. gastroenterology	h.	record of the bile vessels (ducts)
______	9. sclerosing cholangitis	i.	surgical removal of the colon
______	10. anastomosis	j.	presence of a gallstone
______	11. cholelithiasis	k.	study of the stomach and intestines
______	12. steatorrhea	l.	yellowing of skin, tissue, and fluids caused by increased levels of bilirubin in the blood

EXERCISE 6 *Fill in the blanks.*

1. Using the data recorded in the patient's GI consult note, fill in the following blanks.
   a. T: ______________________________
   b. HR: ______________________________
   c. RR: ______________________________
   d. BP: ______________________________
   e. CV: (give definition for abbreviation: ______________________________): RRR (give definition for abbreviation: ______________________________ and ______________________________)
   f. Abd: *hepatomegaly* (give definition: ______________________________), no ______________________________ (enlarged spleen)
2. The patient reports some history of ______________________________ (excessive fat discharged in the feces).
3. Past surgical history: Total *colectomy* (give definition: ______________________________) with *ileorectal anastomosis* (creation of an opening between the ______________________________ and ______________________________).
4. Ms. Mendel's symptoms are concerning for primary *sclerosing cholangitis* (give definition: ______________________________).
5. Other possible diagnoses include *hepatitis* (inflammation of the ______________________________), *cholelithiasis* (presence of ______________________________), and biliary obstruction.
6. Given the less invasive nature, Dr. Marsden recommends an MR *cholangiogram* (give definition: ______________________________).

Learning Outcome 11.7 Exercises

EXERCISE 7 *True or false questions. Indicate true answers with a T and false answers with an F.*

1. Ms. Mendel has an enlarged spleen and liver. ________
2. Ms. Mendel experienced pain in the lower left quadrant of her abdomen. ________
3. Ms. Mendel has too much bilirubin in her blood. ________
4. Ms. Mendel presented to her PCP with an Hx of hematemesis. ________
5. Ms. Mendel will undergo medical treatment and then will be scheduled for a biopsy of her liver. ________

EXERCISE 8 *Multiple-choice questions. Select the correct answer.*

1. Which of the following is NOT a possible diagnosis?
   a. enlarged liver and spleen
   b. inflammation and hardening of the bile vessels (ducts)
   c. inflammation of the liver
   d. the presence of a gallstone
   e. yellowing of skin, tissue, and fluids caused by increased levels of bilirubin in the blood

2. The conjunctivas of the eye are among the first tissues to change color as bilirubin levels rise. This is sometimes referred to as *scleral icterus.* The yellowing of skin, tissue, and fluids caused by increased levels of bilirubin in the blood is commonly known as
   a. cholangitis
   b. hepatitis
   c. icterus
   d. jaundice
   e. jejunitis

3. The patient developed *toxic megacolon.* Which of the following descriptions is a correct breakdown of the term?
   a. damaging (*toxic*) + enlarged (*mega-*) + colon (*colon*)
   b. damaging (*toxic*) + small (*mega-*) + colon (*colon*)
   c. harmless (*toxic*) + enlarged (*mega-*) + colon (*colon*)
   d. harmless (*toxic*) + small (*mega-*) + colon (*colon*)

4. The patient's laboratory data revealed *hypoalbuminemia.* Which of the following descriptions is a correct breakdown of the term?
   a. high (*hypo*) + albumin (*albumin*) + blood condition (*-emia*)
   b. high (*hypo*) + albumin (*albumin*) + urine condition (*-emia*)
   c. low (*hypo*) + albumin (*albumin*) + blood condition (*-emia*)
   d. low (*hypo*) + albumin (*albumin*) + urine condition (*-emia*)

5. The medical professional writing this GI consult recommends an ERCP or an MRCP. *MRCP* stands for *magnetic resonance cholangiopancreatogram.* Which of the following descriptions is a correct definition for *cholangiopancreatogram?*
   a. procedure for mapping the bile vessels (ducts) and pancreas
   b. record of the bile vessels (ducts) and pancreas
   c. procedure for mapping the gallbladder and pancreas
   d. record of the gallbladder and pancreas

Discharge Summary

Date of Admission: 4/13/2015
Date of Discharge: 4/16/2015

Admission Diagnosis

1. Acute abdominal pain
2. Pancreatitis

Discharge Diagnosis

1. Choledocholithiasis
2. S/p choledocholithectomy and cholecystectomy
3. Pancreatitis, resolved

Discharge Condition
Stable

Consultations
General surgery

Procedures

1. Laparoscopic choledocholithectomy and cholecystectomy

Labs
Admission labs: Elevated LFTs, hyperbilirubinemia, leukocytosis, elevated amylase and lipase.
Discharge labs: Everything had returned to normal levels.
Imaging
Ultrasound of the upper abdomen revealed cholelithiasis and choledocholithiasis with bile duct dilation.

HPI
Mrs. Roxana Collach presented to the ED with a 2-day history of increasing epigastric pain. She described the pain as constant and dull with radiation to her back. She also had progressive anorexia. She denied nausea, emesis, or diarrhea. She was febrile in the ED and had marked epigastric tenderness on exam with guarding. Her abdomen was slightly distended and she was mildly jaundiced. Her elevated amylase and lipase confirmed the suspicion of acute pancreatitis. She was admitted for pain control and IVF.

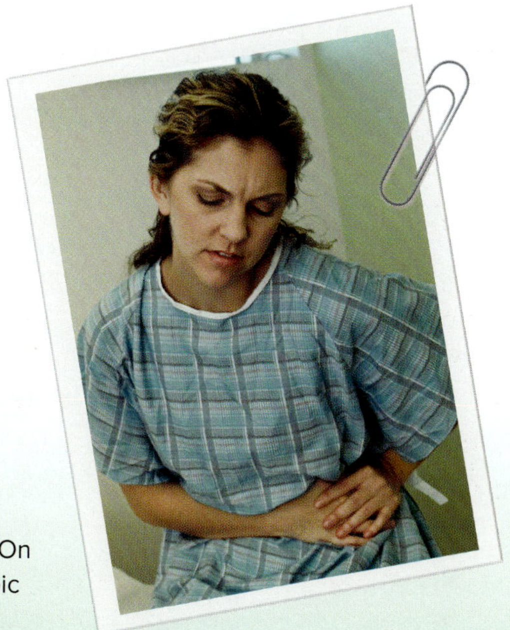

Hospital Course
Mrs. Collach was admitted to the medical service. She was placed on NPO status and given IVF and analgesics. An ultrasound revealed gallstones in the common bile duct as the etiology for Mrs. Collach's pancreatitis. Surgery was consulted. On hospital day 2, Mrs. Collach was taken to the OR for laparoscopic choledocholithectomy and cholecystectomy. She tolerated

Discharge Summary *(continued)*

the procedure well. She began a postoperative refeeding plan with a low-protein, low-fat diet. She tolerated advancing the diet, and 2 days after her surgery, her pain had improved enough that she was discharged home.

Discharge Physical Examination
Temp: 98.6; RR: 24; HR: 86; BP: 100/64.
Gen: WDWN. Alert.
CV: RRR.
Resp: CTA.
GI: Abdomen soft, nondistended, mild tenderness to palpation over the surgical incisions.
Three small horizontal surgical wounds in her abdomen. Wounds clean, dry, and intact.

Activity
No restrictions.

Diet
Low protein, low fat.

Meds
Analgesics prn.

Follow-Up Appointments
Primary care provider: Dr. Primo, 1 week.
Surgery: Dr. Sleiss, 1 month.

Learning Outcome 11.7 Exercises

EXERCISE 9 *Match the term on the left with its definition on the right.*

_____	1. diarrhea	a.	inflammation of the pancreas
_____	2. pancreatitis	b.	passing of fluid or unformed feces
_____	3. jaundice	c.	surgical removal of a stone from the (common) bile duct
_____	4. emesis	d.	surgical removal of the bile (gall) bladder
_____	5. laparascopic	e.	presence of a gallstone
_____	6. epigastric	f.	presence of a stone in the (common) bile duct
_____	7. cholecystectomy	g.	use of a laparoscope to perform minimally invasive surgery
_____	8. choledocholithectomy	h.	upper center portion of the abdomen
_____	9. choledocholithiasis	i.	vomiting
_____	10. cholelithiasis	j.	yellowing of skin, tissue, and fluids caused by increased levels of bilirubin in the blood

EXERCISE 10 *Fill in the blanks.*

1. Using the data recorded in Mrs. Collach's discharge summary, fill in the following blanks.
   a. ____________________ (the presence of a stone in the [common] bile duct).
   b. S/p *choledocholithectomy* (surgical removal of a(n) ____________________ from the ____________________) and *cholecystectomy* (surgical removal of the ____________________).
   c. ____________________ (inflammation of the pancreas), resolved.
2. Using the data recorded for the history of the present illness, fill in the following blanks.
   a. Mrs. Collach presented to the ED (give definition for abbreviation: ____________________) with a 2-day history of increasing *epigastric* (give definition: ____________________) pain.
   b. Mrs. Collach was admitted for pain control and IVF (give definition for abbreviation: ____________________).
3. Using the data recorded at Mrs. Collach's discharge physical examination, fill in the following blanks.
   a. Mrs. Collach's temperature: ____________________
   b. Mrs. Collach's heart rate: ____________________
   c. Mrs. Collach's respiratory rate: ____________________
   d. Mrs. Collach's blood pressure: ____________________

EXERCISE 11 *True or false questions. Indicate true answers with a T and false answers with an F.*

1. Mrs. Collach presented to the emergency department with nausea, vomiting, and diarrhea. _____
2. Mrs. Collach had a fever upon admission. _____
3. Mrs. Collach still has pancreatitis. _____
4. Mrs. Collach was admitted with enterodynia. _____
5. Mrs. Collach had a gallstone removed using a celiotomy. _____
6. As part of the hospital course, Mrs. Collach was given a regular diet of food and drink. _____

Learning Outcome 11.7 Exercises

EXERCISE 12 *Multiple-choice questions. Select the correct answer.*

1. Mrs. Collach's laboratory data revealed *hyperbilirubinemia*. Which is a correct breakdown of the term?
   a. high (*hyper*) + bilirubin (*bilirubin*) + blood condition (*-emia*)
   b. high (*hyper*) + bilirubin (*bilirubin*) + urine condition (*-emia*)
   c. low (*hyper*) + bilirubin (*bilirubin*) + blood condition (*-emia*)
   d. low (*hyper*) + bilirubin (*bilirubin*) + urine condition (*-emia*)
2. Which of the following is the correct definition for the term *laparoscopic choledocholithectomy*?
   a. surgical removal of a stone from the (common) bile duct with the use of a laparoscope to perform minimally invasive surgery
   b. surgical removal of the bile (gall) bladder with the use of a laparoscope to perform minimally invasive surgery
   c. surgical removal of a stone from the (common) bile duct with the use of a laparoscope to create a large incision in the abdomen
   d. surgical removal of the bile (gall) bladder with the use of a laparoscope to create a large incision in the abdomen
3. The abbreviation NPO means
   a. nihil per os
   b. nothing by mouth
   c. the patient shouldn't eat
   d. all of these

Quick Reference

quick reference glossary of roots

Root	Definition	Root	Definition
abdomin/o	abdomen	**hepatic/o**	liver
an/o	anus	**hepat/o**	liver
bil/i	bile (gall)	**ile/o**	ileum
celi/o	abdomen	**jejun/o**	jejunum
chol/e	bile (gall)	**lapar/o**	abdomen
col/o	colon (large intestine)	**lingu/o**	tongue
colon/o	colon (large intestine)	**odont/o**	tooth
cyst/o	bladder	**or/o**	mouth
dent/o	tooth	**pancreat/o**	pancreas
doch/o	duct	**peritone/o**	peritoneum
duoden/o	duodenum	**proct/o**	anus and rectum
enter/o	intestines	**rect/o**	rectum
esophag/o	esophagus	**sial/o**	saliva
gastr/o	stomach	**sigmoid/o**	sigmoid colon
gingiv/o	gums	**stomat/o**	mouth
gloss/o	tongue		

quick reference glossary of terms

Term	Definition
abdominocentesis	puncture of the abdomen (usually for the purpose of withdrawing fluid)
abdominoplasty	surgical reconstruction of the abdomen
aerodontalgia	tooth pain caused by exposure to air
anal fistula	abnormal opening between the rectum and the exterior perianal skin
anastomosis	creation of an opening; a surgical procedure connecting two previously unconnected hollow tubes
anophony	sound from the anus
anoplasty	surgical reconstruction of the anus
anosigmoidoscopy	procedure for looking at the anus and sigmoid colon
antacid	agent that neutralizes acid
antiemetic	agent that prevents/relieves nausea or vomiting
aphagia	inability to eat

quick reference glossary of terms *continued*

Term	Definition
ascites	retention of fluid in the peritoneum
bariatrics	branch of medicine dealing with weight issues
biligenesis	formation of bile
cathartic	agent that produces bowel movements
celiomyositis	inflammation of the abdominal muscle
celiopathy	disease of the abdomen
celiotomy	incision into the abdomen
cholangiogram	record of the bile vessels (ducts)
cholangiography	procedure for mapping the bile vessels (ducts)
cholangioma	tumor of the bile vessels (ducts)
cholangiopancreatography	procedure for mapping the bile vessels (ducts) and pancreas
cholangitis	inflammation of the bile vessels (ducts)
choleangiogastrostomy	creation of an opening between the bile vessel (ducts) and the stomach
cholecystalgia	pain in the gallbladder
cholecystectomy	surgical removal of the bile (gall) bladder
cholecystitis	inflammation of the bile (gall) bladder
cholecystogram	record of the bile (gall) bladder
choledochocele	hernia of the (common) bile duct
choledochoenterostomy	creation of an opening between (common) bile duct and the intestines
choledocholithectomy	surgical removal of a stone from the (common) bile duct
choledocholithiasis	presence of a stone in the (common) bile duct
choledochotomy	incision into the (common) bile duct
cholelith	gallstone; literally, a stone in the bile
cholelithiasis	presence of a gallstone
cholelithotomy	incision to remove bile (gall) stones
cholelithotripsy	crushing of bile (gall) stones
cholemesis	vomiting bile
cirrhosis	liver disease named for the change of color in the liver
colectomy	surgical removal of the colon
colitis	inflammation of the colon
colonoscopy	procedure for looking at the colon
colorectal carcinoma	cancerous tumor of the colon or rectum
colostomy	creation of an opening in the colon

quick reference glossary of terms *continued*

Term	Definition
colovaginal fistula	abnormal opening between the colon and vagina
constipation	difficulty passing feces
dentalgia	tooth pain
dentifrice	toothpaste
dentist	specialist in teeth
dentistry	branch of medicine dealing with teeth
diarrhea	passing of fluid or unformed feces
duodenectomy	surgical removal of the duodenum
duodenitis	inflammation of the duodenum
dysentery	another name for diarrhea
dyspepsia	bad digestion
endoscope	instrument used to look inside
endoscopy	procedure of looking inside
enterectomy	surgical removal of the intestines
enterocele	hernia of the intestines
enterodynia	pain in the intestines
enteropathy	disease of the intestines
enterorrhaphy	suture of the intestines
enterotomy	incision into the intestines
epigastric	upper center portion of the abdomen
esophagalgia	pain in the esophagus
esophageal carcinoma	cancerous tumor of the esophagus
esophagectomy	surgical removal of the esophagus
esophagitis	inflammation of the esophagus
esophagogastroduodenoscopy	procedure for looking inside the esophagus, stomach, and duodenum
esophagogastroplasty	surgical reconstruction of the esophagus and stomach
esophagoscopy	procedure for looking inside the esophagus
eupepsia	good digestion
fecal occult blood test (FOBT)	test of feces to discover blood not visibly apparent
fistula	any abnormal passageway in the body that shouldn't be there
flatus	medical term for passing gas
gastralgia	stomach pain
gastrectomy	surgical removal of the stomach

quick reference glossary of terms *continued*

Term	Definition
gastritis	inflammation of the stomach
gastroduodenostomy	creation of an opening between the stomach and the duodenum
gastrodynia	stomach pain
gastroenteritis	inflammation of the stomach and intestines
gastroenterocolitis	inflammation of the stomach, intestine, and colon
gastroenterologist	specialist in the stomach and intestines
gastroenterology	study of the stomach and intestines
gastroenterostomy	creation of an opening between the stomach and the intestines
gastroesophageal reflux disease (GERD)	disease in which acid comes up from the stomach and damages the esophagus
gastrojejunostomy	creation of an opening between the stomach and the jejunum
gastromalacia	softening of the stomach
gastroparesis	partial paralysis of the stomach
gastropexy	surgical fixation of the stomach
gastroplasty	surgical reconstruction of the stomach
gastroscope	instrument for looking at the stomach
gastroscopy	procedure for looking at the stomach
gingival hyperplasia	overformation of gum tissue
gingivalgia	gum pain
gingivectomy	surgical removal of gum tissue
gingivitis	inflammation of the gums
gingivoglossitis	inflammation of the gums and tongue
gingivoplasty	surgical reconstruction of gum tissue
gingivostomatitis	inflammation of the mouth and gums
glossopathy	disease of the tongue
glossoplasty	surgical reconstruction of the tongue
glossoplegia	paralysis of the tongue
glossorrhaphy	suture of the tongue
glossotomy	incision into the tongue
glossotrichia	overdevelopment of bumps on the tongue, making the tongue appear to be hairy
hematemesis	vomiting blood
hemicolectomy	surgical removal of half (a portion) of the colon
hemorrhoid	inflammation of the veins surrounding the anus

quick reference glossary of terms *continued*

Term	Definition
hemorrhoidectomy	surgical removal of hemorrhoids
hepatectomy	surgical removal of the liver
hepaticogastrostomy	creation of an opening between the liver and the stomach
hepaticotomy	incision into the liver
hepatitis	inflammation of the liver
hepatocarcinoma	cancerous tumor of the liver
hepatoma	tumor of the liver
hepatomalacia	softening of the liver
hepatomegaly	enlargement of the liver
hepatopexy	surgical fixation of the liver
hepatoptosis	downward displacement of the liver
hepatosclerosis	hardening of the liver
hernia	rupture or protrusion of an organ through the wall that normally contains it
herniorrhaphy	suture of a hernia
hyperemesis	excessive vomiting
hypochondriac	upper side portions of the abdomen
hypogastric	lower center portion of the abdomen
icterus	another name for jaundice
ileitis	inflammation of the ileum
ileocolitis	inflammation of the ileum and colon
ileocolostomy	creation of an opening between the ileum and colon
ileorrhaphy	suture of the ileum
ileostomy	creation of an opening in the ileum
ileotomy	incision into the ileum
inguinal	lower side portions of the abdomen
jaundice (icterus)	yellowing of skin, tissue, and fluids caused by increased levels of bilirubin in the blood
jejunitis	inflammation of the jejunum
jejunoileitis	inflammation of the jejunum and ileum
jejunorrhaphy	suture of the jejunum
jejunostomy	creation of an opening in the jejunum
jejunotomy	incision into the jejunum

quick reference glossary of terms *continued*

Term	Definition
laparocele	abdominal hernia
laparoenterostomy	creation of an opening between the abdomen and the intestines
laparoscope	instrument for looking inside the abdomen
laparoscopic surgery	use of a laparoscope to perform minimally invasive surgery
laparoscopy	procedure for looking inside the abdomen
laparotomy	incision into the abdomen
lumbar	middle side portions of the abdomen
nasogastric tube	tube inserted through the nose into the stomach
odontalgia	tooth pain
odontectomy	surgical removal of a tooth
odontoclasis	breaking of a tooth
odontodynia	tooth pain
orthodontics	branch of medicine dealing with the straightening of teeth
orthodontist	specialist in straightening teeth
pancreatectomy	surgical removal of the pancreas
pancreatitis	inflammation of the pancreas
pancreatoduodenectomy	surgical removal of the pancreas and duodenum
pancreatography	procedure for mapping the pancreas
pancreatolith	stone in the pancreas
pancreatolithectomy	surgical removal of stones in the pancreas
pancreatolithiasis	presence of a stone in the pancreas
periodontitis	inflammation of region around the teeth
peritoneoscopy	procedure for looking at the peritoneum
peritonitis	inflammation of the peritoneum
proctitis	inflammation of the anus and rectum
proctologist	specialist in the anus, rectum, and colon
proctology	branch of medicine dealing with the anus, rectum, and colon
proctoplasty	surgical reconstruction of the anus and rectum
proctoptosis	downward displacement of the rectum and anus
proctoscope	instrument for looking at the anus and rectum
proctoscopy	procedure for looking at the anus and rectum
pyloric stenosis	narrowing of the sphincter at the base of the stomach
rectalgia	rectum pain

quick reference glossary of terms *continued*

Term	Definition
rectitis	inflammation of the rectum
rectopexy	surgical fixation of the rectum
sclerosing cholangitis	inflammation and hardening of the bile vessels (ducts)
sialagogic	agent that causes salivation
sialoadenectomy	surgical removal of a salivary gland
sialoadenitis	inflammation of the salivary glands
sialoadenosis	condition of the salivary glands
sialoangiectasis	overexpansion of the salivary vessels
sialolith	stone in the saliva
sialolithiasis	presence of salivary stones
sialolithotomy	incision to removal salivary stones
sialorrhea	excessive salivation
sialostenosis	narrowing of the salivary glands
sigmoidoscope	instrument for looking at the sigmoid colon
sigmoidoscopy	procedure for looking at the sigmoid colon
steatorrhea	excessive fat discharged in the feces
stomatitis	inflammation of the mouth
stomatodynia	mouth pain
stomatogastric	pertaining to the mouth and stomach
stomatomycosis	fungus condition of the mouth
stomatoplasty	surgical reconstruction of the mouth
stomatosis	mouth condition
umbilical	middle center portion of the abdomen

review of terms by roots

Root	Term(s)	
abdomin/o	abdominocentesis abdominoplasty	
an/o	anal fistula anophony	anoplasty anosigmoidoscopy
bil/i	biligenesis	
celi/o	celiomyositis celiopathy	celiotomy

review of terms by roots *continued*

Root	Term(s)	
chol/e	cholangiogram	choledochoenterostomy
	cholangiography	choledocholithectomy
	cholangioma	choledocholithiasis
	cholangiopancreatography	choledochotomy
	cholangitis	cholelith
	choleangiogastrostomy	cholelithiasis
	cholecystalgia	cholelithotomy
	cholecystectomy	cholelithotripsy
	cholecystitis	cholemesis
	cholecystogram	sclerosing cholangitis
	choledochocele	
col/o, colon/o	colectomy	colovaginal fistula
	colitis	gastroenterocolitis
	colonoscopy	hemicolectomy
	colorectal carcinoma	ileocolitis
	colostomy	ileocolostomy
cyst/o	cholecystalgia	cholecystitis
	cholecystectomy	cholecystogram
dent/o	dentalgia	dentist
	dentifrice	dentistry
doch/o	choledochocele	choledocholithiasis
	choledochoenterostomy	choledochotomy
	choledocholithectomy	
duoden/o	duodenectomy	gastroduodenostomy
	duodenitis	pancreatoduodenectomy
	esophagogastroduodenoscopy	
enter/o	choledochoenterostomy	enterotomy
	dysentery	gastroenteritis
	enterectomy	gastroenterocolitis
	enterocele	gastroenterologist
	enterodynia	gastroenterology
	enteropathy	gastroenterostomy
	enterorrhaphy	laparoenterostomy

review of terms by roots *continued*

Root	Term(s)	
esophag/o	esophagalgia	esophagogastroplasty
	esophageal carcinoma	esophagogastroduodenoscopy
	esophagectomy	esophagoscopy
	esophagitis	gastroesophageal reflux disease (GERD)
gastr/o	cholangiogastrostomy	gastroenterostomy
	epigastric	gastroesophageal reflux disease (GERD)
	esophagogastroduodenoscopy	gastrojejunostomy
	esophagogastroplasty	gastromalacia
	gastralgia	gastroparesis
	gastrectomy	gastropexy
	gastritis	gastroplasty
	gastroduodenostomy	gastroscope
	gastrodynia	gastroscopy
	gastroenteritis	hepaticogastrostomy
	gastroenterocolitis	hypogastric
	gastroenterologist	nasogastric tube
	gastroenterology	stomatogastric
gingiv/o	gingival hyperplasia	gingivoglossitis
	gingivalgia	gingivoplasty
	gingivectomy	gingivostomatitis
	gingivitis	
gloss/o	gingivoglossitis	glossorrhaphy
	glossopathy	glossotomy
	glossoplasty	glossotrichia
	glossoplegia	
hepat/o	hepatectomy	hepatomalacia
	hepaticogastrostomy	hepatomegaly
	hepaticotomy	hepatopexy
	hepatitis	hepatoptosis
	hepatocarcinoma	hepatosclerosis
	hepatoma	

review of terms by roots *continued*

Root	Term(s)	
ile/o	ileitis	ileostomy
	ileocolitis	ileotomy
	ileocolostomy	jejunoileitis
	ileorrhaphy	
jejun/o	gastrojejunostomy	jejunorrhaphy
	jejunitis	jejunostomy
	jejunoileitis	jejunotomy
lapar/o	laparocele	laparoscopic surgery
	laparoenterostomy	laparoscopy
	laparoscope	laparotomy
odont/o	aerodontalgia	odontodynia
	odontalgia	orthodontics
	odontectomy	orthodontist
	odontoclasis	periodontitis
pancreat/o	cholangiopancreatography	pancreatography
	pancreatectomy	pancreatolith
	pancreatitis	pancreatolithectomy
	pancreatoduodenectomy	pancreatolithiasis
peritone/o	peritoneoscopy	
	peritonitis	
proct/o	proctitis	proctoptosis
	proctologist	proctoscope
	proctology	proctoscopy
	proctoplasty	
rect/o	colorectal carcinoma	rectitis
	rectalgia	rectopexy
sial/o	sialagogic	sialolith
	sialoadenectomy	sialolithiasis
	sialoadenitis	sialolithotomy
	sialoadenosis	sialorrhea
	sialoangiectasis	sialostenosis
sigmoid/o	anosigmoidoscopy	sigmoidoscopy
	sigmoidoscope	

review of terms by roots *continued*

Root	Term(s)	
stomat/o	anastomosis	jejunostomy
	choledochoenterostomy	laparoenterostomy
	colostomy	stomatitis
	gastroduodenostomy	stomatodynia
	gastroenterostomy	stomatogastric
	gastrojejunostomy	stomatomycosis
	gingivostomatitis	stomatoplasty
	hepaticogastrostomy	stomatosis
	ileocolostomy	
	ileostomy	

other terms

antacid	flatus
antiemetic	hematemesis
aphagia	hemorrhoid
ascites	hemorrhoidectomy
bariatrics	hernia
cathartic	herniorrhaphy
cirrhosis	hyperemesis
constipation	hypochondriac
diarrhea	icterus
dyspepsia	inguinal
endoscope	jaundice (icterus)
endoscopy	lumbar
eupepsia	pyloric stenosis
fecal occult blood test (FOBT)	steatorrhea
fistula	umbilical

The Urinary and Male Reproductive Systems—Urology

12

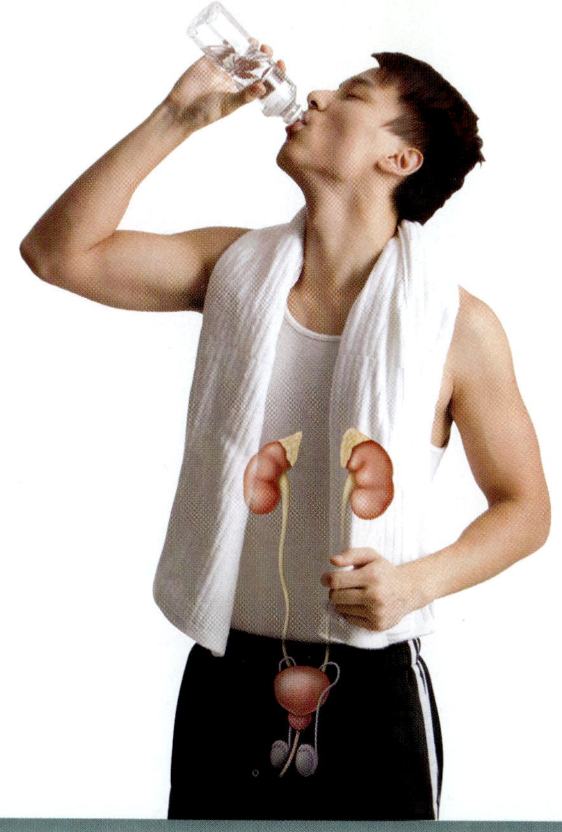

Introduction and Overview of the Urinary and Male Reproductive Systems

So far, we have addressed body systems that are identical in men and women. What separates the sexes, of course, is their reproductive systems. Both men and women produce half the blueprints for new life, which are found in *sperm* and *eggs*. The reproductive systems are responsible for making these code carriers and also for helping to bring the two together.

In medicine, the male and female reproductive systems are cared for by different specialties. The next two chapters deal with those specialties. This chapter deals

learning outcomes

Upon completion of this chapter, you will be able to:

12.1 Identify the **roots/word parts** associated with the **urinary system.**

12.2 Identify the **roots/word parts** associated with the **male reproductive system.**

S **12.3** Translate the **Subjective** terms associated with the **urinary and male reproductive systems.**

O **12.4** Translate the **Objective** terms associated with the **urinary and male reproductive systems.**

A **12.5** Translate the **Assessment** terms associated with the **urinary and male reproductive systems.**

P **12.6** Translate the **Plan** terms associated with the **urinary and male reproductive systems.**

12.7 Use **abbreviations** associated with the **urinary and male reproductive systems.**

12.8 Distinguish terms associated with the **urinary and male reproductive systems** in the context of **electronic health records.**

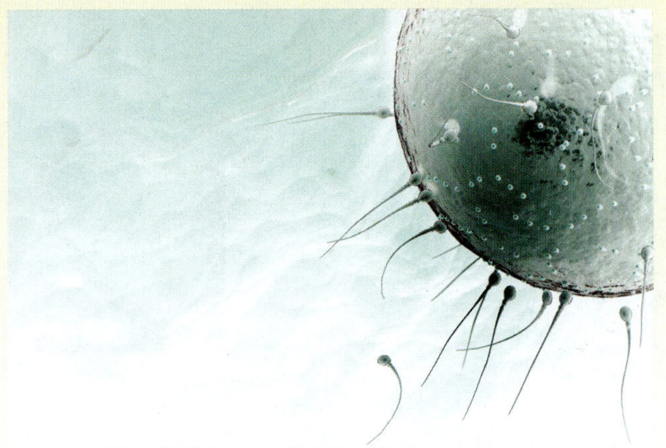

Sperm attempting to fertilize an egg.

with the specialty of *urology.* Since the male reproductive system shares structures with the urinary system, urology deals with both the urinary tract and the male reproductive system. The next chapter deals with the specialty of *obstetrics* and *gynecology,* which focuses specifically on the female reproductive system.

12.1 Word Parts of the Urinary System

Many homes and businesses have aquariums. People enjoy watching fish swim peacefully around in the water. In fact, some studies have shown that watching fish in an aquarium can lower a person's blood pressure.

While the fish are the main attraction, a great deal of hard work goes into keeping the water in their tank just right. The water must be cleaned and maintained with a balance of chemicals to keep a safe and clean environment for the fish to live in. Otherwise, the water becomes unsuitable for life.

The kidneys, the unsung heroes of the body, perform a similar function for the blood. The cells of the body are in constant contact with the blood, just like fish are always in contact with the water in an aquarium. Cells require just the right balance of pH, minerals, water, and sugar, and the kidneys monitor and regulate these levels. If they did not perform their job, blood would soon become toxic.

The basic working unit of the kidney is called the *nephron.* There are more than two million nephrons in a single kidney. Blood passes through the kidneys into a cluster of small blood vessels known as the *glomerulus.* Here, the blood is filtered, with water and nutrients being forced into the surrounding capsule around

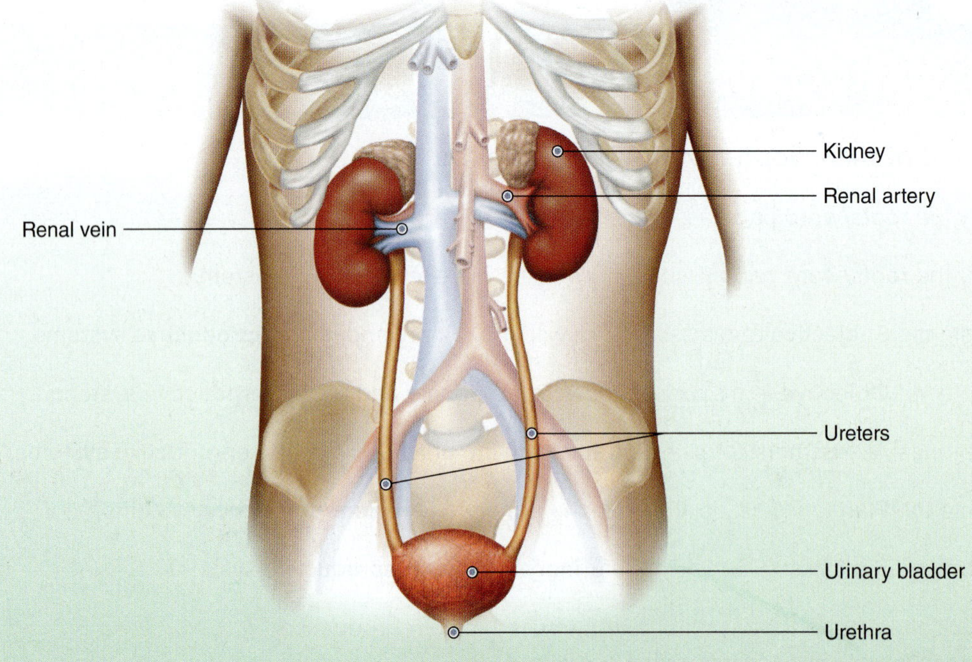

the glomerulus. This filtered liquid (filtrate) then flows through a series of small tubes.

These tubes flow next to blood vessels. As the filtrate passes through this series of tubes, much of the water and nutrients in it are reabsorbed back into the bloodstream. At the same time, the remaining unfiltered waste is forced into the last part of the tubes.

These tubes containing waste dump into a basin known as the *renal pelvis*. Long vessels from each kidney, called *ureters*, drain these collecting areas into the *bladder*, a large holding bag for urine. When the bladder becomes full, a signal is sent to the muscle that is holding the urine in the bladder. When this muscle relaxes, the urine empties out of the body through the *urethra*.

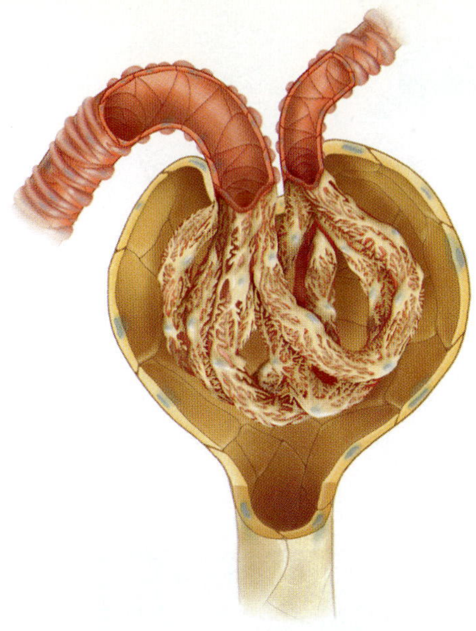

glomerulus (plural: glomeruli)

ROOT: ***glomerul/o***

EXAMPLES: glomerulopathy, glomerulonephritis

NOTES: *Glomerulus* comes from a Latin word meaning *little ball* and refers to the little balls of blood vessels inside the kidney. These serve as the primary place for filtering the blood to form urine.

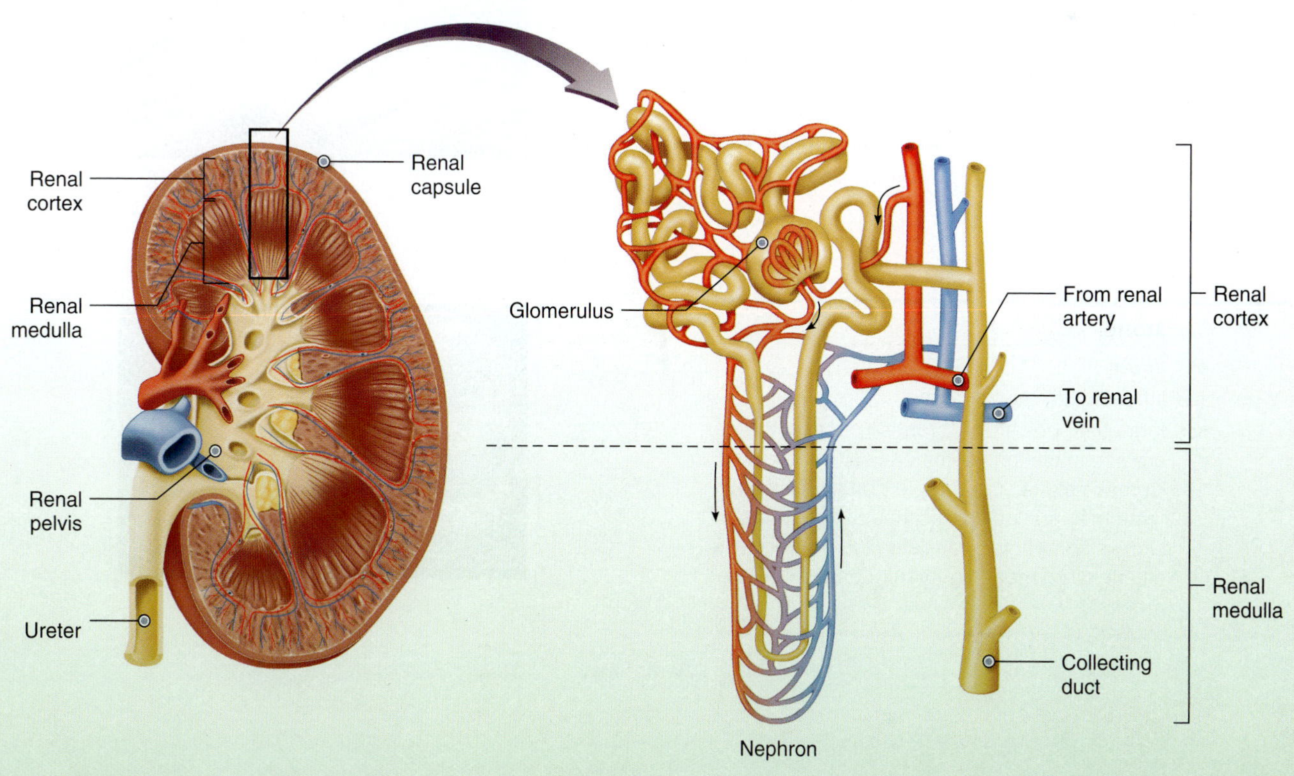

kidney

ROOTS: ***nephr/o, ren/o***

EXAMPLES: nephrology, nephritis, renal failure

NOTES: Kidneys perform the necessary task of filtering the blood—at a rate of 200 quarts per day. If you lose or donate a kidney, your remaining kidney can adjust and perform the work of two by increasing the amount it filters and by increasing in size. If you are born with only one kidney, your kidney may grow to be the size of two normal kidneys.

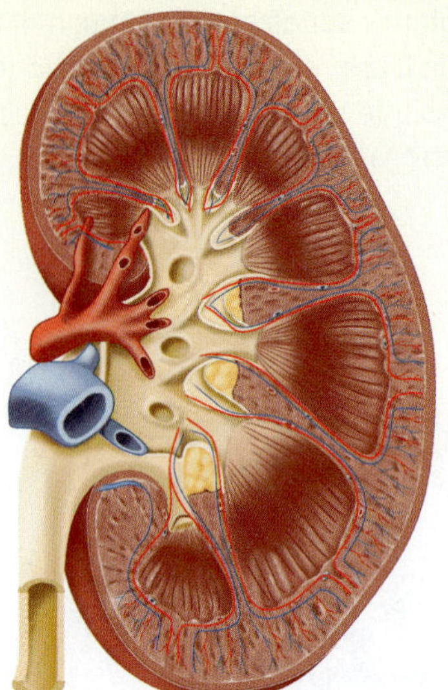

renal pelvis

ROOT: ***pyel/o***

EXAMPLES: pyelonephritis, pyelitis

NOTES: *Pyelo* is a root meaning *pelvis.* There are two things that the word *pelvis* can apply to: the *skeletal pelvis,* which is where your legs and your spine attach to one another; and the *renal pelvis,* which is a series of tubes that funnel urine out of the kidneys and into the ureters and on to the bladder. *Pyelo* is used most commonly for the renal pelvis.

urine

ROOTS: ***ur/o, urin/o***

EXAMPLES: urology, hematuria

NOTES: Healthy urine is completely sterile and contains ammonia molecules. This latter fact led the ancient Romans to use urine in two odd ways: to wash clothes (in fact, Romans set up large urinals outside laundries to gather urine free of charge) and to whiten teeth. It served both functions really well . . . but *gross.*

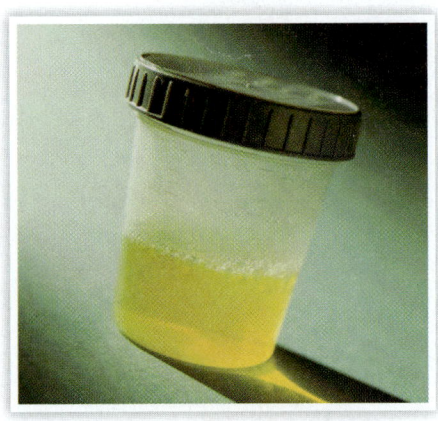

stone

ROOT: ***lith/o***

EXAMPLES: lithiasis, lithotripsy

NOTES: Kidney stones aren't "stones"; instead, they are accumulations of mineral salts and calcium. To make sure people don't mistakenly think they are little rocks, health care professionals sometimes translate *litho* as *calculus,* a Latin word meaning—you guessed it—*little rocks.*

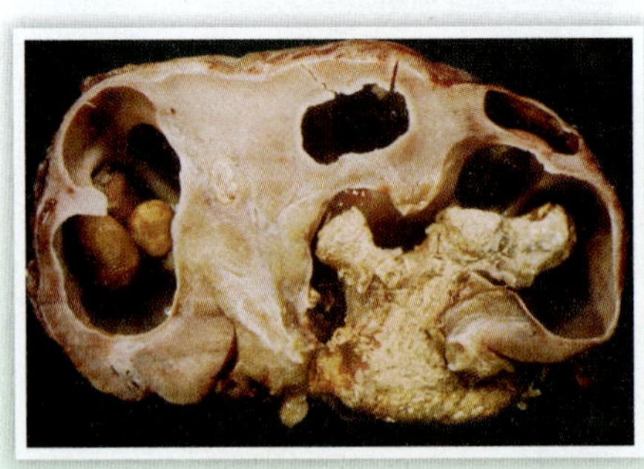

bladder

ROOTS: ***cyst/o, vesic/o***

EXAMPLES: cystotomy, cystitis, vesiculotomy, vesiculitis

NOTES: When completely full, the urinary bladder is roughly the size of a softball and can hold about 18 ounces of liquid. But it rarely reaches capacity. When the bladder is only about a quarter full, most people can't "hold it" anymore and feel an urgent need to urinate.

urethra

ROOT: ***urethr/o***

EXAMPLES: urethrostenosis, urethritis

NOTES: The length of the urethra differs depending on sex. The average male urethra is about 8 inches long, and the average female urethra is 1.5 to 2 inches long. This difference is sometimes mentioned as the reason why kidney stones are more painful for men than women; in fact, some say that the pain of kidney stones is the closest men can come to the pain of giving birth. Others argue that men are just big babies. You be the judge.

ureter

ROOT: ***ureter/o***

EXAMPLES: ureterocele, ureterectomy

NOTES: *Ureters* are the thick-walled tubes about 10 inches in length that carry urine from the kidneys to the bladder. Don't confuse ureters with the *urethra,* a tube that runs from the bladder to the outside world. You have two ureters, but only one urethra.

opening

ROOT: ***meat/o***

EXAMPLES: meatoscope, meatal stenosis

NOTES: *Meatus* comes from a word meaning *to go through;* it means *opening.* The English word *permeate* comes from the same term. There are meatuses in several places in body: nasal meatuses, aural meatuses, and a urethral meatus.

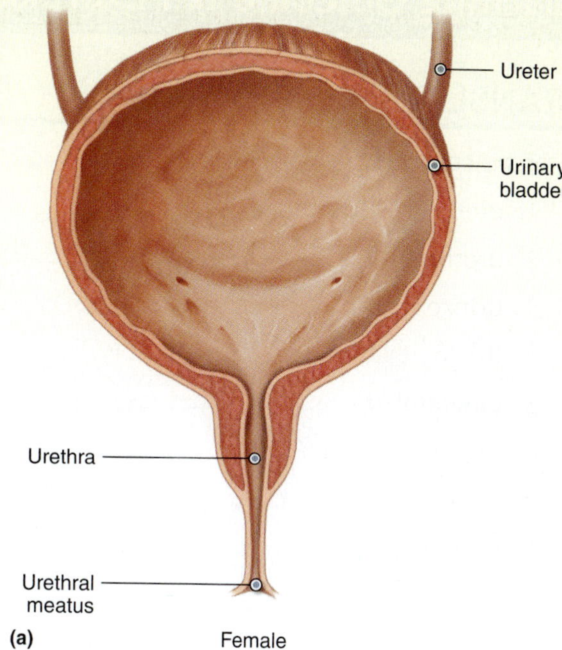

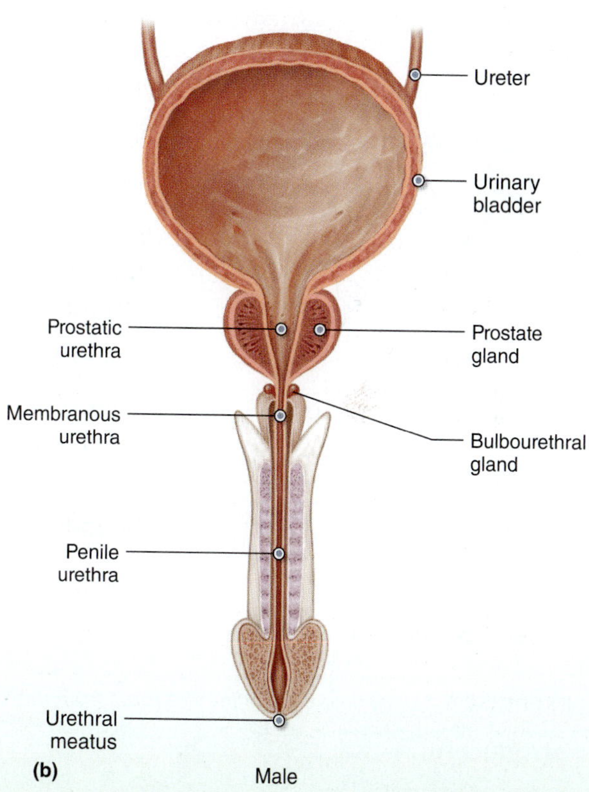

Learning Outcome 12.1 Exercises

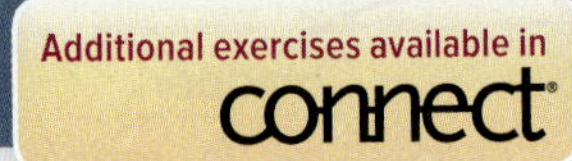

TRANSLATION

EXERCISE 1 *Translate the following roots.*

1. ureter/o ______
2. urethr/o ______
3. urin/o ______
4. lith/o ______
5. glomerul/o ______
6. nephr/o ______
7. ur/o ______
8. cyst/o ______
9. vesic/o ______
10. ren/o ______
11. pyel/o ______
12. meat/o ______

EXERCISE 2 *Match the root on the left with its definition on the right. Some definitions will be used more than once.*

____ 1. cyst/o
____ 2. vesic/o
____ 3. ur/o
____ 4. pyel/o
____ 5. glomerul/o
____ 6. ren/o
____ 7. ureter/o
____ 8. meat/o

a. bladder
b. comes from a word meaning *to go through*
c. from Latin, for *little ball;* refers to little balls of blood vessels inside the kidney that serve as the primary place for filtering the blood to form urine
d. organ that filters the blood
e. series of tubes that funnel urine out of the kidneys and into the ureter and on to the bladder
f. thick-walled tubes about 10 inches in length that carry urine from the kidneys to the bladder
g. urine

EXERCISE 3 *Underline and define the roots from this chapter in the following terms.*

1. glucosuria ______
2. cystodynia ______
3. ureterocele ______
4. urethroscopy ______
5. renal angiogram ______
6. pyelogram ______
7. vesicocele ______
8. meatal stenosis ______
9. uroxanthin ______
10. glomerulosclerosis ______
11. laparonephrectomy ______
12. cystolithectomy (2 roots) ______
13. nephroureterectomy (2 roots) ______

Learning Outcome 12.1 Exercises

EXERCISE 4 *Fill in the blanks.*

1. *ureteralgia:* pain in the ______
2. *urethroplasty:* surgical reconstruction of the ______
3. *nephralgia:* pain in the ______
4. *lithectomy:* removal of a(n) ______
5. *glomerulopathy:* disease of the ______
6. *cystalgia:* pain in the ______
7. *uropathy:* disease of the ______
8. *meatoscope:* device for examining the ______ of the urethra
9. *pyeloplasty:* surgical reconstruction of the ______
10. *renal ischemia:* deficiency of blood in the ______

EXERCISE 5 *Break down the following words into their component parts and translate.*

EXAMPLE: sinusitis *sinus | itis* *inflammation of the sinuses*

1. urologist ______
2. ureteroplasty ______
3. urethrectomy ______
4. cystostomy ______
5. nephrologist ______
6. renal failure ______
7. pyeloplasty ______
8. vesicotomy ______
9. meatotomy ______
10. nephrolithotomy ______

Learning Outcome 12.1 Exercises

GENERATION

EXERCISE 6 *Identify the roots for the following definitions.*

1. ureter ______
2. urethra ______
3. glomerulus ______
4. stone ______
5. opening ______
6. urine (2 roots) ______
7. bladder (2 roots) ______
8. kidney (2 roots) ______

EXERCISE 7 *Build a medical term from the information provided.*

EXAMPLE: inflammation of the sinuses *sinusitis*

1. inflammation of the bladder (use *cyst/o*) ______
2. inflammation of the kidney (use *nephr/o*) ______
3. inflammation of the urethra ______
4. inflammation of the ureter ______
5. inflammation of the renal pelvis ______
6. inflammation of a stone in the kidney (use *nephr/o*) ______
7. inflammation of the glomerulus and kidney (use *nephr/o*) ______
8. inflammation of the renal pelvis and bladder (use *cyst/o*) ______
9. inflammation of the urethra and bladder (use *cyst/o*) ______
10. inflammation of the bladder and ureter (use *cyst/o*) ______
11. inflammation of the ureter and renal pelvis ______
12. stone in the bladder (use *cyst/o)* ______
13. surgical reconstruction of the opening (of the urethra) ______

12.2 Word Parts of the Male Reproductive System

The male reproductive system shares structures with the urinary system. For this reason, *urologists* deal with both urinary tract problems and male genital problems. The male reproductive system is made up of the *testicles,* the *epididymis,* the *seminiferous tubules,* the *prostate gland,* and the *penis.*

The structures of the male genital system can be divided by their function into three categories: those that make and store *sperm,* those that make special carrier fluid for sperm, and the outer parts. The first category makes and stores sperm. Each sperm carries half of the blueprint for a human life (23 chromosomes). The organ that makes these blueprint carriers is called a *gonad.* The male gonads are testicles and the female gonads are the *ovaries.*

In addition to making sperm, the testicles also produce *testosterone,* the male hormone that causes male character traits like muscle growth and facial hair. While sperm cells are made in the testicles, they are stored in the *epididymis.* During sexual intercourse, the sperm cells travel out of the epididymis via ducts called the *vas deferens.* Sperm cells mix with a carrier fluid known as *semen.*

The majority of this fluid is made in the *seminal vesicles* and the prostate gland. At climax, the semen is ejected out of the body *(ejaculation)* through the penis.

The third category of structures is the visible parts of the male reproductive system: the penis and the *scrotum.* These are also known as the male *genitals.* The penis is the organ for directing urine and sperm outside the body, and the scrotum is the external sac that holds the testicles in place outside the body.

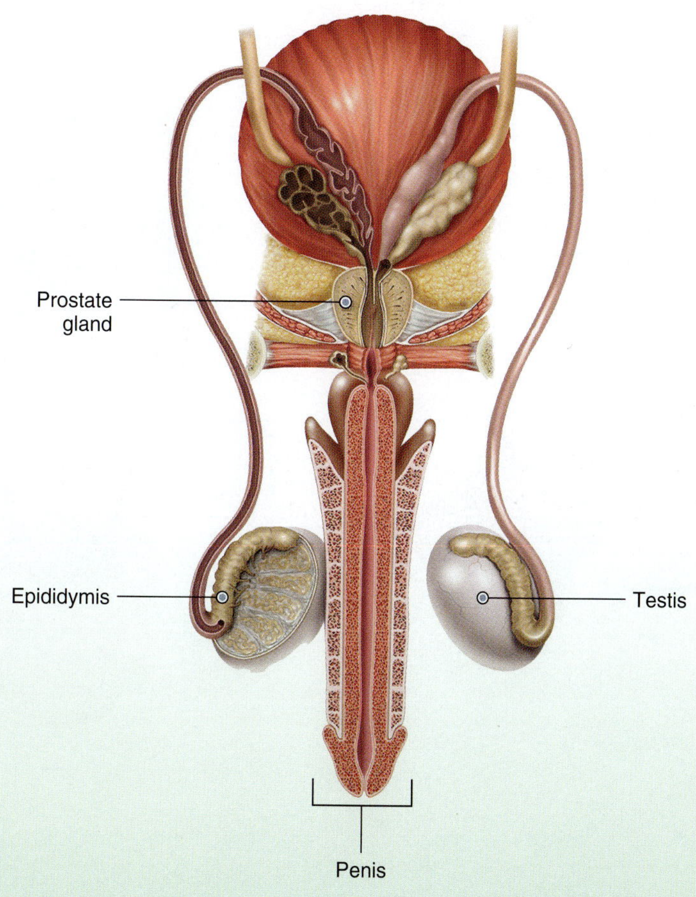

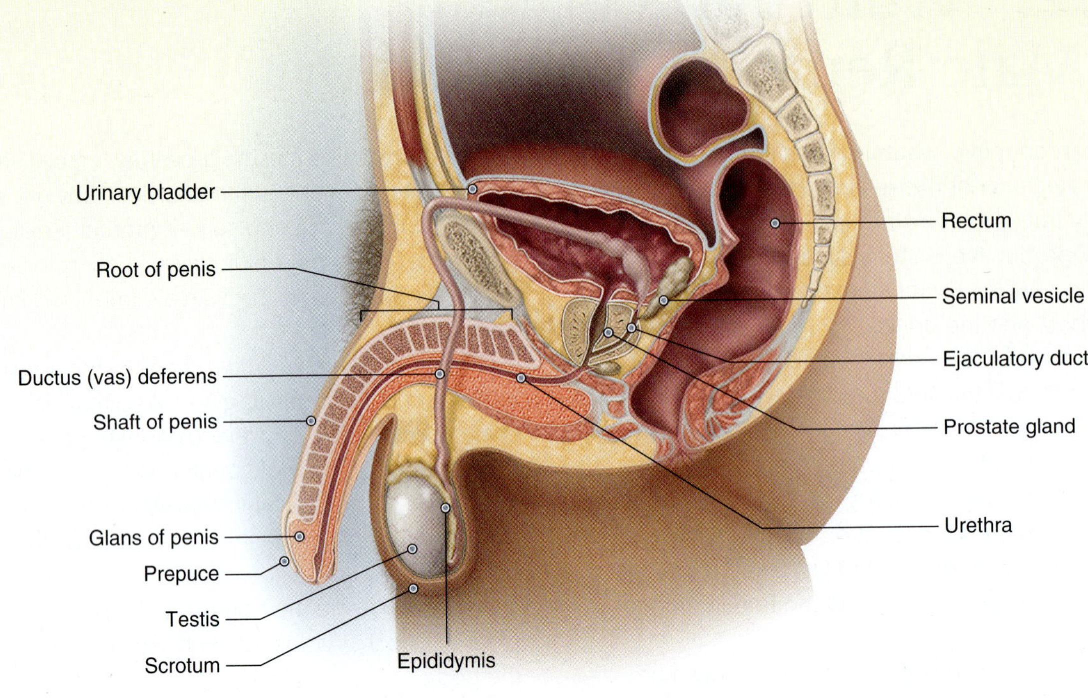

penis

ROOT: ***balan/o***

EXAMPLES: balanorrhea, balanitis

NOTES: The root *balano* comes from a Greek word meaning *acorn;* this is an allusion to the shape of the tip of the penis. It was also the word the Greeks used to refer to a deadbolt lock on a door.

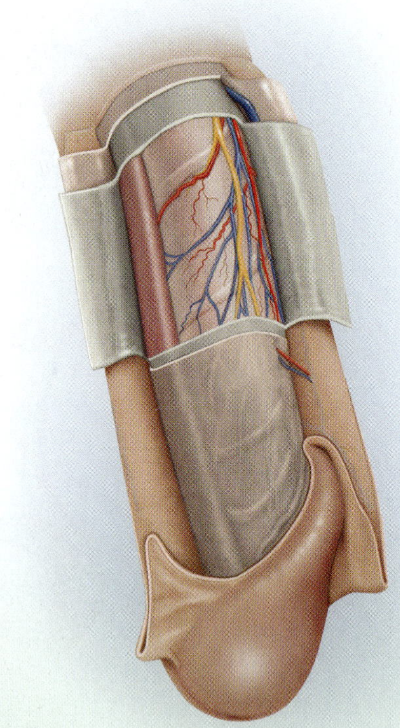

epididymis

ROOT: ***epididym/o***

EXAMPLES: epididymotomy, epididymectomy

NOTES: The *epididymis,* an oblong organ that sits on top of each testicle, is the place where sperm cells complete their final level of development and are stored. Interestingly, the root *didymis* means *twins,* so the name of this organ is literally *upon the twins.*

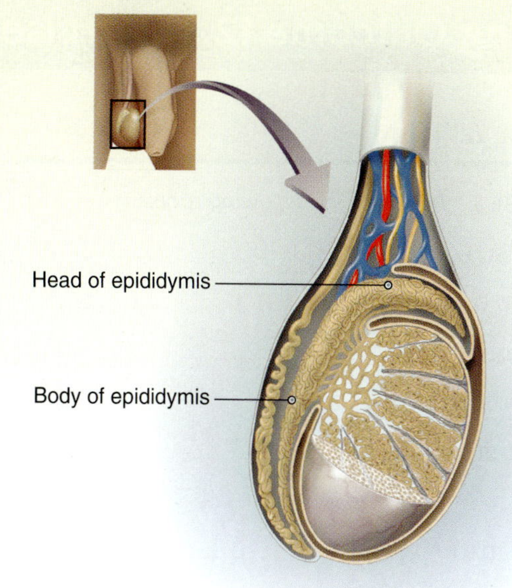

testicle

ROOTS: ***orch/o, orchi/o, orchid/o, test/o***

EXAMPLES: orchitis, orchiopexy, anorchidism, testitis

NOTES: You likely noticed right away that one of the main roots for *testicle* is similar to the word *orchid.* Believe or not, the flower is named for the organ, and not the other way around. The plant was called an *orchid* because some believed that its roots looked like a pair of testicles.

prostate

ROOT: ***prostat/o***

EXAMPLES: prostatitis, prostatomegaly

NOTES: The *prostate* is an organ in the male reproductive tract that surrounds the urethra. The name *prostate* breaks down into *pro (before)* and *state (stand)* and literally translates to mean *the one that stands before or in front of.* It was so named because of its position in front of the urinary bladder.

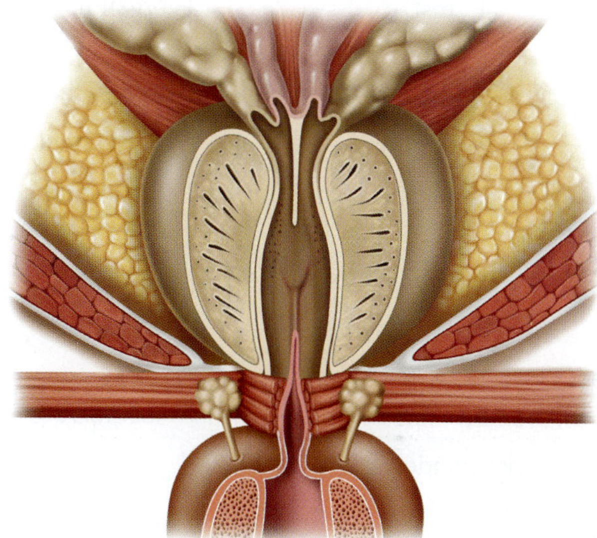

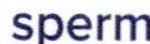

sperm

ROOTS: ***sperm/o, spermat/o, sperm/i***

EXAMPLES: aspermia, spermicide, spermatocele

NOTES: *Sperm* (from Greek, for *seed*) is produced in the testicles. It takes roughly 10 weeks to produce a single sperm. Sperm can sit in the epididymis for as long as 2 weeks before being ejaculated. These sperm can survive in the female reproductive tract for as long as 5 days. Because the male's sperm determines the sex of a baby, sperm can be either male or female. Male sperm are faster swimmers, but weaker. Female sperm are slower, but stronger.

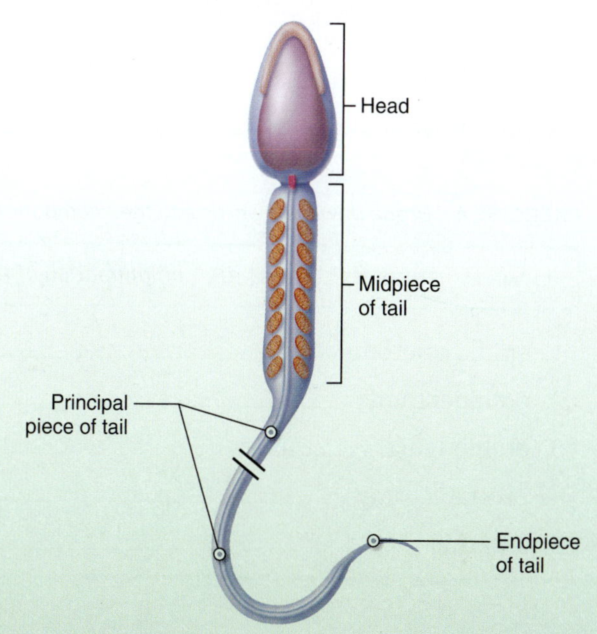

Learning Outcome 12.2 Exercises

TRANSLATION

EXERCISE 1 *Translate the following roots.*

1. prostat/o ____________________
2. test/o ____________________
3. spermat/o ____________________
4. epididym/o ____________________
5. orchid/o ____________________
6. orch/o ____________________
7. balan/o ____________________

EXERCISE 2 *Match the root on the left with its definition on the right. Some definitions will be used more than once.*

e	1. test/o	a. organ in the male reproductive tract surrounding the urethra; the name literally translates into *the one that stands before or in front of*
a	2. prostat/o	b. from Greek, for *acorn,* an allusion to the shape of its tip
c	3. sperm/o	c. from Greek, for *seed;* produced in the testicles
b	4. balan/o	d. organ that sits on top of each testicle; the place where sperm cells complete their final level of development and are stored
e	5. orchi/o	e. testicle
d	6. epididym/o	

EXERCISE 3 *Underline and define the roots from this chapter in the following terms.*

1. spermicide ____________________
2. testicular carcinoma ____________________
3. epididymectomy ____________________
4. balanorrhea ____________________
5. anorchidism ____________________
6. prostatovesiculectomy (2 roots) ____________________

EXERCISE 4 *Break down the words into their component parts and translate.*

EXAMPLE: sinusitis *sinus | itis* *inflammation of the sinuses*

1. epididymotomy ____________________
2. orchidectomy ____________________
3. orchiodynia ____________________
4. prostatectomy ____________________
5. aspermia ____________________

Learning Outcome 12.2 Exercises

GENERATION

EXERCISE 5 *Identify the roots for the following definitions.*

1. prostate ______________________
2. epididymis ______________________
3. penis ______________________
4. sperm (2 roots) ______________________
5. testicle (4 roots) ______________________

EXERCISE 6 *Fill in the blanks.*

1. *testitis:* inflammation of the ______________________
2. *prostatorrhea:* discharge from the ______________________
3. *spermatogenesis:* creation of ______________________
4. *orchitis:* inflammation of the ______________________
5. *balanoplasty:* surgical reconstruction of the ______________________
6. *epididymo-orchitis:* inflammation of the ______________ and ______________

EXERCISE 7 *Build a medical term from the information provided.*

1. inflammation of the testicle (use *orchid/o*) ______________________
2. inflammation of a testicle (use *test/o*) ______________________
3. inflammation of the prostate ______________________
4. inflammation of the epididymis ______________________
5. inflammation of the penis ______________________
6. inflammation of the prostate and bladder (use *cyst/o*) ______________________
7. inflammation of the testicle (use *orch/o*) and epididymis ______________________

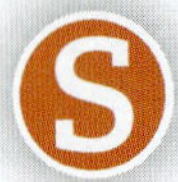

Subjective

Patient History, Problems, Complaints

Urinary Tract

Male Genitalia

Objective

Observation and Discovery

Urinary Tract

Diagnostic Procedures

Professional Terms

Male Genitalia

Diagnostic Procedures

Professional Terms

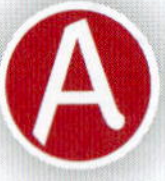

Assessment

Diagnosis and Pathology

Urinary Tract

Male Genitalia

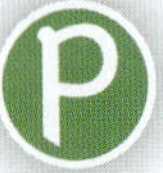

Plan

Treatments and Therapies

Urinary Tract

Male Genitalia

This section contains medical terms built from the roots presented in the previous section. The purpose of this section is to expose you to words used in urology that are built from the word roots presented earlier. The focus of this book is to teach you the process of learning roots and translating them in context. Each term is presented with the correct pronunciation, followed by a word analysis that breaks down the word into its component parts, a definition that provides a literal translation of the word, as well as supplemental information if the literal translation deviates from its medical use. The terms are organized using a health care professional's SOAP note (first introduced in Chapter 2) as a model.

SUBJECTIVE

12.3 Patient History, Problems, Complaints

Patients with urinary system problems frequently seek medical care with one of two types of problems: pain or problems with urinating. Pain is a very common symptom of infections of the urinary system.

Pain with urination *(dysuria)* is the most common symptom of an infection in the urinary tract. A simple urinary tract infection also may cause pain in the bladder *(cystalgia)*. If the infection spreads to the kidney(s), the patient may have kidney pain *(nephralgia)*. Severe kidney pain that comes in waves *(renal colic)* is a very good indicator of a kidney stone. The urethra is also a common source of pain *(urethralgia)* when infected or irritated by chemicals. Difficulty with urination may present with inability to hold urine in *(incontinence, enuresis)*. Patients may also urinate too frequently *(polyuria)* or not enough *(oliguria)*. Complete lack of urination *(anuria)* is a serious symptom that represents either a blockage or kidney failure. A patient's urine itself may be a concern, as he or she may notice blood *(hematuria)* or pus *(pyuria)* in the urine.

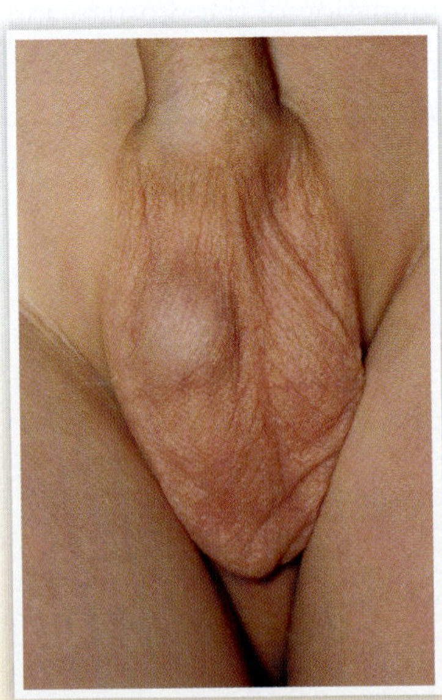

Though a patient might notice only one testicle, usually a medical exam is required to determine whether the missing testicle is not there *(anorchidism)* or is hidden *(cryptorchidism)*.

12.3 Patient History, Problems, Complaints

Male patients may have special genitourinary issues that are unique to them. When genital pain is a concern, the testicle (*orchialgia, orchiodynia*) is the most common site. Male patients may also have problems with erections. They can be painful and prolonged (*priapism*) or may not last long enough for sexual intercourse (*impotence*). Finally, a male patient may have concerns with penile discharge (*balanorrhea, urethrorrhea*). This is often an indicator of a sexually transmitted infection.

urinary tract

Term	Word Analysis
anuria an-YUR-ee-ah **Definition** lack of urination	an / ur / ia no / urine / condition
cystalgia sis-TAL-jah **Definition** pain in the bladder	cyst / algia bladder / pain
cystodynia SIS-toh-DAI-nee-ah **Definition** pain in the bladder	cysto / dynia bladder / pain
cystoplegia SIS-toh-PLEE-jah **Definition** bladder paralysis	cysto / plegia bladder / paralysis
dysuria dis-YUR-ee-ah **Definition** painful urination	dys / ur / ia bad / urine / condition
enuresis EN-yur-EE-sis **Definition** involuntary urination	from Greek, for *to urinate*
hematuria HEE-mah-TUR-ee-ah **Definition** bloody urination	hemat / ur / ia blood / urine / condition
incontinence in-CON-tih-nentz **Definition** inability to control urination	in / con / tinence not / together / hold
nephralgia neh-FRAL-jah **Definition** pain in the kidney	nephr / algia kidney / pain

12.3 Patient History, Problems, Complaints

urinary tract *continued*

Term	Word Analysis
nocturnal enuresis nok-TIR-nal EN-yur-EE-sis **Definition** nighttime involuntary urination	nocturnal enuresis nighttime involuntary urination
nocturia nok-TUR-ee-ah **Definition** nighttime urination	noct / ur / ia night / urine / condition
oliguria aw-lih-GYIR-ee-ah **Definition** low urine output	olig / ur / ia few / urine / condition
polydipsia PAW-lee-DIP-see-ah **Definition** excessive thirst	poly / dips / ia many / thirst / condition
polyuria PAW-lee-YUR-ee-ah **Definition** excessive urination	poly / ur / ia many / urine / condition
pyuria pai-YUR-ee-ah **Definition** pus in the urine	py / ur / ia pus / urine / condition
ureteralgia yur-EE-ter-AL-jah **Definition** pain in the ureter	ureter / algia ureter / pain
urethrodynia yoo-REE-throh-DAI-nee-ah **Definition** pain in the urethra	urethro / dynia urethra / pain
urethrorrhea yoo-REE-throh-REE-ah **Definition** discharge from the urethra	urethro / rrhea urethra / discharge
urocyanosis YUR-oh-SAI-ah-NOH-sis **Definition** blue urine	uro / cyan / osis urine / blue / condition
urodynia YUR-oh-DAI-nee-ah **Definition** painful urination	uro / dynia urine / pain

12.3 Patient History, Problems, Complaints

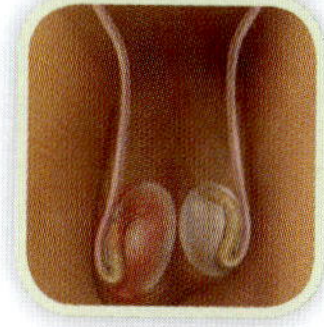
orchialgia

male genitalia

Term	Word Analysis
balanorrhea BAL-ah-noh-REE-ah **Definition** discharge from the penis	balano / rrhea penis / discharge
orchialgia OR-kee-AL-jah **Definition** testicle pain	orchi / algia testicle / pain
orchichorea OR-kee-kor-EE-ah **Definition** involuntary jerking movement of the testicles	orchi / chorea testicle / dance
orchidoptosis OR-kih-dop-TOH-sis **Definition** downward displacement of a testicle	orchido / pt / osis testicle / droop / condition
orchiodynia OR-kee-oh-DAI-nee-ah **Definition** testicle pain	orchio / dynia testicle / pain
priapism PREE-ap-izm **Definition** persistent and painful erection	from ancient Greek minor fertility god named Priapus, who is always shown with a large and permanently erect penis

S Learning Outcome 12.3 Exercises

PRONUNCIATION

EXERCISE 1 *Break down the following words into syllables.*

EXAMPLE: synesthesia *syn | es | the | sia*

1. polyuria ______
2. urodynia ______
3. pyuria ______
4. enuresis ______
5. orchialgia ______
6. ureteralgia ______
7. oliguria ______
8. orchiodynia ______

EXERCISE 2 *Indicate which syllable is emphasized when pronounced.*

EXAMPLE: bronchitis bron**chi**tis

1. incontinence ______
2. cystalgia ______
3. nephralgia ______
4. nocturia ______
5. dysuria ______
6. pyuria ______
7. oliguria ______
8. priapism ______

TRANSLATION

EXERCISE 3 *Break down the following words into their component parts.*

EXAMPLE: nasopharyngoscope *naso | pharyngo | scope*

1. anuria ______
2. dysuria ______
3. nocturia ______
4. cystodynia ______
5. orchiodynia ______
6. urocyanosis ______
7. incontinence ______

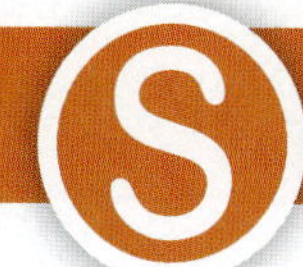

Learning Outcome 12.3 Exercises

EXERCISE 4 *Underline and define the root from this chapter in the following terms.*

1. cystoplegia ______________________
2. urethrorrhea ______________________
3. orchichorea ______________________
4. balanorrhea ______________________
5. ureteralgia ______________________
6. nephralgia ______________________
7. orchidoptosis ______________________
8. enuresis ______________________

EXERCISE 5 *Match the term on the left with its definition on the right.*

	Term	Definition
b	1. incontinence	a. bloody urination
a	2. hematuria	b. inability to control urination
g	3. pyuria	c. low urine output
d	4. nocturnal enuresis	d. nighttime involuntary urination
c	5. oliguria	e. pain in the bladder
e	6. cystodynia	f. persistent and painful erection
f	7. priapism	g. pus in the urine

EXERCISE 6 *Fill in the blanks.*

1. *cystalgia:* pain in the ______________________
2. *orchialgia:* pain in the ______________________
3. *urethrodynia:* pain in the ______________________
4. *urodynia:* pain in ______________________
5. *polydipsia:* excessive ______________________
6. *polyuria:* excessive ______________________

EXERCISE 7 *Translate the following terms as literally as possible.*

EXAMPLE: nasopharyngoscope *an instrument for looking at the nose and throat*

1. cystalgia ______________________
2. hematuria ______________________
3. oliguria ______________________
4. pyuria ______________________
5. urocyanosis ______________________
6. orchialgia ______________________
7. orchichorea ______________________

Learning Outcome 12.3 Exercises

GENERATION

EXERCISE 8 *Build a medical term from the information provided.*

EXAMPLE: inflammation of the sinuses *sinusitis*

1. pain in the ureter ______
2. discharge from the urethra ______
3. discharge from the penis ______
4. downward displacement of a testicle ______
5. bladder paralysis ______
6. pain in the kidney ______
7. nighttime urination ______

EXERCISE 9 *Briefly describe the difference between each pair of terms.*

1. urethrodynia, urodynia ______
2. anuria, dysuria ______
3. polydipsia, polyuria ______
4. enuresis, nocturnal enuresis ______
5. orchiodynia, priapism ______

OBJECTIVE

12.4 Observation and Discovery

When evaluating a patient with urinary concerns, the examiner will first need to determine whether the patient is alert and oriented. Kidney failure can cause confusion and delirium and may also cause swelling (*edema*) in the feet.

The abdominal exam may uncover pain in the lower abdomen (*suprapubic tenderness*), which may be an indication of inflammation of the bladder. Pain when pushing on the lower back (*costovertebral angle*) can warn of kidney infection.

When examining male patients, the examiner will inspect the head of the penis. Does the foreskin pull back normally, or is it stuck (*phimosis*)? The exam also includes visualizing the hole through which the urine comes out (*urethral meatus*). The hole may be too small (*meatal stenosis*) or in the wrong position (*hypospadias*).

A testicular exam includes ensuring that both testes are present in the scrotum. If one is absent, it could mean that the patient is missing a testicle (*anorchid*) or that the testicle is hidden (*cryptorchid*). Palpation of the testicles may reveal a mass which could be fluid (*hydrocele*), misplaced intestines (*hernia*), or a tumor.

The last part of a urologist's physical exam is the insertion of a finger in the patient's anus to feel his prostate (*digital rectal exam*). While unpleasant, this exam is very important in detecting an enlarged prostate.

Not surprisingly, laboratory testing for urinary problems focuses mostly on testing the urine directly (*urinalysis*). A routine urinalysis reveals a lot about a patient. For example, how concentrated the urine is reveals how well hydrated the patient is.

Urinalysis can also show things that are in the urine that don't belong there. Protein in the urine (*proteinuria*) is always abnormal. One specific protein that may show up in the urine is albumin (*albuminuria*). Protein spilling into the urine is a sign that the kidneys are not functioning properly. The presence of sugar (*glucosuria/glycosuria*) is also always abnormal; usually, sugar in the urine indicates that the patient has diabetes. If the patient's diabetes is severe or if he or she is dehydrated, the urine may include a by-product of fat breakdown called *ketones (ketonuria)*. This can also happen in fasting states. Blood in the urine (*hematuria*) may not have been noticed by the patient but can be seen with lab testing. This type of hematuria is called *microscopic hematuria*

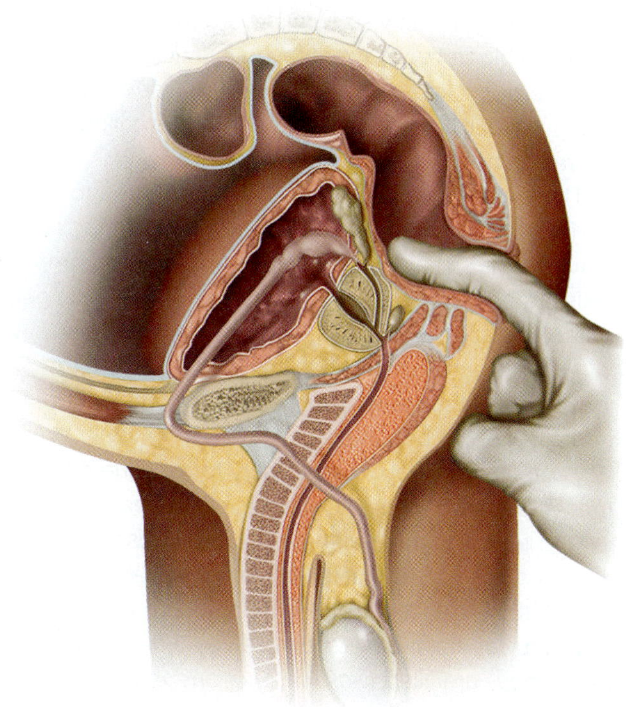

The principal way to examine the prostate is with a digital rectal exam (DRE).

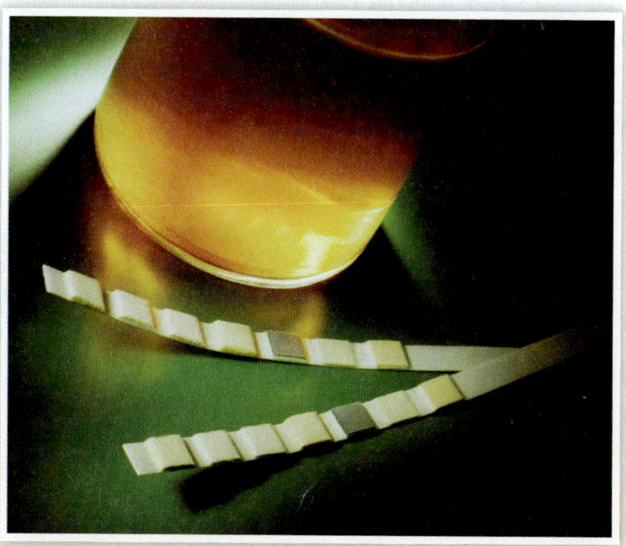

Test strips help in analyzing urine samples.

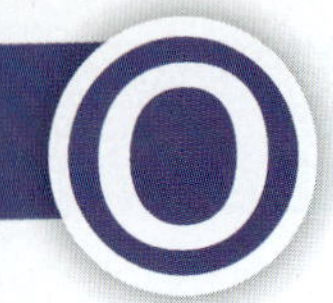

12.4 Observation and Discovery

(as opposed to *gross hematuria,* which can be seen by the naked eye).

When a patient's kidneys do not work properly, there may be some abnormalities in his or her blood work, too. The patient's blood may have high potassium (*hyperkalemia*) or low sodium (*hyponatremia*) levels. Also, the blood may have an overaccumulation of a waste product known as *blood urea nitrogen (BUN).* When the BUN is too high, the condition is called *azotemia.*

There are also a few laboratory tests related to genital function. The main male-specific lab test in the field of urology is *sperm count,* a test of how many sperm cells are present in a patient's *semen.* This test can help detect low sperm counts (*azoospermia/oligospermia*) in an infertile male or confirm that there is no sperm (*aspermia*) in the semen of a patient who has undergone surgery to become sterile.

Sometimes, it may be necessary to examine parts of the urinary tract either with images or a camera to get a clearer understanding of the problem. *Ultrasound* offers the least invasive way of looking at many parts of the urinary system. A renal ultrasound, or *nephrosonography,* is a very common test that can help determine if the kidneys are filled with fluid (*hydronephrosis*). This is often a good indicator of an anatomical problem of the urinary tract. A bladder ultrasound can be helpful to show if a patient is retaining urine.

Among the most common types of images of the urinary tract is an *intravenous pyelogram.* In this test, the patient receives an intravenous injection of a special dye and then undergoes a CT scan of the urinary tract. This test can be very useful in showing kidney stones (*nephrolithiasis*) or problems with the anatomy of the urinary tract. For example, the CT may show that the patient's ureter is narrowing (*ureterostenosis*) or that the ureter has developed a pouch (*ureterocele*). Some patients are allergic to the special dye used in the intravenous pyelogram. In such a case, it may be necessary to insert a special camera into the bladder (*cystoscope*) or ureter (*uretoscope*).

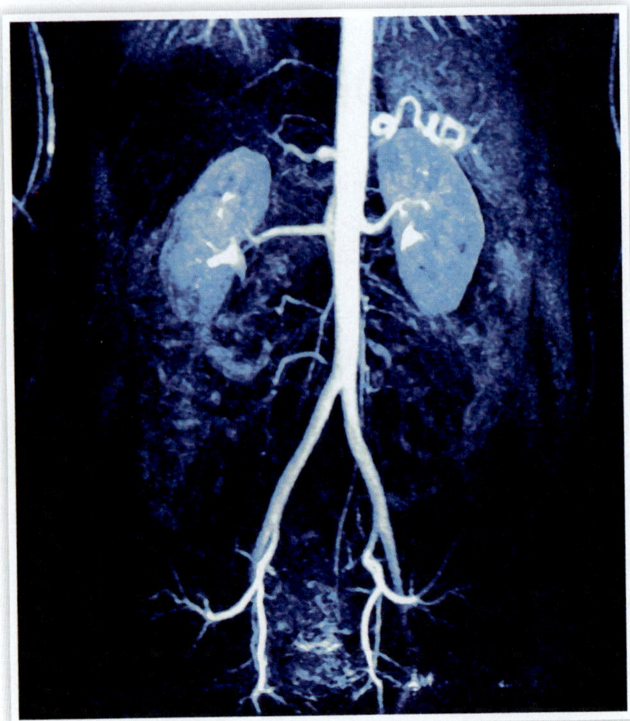

An image of the abdomen with the kidneys and bladder prominent.

At times, a physician may want to watch the flow of urine (*urodynamic testing*). The most common of these types of tests involves putting dye in the patient's bladder and watching the direction of the urine as the patient urinates (*voiding cystourethrogram*).

urinary tract

Term	Word Analysis
albuminuria al-byoo-mih-NUR-ee-ah **Definition** protein in the urine	**albumin / ur / ia** protein / urine / condition
azotemia AZ-oh-TEE-mee-ah **Definition** excess nitrogen in the blood	**azot / emia** nitrogen / blood condition

Note: The *azot* root comes from the two roots *a* (not) and *zo* (living). It was applied to nitrogen because things cannot live in it.

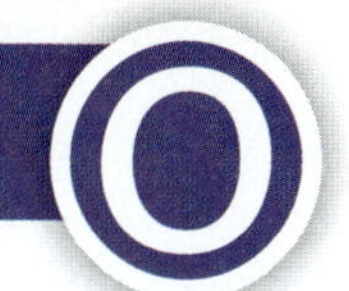

12.4 Observation and Discovery

cystorrhexis

urinary tract *continued*

Term	Word Analysis
azotorrhea AZ-oh-toh-REE-ah **Definition** excessive discharge of nitrogen	azoto / rrhea nitrogen / discharge
azoturia AZ-oh-TUR-ee-ah **Definition** excess nitrogen in the urine	azot / ur / ia nitrogen / urine / condition
cystorrhexis SIS-toh-REK-sis **Definition** rupture of the bladder	cysto / rrhexis bladder / rupture
dipsogenic DIP-soh-JIN-ik **Definition** creating thirst	dipso / genic thirst / creating
glucosuria GLOO-koh-shur-EE-ah **Definition** sugar in the urine	glucos / ur / ia sugar / urine / condition
glycosuria GLAI-koh-shur-EE-ah **Definition** sugar in the urine	glycos / ur / ia sugar / urine / condition
hyperkalemia HAI-per-kah-LEE-mee-ah **Definition** excessive potassium in the blood	hyper / kal / emia over / potassium / blood condition
hyponatremia HAI-poh-nah-TREE-mee-ah **Definition** low sodium in the blood	hypo / natr / emia under / sodium / blood condition
ketolysis kee-TAW-lih-sis **Definition** breakdown of ketones	keto / lysis ketones / loose
ketonuria kee-toh-NUR-ee-ah **Definition** presence of ketones in the urine	keton / ur / ia ketones / urine / condition
meatal stenosis mee-AY-tal steh-NOH-sis **Definition** narrowing of the opening of the urethra	meat / al sten / osis opening / pertaining to narrow / condition
nephroptosis nef-rop-TOH-sis **Definition** downward displacement of a kidney	nephro / pt / osis kidney / drooping / condition
nephrosis neh-FROH-sis **Definition** kidney condition	nephr / osis kidney / condition

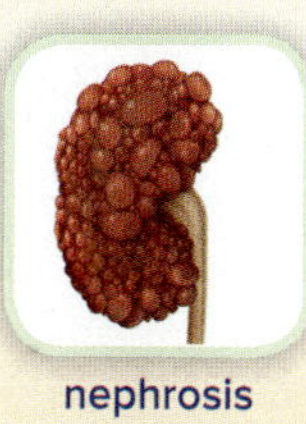

nephrosis

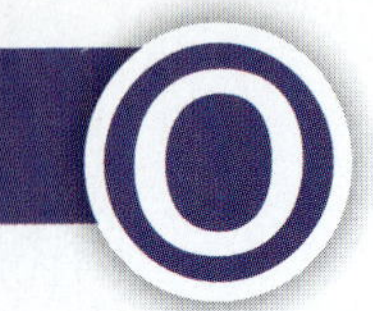

12.4 Observation and Discovery

urinary tract *continued*

Term	Word Analysis
uremia ur-EE-mee-ah **Definition** urine in the blood	ur / emia urine / blood condition
ureterocele yoo-REE-ter-oh-SEEL **Definition** hernia of a ureter	uretero / cele ureter / hernia
ureterolithiasis yoo-REE-ter-oh-lih-THAI-ah-sis **Definition** presence of stones in a ureter	uretero / lith / iasis ureter / stone / presence
ureterostenosis yoo-REE-ter-oh-steh-NOH-sis **Definition** narrowing of a ureter	uretero / sten / osis ureter / narrow / condition
urethrospasm yoo-REE-throh-SPAZ-um **Definition** involuntary contraction of the urethra	urethro / spasm urethra / involuntary contraction
urethrostenosis yoo-REE-throh-steh-NOH-sis **Definition** narrrowing of the urethra	urethro / sten / osis urethra / narrowing / condition

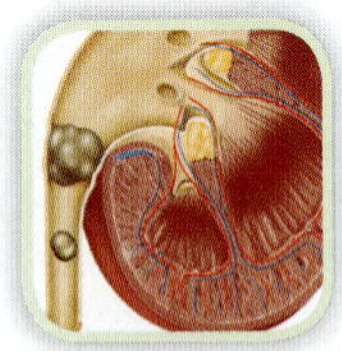

ureterolithiasis

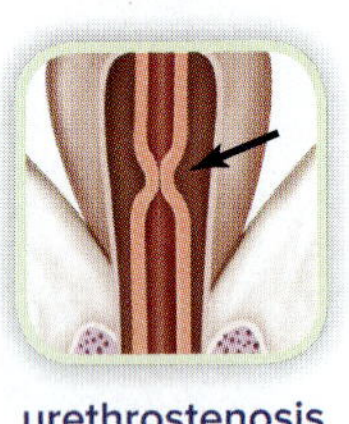

urethrostenosis

diagnostic procedures

Term	Word Analysis
cystogram SIS-toh-gram **Definition** image of the bladder	cysto / gram bladder / record
cystography sis-TAW-grah-fee **Definition** process for recording/imaging the bladder	cysto / graph / y bladder / writing / procedure
cystoscopy sis-TAWS-koh-pee **Definition** process for examining the bladder	cysto / scop / y bladder / looking / procedure
meatoscope mee-AT-oh-SKOHP **Definition** instrument for examining the opening of the urethra	meato / scope opening / instrument to look

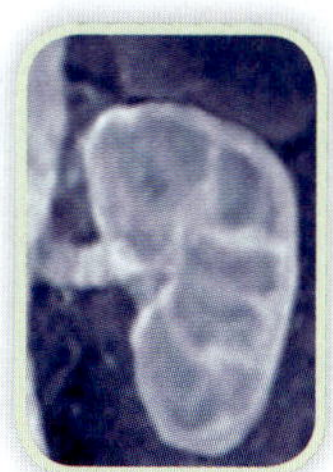
nephrogram

diagnostic procedures *continued*

Term	Word Analysis
meatoscopy MEE-ah-TAW-skoh-pee	meato / scop / y opening / looking / procedure
Definition process for examining the opening of the urethra	
nephrogram NEF-roh-gram	nephro / gram kidney / record
Definition image of a kidney	
nephrography neh-FRAW-grah-fee	nephro / graph / y kidney / writing / procedure
Definition procedure for imaging a kidney	
nephroscopy ne-FRAW-skoh-pee	nephro / scop / y kidney / looking / procedure
Definition procedure for examining a kidney	
nephrosonography NEF-roh-soh-NAW-grah-fee	nephro / sono / graph / y kidney / sound / writing / procedure
Definition procedure for imaging a kidney using sound waves	
pyelogram PAI-el-oh-GRAM	pyelo / gram pelvis / record
Definition image of the renal pelvis	
renal angiogram REE-nal AN-jee-oh-GRAM	ren / al angio / gram kidney / pertaining to vessel / record
Definition image of a kidney blood vessel	
renal angiography REE-nal AN-jee-AW-grah-fee	ren / al angio / graph / y kidney / pertaining to vessel / recording / process
Definition process of imaging a kidney blood vessel	
renal arteriogram REE-nal ar-TER-ee-oh-GRAM	ren / al arterio / gram kidney / pertaining to artery / record
Definition image of a kidney artery	
resectoscope rih-SEK-toh-SKOHP	re / secto / scope back / cut / instrument to look
Definition instrument for examining and cutting (usually the prostate)	
retrograde pyelogram REH-troh-grayd PAI-el-oh-GRAM	retro / grade pyelo / gram backward / walk pelvis / record
Definition image of the renal pelvis produced by injecting a contrast dye from the bladder to the kidney **NOTE:** The term *retrograde* is used because the contrast goes in the opposite direction of normal urine flow.	

12.4 Observation and Discovery

diagnostic procedures *continued*

Term	Word Analysis
ultrasonography UL-trah- soh-NAW-grah-fee **Definition** imaging procedure using high-frequency sound waves	**ultra / sono / graph / y** high / sound / writing / procedure
ureteroscopy yoo-REE-ter-AW-skoh-pee **Definition** process of examining a ureter	**uretero / scop / y** ureter / looking / procedure
urethroscope yoo-REE-throh-SKOHP **Definition** instrument for examining the urethra	**urethro / scope** urethra / instrument to look
urethroscopy yoo-ree-THRAW-skoh-pee **Definition** process of examining the urethra	**urethro / scop / y** urethra / looking / procedure
urinalysis YUR-ih-NAL-ih-sis **Definition** analysis of the urine **NOTE:** The *-in* sound at the end of *urine* combines with an *an-* sound at the beginning of *analysis* to make a single sound.	*urinalysis* is actually a shortened form of *urine analysis*
voiding cystourethrogram VOI-ding SIS-toh-yoo-REE-throh-GRAM **Definition** imaging procedure of the bladder and urethra produced during urination	**voiding cysto / urethro / gram** urinating bladder / urethra / record

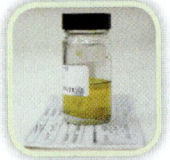

urinalysis

professional terms

Term	Word Analysis
blood urea nitrogen (BUN) blud yoo-REE-ah NAI-troh-jun **Definition** nitrogen in the blood in the form of urea; it is the product of the breakdown of amino acids for energy **NOTE:** The level of urea in the blood can be an indicator of kidney function.	**blood urea nitrogen**
diuresis DAI-yur-EE-sis **Definition** excessive urination **NOTE:** The prefix for this word is actually *dia*, but when the next word part starts with a vowel (as does *uresis*), the *dia* shortens to *di*.	**di / uresis** through / urination
nephrologist neh-FRAW-loh-jist **Definition** specialist in the kidneys	**nephro / logist** kidney / specialist

12.4 Observation and Discovery

professional terms *continued*

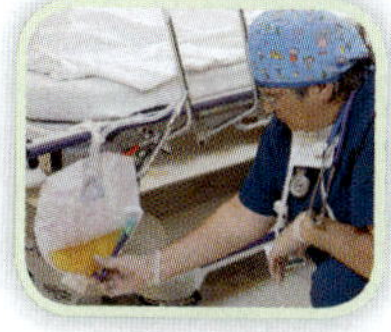
urologist

Term	Word Analysis
nephrology neh-FRAW-loh-jee **Definition** study of the kidneys	nephro / logy kidney / study
urologist yur-AW-loh-jist **Definition** specialist in the urinary tract	uro / logist urine / specialist
urology yur-AW-loh-jee **Definition** study of the urinary tract	uro / logy urine / study
uropoesis YUR-oh-poh-EE-sis **Definition** formation of urine	uro / poesis urine / formation
uroxanthin YUR-oh-ZAN-thin **Definition** substance in urine that makes it yellow	uro / xanthin urine / yellow
voiding VOI-ding **Definition** another term for urination	from a term meaning *empty*

male genitalia

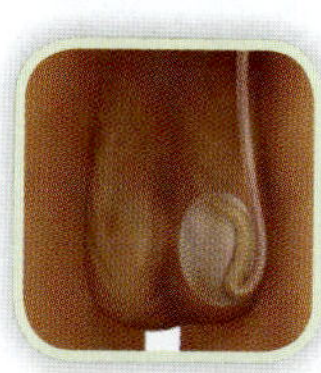
anorchidism

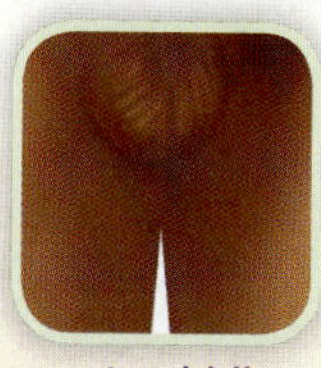
cryptorchidism

Term	Word Analysis
anorchidism an-OR-kih-DIZ-um **Definition** lack of a testicle	an / orchid / ism no / testicle / condition
aspermia ay-SPER-mee-ah **Definition** condition characterized by lack of sperm	a / sperm / ia no / sperm / condition
azoospermia ay-ZOH-aw-SPER-mee-ah **Definition** condition characterized by lack of living sperm	a / zoo / sperm / ia no / living / sperm / condition
cryptorchidism krip-TOR-kih-DIZ-um **Definition** hidden testicle	crypt / orchid / ism hidden / testicle / condition

12.4 Observation and Discovery

male genitalia *continued*

Term	Word Analysis
hydrocele HAI-droh-SEEL **Definition** fluid-filled mass in a testicle	**hydro / cele** water / hernia
hypospadias HAI-poh-SPAY-dee-as **Definition** birth defect in which the opening of the urethra is on the underside, instead of the end, of the penis	**from Greek, for** ***to tear underneath***
oligospermia AW-lih-goh-SPER-mee-ah **Definition** condition characterized by low sperm production	**oligo / sperm / ia** low / sperm / condition
phimosis fih-MOH-sis **Definition** contraction of the foreskin of the penis, preventing it from being retracted	**from Greek, for** ***muzzle***
prostatolith pros-TAT-oh-lith **Definition** stone in the prostate	**prostato / lith** prostate / stone
prostatomegaly PROS-ta-toh-MEH-gah-lee **Definition** abnormal enlargement of the prostate	**prostato / megaly** prostate / enlargement
prostatorrhea PROS-ta-toh-REE-ah **Definition** discharge from the prostate	**prostato / rrhea** prostate / discharge
seminoma SEM-oh-NOH-mah **Definition** type of testicular cancer arising from sperm-forming tissue	**semin / oma** sperm / tumor
spermatocele sper-MAT-oh-SEEL **Definition** hernia or distention of the epididymis caused by sperm cells	**spermato / cele** sperm / hernia
spermatolysis SPER-mah-TAW-lih-sis **Definition** destruction of sperm cells	**spermato / lysis** sperm / loose

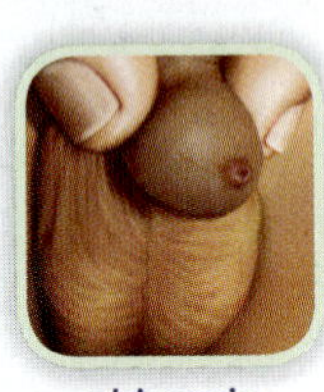
phimosis

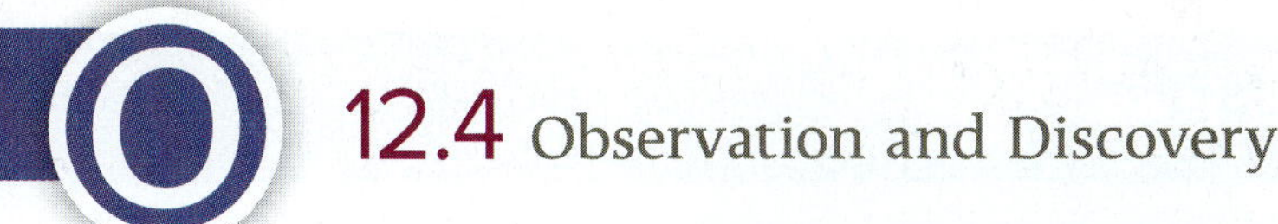

12.4 Observation and Discovery

diagnostic procedures

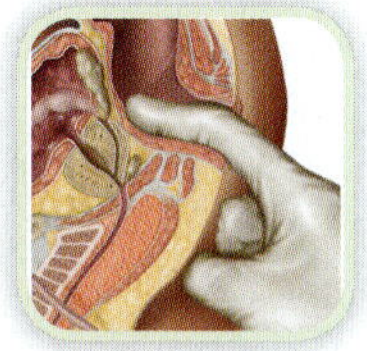
digital rectal exam

Term	Word Analysis
digital rectal exam DIJ-ih-tal REK-tal ek-ZAM	digit / al rect / al exam finger / pertaining to rectum / pertaining to exam
Definition examination of the prostate using a finger inserted into the rectum	
transrectal ultrasonography TRANZ-REK-tal UL-trah-soh-NAW-grah-fee	trans / rect / al ultra / sono / graph / y through / rectum / pertaining to high / sound / writing / procedure
Definition procedure using a probe inserted into the rectum using high-frequency sound waves to scan through the rectum to nearby tissue (most commonly, the prostate)	
urethrogram yoo-REE-throh-GRAM	urethro / gram urethra / record
Definition image of the urethra	

professional terms

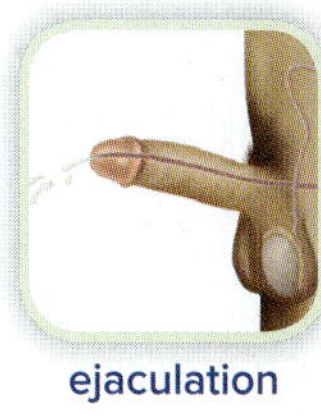
ejaculation

Term	Word Analysis
ejaculation ee-JAK-yoo-LAY-shun	e / jacul / ation out / throw / process
Definition emission of semen from the urethra	
gonads GOH-nadz	gon / ads creation / pair
Definition pair of organs used for sexual reproduction; in males, they are the testicles, and in females, they are the ovaries	
spermatogenesis sper-MAT-oh-JIN-eh-sis	spermato / genesis sperm / creation
Definition creation of sperm	
vas deferens VAS DEH-frenz	vas de / ferens vessel away / carrying
Definition vessel carrying sperm from the testicles **NOTE:** The word "vessel" can cause confusion. Most people hear "vessel" and think "blood vessel." "Vessel" simply means "tube or duct." So the vas deferens is a vessel; it just carries sperm instead of blood.	

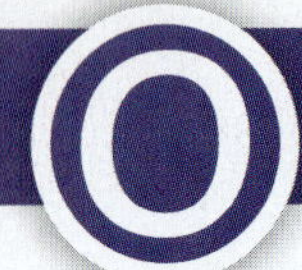

Learning Outcome 12.4 Exercises

PRONUNCIATION

EXERCISE 1 *Break down the following words into syllables.*

EXAMPLE: synesthesia *syn | es | the | sia*

1. hydrocele ______
2. seminoma ______
3. dipsogenic ______
4. glucosuria ______
5. azotemia ______
6. azoturia ______
7. resectoscope ______
8. urinalysis ______
9. urethrospasm ______
10. urethrogram ______
11. spermatocele ______
12. cystorrhexis ______
13. prostatorrhea ______
14. prostatomegaly ______

EXERCISE 2 *Indicate which syllable is emphasized when pronounced.*

EXAMPLE: bronchitis bron**chi**tis

1. gonads ______
2. voiding ______
3. uremia ______
4. aspermia ______
5. nephrosis ______
6. ketolysis ______
7. ketonuria ______
8. meatal stenosis ______
9. prostatolith ______
10. nephroptosis ______
11. cryptorchidism ______
12. urology ______
13. urologist ______
14. nephrology ______
15. nephrologist ______
16. cystography ______
17. cystoscopy ______
18. nephroscopy ______
19. nephrogram ______
20. nephrography ______

TRANSLATION

EXERCISE 3 *Break down the following words into their component parts.*

EXAMPLE: nasopharyngoscope *naso | pharyngo | scope*

1. urology ______
2. nephrology ______
3. nephrogram ______
4. cystogram ______
5. spermatocele ______
6. ureterocele ______
7. hydrocele ______

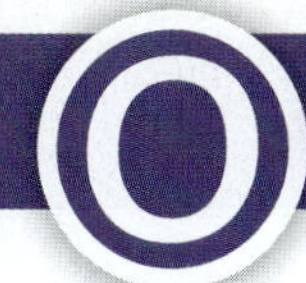

Learning Outcome 12.4 Exercises

8. meatoscope ______
9. urethroscope ______
10. pyelogram ______
11. nephrosis ______
12. prostatomegaly ______
13. urethrospasm ______
14. albuminuria ______
15. dipsogenic ______
16. aspermia ______
17. nephrosonography ______
18. ultrasonography ______
19. resectoscope ______
20. anorchidism ______

EXERCISE 4 *Underline and define the roots from this chapter in the following terms.*

1. urinalysis ______
2. nephrologist ______
3. urologist ______
4. urethrogram ______
5. spermatolysis ______
6. nephroptosis ______
7. cystorrhexis ______
8. meatal stenosis ______
9. ureterostenosis ______
10. urethrostenosis ______
11. oligospermia ______
12. azoospermia ______
13. uroxanthin ______
14. azoturia ______
15. glucosuria ______
16. retrograde pyelogram ______
17. diuresis ______
18. cryptidorchidism ______
19. prostatolith (2 roots) ______
20. ureterolithiasis (2 roots) ______

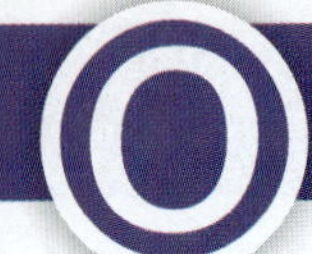

Learning Outcome 12.4 Exercises

EXERCISE 5 *Match the term on the left with its definition on the right.*

h.	1. ejaculation	a.	birth defect in which the opening of the urethra is on the underside, instead of the end, of the penis
i	2. gonads	b.	contraction of the foreskin of the penis, preventing it from being retracted
g	3. blood urea nitrogen	c.	procedure using a probe inserted into the rectum using high-frequency sound waves to scan through the rectum to nearby tissue (most commonly, the prostate)
f	4. digital rectal exam	d.	type of testicular cancer arising from sperm-forming tissue
e	5. voiding	e.	another term for urination
c.	6. transrectal ultrasonography	f.	exam of the prostate using a finger inserted into the rectum
j	7. vas deferens	g.	nitrogen in the blood in the form of urea; can be an indicator of kidney function
d	8. seminoma	h.	emission of semem from the urethra
a.	9. hypospadias	i.	pair of organs used for sexual reproduction (testicles in males; ovaries in females)
b.	10. phimosis	j.	vessel carrying sperm from the testicles

EXERCISE 6 *Underline the correct option for each given translation.*

EXAMPLE: hypoglycemia ***hypo*** **over/under** ***pharyngo*** **salt/sugar** **-emia blood/urine condition**

1. *albuminuria* = *albumin* protein/nitrogen + *uria* urine/blood condition
2. *azotemia* = *azot* protein/nitrogen + *emia* urine/blood condition
3. *glucosuria* = *gluco* sugar/sodium + *uria* urine/blood condition
4. *glycosuria* = *glycos* sugar/potassium + *uria* urine/blood condition
5. *hyperkalemia* = *hyper* over/under + *kal* sugar/potassium + *emia* urine/blood condition
6. *hyponatremia* = *hypo* over/under + *natr* sugar/sodium + *emia* urine/blood condition

EXERCISE 7 *Fill in the blanks.*

1. *ureteroscopy:* process for examining the ______________________________
2. *urethroscopy:* process for examining the ______________________________
3. *cystoscopy:* process for examining the ______________________________
4. *nephroscopy:* process for examining the ______________________________
5. *meatoscopy:* process for examining the ______________________________
6. *cystography:* process for recording/imaging the ______________________________
7. *nephrography:* process for recording/imaging the ______________________________
8. *renal angiogram:* image of a(n) ______________________________

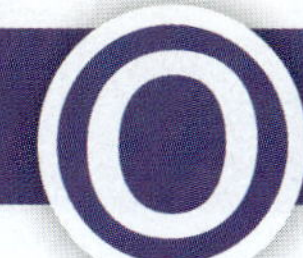

Learning Outcome 12.4 Exercises

9. *renal arteriogram:* image of a(n) ______
10. *renal angiography:* process of imaging a(n) ______

EXERCISE 8 *Translate the following terms as literally as possible.*

EXAMPLE: nasopharyngoscope *an instrument for looking at the nose and throat*

1. nephrology ______
2. cystoscopy ______
3. meatoscope ______
4. urethroscope ______
5. pyelogram ______
6. spermatogenesis ______
7. urinalysis ______
8. prostatorrhea ______
9. cryptorchidism ______
10. glucosuria ______
11. ketonuria ______
12. uropoesis ______
13. uroxanthin ______
14. cystorrhexis ______
15. uremia ______
16. anorchidism ______
17. azoospermia ______
18. resectoscope ______
19. ketolysis ______
20. dipsogenic ______
21. azotorrhea ______

GENERATION

EXERCISE 9 *Build a medical term from the information provided.*

EXAMPLE: inflammation of the sinuses *sinusitis*

1. kidney condition (use *nephr/o*) ______
2. image of the urethra ______
3. procedure for imaging a kidney (use *nephr/o*) ______
4. process for recording/imaging the bladder (use *cyst/o*) ______

Learning Outcome 12.4 Exercises

5. process of imaging a kidney blood vessel (use *ren/o*) ______________________
6. process for examining the opening of the urethra ______________________
7. procedure for examining a kidney ______________________
8. specialist in the kidneys ______________________
9. abnormal enlargement of the prostate ______________________
10. involuntary contraction of the urethra ______________________
11. downward displacement of a kidney ______________________
12. low-sperm condition ______________________
13. urine formation ______________________
14. hernia of a ureter ______________________
15. stone in the prostate ______________________
16. presence of stones in the ureter ______________________
17. low sodium in the blood ______________________
18. excessive potassium in the blood ______________________
19. imaging procedure using high-frequency sound waves ______________________
20. procedure for imaging a kidney using sound waves ______________________

EXERCISE 10 *Multiple-choice questions. Select the correct answer(s).*

1. The emission of semen from the urethra is known as
   - a. aspermia
   - b. ejaculation
   - c. phimosis
   - d. seminoma
   - e. spermatolysis
2. The breakdown of ketones is known as
   - a. azotemia
   - b. azotorrhea
   - c. hyperkalemia
   - d. ketolysis
   - e. ketonuria
3. The narrowing of the opening of the urethra is called
   - a. meatal stenosis
   - b. meatorrhaphy
   - c. ureterostenosis
   - d. urethrospasm
   - e. urethrostenosis
4. Which of the choices below are true of the term *blood urea nitrogen*?
   - a. abbreviated BUN
   - b. nitrogen in the blood in the form of urea
   - c. product of the breakdown of amino acids for energy
   - d. level of urea in the blood can be an indicator of kidney function
   - e. all of these

Learning Outcome 12.4 Exercises

5. The medical term for *excessive urination* is
   a. diuresis
   b. uremia
   c. uropoesis
   d. uroxanthin
   e. voiding
6. A hernia or distention of the epididymis caused by sperm cells is called a(n)
   a. epididymitis
   b. epididymocele
   c. hydrocele
   d. seminoma
   e. spermatocele
7. A *hydrocele* is a fluid-filled mass in the
   a. bladder
   b. kidney
   c. prostate
   d. testicle
   e. none of these
8. The *digital rectal exam* and the *transrectal ultrasonography* are both procedures for examining the
   a. bladder
   b. kidney
   c. prostate
   d. testicle
   e. none of these
9. Which of the statements below are true of the term *retrograde pyelogram* (select all that apply)?
   a. image of the kidney
   b. image of the renal pelvis
   c. image produced by injecting a contrast dye from the bladder to the kidney
   d. image produced by injecting a contrast dye from the bladder to the urethra
   e. literally means *backward walk pelvis record*
10. Which of the statements below are true of the term *seminoma* (select all that apply)?
   a. a type of prostate cancer
   b. a type of testicular cancer
   c. arises from sperm-forming tissue
   d. literally means *sperm condition*
   e. literally means *sperm tumor*
11. Which of the statements below are true of the term *hypospadias* (select all that apply)?
   a. birth defect
   b. from Greek, for *to tear underneath*
   c. literally means *over sperm*
   d. opening of the urethra is on the end of the penis
   e. opening of the urethra is on the underside of the penis

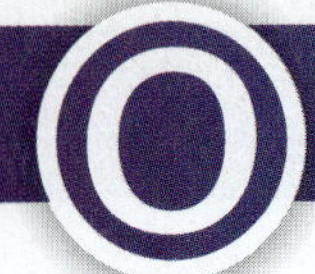

Learning Outcome 12.4 Exercises

12. Select all of the terms below that pertain to male genitalia.
    - a. aspermia
    - b. phimosis
    - c. uremia
    - d. ureterolithiasis
    - e. voiding

13. Select all of the terms below that pertain to the urinary tract.
    - a. aspermia
    - b. phimosis
    - c. uremia
    - d. ureterolithiasis
    - e. voiding

EXERCISE 11 *Briefly describe the difference between each pair of terms.*

1. urologist, urology ______________________________
2. cystogram, nephrogram ______________________________
3. ureteroscopy, urethroscopy ______________________________
4. ureterostenosis, urethostenosis ______________________________
5. spermatolysis, spermatogenesis ______________________________
6. azotorrhea, prostatorrhea ______________________________
7. azotemia, azoturia ______________________________
8. renal angiogram, renal arteriogram ______________________________
9. gonads, vas deferens ______________________________

ASSESSMENT

12.5 Diagnosis and Pathology

Just like all the other body systems, the urinary system can have problems with its anatomy, infection, tumors, and blood supply. On a large scale, the vessels in patients' urinary tracts can have abnormal pouches (for example, *cystoceles*). These pouches can be harmless or cause a blockage of urine. In the case of the ureter (*ureterocele*), this pouching intrudes into the bladder. Patients may also have large cysts in the kidneys (*polycystic kidney disease*). These don't cause blockage, but they can prevent the kidneys from working correctly.

On a microscopic level, the kidneys can have all manner of problems. These general kidney problems (*nephropathy*) fall into two general types with (*nephritis*) or without (*nephrosis*) inflammation. Often, the difference is seen in a urinalysis. Nephritis will most often cause white blood cells and red blood cells to show up in the urine. Both types of diseases can be severe enough to lead to kidney failure. Kidney failure is marked by the kidney's inability to filter waste out of the blood. If this problem is not fixed, the patient will die.

The urinary tract is vulnerable to infection. Urinary tract infections (UTIs) are often divided into lower urinary tract and upper urinary tract, infections, depending on whether the kidneys are involved. Lower urinary tract infections generally refer to infections of the bladder (*cystitis*). They are much more common in females than in males, and they are also frequently seen in patients whose urine flows back toward the kidneys from the bladder (*vesicoureteral reflux*).

When infection spreads to the kidneys (*pyelonephritis*), it generally becomes more severe. A patient with pyelonephritis may have back pain, high fever, and may appear very ill. Another common infection of the urinary tract involves just the urethra (*urethritis*). The usual cause is *gonorrhea,* a sexually transmitted infection.

Tumors of the urinary tract are most common in the larger structures of the tract: the kidney (*nephroma*) or bladder (*cystoma*). The most usual presenting symptom is blood in the urine. By far, the most common cancer of the kidney is *renal cell carcinoma.* Often, there are few early warning symptoms for this cancer.

Kidneys need a constant supply of blood. Poor blood supply to the kidneys (*renal ischemia*) is usually caused by cholesterol deposits in the arteries. Another cause is narrowing of the arteries that lead to the kidney (*renal artery stenosis*). When the blood supply to the kidneys is low, the kidneys release signals to the rest of the body to increase the blood's pressure (*renovascular hypertension*). Any time a patient's high blood pressure doesn't respond to typical medical management, a renal cause should be considered.

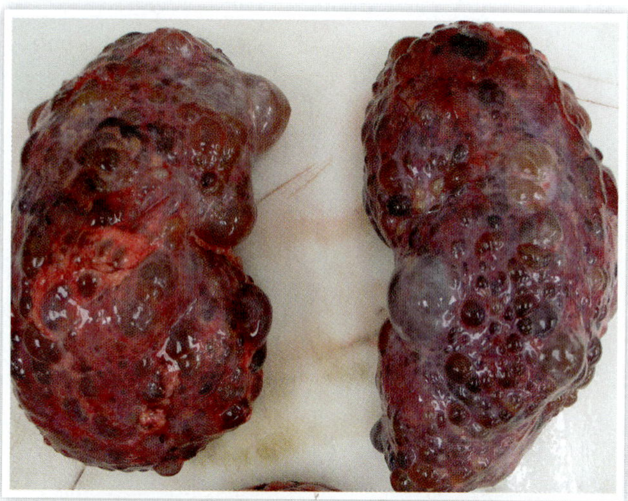

A pair of kidneys with polycystic kidney disease.

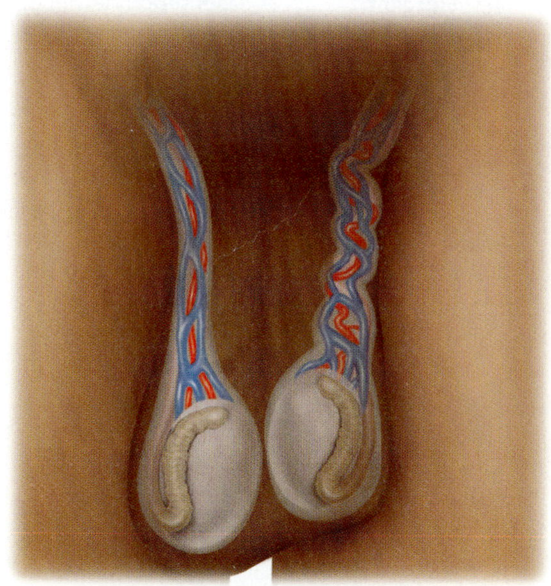

Testicular torsion—when a testicle becomes twisted—is considered a medical emergency.

Male patients can have specific problems with their genitourinary systems. The prostate gland is a common cause of problems in older men. The prostate gland

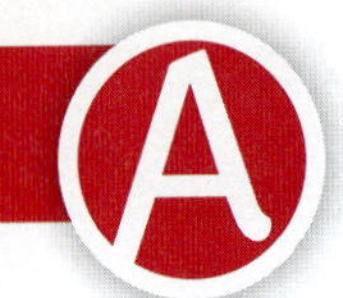

12.5 Diagnosis and Pathology

may become enlarged (*benign prostate hypertrophy*), infected (*prostatitis*), or cancerous. Prostate symptoms include pain and the blocked flow of urine, leading to a weak urine stream or difficulty starting a urine stream at all.

The testicles can cause problems in any age group. *Testicular carcinoma* is the most common form of cancer in young adult men. It usually presents as a painful lump on the testicle. The testicle can also become infected (*orchitis*), a problem usually associated with the mumps.

Since testicles hang from the body, it is possible for one of them to become twisted (*testicular torsion*). This can cut off the blood supply to the testicle and is considered a medical emergency. Concerns in other parts of the reproductive system include infection of the epididymis (*epididymitis*) and swelling of the veins in the scrotum (*varicocele*).

cystocele

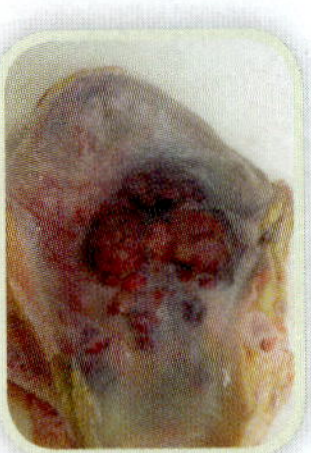

cystoma

urinary tract

Term	Word Analysis
cystitis sis-TAI-tis **Definition** inflammation of the bladder	cyst / itis bladder / inflammation
cystocele SIS-toh-seel **Definition** hernia of the bladder	cysto / cele bladder / tumor
cystolith SIS-toh-lith **Definition** stone in the bladder	cysto / lith bladder / stone
cystoma sis-TOH-mah **Definition** tumor of the bladder	cyst / oma bladder / tumor
cystoptosis sis-TOP-toh-sis **Definition** downward displacement of the bladder	cysto / pt / osis bladder / drooping / condition
cystospasm SIS-toh-SPAZ-um **Definition** involuntary contraction of the bladder	cysto / spasm bladder / involuntary contraction
cystoureteritis SIS-toh-yoo-REE-ter-AI-tis **Definition** inflammation of the bladder and urethra	cysto / ureter / itis bladder / ureter / inflammation
cystourethrocele SIS-toh-yoo-REE-throh-seel **Definition** hernia of the bladder and urethra	cysto / urethro / cele bladder / urethra / hernia

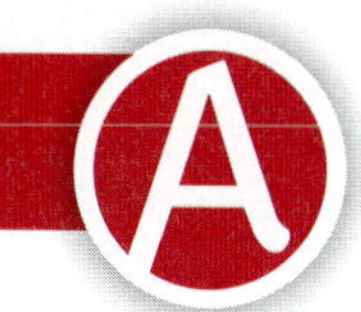

12.5 Diagnosis and Pathology

urinary tract *continued*

Term	Word Analysis
glomerulonephritis gloh-MER-yoo-loh-neh-FRAI-tis	glomerulo / nephr / itis glomerulus / kidney / inflammation
Definition inflammation of the kidneys involving primarily the glomeruli	
glomerulopathy gloh-MER-yoo-LAW-pah-thee	glomerulo / pathy glomerulus / disease
Definition disease of the kidney involving primarily the glomeruli	
glomerulosclerosis gloh-MER-yoo-loh-skleh-ROH-sis	glomerulo / sclerosis glomerulus / hardening
Definition hardening of the glomeruli	
hydronephrosis HAI-droh-neh-FROH-sis	hydro / nephr / osis water / kidney / condition
Definition kidney condition caused by the obstruction of urine flow	
hypernephroma HAI-per-neh-FROH-mah	hyper / nephr / oma over / kidney / tumor
Definition another name for renal cell carcinoma	
lithonephritis LIH-thoh-neh-FRAI-tis	litho / nephr / itis stone / kidney / inflammation
Definition inflammation of the kidneys caused by stones	
nephritis neh-FRAI-tis	nephr / itis kidney / inflammation
Definition inflammation of the kidney	
nephrocele NEH-froh-seel	nephro / cele kidney / hernia
Definition hernia of a kidney	
nephrohypertrophy NEH-froh-hai-PER-troh-fee	nephro / hyper / troph / y kidney / over / nourishment / condition
Definition overdevelopment of the kidney	
nephrolithiasis NEH-froh-lih-THAI-ah-sis	nephro / lith / iasis kidney / stone / presence
Definition presence of stones in the kidney	
nephroma neh-FROH-mah	nephr / oma kidney / tumor
Definition kidney tumor	
nephromalacia NEH-froh-mah-LAY-shah	nephro / malacia kidney / softening
Definition abnormal softening of a kidney	

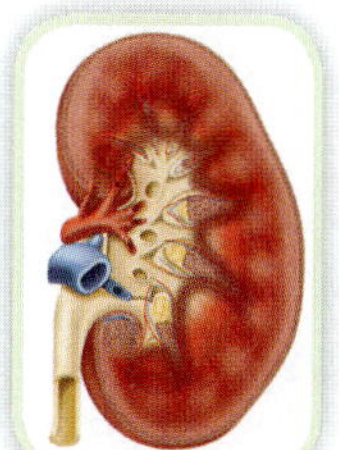
nephritis

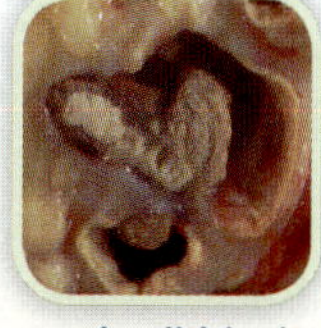
nephrolithiasis

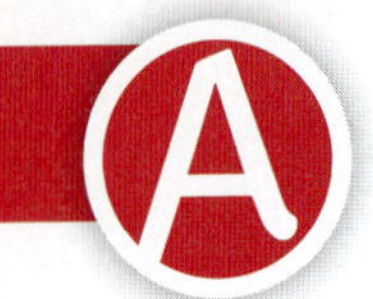

12.5 Diagnosis and Pathology

urinary tract *continued*

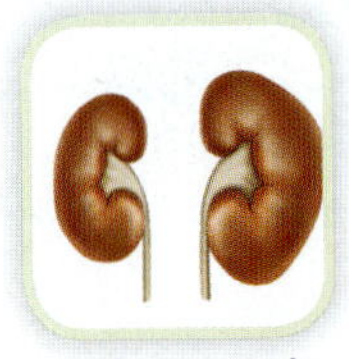

nephromegaly

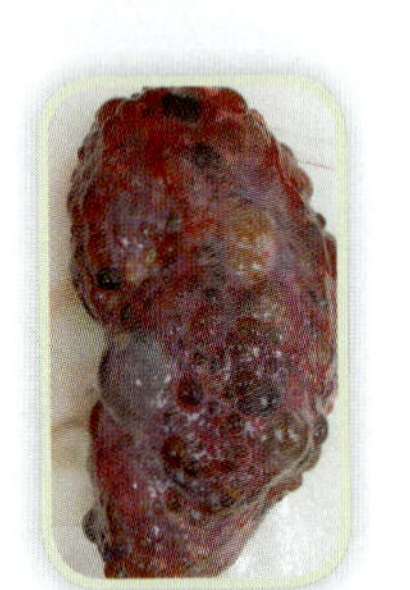

polycystic kidney disease

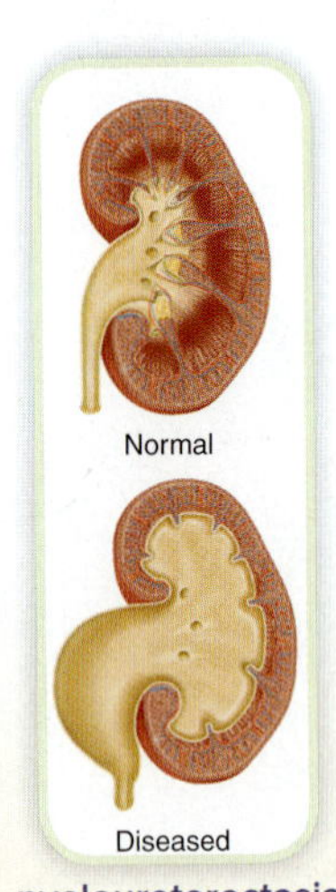

pyeloureterectasia

Term	Word Analysis
nephromegaly NEH-froh-MEG-ah-lee **Definition** abnormal enlargement of a kidney	nephro / megaly kidney / enlargement
nephropathy neh-FRAW-pah-thee **Definition** any kidney disease	nephro / pathy kidney / disease
nephroptosis NEH-frop-TOH-sis **Definition** downward displacement of a kidney	nephro / pt / osis kidney / drooping / condition
nephrosclerosis NEH-froh-skleh-ROH-sis **Definition** abnormal hardening of a kidney	nephro / scler / osis kidney / hardening / condition
polycystic kidney disease PAW-lee-SIS-tik KID-nee dih-ZEEZ **Definition** disease characterized by the formation of many fluid-filled cysts in the kidneys	poly / cyst / ic kidney disease many / cysts / pertaining to
pyelitis PAI-el-AI-tis **Definition** inflammation of the renal pelvis	pyel / itis pelvis / inflammation
pyelocystitis PAI-el-oh-sis-TAI-tis **Definition** inflammation of the renal pelvis and bladder	pyelo / cyst / itis pelvis / bladder / inflammation
pyelocystostomosis PAI-el-oh-SIS-toh-staw-MOH-sis **Definition** creation of an opening between the renal pelvis and bladder	pyelo / cysto / stom / osis pelvis / bladder / mouth / condition
pyelonephritis PAI-el-oh-neh-FRAI-tis **Definition** inflammation of the kidney and renal pelvis	pyelo / nephr / itis pelvis / kidney / inflammation
pyelopathy PAI-el-AW-pah-thee **Definition** disease of the renal pelvis	pyelo / pathy pelvis / disease
pyeloureterectasia PAI-el-oh-yoo-REE-ter-ek-TAY-zhah **Definition** dilation of the renal pelvis and ureter	pyelo / ureter / ectas / ia pelvis / ureter / expansion / condition

urinary tract *continued*

Term	Word Analysis
pyonephritis PAI-oh-neh-FRAI-tis **Definition** inflammation of the kidney caused by pus	pyo / nephr / itis pus / kidney / inflammation
pyonephrolithiasis PAI-oh-NEH-froh-lih-THAI-ah-sis **Definition** presence of pus and stones in the kidney	pyo / nephro / lith / iasis pus / kidney / stone / presence
pyopyeloectasis PAI-oh-PAI-el-oh-EK-tah-sis **Definition** pus in a dilated renal pelvis	pyo / pyelo / ectasis pus / pelvis / expansion
renal cell carcinoma REE-nal SELL KAR-sih-NOH-mah **Definition** cancer of the kidneys	ren / al cell carcin / oma kidney / pertaining to cell cancer / tumor
renal failure REE-nal FAY-el-yur **Definition** kidney failure	ren / al failure kidney / pertaining to failure
renal ischemia REE-nal ih-SKEE-mee-ah **Definition** deficiency of blood in a kidney	ren / al isch / emia kidney / pertaining to hold back / blood condition
stress urinary incontinence (SUI) stress YUR-ih-NAR-ee in-CON-tih-nentz **Definition** loss of bladder control caused by the application of external pressure **Note:** This is the medical term for loss of bladder control due to excessive laughing, a hard cough, or similar motion.	stress urin / ary in / con / tinence stress urine / pertaining to not / together / holding
ureteritis yoo-REE-ter-AI-tis **Definition** inflammation of a ureter	ureter / itis ureter / inflammation
ureteropyelonephritis yoo-REE-ter-oh-PAI-el-oh-neh-FRAI-tis **Definition** inflammation of a kidney, renal pelvis, and ureter	uretero / pyelo / nephr / itis ureter / pelvis / kidney / inflammation
urethritis yoo-ree-THRAI-tis **Definition** inflammation of the urethra	urethr / itis urethra / inflammation
urethrocystitis yoo-REE-throh-sis-TAI-tis **Definition** inflammation of the urethra and bladder	urethro / cyst / itis urethra / bladder / inflammation

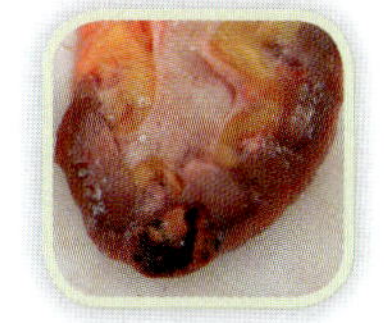
renal cell carcinoma

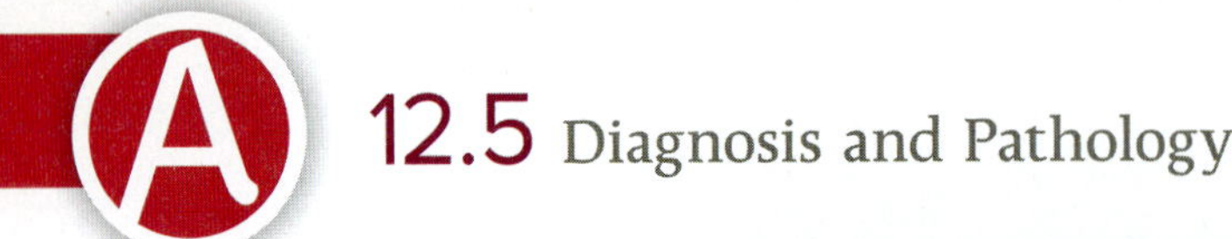

12.5 Diagnosis and Pathology

urinary tract *continued*

Term	Word Analysis
urinary tract infection (UTI) YUR-ih-NAR-ee trakt in-FEK-shun **Definition** infection of the urinary tract	urinary tract infection
uropathy yur-AW-pah-thee **Definition** disease of the urinary tract	uro / pathy urine / disease
vesicocele VES-ih-koh-SEEL **Definition** hernia of the bladder	vesico / cele bladder / hernia
vesicoureteral reflux (VUR) VES-ih-koh-yoo-REE-ter-al REE-fluks **Definition** abnormal flow of urine from the bladder back into the ureters	vesico / ureter / al re / flux bladder / ureter / pertaining to back / flow
ureteropyelitis yoo-REE-ter-oh-PAI-el-AI-tis **Definition** inflammation of a ureter and renal pelvis	uretero / pyel / itis ureter / pelvis / inflammation

male genitalia

Term	Word Analysis
balanitis bal-ah-NAI-tis **Definition** inflammation of the penis	balan / itis penis / inflammation
benign prostate hyperplasia beh-NAIN PROS-tayt HAI-per-PLAY-zhah **Definition** noncancerous overdevelopment of the prostate, also known as *enlarged prostate*	benign prostate hyper / plas / ia friendly prostate over / formation / condition
benign prostate hypertrophy beh-NAIN PROS-tayt hai-PER-troh-fee **Definition** another term for benign prostate hyperplasia	benign prostate hyper / troph / y friendly prostate over / nourishment / condition
epididymitis EP-ih-DID-ih-MAI-tis **Definition** inflammation of the epididymis	epididym / itis epididymis / inflammation
epididymo-orchitis EP-ih-DID-ih-moh-or-KAI-tis **Definition** inflammation of the testicles and epididymis	epididymo / orch / itis epididymis / testicle / inflammation

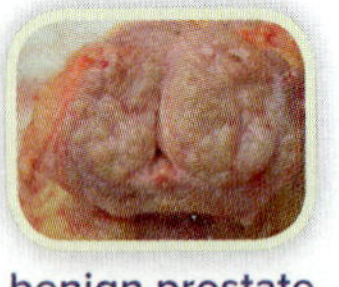

benign prostate hyperplasia

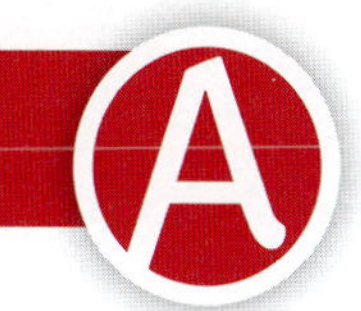

12.5 Diagnosis and Pathology

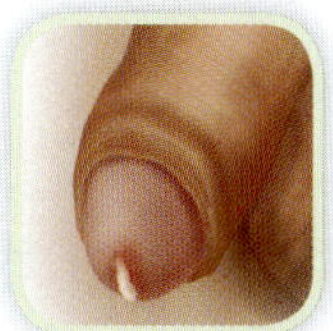

gonorrhea

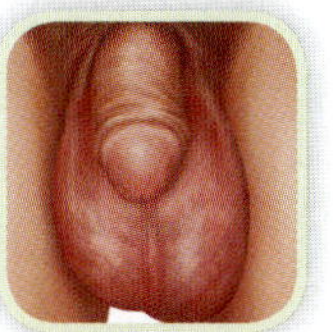

orchitis

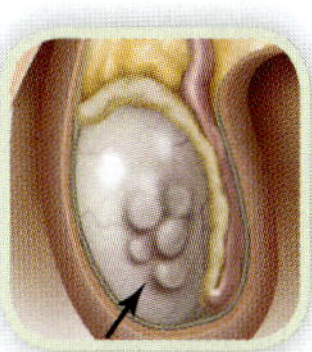

testicular carcinoma

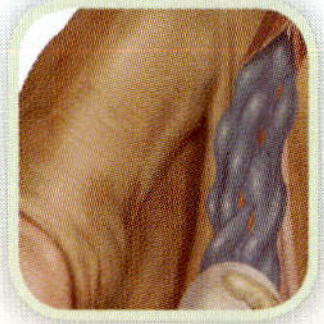

varicocele

male genitalia *continued*

Term	Word Analysis
gonorrhea GAW-noh-REE-ah **Definition** discharge from the gonads	gono / rrhea gonad / discharge
orchiditis OR-kih-DAI-tis **Definition** inflammation of the testicles and epididymis	orchid / itis testicle / inflammation
orchiepididymitis OR-kee-EP-ih-DID-ih-MAI-tis **Definition** inflammation of the testicles and epididymis	orchi / epididym / itis testicle / epididymis / inflammation
orchiopathy OR-kee-AW-pah-thee **Definition** disease of the testicles	orchio / pathy testicle / disease
orchitis or-KAI-tis **Definition** inflammation of the testicles and epididymis	orch / itis testicle / inflammation
prostatitis PRAWS-tah-TAI-tis **Definition** inflammation of the prostate	prostat / itis prostate / inflammation
prostatocystitis PROS-ta-toh-sis-TAI-tis **Definition** inflammation of the prostate and bladder	prostato / cyst / itis prostate / bladder / inflammation
prostatovesiculitis PROS-ta-toh-veh-SIK-yoo-LAI-tis **Definition** inflammation of the prostate and seminal vesicles	prostato / vesicul / itis prostate / bladder / inflammation
testicular carcinoma tes-TIK-yoo-lar KAR-sih-NOH-mah **Definition** testicular cancer	testicul / ar carcin / oma testicle / pertaining to cancer / tumor
testitis tes-TAI-tis **Definition** inflammation of a testicle	test / itis testicle / inflammation
varicocele VAR-ih-koh-SEEL **Definition** overexpansion of the blood vessels of the testicles, leading to a soft tumor	varico / cele twisted / hernia

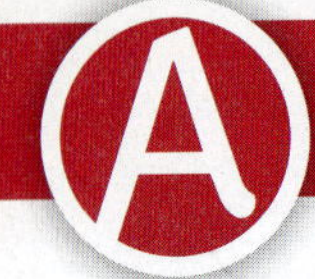

Learning Outcome 12.5 Exercises

PRONUNCIATION

EXERCISE 1 *Break down the following words into syllables.*

EXAMPLE: synesthesia *syn | es | the | sia*

1. cystocele ______
2. nephrocele ______
3. cystolith ______
4. cystospasm ______
5. cystoptosis ______
6. nephroptosis ______
7. pyelitis ______
8. ureteritis ______
9. orchiditis ______
10. prostatitis ______
11. pyonephritis ______
12. pyelopathy ______
13. nephromegaly ______
14. nephrolithiasis ______
15. glomerulonephritis ______
16. pyelocystostomosis ______

EXERCISE 2 *Indicate which syllable is emphasized when pronounced.*

EXAMPLE: bronchitis bron**chi**tis

1. cystitis ______
2. orchitis ______
3. testitis ______
4. nephritis ______
5. balanitis ______
6. urethritis ______
7. cystoma ______
8. nephroma ______
9. uropathy ______
10. nephropathy ______

TRANSLATION

EXERCISE 3 *Break down the following words into their component parts.*

EXAMPLE: nasopharyngoscope *naso | pharyngo | scope*

1. cystitis ______
2. testitis ______
3. nephritis ______
4. vesicocele ______
5. gonorrhea ______
6. orchiopathy ______
7. epididymitis ______
8. nephromalacia ______
9. hydronephritis ______
10. uteropyelitis ______
11. urethrocystitis ______
12. pyelonephritis ______

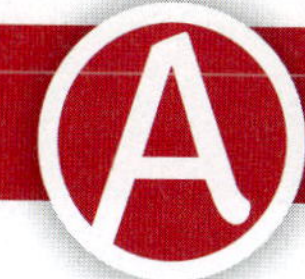

Learning Outcome 12.5 Exercises

13. pyonephritis ______
14. prostatocystitis ______
15. orchiepididymitis ______
16. glomerulosclerosis ______
17. nephrolithiasis ______
18. pyopyeloectasis ______
19. ureteropyelonephritis ______
20. pyelocystostomosis ______

EXERCISE 4 *Underline and define the roots from this chapter in the following terms.*

1. prostatitis ______
2. ureteritis ______
3. urethritis ______
4. orchitis ______
5. orchiditis ______
6. balanitis ______
7. cystocele ______
8. nephrocele ______
9. uropathy ______
10. pyelopathy ______
11. glomerulopathy ______
12. renal failure ______
13. cystoptosis ______
14. nephromegaly ______
15. hypernephroma ______
16. renal cell carcinoma ______
17. testicular carcinoma ______
18. cystourethrocele (2 roots) ______
19. lithonephritis (2 roots) ______
20. pyeloureterectasia (2 roots) ______
21. pyonephrolithiasis (2 roots) ______
22. vesicoureteral reflux (2 roots) ______
23. epididymo-orchitis (2 roots) ______
24. prostatovesiculitis (2 roots) ______

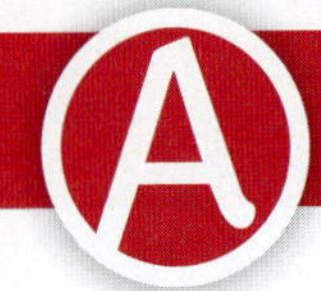

Learning Outcome 12.5 Exercises

EXERCISE 5 *Match the term on the left with its definition on the right.*

____	1. urinary tract infection	a.	deficiency of blood in a kidney
____	2. stress urinary incontinence disease	b.	disease characterized by the formation of many fluid-filled cysts in the kidneys
____	3. polycystic kidney disease	c.	infection of the urinary tract
____	4. benign prostate hypertrophy	d.	kidney condition caused by obstruction of urine flow
____	5. hydronephrosis	e.	literally, *friendly prostate overformation condition;* noncancerous overdevelopment of the prostate or *enlarged prostate*
____	6. benign prostate hyperplasia	f.	literally, *friendly prostate overnourishment condition;* noncancerous overdevelopment of the prostate or enlarged prostate
____	7. nephrohypertrophy	g.	loss of bladder control caused by the application of external pressure
____	8. varicocele	h.	overdevelopment of the kidney
____	9. renal ischemia	i.	overexpansion of the blood vessels of the testicles, leading to a soft tumor

EXERCISE 6 *Fill in the blanks.*

1. *testitis:* inflammation of the ____________________
2. *prostatitis:* inflammation of the ____________________
3. *urethritis:* inflammation of the ____________________
4. *nephritis:* inflammation of the ____________________
5. *ureteritis:* inflammation of the ____________________
6. *orchiditis:* inflammation of the ____________________
7. *cystitis:* inflammation of the ____________________
8. *pyelitis:* inflammation of the ____________________
9. *balanitis:* inflammation of the ____________________
10. *orchitis:* inflammation of the ____________________
11. *epididymitis:* inflammation of the ____________________
12. *cystoureteritis:* inflammation of the ____________ and ____________
13. *urethrocystitis:* inflammation of the ____________ and ____________
14. *ureteropyelitis:* inflammation of the ____________ and ____________
15. *prostatocystitis:* inflammation of the ____________ and ____________
16. *pyelocystitis:* inflammation of the ____________ and ____________

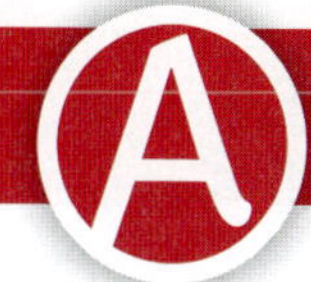

Learning Outcome 12.5 Exercises

17. *pyelonephritis:* inflammation of the ________________ and ________________
18. *epididymo-orchitis:* inflammation of the ________________ and ________________
19. *ureteropyelonephritis:* inflammation of the ________________, ________________ and ________________

EXERCISE 7 *Translate the following terms as literally as possible.*

EXAMPLE: nasopharyngoscope *an instrument for looking at the nose and throat*

1. cystolith ________________
2. pyelopathy ________________
3. gonorrhea ________________
4. glomerulopathy ________________
5. nephromegaly ________________
6. pyonephritis ________________
7. prostatovesiculitis ________________
8. orchiepididymitis ________________
9. nephrolithiasis ________________
10. nephrohypertrophy ________________
11. testicular carcinoma ________________
12. pyelocystostomosis ________________
13. pyeloureterectasia ________________
14. pyopyeloectasis ________________
15. renal ischemia ________________
16. benign prostate hyperplasia ________________

GENERATION

EXERCISE 8 *Build a medical term from the information provided.*

EXAMPLE: inflammation of the sinuses *sinusitis*

1. hernia of the bladder (use *cyst/o*) ________________
2. hernia of the bladder (use *vesic/o*) ________________
3. hernia of a kidney ________________
4. kidney failure (use *ren/o*) ________________
5. kidney tumor (use *nephr/o*) ________________
6. kidney disease (use *nephr/o*) ________________

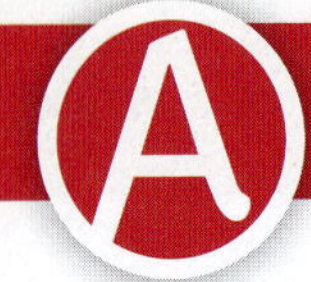

Learning Outcome 12.5 Exercises

7. involuntary contraction of the bladder (use *cyst/o*) ____________
8. disease of the testicles (use *orchi/o*) ____________
9. disease of the urinary tract ____________
10. abnormal hardening of a kidney ____________
11. hardening of the glomeruli ____________
12. downward displacement of a kidney ____________
13. inflammation of the kidneys involving primarily the glomeruli (use *nephr/o*) ____________
14. inflammation of the kidney and renal pelvis ____________
15. inflammation of the kidneys caused by stones ____________
16. inflammation of the bladder and urethra ____________
17. presence of pus and stones in the kidney (use *nephr/o*) ____________

EXERCISE 9 *Multiple-choice questions. Select the correct answer(s).*

1. Select all of the terms below that pertain to the urinary tract.
   - a. cystoma
   - b. cystospasm
   - c. epididymitis
   - d. glomerulopathy
   - e. hypernephroma
   - f. nephroma
   - g. orchitis
   - h. testicular carcinoma
2. Select all of the terms below that pertain to the male genitalia.
   - a. cystoma
   - b. cystospasm
   - c. epididymitis
   - d. glomerulopathy
   - e. hypernephroma
   - f. nephroma
   - g. orchitis
   - h. testicular carcinoma
3. The term *nephropathy* refers to
   - a. any cancer of the kidney
   - b. any cancer of the urinary tract
   - c. any disease of the bladder
   - d. any disease of the kidney
   - e. any disease of the urinary tract
4. Which of the following statements is true of the term *stress urinary incontinence?*
   - a. abbreviated SUI stress urinary incontinence
   - b. loss of bladder control caused by the application of external pressure
   - c. medical term for loss of bladder control due to excessive laughing, a hard cough, or something like that
   - d. would apply to the common phrase "I peed in my pants"
   - e. all of these

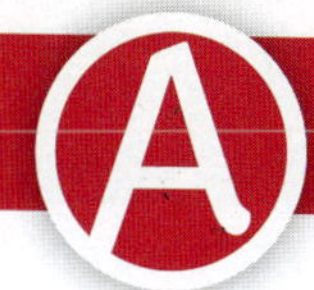

Learning Outcome 12.5 Exercises

5. An infection of the urinary tract is known as a
   a. urinary tract infection
   b. uropathy
   c. UTI
   d. urinary tract infection and UTI
   e. uropathy and UTI
6. A disease characterized by the formation of many fluid-filled cysts in the kidneys is known as
   a. hypernephroma
   b. nephrohypertrophy
   c. nephrolithiasis
   d. polycystic kidney disease
   e. renal cell carcinoma
7. The abnormal flow of urine from the bladder back into the ureter is known as
   a. urethrocystitis
   b. urinary tract infection
   c. uropathy
   d. vesicocele
   e. vesicoureteral reflux
8. The overexpansion of the blood vessels of the testicles, leading to a soft tumor, is called
   a. epididymo-orchitis
   b. pyeloureterectasia
   c. renal ischemia
   d. varicocele
   e. vesicocele
9. Select all of the choices below that pertain to the term *renal cell carcinoma.*
   a. also known as hypernephroma
   b. also known as nephrohypertrophy
   c. also known as polycystic kidney disease
   d. benign growth in the kidneys
   e. cancer of the kidneys
10. Select all of the choices below that pertain to the term *benign prostate hypertrophy.*
    a. also known as benign prostate hyperplasia
    b. also known as enlarged prostate
    c. literally, *friendly prostate overformation condition*
    d. literally, *friendly prostate overnourishment condition*
    e. noncancerous overdevelopment of the prostate

EXERCISE 10 *Briefly describe the difference between each pair of terms.*

1. cystolith, cystoma ______________________
2. cystoptosis, nephroptosis ______________________
3. nephromalacia, nephrosclerosis ______________________
4. pyelitis, pyelocystitis ______________________
5. prostatocystitis, prostatovesiculitis ______________________

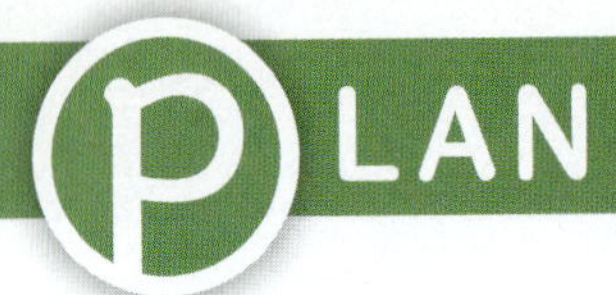

12.6 Treatments and Therapies

The main medicines used to treat the kidneys and urinary tract are focused on helping the patient urinate more (*diuretic*) or less (*antidiuretic*) often. If urinary control is a problem due to twitching of the muscle that holds back urine flow, an *antispasmodic* may be helpful.

Medicines that are specifically for men are very limited. They include medicine to help correct erectile dysfunction and testosterone, the male hormone, which is used in patients with low levels of the hormone. Patients may also choose to use liquids designed to kill sperm (*spermicides*) as a method of birth control; spermicides are available over the counter.

The most common nonsurgical procedure involving the urinary tract is bladder *catheterization*. A *catheter* is a small tube inserted into the bladder to help with urination or to get a urine sample.

The main nonsurgical treatment for the urinary tract is *dialysis*. Dialysis does the work of the kidneys when they have failed. Dialysis must be done regularly or the patient will die. The two types of dialysis involve either the inner lining of the abdomen (*peritoneal dialysis*) or a machine outside the body (*hemodialysis*). Another nonsurgical treatment in the urinary system is the use of sound waves to break up a stone in the urinary tract (*extracorporeal shock wave lithotripsy*).

Often, surgeries of the urinary tract help correct anatomical problems and restore normal urine flow. This can involve direct work on a part of the tract like the ureter (*ureteroplasty*) or urethra (*urethroplasty*). It could also involve making a new connection between two points in the tract, like a connection between the kidney and bladder (*nephrocystanastomosis*).

Another surgery of the kidneys is their complete removal (*nephrectomy*), which is often the main treatment for renal cell carcinoma. In men, the prostate is another organ that can be completely removed (*prostatectomy*) if cancerous. Part of the prostate may be removed through the urethra (*transurethral resection of the prostate*) when the prostate is enlarged and blocking urine flow. Newer, less invasive procedures for this include using a heated needle (*transurethral needle ablation*) to remove part of the prostate.

When a testicle rides high in the scrotum it may need to be fixed (*orchiopexy*) or removed altogether (*orchiectomy*). When removed, a fake testicle (*testicular prosthesis*) is sometimes placed in the scrotum.

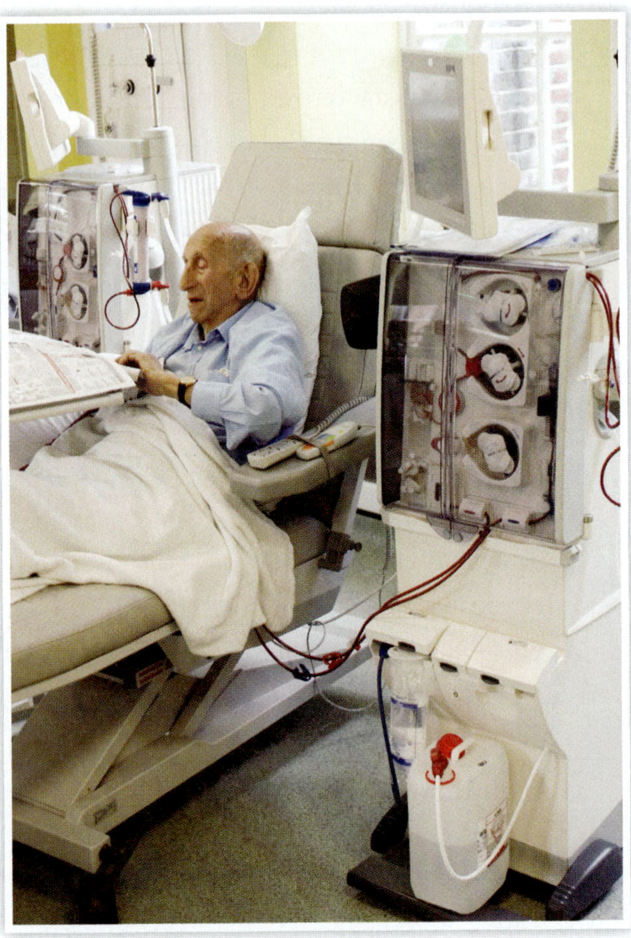

Hemodialysis uses a machine to do the work of kidneys that do not function as they should.

The most common procedure in males is the removal of the foreskin at birth (*circumcision*). While there are small medical benefits, the surgery is generally chosen for cultural or religious reasons. Circumcision is not recommended in patients with hypospadias or epispadias because the foreskin is used to surgically correct those conditions (*balanoplasty*). *Vasectomy* is another very common procedure. In the procedure, a surgeon cuts the vas deferens as a means of birth control. Occasionally, situations change, so a patient may want to reverse the procedure. Doing so is simple—reconnecting the two end of the vas deferens (*vasovasotomy*).

12.6 Treatments and Therapies

cystolithectomy

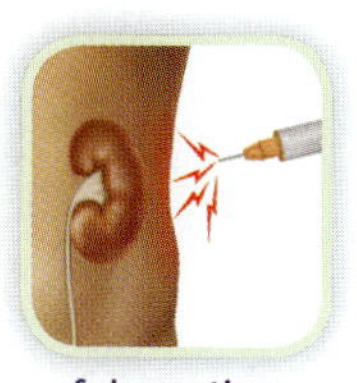

fulguration

urinary tract

Term	Word Analysis
antispasmodic AN-tee-spaz-MAW-dik **Definition** drug used to prevent spasms	anti / spasmod / ic against / involuntary contraction / pertaining to
cystectomy sis-TEK-toh-mee **Definition** surgical removal of the bladder	cyst / ec / tomy bladder / out / cut
cystolithectomy sis-toh-lih-THEK-toh-mee **Definition** surgical removal of a stone in the bladder	cysto / lith / ec / tomy bladder / stone / out / cut
cystostomy sis-TAW-stoh-mee **Definition** creation of an opening in the bladder	cysto / stom / y bladder / mouth / procedure
diuretic DAI-yur-IT-ik **Definition** agent that causes urination	di / uret / ic through / urine / pertaining to
extracorporeal shock wave lithotripsy (ESWL) EKS-trah-cor-POR-ee-al shok wayv LIH-thoh-TRIP-see **Definition** breakdown of kidney stones using sound waves generated outside the body	extra / corpore / al outside / body / pertaining to shock wave litho / tripsy shock wave stone / wear down procedure
fulguration FUL-gur-AY-shun **Definition** use of electric current to destroy tissue	from Latin, for *lightning*
heminephrectomy HEH-mee-neh-FREK-toh-mee **Definition** surgical removal of half a kidney	hemi / nephr / ec / tomy half / kidney / out / cut
heminephroureterectomy HEH-mee-NEH-froh-yoo-REE-ter-EK-toh-mee **Definition** surgical removal of half a kidney and a ureter	hemi / nephro / ureter / ec / tomy half / kidney / ureter / out / cut
hemodialysis HEE-moh-dai-AL-ah-sis **Definition** procedure for removing waste from the bloodstream	hemo / dia / lysis blood / through / loose
intracorporeal lithotripsy IN-trah-cor-POR-ee-al LIH-thoh-TRIP-see **Definition** breakdown of kidney stones using a device placed inside the body	intra / corpore / al litho / tripsy inside / body / pertaining to stone / wear down procedure

12.6 Treatments and Therapies

urinary tract *continued*

Term	Word Analysis
kidney dialysis KID-nee dai-AL-ah-sis	dia / lysis through / loose
Definition procedure for removing waste from the blood (a shorter name for hemodialysis) **Note:** The name comes from the fact that the procedure separates or loses *(lysis)* blood from waste by passing it through *(dia)* an external filter.	
laparonephrectomy LAP-ah-roh-neh-FREK-toh-mee	laparo / nephr / ec / tomy abdomen / kidney / out / cut
Definition surgical removal of a kidney through the abdomen	
lithectomy lih-THEK-toh-mee	lith / ec / tomy stone / out / cut
Definition surgical removal of a stone	
lithocystotomy LIH-thoh-SIS-TAW-toh-mee	litho / cysto / tomy stone / bladder / cut
Definition incision into the bladder to remove a stone	
lithonephrotomy LIH-thoh-nef-FRAW-toh-mee	litho / nephro / tomy stone / kidney / cut
Definition incision into a kidney to remove a stone	
lithotripsy LIH-thoh-TRIP-see	litho / tripsy stone / wear down procedure
Definition breakdown of a stone	
meatoplasty mee-AT-toh-PLAS-tee	meato / plasty opening / reconstruction
Definition surgical reconstruction of the opening of the urethra	
meatorrhaphy MEE-ah-TOR-ah-fee	meato / rrhaphy opening / suture
Definition suture of the opening of the urethra	
meatotomy MEE-ah-TAW-toh-mee	meato / tomy opening / cut
Definition incision into the opening of the urethra	
nephrectomy neh-FREK-toh-mee	nephr / ec / tomy kidney / out / cut
Definition surgical removal of a kidney through the abdomen	
nephrocystanastomosis NEH-froh-SIST-ah-NAS-tah-MOH-sis	nephro / cyst / ana / stom / osis kidney / bladder / up / mouth / condition
Definition opening of a passageway between a kidney and the bladder	
nephrolithotomy NEH-froh-lih-THAW-toh-mee	nephro / litho / tomy kidney / stone / cut
Definition incision into a kidney to remove a stone	

kidney dialysis

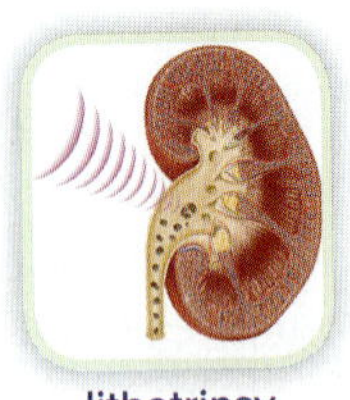

lithotripsy

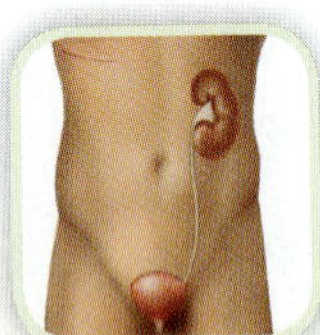

nephrectomy

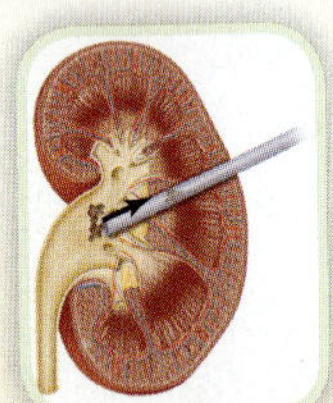

nephrolithotomy

12.6 Treatments and Therapies

urinary tract *continued*

Term	Word Analysis
nephropexy NEH-froh-PEK-see	nephro / pexy kidney / fixation
Definition surgical fixation of a kidney	
nephrorrhaphy neh-FROR-ah-fee	nephro / rrhaphy kidney / suture
Definition suture of a kidney	
nephrostomy neh-FRAW-stoh-mee	nephro / stom / y kidney / mouth / procedure
Definition creation of an opening in a kidney	
nephrotomy neh-FRAW-toh-mee	nephro / tomy kidney / cut
Definition incision into a kidney	
nephrotoxin NEH-froh-TOK-sin	nephro / toxin kidney / poison
Definition agent poisonous to the kidney	
nephroureterectomy NEH-froh-yoo-REE-ter-EK-toh-mee	nephro / ureter / ec / tomy kidney / ureter / out / cut
Definition surgical removal of a kidney and ureter	
pyelolithotomy PAI-el-oh-lih-THAW-toh-mee	pyelo / litho / tomy pelvis / stone / cut
Definition incision into a renal pelvis to remove a stone	
pyeloplasty PAI-el-oh-PLAS-tee	pyelo / plasty pelvis / reconstruction
Definition surgical reconstruction of a renal pelvis	
pyelostomy PAI-el-AW-stoh-mee	pyelo / stom / y pelvis / mouth / procedure
Definition creation of an opening in a renal pelvis	
pyelotomy PAI-el-AW-toh-mee	pyelo / tomy pelvis / cut
Definition incision into a renal pelvis	
renal angioplasty REE-nal AN-jee-oh-PLAS-tee	ren / al angio / plasty kidney / pertaining to vessel / reconstruction
Definition surgical reconstruction of a kidney blood vessel	
ureteroileostomy yoo-REE-ter-oh-IL-ee-AW-stoh-mee	uretero / ileo / stom / y ureter / ileum / mouth / procedure
Definition creation of an opening between a ureter and the ileum (a portion of the small intestine)	
ureteronephrectomy yoo-REE-ter-oh-neh-FREK-toh-mee	uretero / nephr / ec / tomy ureter / kidney / out / cut
Definition surgical removal of a kidney and ureter	

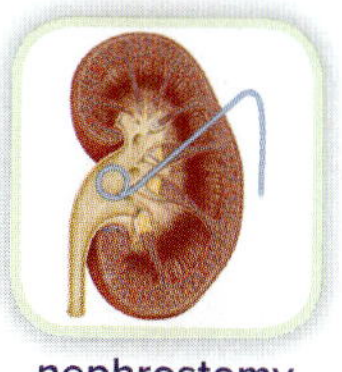
nephrostomy

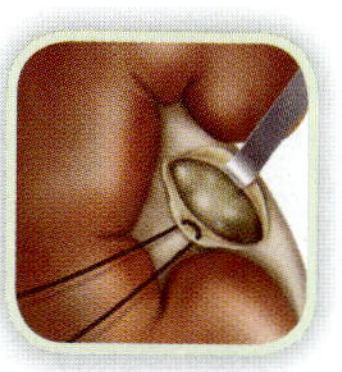
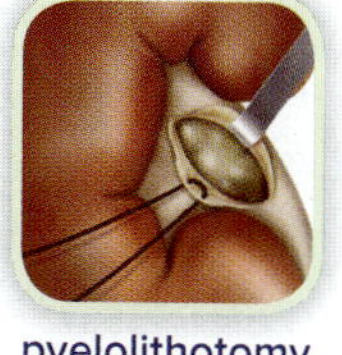
pyelolithotomy

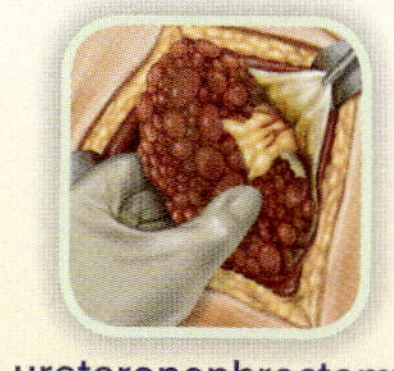
ureteronephrectomy

12.6 Treatments and Therapies

urinary tract *continued*

Term	Word Analysis
ureteroplasty yoo-REE-ter-oh-PLAS-tee **Definition** surgical recontruction of a ureter	uretero / plasty ureter / reconstruction
ureterorrhaphy yoo-REE-ter-OR-ah-fee **Definition** suture of a ureter	uretero / rrhaphy ureter / suture
urethrectomy yoo-ree-THREK-toh-mee **Definition** surgical removal of the urethra	urethr / ec / tomy urethra / out / cut
urethropexy yoo-REE-throh-PEK-see **Definition** surgical fixation of the urethra	urethro / pexy urethra / fixation
urethroplasty yoo-REE-throh-PLAS-tee **Definition** surgical reconstruction of the urethra	urethro / plasty urethra / reconstruction
urethrotomy yoo-ree-THRAW-toh-mee **Definition** incision into the urethra	urethro / tomy urethra / cut
urinary catheterization YUR-ih-NAR-ee KATH-eh-ter-ih-ZAY-shun **Definition** insertion of a catheter into the bladder to drain urine **NOTE:** The word *catheter* comes from Greek, for *to go inside.*	urin / ary — catheter / ization urine / pertaining to — catheter / procedure
urostomy yur-AW-stoh-mee **Definition** creation of an opening in the urinary tract, normally to divert urine flow away from a diseased bladder	uro /stom / y urine / mouth / procedure
vesicostomy VEH-sih-KAW-stoh-mee **Definition** creation of an opening in the bladder	vesico / stom / y bladder / mouth / procedure
vesicotomy VEH-sih-KAW-toh-mee **Definition** incision into the bladder	vesico / tomy bladder / cut

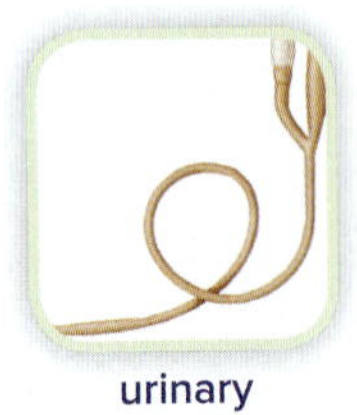
urinary catheterization

12.6 Treatments and Therapies

male genitalia

Term	Word Analysis
balanoplasty BAL-ah-noh-PLAS-tee **Definition** surgical reconstruction of the penis	balano / plasty penis / reconstruction
circumcision SIR-kum-SIH-zhun **Definition** surgical removal of the foreskin of the penis	circum / cision around / cut
epididymectomy EP-ih-DID-ih-MEK-toh-mee **Definition** surgical removal of the epididymis	epididym / ec / tomy epididymis / out / cut
epididymotomy EP-ih-DID-ih-MAW-toh-mee **Definition** incision into the epididymis	epididymo / tomy epididymis / cut
hydrocelectomy HAI-droh-seel-EK-toh-mee **Definition** surgical removal of a hydrocele	hydro / cel / ec / tomy water / hernia / out / cut
orchidectomy OR-kid-EK-toh-mee **Definition** surgical removal of a testicle	orchid / ec / tomy testicle / out / cut
orchidopexy OR-kid-oh-PEK-see **Definition** surgical fixation of a testicle	orchido / pexy testicle / fixation
orchidotomy OR-kid-AW-toh-mee **Definition** incision into a testicle	orchido / tomy testicle / cut
orchiectomy kee-EK-mee **Definition** surgical removal of a testicle	orchi / ec / tomy testicle / out / cut
orchiopexy OR-kee-oh-PEK-see **Definition** surgical fixation of a testicle	orchio / pexy testicle / fixation
orchioplasty OR-kee-oh-PLAS-tee **Definition** surgical reconstruction of a testicle	orchio / plasty testicle / reconstruction

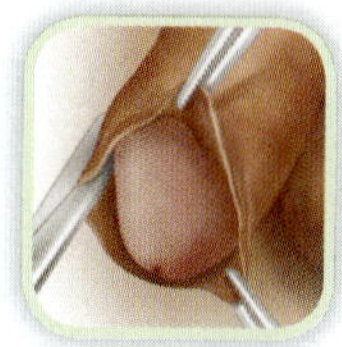
circumcision

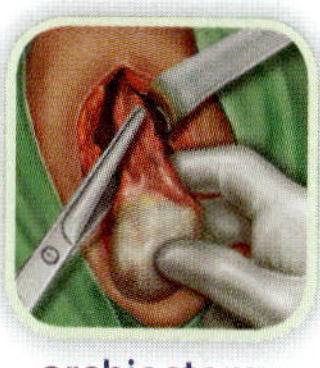
orchiectomy

12.6 Treatments and Therapies

male genitalia *continued*

Term	Word Analysis
prostatectomy PROS-tat-TEK-toh-mee	**prostat / ec / tomy** prostate / out / cut
Definition surgical removal of the prostate	
prostatolithotomy pros-TAT-oh-lih-THAW-toh-mee	**prostato / litho / tomy** prostate / stone / cut
Definition incision into the prostate to remove a stone	
prostatovesiculectomy pros-TAT-oh-veh-SIK-yoo-LEK-toh-mee	**prostato / vesicul / ec / tomy** prostate / bladder / out / cut
Definition surgical removal of the prostate and seminal vesicles **Note:** Here, the root *vesicul* refers *not* to the urinary bladder but instead to the small seminal vesicles, or bladders that hold seminal fluid.	
spermicide SPER-mih-sahyd	**spermi / cide** sperm / kill
Definition agent that kills sperm	
spermolytic SPER-moh-LIH-tik	**spermo / lytic** sperm / loose
Definition agent that kills sperm	
transurethral resection of the prostate (TURP)	**trans / urethr / al re / sect / ion** through / urethra / pertaining to back / cut / procedure
Definition procedure of removing all or part of the prostate by the insertion of a resectoscope into the urethra	
vasectomy vah-SEK-toh-mee	**vas / ec / tomy** vessel / out / cut
Definition surgical removal of the vas deferens	
vasovasostomy VAS-oh-vah-SAW-stoh-mee	**vaso / vaso / stom / y** vessel / vessel / mouth / procedure
Definition creation of an opening between two vessels; this is the technical term for a vasectomy reversal	
vesiculectomy veh-SIK-yoo-LEK-toh-mee	**vesicul / ec / tomy** bladder / out / cut
Definition surgical removal of the seminal vesicles **Note:** See the note for prostatovesiculectomy above to see how *vesiculo* refers not to the bladder but to seminal vesicles.	

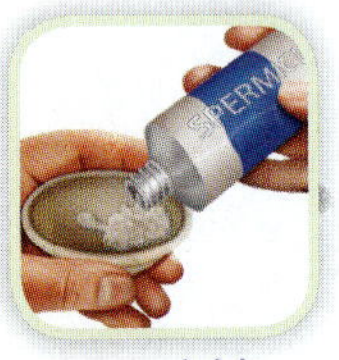
spermicide

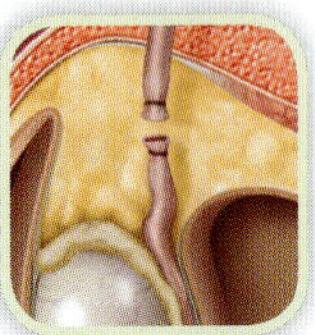
vasectomy

Learning Outcome 12.6 Exercises

PRONUNCIATION

EXERCISE 1 *Break down the following words into syllables.*

EXAMPLE: synesthesia *syn | es | the | sia*

1. orchiopexy ______
2. urethropexy ______
3. nephropexy ______
4. orchidopexy ______
5. lithotripsy ______
6. nephrotoxin ______
7. urethrotomy ______
8. vesicostomy ______
9. ureteroplasty ______
10. balanoplasty ______
11. urethrectomy ______
12. vesiculectomy ______
13. prostatectomy ______
14. kidney dialysis ______
15. heminephrectomy ______
16. nephrolithotomy ______
17. vasovasostomy ______
18. ureteroileostomy ______
19. ureterorrhaphy ______
20. epididymotomy ______
21. intracorporeal lithotripsy ______

EXERCISE 2 *Indicate which syllable is emphasized when pronounced.*

EXAMPLE: bronchitis bron**chi**tis

1. spermicide ______
2. vasectomy ______
3. lithectomy ______
4. cystectomy ______
5. nephrectomy ______
6. urostomy ______
7. cystostomy ______
8. nephrostomy ______
9. nephrotomy ______
10. cystolithectomy ______
11. nephrorrhaphy ______

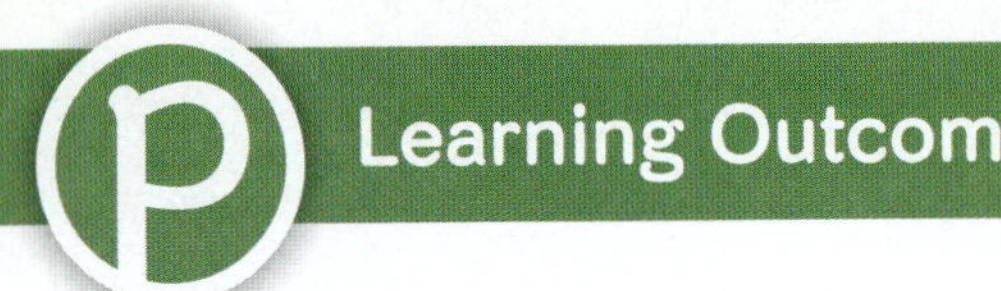

Learning Outcome 12.6 Exercises

TRANSLATION

EXERCISE 3 *Break down the following words into their component parts.*

EXAMPLE: nasopharyngoscope *naso | pharyngo | scope*

1. nephrotoxin ______
2. urostomy ______
3. orchiopexy ______
4. urethroplasty ______
5. antispasmodic ______
6. meatorrhaphy ______
7. nephrorrhaphy ______
8. ureterorrhaphy ______
9. spermolytic ______
10. vesiculectomy ______
11. hydrocelectomy ______
12. vasovasostomy ______
13. pyelolithotomy ______
14. lithonephrotomy ______
15. nephrolithotomy ______
16. prostatolithotomy ______
17. ureteroileostomy ______
18. heminephrectomy ______
19. laparonephrectomy ______
20. cystolithectomy ______
21. hemodialysis ______
22. circumcision ______

EXERCISE 4 *Underline and define the roots from this chapter in the following terms.*

1. spermicide ______
2. lithotripsy ______
3. ureteroplasty ______
4. orchioplasty ______
5. balanoplasty ______
6. meatoplasty ______
7. urethropexy ______
8. nephropexy ______
9. orchidopexy ______

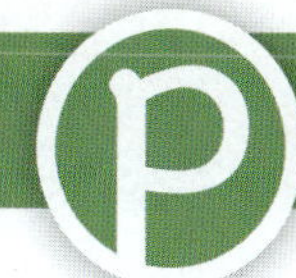

Learning Outcome 12.6 Exercises

10. cystostomy ______________________________
11. nephrostomy ______________________________
12. pyelostomy ______________________________
13. vesicostomy ______________________________
14. epididymotomy ______________________________
15. diuretic ______________________________
16. renal angioplasty ______________________________
17. intracorporeal lithotripsy ______________________________
18. transurethral resection ______________________________
19. urinary catheterization ______________________________
20. extracorporeal shock wave lithotripsy ______________________________
21. heminephroureterectomy (2 roots) ______________________________
22. prostatovesiculectomy (2 roots) ______________________________
23. nephrocystanastomosis (2 roots) ______________________________

EXERCISE 5 *Match the term on the left with its definition on the right.*

Term	Definition
____ 1. circumcision	a. agent that causes urination
____ 2. kidney dialysis	b. insertion of a catheter into the bladder to drain urine
____ 3. urinary catheterization	c. procedure for removing waste from the bloodstream
____ 4. diuretic	d. procedure for removing waste from the blood (a shorter name for hemodialysis)
____ 5. hemodialysis	e. procedure of removing all or part of the prostate by the insertion of a resectoscope into the urethra
____ 6. vasovasostomy	f. surgical removal of the foreskin of the penis
____ 7. transurethral resection of the prostate	g. breakdown of kidney stones using a device placed inside the body
____ 8. intracorporeal lithotripsy	h. breakdown of kidney stones using sound waves generated outside the body
____ 9. extracorporeal shock wave lithotripsy	i. creation of an opening between two vessels; the technical term for a vasectomy reversal
____ 10. fulguration	j. use of electric current to destroy tissue

EXERCISE 6 *Fill in the blanks.*

1. *meatotomy:* incision into ______________________________
2. *nephrotomy:* incision into ______________________________
3. *pyelotomy:* incision into ______________________________
4. *urethrotomy:* incision into ______________________________
5. *vesicotomy:* incision into ______________________________
6. *epididymotomy:* incision into ______________________________

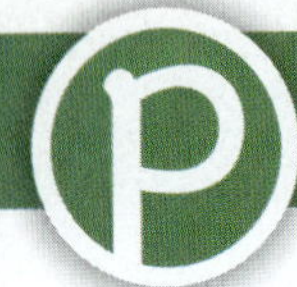

Learning Outcome 12.6 Exercises

7. *orchidotomy:* incision into ______
8. *cystectomy:* surgical removal of the ______
9. *lithectomy:* surgical removal of the ______
10. *nephrectomy:* surgical removal of the ______
11. *urethrectomy:* surgical removal of the ______
12. *epididymectomy:* surgical removal of the ______
13. *orchidectomy:* surgical removal of the ______
14. *orchiectomy:* surgical removal of the ______
15. *prostatectomy:* surgical removal of the ______
16. *vasectomy:* surgical removal of the ______
17. *nephroureterectomy:* surgical removal of a(n) ______ and ______
18. *ureteronephrectomy:* surgical removal of a(n) ______ and ______
19. *prostatovesiculectomy:* surgical removal of a(n) ______ and ______

EXERCISE 7 *Translate the following terms as literally as possible.*

EXAMPLE: nasopharyngoscope *an instrument for looking at the nose and throat*

1. urethrotomy ______
2. vasectomy ______
3. orchidopexy ______
4. meatorrhaphy ______
5. ureterorrhaphy ______
6. pyelostomy ______
7. lithotripsy ______
8. vesiculectomy ______
9. epididymotomy ______
10. spermicide ______
11. antispasmodic ______
12. cystolithectomy ______
13. prostatolithotomy ______
14. prostatovesiculectomy ______
15. renal angioplasty ______
16. hydrocelectomy ______
17. ureteroileostomy ______
18. heminephroureterectomy ______
19. nephrocystanastomosis ______

Learning Outcome 12.6 Exercises

GENERATION

EXERCISE 8 *Build a medical term from the information provided.*

EXAMPLE: inflammation of the sinuses *sinusitis*

1. incision into the bladder (use *vesic/o*) ______________________
2. incision into a testicle (use *orchid/o*) ______________________
3. incision into the opening (of the urethra) ______________________
4. creation of an opening in the bladder (use *cyst/o*) ______________________
5. creation of an opening in the bladder (use *vesic/o*) ______________________
6. surgical removal of the epididymis ______________________
7. surgical removal of the urethra ______________________
8. surgical removal of the prostate ______________________
9. surgical removal of a kidney and ureter ______________________
10. surgical reconstruction of a ureter ______________________
11. surgical reconstruction of the opening (of the urethra) ______________________
12. surgical reconstruction of a renal pelvis ______________________
13. surgical reconstruction of the penis ______________________
14. surgical fixation of the urethra ______________________

EXERCISE 9 *Multiple-choice questions. Select the correct answer(s).*

1. The surgical removal of a kidney through the abdomen is known as
   a. abdominonephrectomy
   b. fulguration
   c. heminephrectomy
   d. laparonephrectomy
   e. meatonephrectomy
2. An incision into the renal pelvis is called a
   a. renal incision
   b. pyelectomy
   c. pyelotomy
   d. nephrotomy
   e. nephrectomy
3. A *spermolytic* is
   a. an agent that assists in conception by making sperm meet with an egg for fertilzation
   b. an agent that assists the testicles in the formation of sperm
   c. an agent that creates sperm
   d. an agent that kills sperm
   e. none of these

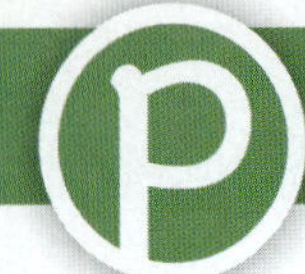

Learning Outcome 12.6 Exercises

4. Which of the following statements is true of the term *kidney dialysis*?
   a. procedure for removing waste from the blood
   b. shorter name for hemodialysis
   c. its name comes from the fact that the procedure separates or looses (*lysis*) blood from waste by passing it through *(dia)* an external filter
   d. all of these
   e. none of these
5. Select all of the following choices that pertain to the term *urostomy*.
   a. creation of an opening in the bladder
   b. creation of an opening in the urinary tract
   c. literally, *bladder mouth procedure*
   d. literally, *urine mouth procedure*
   e. procedure normally used to divert urine flow away from a diseased bladder
6. Select all of the following choices that pertain to the term *fulguration*.
   a. from Latin, for *coffee*
   b. from Latin, for *lightning*
   c. the use of electric current to destroy tissue
   d. the use of electric current to repair tissue
   e. none of these
7. Select all of the following terms that pertain to the urinary tract.
   a. cystectomy
   b. epididymectomy
   c. lithectomy
   d. nephrectomy
   e. orchidectomy
   f. prostatectomy
   g. urethrectomy
   h. vesicotomy
8. Select all of the following terms that pertain to the male genitalia.
   a. cystectomy
   b. epididymectomy
   c. lithectomy
   d. nephrectomy
   e. orchidectomy
   f. prostatectomy
   g. urethrectomy
   h. vesicotomy

EXERCISE 10 *Briefly describe the difference between each pair of terms.*

1. ureteroplasty, urethroplasty ____________________
2. balanoplasty, orchioplasty ____________________
3. nephrostomy, nephrotomy ____________________
4. orchiectomy, orchiopexy ____________________
5. heminephrectomy, nephrectomy ____________________
6. lithocystotomy, lithonephrotomy ____________________
7. nephrolithotomy, pyelolithotomy ____________________

12.7 Abbreviations

Abbreviations provide a shorthand way of referring to things that either recur often or are too long to write out. When dealing with the urinary tract and male genitalia, these terms can include lab work (UA), diagnostic procedures (DRE), common complaints (SUI), diagnoses (UTI, BPH), or treatments (ESWL, TURP).

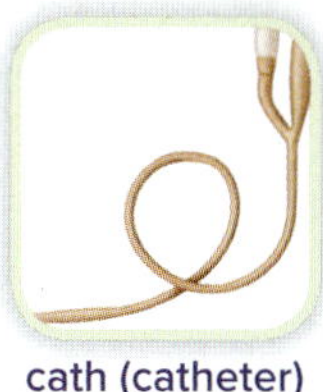

cath (catheter)

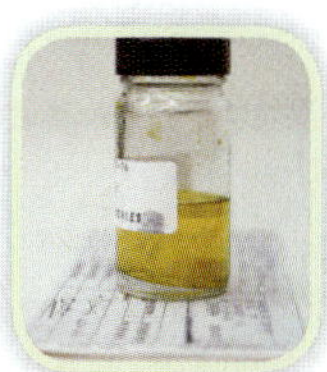

UA (urinalysis)

urinary tract

Abbreviation	Definition
BUN	blood urea nitrogen
Bx	biopsy
cath	catheter
ESWL	extracorporeal shock wave lithotripsy
HD	hemodialysis
I&O	intake and output
IVP	intravenous pyelogram
IVU	intravenous urogram
KUB	kidneys, ureters, bladder
OAB	overactive bladder
PKD	polycystic kidney disease
RP	retrograde pyelogram
SUI	stress urinary incontinence
UA	urinalysis
UTI	urinary tract infection
VCUG	voiding cystourethrogram
VUR	vesicoureteral reflux

DRE (digital rectal exam)

male genitalia

Abbreviation	Definition
BPH	benign prostate hyperplasia
DRE	digital rectal exam
ED	erectile dysfunction
PSA	prostate-specific antigen
STD/STI	sexually transmitted disease, sexually transmitted infection
TURP	transurethral resection of the prostate

Learning Outcome 12.7 Exercises

EXERCISE 1 *Define the following abbreviations.*

1. STD ______
2. STI ______
3. cath ______
4. ED ______
5. UTI ______
6. IVP ______
7. IVU ______
8. UA ______
9. HD ______
10. KUB ______
11. RP ______
12. VCUG ______
13. PSA ______
14. OAB ______

EXERCISE 2 *Give the abbreviations for the following definitions.*

1. biopsy ______
2. catheter ______
3. digital rectal exam ______
4. blood urea nitrogen ______
5. intravenous urogram ______
6. kidneys, ureters, bladder ______
7. polycystic kidney disease ______
8. stress urinary incontinence ______
9. benign prostate hyperplasia ______
10. transurethral resection of the prostate ______
11. voiding cystourethrogram ______
12. extracorporeal shock wave lithotripsy ______
13. intake and output ______

Learning Outcome 12.7 Exercises

EXERCISE 3 *Match the abbreviation on the left with its full definition on its right.*

______	1. UTI	a. abnormal flow of urine from the bladder back into the ureters
______	2. UA	b. analysis of the urine
______	3. DRE	c. disease characterized by the formation of many fluid-filled cysts in the kidneys
______	4. HD	d. examination of the prostate using a finger inserted into the rectum
______	5. BPH	e. image of the renal pelvis produced by injecting a contrast dye from the bladder to the kidney
______	6. PKD	f. infection of the urinary tract
______	7. BUN	g. loss of bladder control caused by the application of external pressure
______	8. RP	h. nitrogen in the blood in the form of urea; it is the product of the breakdown of amino acids for energy
______	9. SUI	i. noncancerous overdevelopment of the prostate, also known as an enlarged prostate
______	10. VUR	j. procedure for removing waste from the bloodstream

EXERCISE 4 *Multiple-choice questions. Select the correct answer(s).*

1. IVP stands for *intravenous pyelogram.* Which is the correct breakdown of the term?
   a. *intra* (inside) + *venous* (vein) + *pyelo* (renal pelvis) + *gram* (record)
   b. *intra* (outside) + *venous* (vein) + *pyelo* (renal pelvis) + *gram* (record)
   c. *intra* (outside) + *venous* (vein) + *pyelo* (bladder) + *gram* (record)
   d. *intra* (inside) + *venous* (vein) + *pyelo* (bladder) + *gram* (record)
   e. *intra* (inside) + *venous* (vein) + *pyelo* (kidney) + *gram* (record)

2. VUR stands for *vesicoureteral flux.* Which is the correct breakdwn of the term?
   a. *vesico* (bladder) + *ureteral* (testicle) + *reflux* (flow back)
   b. *vesico* (bladder) + *ureteral* (ureter) + *reflux* (flow back)
   c. *vesico* (kidney) + *ureteral* (ureter) + *reflux* (flow back)
   d. *vesico* (seminal vesicle) + *ureteral* (testicle) + *reflux* (flow back)
   e. *vesico* (seminal vesicle) + *ureteral* (ureter) + *reflux* (flow back)

3. TURP stands for
   a. topographical ureteral retrograde procedure
   b. topographical urethral retrograde procedure
   c. transureteral resection of the prostate
   d. transurethral resection of the prostate
   e. transurethral retrograde pyelogram

12.8 Electronic Health Records

Consult Note

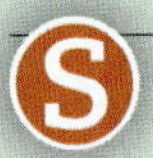
Subjective

Reason for Consult: **urinary retention**

HPI: Mr. Johnson is a 57-year-old male with a 2-month history of difficulty **voiding.** He reports **urgency** and **frequency.** He has had increasing problems with a weak urinary stream. The symptoms have progressed to include mild abdominal discomfort and **erectile dysfunction**. He denies any **incontinence, hematuria, balanorrhea, orchiodynia,** or trauma. He has not tried any medicines at this point.

PMHx: Hypercholestrolemia–currently controlled with diet. Positive history of gonococcal **urethritis** 3 years previously. No history of **urolithiasis.**

Objective

Physical Exam

Vitals: T 98.6; HR: 84; RR: 24; BP: 124/90.

Gen: Alert, well-appearing man in no apparent distress.

HEENT: Normocephalic. Pupils equal, round, and reactive to light and accommodation. Tympanic membranes normal. Mucous membranes moist and pink.

Neck: Supple. No lymphadenopathy. No jugulovenous distention.

Cardiovascular: Regular in rate and rhythm without murmur, gallops, or rubs.

Resp: Clear to auscultation bilaterally.

Abd: Mild distention. Fullness and discomfort of **suprapubic** area.

Neuro: Normal reflexes and strength of the lower extremities, normal sphincter tone.

Gross appearance of penis: No **meatal stenosis,** easily retractable foreskin, no penile ulcers.

DRE: Enlarged prostate of 3 finger breadths. No **prostatorrhea.**

Labs: Elevated PSA. UA normal. UCx negative. BMP normal.

Imaging:

Transabdominal ultrasound revealed significant **postvoid** residual. Consistent with **bladder outlet obstruction.**

Cystoscopy to r/o **urethral stricture** was normal.

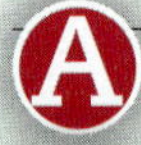
Assessment

Mr. Johnson has **benign prostatic hyperplasia**.

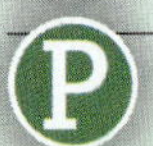
Plan

Plan:

We will be starting initial treatment of fluid intake restriction and medicine. I explained to Mr. Johnson that if he fails this therapy, the next step would be surgical. There are several options available. I discussed these options, including **TURP** versus open **prostatectomy** versus **transurethral incision of prostate** (TUIP). Mr. Johnson will return to my clinic for follow-up in 6 weeks.

–Jonas Wallin, MD

Learning Outcome 12.8 Exercises

EXERCISE 1 *Match the term on the left with its definition on the right.*

____ 1. urethritis
____ 2. prostatomegaly
____ 3. voiding
____ 4. incontinence
____ 5. prostatectomy
____ 6. orchiodynia
____ 7. benign prostate hyperplasia
____ 8. hematuria
____ 9. balanorrhea
____ 10. meatal stenosis

a. abnormal enlargement of the prostate
b. another term for urination
c. bloody urination
d. discharge from the penis
e. inability to control urination
f. inflammation of the urethra
g. narrowing of the opening of the urethra
h. noncancerous overdevelopment of the prostate, also known as an enlarged prostate
i. surgical removal of the prostate
j. testicle pain

EXERCISE 2 *Match the abbreviation on the left with its definition on the right.*

____ 1. ED
____ 2. UA
____ 3. BPH
____ 4. DRE
____ 5. TURP

a. benign prostate hyperplasia
b. digital rectal exam
c. erectile dysfunction
d. transurethral resection of the prostate
e. urinalysis

EXERCISE 3 *Fill in the blanks.*

1. ____ ____ ____: History of present illness
   a. The patient's name: ____
   b. The patient's age: ____
   c. The patient's gender: ____
   d. The patient's CC: difficulty ____ (urinating), the symptoms of which have progressed to include abdominal discomfort and *erectile dysfunction* (give abbreviation: ____)
   e. The patient denies *incontinence* (give definition: ____), *hematuria* (give definition: ____), *balanorrhea* (give definition: ____), or *orchiodynia* (give definition: ____)
2. PMHx: Past Medical ____
   a. Positive history of gonococcal *urethritis* (inflammation of the ____)
   b. No history of *urololithiasis* (presence of ____ in the urinary system)
3. PE: ____ Exam
   a. DRE: (define abbreviation: ____ ____ ____)
   b. No ____ (discharge from the prostate)

Learning Outcome 12.8 Exercises

EXERCISE 4 *True or false questions. Indicate true answers with a T and false answers with an F.*

1. Mr. Johnson is experiencing ED. ________
2. Mr. Johnson complains of blood in the urine as well as an inability to control his urination. ________
3. Mr. Johnson's prostate is a normal size. ________
4. The patient's urinalysis was abnormal. ________
5. The patient has BPH. ________
6. The patient has cancer and will need to have his prostate removed. ________

EXERCISE 5 *Multiple-choice questions. Select the correct answer(s).*

1. A *cystoscopy* is a
   a. procedure for examining the bladder
   b. procedure for examining the urinary tract
   c. recording or image of the bladder
   d. recording or image of the urinary tract
2. Mr. Johnson's imaging revealed "significant *postvoid* residual." The term *postvoid* refers to
   a. after urination
   b. before urination
   c. the urinary tract
   d. the urine itself
3. The patient does not have a past medical history of *urolithiasis.* Which of the following is a correct breakdown of this term?
   a. *uro* (urinary tract) + *lith* (stones) + *iasis* (inflammation)
   b. *uro* (urinary tract) + *lith* (stones) + *iasis* (presence)
   c. *uro* (urinary tract) + *lith* (tumor) + *iasis* (inflammation)
   d. *uro* (urinary tract) + *lith* (tumor) + *iasis* (presence)
4. One of the patient's surgical options includes a *transurethral incision of prostate* (TUIP). Which of the following is a correct breakdown of the term *transurethral?*
   a. *trans* (through) + *urethra* (urethra)
   b. *trans* (around) + *urethra* (urethra)
   c. *trans* (out) + *urethra* (urethra)
   d. *trans* (inside) + *urethra* (urethra)
5. The patient has a history of *hypercholesterolemia.* Which of the following is a correct breakdown of this term?
   a. *hyper* (over) + *cholesterol* (cholesterol) + *emia* (blood condition)
   b. *hyper* (over) + *cholesterol* (cholesterol) + *emia* (urine condition)
   c. *hyper* (under) + *cholesterol* (cholesterol) + *emia* (blood condition)
   d. *hyper* (under) + *cholesterol* (cholesterol) + *emia* (urine condition)

Urology Clinic Note

Subjective:

Mr. Hector Joules presents to the office today for swelling in his right testicle. The swelling has been present for the past month. He reports **orchialgia,** described as a dull ache in the testicle. He also has had a feeling of heaviness in his abdomen. He hasn't had any recent injury to the area. He denies risky sexual behavior, **urethrorrhea, dysuria, nocturia, polyuria.**

PMHx: **Cryptorchidism** as a child.

PSHx: **Orchipexy** at 4 years.

Objective:

Vital signs: Temp: 100.0; HR: 62; RR: 22; BP: 102/72.

General: Well developed, well nourished, in no acute distress. Alert and oriented.

HEENT: Normocephalic atraumatic. Pupils equal, round, and reactive to light and accommodation. Mucous membranes moist and pink. Nares patent. Normal ear canals and tympanic membranes.

CV: Regular in rate and rhythm without murmurs.

Resp: Clear to auscultation bilaterally. No wheezes, rales, or rhonchi.

Abd: Soft, nontender, nondistended. Hepatomegaly 2 cm below costal margin. No splenomegaly.

GU: Right-sided 2.5 cm solid, firm testicular mass. Immobile and fixed to testicle. Nontender to palpation.

Lymph nodes: Enlarged supraclavicular and inguinal nodes.

Tests: Testicular U/S.

Assessment:

This is a 24-year-old male with a right-sided testicular mass. Given the u/s results, this is most likely testicular carcinoma. The differential diagnosis also includes **epididymitis, testicular torsion, hydrocele, spermatocele,** and **varicocele.**

Plan:

Since there is significant risk for cancer, we will schedule Mr. Joules for a radical **orchidectomy.** We will send samples to Pathology to confirm the diagnosis and staging. I outlined the general treatment and follow-up plan with Mr. Joules. Today, we will check a sperm count to establish a baseline, as **azoospermia/oligospermia** are risks of surgery.

–Priscilla Pascal, MD

Learning Outcome 12.8 Exercises

EXERCISE 6 *Match the term on the left with its definition on the right.*

_____ 1. testicular carcinoma
_____ 2. orchialgia
_____ 3. orchidectomy
_____ 4. urethrorrhea
_____ 5. epididymitis
_____ 6. dysuria
_____ 7. nocturia
_____ 8. polyuria
_____ 9. cryptorchidism
_____ 10. orchiopexy
_____ 11. hydrocele
_____ 12. varicocele
_____ 13. spermatocele
_____ 14. azoospermia
_____ 15. oligospermia

a. fluid-filled mass in a testicle
b. hernia or distention of the epididymis caused by sperm cells
c. condition characterized by lack of living sperm
d. condition characterized by low sperm production
e. discharge from the urethra
f. excessive urination
g. hidden testicle
h. inflammation of the epididymis
i. nighttime urination
j. overexpansion of the blood vessels of the testicles, leading to a soft tumor
k. painful urination
l. surgical fixation of a testicle
m. surgical removal of a testicle
n. testicle pain
o. testicular cancer

EXERCISE 7 *Fill in the blanks.*

1. The patient's name: ____________________
2. The patient's age: ____________________
3. The patient's gender: ____________________
4. The patient's temperature: ____________________
5. Subjective
   a. The patient reports *orchialgia* (give definition: ____________________)
   b. The patient denies *urethrorrhea* (give definition: ____________________), *dysuria* (give definition: ____________________), *nocturia* (give definition: ____________________), or *polyuria* (give definition: ____________________)
6. PMHx: Past Medical ____________________
   a. ____________________ (hidden testicle) as a child
7. PSHX: Past ____________________ History
   a. *orchiopexy* (give definition: ____________________) at 4 years

Learning Outcome 12.8 Exercises

EXERCISE 8 *True or false questions. Indicate true answers with a T and false answers with an F.*

1. The patient does not have painful or excessive urination. ________
2. Mr. Joules most likely has testicular cancer. ________
3. The patient will be able to keep both of his testicles. ________
4. Lack of living sperm is one risk of the recommended surgery. ________

EXERCISE 9 *Multiple-choice questions. Select the correct answer(s).*

1. Which of the following symptoms is the patient reporting?
   a. discharge from the urethra
   b. excessive urination
   c. nighttime urination
   d. pain in the testicle
   e. painful urination
2. Which of the following choices is NOT part of the differential diagnosis?
   a. fluid-filled mass in the testicle
   b. hernia or distention of the epididymis caused by sperm cells
   c. inflammation of the epididymis
   d. noncancerous overdevelopment of the prostate
   e. overexpansion of the blood vessels of the testicles, leading to a soft tumor
3. Which of the following choices is NOT part of the patient's plan?
   a. a test to determine the patient's live sperm count
   b. a test to determine the patient's sperm production
   c. biopsy of a testicle
   d. surgical removal of a testicle
   e. none of these

Discharge Summary

Patient: Susan Nesbit
Date of Admission: 7/7/2015
Date of Discharge: 7/17/2015

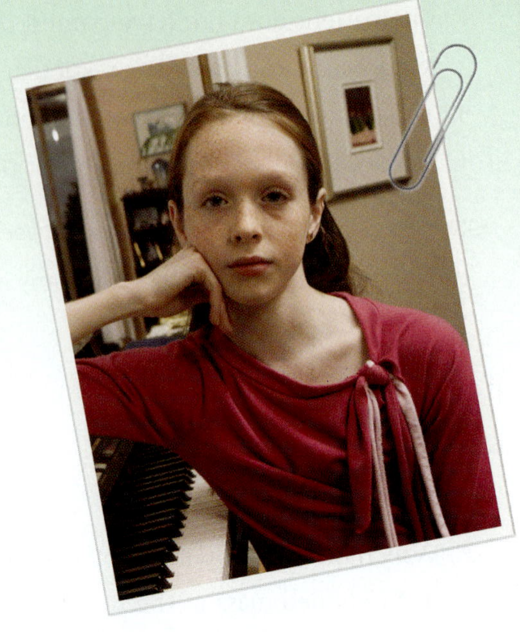

Admission Diagnosis

1. **Dysuria**
2. Fever

Discharge Diagnosis

1. **Pyelonephritis**
2. **Perinephric Abscess**

Discharge Condition:
Stable

Consultations
Nephrology
Urology

Procedures

1. U/S guided percutaneous **renal** needle aspiration with drain placement.

Labs
Admission labs: UA: **Pyuria:** >20 wbcs; **Hematuria:** 3+ blood; **Albuminuria:** 1+ protein.
Urine culture: *E. coli.*
Blood culture: *E. coli.*
Discharge labs: UA normal. Urine culture normal.

Imaging
VCUG: No **vesicoureteral reflux** noted.
RUS: No **hydronephrosis** noted. Normal.
Spiral CT of kidneys on day 3 of admission revealed perinephric abscess formation of the left kidney.

HPI
Miss Susan Nesbit is a 12-year-old female who first visited her primary care provider for **dysuria.** A **UA** was ordered, but the patient could not urinate in the office. She took the UA cup home, but did not return with the sample. The next day, Susan's dysuria worsened, and she developed a fever of 102.3°F, as well as vomiting and **hematuria,** so she returned to the clinic. A urinalysis performed in the office revealed significant **pyuria, hematuria,** and **albuminuria.** Since Susan was not able to keep any fluids down, her primary care provider sent her to the emergency department for evaluation for admission.

Discharge Summary *continued*

Hospital Course

On arrival to the ED, Susan was alert and oriented, but she looked a little pale and tired. She was treated with IVF for dehydration and given antipyretics for her fever. Within an hour, she had improved some, but given her inability to tolerate PO, the pediatric on-call physician recommended that she be admitted. She was admitted for a UTI and treated with IV antibiotics, and a urine culture was sent. On hospital day 2, her fever had improved, and she was looking better overall. Unfortunately, on hospital day 3, Susan's fever returned, and she looked acutely ill.

A spiral CT of Susan's abdomen and pelvis showed a developing perinephric abscess. Both nephrology and urology were consulted at that time, and they both agreed that the best treatment option would be needle aspiration with drain placement. She was taken to the OR, and the drain was placed. Fluid collection from the abscess was sent for culture.

Susan tolerated the procedure well and was admitted to the PICU. She continued IV antibiotics through her PICU course. After 5 days with the drain, the discharge had decreased significantly, so we repeated a spiral CT to confirm clearing of the abscess. The CT was normal, so the drain was removed and Susan was transferred to the regular pediatric wing. A renal ultrasound was also normal, as was a vesicocystourethrogram. Susan switched to oral antibiotcs and was discharged home.

Discharge Physical Examination
VS
Temp: 98.6; RR: 24; HR: 86; BP: 100/64.
General: WDWN. Alert.
HEENT: PERRLA, TMs normal. Mucous membranes moist and pink.
CV: RRR.
RESP: CTA.
Abdomen: Soft, nondistended, no CVA tenderness. No suprapubic tenderness.
Skin: Warm, pink.

Activity

No restrictions. Diet No restrictions.

Meds

Antibiotics.

Follow-Up Appointments
Primary care provider: 1 week
Urology: 2 weeks
Nephrology: 1 month

–Dictated by Jennifer Wong, DO

Learning Outcome 12.8 Exercises

EXERCISE 10 *Match the term on the left with its definition on the right.*

_____	1. urology	a.	abnormal flow of urine from the bladder back into the ureters
_____	2. nephrology	b.	bloody urination
_____	3. dysuria	c.	inflammation of the kidney and renal pelvis
_____	4. hematuria	d.	kidney condition caused by the obstruction of urine flow
_____	5. pyuria	e.	painful urination
_____	6. albuminuria	f.	protein in the urine
_____	7. pyelonephritis	g.	pus in the urine
_____	8. hydronephrosis	h.	study of the kidneys
_____	9. vesicoureteral reflux	i.	study of the urinary tract

EXERCISE 11 *Fill in the blanks.*

1. Admission diagnosis
   a. *Dysuria* (give definition: ____)
2. Discharge diagnosis
   a. *Pyelonephritis* (give definition: ____)
3. Consultations
   a. *Nephrology* (study of the ____)
   b. *Urology* (study of the ____)
4. Labs: UA (give definition for abbreviation: _______________________________________)
   a. *pyuria* (_______________________ in urine)
   b. *hematuria* (_______________________ in urine)
   c. *albuminuria* (_______________________ in urine)

EXERCISE 12 *True or false questions. Indicate true answers with a T and false answers with an F.*

1. Susan's imaging revealed that she has vesicoureteral reflux. _________
2. On arrival to the ED, Susan was treated with intravenous fluids. _________
3. Susan could tolerate oral food and drink upon her arrival to the ED. _________
4. Susan was admitted to the hospital for a urinary tract infection. _________
5. Susan's imaging revealed a kidney condition caused by the obstruction of urine flow. _________

EXERCISE 13 *Multiple-choice questions. Select the correct answer(s).*

1. According to the in-clinic urinalysis, which of the following was NOT present in Susan's urine?
   a. blood
   b. protein
   c. pus
   d. sugar
   e. all of these were present in Susan's urine

Learning Outcome 12.8 Exercises

2. According to the discharge diagnosis, Susan had a *perinephric abscess*. Which of the following choices is a correct breakdown of the term *perinephric*?
   a. *peri* (around) + *nephric* (bladder)
   b. *peri* (around) + *nephric* (kidney)
   c. *peri* (inside) + *nephric* (bladder)
   d. *peri* (inside) + *nephric* (kidney)
   e. *peri* (outside) + *nephric* (kidney)
3. The hospital course reports that Susan's *renal ultrasound* was normal. A *renal ultrasound* is an
   a. image of the bladder using high frequency sound waves
   b. image of the kidney using high frequency sound waves
   c. image of the renal pelvis using high frequency sound waves
   d. image of the urinary tract using high frequency sound waves
   e. none of these

Urology Consult

Chief Complaint: **Hematuria.**

History of Present Illness: Doug Harper is a 5-year-old boy with a 2-day history of gross **hematuria.** Doug's parents noted that Doug had had **oliguria** the past 2 days and had very dark, tea-colored urine. They took Doug to his primary care provider, Nelda Lopez, NP. Ms. Lopez tested a **urinalysis,** and the results showed **hematuria** and **albuminuria.** She also noted Doug had periorbital edema and that he was **hypertensive** in the office. The parents report that Doug had a recent throat infection (last week) that resolved on its own.

Review of Systems: Positive for nausea, but no emesis. Otherwise negative.

Medications: None.

Allergies: No known drug allergies.

Past Medical History: Noncontributory.

Past Surgical History: **Balanoplasty** for **hypospadias** at age 1.

Social History: Doug lives with his parents and older sister. He is going into kindergarten in the fall.

Family History: Paternal grandfather with **polycystic kidney disease.**

Vital Signs

Temp: 98.6; Heart Rate: 100; Respiratory Rate: 24; Blood Pressure: 118/86.

Physical Exam

General: WDWN. Nontoxic. NAD.

Head: PERRLA. EOMI bilaterally. Periorbital edema. No erythema. No proptosis. Mucous membranes moist and pink. TMs normal.

Cardiovascular: Regular in rate and rhythm without murmurs, gallop, or rubs. No JVD.

Respiratory: Clear to auscultation.

Abdomen: Soft, nontender, nondistended, no hepatosplenomegaly. No **CVA tenderness.**

Neurologic: Alert, oriented.

Skin: Pink, warm.

Extremities: Edema of feet. Dorsal pedal pulses present.

Labs: Elevated BUN and creatinine. **Hypocomplementemia.** Antistreptolysin O and antiDNAase B.

Imaging: None.

Assessment/Plan

1. Hematuria/albuminuria: Doug clearly has a **nephropathy.** The differential diagnosis includes **post streptococcal glomerulonephritis,** basement membrane disease, lupus **nephritis, membranoproliferative glomerulonephritis.** Since he had a recent throat infection, post streptococcal glomerulonephritis is the most likely cause. We will wait for the labs to confirm a recent strep infection.
2. Hypertension, edema: We will begin Doug on **diuretics** and **fluid restriction,** as well as a low-sodium diet.

–William Hunter, MD

Learning Outcome 12.8 Exercises

EXERCISE 14 *Match the term on the left with its definition on the right.*

_____	1. nephritis	a.	birth defect in which the opening of the urethra is on the underside, instead of the end, of the penis
_____	2. nephropathy	b.	agent that causes urination
_____	3. urinalysis	c.	analysis of the urine
_____	4. diuretic	d.	any kidney disease
_____	5. polycystic kidney disease	e.	bloody urination
_____	6. hematuria	f.	disease characterized by the formation of many fluid-filled cysts in the kidneys
_____	7. albuminuria	g.	inflammation of the kidney
_____	8. oliguria	h.	inflammation of the kidneys, involving primarily the glomeruli
_____	9. glomerulonephritis	i.	low urine output
_____	10. balanoplasty	j.	protein in the urine
_____	11. hypospadias	k.	surgical reconstruction of the penis

EXERCISE 15 *Fill in the blanks.*

1. HPI (define abbreviation: ____________________ of ____________________)
   a. Patient's name: ____________________
   b. Patient's age: ____________________
   c. Patient's gender: ____________________
   d. 2-day history of *hematuria* (give definition: ____________________)
   e. Patient had ____________________ (low urine output)
   f. *Urinalysis* (give abbreviation: ____________) showed ____________ (blood in the urine) and *albuminuria* (give definition: ____________________)
2. PMHx (define abbreviation: ____________ ____________ ____________ ____________): noncontributory
3. ____________ ____________ ____________(Past Surgical History)
   a. *Balanoplasty* (give definition: ____________________) for ____________________ (a birth defect in which the opening of the urethra is on the underside, instead of the end, of the penis).
4. Assessment/Plan
   a. The patient clearly has a(n) ____________________ (disease of the kidney)
   b. The patient will begin fluid restriction and the use of ____________________ (agent that causes urination)

EXERCISE 16 *True or false questions. Indicate true answers with a T and false answers with an F.*

1. According to Dr. Hunter, Doug has a disease of the kidney. ________
2. Doug's CC is PKD. ________
3. Doug is nauseus and vomiting. ________

Learning Outcome 12.8 Exercises

EXERCISE 17 *Multiple-choice questions. Select the correct answer(s).*

1. Doug's grandfather has which of the following medical conditions?
   a. disease characterized by the formation of many fluid-filled cysts in the kidneys
   b. PKD
   c. polycystic kidney disease
   d. all of these
   e. none of these
2. Doug's physical exam revealed *hepatosplenomegaly*. Which of the following is a correct breakdown of the term *hepatosplenomegaly*?
   a. *hepato* (bladder) + *spleno* (spleen) + *megaly* (enlarged)
   b. *hepato* (kidney) + *spleno* (spleen) + *megaly* (reduced)
   c. *hepato* (liver) + *spleno* (spleen) + *megaly* (enlarged)
   d. *hepato* (prostate) + *spleno* (spleen) + *megaly* (enlarged)
   e. *hepato* (testicle) + *spleno* (spleen) + *megaly* (reduced)
3. According to Dr. Hunter's differential diagnosis, Doug may have a form of *glomerulonephritis*. Which of the following is a correct breakdown of the term?
   a. *glomerulo* (glomerulus) + *nephro* (bladder) + *itis* (disease)
   b. *glomerulo* (glomerulus) + *nephro* (bladder) + *itis* (inflammation)
   c. *glomerulo* (glomerulus) + *nephro* (kidney) + *itis* (disease)
   d. *glomerulo* (glomerulus) + *nephro* (kidney) + *itis* (inflammation)
   e. *glomerulo* (glomerulus) + *nephro* (kidney) + *itis* (tumor)

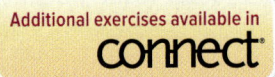

Chapter Review exercises, along with additional practice items, are available in Connect!

Quick Reference

quick reference glossary of roots

Root	Definition	Root	Definition
balan/o	penis	**pyel/o**	renal pelvis
cyst/o	bladder	**ren/o**	kidney
epididym/o	epididymis	**sperm/o, spermat/o**	sperm
glomerul/o	glomerulus	**test/o**	testicle
lith/o	stone	**ur/o, urin/o**	urine
meat/o	opening	**ureter/o**	ureter
nephr/o	kidney	**urethr/o**	urethra
orch/o, orchi/o, orchid/o	testicle	**vesic/o**	bladder
prostat/o	prostate		

quick reference glossary of terms

Term	Definition
albuminuria	protein in the urine
anorchidism	absence of a testicle
antispasmodic	drug used to prevent spasms
anuria	lack of urination
aspermia	condition characterized by a lack of sperm
azoospermia	condition characterized by lack of living sperm
azotemia	excess nitrogen in the blood
azotorrhea	excessive discharge of nitrogen
azoturia	excess nitrogen in the urine
balanitis	inflammation of the penis
balanoplasty	surgical reconstruction of the penis
balanorrhea	discharge from the penis
benign prostate hyperplasia	noncancerous overdevelopment of the prostate; also known as *enlarged prostate*
benign prostate hypertrophy	another term for benign prostate hyperplasia
blood urea nitrogen	nitrogen in the blood in the form of urea; it is the product of the breakdown of amino acids for energy
circumcision	surgical removal of the foreskin of the penis
cryptorchidism	hidden testicle

quick reference glossary of terms *continued*

Term	Definition
cystalgia	pain in the bladder
cystectomy	surgical removal of the bladder
cystitis	inflammation of the bladder
cystocele	hernia of the bladder
cystodynia	pain in the bladder
cystogram	image of the bladder
cystography	process for recording/imaging the bladder
cystoliith	stone in the bladder
cystolithectomy	surgical removal of a stone in the bladder
cystoma	tumor of the bladder
cystoplegia	bladder paralysis
cystoptosis	downward displacement of the bladder
cystorrhexis	rupture of the bladder
cystoscopy	process for examining the bladder
cystospasm	involuntary contraction of the bladder
cystostomy	creation of an opening in the bladder
cystoureteritis	inflammation of the bladder and urethra
cystourethrocele	hernia of the bladder and urethra
digital rectal exam	examination of the prostate using a finger inserted into the rectum
dipsogenic	creating thirst
diuresis	excessive urination
diuretic	agent that causes urination
dysuria	painful urination
ejaculation	emission of semen from the urethra
enuresis	involutary urination
epididymectomy	surgical removal of the epididymis
epididymitis	inflammation of the epididymis
epididymo-orchitis	inflammation of the testicles and epididymis
epididymotomy	incision into the epididymis
extracorporeal shock wave lithotripsy (ESWL)	breakdown of kidney stones using sound waves generated outside the body
fulguration	use of electric current to destroy tissue
glomerulonephritis	inflammation of the kidneys involving primarily the glomeruli

quick reference glossary of terms *continued*

Term	Definition
glomerulopathy	disease of the kidney involving primarily the glomeruli
glomerulosclerosis	hardening of the glomeruli
glucosuria	sugar in the urine
glycosuria	sugar in the urine
gonads	the pair of organs used for sexual reproduction; testicles in males and ovaries in females
gonorrhea	discharge from the gonads
hematuria	bloody urination
heminephrectomy	surgical removal of half a kidney
heminephroureterectomy	surgical removal of half a kidney and a ureter
hemodialysis	procedure for removing waste from the bloodstream
hydrocele	fluid-filled mass in a testicle
hydrocelectomy	surgical removal of a hydrocele
hydronephrosis	kidney condition caused by the obstruction of urine flow
hyperkalemia	excessive potassium in the blood
hypernephroma	cancer of the kidneys
hyponatremia	low sodium in the blood
hypospadias	birth defect in which the opening of the urethra is on the underside, instead of the end, of the penis
incontinence	inability to control urination
intracorporeal lithotripsy	breakdown of kidney stones using a device placed inside the body
ketolysis	breakdown of ketones
ketonuria	presence of ketones in the urine
kidney dialysis	procedure for removing waste from the blood (a shorter name for hemodialysis)
laparonephrectomy	surgical removal of a kidney through the abdomen
lithectomy	surgical removal of a stone in the bladder
lithocystotomy	incision into the bladder to remove a stone
lithonephritis	inflammation of the kidneys caused by stones
lithonephrotomy	incision into a kidney to remove a stone
lithotripsy	breakdown of a stone
meatal stenosis	narrowing of the opening of the urethra
meatoplasty	surgical reconstruction of the opening of the urethra
meatorrhaphy	suture of the opening of the urethra

quick reference glossary of terms *continued*

Term	Definition
meatoscope	instrument for examining the opening of the urethra
meatoscopy	process for examining the opening of the urethra
meatotomy	incision into the opening of the urethra
nephralgia	pain in the kidney
nephrectomy	surgical removal of a kidney
nephritis	inflammation of the kidney
nephrocele	hernia of a kidney
nephrocystanastomosis	opening of a passageway between kidney and bladder
nephrogram	image of a kidney
nephrography	procedure for imaging a kidney
nephrohypertrophy	overdevelopment of the kidney
nephrolithiasis	the presence of stones in the kidney
nephrolithotomy	incision into a kidney to remove a stone
nephrologist	specialist in the kidneys
nephrology	study of the kidneys
nephroma	kidney timor
nephromalacia	abnormal softening of a kidney
nephromegaly	abnormal enlargement of a kidney
nephropathy	any kidney disease
nephropexy	surgical fixation of a kidney
nephroptosis	downward displacement of a kidney
nephrorrhaphy	suture of a kidney
nephrosclerosis	abnormal hardening of a kidney
nephroscopy	procedure for examining a kidney
nephrosis	kidney condition
nephrosonography	procedure for imaging a kidney using sound waves
nephrostomy	creation of an opening in a kidney
nephrotomy	incision into a kidney to remove a stone
nephrotoxin	an agent poisonous to the kidney
nephroureterectomy	surgical removal of a kidney and ureter
nocturia	nighttime urination
nocturnal enuresis	nighttime involuntary urination

quick reference glossary of terms *continued*

Term	Definition
oligospermia	condition characterized by low sperm production
oliguria	low urine output
orchialgia	testicle pain
orchichorhea	involuntary jerking movement of the testicles
orchidectomy	surgical removal of a testicle
orchiditis	inflammation of the testicles and epididymis
orchidopexy	surgical fixation of a testicle
orchidoptosis	downward displacement of a testicle
orchidotomy	incision into a testicle
orchiectomy	surgical removal of a testicle
orchiepididymitis	inflammation of the testicles and epididymis
orchiodynia	testicle pain
orchiopathy	disease of the testicles
orchiopexy	surgical fixation of a testicle
orchioplasty	surgical reconstruction of a testicle
orchitis	inflammation of the testicles and epididymis
phimosis	contraction of the foreskin of the penis, preventing it from being retracted
polycystic kidney disease	disease characterized by the formation of many fluid-filled cysts in the kidneys
polydipsia	excessive thirst
polyuria	excessive urination
priapism	persistent and painful erection
prostatectomy	surgical removal of the prostate
prostatitis	inflammation of the prostate
prostatocystitis	inflammation of the prostate and bladder
prostatolith	a stone in the prostate
prostatolithotomy	incision into a prostate to remove a stone
prostatomegaly	abnormal enlargement of the prostate
prostatorrhea	discharge from the prostate
prostatovesiculectomy	surgical removal of the prostate and seminal vesicles
prostatovesiculitis	inflammation of the prostate and seminal vesicles
pyelitis	inflammation of the renal pelvis
pyelocystitis	inflammation of the renal pelvis and bladder

quick reference glossary of terms *continued*

Term	Definition
pyelocystostomosis	creation of an opening between the renal pelvis and bladder
pyelogram	image of the renal pelvis
pyelolithotomy	incision into a renal pelvis to remove a stone
pyelonephritis	inflammation of the kidney and renal pelvis
pyelopathy	disease of the renal pelvis
pyeloplasty	surgical reconstruction of a renal pelvis
pyelostomy	creation of an opening in a renal pelvis
pyelotomy	incision into a renal pelvis
pyeloureterectasia	dilation of the renal pelvis and ureter
pyonephritis	inflammation of the kidney caused by pus
pyonephrolithiasis	the presence of pus and stones in the kidney
pyopyeloectasis	pus in a dilated renal pelvis
pyuria	pus in the urine
renal angiogram	image of a kidney blood vessel
renal angiography	process of imaging a kidney blood vessel
renal angioplasty	surgical reconstruction of a kidney blood vessel
renal arteriogram	image of a kidney artery
renal cell carcinoma (hypernephroma)	cancer of the kidneys
renal failure	kidney failure
renal ischemia	deficiency of blood in a kidney
resectoscope	instrument for examining and cutting (usually the prostate)
retrograde pyelogram	image of the renal pelvis produced by injecting a contrast dye from the bladder to the kidney
seminoma	type of testicular cancer arising from sperm-forming tissue
spermatocele	hernia or distention of the epididymis caused by sperm cells
spermatogenesis	creation of sperm
spermatolysis	destruction of sperm cells
spermicide	agent that kills sperm
spermolytic	agent that kills sperm
stress urinary incontinence (SUI)	loss of bladder control caused by the application of external pressure
testicular carcinoma	testicular cancer

quick reference glossary of terms *continued*

Term	Definition
testitis	inflammation of the testicles and epididymis
transrectal ultrasonography	procedure involving a probe inserted into the rectum using high-frequency sound waves to scan through the rectum to nearby tissue (most commonly, the prostate)
transurethral resection of the prostate (TURP)	procedure of removing all or part of the prostate by the insertion of a resectoscope into the urethra
ultrasonography	imaging procedure using high-frequency sound waves
uremia	urine in the blood
ureteralgia	pain in the ureter
ureteritis	inflammation of a ureter
ureterocele	hernia of the ureter
ureteroileostomy	creation of an opening between a ureter and the ileum, a portion of the small intestine
ureterolithiasis	presence of stones in a ureter
ureteronephrectomy	surgical removal of a kidney and ureter
ureteroplasty	surgical reconstruction of a ureter
ureteropyelitis	inflammation of a ureter and renal pelvis
ureteropyelonephritis	inflammation of a kidney, renal pelvis, and ureter
ureterorrhaphy	suture of the ureter
ureteroscopy	process of examining a ureter
ureterostenosis	narrowing of a ureter
urethrectomy	surgical removal of the urethra
urethritis	inflammation of the urethra
urethrocystitis	inflammation of the urethra and bladder
urethrodynia	pain in the urethra
urethrogram	image of the urethra
urethropexy	surgical fixation of the urethra
urethroplasty	surgical reconstruction of the urethra
urethrorrhea	discharge from the urethra
urethroscope	instrument for examining the urethra
urethroscopy	process of examining the urethra
urethrospasm	involuntary contraction of the urethra
urethrostenosis	narrrowing of the urethra
urethrotomy	incision into the urethra

quick reference glossary of terms *continued*

Term	Definition
urinalysis	analysis of the urine
urinary catheterization	insertion of a catheter into the bladder to drain urine
urinary tract infection (UTI)	infection of the urinary tract
urocyanosis	blue urine
urodynia	painful
urologist	specialist in the urinary tract
urology	study of the urinary tract
uropathy	disease of the urinary tract
uropoesis	formation of urine
urostomy	creation of an opening in the urinary tract, normally to divert urine flow away from a diseased bladder
uroxanthin	substance in urine that makes it yellow
varicocele	overexpansion of the blood vessels of the testicles, leading to a soft tumor
vas deferens	vessel carrying sperm from the testicles
vasectomy	surgical removal of the vas deferens
vasovasostomy	creation of an opening between two vessels; technical term for a vasectomy reversal
vesicocele	hernia of the bladder
vesicostomy	creation of an opening in the bladder
vesicotomy	incision into the bladder
vesicoureteral reflux	abnormal flow of urine from the bladder back into the ureters
vesiculectomy	surgical removal of the seminal vesicles
voiding	another term for urination

review of terms by roots

Root	Term(s)	
balan/o	balanitis	balanorrhea
	balanoplasty	
cyst/o	cystalgia	cystoscopy
	cystectomy	cystospasm
	cystitis	cystostomy
	cystocele	cystoureteritis
	cystodynia	cystourethrocele
	cystogram	lithocystotomy
	cystography	nephrocystanastomosis
	cystolith	polycystic kidney disease
	cystolithectomy	prostatocystitis
	cystoma	pyelocystitis
	cystoplegia	pyelocystostomosis
	cystoptosis	urethrocystitis
	cystorrhexis	voiding cystourethrogram
epididym/o	epididymectomy	epididymotomy
	epididymitis	orchiepididymitis
	epididymo-orchitis	
glomerul/o	glomerulonephritis	glomerulosclerosis
	glomerulopathy	
lith/o	cystolith	lithotripsy
	cystolithectomy	nephrolithiasis
	extracorporeal shock wave lithotripsy (ESWL)	nephrolithotomy
	intracorporeal lithotripsy	prostatolithotomy
	lithectomy	pyelolithotomy
	lithocystotomy	pyonephrolithiasis
	lithonephritis	ureterolithiasis
	lithonephrotomy	

review of terms by roots *continued*

Root	Term(s)	
meat/o	meatal stenosis	meatoscope
	meatoplasty	meatoscopy
	meatorrhaphy	meatotomy
nephr/o	glomerulonephritis	nephroma
	heminephrectomy	nephromalacia
	heminephroureterectomy	nephromegaly
	hydronephrosis	nephropathy
	hypernephroma	nephropexy
	laparonephrectomy	nephroptosis
	lithonephritis	nephrorrhaphy
	lithonephrotomy	nephrosclerosis
	nephralgia	nephroscopy
	nephrectomy	nephrosis
	nephritis	nephrosonography
	nephrocele	nephrostomy
	nephrocystanastomosis	nephrotomy
	nephrogram	nephrotoxin
	nephrography	nephroureterectomy
	nephrohypertrophy	pyelonephritis
	nephrolithiasis	pyonephritis
	nephrolithotomy	pyonephrolithiasis
	nephrologist	ureteronephrectomy
	nephrology	ureteropyelonephritis
orch/o, orchi/o, orchid/o	anorchidism	orchidotomy
	cryptorchidism	orchiectomy
	epididymo-orchitis	orchiepididymitis
	orchialgia	orchiodynia
	orchichorea	orchiopathy
	orchidectomy	orchiopexy

review of terms by roots *continued*

Root	Term(s)	
	orchiditis	orchioplasty
	orchidopexy	orchitis
	orchidoptosis	
prostat/o	benign prostate hyperplasia	prostatolithotomy
	benign prostate hypertrophy	prostatomegaly
	prostatectomy	prostatorrhea
	prostatitis	prostatovesiculectomy
	prostatocystitis	prostatovesiculitis
	prostatolith	transurethral resection of the prostate (TURP)
pyel/o	pyelitis	pyelostomy
	pyelocystitis	pyelotomy
	pyelocystostomosis	pyeloureterectasia
	pyelogram	pyopyeloectasis
	pyelolithotomy	retrograde pyelogram
	pyelonephritis	ureteropyelitis
	pyelopathy	ureteropyelonephritis
	pyeloplasty	
ren/o	renal angiogram	renal cell carcinoma (hypernephroma)
	renal angiography	renal failure
	renal angioplasty	renal ischemia
	renal arteriogram	
sperm/o, spermat/o	aspermia	spermatogenesis
	azoospermia	spermatolysis
	oligospermia	spermicide
	spermatocele	spermolytic
test/o	testicular carcinoma	
	testitis	

review of terms by roots *continued*

Root	Term(s)	
ureter/o	cystoureteritis	ureteronephrectomy
	heminephroureterectomy	ureteroplasty
	nephroureterectomy	ureteropyelitis
	pyeloureterectasia	ureteropyelonephritis
	ureteralgia	ureterorrhaphy
	ureteritis	ureteroscopy
	ureterocele	ureterostenosis
	ureteroileostomy	vesicoureteral reflux
	ureterolithiasis	
urethr/o	cystourethrocele	urethroplasty
	transurethral resection of the prostate (TURP)	urethrorrhea
	urethrectomy	urethroscope
	urethritis	urethroscopy
	urethrocystitis	urethrospasm
	urethrodynia	urethrostenosis
	urethrogram	urethrotomy
	urethropexy	
ur/o	albuminuria	pyuria
	anuria	stress urinary incontinence
	azoturia	uremia
	diuresis	urinalysis
	diuretic	urinary catheterization
	dysuria	urinary tract infection
	enuresis	urocyanosis
	glucosuria	urodynia
	glycosuria	urologist
	hematuria	urology
	ketonuria	uropathy
	nocturia	uropoesis
	nocturnal enuresis	urostomy
	oliguria	uroxanthin
	polyuria	

review of terms by roots *continued*

Root	Term(s)	
vesic/o	prostatovesiculectomy	vesicotomy
	prostatovesiculitis	vesicoureteral reflux
	vesicocele	vesiculectomy
	vesicostomy	

other terms

antispasmodic	hypospadias
azotemia	incontinence
azotorrhea	ketolysis
blood urea nitrogen	kidney dialysis
circumcision	phimosis
digital rectal exam	polydipsia
dipsogenic	priapism
ejaculation	resectoscope
fulguration	seminoma
gonads	transrectal ultrasonography
gonorrhea	ultrasonography
hemodialysis	varicocele
hydrocele	vas deferens
hydrocelectomy	vasectomy
hyperkalemia	vasovasostomy
hyponatremia	voiding

The Female Reproductive System—Gynecology, Obstetrics, and Neonatology 13

Introduction and Overview of the Female Reproductive System

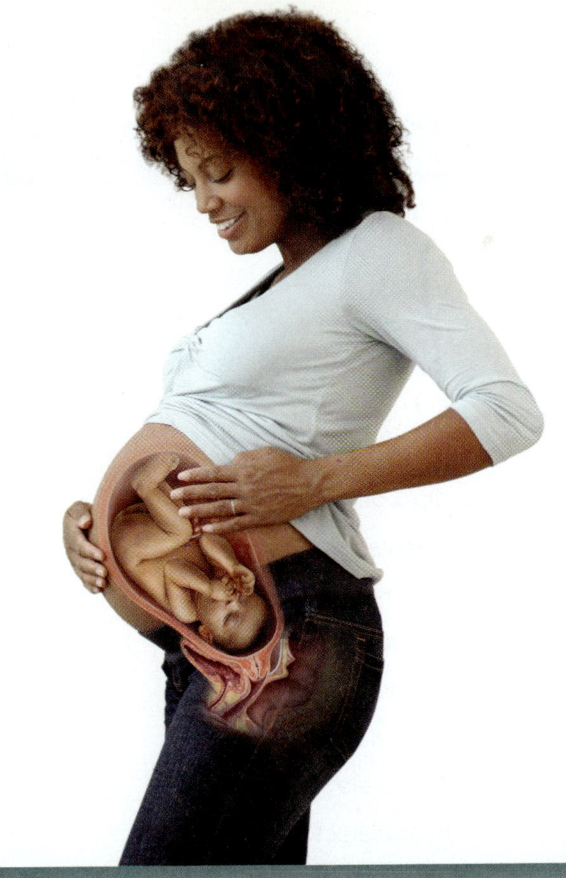

With few exceptions, everyone is born with the basic equipment to help bring new life into the world. Both sexes contain reproductive organs that produce half the code for a human life. The female reproductive system is much more active and complex. While the main function of the male reproductive system is the production and the delivery of sperm cells, the female reproductive system is responsible for much more. Females not only provide half the code for a human life, but they also provide the environment and nutrition to sustain and grow that life until birth.

learning outcomes

Upon completion of this chapter, you will be able to:

13.1 Identify the **roots/word parts** associated with the **female reproductive system.**

S **13.2** Translate the **Subjective** terms associated with the **female reproductive system.**

O **13.3** Translate the **Objective** terms associated with the **female reproductive system.**

A **13.4** Translate the **Assessment** terms associated with the **female reproductive system.**

P **13.5** Translate the **Plan** terms associated with the **female reproductive system.**

13.6 Use **abbreviations** associated with the **female reproductive system.**

13.7 Distinguish terms associated with the **female reproductive system** in the context of **electronic health records.**

13.1 Word Parts of the Female Reproductive System

Gynecology, External

The outer structures of the female reproductive system are collectively known as the *vulva*. The vulva includes the clitoris, the labia majora and labia minora, the urethral meatus, and the vaginal opening.

The *clitoris* is the most sensitive part of a woman's anatomy. In this way, it is similar to the head of a man's penis. The *labia* are the folds of tissue around the opening of the vagina. The outer folds, which are larger, are the *labia majora*, and the inner folds, which are thinner, are the *labia minora*. The urethra opens out into the vagina.

While not directly connected to the rest of the reproductive parts, the *breasts* are a very important outside structure. While they are very sensitive and provide stimulation that plays a part in sexual intercourse, their main purpose is to provide a food supply for a newborn baby.

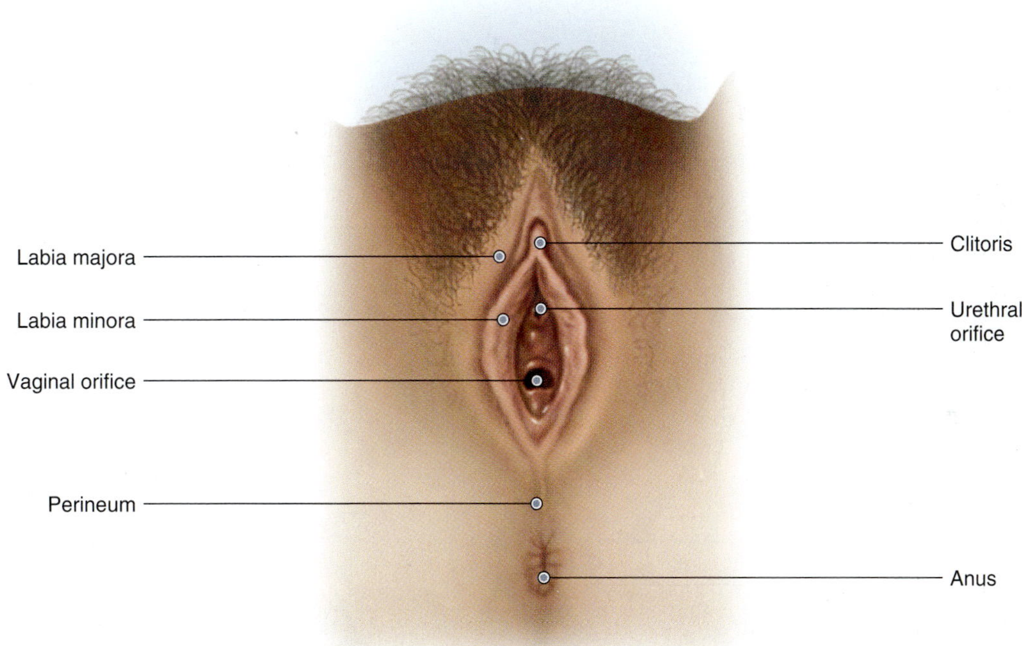

vagina

ROOTS: ***colp/o, vagin/o***

EXAMPLES: colposcope, vaginitis

NOTES: The word *vagina* comes from Latin and means the *sheath* or *scabbard of a sword.*

vulva

ROOTS: ***episi/o, vulv/o***

EXAMPLES: episiotomy, vulvodynia

NOTES: *Vulva* is the term for the external genital organs of a female.

perineum

ROOT: ***perine/o***

EXAMPLES: perineoplasty, perineorrhaphy

NOTES: *Perineum* is the term for the region between the genital organs and the anus. No one is really sure where the term came from, but one easy way to remember what it means is to think *peri* (*around*) + *anus* = *region around the anus.* It's not 100 percent accurate, but it's enough to help you remember.

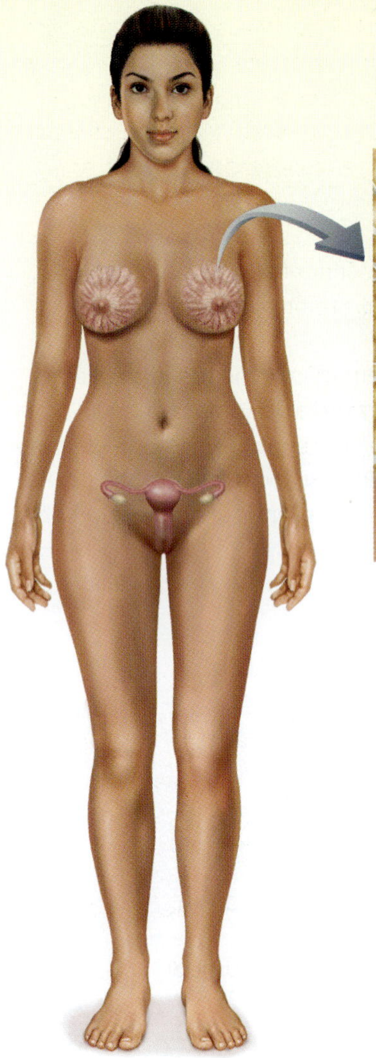

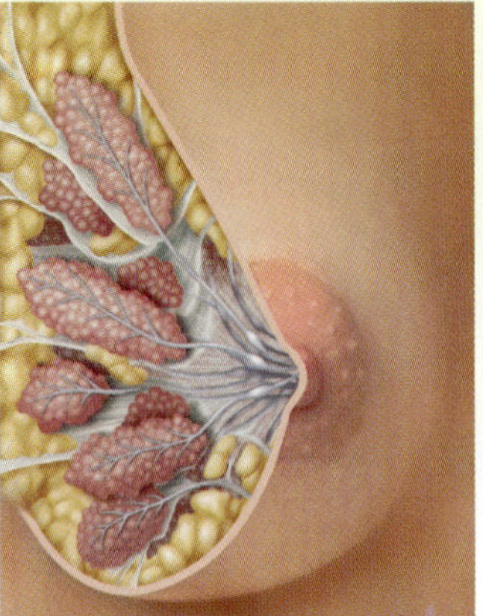

woman

ROOTS: ***gynec/o, gyn/o***

EXAMPLES: gynecology, gynecologist

NOTES: This root comes from Greek, for *woman.* If you are afraid of women, you have *gynophobia.* Believe it or not, this root is where the English words *queen* and *goon* come from.

breast

ROOTS: ***mast/o, mamm/o***

EXAMPLES: mastopexy, mastectomy, mammogram

NOTES: Believe it or not, the name of the *mastodon,* a long-extinct type of elephant similar to a mammoth, actually breaks down as *mast* (*breast*) and *odon* (*tooth*). The mastodon got its name from a scientist who thought that the animal's molar teeth had nipple-like tops, which gave them the appearance of breasts.

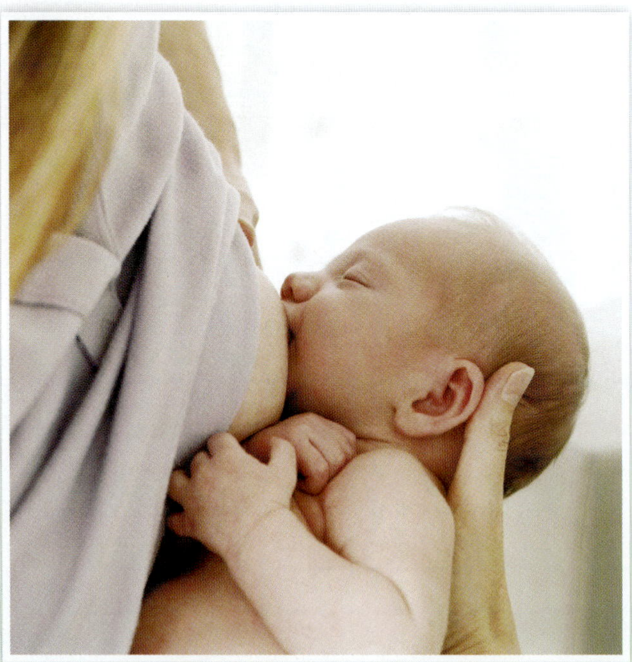

milk

ROOT: ***lact/o***

EXAMPLES: lactation, lactorrhea

NOTES: The root for milk, *lacto,* is also the root for the English word *galaxy.* Have you ever looked at the stars from a really dark spot out in the country? If so, you've seen stars that you'd never be able to see near a city. One thing you can see is the Milky Way, the thick band of stars that makes up our galaxy. It's called the Milky Way because the ancient Greeks thought the dense cloud of stars looked like milk sprayed in the night sky. A Greek myth tells how the hero Hercules, who was breast-fed by the goddess Hera, once bit down so hard that milk sprayed everywhere—creating the Milky Way.

Gynecology, Internal

A woman's inner reproductive system is shaped like a capital "T." On either end of the horizontal part of the "T" rest the ovaries. The *ovaries* hold all of the woman's eggs (*ova*). Roughly every 28 to 30 days during a woman's adult years, an ovary will allow an egg to mature and then releases it (*ovulation*). The ova travel along tubes (*fallopian tubes*) to the uterus.

The *uterus* is a pear-shaped organ in the vertical part of the "T," along with the vagina. The uterus is the incubator for growing and developing new life. Every month, the walls of the uterus grow and become rich in blood supply. If the woman's egg is fertilized by a sperm, it travels to the uterus and implants itself in the walls. If a new life is not implanted in the walls of the uterus, the tissues are shed and the process starts all over again. This cycle of building and shedding nutritive tissues in the uterus is known as the *menstrual cycle*. It is driven by the female hormones *estrogen* and *progesterone*. Both of these hormones are made in the ovaries.

At the end of the uterus is a connection to the vagina known as the *cervix*. It is smaller and thicker than the rest of the uterus. Further down the vertical part of the "T" is the vagina, the reproductive system's main point of contact with the outside world. It is the part of a woman's body that is involved in sexual intercourse. Additionally, the opening of the urethra, which drains the bladder, is found in the anterior wall of the vagina.

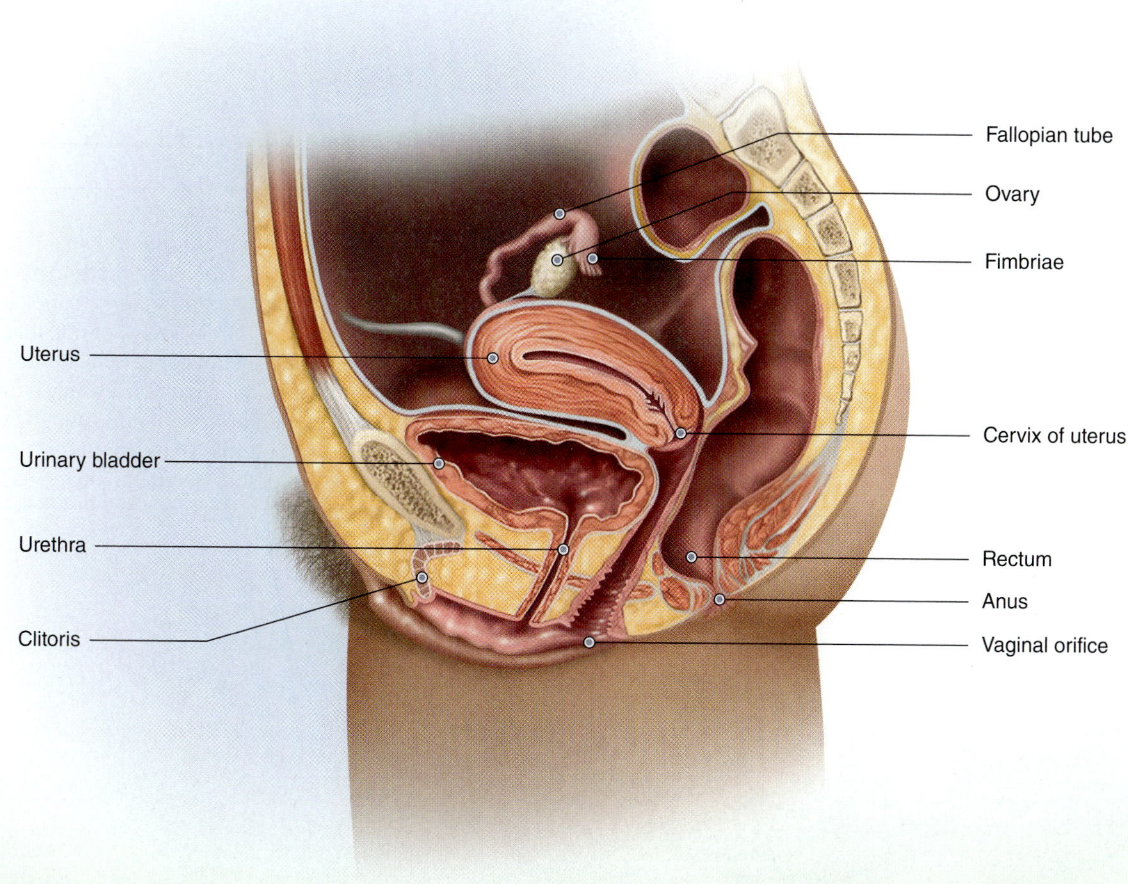

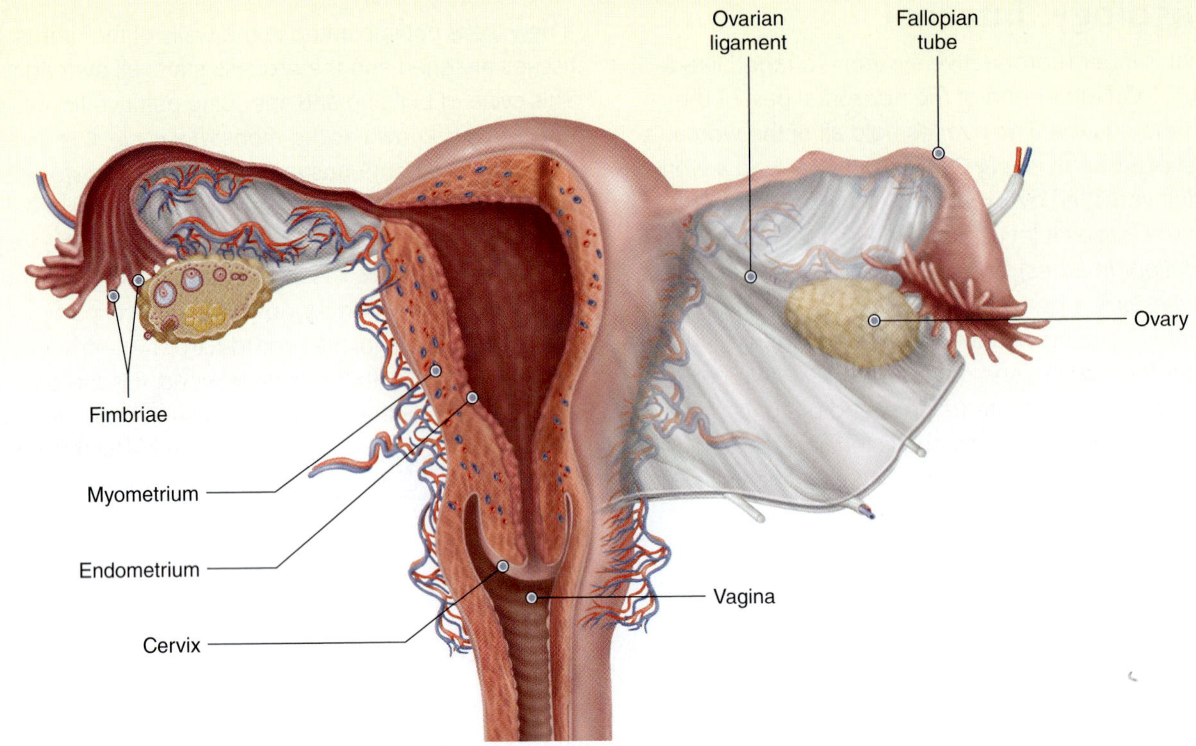

cervix

ROOT: ***cervic/o***

EXAMPLES: cervicodynia, cervicitis

NOTES: *Cervix* means *neck* and refers not to the neck connecting your head to your body but to the opening between the uterus and the vagina.

REMEMBER: The letter *c* changes sounds depending on what vowel follows it. Before *e* or *i*, the letter *c* makes an *s* sound (**ce**rvi**ci**tis—**SE**R-vih-**SAI**-tis). Before *a, o,* or *u,* the letter *c* makes a *k* sound (**ce**rvi**co**dynia—**SE**R-vih-**ko**h-DAI-nee-ah).

uterus

ROOTS: ***hyster/o, metr/o, uter/o***

EXAMPLES: hysterectomy, endometrium, uterus

NOTES: Break down the word *hysteria* as a medical term. It means a *uterus condition,* right (*hyster* + *ia*)? Believe it or not, that is exactly where the term came from. It was used to refer to a medical condition (usually neurological) occurring in women and caused by a malfunctioning uterus. Think about that the next time you refer to a friend or a movie as "hysterical."

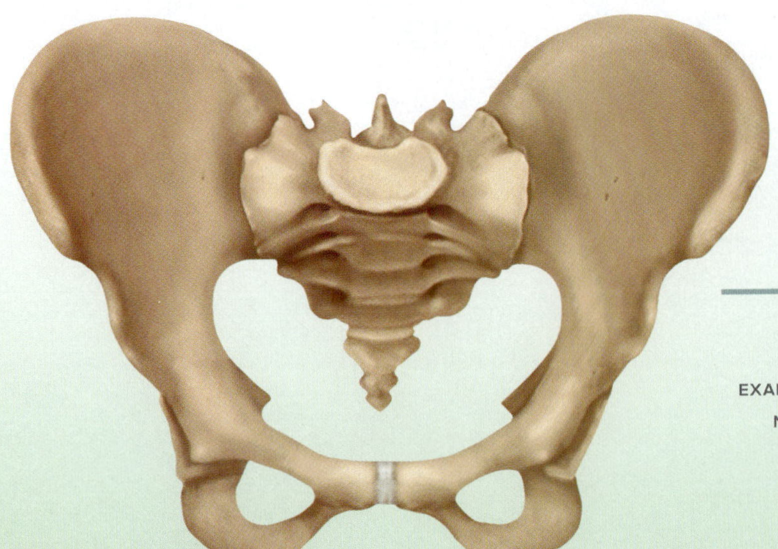

pelvis

ROOT: ***pelv/i***

EXAMPLES: pelvimetry, pelvic sonography

NOTES: *Pelvis* comes from a Latin word meaning *basin* or *washtub* and refers to the shape of the bones that make up the pelvis. Another root, *pyelo,* also means *pelvis,* but this root is used exclusively for the portion of the kidney called the *renal pelvis.*

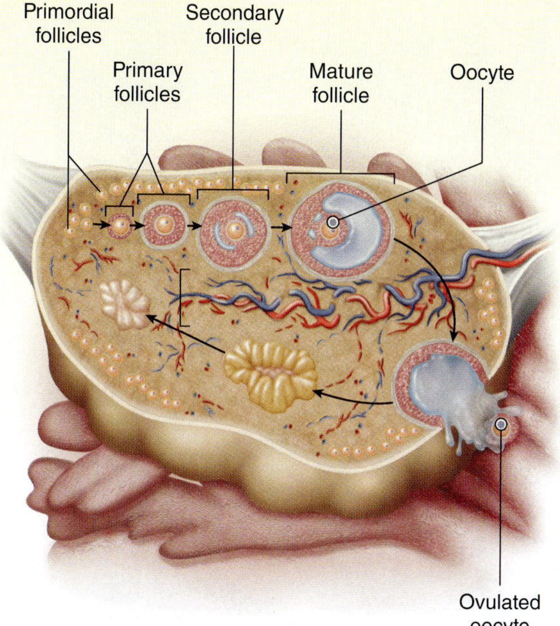

ovary

ROOTS: ***oophor/o, ovari/o***

EXAMPLES: oophorectomy, ovariocentesis

NOTES: *Oophoro* can be broken down into two words: *oo,* meaning *egg,* and *phor,* meaning *to carry.* Thus, *oophor* literally means *the thing that carries the eggs.*

menstruation

ROOT: ***men/o***

EXAMPLES: menorrhea, menopause

NOTES: *Meno* comes from Greek, for *month,* and refers to the standard 28-day recurrence of menstrual cycles. It is no wonder that in ancient Greece, Artemis was both the goddess who watched over young girls entering womanhood and the goddess associated with the moon, which goes through its phases every 28 days.

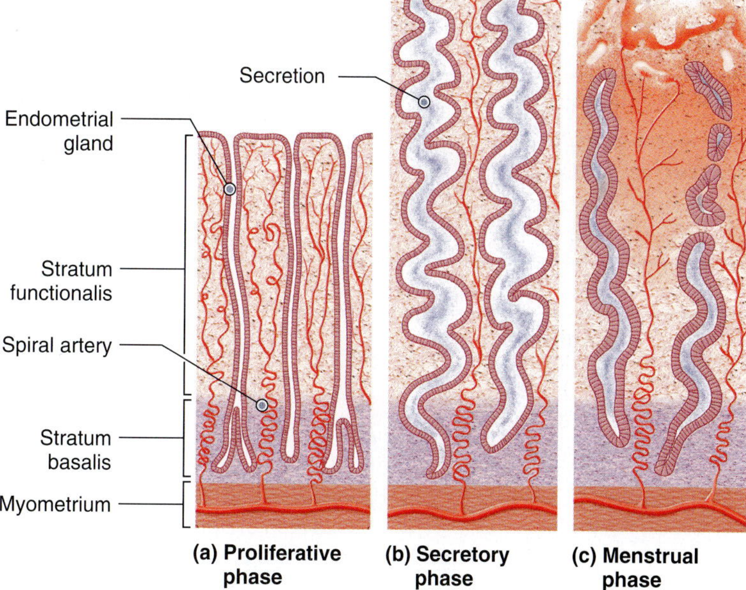

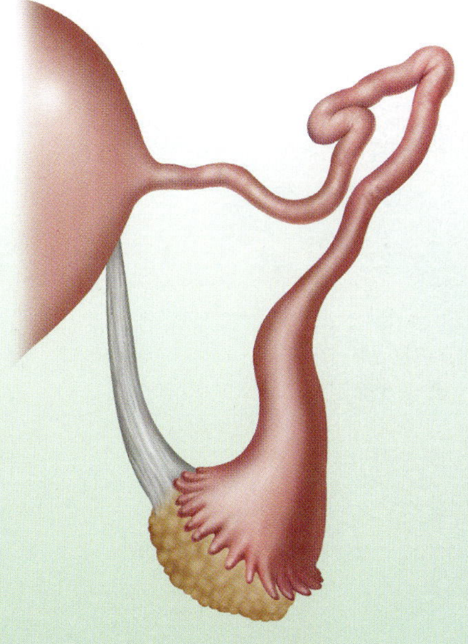

fallopian tube

ROOT: ***salping/o***

EXAMPLES: salpingectomy, salpingoscope

NOTES: *Salpingo* comes from the Latin word for *trumpet.* Four sites in the body use this term due to their resemblance to a long, straight Roman trumpet: the ear canals and the fallopian tubes, which connect the ovaries to the uterus. The fallopian tubes are named for Gabriello Fallopio, an Italian specialist in anatomy who first described them in the 1500s.

REMEMBER: The letter *g* changes sounds depending on what vowel follows it. Before *e* or *i,* the letter *g* makes a *j* sound (salpin**gi**tis—SAL-pin-**JAI**-tis). Before *a, o,* or *u,* the letter *g* makes a *g* sound (salpin**go**scope—sal-PING-**goh**-SKOHP).

Obstetrics

Pregnancy is the amazing process of a human life growing inside a woman. During pregnancy, a baby is called a *fetus.* The fetus grows and develops in the mother's *uterus.* The fetus is connected to the uterus via the *placenta.* The placenta is an important source for feeding the fetus. There, nutrients provided by the mother's blood vessels cross into the blood vessels of the fetus.

The fetus is attached to the placenta through the *umbilical cord,* which is cut at birth. This is where the belly button comes from. The fetus is surrounded by a fluid-filled sac (*amnion* or *amniotic sac*) that helps act as a shock absorber to protect it. Outside the amnion is another membrane, the *chorion,* which helps anchor the baby to the walls of the uterus and provides nutrition.

When the fetus is ready for birth, the woman's body goes through the painful process known as *labor.* During labor, the woman's *cervix* widens and the muscles of the uterus squeeze to push the baby out.

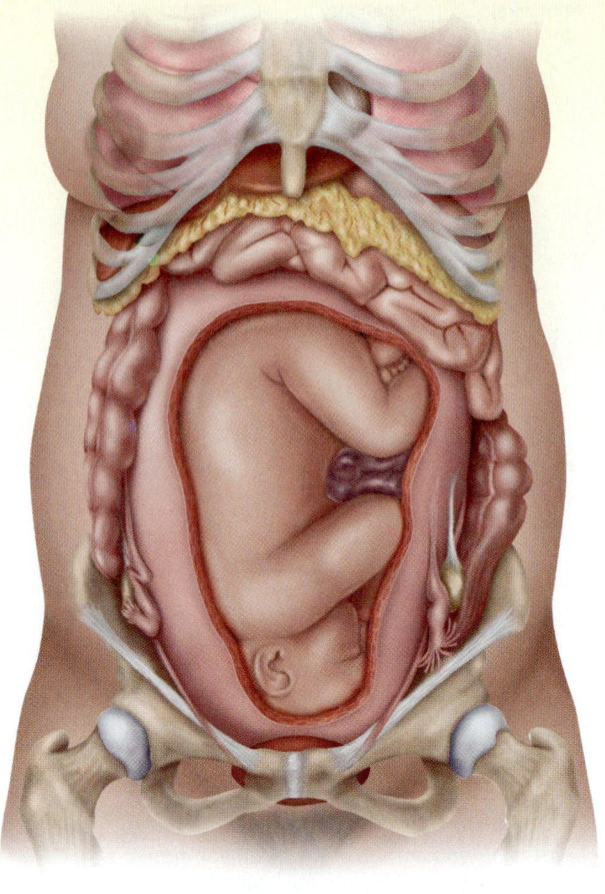

amnion

ROOT: ***amni/o***

EXAMPLE: amniocentesis

NOTES: The *amnion* is the innermost membrane covering the fetus.

pregnancy

SUFFIX: ***-cyesis***

EXAMPLE: pseudocyesis

NOTES: Although women experience pregnancy firsthand, there is a documented medical condition called Couvade syndrome, or sympathetic pregnancy, in which a man experiences some of the symptoms of pregnancy, including weight gain, morning sickness, and, in some cases, labor "pains."

chorion

ROOTS: ***chori/o, chorion/o***

EXAMPLE: choriocarcinoma, chorionitis

NOTES: The *chorion* is the outer membrane covering the fetus. It connects the fetus to the wall of the uterus.

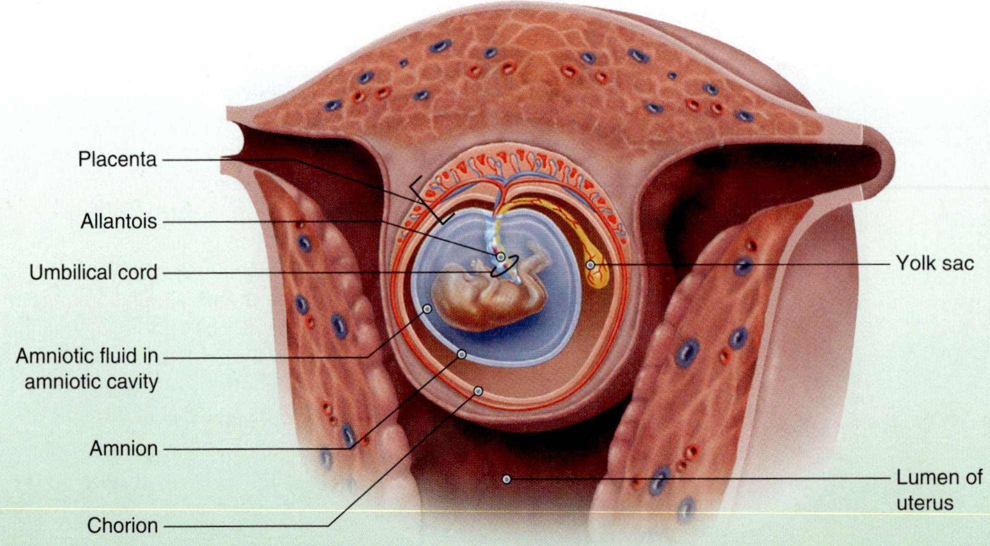

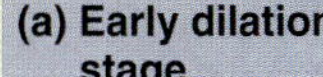

(a) Early dilation stage

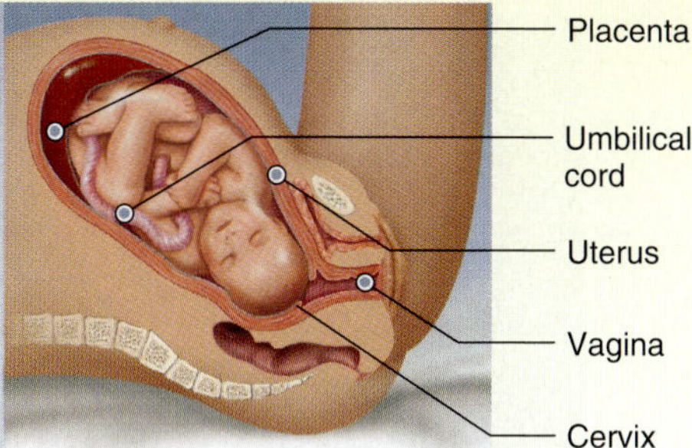

(b) Late dilation stage

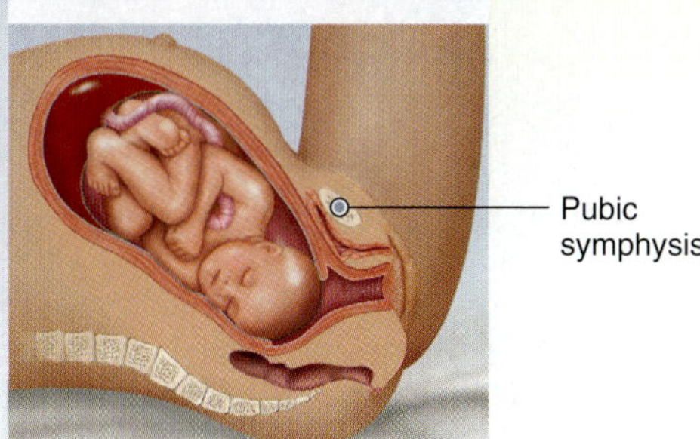

(c) Expulsion stage

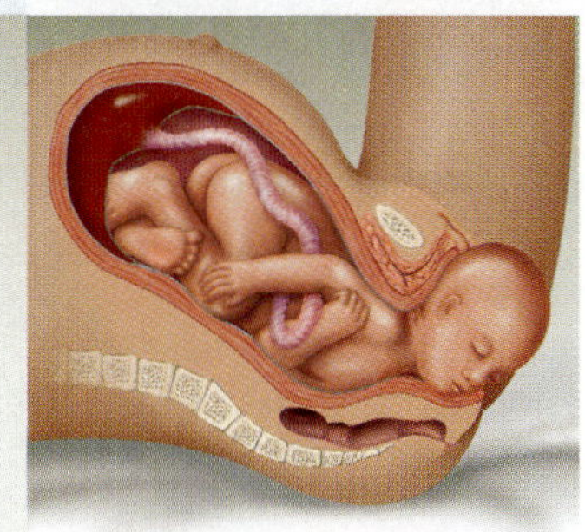

(d) Placental stage

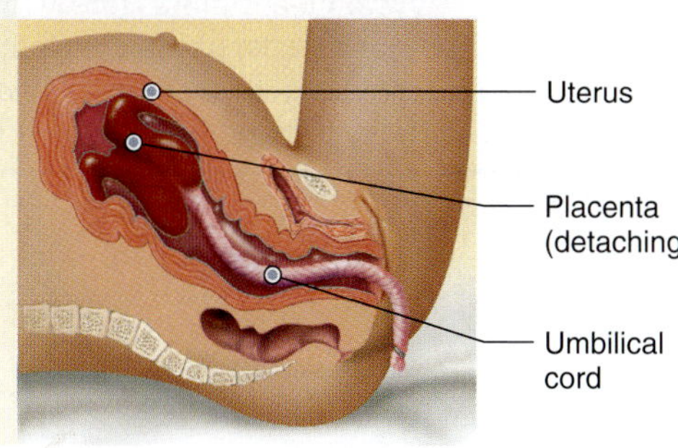

labor

ROOT: *toc/o*

EXAMPLES: dystocia, tocograph

NOTES: In the United States, there are more boy babies born than girl babies. For the past 60 years, the ratio has been about the same: 105 male births for every 100 female births. Also, according to some statistics, Tuesday is the most popular day to give birth. One more fun fact: Jimmy Carter was the first U.S. president to be born in a hospital.

fetus

ROOT: ***fet/o***

EXAMPLE: fetometry

NOTES: *Fetus* is a Latin word that means *offspring.* The Greek word is *embryo.* In current medical usage, a fetus is an unborn child after the eighth week of pregnancy. Before that time, it is referred to as an embryo. Before the fertilization of an egg, the sperm and egg are called *gametes* (Greek for *husband* and *wife*). Once they join, a separate, distinct, and genetically unique creature is created that is called a *zygote* (Greek for *joined together*). Once the unborn child becomes implanted in the wall of the uterus, it is called an embryo.

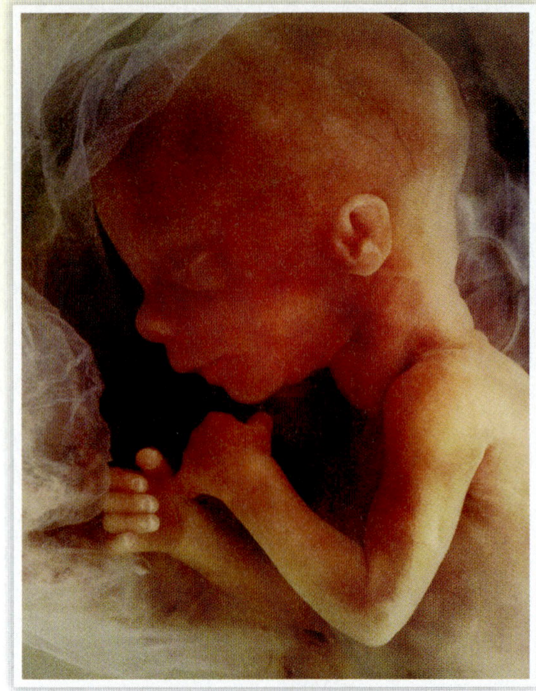

birth

ROOTS: ***part/o, nat/o***

EXAMPLES: postpartum, neonatal

NOTES: Both roots mean *birth,* but their focus is different. *Parto* means more accurately *to give birth* and therefore focuses on the mother. *Nato* means more literally *to be born* and therefore focuses on the baby. Hence, a mother gets *postpartum depression* and a baby is cared for by a *neonatologist.*

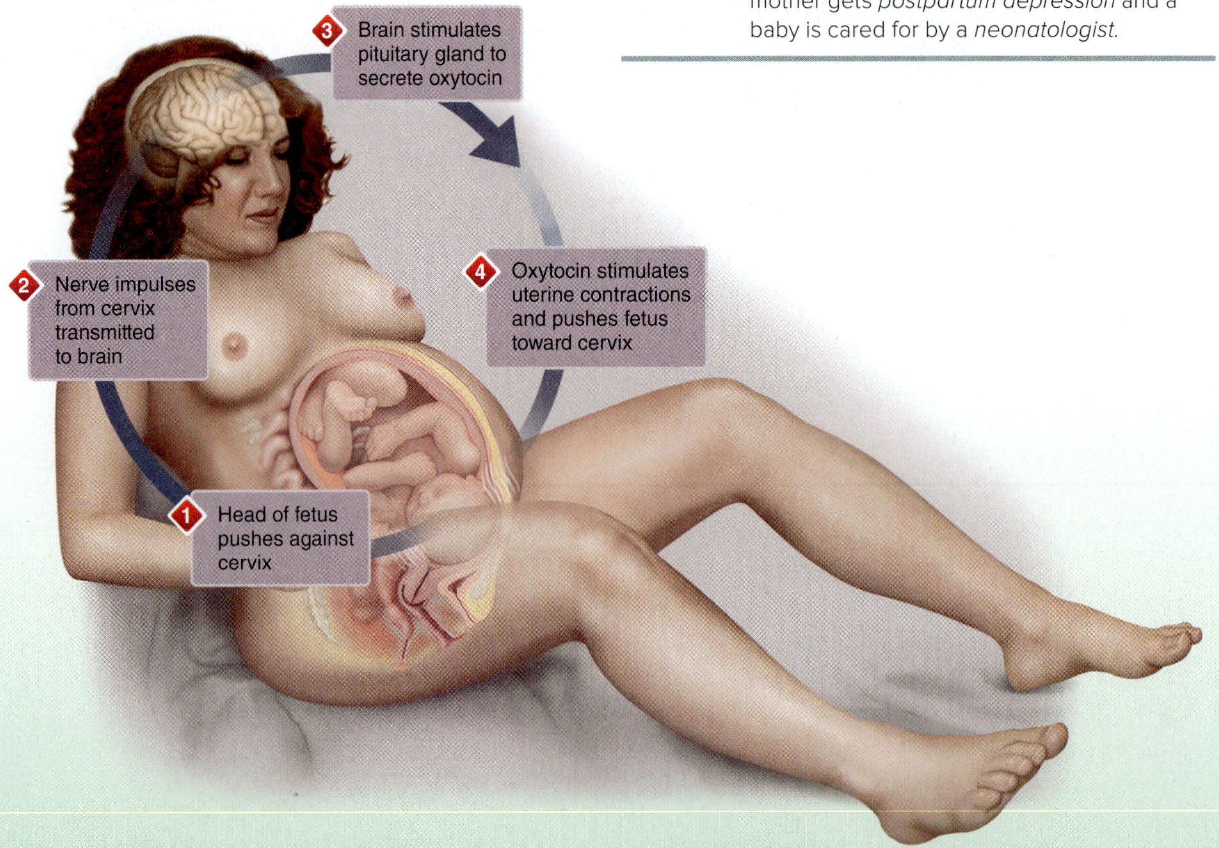

1 Head of fetus pushes against cervix
2 Nerve impulses from cervix transmitted to brain
3 Brain stimulates pituitary gland to secrete oxytocin
4 Oxytocin stimulates uterine contractions and pushes fetus toward cervix

Learning Outcome 13.1 Exercises

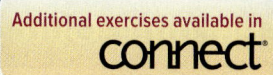

TRANSLATION

EXERCISE 1 *Match the root on the left with its definition on the right. Some definitions will be used more than once.*

Answer	Root		Definition
e	1. vagin/o	a.	breast
b	2. vulv/o	b.	external genital organs of a female
a	3. mamm/o	c.	milk
c	4. lact/o	d.	region between the genital organs and the anus
f	5. gynec/o	e.	vagina
d	6. perine/o	f.	woman
f	7. gyn/o		
e	8. colp/o		
b	9. episi/o		
a	10. mast/o		

EXERCISE 2 *Translate the following roots.*

1. vagin/o __________
2. vulv/o __________
3. gynec/o __________
4. lact/o __________
5. perine/o __________
6. mamm/o __________
7. gyn/o __________
8. episi/o __________
9. mast/o __________
10. colp/o __________

EXERCISE 3 *Underline and define the roots from this chapter in the following terms.*

1. vulvitis __________
2. lactation __________
3. perineocele __________
4. colpocystitis __________
5. mammoplasty __________
6. mastoptosis __________
7. episiorrhaphy __________
8. vaginomycosis __________
9. gynecomastia (2 roots) __________
10. vaginoperineorrhaphy (2 roots) __________

EXERCISE 4 *Break down the following words into their component parts and translate.*

> EXAMPLE: sinusitis *sinus | itis* *inflammation of the sinuses*

1. vaginitis __________
2. vulvitis __________
3. mastitis __________
4. colpitis __________
5. gynecologist __________

6. mammogram ________________
7. lactogenic ________________
8. perineorrhaphy ________________
9. episiostenosis ________________
10. vulvovaginitis ________________

EXERCISE 5 *Match the root on the left with its definition on the right. Some definitions will be used more than once.*

f	1. uter/o	a.	fallopian tube
d	2. ovari/o	b.	menstruation
c	3. cervic/o	c.	opening between the uterus and the vagina
e	4. pelv/i	d.	ovary
b	5. men/o	e.	pelvis
f	6. hyster/o	f.	uterus
f	7. metr/o		
d	8. oophor/o		
a	9. salping/o		

EXERCISE 6 *Translate the following roots.*

1. ovari/o ________________
2. cervic/o ________________
3. pelv/i ________________
4. uter/o ________________
5. men/o ________________
6. hyster/o ________________
7. salping/o ________________
8. oophor/o ________________
9. metr/o ________________

EXERCISE 7 *Underline and define the roots from this chapter in the following terms.*

1. ovariocentesis ________________
2. uterine prolapse ________________
3. cervical dysplasia ________________
4. menorrhagia ________________
5. salpingectomy ________________
6. endometritis ________________
7. hysteroptosis ________________
8. oophorocystectomy ________________

Learning Outcome 13.1 Exercises

9. cephalopelvic disproportion ______________________________
10. metromenorrhagia (2 roots) ______________________________
11. metrocolpocele (2 roots) ______________________________
12. salpingo-oophorectomy (2 roots) ______________________________
13. hysterosalpingectomy (2 roots) ______________________________

EXERCISE 8 *Break down the following words into their component parts and translate.*

> EXAMPLE: sinusitis *sinus | itis* *inflammation of the sinuses*

1. ovaritis ______________________________
2. cervicography ______________________________
3. hysterography ______________________________
4. oophoroma ______________________________
5. perimetritis ______________________________
6. dysmenorrhea ______________________________
7. hysterosalpingogram ______________________________
8. sonohysterography ______________________________

EXERCISE 9 *Match the word part on the left with its definition on the right. Some definitions will be used more than once.*

Answer	Word part		Definition
g	1. fet/o	a.	*to be born;* focus on the baby
a	2. nat/o	b.	*to give birth;* focus on the mother
c	3. amni/o	c.	innermost membrane covering the fetus
a	4. part/o	d.	labor
e	5. chorion/o	e.	outer membrane covering the fetus; connects the fetus to the wall of the uterus
c.	6. chori/o	f.	pregnancy
f.	7. -cyesis	g.	unborn child after the eighth week of pregnancy
d.	8. toc/o		

EXERCISE 10 *Translate the following word parts.*

1. amni/o ______________________________
2. chori/o, chorion/o ______________________________
3. fet/o ______________________________
4. nat/o ______________________________
5. part/o ______________________________
6. toc/o ______________________________
7. -cyesis ______________________________

Learning Outcome 13.1 Exercises

EXERCISE 11 *Underline and define the word parts from this chapter in the following terms.*

1. fetometry ____
2. amniorrhexis ____
3. choriocarcinoma ____
4. pseudocyesis ____
5. perinatologist ____
6. intrapartum ____
7. eutocia ____

EXERCISE 12 *Break down the following words into their component parts and translate.*

EXAMPLE: sinusitis *sinus | itis* *inflammation of the sinuses*

1. amnioscopy ____
2. chorioamnionitis ____
3. ovariocyesis ____
4. fetometry ____
5. neonatal ____
6. antepartum ____
7. tocography ____

GENERATION

EXERCISE 13 *Identify the roots for the following definitions.*

1. perineum ____
2. milk ____
3. woman (2 roots) ____
4. breast (2 roots) ____
5. vagina (2 roots) ____
6. vulva (2 roots) ____

EXERCISE 14 *Build a medical term from the information provided.*

EXAMPLE: inflammation of the sinuses *sinusitis*

1. pain in the vulva (use *vulv/o*) ____
2. surgical removal of a breast (use *mast/o*) ____
3. incision into the vulva (use *episi/o*) ____
4. the discharge of milk (use *-rrhea*) ____
5. surgical reconstruction of a breast (use *mamm/o*) ____

Learning Outcome 13.1 Exercises

6. surgical reconstruction of the vagina (use *vagin/o*) ____________________
7. surgical reconstruction of the vagina (use *colp/o*) ____________________
8. surgical reconstruction of the perineum ____________________
9. the study of medical issues specific to women ____________________
10. surgical reconstruction of the vagina and perineum (use *vagin/o*) ____________________

EXERCISE 15 *Identify the roots for the following definitions.*

1. cervix ____________________
2. pelvis ____________________
3. menstruation ____________________
4. fallopian tube ____________________
5. ovary (2 roots) ____________________
6. uterus (3 roots) ____________________

EXERCISE 16 *Build a medical term from the information provided.*

1. instrument for examining the uterus (use *hyster/o*) ____________________
2. inflammation of an ovary (use *oophor/o*) ____________________
3. pain in the ovary (use *ovari/o*) ____________________
4. inflammation of the cervix ____________________
5. procedure for measuring the pelvis ____________________
6. inflammation of the fallopian tube ____________________
7. inflammation of the fallopian tube and ovary (use *oophor/o*) ____________________

EXERCISE 17 *Identify the roots for the following definitions.*

1. fetus ____________________
2. amnion ____________________
3. pregnancy ____________________
4. labor ____________________
5. chorion (2 roots) ____________________
6. birth (2 roots) ____________________

EXERCISE 18 *Build a medical term from the information provided.*

1. pertaining to after the birth (use *nat/o*) ____________________
2. pertaining to after the birth (use *part/o*) ____________________
3. inflammation of the chorion ____________________
4. instrument for examining the amnion ____________________
5. instrument for recording the strength of labor (contractions) ____________________
6. pregnancy in a fallopian tube ____________________

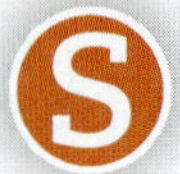

Subjective

Patient History, Problems, Complaints

Gynecology

Obstetrics

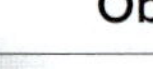

Objective

Observation and Discovery

Gynecology

Gynecology—Diagnostic Procedures

Gynecology—Professional Terms

Obstetrics

Obstetrics—Diagnostic Procedures

Obstetrics—Professional Terms

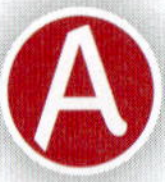

Assessment

Diagnosis and Pathology

Gynecology

Obstetrics

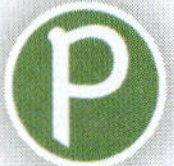

Plan

Treatments and Therapies

Gynecology

Obstetrics

This section contains medical terms built from the roots presented in the previous section. The purpose of this section is to expose you to words used in gynecology, obstetrics, and neonatology that are built from the word roots presented earlier. The focus of this book is to teach you the process of learning roots and translating them in context. Each term is presented with the correct pronunciation, followed by a word analysis that breaks down the word into its component parts, a definition that provides a literal translation of the word, as well as supplemental information if the literal translation deviates from its medical use.

The terms are organized using a health care professional's SOAP note (first introduced in Chapter 2) as a model.

SUBJECTIVE

13.2 Patient History, Problems, Complaints

Pain is always a common symptom in medicine, and the female reproductive system is no exception. The nerve fibers of the interior reproductive system share nerves with the lower gastrointestinal tract, so pain originating from this area can be hard to distinguish from gastrointestinal pain.

Pain in the vulva (*vulvodynia*) is often a condition without a known cause. Pain in the vagina (*vaginodynia*) is a common complication of infections, including fungal infections. More commonly, women will present to a medical office with pain that recurs at specific times, such as during menses (*dysmenorrhea*) or sexual intercourse (*dyspareunia*). Many times, women have both symptoms. These can be complications of *endometriosis* or *pelvic inflammatory disorder.*

Both females and males can present with pain in the breast (*mastalgia*). Women often suffer from this condition during breastfeeding. In males, this usually happens during puberty, when they may develop a small amount of breast tissue (*gynecomastia*).

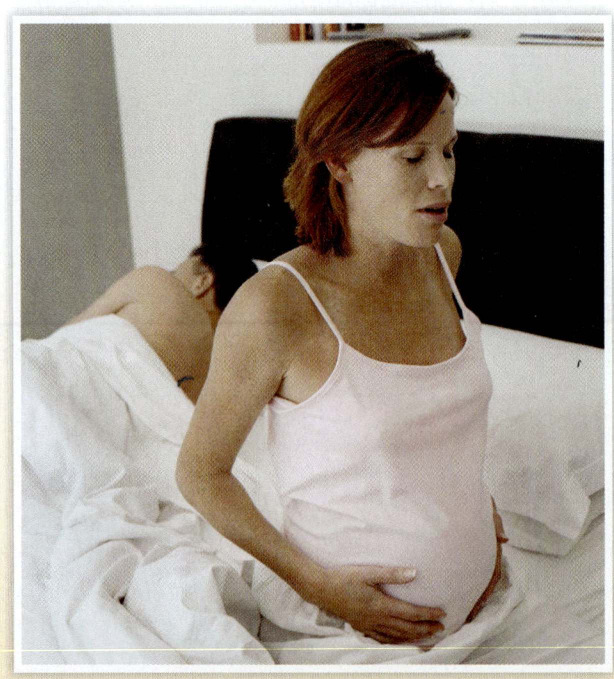

Contractions are a specific type of pain felt during pregnancy.

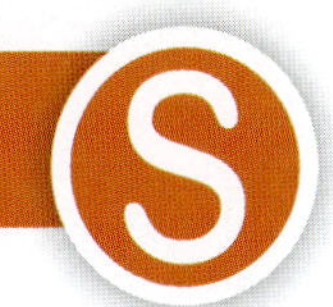

13.2 Patient History, Problems, Complaints

Women often come to health care providers with problems with menses. Their menses can be too frequent (*metrorrhagia*), too heavy (*menorrhagia*), or both (*metromenorrhagia*). Patients also may experience skipped periods (*oligomenorrhea*) or none at all (*amenorrhea*).

Women may also present with complaints of *abnormal discharge*. The discharge's odor and color can be good indicators of its cause. Sexually transmitted infections, such as *gonorrhea,* are a common cause of abnormal discharge.

During pregnancy, a woman's "water" breaking is also a discharge (*amniorrhea*). It is a good indicator that delivery is near.

gynecology

Term	Word Analysis
amenorrhea AY-men-oh-REE-ah **Definition** no menstruation	a / meno / rrhea no / menstruation / discharge
colpostenosis KOL-poh-steh-NOH-sis **Definition** narrowing in the vaginal opening	colpo / sten / osis vagina / narrow / condition
dysmenorrhea DIS-men-oh-REE-ah **Definition** painful menstruation	dys / meno / rrhea bad / menstruation / discharge
dyspareunia dis-pah-ROO-nee-ah **Definition** painful sexual intercourse	dys / par / eun / ia bad / alongside / couch / condition
gynecomastia GAI-neh-koh-MAS-tee-a **Definition** development of breast tissue in males **Note:** This term applies to men and not women, but it is included in this chapter because of the root it uses.	gyneco / mast / ia woman / breast / condition
hysteralgia HIS-ter-AL-jah **Definition** pain in the uterus	hyster / algia uterus / pain
hysterodynia HIS-ter-oh-DAI-nee-ah **Definition** pain in the uterus	hystero / dynia uterus / pain
leukorrhea LOO-koh-REE-ah **Definition** white vaginal discharge	leuko / rrhea white / discharge
mastalgia mas-TAL-jah **Definition** breast pain	mast / algia breast / pain
mastoptosis MAS-top-TOH-sis **Definition** downward displacement (drooping) of the breast	masto / pt / osis breast / droop / condition

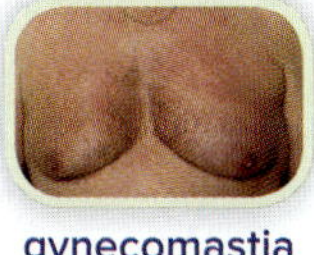

gynecomastia

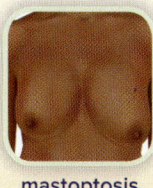

mastoptosis

13.2 Patient History, Problems, Complaints

gynecology *continued*

Term	Word Analysis
menorrhagia MEN-oh-RAY-jah **Definition** excessive menstrual flow	**meno / rrhagia** menstruation / excessive discharge
menorrhalgia MEN-oh-RAL-jah **Definition** painful menstruation **NOTE:** The difference between the last two words is only one letter—but that one letter makes a big difference.	**meno / rrh / algia** uterus / discharge / pain
metromenorrhagia MEH-troh-MEN-oh-RAY-jah **Definition** excessive menstrual bleeding at irregular intervals	**metro / meno / rrhagia** uterus / menstruation / excessive discharge
metrorrhagia MEH-troh-RAY-jah **Definition** menstrual bleeding at irregular times	**metro / rrhagia** uterus / excessive discharge
oligomenorrhea AW-lih-goh-MEN-oh-REE-ah **Definition** infrequent or light menstrual periods	**oligo / meno / rrhea** few / menstruation / discharge
ovaralgia OH-var-AL-jah **Definition** pain of the ovaries	**ovar / algia** ovary / pain
ovarialgia oh-VAR-ee-AL-jah **Definition** pain of the ovaries **NOTE:** Both ovaralgia and ovarialgia are acceptable spellings and mean the same thing.	**ovari / algia** ovary / pain
perineocele PER-ih-NEE-oh-seel **Definition** hernia in the perineal region	**perineo / cele** perineum / pouch / tumor / hernia
polymenorrhea PAW-lee-MEN-oh-REE-ah **Definition** menstrual periods occurring with greater than normal frequency	**poly / meno / rrhea** many / menstruation / discharge
vaginodynia VAJ-ih-noh-DAI-nee-ah **Definition** vaginal pain	**vagino / dynia** vagina / pain
vulvodynia VUL-voh-DAI-nee-ah **Definition** pain in the vulva	**vulvo / dynia** vulva / pain

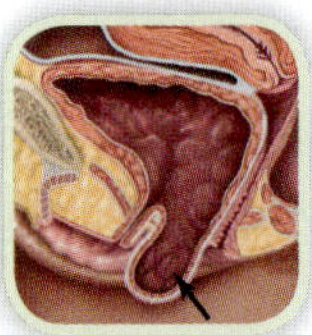
perineocele

13.2 Patient History, Problems, Complaints

obstetrics

Term	Word Analysis
amniorrhea AM-nee-oh-REE-ah **Definition** discharge of amniotic fluid	amnio / rrhea amnion / discharge
amniorrhexis AM-nee-oh-REK-sis **Definition** rupture of the amniotic sac	amnio / rrhexis amnion / rupture
Braxton Hicks contraction BRAKS-ton HIKS con-TRAK-shun **Definition** sporadic contractions of the uterine muscles of women not in labor; also known as false labor	*named after John Braxton Hicks, the doctor who first noted them, in 1872*
contraction con-TRAK-shun **Definition** shortening or tightening of a muscle; during labor, the uterine muscles contract	from Latin, for *to draw together* or *shorten*

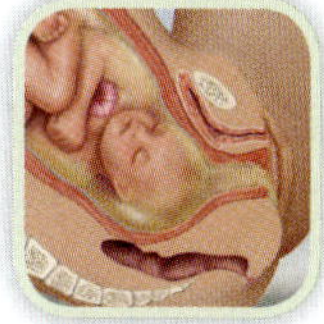
amniorrhexis

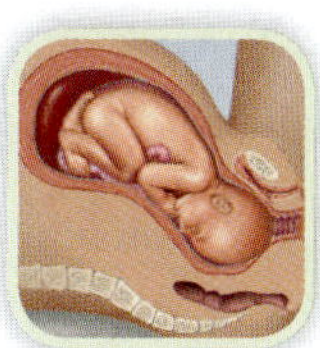
contraction

Learning Outcome 13.2 Exercises

PRONUNCIATION

EXERCISE 1 *Break down the following words into syllables.*

EXAMPLE: synesthesia *syn | es | the | sia*

1. mastoptosis ______
2. hysterodynia ______
3. colpostenosis ______
4. metrorrhagia ______
5. menorrhalgia ______
6. perineocele ______
7. metromenorrhagia ______

EXERCISE 2 *Indicate which syllable is emphasized when pronounced.*

EXAMPLE: bronchitis bron**chi**tis

1. dyspareunia ______
2. mastalgia ______
3. contraction ______
4. menorrhagia (2) ______
5. ovarialgia (2) ______
6. ovaralgia (2) ______
7. amenorrhea (2) ______
8. amniorrhexis (2) ______

TRANSLATION

EXERCISE 3 *Break down the following words into their component parts.*

EXAMPLE: nasopharyngoscope *naso | pharyngo | scope*

1. ovaralgia ______
2. leukorrhea ______
3. hysterodynia ______
4. menorrhagia ______
5. menorrhalgia ______
6. perineocele ______
7. amniorrhexis ______
8. gynecomastia ______
9. mastoptosis ______
10. amenorrhea ______

Learning Outcome 13.2 Exercises

EXERCISE 4 *Underline and define the word parts from this chapter in the following terms.*

1. ovarialgia ______
2. vaginodynia ______
3. vulvodynia ______
4. amniorrhea ______
5. hysteralgia ______
6. mastalgia ______
7. metrorrhagia ______
8. colpostenosis ______
9. dysmenorrhea ______
10. oligomenorrhea ______
11. metromenorrhagia (2 roots) ______

EXERCISE 5 *Match the term on the left with its definition on the right.*

Answer	Term		Definition
i	1. contraction	a.	discharge of amniotic fluid
h	2. Braxton Hicks contraction	b.	excessive menstrual bleeding at irregular intervals
e	3. amenorrhea	c.	infrequent or light menstrual periods
j	4. leukorrhea	d.	menstrual periods occurring with greater than normal frequency
a	5. amniorrhea	e.	no menstruation
d	6. polymenorrhea	f.	painful menstruation
f	7. dysmenorrhea	g.	painful sexual intercourse
c	8. oligomenorrhea	h.	sporadic contraction of the uterine muscles of women in labor; also known as false labor
___	9. dyspareunia	i.	shortening or tightening of a muscle
b	10. metromenorrhagia	j.	white vaginal discharge

EXERCISE 6 *Translate the following terms as literally as possible.*

EXAMPLE: nasopharyngoscope *an instrument for looking at the nose and throat*

1. vaginodynia ______
2. vulvodynia ______
3. hysterodynia ______
4. ovaralgia ______
5. hysteralgia ______
6. mastalgia ______

Learning Outcome 13.2 Exercises

7. colpostenosis ____________
8. perineocele ____________
9. amniorrhexis ____________
10. metrorrhagia ____________
11. oligomenorrhea ____________

GENERATION

EXERCISE 7 *Build a medical term from the information provided.*

EXAMPLE: inflammation of the sinuses *sinusitis*

1. discharge of amniotic fluid ____________
2. no menstruation ____________
3. excessive menstrual flow ____________
4. painful menstruation ____________
5. white discharge ____________
6. downward displacement (drooping) of the breast ____________
7. development of breast tissue in males ____________
8. menstrual periods occurring with greater than normal frequency ____________

EXERCISE 8 *Multiple-choice questions. Select the correct answer.*

1. Sporadic contractions of the uterine muscles of women not in labor are known as
   a. Braxton Hicks contractions
   b. dyspareunia
   c. pseudocyesis
   d. pseudotocoria
2. Which of the following statements about the term *contraction* is FALSE?
   a. from Greek, for *to ball up*
   b. from Latin, for *to draw together* or *shorten*
   c. means the shortening or tightening of a muscle
   d. occurs during labor
3. The term *dyspareunia* means
   a. painful menstruation
   b. painful sexual intercourse
   c. unusual menstruation
   d. unusual sexual intercourse
4. Which of the following words is the correct medical term for *pain in the ovaries*?
   a. oopharalgia
   b. oophorodynia
   c. ovarialgia
   d. ovariodynia

OBJECTIVE

13.3 Observation and Discovery

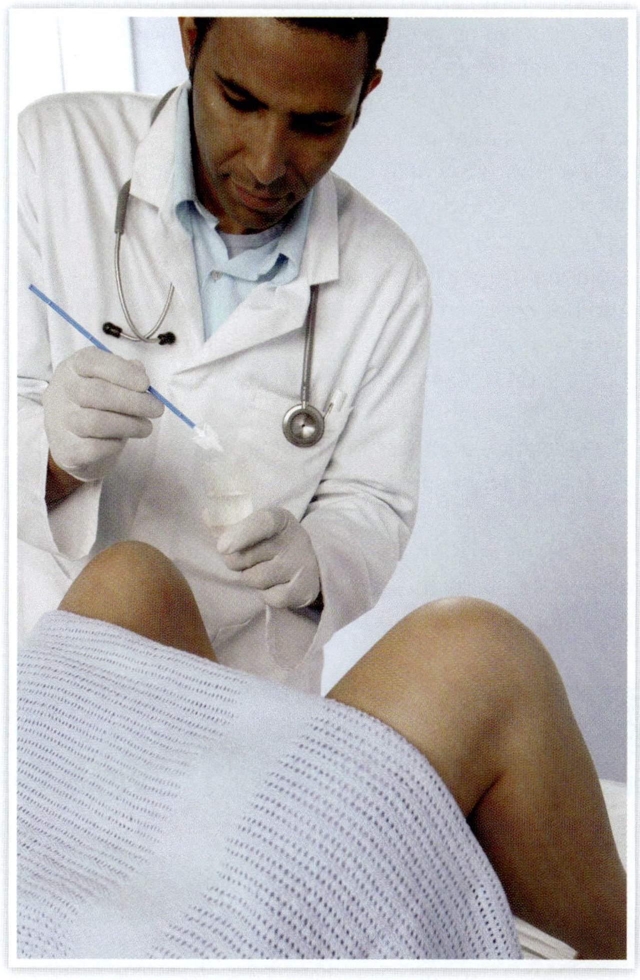

Pelvic exams and mammograms provide vital information for diagnosing gynecological issues.

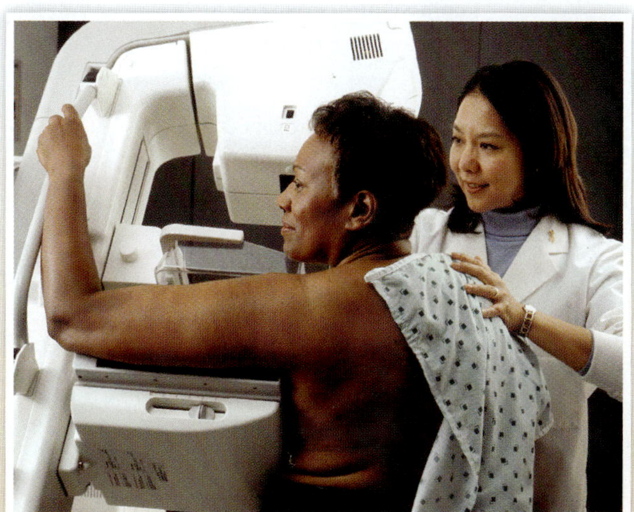

A physical exam of the female reproductive system includes a breast exam, an external genital exam, and a pelvic exam. When examining a patient's breast, the examiner must pay close attention to color changes, skin texture, any lumps in the breast, and the nipple. In an external genital exam, examiners must take into consideration the patient's developmental stage (if she is a child) and the general appearance of the vulvar area.

The most important part of a female reproductive (*gynecologic*) exam is the pelvic exam. This involves placing an instrument called a *speculum* in the opening of the vagina. This instrument spreads open the walls of the vagina to make it easier to visualize the cervix.

An exam of the cervix (*colposcopy*) is a routine exam for all adult females. A critical part of this exam is the Pap smear, which involves removing a sample of tissue from the cervix and examining it with a microscope to screen for cancer.

Feeling the uterus and ovaries requires a *bimanual* exam, which involves placing fingers from one hand inside the vagina and one hand on the abdomen and feeling the structures between both hands. This type of exam aids in detecting any lumps or painful areas.

Finally, the examiner may need to perform a *rectovaginal* exam to best feel the walls of the vagina. The exam involves placing one or two fingers in the patient's rectum and the other in her vagina to search for any abnormalities.

Two common types of imaging studies are used to analyze a woman's reproductive system. One is the *mammogram,* a special x-ray that looks for cancer in the breast. The other common image type is an *ultrasound.* An ultrasound placed inside the vagina (*transvaginal ultrasound*) is a common way of looking at the ovaries, uterus, and cervix. During pregnancy, ultrasound is commonly used to screen the health of the uterus and baby (*prenatal ultrasound*). Many times, a more direct visual inspection of a patient's reproductive tract can help a physician determine the nature of a patient's problem. For a more in-depth view of the vulva, vagina, and cervix, the physician may need to use a special magnifying instrument *(colposcope).* This procedure is known as *colposcopy.* Similarly, he or she may use a special device to visualize the inside of the uterus *(hysteroscopy).*

13.3 Observation and Discovery

Women frequently see health care providers for *prenatal care* throughout a pregnancy. Just prior to delivery (*antepartum*), it is important to determine how the baby is positioned inside the mother (*presentation*). By the time the baby is ready for delivery, its head should be facing downward (*cephalic*), but at times a baby's bottom or legs will be near the birth canal (*breech*). Because it is harder to deliver a baby in breech presentation, most obstetricians will choose to deliver the baby surgically (*cesarean section*).

During the antepartum visits, a health care worker will also need to determine the baby's size (*fetometry*), whether or not any birth defects (*congenital anomalies*) are present, and the womb's fluid (*amniotic fluid*) level. A large (*macrocephaly*) or small (*microcephaly*) head could indicate a problem with the brain. Too little amniotic fluid (*oligohydramnios*) generally indicates kidney problems in the baby. Too much fluid (*polyhydramnios*) can have numerous causes, including diabetes in the mother or gastrointestinal or urinary problems in the baby.

During delivery, the goal is a normal, uncomplicated delivery (*eutocia*). However, the delivery can be unusually painful (*dystocia*), perhaps if the baby's head is larger than the delivery canal (*cephalopelvic disproportion*). This condition is another common reason for a cesarean section delivery.

After delivery (*postpartum*), the mother will have follow-up exams to ensure that she is recovering well and to determine whether she has begun producing breast milk (*lactorrrhea*). This usually happens by three to four days after delivery.

The laboratory data collected when diagnosing female reproductive problems include results from a test called the *Pap smear,* which screens for cancer. It is among the most common labs specific to females. Another common lab is the wet mount. A *wet mount* involves collecting some vaginal discharge and putting it on a slide to examine with a microscope and look for signs of infection.

Pregnant patients often need lab tests to evaluate the fluid that surrounds the baby (*amniocentesis*). The test's results can reveal information on the baby's lung maturity, the presence of certain birth defects involving the spinal cord, and certain genetic conditions.

gynecology

Term	Word Analysis
amastia ay-MAS-tee-ah **Definition** absence of breast	a / mast / ia no / breast / condition
cervical dysplasia SER-vih-kal dis-PLAY-zhah **Definition** bad formation of cervical cells	cervic / al dys / plasia cervix / pertaining to bad / formation
colpoptosis KOL-pawp-TOH-sis **Definition** downward displacement of the vagina	colpo / pt / osis vagina / droop / condition
episiostenosis eh-PEE-zee-oh-stih-NOH-sis **Definition** narrowing of the vulvar opening	episio / sten / osis vulva / narrow / condition
hematosalpinx heh-MAT-oh-SAL-pinks **Definition** blockage in a fallopian tube caused by blood	hemato / salpinx blood / fallopian tube
hydrosalpinx HAI-droh-SAL-pinks **Definition** blockage in a fallopian tube caused by water (or any clear fluid)	hydro / salpinx water / fallopian tube

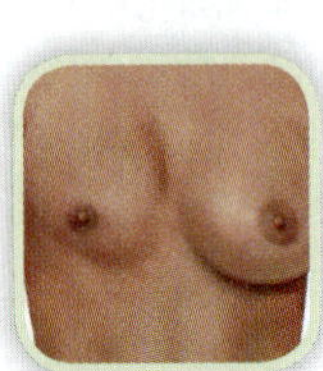
amastia

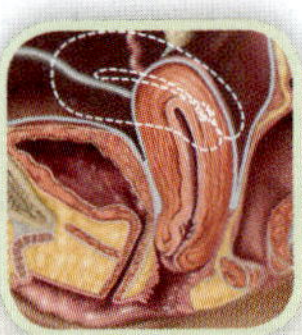
colpoptosis

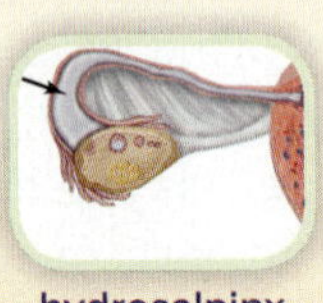
hydrosalpinx

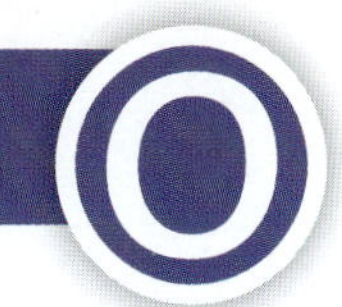

13.3 Observation and Discovery

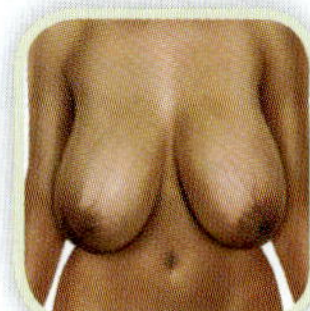

hypermastia

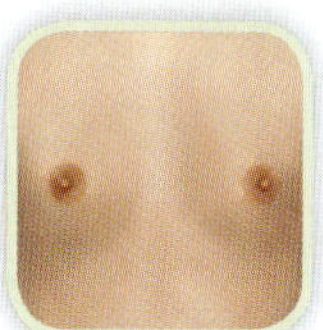

hypomastia

gynecology *continued*

Term	Word Analysis
hypermastia HAI-per-MAS-tee-ah **Definition** excessively large breasts **Note:** This term can also refer to an abnormal number of breasts.	hyper / mast / ia over / breast / condition
hypomastia HAI-poh-MAS-tee-ah **Definition** abnormally small breasts	hypo / mast / ia under / breast / condition
hysteroptosis HIS-ter-awp-TOH-sis **Definition** downward displacement of the uterus into the vagina	hystero / pt / osis uterus / droop / condition
macromastia MAK-roh-MAS-tee-ah **Definition** abnormally large breasts	macro / mast / ia big / breast / condition
micromastia MAI-kroh-MAS-tee-ah **Definition** abnormally small breasts	micro / mast / ia small / breast / condition
oophorocystosis OH-aw-FOR-oh-SIS-toh-sis **Definition** ovarian cysts	oophoro / cyst / osis ovary / cyst / condition
pyosalpinx PAI-oh-SAL-pinks **Definition** blockage in a fallopian tube caused by pus	pyo / salpinx pus / fallopian tube
uterine prolapse YOO-ter-in PROH-laps **Definition** downward displacement of the uterus into the vagina	uter / ine pro / lapse uterus / pertaining to forward / fall

gynecology—diagnostic procedures

Term	Word Analysis
cervicography SER-vih-KAW-grah-fee **Definition** procedure for imaging the cervix	cervico / graph / y cervix / recording / process
colposcope KOL-poh-SKOHP **Definition** instrument used to examine the vagina	colpo / scope vagina / instrument to look
colposcopy kol-PAW-skoh-pee **Definition** procedure for examining the vagina	colpo / scopy vagina / procedure to look

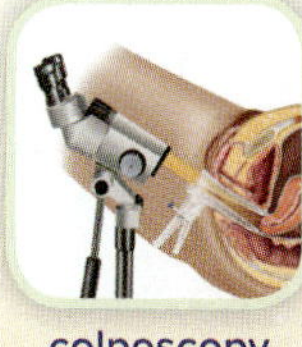

colposcopy

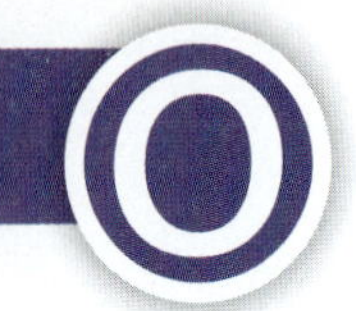

13.3 Observation and Discovery

mammogram

Pap smear

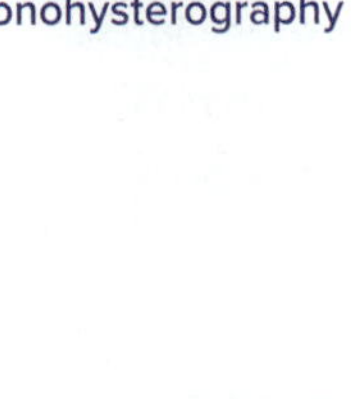

sonohysterography

gynecology—diagnostic procedures *continued*

Term	Word Analysis
hysterosalpingogram HIS-ter-oh-sal-PING-goh-gram	**hystero / salpingo / gram** uterus / fallopian tube / record
Definition record of the uterus and fallopian tubes	
hysteroscope HIS-ter-oh-SKOHP	**hystero / scope** uterus / instrument to look
Definition instrument for examining the uterus	
hysteroscopy HIS-ter-AW-skoh-pee	**hystero / scopy** uterus / procedure to look
Definition procedure for examining the uterus	
mammogram MAM-oh-GRAM	**mammo / gram** breast / record
Definition record of a breast exam	
Pap smear PAP SMEER	*named after the inventor of the procedure, Dr. Georgios Papanicolaou*
Definition test used to detect cancer cells, most commonly in the cervix	
sonohysterography SOH-noh-HIS-ter-AW-grah-fee	**sono / hystero / graph / y** sound / uterus / recording / process
Definition procedure using sound waves to examine the uterus	
transvaginal sonography TRANZ-VAJ-ih-nal soh-NAW-grah-fee	**trans / vagin / al sono / graph / y** through / vagina / pertaining to sound / recording / process
Definition imaging procedure using sound waves emitted from a device inserted in the vagina	
vaginoscope VAJ-ih-noh-SKOHP	**vagino / scope** vagina / instrument to look
Definition instrument used to examine the vagina	

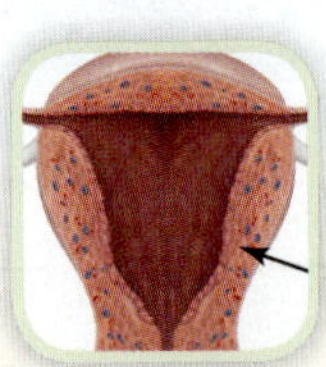

endometrium

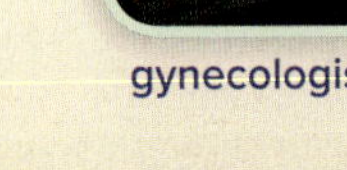

gynecologist

gynecology—professional terms

Term	Word Analysis
endometrium EN-doh-MEE-tree-um	**endo / metr / ium** inside / uterus / tissue
Definition inner layer of uterine tissue	
gynecologist GAI-neh-KAW-loh-jist	**gyneco / logist** woman / specialist
Definition specialist in medical issues specific to women	
gynecology GAI-neh-KAW-loh-jee	**gyneco / logy** woman / study
Definition study of medical issues specific to women	
menarche MEN-ar-kee	**men / arche** menstruation / beginning
Definition beginning or first menstruation	

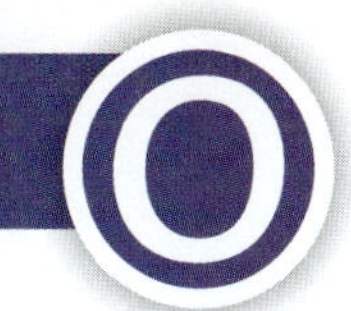

13.3 Observation and Discovery

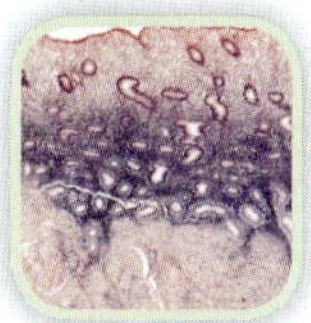
myometrium

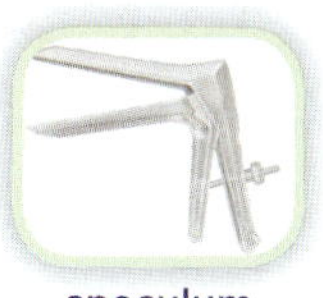
speculum

gynecology—professional terms *continued*

Term	Word Analysis
myometrium MAI-oh-MEE-tree-um **Definition** middle layer of uterine muscle tissue	myo / metr / ium muscle / uterus / tissue
perimetrium PER-ee-MEE-tree-um **Definition** tissue on the outside of the uterus, the outer layer of the uterus	peri / metr / ium around / uterus / tissue
speculum SPEH-kyoo-lum **Definition** device for examining a body cavity, most commonly the vagina	from Latin, for *mirror*

obstetrics

Term	Word Analysis
bradytocia BRAY-dih-TOH-shee-ah **Definition** slow labor	brady / toc / ia slow / birth / condition
cephalopelvic disproportion (CPD) SEE-fah-loh-PEL-vik DIS-proh-POR-shun **Definition** condition characterized by the inability of the mother's pelvis to allow the baby to pass through the birth canal **NOTE:** This can be caused by either a small pelvis or a large baby, or both.	cephalo / pelv / ic disproportion head / pelvic / pertaining to
congenital anomaly con-JIN-ih-tal ah-NAW-moh-lee **Definition** irregular condition that is present at the time of birth	con / genit / al anomaly with / birth / pertaining to irregularity
dystocia dis-TOH-shee-ah **Definition** difficult labor	dys / toc / ia bad / birth / condition
eutocia yoo-TOH-shee-ah **Definition** normal labor	eu / toc / ia good / birth / condition
gravida GRAH-vid-ah **Definition** another term for pregnant **NOTE:** This word, which is also where the word gravity comes from, means heavy and is similar to an old expression about pregnancy that a woman is "great with child."	gravida heavy
hysterocele HIS-ter-oh-SEEL **Definition** hernia of the uterus	hystero / cele uterus / pouch / tumor / hernia
hysterorrhexis HIS-ter-oh-REK-sis **Definition** rupture of the uterus	hystero / rrhexis uterus / rupture

obstetrics *continued*

Term	Word Analysis
lactogenic LAK-toh-JIN-ik **Definition** causing the formation of milk	lacto / gen / ic milk / creation / pertaining to
lactorrhea LAK-toh-REE-ah **Definition** discharge of milk	lacto / rrhea milk / discharge
macrosomia MAK-roh-SOH-mee-ah **Definition** baby with a large body	macro / som / ia large / body / condition
microcephalus MAI-kroh-SEF-ah-lus **Definition** baby with a small head	micro / cephalus small / head
oligohydramnios AW-lih-goh-hai-DRAM-nee-ohs **Definition** not enough amniotic fluid	oligo / hydr / amnios few / water / amnion
polyhydramnios PAW-lee-hai-DRAM-nee-ohs **Definition** excessive amniotic fluid	poly / hydr / amnios a lot / water / amnion
teratogenic TER-ah-toh-JIN-ik **Definition** causing the formation of birth defects	terato / gen / ic monster / creation / pertaining to

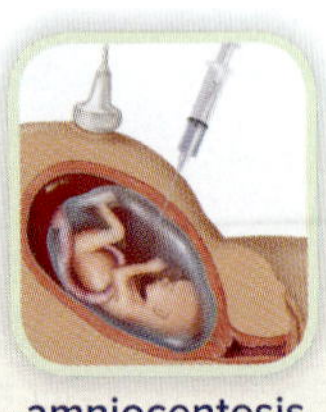

amniocentesis

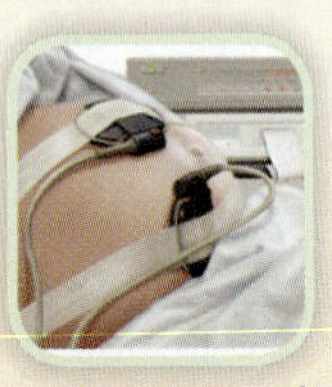

cardiotocograph

obstetrics—diagnostic procedures

Term	Word Analysis
amniocentesis AM-nee-oh-sin-TEE-sis **Definition** surgical puncture of the amnion	amnio / centesis amnion / puncture
amnioscope AM-nee-oh-SKOHP **Definition** instrument for examining the amnion	amnio / scope amnion / instrument to look
amnioscopy AM-nee-AW-skoh-pee **Definition** procedure for examining the amnion	amnio / scop / y amnion / look / procedure
cardiotocograph KAR-dee-oh-TOH-koh-GRAF **Definition** instrument for recording the baby's heart rate during contractions; also known as a fetal heart monitor	cardio / toco / graph heart / birth / instrument to record

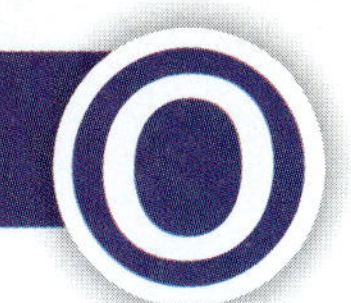

13.3 Observation and Discovery

obstetrics—diagnostic procedures *continued*

Term	Word Analysis
fetometry fee-TAW-meh-tree **Definition** procedure for measuring the fetus	feto / metr / y fetus / measure / procedure
hysterography HIS-ter-AW-grah-fee **Definition** procedure for imaging the uterus	hystero / graph / y uterus / writing / procedure
pelvic sonograph PEL-vik SAW-noh-GRAF **Definition** instrument for imaging the pelvis using sound waves	pelv / ic sono / graph pelvis / pertaining to sound / instrument to record
pelvicephalometry PEL-vih-SEF-eh-LAW-meh-tree **Definition** procedure for measuring the head size of the baby and the pelvis size of the mother	pelvi / cephalo / metr / y pelvis / head / measure / procedure
pelvimetry pel-VIM-eh-tree **Definition** procedure for measuring the pelvis	pelvi / metr / y pelvis / measure / procedure
tocodynagraph TOH-koh-DAI-nah-GRAF **Definition** instrument for recording the strength of labor contractions	toco / dyna / graph birth / power / instrument to record
tocography toh-KAW-grah-fee **Definition** procedure for recording the strength of labor contractions	toco / graph / y birth / recording / procedure

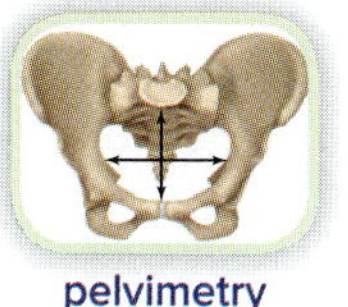
pelvimetry

obstetrics—professional terms

Term	Word Analysis
antepartum AN-tee-PAR-tum **Definition** time before birth	ante / partum before / birth
intrapartum IN-trah-PAR-tum **Definition** time during birth	intra / partum during / birth
lactation lak-TAY-shun **Definition** production of milk	lact / ation milk / formation
natal NAY-tal **Definition** pertaining to birth	nat / al birth / pertaining to

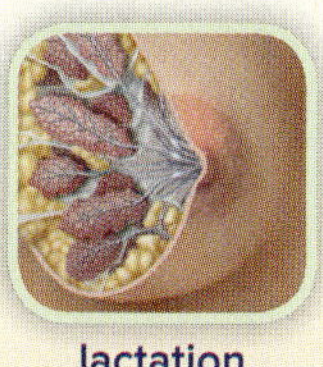
lactation

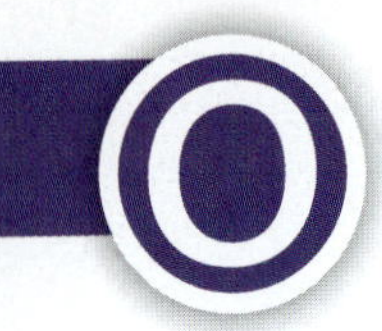

13.3 Observation and Discovery

obstetrics—professional terms *continued*

Term	Word Analysis
neonatal NEE-oh-NAY-tal **Definition** pertaining to new birth; normally the first 28 days after birth	neo / nat / al new / birth / pertaining to
neonatologist NEE-oh-nay-TAW-loh-jist **Definition** specialist in the neonatal period	neo / nato / logist new / birth / specialist
neonatology NEE-oh-nay-TAW-loh-jee **Definition** study of the neonatal period	neo / nato / logy new / birth / study
obstetrician OB-steh-TRIH-shun **Definition** specialist in pregnancy, labor, and delivery of newborns	from Latin, for *midwife* or literally *one who stands beside*
obstetrics ob-STEH-triks **Definition** branch of medicine dealing with pregnancy, labor, and delivery of newborns	from Latin, for *midwife* or literally *one who stands beside*
perinatal PEH-ree-NAY-tal **Definition** time around the birth, normally ranging from 28 weeks of pregnancy to 28 days after pregnancy	peri / nat / al around / birth / pertaining to
perinatologist PEH-ree-nay-TAW-loh-jist **Definition** specialist in the perinatal period	peri / nato / logist around / birth / specialist
perinatology PER-ee-nay-TAW-loh-jee **Definition** branch of medicine dealing with the perinatal period	peri / nato / logy around / birth / study
postnatal post-NAY-tal **Definition** pertaining to after birth	post / nat / al after / birth / pertaining to
postpartum POST-PAR-tum **Definition** pertaining to after birth NOTE: The difference between this word and *postnatal* is the focus. Normally, *nato* words focus on the baby and *partum* words focus on the mother.	post / partum after / birth
prenatal pree-NAY-tal **Definition** pertaining to before birth	pre / natal before / birth
teratology TER-ah-TAW-loh-jee **Definition** branch of medicine dealing with the study of birth defects and their causes	terato / logy monster / study

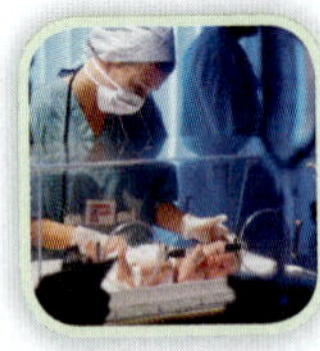
neonatology

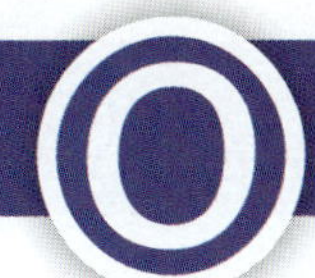

Learning Outcome 13.3 Exercises

PRONUNCIATION

EXERCISE 1 *Break down the following words into syllables.*

EXAMPLE: synesthesia *syn | es | the | sia*

1. amastia ______
2. perinatal ______
3. hypomastia ______
4. macromastia ______
5. micromastia ______
6. macrosomia ______
7. antepartum ______
8. intrapartum ______
9. endometrium ______
10. perimetrium ______
11. teratogenic ______
12. amnioscope ______
13. amnioscopy ______
14. hysterography ______
15. cardiotocograph ______
16. neonatology ______
17. obstetrician ______
18. hysterorrhexis ______
19. oligohydramnios ______
20. polyhydramnios ______

EXERCISE 2 *Indicate which syllables are emphasized when pronounced.*

EXAMPLE: bronchitis bron**chi**tis

1. natal ______
2. postnatal ______
3. prenatal ______
4. speculum ______
5. dystocia ______
6. eutocia ______
7. fetometry ______
8. pelvimetry ______
9. tocography ______

10. lactation ____________________
11. obstetrics ____________________
12. gravida ____________________
13. amastia ____________________
14. menarche ____________________
15. colposcopy ____________________
16. colposcope (2) ____________________
17. hysteroscopy (2) ____________________
18. hysteroscope (2) ____________________

TRANSLATION

EXERCISE 3 *Break down the following words into their component parts.*

EXAMPLE: nasopharyngoscope *naso | pharyngo | scope*

1. vaginoscope ____________________
2. fetometry ____________________
3. lactorrhea ____________________
4. hysterocele ____________________
5. gynecology ____________________
6. neonatal ____________________
7. postnatal ____________________
8. intrapartum ____________________
9. dystocia ____________________
10. eutocia ____________________
11. amniocentesis ____________________
12. cervical dysplasia ____________________
13. pelvic sonograph ____________________
14. neonatology ____________________
15. perinatologist ____________________
16. hematosalpinx ____________________
17. pyosalpinx ____________________
18. colpoptosis ____________________
19. hysteroptosis ____________________
20. sonohysterography ____________________
21. tocodynagraph ____________________

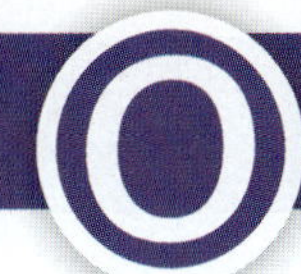

Learning Outcome 13.3 Exercises

22. polyhydramnios ______
23. teratology ______
24. microcephalus ______

EXERCISE 4 *Underline and define the word parts from this chapter in the following terms.*

1. natal ______
2. amnioscope ______
3. cervicography ______
4. gynecologist ______
5. lactogenic ______
6. mammogram ______
7. pelvimetry ______
8. prenatal ______
9. postpartum ______
10. cardiotocograph ______
11. perinatal ______
12. colposcope ______
13. hysteroscope ______
14. episiostenosis ______
15. neonatologist ______
16. antepartum ______
17. amastia ______
18. perinatology ______
19. bradytocia ______
20. menarche ______
21. oligohydramnios ______
22. hysterorrhexis ______
23. hydrosalpinx ______
24. myometrium ______
25. oophorocystosis ______
26. transvaginal sonography ______
27. pelvicephalometry ______
28. hysterosalpingogram (2 roots) ______

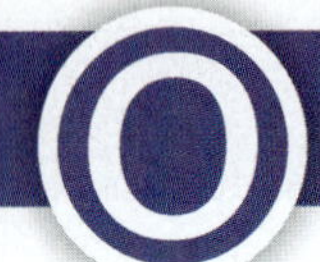

Learning Outcome 13.3 Exercises

EXERCISE 5 *Match the term on the left with its definition on the right.*

e	1. Pap smear	a.	baby with a large body
g	2. obstetrics	b.	condition characterized by the inability of the mother's pelvis to allow the baby to pass through the birth canal
d	3. obstetrician	c.	device for examining a body cavity, most commonly the vagina
c	4. speculum	d.	specialist in pregnancy, labor, and delivery of newborns
f	5. congenital anomaly	e.	test used to detect cancer cells, most commonly in the cervix
b	6. cephalopelvic disproportion	f.	irregular condition that is present at the time of birth
i	7. uterine prolapse	g.	branch of medicine dealing with pregnancy, labor, and delivery of newborns
a	8. macrosomia	h.	causing the formation of birth defects
h	9. teratogenic	i.	downward displacement of the uterus into the vagina
j	10. gravida	j.	pregnant

EXERCISE 6 *Fill in the blanks.*

1. *amnioscopy:* procedure for examining the ____________________
2. *cervicography:* procedure for imaging the ____________________
3. *hysterography:* procedure for imaging the ____________________
4. *colposcopy:* procedure for examining the ____________________
5. *hysteroscopy:* procedure for examining the ____________________
6. *tocography:* procedure for recording the strength of ____________________
7. *mammography:* procedure for imaging the ____________________
8. *vaginoscopy:* procedure for examining the ____________________

EXERCISE 7 *Translate the following terms as literally as possible.*

> EXAMPLE: nasopharyngoscope *an instrument for looking at the nose and throat*

1. natal ____________________
2. lactation ____________________
3. gynecology ____________________
4. tocograph ____________________
5. colposcope ____________________
6. hysteroscope ____________________

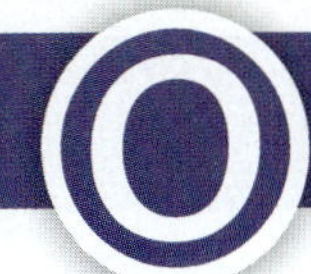

Learning Outcome 13.3 Exercises

7. hysterocele ______
8. lactorrhea ______
9. pyosalpinx ______
10. hypomastia ______
11. micromastia ______
12. amniocentesis ______
13. perinatology ______
14. hysterorrhexis ______
15. perimetrium ______
16. colpoptosis ______
17. oophorocystosis ______
18. cervical dysplasia ______
19. tocodynograph ______
20. cardiotocograph ______
21. transvaginal sonography ______
22. pervicephalometry ______
23. macrosomia ______
24. teratology ______

GENERATION

EXERCISE 8 *Build a medical term from the information provided.*

EXAMPLE: inflammation of the sinuses *sinusitis*

1. instrument used to examine the vagina (use *vagin/o*) ______
2. procedure for examining the vagina (use *colp/o*) ______
3. procedure for imaging the uterus (use *hyster/o*) ______
4. procedure for examining the uterus (use *hyster/o*) ______
5. procedure using sound waves to examine the uterus (use *hyster/o*) ______
6. record of a breast exam (use *mamm/o*) ______
7. procedure for examining the amnion ______
8. procedure for measuring the fetus ______
9. instrument for imaging the pelvis using sound waves ______
10. study of the neonatal period ______
11. specialist in medical issues specific to women ______
12. slow labor ______

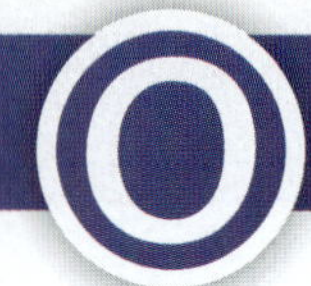

Learning Outcome 13.3 Exercises

13. narrowing of the vulvar opening (use *episi/o*) ______________________
14. causing the formation of milk ______________________
15. absence of breasts (use *mast/o*) ______________________
16. beginning or first menstruation ______________________
17. excessively large breasts (use *hyper-*) ______________________
18. downward displacement of the uterus ______________________
19. inner layer of uterine tissue ______________________
20. time during birth (use *part/o*) ______________________
21. record of the uterus and fallopian tubes ______________________
22. procedure for recording the strength of labor contractions ______________________
23. baby with a small head ______________________

EXERCISE 9 *Multiple-choice questions. Select the correct answer(s).*

1. The production of milk is called
   a. intrapartum
   b. lactation
   c. lactogenic
   d. lactorrhea
   e. none of these
2. The downward displacement of the uterus into the vagina is known as
   a. uterine prolapse
   b. hysteroptosis
   c. vesicovaginal fistula
   d. uterine prolapse and hysteroptosis
   e. hysteroptosis and vesicovaginal fistula
3. The middle layer of uterine muscle tissue is the
   a. endometrium
   b. intrametrium
   c. myometrium
   d. perimetrium
   e. none of these
4. A condition characterized by the inability of the mother's pelvis to allow the baby to pass through the birth canal is known as
   a. cephalopelvic disproportion
   b. microcephalus
   c. pelvicephalometry
   d. teratogenic
   e. none of these
5. Another term for *pregnant* is
   a. amastia
   b. gravida
   c. menarche
   d. prenatal
   e. teratogenic

-cyesis

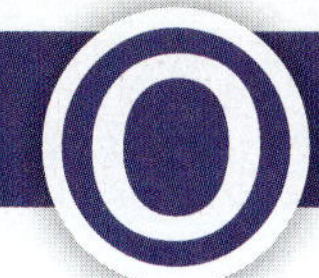

Learning Outcome 13.3 Exercises

6. Select all of the following statements that apply to the term *Pap smear.*
   a. a diagnostic procedure used in gynecology
   b. a diagnostic procedure used in obstetrics
   c. a test used to detect cancer cells, most commonly in the cervix
   d. a test used to detect cancer cells, most commonly in the vulva
   e. named after the inventor of the procedure, Dr. Georgios Papanicolaou
7. A device for examining a body cavity, most commonly the vagina, is called a(n)
   a. episiostenosis
   b. gravida
   c. hysterocele
   d. mammogram
   e. speculum
8. Select all of the following terms that pertain to obstetrics.
   a. amnioscope
   b. colposcope
   c. hysteroscope
   d. pelvimetry
   e. tocodynograph
   f. vaginoscope
9. Select all of the following terms that pertain to gynecology.
   a. amnioscope
   b. colposcope
   c. hysteroscope
   d. pelvimetry
   e. tocodynograph
   f. vaginoscope

EXERCISE 10 *Briefly describe the difference between each pair of terms.*

1. postnatal, prenatal ______
2. obstetrics, obstetrician ______
3. macromastia, micromastia ______
4. hypermastia, hypomastia ______
5. antepartum, postpartum ______
6. endometrium, perimetrium ______
7. neonatal, perinatal ______
8. neonatologist, perinatologist ______
9. dystocia, eutocia ______
10. hematosalpinx, hydrosalpinx ______
11. congenital anomaly, teratogenic ______

ASSESSMENT

13.4 Diagnosis and Pathology

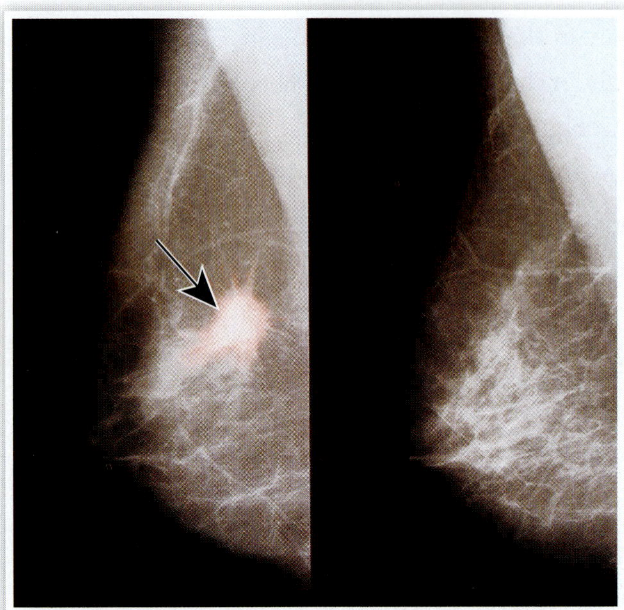
Mammogram of a breast with a tumor at the arrow (left), compared with the appearance of normal fibrous connective tissue of the breast (right).

Problems with periods are very routine causes for females to seek medical help. The normal range for a female's first period (*menarche*) is 10 to 16 years of age. An early or delayed start for periods may indicate an underlying problem. Missing one or more periods (*amenorrhea*) is a common reason for a medical visit. This can be caused by pregnancy, hormone problems, or problems with anatomy.

Unfortunately, cancers of the female reproductive system are common problems. Breast cancer (*adenocarcinoma of the breast*) is the most common cancer in women. For this reason, routine exams and mammograms are very important in female health care.

The uterus, cervix, and ovaries are also common areas for cancer. The Pap smear helps detect early evidence of cancer or precancerous changes in the cervix (*cervical intraepithelial neoplasia*).

Infection or inflammation of the female reproductive system happens more frequently in the outer parts of the reproductive system. Irritation of the vagina (*vaginitis*) or the vagina and its surrounding area (*vulvovaginitis*) can present with pain and/or itching. Both bacteria (*bacterial vaginosis*) and fungi (*vaginomycosis*) are frequent causes.

Many bacterial and viral infections of the female reproductive tract are spread through sexual intercourse. If infection spreads higher into the reproductive tract, such as to the fallopian tubes (*salpingitis*) and cervix (*cervicitis*), the patient may become quite ill; these infections can even lead to scarring and infertility. Another common infection in females is infection of the breast (*mastitis*), particularly in nursing mothers. Mastitis can make the breastfeeding process very painful.

Pregnancy can cause its own set of medical issues. A fertilized egg that implants anywhere other than the uterus is known as an *ectopic pregnancy.* Examples of ectopic locations include the fallopian tubes (*salpingocyesis*) and ovaries (*ovariacyesis*). Ectopic pregnancies are not viable, and they can cause pain and bleeding, infertility, and even death in some extreme circumstances.

During pregnancy, many women experience nausea and vomiting, a condition commonly known as *morning sickness.* In some cases, the vomiting can become quite severe (*hyperemesis gravidum*) and need medical treatment.

Another problem encountered by some women during pregnancy is *preeclampsia.* This condition is marked by high blood pressure and protein in the urine. It can progress to include seizures (*eclampsia*).

The connection point between the mother and the baby (*placenta*) can also be a source of medical problems. A placenta in the wrong position can block the opening in the uterus (*placenta previa*), making delivery problematic. If the blood supply to the placenta is interrupted (*abruptio placentae*), the baby may be at risk of not getting enough blood, and the mother could suffer severe blood loss.

The membranes of the womb can develop tumors or infection. Tumors of the womb actually arise from fetal tissue. Rarely, this can become cancerous (*choriocarcinoma*). Infections in the womb (*chorioamnionitis*) routinely occur just prior to delivery and are treated with antibiotics.

Not every pregnancy produces a baby capable of survival. In fact, upward of 25 percent of all known pregnancies result in the mother's body ending the pregnancy. This is mainly the mother's body's response

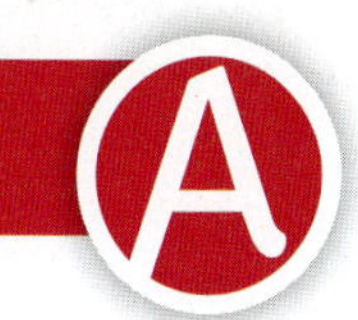

to a fetus with severe problems that would prevent survival. Commonly known as a *miscarriage,* the medical term is *spontaneous abortion.* This is opposed to common lay use of the term *abortion,* which usually refers to an *induced abortion.* An induced abortion is when a pregnancy is deliberately ended by artificial means. Induced abortions can be performed by taking a medication or via surgery.

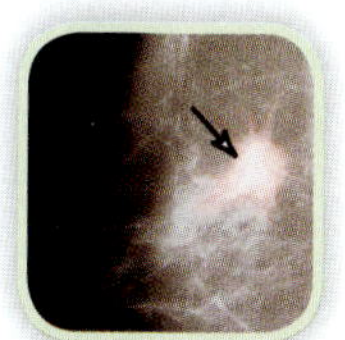

adenocarcinoma

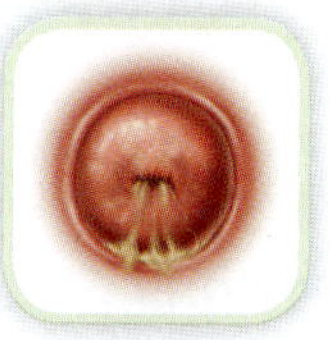

cervicitis

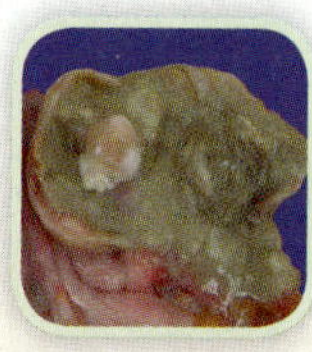

dermoid cyst

gynecology

Term	Word Analysis
adenocarcinoma of the breast AD-en-oh-KAR-sih-NOH-mah **Definition** glandular tumor in the breast	adeno / carcin / oma of the breast gland / cancer / tumor
cervical intraepithelial neoplasia SER-vih-kal IN-trah-EP-ih-THEE-lee-al NEE-oh-PLAY-zhah **Definition** abnormal growth of cervical cells NOTE: Epithelial cells are a type of tissue that lines the surface of the skin and other membranes.	cervic /al intra / epithelial neo / plasia cervix / pertaining to inside / epithelial new / formation
cervicitis SER-vih-SAI-tis **Definition** inflammation of the cervix	cervic / itis cervix / inflammation
cervicocolpitis SER-vih-koh-kol-PAI-tis **Definition** inflammation of the cervix and vagina	cervico / colp / itis cervix / vagina / inflammation
cervicovaginitis SER-vih-koh-VAJ-ih-NAI-tis **Definition** inflammation of the cervix and vagina	cervico / vagin / itis cervix / vagina / inflammation
colpitis kol-PAI-tis **Definition** inflammation of the vagina	colp / itis vagina / inflammation
colpocystitis KOL-poh-sis-TAI-tis **Definition** inflammation of the vagina and urinary bladder	colpo / cyst / itis vagina / bladder / inflammation
cystocele SIS-toh-seel **Definition** hernia of the urinary bladder into the vagina	cysto / cele bladder / pouch / tumor / hernia
dermoid cyst DER-moyd SIST **Definition** ovarian cyst containing skin and sometimes hair, teeth, bone, or cartilage	derm / oid cyst skin / resembling cyst
teratoma TER-ah-TOH-mah **Definition** another term for a dermoid cyst; the name derives from the contents of the cyst	terat / oma monster / tumor

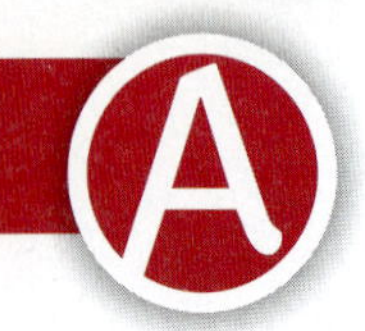

13.4 Diagnosis and Pathology

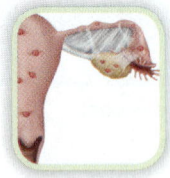

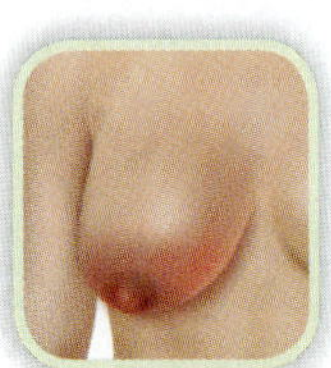
endometriosis

mastitis

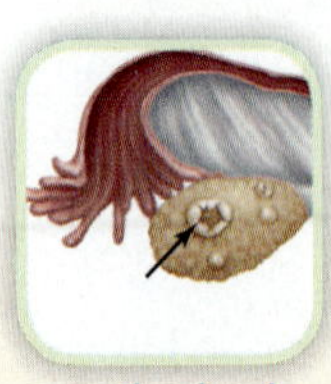
ovariorrhexis

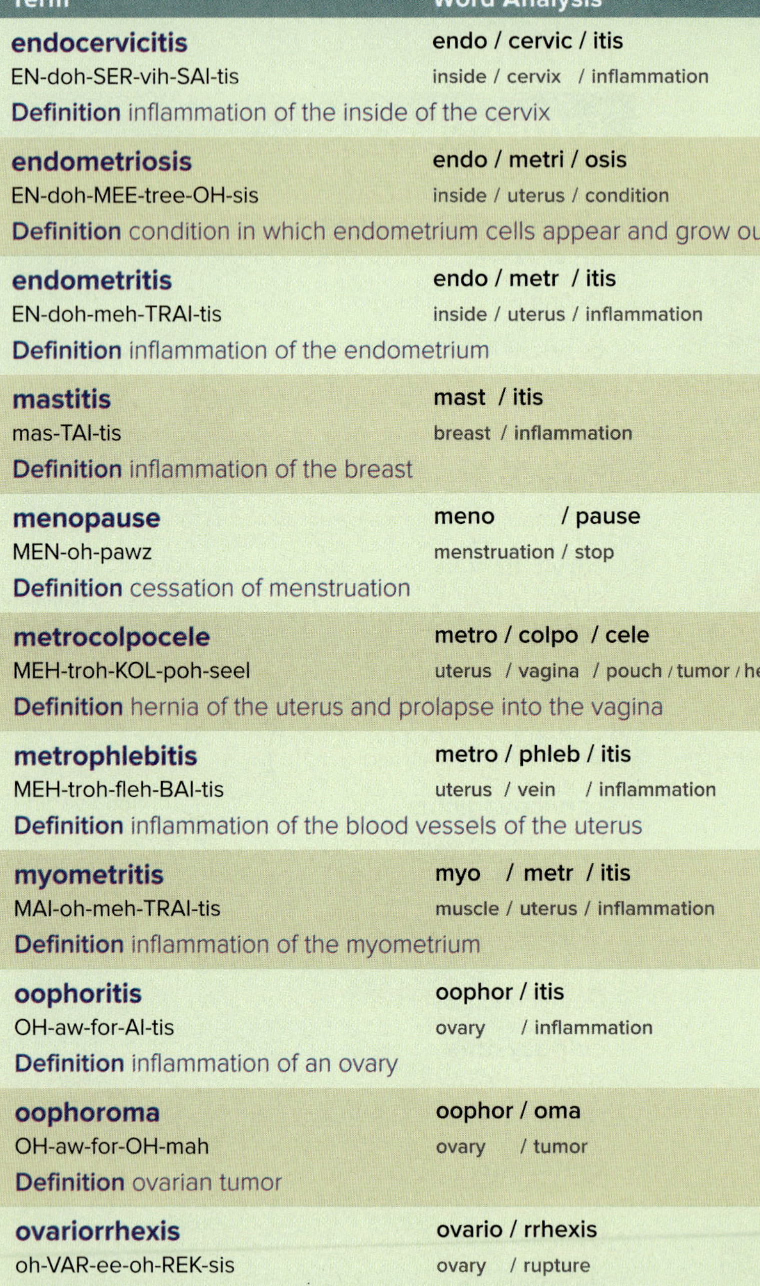

gynecology *continued*

Term	Word Analysis
endocervicitis	endo / cervic / itis
EN-doh-SER-vih-SAI-tis	inside / cervix / inflammation
Definition inflammation of the inside of the cervix	
endometriosis	endo / metri / osis
EN-doh-MEE-tree-OH-sis	inside / uterus / condition
Definition condition in which endometrium cells appear and grow outside the uterus	
endometritis	endo / metr / itis
EN-doh-meh-TRAI-tis	inside / uterus / inflammation
Definition inflammation of the endometrium	
mastitis	mast / itis
mas-TAI-tis	breast / inflammation
Definition inflammation of the breast	
menopause	meno / pause
MEN-oh-pawz	menstruation / stop
Definition cessation of menstruation	
metrocolpocele	metro / colpo / cele
MEH-troh-KOL-poh-seel	uterus / vagina / pouch / tumor / hernia
Definition hernia of the uterus and prolapse into the vagina	
metrophlebitis	metro / phleb / itis
MEH-troh-fleh-BAI-tis	uterus / vein / inflammation
Definition inflammation of the blood vessels of the uterus	
myometritis	myo / metr / itis
MAI-oh-meh-TRAI-tis	muscle / uterus / inflammation
Definition inflammation of the myometrium	
oophoritis	oophor / itis
OH-aw-for-AI-tis	ovary / inflammation
Definition inflammation of an ovary	
oophoroma	oophor / oma
OH-aw-for-OH-mah	ovary / tumor
Definition ovarian tumor	
ovariorrhexis	ovario / rrhexis
oh-VAR-ee-oh-REK-sis	ovary / rupture
Definition rupture of an ovary	
ovaritis	ovar / itis
OH-var-AI-tis	ovary / inflammation
Definition inflammation of an ovary	
perimetritis	peri / metr / itis
PEH-ree-meh-TRAI-tis	around / uterus / inflammation
Definition inflammation of the perimetrium	

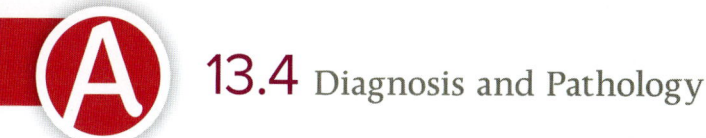

gynecology *continued*

Term	Word Analysis
rectocele REK-toh-seel	recto / cele rectum / pouch / tumor / hernia
Definition hernia or protrusion of the rectum into the vagina	
salpingitis SAL-pin-JAI-tis	salping / itis tube / inflammation
Definition inflammation of a fallopian tube	
salpingocele sal-PING-goh-seel	salpingo / cele tube / pouch / tumor / hernia
Definition hernia of a fallopian tube	
salpingo-oophoritis sal-PIN-goh- OH-aw-for-AI-tis	salpingo / oophor / itis tube / ovary / inflammation
Definition inflammation of a fallopian tube and ovary	
urethrocele yur-EE-throh-seel	urethro / cele urethra / pouch / tumor / hernia
Definition hernia or prolapse of the urethra into the vagina	
vaginitis VAJ-ih-NAI-tis	vagin / itis vagina / inflammation
Definition inflammation of the vagina	
vaginomycosis VAJ-ih-noh-MAI-koh-sis	vagino / myc / osis vagina / fungus / condition
Definition fungal condition of the vagina	
vaginosis VAJ-ih-NOH-sis	vagin / osis vagina / condition
Definition condition of the vagina	
vesicovaginal fistula VES-ih-koh-VAJ-ih-nal FIS-tyoo-lah	vesico / vagin / al fistula bladder / vagina / pertaining to pipe
Definition abnormal opening between the urinary bladder and the vagina	
vulvitis vul-VAI-tis	vulv / itis vulva / inflammation
Definition inflammation of the vulva	
vulvovaginitis VUL-voh-VAJ-ih-NAI-tis	vulvo / vagin / itis vulva / vagina / inflammation
Definition inflammation of the vulva and vagina	

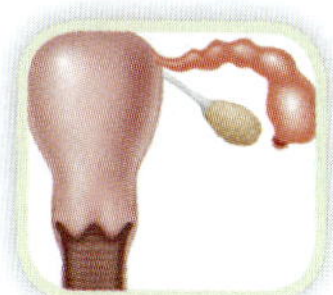
salpingitis

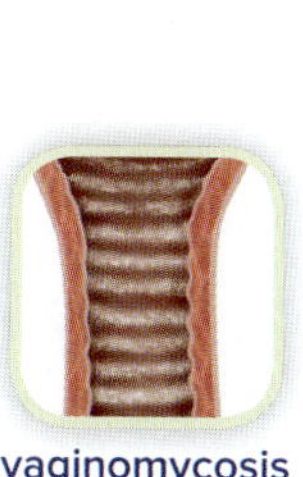
vaginomycosis

obstetrics

Term	Word Analysis
abortion ah-BOR-shun	from Latin, for *an untimely birth or miscarriage*

Definition termination of pregnancy

NOTE: There are two general categories of abortion: *spontaneous* (when the body does it of its own accord) and *induced* (when there is an external cause). Outside the medical world, many people commonly use the term "miscarriage" to refer to a spontaneous abortion and "abortion" to refer exclusively to an induced abortion.

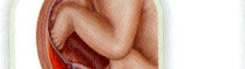

abruptio placentae

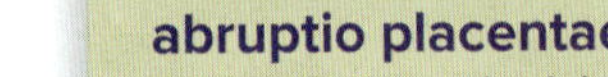

Term	Word Analysis
abruptio placentae ah-BRUP-shee-oh plah-SIN-tee	abruptio placentae tear away placenta

Definition separation of the placenta from the wall of the uterus

Term	Word Analysis
chorioamnionitis KOR-ee-oh-AM-nee-oh-NAI-tis	chorio / amnion / itis chorion / amnion / inflammation

Definition inflammation of the chorion and amnion

Term	Word Analysis
chorioangioma KOR-ee-oh-AN-jee-OH-mah	chorio / angi / oma chorion / vessel / tumor

Definition blood vessel tumor of the chorion

Term	Word Analysis
choriocarcinoma KOR-ee-oh-KAR-sih-NOH-mah	chorio / carcin / oma chorion / cancer / tumor

Definition cancerous tumor of the chorion

Term	Word Analysis
chorionitis KOR-ee-aw-NAI-tis	chorion / itis chorion / inflammation

Definition inflammation of the chorion

Term	Word Analysis
eclampsia eh-KLAMP-see-ah	from Greek, for *to shine or lightning*

Definition severe, life-threatening complication of pregnancy characterized by seizures

NOTE: The term probably comes from the fact that seizures strike suddenly, like lightning.

Term	Word Analysis
ectopic pregnancy ek-TOP-ik PREG-nan-see	ec / top / ic pregnancy outside / place / pertaining to pregnancy

Definition implantation of a fertilized egg in a place other than the uterus

Term	Word Analysis
hyperemesis gravidarum HAI-per-eh-MEE-sis GRAV-ih-DAR-um	hyper / emesis gravidarum over / vomit pregnancy

Definition pregnancy-related vomiting; an extreme form of the more common *morning sickness*

Term	Word Analysis
hysterorrhexis HIS-ter-oh-REK-sis	hystero / rrhexis uterus / rupture

Definition rupture of the uterus

Term	Word Analysis
ovariocyesis oh-VAR-ee-oh-sai-EE-sis	ovario / cyesis ovary / pregnancy

Definition ectopic pregnancy in an ovary

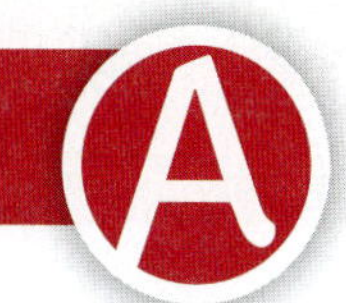

13.4 Diagnosis and Pathology

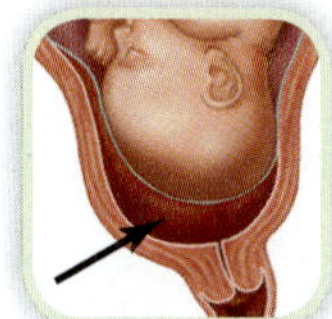
placenta previa

obstetrics *continued*

Term	Word Analysis
placenta previa plah-SIN-tah PREE-vee-ah	placenta previa placenta first
Definition condition in which the placenta is attached to the uterus near the cervix	
preeclampsia PREE-eh-KLAMP-see-ah	pre / eclampsia before / eclampsia
Definition condition characterized by high blood pressure and high protein in the urine **NOTE:** See *eclampsia* for the origin of the term. The term comes from the fact that without proper treatment, a patient will develop eclampsia.	
pseudocyesis SOO-doh-sai-EE-sis	pseudo / cyesis false / pregnancy
Definition false pregnancy	
salpingocyesis sal-PING-goh-sai-EE-sis	salpingo / cyesis tube / pregnancy
Definition ectopic pregnancy in a fallopian tube	
spontaneous abortion spawn-TAY-nee-is ah-BOR-shun	
Definition naturally occurring termination of pregnancy; also known as a *miscarriage* **NOTE:** See *abortion* for the origin of the term.	

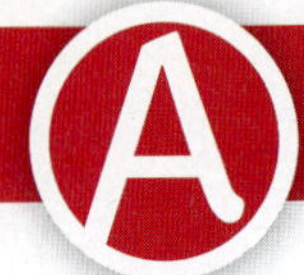

Learning Outcome 13.4 Exercises

PRONUNCIATION

EXERCISE 1 *Break down the following words into syllables.*

EXAMPLE: synesthesia *syn | es | the | sia*

1. teratoma ______
2. ovaritis ______
3. vaginitis ______
4. vaginosis ______
5. chorionitis ______
6. myometritis ______
7. perimetritis ______
8. endometriosis ______
9. metrocolpocele ______
10. hysterorrhexis ______
11. ovariorrhexis ______
12. preeclampsia ______
13. pseudocyesis ______
14. salpingocyesis ______
15. vulvovaginitis ______
16. salpingo-oophoritis ______

EXERCISE 2 *Indicate which syllable is emphasized when pronounced.*

EXAMPLE: bronchitis bron**chi**tis

1. colpitis ______
2. mastitis ______
3. vulvitis ______
4. salpingitis ______
5. cystocele ______
6. rectocele ______
7. urethrocele ______
8. menopause ______
9. eclampsia ______
10. placenta ______
11. previa ______
12. hyperemesis (2) ______
13. gravidarum (2) ______

TRANSLATION

EXERCISE 3 *Break down the following words into their component parts.*

EXAMPLE: nasopharyngoscope *naso | pharyngo | scope*

1. vaginosis ______
2. cystocele ______
3. rectocele ______
4. teratoma ______
5. urethrocele ______
6. pseudocyesis ______
7. ovariorrhexis ______
8. hysterorrhexis ______

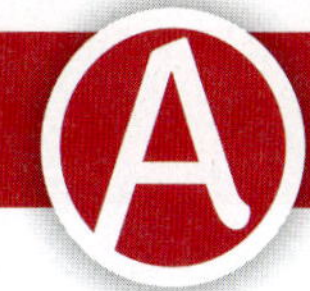

Learning Outcome 13.4 Exercises

9. colpocystitis ______
10. endocervicitis ______
11. metrocolpocele ______
12. myometritis ______
13. choriocarcinoma ______
14. vaginomycosis ______

EXERCISE 4 *Underline and define the word parts from this chapter in the following terms.*

1. chorioangioma ______
2. menopause ______
3. metrophlebitis ______
4. cervical intraepithelial neoplasia ______
5. oophoroma ______
6. salpingocele ______
7. endometriosis ______
8. vesicovaginal fistula ______
9. vulvovaginitis (2 word parts) ______
10. ovariocyesis (2 word parts) ______
11. salpingocyesis (2 word parts) ______

EXERCISE 5 *Match the term on the left with its definition on the right.*

h	1. abortion	a.	condition characterized by high blood pressure and high level of protein in the urine
i	2. spontaneous abortion	b.	condition in which the placenta is attached to the uterus near the cervix
g	3. ectopic pregnancy	c.	glandular tumor in the breast
c	4. adenocarcinoma of the breast	d.	ovarian cyst containing skin and sometimes hair, teeth, bone, or cartilage
d	5. dermoid cyst	e.	characterized by seizures
j	6. abruptio placentae (tear away)	f.	pregnancy-related vomiting; an extreme form of the more common *morning sickness*
b	7. placenta previa	g.	implantation of a fertilized egg in a place other than the uterus
e	8. eclampsia	h.	termination of pregnancy
f	9. hyperemesis gravidarum	i.	naturally occurring termination of pregnancy; also known as a *miscarriage*
a	10. preeclampsia	j.	separation of the placenta from the wall of the uterus

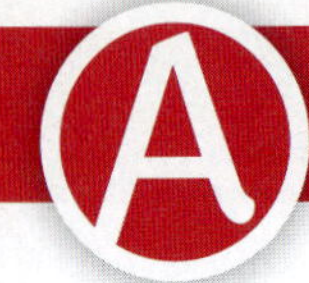

Learning Outcome 13.4 Exercises

EXERCISE 6 *Fill in the blanks.*

1. *vaginitis:* inflammation of the ______________________
2. *vulvitis:* inflammation of the ______________________
3. *cervicitis:* inflammation of the ______________________
4. *ovaritis:* inflammation of the ______________________
5. *chorionitis:* inflammation of the ______________________
6. *mastitis:* inflammation of the ______________________
7. *colpitis:* inflammation of the ______________________
8. *endometritis:* inflammation of the ______________________
9. *perimetritis:* inflammation of the ______________________
10. *oophoritis:* inflammation of the ______________________
11. *salpingitis:* inflammation of the ______________________
12. *cervicocolpitis:* inflammation of the ______________ and ______________
13. *cervicovaginitis:* inflammation of the ______________ and ______________
14. *chorioamnionitis:* inflammation of the ______________ and ______________
15. *salpingo-oophoritis:* inflammation of the ______________ and ______________
16. *vulvovaginitis:* inflammation of the ______________ and ______________

EXERCISE 7 *Translate the following terms as literally as possible.*

EXAMPLE: nasopharyngoscope *an instrument for looking at the nose and throat*

1. chorionitis ______________________
2. oophoritis ______________________
3. salpingitis ______________________
4. ovariorrhexis ______________________
5. menopause ______________________
6. myometritis ______________________
7. colpocystitis ______________________
8. endocervicitis ______________________
9. cervicocolpitis ______________________
10. cervicovaginitis ______________________
11. salpingo-oophoritis ______________________
12. adenocarcinoma of the breast ______________________

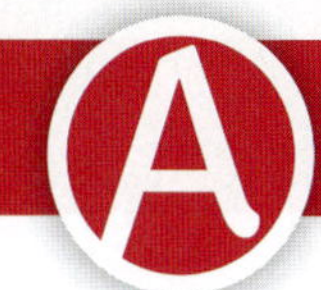

Learning Outcome 13.4 Exercises

GENERATION

EXERCISE 8 *Build a medical term from the information provided.*

EXAMPLE: inflammation of the sinuses *sinusitis*

1. inflammation of the vagina (use *vagin/o*) ______
2. inflammation of the vulva (use *vulv/o*) ______
3. inflammation of the ovary (use *ovari/o*) ______
4. inflammation of the vagina (use *colp/o*) ______
5. inflammation of the cervix ______
6. false pregnancy ______
7. rupture of the uterus ______
8. hernia of a fallopian tube ______
9. tumor of the ovary ______
10. inflammation of the breast ______
11. inflammation of the chorion and amnion ______
12. inflammation of the blood vessels of the uterus (use *metr/o*) ______
13. a blood vessel tumor of the chorion ______
14. cancerous tumor of the chorion ______

EXERCISE 9 *Multiple-choice questions. Select the correct answer(s).*

1. The implantation of a fertilized egg in a place other than the uterus is called a(n)
   a. ectopic pregnancy
   b. ovariocyesis
   c. pseudocyesis
   d. salpingocyesis
   e. none of these
2. Which of the following options is the correct breakdown of the term *hyperemesis gravidarum*?
   a. over (*hyper*) + throw up (*emesis*) + pregnancy (*gravidarum*)
   b. under (*hyper*) + throw up (*emesis*) + pregnancy (*gravidarum*)
   c. over (*hyper*) + grow (*emesis*) + pregnancy (*gravidarum*)
   d. under (*hyper*) + grow (*emesis*) + pregnancy (*gravidarum*)
   e. none of these

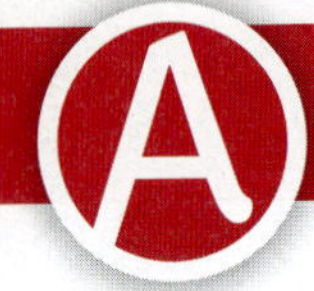

Learning Outcome 13.4 Exercises

3. Which of the following statements is the correct definition of the term *rectocele?*
   a. hernia or protrusion of the rectum into the vagina
   b. hernia or protrusion of the uterus into the rectum
   c. abnormal opening between the vagina and the rectum
   d. abnormal opening between the uterus and rectum
   e. none of these
4. Which of the following statements is the correct definition of the term *cervical intraepithelial neoplasia?*
   a. abnormal growth of cervical cells
   b. abnormal growth of ovarian cells
   c. abnormal growth of uterine cells
   d. new growth in the ovaries that extends into the uterus
   e. new growth in the uterus that extends into the cervix
5. Which of the following statements is the correct definition of *endometriosis?*
   a. a condition in which endometrium cells appear and grow outside the uterus
   b. condition of the inside of the cervix
   c. inflammation of the endometrium
   d. inflammation of the inside of the cervix
   e. none of these
6. Which of the following statements is the correct definition of the term *metrocolpocele?*
   a. an abnormal opening between the urinary bladder and the vagina
   b. hernia of the uterus and prolapse into the vagina
   c. an abnormal opening between the uterus and the vagina
   d. hernia of the urinary bladder into the vagina
   e. none of these
7. Which of the following statements is the correct definition of the term *vesicovaginal fistula?*
   a. an abnormal opening between the urinary bladder and the vagina
   b. hernia of the uterus and prolapse into the vagina
   c. an abnormal opening between the uterus and the vagina
   d. hernia of the urinary bladder into the vagina
   e. none of these

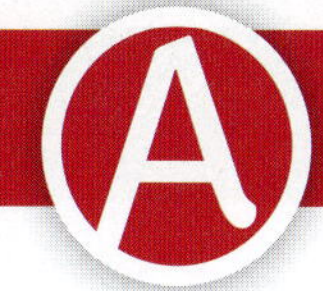

Learning Outcome 13.4 Exercises

8. Select all of the following that apply to the term *dermoid cyst*.
    a. a uterine cyst
    b. also called a *teratoma*
    c. an ovarian cyst
    d. contains skin and sometimes hair, teeth, bone, or cartilage
    e. literally means *monster tumor*
    f. literally means *skin resembling cyst*
9. Select all of the following that apply to the term *teratoma*.
    a. a uterine cyst
    b. also called a *dermoid cyst*
    c. an ovarian cyst
    d. contains skin and sometimes hair, teeth, bone, or cartilage
    e. literally means *monster tumor*
    f. literally means *skin resembling cyst*

EXERCISE 10 *Briefly describe the difference between each pair of terms.*

1. induced abortion, spontaneous abortion ______________________
2. endometritis, perimetritis ______________________
3. vaginomycosis, vaginosis ______________________
4. ovariocyesis, salpingocyesis ______________________
5. cystocele, urethrocele ______________________
6. eclampsia, preeclampsia ______________________
7. abruptio placentae, placenta previa ______________________

PLAN

13.5 Treatments and Therapies

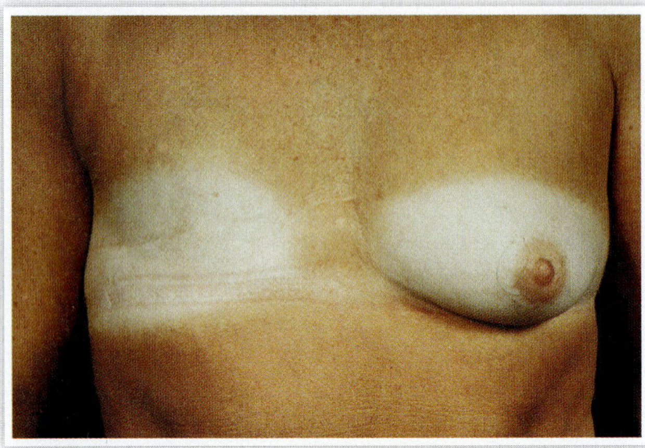

Breast cancer is a common reason a doctor might recommend a mastectomy.

One unique attribute of physicians trained in obstetrics and gynecology is that they are primary care providers for many women's health issues, but they are also surgeons. *Gynecologic surgeries* involve the interior structures of the female reproductive tract, such as the ovaries, fallopian tubes, and uterus. Ovarian surgeries can include the removal of an ovary (*oophorectomy*) to treat ovarian cancer or just the removal of a cyst on the ovary (*ovarian cystectomy*). At times, a fallopian tube is removed along with an ovary (*salpingo-oophorectomy*).

The fallopian tubes are common sites for ectopic pregnancies, and their standard treatment involves surgically opening the fallopian tube (*salpingotomy*) and removing the developing embryo. This procedure can maintain fertility and proper function of the reproductive system, but sometimes, as with a ruptured ectopic pregnancy, the tube must be removed altogether (*salpingectomy*). Another procedure involving the fallopian tubes involves blocking them (*tubal ligation*) as a means of preventing future pregnancies (*sterilization*).

Among the most frequently performed surgeries in gynecology is removal of the uterus (*hysterectomy*). Numerous medical problems are treated with hysterectomy, including cancer, fibroid tumors, and endometriosis. Prolapse of the uterus can be treated by surgically securing the uterus to another structure (*hysteropexy* or *colpopexy*).

Another very common procedure involving the uterus is *dilation and curettage* (commonly referred to as *D&C*). In this procedure, the opening of the cervix is gradually dilated with special instruments. Then, tissues lining the uterus are removed. D&C is commonly used to evaluate and treat problems of the uterus, such as abnormal bleeding. This may be due to benign problems, such as polyps, or fibroid tumors, which can be removed by cutting them out of the muscular wall of the uterus (*myomectomy.*) D&C is also utilized following a miscarriage when the uterus fails to fully shed the nonviable tissue.

Defects of the vagina, whether they originate from birth or from abuse, can be corrected by a plastic surgeon (*vaginoplasty*).

Surgeries involving the breast are much more common procedures, with breast cancer being the leading reason. In some instances, the breast can be spared and just the cancer is removed (*mastotomy* with *lumpectomy*). Many times, the entire breast is removed (*mastectomy*). In these cases, breast reconstruction surgery can help restore the normal appearance of the breast. Other breast surgeries include breast reduction (*mammoplasty*) and breast lift (*mastopexy*).

The science of obstetrics is focused on keeping both mother and baby healthy during pregnancy. One important aspect is making sure that the mother avoids substances that can harm the growth of the baby (*teratogen*).

In a healthy pregnancy, delivery involves the muscles of the uterus squeezing to push the baby through the canal. If her contractions come too early, before her baby is ready to be born, a patient can take medicines that can help stop them (*tocolytic*). There are also medicines, such as oxytocin, that can be used to bring on contractions and induce labor.

13.5 Treatments and Therapies

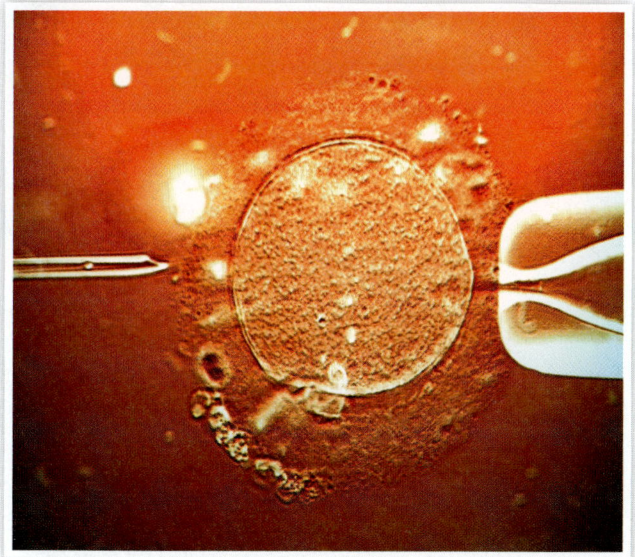

For couples struggling with fertility issues, in vitro fertilization provides possibility.

Once it is time for delivery, there are two possibilities. The most common is a vaginal delivery, which involves delivering the baby naturally through the birth canal. It may be necessary to make a small cut in the mother's perineum (*episiotomy*) to help prevent tearing of skin during delivery. In cases where a baby is positioned in the wrong direction or is not moving quickly through the birth canal, the baby might need to be delivered surgically (*cesarean section*). This surgery, the most common one in medicine, involves first cutting the abdomen of the mother (*laparotomy*) and then cutting open her uterus (*hysterotomy*) to gain access to the baby.

Another procedure unique to women's health is in vitro fertilization, the fertilization of a female's egg by a male's sperm outside the body (*in vitro*). After the fertilization is complete, the *zygote* is then transferred into the woman's uterus.

gynecology

Term	Word Analysis
cervicectomy SER-vih-SEK-toh-mee **Definition** surgical removal of the cervix	cervic / ec / tomy cervix / out / cut
colpopexy KOL-poh-PEK-see **Definition** surgical fixation of the vagina	colpo / pexy vagina / fixation
colpoplasty KOL-poh-PLAS-tee **Definition** surgical reconstruction of the vagina	colpo / plasty vagina / reconstruction
episiorrhaphy eh-PEE-zee-OR-ah-fee **Definition** suture of the vulva	episio / rrhaphy vulva / suture
hysterectomy HIS-ter-EK-toh-mee **Definition** surgical removal of the uterus	hyster / ec / tomy uterus / out / cut
hysteropexy HIS-ter-oh-PEK-see **Definition** surgical fixation of the uterus	hystero / pexy uterus / fixation
hysterosalpingectomy HIS-ter-oh-SAL-pin-JEK-toh-mee **Definition** surgical removal of the uterus and fallopian tube(s)	hystero / salping / ec / tomy uterus / tube / out / cut

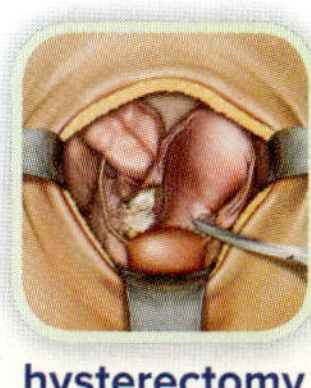

hysterectomy

13.5 Treatments and Therapies

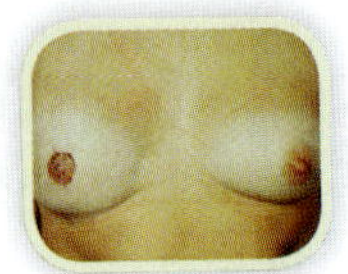
mammoplasty

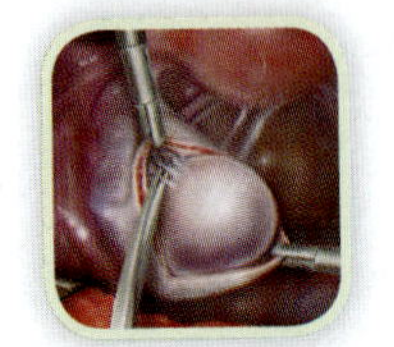
ovarian cystectomy

gynecology *continued*

Term	Word Analysis
mammoplasty MAM-oh-PLAS-tee **Definition** surgical reconstruction of a breast	mammo / plasty breast / reconstruction
mastectomy mas-TEK-toh-mee **Definition** surgical removal of a breast	mast / ec / tomy breast / out / cut
mastopexy MAS-toh-PEK-see **Definition** surgical fixation of a breast	masto / pexy breast / fixation
myomectomy MAI-oh-MEK-toh-mee **Definition** surgical removal of a tumor in the muscle (usually refers to the muscle of the uterine wall)	my / om / ec / tomy muscle / tumor / out / cut
oophorectomy OH-aw-for-EK-toh-mee **Definition** surgical removal of an ovary	oophor / ec / tomy ovary / out / cut
oophorocystectomy oh-AW-for-oh-sis-TEK-toh-mee **Definition** surgical removal of an ovarian cyst	oophoro / cyst / ec / tomy ovary / cyst / out / cut
oophorotomy oh-AW-for-AW-toh-mee **Definition** incision into an ovary	oophoro / tomy ovary / cut
ovarian cystectomy oh-VEH-ree-an sis-TEK-toh-mee **Definition** surgical removal of an ovarian cyst	ovari / an cyst / ec / tomy ovary / pertaining to cyst / out / cut
ovariocentesis oh-VAW-ree-oh-sin-TEE-sis **Definition** surgical puncture of an ovary	ovario / centesis ovary / puncture
ovariostomy oh-VAW-ree-AW-stoh-me **Definition** creation of an opening into an ovary	ovario / stom / y ovary / mouth / procedure

gynecology *continued*

Term	Word Analysis
perineorrhaphy PER-ih-nee-OR-ah-fee **Definition** suture of the perineum	perineo / rrhaphy perineum / suture
salpingectomy SAL-pin-JEK-toh-mee **Definition** surgical removal of a fallopian tube	salping / ec / tomy tube / out / cut
salpingo-oophorectomy sal-PING-goh-OH-aw-for-EK-toh-mee **Definition** surgical removal of a fallopian tube and ovary	salpingo / oophor / ec / tomy tube / ovary / out / cut
salpingopexy sal-PING-goh-PEK-see **Definition** surgical fixation of a fallopian tube	salpingo / pexy tube / fixation
perineoplasty PER-ih-NEE-oh-PLAS-tee **Definition** surgical reconstruction of the perineum	perineo / plasty perineum / reconstruction
perineotomy PER-ih-nee-AW-toh-mee **Definition** incision into the perineum	perineo / tomy perineum / cut
vaginoperineorrhaphy VAJ-ih-noh-PER-ih-nee-OR-ah-fee **Definition** suture of the vagina and perineum	vagino / perineo / rrhaphy vagina / perineum / suture
vaginoperineoplasty VAJ-ih-noh-PER-ih-NEE-oh-PLAS-tee **Definition** surgical reconstruction of the vagina and perineum	vagino / perineo / plasty vagina / perineum / reconstruction
vaginoperineotomy VAJ-ih-noh-PER-ih-nee-AW-toh-mee **Definition** incision into the vagina and perineum	vagino / perineo / tomy vagina / perineum / cut
vaginoplasty vah-JI-noh-PLAS-tee **Definition** surgical reconstruction of the vagina	vagino / plasty vagina / reconstruction

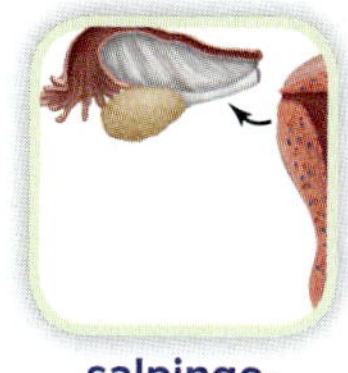

salpingo-oophorectomy

13.5 Treatments and Therapies

obstetrics

Term	Word Analysis
abortifacient ah-BOR-tih-FAY-shunt **Definition** drug or device that causes the termination of pregnancy	aborti / facient abortion / do
amniotomy AM-nee-AW-toh-mee **Definition** incision into the amnion	amnio / tomy amnion / cut
cesarean section sih-SER-ee-an SEK-shun **Definition** delivery of a baby through an incision made in the uterus **Note:** This term does *not* refer to Julius Caesar's method of delivery. Rather, it refers to an ancient Roman law that required a child to be cut from a mother's womb if the mother died in childbirth.	cesarean section
episiotomy eh-PEE-zee-AW-toh-mee **Definition** incision into the vulva	episio / tomy vulva / cut
hysterotomy HIS-ter-AW-toh-mee **Definition** incision into the uterus	hystero / tomy uterus / cut
induced abortion in-DOOST ah-BOR-shun **Definition** intentional termination of pregnancy	*see note on abortion*
in vitro fertilization in VEE-troh FER-tih-lih-ZAY-shun **Definition** fertilization of an egg done in a test tube	in vitro fertilization in glass fertilization
oxytocin OK-see-TOH-sin **Definition** agent that stimulates uterine contractions and accelerates labor	oxy / toc / in swift / birth / agent
tocolytic TOH-koh-LIH-tik **Definition** agent that stops or delays premature labor and contractions	toco / lyt / ic labor / loosing / agent

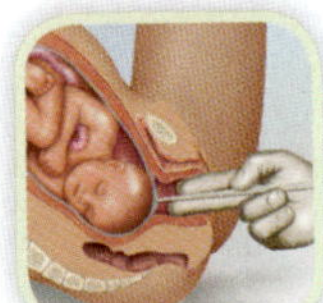

amniotomy

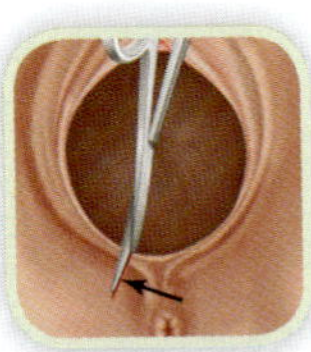

episiotomy

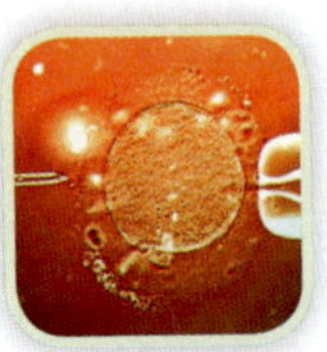

in vitro fertilization

Learning Outcome 13.5 Exercises

PRONUNCIATION

EXERCISE 1 *Break down the following words into syllables.*

EXAMPLE: synesthesia *syn | es | the | sia*

1. colpopexy ______
2. mastopexy ______
3. colpoplasty ______
4. episiotomy ______
5. amniotomy ______
6. mastectomy ______
7. hysterotomy ______
8. vaginoplasty ______
9. hysteropexy ______
10. hysterectomy ______
11. salpingectomy ______
12. mammoplasty ______
13. perineorrhaphy ______
14. perineoplasty ______

EXERCISE 2 *Indicate which syllables are emphasized when pronounced.*

EXAMPLE: bronchitis bron**chi**tis

1. cervicectomy (2) ______
2. oophorotomy (2) ______
3. ovariostomy (2) ______
4. salpingectomy (2) ______
5. perineotomy (2) ______
6. oxytocin (2) ______

TRANSLATION

EXERCISE 3 *Break down the following words into their component parts.*

EXAMPLE: nasopharyngoscope *naso | pharyngo | scope*

1. mammoplasty ______
2. ovariocentesis ______
3. perineotomy ______

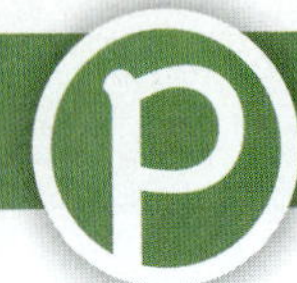

Learning Outcome 13.5 Exercises

4. hysterotomy ______
5. colpoplasty ______
6. episiorrhaphy ______
7. vaginoperineorrhaphy ______
8. oophorocystectomy ______

EXERCISE 4 *Underline and define the word parts from this chapter in the following terms.*

1. amniotomy ______
2. vaginoplasty ______
3. cervicectomy ______
4. ovariostomy ______
5. perineoplasty ______
6. colpopexy ______
7. episiotomy ______
8. hysteropexy ______
9. mastopexy ______
10. salpingopexy ______
11. oophorotomy ______
12. vaginoperineoplasty (2 roots) ______

EXERCISE 5 *Match the term on the left with its definition on the right.*

c	1. cesarean section	a. drug or device that causes the termination of a pregnancy
d.	2. in vitro fertilization	b. agent that stimulates uterine contractions and accelerates labor
g	3. induced abortion	c. delivery of a baby through an incision made in the uterus
f.	4. perineorrhaphy	d. fertilization of an egg done in a test tube
e	5. vaginoperineotomy	e. incision into the vagina and perineum
a	6. abortifacient	f. suture of the perineum
b	7. oxytocin	g. intentional termination of pregnancy

EXERCISE 6 *Fill in the blanks.*

1. *cervicectomy:* surgical removal of the ______
2. *hysterectomy:* surgical removal of the ______
3. *mastectomy:* surgical removal of a(n) ______
4. *oophorectomy:* surgical removal of a(n) ______
5. *salpingectomy:* surgical removal of a(n) ______
6. *oophorcystectomy:* surgical removal of a(n) ______
7. *ovarian cystectomy:* surgical removal of a(n) ______

8. *salpingo-oophorectomy:* surgical removal of a(n) ______________ and ______________
9. *hysterosalpingectomy:* surgical removal of the ______________ and ______________
10. *myomectomy:* surgical removal of a(n) ______________

EXERCISE 7 *Translate the following terms as literally as possible.*

EXAMPLE: nasopharyngoscope *an instrument for looking at the nose and throat*

1. vaginoplasty ______________
2. perineoplasty ______________
3. colpoplasty ______________
4. episiotomy ______________
5. mastectomy ______________
6. ovariocentesis ______________
7. hysteropexy ______________
8. salpingopexy ______________
9. oophorocystectomy ______________
10. ovarian cystectomy ______________
11. vaginoperineorrhaphy ______________
12. myomectomy ______________
13. in vitro fertilization ______________

GENERATION

EXERCISE 8 *Build a medical term from the information provided.*

EXAMPLE: inflammation of the sinuses *sinusitis*

1. surgical removal of the uterus (use *hyster/o*) ______________
2. surgical removal of an ovary (use *oophor/o*) ______________
3. surgical removal of the cervix ______________
4. surgical removal of the fallopian tube ______________
5. surgical reconstruction of a breast (use *mamm/o*) ______________
6. surgical fixation of the vagina (use *colp/o*) ______________
7. surgical fixation of a breast (use *mast/o*) ______________
8. incision into the amnion ______________
9. suture of the vulva (use *episi/o*) ______________
10. suture of the perineum ______________
11. creation of an opening into an ovary (use *ovari/o*) ______________

Learning Outcome 13.5 Exercises

12. suture of the vagina and perineum ______
13. surgical removal of a fallopian tube and ovary ______
14. surgical removal of the uterus and fallopian tube ______

EXERCISE 9 *Multiple-choice questions. Select the correct answer(s).*

1. A drug or device that causes the termination of a pregnancy is called a(n)
   a. abortifacient
   b. oxytocin
   c. amniotomy
   d. cesarean section
   e. episiorrhaphy
2. An *induced abortion* is
   a. the intentional termination of pregnancy
   b. the naturally occurring termination of pregnancy
   c. a drug or device that causes the termination of a pregnancy
   d. the separation of the placenta from the wall of the uterus
   e. none of these
3. Select all of the following statements that apply to the term *cesarean section.*
   a. a term common in obstetrics
   b. delivery of a baby through an incision in the perineum
   c. delivery of a baby through an incision made in the uterus
   d. refers to an ancient Roman law that required a child to be cut from its mother's womb if the mother died in childbirth
   e. the way in which Julius Caesar was delivered
4. Select all of the following terms that pertain to internal gynecology.
   a. amniotomy
   b. episiotomy
   c. hysterotomy
   d. oophorotomy
   e. oxytocin
   f. perineotomy
   g. vaginoperineotomy
5. Select all of the following terms that pertain to external gynecology.
   a. amniotomy
   b. episiotomy
   c. hysterotomy
   d. oophorotomy
   e. oxytocin
   f. perineotomy
   g. vaginoperineotomy
6. Select all of the following terms that pertain to obstetrics.
   a. amniotomy
   b. episiotomy
   c. hysterotomy
   d. oophorotomy
   e. oxytocin
   f. perineotomy
   g. vaginoperineotomy

13.6 Abbreviations

Abbreviations provide a shorthand way of referring to things that either recur often or are too long to write out. When dealing with gynecology and obstetrics, these abbreviations can refer to things ranging from body parts (Cx) to diagnostic procedures (SHG, TVS), diagnoses (CIPP, PMS, TSS), and treatments (LEEP, HRT, TAH).

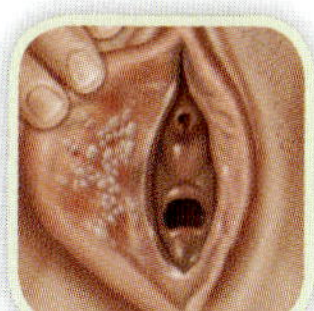
HPV (human papillomavirus)

gynecology

Abbreviation	Definition
CIPP	chronic idiopathic pelvic pain
Cx	cervix
GYN	gynecology
HPV	human papillomavirus
HRT	hormone replacement therapy
HSG	hysterosalpingogram
LEEP	loop electrosurgical excision procedure
PID	pelvic inflammatory disease
PMS	premenstrual syndrome
SHG	sonohysterography
STD/STI	sexually transmitted disease/infection
TAH/BSO	total abdominal hysterectomy/bilateral salpingo-oophorectomy
TSS	toxic shock syndrome
TVS	transvaginal sonography
VH	vaginal hysterectomy

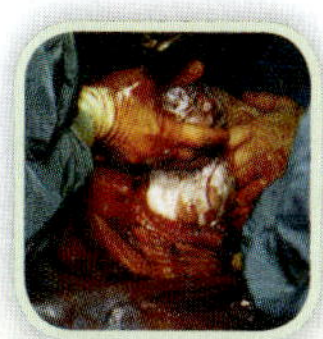
CS, C-section (cesarean section)

P (births)

obstetrics

Abbreviation	Definition
CPD	cephalopelvic disproportion
CS, C-section	cesarean section
DOB	date of birth
EDD	expected date of delivery
FAS	fetal alcohol syndrome
FOB	father of the baby (or fecal occult blood)
G	gravida
IVF	in vitro fertilization
LGA	large for gestational age
LMP	last menstrual period
P	births (comes from the word *para,* which means *birth)*
RDS	respiratory distress syndrome
SGA	small for gestational age

Learning Outcome 13.6 Exercises

EXERCISE 1 *Define the following abbreviations.*

1. HRT ______
2. PID ______
3. PMS ______
4. TSS ______
5. HPV ______
6. STD ______
7. DOB ______
8. EDD ______
9. FAS ______
10. LMP ______
11. CPD ______
12. CS ______
13. G ______
14. FOB ______
15. HSG ______

EXERCISE 2 *Give the abbreviations for the following definitions.*

1. chronic idiopathic pelvic pain ______
2. loop electrosurgical excision procedure ______
3. respiratory distress syndrome ______
4. small for gestational age ______
5. large for gestational age ______
6. para ______
7. father of the baby ______
8. sexually transmitted infection ______
9. cesarean section ______
10. total abdominal hysterectomy ______
11. bilateral salpingo-oophorectomy ______
12. transvaginal sonography ______
13. sonohysterography ______
14. vaginal hysterectomy ______
15. in vitro fertilization ______

Learning Outcome 13.6 Exercises

EXERCISE 3 *Match the abbreviation on the left with its full definition on the right.*

____ 1. GYN		a. condition characterized by the inability of the mother's pelvis to allow the baby to pass through the birth canal
____ 2. CS		b. delivery of a baby through an incision made in the uterus
____ 3. Cx		c. imaging procedure using sound waves emitted from a device inserted in the vagina
____ 4. CPD		d. pregnant
____ 5. TVS		e. opening between the uterus and the vagina
____ 6. G		f. procedure using sound waves to examine the uterus
____ 7. TAH		g. surgical removal of both of the ovaries and adjacent fallopian tubes; often performed as part of a total abdominal hysterectomy
____ 8. VH		h. surgical removal of the uterus through an incision in the abdomen; usually includes the removal of both ovaries and fallopian tubes
____ 9. BSO		i. surgical removal of the uterus through an incision in the vagina
____ 10. SHG		j. study of medical issues specific to women

EXERCISE 4 *Multiple-choice questions. Select the correct answer(s).*

1. HPV is a type of

   a. STD b. STI c. sexually transmitted disease
   d. sexually transmitted infection e. all of these

2. Pelvic pain that persists for a period of more than 3 months and has arisen spontaneously or from an obscure or unknown cause is known as

   a. CIPP b. CPD c. EDD
   d. RDS e. SGA

3. Which of the following abbreviations does NOT pertain to obstetrics?

   a. DOB b. EDD c. G
   d. GYN e. LGA

4. A baby whose birth weight lies above the 90th percentile for its *gestational age*, or the length of time the baby has been in the womb, would be considered

   a. CPD b. EDD c. LGA
   d. LMP e. SGA

5. The term *para* comes from the Latin term *parere*, meaning *to bring forth* or *to bear*. In medical terminology, this refers to a woman who has given birth to a viable infant (weighing at least 1 pound or of more than 20 weeks' gestation), regardless of whether that infant was alive at birth. The abbreviation for *para* is

   a. P b. PAR c. PR
   d. PRA e. none of these

6. EDD stands for

   a. electrodilator development b. expected date of delivery c. expected developmental delay
   d. expected due date e. none of these

13.7 Electronic Health Records

Postoperative Note

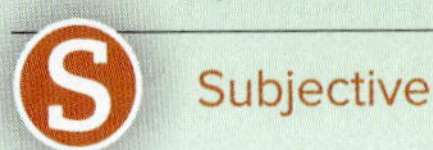

Subjective

Preoperative Diagnosis:

1. **Abruptio placentae**
2. **Chorioamnionitis**
3. **Fetal distress**

Postoperative Diagnosis:

1. Abruptio placentae
2. Chorioamnionitis
3. Fetal distress

Procedure: Emergency cesarean section

Anesthesia: General

Estimated blood loss: 750 mL

Complications: None

Findings: Male infant with cephalic presentation. Normal uterus, fallopian tubes, and ovaries.

Indications: The patient, Mrs. Jenna Friedman, is a 23-year-old **gravida** 2 **para** 1 female who presents at 37 4/7 weeks' **gestation** with ***bleeding*** and painful **uterine contractions** for 4 hours. An emergent ultrasound was performed to rule out **placenta previa**. The ultrasound showed a **retroplacental** hematoma. She was admitted for evaluation and treatment for **abruptio placentae**. Her physical exam on admission was significant for fever to 101.2°F, as well as abdominal and uterine tenderness.

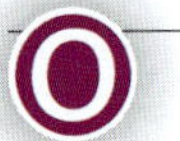

Objective

She was 3 cm ***dilated and effaced***. Initial lab work included a CBC that showed an elevated white blood cell count but no anemia. Fibrinogen and PT/PTT were all normal, which reassured us that she did not have DIC or a coagulopathy. The patient was placed on IV fluids and antibiotics for presumed **chorioamnionitis** and was placed under continuous monitoring. Two hours after admission, fetal heart rate monitors alerted us to **fetal bradycardia** and late decelerations. The decision was made to proceed with **emergency cesarean section**.

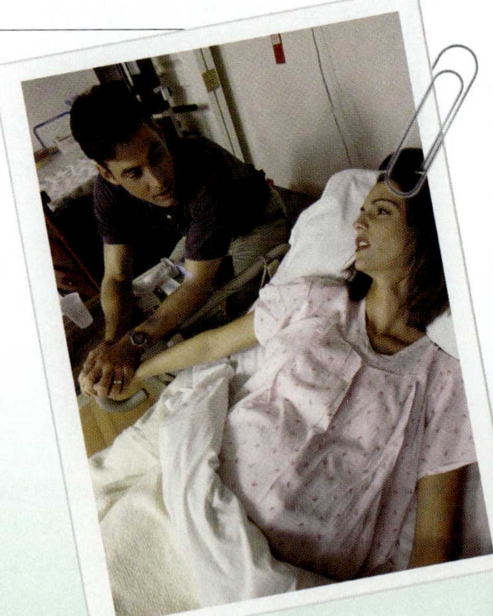

Input: 2 L normal saline via peripheral IV.

Output: 750 mL blood, 500 mL urine.

Postoperative Note *(continued)*

HR: 76; RR: 22; BP: 102/72.

General: Sedated. Nasal cannula O_2 at 0.5 lpm.

HEENT: PERRLA. Mucous membranes moist and pink. Nares patent. No nasal flaring.

CV: RRR with murmur.

Resp: CTA.

Abd: Midline surgical wound. Dressing is clean, dry, and intact.

GU: Grossly normal, no bleeding.

Assessment

1. Postop cesarean section–stable.
2. Chorioamnionitis.
3. Abruptio placentae–resolved. Hemodynamically stable.

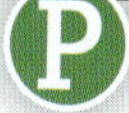

Plan

1. Continue IV fluids and progress to PO as patient becomes more alert.
2. Continue IV antibiotics.
3. Monitor blood pressure. Follow-up CBC.

–Patricia Collingsworth, PA

Learning Outcome 13.7 Exercises

EXERCISE 1 *Match the term on the left with its definition on the right.*

______	1. cesarean section	a. condition in whch the placenta is attached to the uterus near the cervix
______	2. contraction	b. another term for pregnant
______	3. choriamnionitis	c. delivery of a baby through an incision made in the uterus
______	4. abruptio placentae	d. inflammation of the chorion and amnion
______	5. placenta previa	e. separation of the placenta from the wall of the uterus
______	6. gravida	f. shortening or tightening of a muscle

EXERCISE 2 *Fill in the blanks.*

1. Using the data recorded at the patient's physical examination, fill in the following blanks.
   a. Mrs. Friedman's heart rate: ______
   b. Mrs. Friedman's respiratory rate: ______
   c. Mrs. Friedman's blood pressure: ______
2. Preoperative diagnois:
   a. *Abruptio placentae*–give definition: ______
   b. ______: inflammation of the chorion and amnion
   c. *Fetal distress:* presence of signs in a pregnant woman either *prepartum* (give definition: ______) or *intrapartum* (give definition: ______) that suggest the fetus may not be well.
3. Plan:
   a. Continue IV fluids (give definition for abbreviation: ______) and progress to ______ (*per os*–give definition: ______) as patient becomes more alert.
   b. Continue ______ (intravenous) antibiotics.
   c. Monitor BP (give definition for abbreviation: ______). Follow-up ______ (complete blood count).

EXERCISE 3 *True or false questions. Indicate true answers with a T and false answers with an F.*

1. Mrs. Friedman is a 23-year-old pregnant woman. ______
2. Mrs. Friedman is afebrile. ______
3. Mrs. Friedman has placenta previa. ______
4. Mrs. Friedman was placed on intravenous antibiotics. ______
5. Mrs. Friedman had a vaginal birth. ______
6. Mrs. Friedman was given 2 L of saline through an IV. ______

Learning Outcome 13.7 Exercises

EXERCISE 4 *Multiple-choice questions. Select the correct answer.*

1. The ultrasound performed on Mrs. Friedman showed *retroplacental hematoma*. Which of the following options is the correct breakdown of this term?
   a. *retro* (behind) + *placental* (placenta) + *hema* (blood) + *toma* (tumor)
   b. *retro* (behind) + *placental* (position) + *hema* (blood) + *toma* (tumor)
   c. *retro* (behind) + *placental* (position) + *hema* (urine) + *toma* (tumor)
   d. *retro* (behind) + *placental* (uterus) + *hema* (blood) + *toma* (hole)
   e. *retro* (behind) + *placental* (uterus) + *hema* (urine) + *toma* (hole)
2. Two hours after admission, heart rate monitors alerted the medical staff to *fetal bradycardia*. Which of the following options is the correct breakdown of this term?
   a. *fetal* (pertaining to the fetus) + *brady* (fast) + *cardia* (blood flow)
   b. *fetal* (pertaining to the fetus) + *brady* (fast) + *cardia* (heartbeat)
   c. *fetal* (pertaining to the fetus) + *brady* (slow) + *cardia* (heartbeat)
   d. *fetal* (pertaining to the uterus) + *brady* (fast) + *cardia* (blood flow)
   e. *fetal* (pertaining to the uterus) + *brady* (slow) + *cardia* (heartbeat)
3. Which of the following options is the correct abbreviation for *cesarean section*?
   a. CS
   b. C-sec
   c. C-section
   d. CS and C-sec
   e. CS and C-section

Emergency Department Note

Chief Complaint: Abdominal pain, fever.

History of Present Illness

Ms. Sara Miller, a 25-year-old woman, has had a 3-day history of worsening lower abdominal pain. The pain is a constant dull ache. The pain began a few days after her last **menstrual** cycle ended. The pain worsens with movement. Ms. Miller also reports **dyspareunia** and purulent **vaginal discharge.** She has tried over-the-counter ibuprofen, which yielded mild relief of the pain. The pain has worsened and now she also has nausea. She denies vomiting, diarrhea, or dysuria.

Past Medical History: Recent treatment for chlamydia **vulvovaginitis. Menarche** at 13 years of age. **LMP** 1 week ago.

Past Surgical History: None.

Social History: High-risk sexual behavior. Sexually active with multiple partners, inconsistent use of protection via condoms with her partners. 1-pack-per-day smoker.

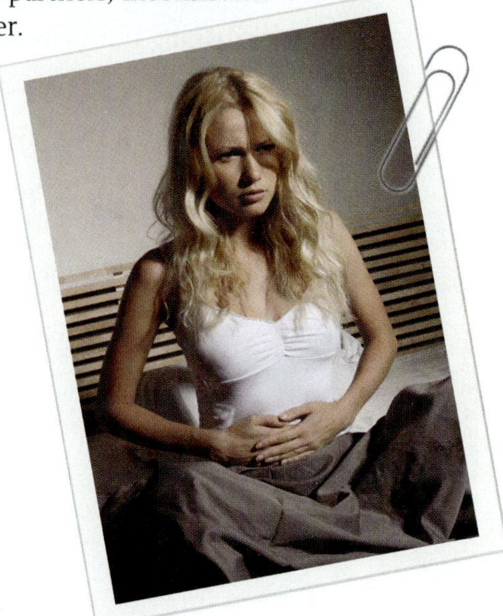

Family History: Noncontributory.

Medications: None.

Allergies: No known drug allergies.

Physical Exam

Vital Signs: Temperature: 102.3; Heart Rate: 90; Respiratory Rate: 20; BP: 112/84.

General: Well developed and nourished, in mild discomfort. Alert and oriented x 3.

Head: Normocephalic atraumatic, slightly dry mucous membranes. Pupils equal, round, and reactive to light. TMs normal.

Neck: Supple.

Cardiovascular: Mild tachycardia. No murmur, gallop, or rub.

Respiratory: Normal effort. Clear to auscultation. No retractions.

Abdomen: Generalized tenderness to palpation. Rebound and guarding present, especially over suprapubic region. Spleen and liver edge not palpable.

Skin: Dry. Cap refill 2 seconds.

Extremities: No cyanosis, clubbing, or edema.

Pelvic exam: Adnexal tenderness and cervical motion tenderness.

Emergency Department Course

Ms. Miller arrived at the emergency department in mild discomfort. An IV was started, and she was treated with IV fluids for mild dehydration. Ms. Miller was also given an antiemetic and ibuprofen. A rapid **hCG** test to rule out **ectopic pregnancy** was negative. A swab of Ms. Miller's purulent vaginal discharge revealed **leukorrhea.** We performed a **transvaginal sonography.** Suspicion for **pelvic inflammatory disorder** was confirmed by findings of enlarged ovaries consistent with **oophoritis, endometritis,** and **hydrosalpinx.** Results for chlamydia reinfection and gonorrhea are still pending.

Ms. Miller tolerated PO fluids and looked a little better. We educated Ms. Miller on the risks of **STIs** and the need for barrier protection. We also explained the complications of **PID,** including **tubo-ovarian abscess** and tubal **infertility.** She was sent home for outpatient management.

Disposition

Discharge to home with prescription for oral antibiotics.

–Sal Kaye, MD

Learning Outcome 13.7 Exercises

EXERCISE 5 *Match the term on the left with its definition on the right.*

______	1. menarche	a.	blockage in a fallopian tube caused by water or any clear fluid
______	2. ectopic pregnancy	b.	imaging procedure using sound waves emitted from a device inserted in the vagina
______	3. transvaginal sonography	c.	inflammation of an ovary
______	4. vulvovaginitis	d.	inflammation of the endometrium
______	5. leukorrhea	e.	inflammation of the vulva and vagina
______	6. endometritis	f.	painful sexual intercourse
______	7. oophoritis	g.	beginning or first menstruation
______	8. dyspareunia	h.	implantation of a fertilized egg in a place other than the uterus
______	9. hydrosalpinx	i.	white vaginal discharge

EXERCISE 6 *Fill in the blanks.*

1. Using the data recorded at Ms. Miller's physical examination, fill in the following blanks.
   a. T: ______________________________
   b. HR: ______________________________
   c. RR: ______________________________
   d. BP: ______________________________
   e. General: well developed, well nourished (give abbreviation: ______________________)
2. Past Medical History:
   a. Recent treatment for chlamydia *vulvovaginitis* (inflammation of the ______________________ and ______________________)
   b. *Menarche* (give definition: ______________________) at 13 years of age
   c. *LMP* (define abbreviation: ______________________)
3. Emergency Department Course:
   a. A rapid hCG test to rule out ______________________ (the implantation of a fertilized egg in a place other than the uterus) was negative.
   b. Suspicion for *pelvic inflammatory disorder* (give abbreviation: ______________________) was confirmed by findings of enlarged ovaries consistent with *oophoritis* (inflammation of ______________________), *endometritis* (inflammation of the tissue on the ______________________ of the ______________________), and ______________________ (blockage in a fallopian tube caused by water [or any clear fluid]).

Learning Outcome 13.7 Exercises

EXERCISE 7 *True or false questions. Indicate true answers with a T and false answers with an F.*

1. Ms. Miller is experiencing painful sexual intercourse. ________
2. Ms. Miller has trouble urinating. ________
3. Ms. Miller has a slightly faster heart rate than normal. ________
4. Ms. Miller arrived to the ED in mild discomfort. ________
5. Ms. Miller was given a medication to help prevent nausea. ________
6. The TVS confirmed PID. ________
7. Ms. Miller could not hold down any fluids. ________

EXERCISE 8 *Multiple-choice questions. Select the correct answer.*

1. A swab of Ms. Miller's vaginal discharge revealed
   a. leukorrhea
   b. lactorrhea
   c. amenorrhea
   d. none of these
2. The root word in *menstrual cycle* is the Greek word *meno*, which refers to
   a. fallopian tubes
   b. menstruation
   c. ovaries
   d. the uterus
3. *Pelvic inflammatory disorder* is a generic term for inflammation of the uterus, fallopian tubes, and/or ovaries. Which of the following medical terms is NOT included in this definition?
   a. colpitis
   b. endometritis
   c. oophoritis
   d. salpingitis

Gynecology Clinic Note

Subjective

Mrs. Lana Pecos is a 47-year-old **premenopausal** woman with a chief complaint of heavy **menses.** For more than a year, she has experienced menstrual flow for 9 to 10 days every 2 to 3 weeks. She denies vaginal discharge and bleeding from her gums or in her stool. No easy bruising.

PMHx: Last **mammogram** 6 years ago, normal. Pap smear 10 years ago: **cervical intraepithelial neoplasia** II treated with **LEEP.** Last **Pap smear** 5 years ago: Normal.

ROS: She denies visual changes.

Objective

Physical Exam

Weight: 270 lbs; Temp: 98.6; HR: 62; BP: 102/74; RR: 22.

General: Obese, pale. Alert and in NAD.

HEENT: Pale conjunctiva. PERRLA. TMs normal. Normal dentition. Mucous membranes moist.

Neck: Supple. No goiter.

CV: RRR without murmur.

Resp: CTA.

Skin: Acanthosis nigricans. Abdominal striae.

Abdomen: Soft, nontender, nondistended.

Pelvic: Uniformly large **uterus.**

Labs: Hgb 10.4. Microcytosis. Hypochromia. Otherwise normal CBC, PT/PTT.

Endometrial Bx: Hyperplasia with atypia.

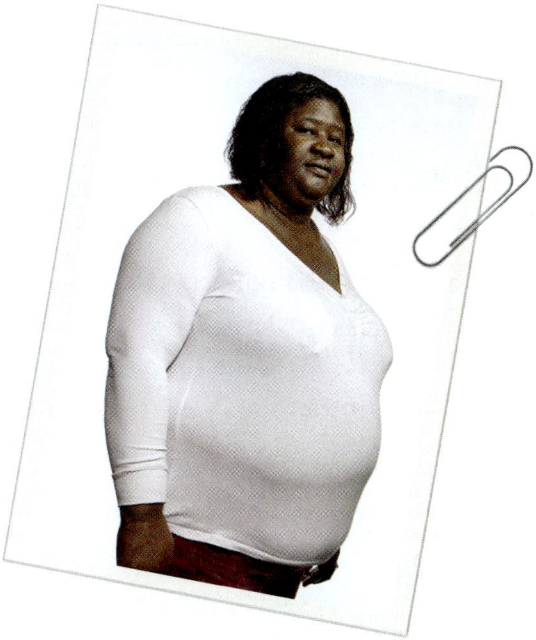

Assessment

Given her preliminary **endometrial biopsy** results, Mrs. Pecos's **metromenorrhagia** is due to **endometrial hyperplasia.** We will send the tissue sample to pathology to confirm the finding of atypia, but it is likely that she also has **myoinvasive endometrioid adenocarcinoma.**

Plan

Mrs. Pecos will need a **hysterectomy** and a referral to oncology. I will also begin her on iron supplementation.

–Mary Clary, DO

Learning Outcome 13.7 Exercises

EXERCISE 9 *Match the term on the left with its definition on the right.*

_____ 1. Pap smear
_____ 2. menopause
_____ 3. mammogram
_____ 4. hysterectomy
_____ 5. endometrium
_____ 6. cervical intraepithelial neoplasia
_____ 7. metromenorrhagia

a. record of a breast exam
b. test used to detect cancer cells, most commonly in the cervix
c. abnormal growth of cervical cells
d. cessation of menstruation
e. excessive menstrual bleeding at irregular intervals
f. surgical removal of the uterus
g. inner layer of uterine tissue

EXERCISE 10 *Fill in the blanks.*

1. Subjective
   a. PMHx (define abbreviation: _____________________): last *mammogram* (give definition: _____________________) 6 years ago: normal
   b. _____________(a test used to detect cancer cells, most commonly in the cervix): 10 years ago: *cervical intraepithelial neoplasia* II (give definition: _____________________) treated with LEEP (define abbreviation: _____________________)
2. Objective
   a. Mrs. Pecos's temperature: _____________________
   b. Mrs. Pecos's heart rate: _____________________
   c. Mrs. Pecos's respiratory rate: _____________________
   d. Mrs. Pecos's blood pressure: _____________________
3. Assessment
   a. Mrs. Pecos has *metromenorrhagia* (give definition: _____________________)
4. Plan
   a. Mrs. Pecos will need a *hysterectomy* (give definition: _____________________) and a likely referral to _____________________ (the branch of medicine dealing with tumors).

EXERCISE 11 *True or false questions. Indicate true answers with a T and false answers with an F.*

1. Mrs. Pecos is also experiencing leukorrhea. _______
2. According to her pelvic exam, Mrs. Pecos has macromastia. _______
3. Mrs. Pecos was given a biopsy. _______
4. Mrs. Pecos will likely have her uterus removed. _______

Learning Outcome 13.7 Exercises

EXERCISE 12 *Multiple-choice questions. Select the correct answer.*

1. *Menses* is the term for a woman's monthly flow during her menstrual cycle. In this health record, the patient's chief complaint is
   a. heavy menses
   b. irregular menses
   c. lack of menses
   d. light menses
   e. none of these
2. The *endometrium* is
   a. another term for *uterus*
   b. the middle layer of uterine tissue
   c. the muscular layer of the uterus
   d. the inner layer of uterine tissue
   e. the tissue on the outside of the uterus
3. Mrs. Pecos is a 47-year-old *premenopausal* woman, which means that
   a. her menstrual flow has not ceased
   b. her menstrual flow is heavy
   c. her menstrual flow is irregular
   d. her menstrual flow is just beginning
   e. none of these
4. The medical professional believes the patient has *endometrial hyperplasia.* Which of the following options is a correct breakdown of this term?
   a. *endo* (inside) + *metrial* (fallopian tube) + *hyper* (under) + *plasia* (new formation)
   b. *endo* (inside) + *metrial* (pelvis) + *hyper* (over) + *plasia* (new formation)
   c. *endo* (inside) + *metrial* (uterus) + *hyper* (over) + *plasia* (new formation)
   d. *endo* (outside) + *metrial* (cervix) + *hyper* (under) + *plasia* (new formation)
   e. *endo* (outside) + *metrial* (perineum) + *hyper* (over) + *plasia* (new formation)

Quick Reference

quick reference glossary of roots

Root	Definition	Root	Definition
amni/o	amnion	**men/o**	menstruation
cervic/o	cervix	**metr/o**	uterus
chori/o	chorion	**nat/o**	birth
chorion/o	chorion	**oophor/o**	ovary
colp/o	vagina	**ovari/o**	ovary
-cyesis	pregnancy	**part/o**	birth
episi/o	vulva	**pelv/i**	pelvis
fet/o	fetus	**perine/o**	perineum
gyn/o	woman	**toc/o**	labor
gynec/o	woman	**salping/o**	fallopian tube
hyster/o	uterus	**uter/o**	uterus
lact/o	milk	**vagin/o**	vagina
mamm/o	breast	**vulv/o**	vulva
mast/o	breast		

quick reference glossary of terms

Term	Definition
abortifacient	drug or device that causes the termination of a pregnancy
abortion	termination of pregnancy
abruptio placentae	separation of the placenta from the wall of the uterus
adenocarcinoma of the breast	glandular tumor in the breast
amastia	absence of breasts
amenorrhea	no menstruation
amniocentesis	surgical puncture of the amnion
amniorrhea	discharge of amniotic fluid
amniorrhexis	rupture of the amniotic sac

quick reference glossary of terms *continued*

Term	Definition
amnioscope	instrument for examining the amnion
amnioscopy	procedure for examining the amnion
amniotomy	incision into the amnion
antepartum	time before birth
bradytocia	slow labor
Braxton Hicks contraction	sporadic contractions of the uterine muscles of women in labor; also known as false labor
cardiotocograph	instrument for recording the fetal heart rate during labor
cephalopelvic disproportion (CPD)	condition characterized by the inability of the mother's pelvis to allow the baby to pass through the birth canal
cervical dysplasia	bad formation of cervical cells
cervical intraepithelial neoplasia	abnormal growth of cervical cells
cervicectomy	surgical removal of the cervix
cervicitis	inflammation of the cervix
cervicocolpitis	inflammation of the cervix and vagina
cervicography	procedure for imaging the cervix
cervicovaginitis	inflammation of the cervix and vagina
cesarean section	delivery of a baby through an incision made in the uterus
chorioamnionitis	inflammation of the chorion and amnion
chorioangioma	blood vessel tumor of the chorion
choriocarcinoma	cancerous tumor of the chorion
chorionitis	inflammation of the chorion
colpitis	inflammation of the vagina
colpocystitis	inflammation of the vagina and urinary bladder
colpopexy	surgical fixation of the vagina
colpoplasty	surgical reconstruction of the vagina
colpoptosis	downward placement of the vagina
colposcope	instrument used to examine the vagina

quick reference glossary of terms *continued*

Term	Definition
colposcopy	procedure for examining the vagina
colpostenosis	narrowing in the vaginal opening
congenital anomaly	irregular condition that is present at the time of birth
contraction	shortening or tightening of a muscle (during labor, uterine muscles contract)
cystocele	hernia of the urinary bladder into the vagina
dermoid cyst	ovarian cyst containing skin and sometimes hair, teeth, bone, or cartilage
dysmenorrhea	painful menstruation
dyspareunia	painful sexual intercourse
dystocia	difficult labor
eclampsia	severe, life-threatening complication of pregnancy characterized by seizures
ectopic pregnancy	implantation of a fertilized egg in a place other than the uterus
endocervicitis	inflammation of the inside of the cervix
endometriosis	condition in which endometrium cells appear and grow outside the uterus
endometritis	inflammation of the endometrium
endometrium	inner layer of uterine tissue
episiorrhaphy	suture of the vulva
episiostenosis	narrowing of the vulvar opening
episiotomy	incision into the vulva
eutocia	normal labor
fetometry	procedure for measuring the fetus
gravida	another term for *pregnant*
gynecologist	specialist in medical issues specific to women
gynecology	study of medical issues specific to women
gynecomastia	development of breast tissue in males
hematosalpinx	blockage in a fallopian tube caused by blood
hydrosalpinx	blockage in a fallopian tube caused by water (or any clear fluid)
hyperemesis gravidarum	pregnancy-related vomiting; an extreme form of the more common *morning sickness*

quick reference glossary of terms *continued*

Term	Definition
hypermastia	excessively large breasts (can also refer to an abnormal number of breasts)
hypomastia	abnormally small breasts
hysteralgia	pain in the uterus
hysterectomy	surgical removal of the uterus
hysterocele	hernia of the uterus
hysterodynia	pain in the uterus
hysterography	procedure for imaging the uterus
hysteropexy	surgical fixation of the uterus
hysteroptosis	downward displacement of the uterus into the vagina
hysterorrhexis	rupture of the uterus
hysterosalpingectomy	surgical removal of the uterus and fallopian tube
hysterosalpingogram	record of the uterus and fallopian tubes
hysteroscope	instrument for examining the uterus
hysteroscopy	procedure for examining the uterus
hysterotomy	incision into the uterus
in vitro fertilization	fertilization of an egg done in a test tube
induced abortion	intentional termination of pregnancy
intrapartum	time during birth
lactation	production of milk
lactogenic	causing the formation of milk
lactorrhea	discharge of milk
leukorrhea	white vaginal discharge
macromastia	abnormally large breasts
macrosomia	baby with a large body
mammogram	record of a breast exam
mammoplasty	surgical reconstruction of a breast
mastalgia	breast pain
mastectomy	surgical removal of a breast

quick reference glossary of terms *continued*

Term	Definition
mastitis	inflammation of the breast
mastopexy	surgical fixation of a breast
mastoptosis	downward displacement (drooping) of the breast
menarche	beginning or first menstruation
menopause	cessation of menstruation
menorrhagia	excessive menstrual flow
menorrhalgia	painful menstruation
metrocolpocele	hernia of the uterus and prolapse into the vagina
metromenorrhagia	excessive menstrual bleeding at irregular intervals
metrophlebitis	inflammation of the blood vessels of the uterus
metrorrhagia	menstrual bleeding at irregular times
microcephalus	baby with a small head
micromastia	abnormally small breasts
myomectomy	surgical removal of a tumor in the muscle (usually refers to the muscle of the uterine wall)
myometritis	inflammation of the myometrium
myometrium	middle layer of uterine muscle tissue
natal	pertaining to birth
neonatal	pertaining to new birth (normally the first 28 days after birth)
neonatologist	specialist in the neonatal period
neonatology	study of the neonatal period
obstetrician	specialist in pregnancy, labor, and delivery of newborns
obstetrics	branch of medicine dealing with pregnancy, labor, and delivery of newborns
oligohydramnios	not enough amniotic fluid
oligomenorrhea	infrequent or light menstrual periods
oophorectomy	surgical removal of an ovary
oophoritis	inflammation of an ovary
oophorocystectomy	surgical removal of an ovarian cyst

quick reference glossary of terms *continued*

Term	Definition
oophorocystosis	ovarian cysts
oophoroma	ovarian tumor
oophorotomy	incision into an ovary
ovaralgia	pain in the ovaries
ovarialgia	pain in the ovaries
ovarian cystectomy	surgical removal of an ovarian cyst
ovariocentesis	surgical puncture of an ovary
ovariocyesis	ectopic pregnancy in an ovary
ovariorrhexis	rupture of an ovary
ovariostomy	creation of an opening into an ovary
ovaritis	inflammation of an ovary
oxytocin	agent that stimulates uterine contractions and accelerates labor
Pap (Papanicolaou) smear	test used to detect cancer cells, most commonly in the cervix
pelvic sonograph	instrument for imaging the pelvis using sound waves
pelvicephalometry	procedure for measuring the head size of the baby and the pelvis size of the mother
pelvimetry	procedure for measuring the pelvis
perimetritis	inflammation of the perimetrium
perimetrium	tissue on the outside of the uterus, the outer layer of the uterus
perinatal	time around birth (normally ranging from 28 weeks of pregnancy to 28 days after pregnancy)
perinatologist	specialist in the perinatal period
perinatology	branch of medicine dealing with the perinatal period
perineocele	hernia in the perineum region
perineoplasty	surgical reconstruction of the perineum
perineorrhaphy	suture of the perineum
perineotomy	incision into the perineum
placenta previa	condition in whch the placenta is attached to the uterus near the cervix

quick reference glossary of terms *continued*

Term	Definition
polyhydramnios	excessive amniotic fluid
polymenorrhea	menstrual periods occurring with greater than normal frequency
postnatal	pertaining to after birth
postpartum	pertaining to after birth
preeclampsia	condition characterized by high blood pressure and high protein levels in the urine
prenatal	pertaining to before birth
pseudocyesis	false pregnancy
pyosalpinx	blockage in a fallopian tube caused by pus
rectocele	hernia or protrusion of the rectum into the vagina
salpingectomy	surgical removal of a fallopian tube
salpingitis	inflammation of a fallopian tube
salpingocele	hernia of a fallopian tube
salpingocyesis	ectopic pregnancy in a fallopian tube
salpingo-oophorectomy	surgical removal of a fallopian tube and ovary
salpingo-oophoritis	inflammation of a fallopian tube and ovary
salpingopexy	surgical fixation of a fallopian tube
sonohysterography	procedure using sound waves to examine the uterus
speculum	device for examining a body cavity, most commonly the vagina
spontaneous abortion	the naturally occurring termination of pregnancy; also known as a *miscarriage*
teratogenic	causing the formation of birth defects
teratology	branch of medicine dealing with the study of birth defects and their causes
teratoma	see *dermoid cyst*
tocodynagraph	instrument for recording the strength of labor contractions
tocography	procedure for recording the strength of labor contractions
transvaginal sonography	imaging procedure using sound waves emitted from device inserted in the vagina
urethrocele	hernia or prolapse of the urethra into the vagina
uterine prolapse	downward displacement of the uterus into the vagina

quick reference glossary of terms *continued*

Term	Definition
vaginitis	inflammation of the vagina
vaginodynia	vaginal pain
vaginomycosis	fungal condition of the vagina
vaginoperineoplasty	suture of the vagina and perineum
vaginoperineorrhaphy	suture of the vagina and perineum
vaginoperineotomy	incision into the vagina and perineum
vaginoplasty	surgical reconstruction of the vagina
vaginoscope	instrument used to examine the vagina
vaginosis	condition of the vagina
vesicovaginal fistula	abnormal opening between the urinary bladder and the vagina
vulvitis	inflammation of the vulva
vulvodynia	pain in the vulva
vulvovaginitis	inflammation of the vulva and vagina

review of terms by roots

Root	Term(s)	
amni/o	amniocentesis	amniotomy
	amniorrhea	chorioamnionitis
	amniorrhexis	oligohydramnios
	amnioscope	polyhydramnios
	amnioscopy	
cervic/o	cervical dysplasia	cervicocolpitis
	cervical intraepithelial neoplasia	cervicography
	cervicectomy	cervicovaginitis
	cervicitis	endocervicitis
chori/o	chorioamnionitis	choriocarcinoma
	chorioangioma	chorionitis

review of terms by roots *continued*

Root	Term(s)	
colp/o	cervicocolpitis	colpoptosis
	colpitis	colposcope
	colpocystitis	colposcopy
	colpopexy	colpostenosis
	colpoplasty	metrocolpocele
-cyesis	ovariocyesis	salpingocyesis
	pseudocyesis	
episi/o	episiorrhaphy	episiotomy
	episiostenosis	
fet/o	fetometry	
gynec/o	gynecologist	
	gynecology	
hyster/o	hysteralgia	hysterorrhexis
	hysterectomy	hysterosalpingectomy
	hysterocele	hysterosalpingogram
	hysterodynia	hysteroscope
	hysterography	hysteroscopy
	hysteropexy	hysterotomy
	hysteroptosis	sonohysterography
lact/o	lactation	lactorrhea
	lactogenic	
mamm/o	mammogram	mammoplasty
mast/o	amastia	mastectomy
	gynecomastia	mastitis
	hypermastia	mastopexy
	hypomastia	mastoptosis
	macromastia	micromastia
	mastalgia	

review of terms by roots *continued*

Root	Term(s)	
men/o	amenorrhea	menorrhagia
	dysmenorrhea	menorrhalgia
	menarche	metromenorrhagia
	menopause	oligomenorrhea
metr/o	endometriosis	metrorrhagia
	endometritis	myometritis
	endometrium	myometrium
	metrocolpocele	perimetritis
	metromenorrhagia	perimetrium
	metrophlebitis	
nat/o	natal	perinatologist
	neonatal	perinatology
	neonatologist	postnatal
	neonatology	prenatal
	perinatal	
oophor/o	oophorectomy	oophoroma
	oophoritis	oophorotomy
	oophorocystectomy	salpingo-oophorectomy
	oophorocystosis	salpingo-oophoritis
ovari/o	ovaralgia	ovariocyesis
	ovarialgia	ovariorrhexis
	ovarian cystectomy	ovariostomy
	ovariocentesis	ovaritis
part/o	antepartum	postpartum
	intrapartum	
pelv/i	cephalopelvic disproportion	pelvicephalometry
	pelvic sonograph	pelvimetry

review of terms by roots *continued*

Root	Term(s)	
perine/o	perineocele	vaginoperineoplasty
	perineoplasty	vaginoperineorrhaphy
	perineorrhaphy	vaginoperineotomy
	perineotomy	
salping/o	hematosalpinx	salpingitis
	hydrosalpinx	salpingocele
	hysterosalpingectomy	salpingocyesis
	hysterosalpingogram	salpingo-oophorectomy
	pyosalpinx	salpingo-oophoritis
	salpingectomy	salpingopexy
toc/o	bradytocia	oxytocin
	cardiotocograph	tocodynagraph
	dystocia	tocography
	eutocia	
uter/o	uterine prolapse	
vagin/o	cervicovaginitis	vaginoperineotomy
	transvaginal sonography	vaginoplasty
	vaginitis	vaginoscope
	vaginodynia	vaginosis
	vaginomycosis	vesicovaginal fistula
	vaginoperineoplasty	vulvovaginitis
	vaginoperineorrhaphy	
vulv/o	vulvitis	vulvovaginitis
	vulvodynia	

other terms

abortifacient	leukorrhea
abortion	macrosomia
abruptio placentae	microcephalus
adenocarcinoma of the breast	myomectomy
Braxton Hicks contraction	obstetrician
cesarean section	obstetrics
congenital anomaly	Pap smear (Papanicolaou)
contraction	placenta previa
cystocele	preeclampsia
dermoid cyst	rectocele
dyspareunia	speculum
eclampsia	spontaneous abortion
ectopic pregnancy	teratogenic
gravida	teratology
hyperemesis gravidarum	teratoma
in vitro fertilization	urethrocele
induced abortion	

appendix A: prefixes

Prefix	Definition
A	
a-, an-	not
ab-	away
ad-, af-	toward
ambi-	both
ambly-	dull
ante-	before
anti-	against
auto-	self
B	
bi-	two
brady-	slow
C	
cata-	down
circum-	around
con-	with, together
contra-	against
crypto-	hidden
D	
de-	down, away from
dia-	through
dipl-	double
dys-	bad
E	
e-	out
ec-	out
ecto-	outside
ef-	out
em-, en-	in, inside
endo-	in, inside
epi-	upon
eso-	inward
eu-	good, normal
ex-	out
exo-	outside
extra-	outside
H	
hemi-	half
hetero-	different
homo-	similar
hyper-	over
hypo-	under

Prefix	Definition
I	
idio-	private
inter-	between
intra-	in, inside
iso-	equal
M	
macro-	large
meta-	after, other, beyond
micro-	small
mono-	one
multi-	many
N	
neo-	new
O	
ob-	in the way
oligo-	few
ortho-	straight
P	
pan-	all
par-, para-	around, beside
per-	through
peri-	around
poly-	many
post-	after
pre-	before
presby-	old
pro-	before, on behalf of
pros-	to, toward
pseud-, pseudo-	false
R	
re-	again
S	
schizo-	divided
semi-	half
sub-	beneath
sym-, syn-	with, together
T	
tachy-	fast
trans-	through, across
U	
uni-	one

appendix B: suffixes

Suffix	Definition
A	
-acusis	hearing condition
-agon	to lead
-ant	agent
-arche	beginning
-asthenia	weakness
-ation	process, procedure
C	
-cide	to kill
-cision	cut
-clasia	breaking
-clasis	breaking
D	
-drome	run
E	
-ectasia	expansion, dilation
-ectasis	expansion, dilation
-edema	swelling
-emia	blood condition
G	
-genic	beginning in, producing
-graft	transplant
I	
-iasis	presence
-icle	little
-ictal	seizure
-ive	agent
L	
-listhesis	slipping
-lith	stone
-loqui	speak
-luxation	dislocation
-lytic	break down
M	
-malacia	abnormal softening
-megaly	abnormal enlargement
O	
-opia	vision condition
-opsia	vision condition

Suffix	Definition
P	
-paresis	slight or partial paralysis
-pareunia	sexual intercourse
-pathy	disease/condition
-penia	deficiency
-phagia	eating
-philia	abnormal liking for or tendency toward
-phoria	carry condition
-plasia	formation
-plasm	formation
-plastic	formation
-plasty	surgical reconstruction
-plegia	paralysis
-pnea	breathing
-poesis	formation
-ptosis	drooping
-ptysis	cough
R	
-rrhage, -rrhagia	excessive flow
-rrhaphy	suture
-rrhea	flow
-rrhexis	rupture
S	
-sclerosis	hardening condition
-scope	instrument used to look
-scopy	process of looking
-spasm	involuntary contraction
-stenosis	narrowing
-stomy	creation of an opening
T	
-thesis	place
-tomy	incision
-toxic	poisonous
-toxin	a substance poisonous to
-tripsy	wear down procedure, surgical crushing
-trophy	nourishment condition
-tropin	stimulating hormone
U	
-ula	small
-uria	urine condition
Y	
-y	condition or process

appendix C: roots only mentioned in word analysis

Root	Definition
A	
acr/o	extremity, top, heights
aer/o	air
ambul/o	walk
B	
bi/o	life
C	
carcin/o	cancer
chem/o	chemical
chron/o	time
chyl/o	chyle
coni/o	dust
cry/o	cold
cyan/o	blue
D	
desicc/o	drying
dips/o	thirst
E	
electr/o	electricity
eury/o	wide
F	
fibr/o	fiber
G	
galact/o	milk
gen/o	generation/cause
gnosi/o	knowledge
graph/o	write
H	
hem/o, hemat/o	blood
hepat/o	liver
hydr/o	water
I	
isch/o	hold back
K	
kel/o	tumor
klept/o	theft
kyph/o	bent

Root	Definition
L	
lex/o	reading
lord/o	bend backward
M	
morph/o	change
muc/o	mucus
myc/o	fungus
N	
narc/o	sleep
necr/o	death
neur/o	nerve
noct/o	night
O	
orth/o	straight
osm/o	smelling
P	
path/o	suffering/disease
phag/o	eat
pharmac/o	drug
phas/o	speaking
phil/o	love
phon/o	sound/voice
plas/o	formation
poli/o	gray
por/o	pore
prosop/o	face
py/o	pus
pylor/o	gatekeeper
pyr/o	fire
S	
sarc/o	flesh
scler/o	hard
scoli/o	crooked
sept/i	rotting
sept/o	wall, partition
somat/o	body
son/o	sound
spin/o	spine
stigmat/o	point
stom/o	mouth

Root	Definition
T	
tel/o	complete, end
thel/o	breast
thromb/o	clot
tom/o	cut
top/o	place
trich/o	hair
trop/o	turn
troph/o	nourishment/development
tuss/o	cough
X	
xen/o	foreign
xer/o	dry

A

abdominocentesis (ab-DAW-min-oh-sin-TEE-sis) puncture of the abdomen (usually for the purpose of withdrawing fluid)

abdominoplasty (ab-DAW-min-oh-PLAS-tee) surgical reconstruction of the abdomen

abortifacient (ah-BOR-tih-FAY-shunt) drug or device that causes the termination of a pregnancy

abortion (ah-BOR-shun) termination of pregnancy

abrasion (ah-BRAY-zhun) a scraping away of skin

abruptio placentae (ah-BRUP-shee-oh plah-SIN-tee) separation of the placenta from the wall of the uterus

abscess (AB-ses) a localized collection of pus in the body

achondroplasia (AY-kawn-droh-PLAY-zhah) a defect in the formation of cartilage

acidemia (A-sih-DEE-mee-ah) abnormal acidity of the blood

acne vulgaris (AK-nee vul-GAR-is) common acne; an inflammation of the skin follicles

acoustic neuroma (ah-KOO-stik nir-OH-mah) a tumor on the acoustic nerve

acromegaly (AK-roh-MEH-gah-lee) abnormal enlargement of the extremities

acrophobia (AK-roh-FOH-bee-ah) fear of heights

actinic dermatitis (ak-TIN-ik der-mah-TAI-tis) inflammation of the skin caused by sun exposure

actinic keratosis (ak-TIN-ik keh-rah-TOH-sis) horny skin condition caused by sun exposure

adenalgia (AD-en-AL-jah) pain in a gland

adenectomy (AD-en-EK-toh-mee) removal of a gland

adenitis (AD-en-AI-tis) inflammation of a gland

adenocarcinoma (ad-EN-oh-KAR-sih-NOH-mah) cancerous tumor of a gland

adenocarcinoma of the breast (AD-en-oh-KAR-sih-NOH-mah) glandular tumor in the breast

adenoidectomy (a-din-oid-EK-toe-mee) removal of the adenoids

adenoma (AD-eh-NOH-mah) glandular tumor

adenomegaly (ah-DEN-oh-MEH-gah-lee) abnormal enlargement of a gland

adenopathy (AD-en-AW-pah-thee) gland disease

adenosis (AD-en-OH-sis) gland condition

adipocele (a-dih-poh-SEEL) hernia filled with fatty tissue

adrenal adenoma (ad-REE-nal AD-en-OH-mah) tumor of the adrenal gland

adrenal insufficiency (ad-REE-nal IN-suh-FIH-shun-see) condition in which the adrenal glands underproduce necessary hormones

adrenal virilism (ad-REE-nal VIR-il-izm) development of male secondary sexual characteristics caused by excessive secretion of the adrenal gland

adrenalectomy (ad-REE-nal-EK-toh-mee) removal of the adrenal gland

adrenaline (ad-REN-ah-lin) hormone secreted by the adrenal gland (from Latin; see also *epinephrine*)

adrenalitis (ad-REE-nah-LAI-tis) inflammation of the adrenal gland

adrenarche (AD-ren-AR-kay) beginning of adrenal secretion (at puberty)

adrenocortical carcinoma (ad-REE-noh-KOR-tih-kal KAR-sih-NOH-mah) cancerous tumor originating in the cortex of the adrenal gland

adrenocortical insufficiency (ad-REE-noh-KOR-tih-kal IN-suh-FIH-shun-see) condition in which the adrenal cortex underproduces necessary hormones

adrenocorticohyperplasia (ad-REE-noh-KOR-tih-koh-HAI-per-PLAY-zhah) overdevelopment of the cortex of the adrenal gland

adrenocorticotropic hormone (ACTH) (ah-DREH-noh-KOR-tih-koh-TROH-pik HOR-mohn) hormone secreted by the pituitary gland that stimulates the cortex of the adrenal gland

adrenomegaly (ad-REN-oh-MEH-gah-lee) abnormal enlargement of the adrenal gland

aerodontalgia (ER-oh-dawn-TAL-jah) tooth pain caused by exposure to air

aerotitis (AIR-oh-TAI-tis) inflammation of the ear caused by air

afferent nerve (A-fir-ent nirv) a nerve that carries impulses toward the central nervous system

agnosia (AG-noh-zhah) inability to comprehend

agoraphobia (ah-GOR-ah-FOH-bee-ah) fear of outdoor spaces

akinetopsia (ah-KEE-nah-TOP-see-ah) the inability to see objects in motion

albinism (AL-bin-ism) lack of pigment in skin causing the patient to look white

albino (al-BAY-noh) a person afflicted with albinism

albuminuria (al-byoo-mih-NUR-ee-ah) protein in the urine

alkalemia (AL-kah-LEE-mee-ah) abnormal alkalinity (opposite of acidity) of the blood

allograft (A-loh-GRAFT) see *homograft*

alopecia (a-loh-PEE-sha) baldness

amastia (ay-MAS-tee-ah) absence of breasts

ambiopia (AM-bee-OH-pee-ah) double vision

amblyopia (AM-blih-OH-pee-ah) decreased vision (when it occurs in one eye, it is referred to as lazy eye)

amenorrhea (AY-men-oh-REE-ah) no menstruation

amniocentesis (AM-nee-oh-sin-TEE-sis) surgical puncture of the amnion

amniorrhea (AM-nee-oh-REE-ah) discharge of amniotic fluid

amniorrhexis (AM-nee-oh-REK-sis) rupture of the amniotic sac

amnioscope (AM-nee-oh-SKOHP) instrument for examining the amnion

amnioscopy (AM-nee-AW-skoh-pee) procedure for examining the amnion

amniotomy (AM-nee-AW-toh-mee) incision into the amnion

amytrophic lateral sclerosis (ALS) (a-MAI-aw-TROH-fik LAT-tih-ral skleh-ROH-sis) a degenerative disease of the central nervous system causing loss of muscle control; also known as Lou Gehrig's disease

anal fistula (AY-nal FIS-tyoo-la) abnormal opening between the rectum and the exterior perianal skin

analgesic (an-al-JEE-zik) a drug that relieves pain

anastomosis (ah-NAS-toh-moh-sis) creation of an opening; a surgical procedure connecting two previously unconnected hollow tubes.

anemia (ah-NEE-mee-ah) reduction of red blood cells noticed by the patient by weakness and fatigue

anesthesiologist (A-neh-STHEE-zee-AW-loh-jist) doctor who specializes in anesthesiology

anesthetic (an-es-THET-ik) a drug that causes loss of sensation

aneurysm (AN-yir-IZ-um) bulge in a blood vessel

aneurysmectomy (AN-yir-IZ-um-EK-toh-mee) surgical removal of an aneurysm

angina pectoris (an-JAI-nah PEK-tor-is) oppressive pain in the chest caused by irregular blood flow to the heart

angiocarditis (AN-jee-oh-kar-DAI-tis) inflammation of the heart vessels

angioedema (AN-jee-oh-eh-DEE-mah) swelling of the blood vessels

angiogenesis (AN-jee-oh-JIN-eh-sis) development of blood vessels

angiogram (AN-jee-oh-GRAM) record of the blood vessels

angiography (AN-jee-AW-grah-fee) procedure to describe the blood vessels

angiolith (AN-jee-oh-LITH) stone forming in the wall of a blood vessel

angioma (AN-jee-OH-mah) blood vessel tumor

angioplasty (AN-jee-oh-PLAS-tee) surgical reconstruction of a vessel

angiopoiesis (AN-jee-oh-poh-EE-sis) formation of blood vessels

angiorrhaphy (AN-jee-OR-ah-fee) suture of a vessel

angiosclerosis (AN-jee-oh-skleh-ROH-sis) hardening of a blood vessel

angioscope (AN-jee-oh-SKOWP) device for looking into a blood vessel

anhidrosis (an-ih-DROH-sis) lack of sweating

aniridia (AN-ih-RIH-dee-ah) absence of an iris

anisocytosis (AN-ai-soh-SAI-toh-sis) condition characterized by a great inequality in the size of red blood cells

ankylosing spondylitis (an-kih-LOH-sing spawn-dih-LAI-tis) a stiffening inflammation of the vertebrae

ankylosis (an-kih-LOH-sis) joint stiffness

anophony (an-AW-foh-nee) sound from the anus

anoplasty (AN-noh-PLAS-tee) surgical reconstruction of the anus

anorchidism (an-OR-kih-DIZ-um) absence of a testicle

anorexia (a-noh-REK-see-ah) an eating disorder characterized by the patient's refusal to eat

anosigmoidoscopy (AN-oh-SIG-moid-AW-skoh-pee) procedure for looking at the anus and sigmoid colon

anosmia (an-AWZ-mee-ah) lack of a sense of smell

antacid (ant-AS-id) agent that neutralizes acid

antepartum (AN-tee-PAR-tum) time before birth

antianginal (AN-tee-AN-jih-nal) a drug that prevents or relieves the symptoms of angina pectoris

antiarrhythmic (AN-tee-a-RITH-mik) a drug that opposes an irregular heartbeat

antiarthritic (AN-tee-ar-THRIH-tik) a drug that opposes joint inflammation

antibiotic (an-tai-bai-OH-tik) a drug that destroys or opposes the growth of microorganisms

antibody (AN-tih-BAW-dee) substance produced by the body in response to an antigen

anticoagulant (AN-tee-coh-AG-yoo-lant) drug that prevents the coagulation of blood

anticonvulsant (AN-tee-kon-VUL-sant) a drug that opposes convulsions

antidepressant (AN-tee-deh-PREH-sant) a drug that opposes depression

antiemetic (AN-tih-EE-met-ik) agent that prevents/relieves nausea or vomiting

antigen (AN-tih-JIN) substance that causes the body to produce antibodies

antihistamine (an-tee-HIS-tah-meen) a drug that opposes the effects of histamine

antihypertensive (AN-tee-HAI-per-TEN-siv) drug that opposes high blood pressure

anti-inflammatory (AN-tee-in-FLA-mah-TOR-ee) a drug that opposes inflammation

antipruritic (an-tee-pruh-RIH-tik) a drug that prevents or relieves itching

antipsychotic (AN-tee-sai-KAW-tik) a drug that opposes psychosis

antipyretic (AN-tee-pir-ih-tik) a drug that opposes fever

antiseptic (an-tee-SEP-tik) a drug that prevents sepsis (rotting of flesh) by killing microorganisms

antispasmodic (AN-tee-spaz-MAW-dik) drug used to prevent spasms

antitussive (an-tee-TUSS-iv) a drug that prevents coughing

anuria (an-YUR-ee-ah) lack of urination

anxiolytic (ANG-zee-oh-LIH-tik) a drug that lessens anxiety

aortalgia (AY-or-TAL-jah) pain in the aorta

aortectasia (ay-OR-tek-TAY-zhah) dilation of the aorta

aortic aneurysm (ay-OR-tik AN-yir-IZ-um) bulging or swelling of the aorta

aortic regurgitation (ay-OR-tik ree-GIR-jih-TAY-shun) flow of blood backward from the aorta into the heart; caused by a weak heart valve

aortic stenosis (ay-OR-tik stih-NOH-sis) narrowing of the aorta

aortitis (ay-or-TAI-tis) inflammation of the aorta

aortogram (ay-OR-tah-GRAM) record of the aorta

aortolith (ay-OR-toh-LITH) stone deposit in the wall of the aorta

aortorrhaphy (ay-or-TOR-ah-fee) suture of the aorta

aortotomy (ay-or-TAW-toh-mee) incision into the aorta

apathy (A-pah-thee) lack of emotion

aphagia (a-FAY-jah) inability to eat

aphakia (ah-FAY-kee-ia) absence of a lens

aphasia (ah-FAY-zhah) inability to speak

apheresis (AH-fer-EE-sis) general term for a process, similar to dialysis, that draws blood, removes something from it, then returns the rest of the blood to the patient

aplastic anemia (AY-plas-tik ah-NEE-mee-ah) anemia caused by red blood cells not being formed in sufficient quantities

apnea (AP-nee-yah) cessation of breathing

arrhythmia (ay-RITH-mee-ah) irregular heartbeat

arteriectomy (ar-TER-ee-EK-toh-mee) surgical removal of an artery

arteriogram (ar-TER-ee-oh-GRAM) record of an artery

arteriolith (ar-TER-ee-oh-LITH) stone in an artery

arteriopathy (ar-TER-ee-AW-pah-thee) disease of the arteries

arterioplasty (ar-TER-ee-oh-PLAS-tee) surgical reconstruction of an artery

arteriorrhaphy (ar-TER-ee-OR-ah-fee) suture of an artery

arteriorrhexis (ar-TER-ee-oh-REK-sis) rupture of an artery

arteriosclerosis (ar-TER-ee-oh-skleh-ROH-sis) hardening of an artery

arteritis (AR-ter-AI-tis) inflammation of the arteries

arthralgia (ar-THRAL-jah) joint pain

arthrectomy (ar-THREK-toh-mee) removal of a joint

arthritis (ar-THRAI-tis) joint inflammation

arthrocele (AR-throh-seel) hernia of a joint

arthrocentesis (ar-throh-sin-TEE-sis) puncture of a joint

arthroclasia (AR-throh-KLAY-zhah) the therapeutic breaking of a joint to allow for increased mobility

arthrodesis (AR-throh-DEE-sis) the surgical fixation of a joint

arthrodynia (ar-throh-DAI-nee-ah) joint pain

arthrodysplasia (AR-throh-dis-PLAY-zhah) abnormal joint development

arthrogram (AR-throh-gram) visual record of a joint

arthrography (ar-THRAW-grah-fee) procedure used to examine a joint

arthrolysis (ar-THRAW-lih-sis) loosening a stiff joint

arthropathy (ar-THRAW-pah-thee) joint disease

arthroplasty (AR-throh-PLAS-tee) reconstruction of a joint

arthrosclerosis (AR-throh-skleh-ROH-sis) hardening of the joints

arthroscope (AR-throh-skohp) instrument for looking into a joint

arthroscopy (ar-THRAW-skoh-pee) procedure of looking into a joint

arthrotomy (ar-THRAW-toh-mee) incision into a joint

ascites (ah-SAI-teez) retention of fluid in the peritoneum

aspermia (ay-SPER-mee-ah) condition characterized by a lack of sperm

asplenia (ah-SPLEE-nee-ah) absence of a spleen or of spleen function

asthenopia (AS-then-OH-pee-ah) weak vision (i.e., eye strain)

asthma (AZ-ma) a disease caused by episodic narrowing and inflammation of the airway

astigmatism (ah-STIG-mah-TIZ-um) vision problem caused by the fact that light rays entering the eye aren't focused on a single point in the back of the eye

ataxia (ah-TAK-see-ah) lack of coordination

atelectasis (ah-tel-EK-ta-sis) incomplete expansion

atherectomy (A-ther-EK-toh-mee) surgical removal of fatty plaque within an artery

atherogenesis (A-ther-oh-JIN-eh-sis) formation of fatty plaque on the wall of an artery

atherosclerosis (A-ther-oh-skleh-ROH-sis) hardening of an artery due to build-up of fatty plaque

atopic dermatitis (AY-taw-pik der-mah-TAI-tis) an unusual inflammation of the skin (atopic usually means not in the right place)

atopognosis (AY-top-aw-GNOH-sis) inability to locate a sensation

atrial fibrillation (AY-tree-al FIB-rih-LAY-shun) quivering or spontaneous contraction of muscle fibers in the heart's atrium

atrial septal defect (AY-tree-al SEP-tal DEE-fekt) flaw in the septum that divides the two atria of the heart

atrophy (A-troh-fee) underdevelopment, decrease, or loss of muscle tissue

audiogram (AW-dee-oh-GRAM) record produced by an audiometer

audiologist (aw-dee-AW-loh-jist) hearing specialist

audiometer (aw-dee-AW-meh-ter) instrument for measuring hearing

audiometry (aw-dee-AW-meh-tree) procedure for measuring hearing

auditory prosthesis (AW-dih-TOR-ee praws-THEE-sis) hearing aid

aural (AW-ral) pertaining to the ear

auscultation (ah-skul-TAY-shun) from the Latin word *ausculto,* meaning *to listen;* a doctor using a stethoscope is performing an auscultation

autism (AH-tiz-um) a psychiatric disorder characterized by the withdrawal from communication with others. The patient is focused only on the self

autograft (AW-toh-GRAFT) skin transplant taken from a different place on the patient's body

autoimmune disease (AW-toh-ih-MYOON dih-ZEEZ) a disease caused by the body's immune system attacking the body's own healthy tissue

azoospermia (ay-ZOH-aw-SPER-mee-ah) a condition characterized by lack of living sperm

azotemia (AZ-oh-TEE-mee-ah) excess nitrogen in the blood

azotorrhea (AZ-oh-toh-REE-ah) excessive discharge of nitrogen

azoturia (AZ-oh-TUR-ee-ah) excess nitrogen in the urine

B

balanitis (bal-ah-NAI-tis) inflammation of the penis

balanoplasty (BAL-ah-noh-PLAS-tee) surgical reconstruction of the penis

balanorrhea (BAL-ah-noh-REE-ah) discharge from the penis

bariatrics (BAR-ee-ah-triks) branch of medicine dealing with weight issues

basal cell carcinoma (BAY-zul sell kar-sih-NOH-mah) cancerous tumor of basal skin cells

benign prostate hyperplasia (beh-NAIN PROS-tayt HAI-per-PLAY-zhah) noncancerous overdevelopment of the prostate; also known as enlarged prostate

benign prostate hypertrophy (beh-NAIN PROS-tayt hai-PER-troh-fee) another term for benign prostate hyperplasia

biligenesis (blh-lih-JIN-eh-sis) formation of bile

bilirubinemia (BIH-lee-ROO-bin-EE-mee-ah) the presence of bilirubin (red bile; a substance derived from red blood cells that have completed their life span) in the blood

binocular (bai-NAW-kyoo-lar) pertaining to both eyes

biopsy (BAI-op-see) removal of tissue in order to examine it

blepharedema (BLEF-ar-eh-DEE-mah) eyelid swelling

blepharitis (BLEF-ah-RAI-tis) eyelid inflammation

blepharoconjunctivitis (BLEF-ah-roh-con-JUNK-tih-VAI-tis) inflammation of the eyelid and conjunctiva

blepharoplasty (BLEF-ah-roh-PLAS-tee) surgical reconstruction of the eyelid

blepharoplegia (BLEF-ah-roh-PLEE-jah) paralysis of the eyelid

blepharoptosis (BLEF-ar-awp-TOH-sis) drooping eyelid

blepharopyorrhea (BLEF-ah-roh-PAI-oh-REE-ah) discharge of pus from the eyelid

blepharospasm (BLEF-ah-roh-SPAZ-um) involuntary contraction of an eyelid

blepharotomy (BLEF-ah-RAW-toh-mee) incision into the eyelid

blood pressure (blud PRESH-ir) force exerted by blood on the walls of blood vessels

blood urea nitrogen (BUN) (blud yoo-REE-ah NAI-troh-jun) nitrogen in the blood in the form of urea; it is the product of the breakdown of amino acids for energy

bradycardia (BRAY-dih-KAR-dee-ah) slow heartbeat

bradykinesia (bray-dih-kih-NEE-zhah) slow movement

bradypnea (brad-ip-NEE-ah) slow breathing

bradytocia (BRAY-dih-TOH-shee-ah) slow labor

Braxton Hicks contraction (BRAKS-ton HIKS con-TRAK-shun) sporadic contractions of the uterine muscles of women in labor; also known as false labor

bronchiectasis (bron-key-EK-ta-sis) expansion of the bronchi

bronchiogenic carcinoma (bron-kee-oh-JEN-ic car-si-NO-ma) a cancerous tumor originating in the bronchi

bronchiolitis (bron-kee-yo-LAI-tis) inflammation of the bronchiole

bronchioplasty (bron-koh-PLAS-tee) reconstruction of a bronchus

bronchitis (bron-KAI-tis) inflammation of the bronchi

bronchodilator (bron-koh-DAI-lay-tor) a drug that expands the walls of the bronchi

bronchorrhea (bron-koh-REE-ah) discharge from the bronchi

bronchoscopy (bron-KOS-koh-pee) a procedure to look inside the bronchi

bronchospasm (BRON-ko-spaz-um) involuntary contraction of the bronchia

bulimia (boo-LEE-mee-ah) an eating disorder characterized by overeating and usually followed by forced vomiting

bulla (BUL-lah) from Latin, for *bubble;* a large blister

bursectomy (bir-SEK-toh-mee) removal of a bursa

bursitis (bur-SAI-tis) inflammation of the bursa

bursolith (BIR-soh-lith) a stone in a bursa

bursopathy (bur-SAW-pah-thee) disease of the bursa

bursotomy (bir-SAW-toh-mee) incision into a bursa

C

calciuria (CAL-sih-YOO-ree-ah) calcium in the urine

capnography (cap-NAH-gra-fee) a procedure to record carbon dioxide levels

capnometer (cap-NOM-eh-ter) instrument to measure carbon dioxide levels

cardiac arrest (KAR-dee-ak ah-REST) cessation of functional circulation

cardiac catheterization (KAR-dee-ak KATH-eh-ter-ih-ZAY-shun) the process of inserting a tube (catheter) into the heart

cardiologist (KAR-dee-AW-loh-jist) heart specialist

cardiology (KAR-dee-AW-loh-jee) branch of medicine dealing with the heart

cardiomegaly (KAR-dee-oh-MEH-gah-lee) enlarged heart

cardiomyopathy (KAR-dee-oh-mai-AW-pah-thee) disease of the heart muscle

cardiomyotomy (KAR-dee-oh-mai-AW-toh-mee) incision into the heart muscle

cardiopulmonary bypass (KAR-dee-oh-PUL-mon-AR-ee BAI-pas) procedure that temporarily circulates and oxygenates a patient's blood during a portion of heart surgery where the heart is stopped

cardiopulmonary resuscitation (CPR) (KAR-dee-oh-PUL-mon-air-ee ree-sus-ih-TAY-shun) a method of artificially maintaining blood flow and airflow when breathing and pulse have stopped

cardiothoracic surgery (KAR-dee-oh-thoh-RA-sik SIR-jir-ee) surgery that involves cutting through the patient's chest to get to the heart

cardiotocograph (KAR-dee-oh-TOH-koh-GRAF) instrument for recording the fetal heart rate during labor

cardiotonic (KAR-dee-oh-TAW-nik) a drug that increases the strength of heart contractions

cardiotoxic (KAR-dee-oh-TOK-sik) poisonous to the heart

cardiovascular (KAR-dee-oh-VAS-kyoo-lar) pertaining to the heart and blood vessels

cardioversion (KAR-dee-oh-VER-zhun) returning a heart to normal rhythm

carditis (kar-DAI-tis) inflammation of the heart

carpectomy (kar-PEK-toh-mee) removal of all or part of the wrist

carpitis (kar-PAI-tis) wrist inflammation

caseous necrosis (KAYZ-ee-us ne-CROW-sis) the death of tissue with a cheeselike appearance

cataract (KAT-ah-RAKT) opacity (cloudiness) of the lens of the eye (from Latin, for *waterfall*)

catatonia (KAT-ah-TOH-nee-ah) condition characterized by reduced muscle tone

cathartic (kah-THAR-tik) agent that produces bowel movements

causalgia (kaw-ZAL-jah) painful sensation of burning

celiomyositis (SEE-lee-oh-MAI-oh-sai-TOH-sis) inflammation of the abdominal muscle

celiopathy (see-lee-AW-pah-thee) disease of the abdomen

celiotomy (SEE-lee-AW-toh-mee) incision into the abdomen

cephalalgia (SEH-ful-AL-jah) head pain

cephalodynia (SEH-fah-loh-DAI-nee-ah) head pain

cephalopelvic disproportion (CPD) (SEE-fah-loh-PEL-vik DIS-proh-POR-shun) condition characterized by the inability of the mother's pelvis to allow the baby to pass through the birth canal

cerebellitis (ser-eh-bell-AI-tis) inflammation of the cerebellum

cerebral aneurysm (seh-REE-bral AN-yir-iz-um) the widening or abnormal dilation of a blood vessel in the brain

cerebral angiography (seih-REE-bral AN-gee-AW-grah-fee) procedure used to examine blood vessels in the brain

cerebral arteriosclerosis (seh-REE-bral ar-TIR-ee-oh-skleh-ROH-sis) the hardening of an artery in the brain

cerebral atherosclerosis (seh-REE-bral A-ther-oh-skleh-ROH-sis) the hardening of an artery in the brain caused by the buildup of fatty plaque

cerebral atrophy (seh-REE-bral A-troh-fee) wasting away of brain tissue

cerebral embolism (seh-REE-bral EM-boh-lih-zum) the blockage of a blood vessel in the brain caused by a foreign object (embolus) such as fat or bacteria

cerebral palsy (seh-REE-bral PAL-zee) paralysis caused by damage to the area of the brain responsible for movement

cerebral thrombosis (seh-REE-bral throm-BOH-sis) the blockage of a blood vessel in the brain caused by a clot

cerebromeningitis (seh-REE-broh-MEN-in-JAI-tis) inflammation of the brain and meninges

cerebrotomy (sih-ree-BRAW-toh-mee) incision into the brain

cerebrovascular accident (CVA) (seh-REE-broh-VAS-kyoo-lar AK-sih-dent) an accident involving the blood vessels of the brain

cerebrovascular disease (seh-REE-broh-VAS-kyoo-lar dih-ZEEZ) a disease of the blood vessels of the brain

cerumen impaction (SEH-roo-men im-PAK-shun) buildup of ear wax blocking the ear canal

ceruminolysis (seh-ROO-min-AW-lih-sis) breakdown of ear wax

ceruminolytic (seh-ROO-min-oh-LIH-tik) drug that aids in the breakdown of ear wax

ceruminoma (seh-ROO-min-OH-mah) benign tumor of the cerumen-secreting glands of the ear

ceruminosis (seh-ROO-min-OH-sis) excessive formation of ear wax

cervical dysplasia (SER-vih-kal dis-PLAY-zhah) bad formation of cervical cells

cervical intraepithelial neoplasia (SER-vih-kal IN-trah-EP-ih-THEE-lee-al NEE-oh-PLAY-zhah) abnormal growth of cervical cells

cervicectomy (SER-vih-SEK-toh-mee) surgical removal of the cervix

cervicitis (SER-vih-SAI-tis) inflammation of the cervix

cervicocolpitis (SER-vih-koh-kol-PAI-tis) inflammation of the cervix and vagina

cervicodynia (sir-vih-koh-DAI-nee-ah) neck pain

cervicography (SER-vih-KAW-grah-fee) procedure for imaging the cervix

cervicovaginitis (SER-vih-koh-VAJ-ih-NAI-tis) inflammation of the cervix and vagina

cesarean section (sih-SER-ee-an SEK-shun) delivery of a baby through an incision made in the uterus

chemosurgery (KEE-moh-SIR-juh-ree) removal of tissue that has been destroyed using chemicals

chemotherapy (KEE-moh-THER-ah-pee) treatment using chemicals

cherry angioma (CHEH-ree an-gee-OH-mah) a small blood vessel tumor

chloremia (klor-EE-mee-ah) increased chloride in the blood

cholangiogastrostomy (koh-LAN-jee-oh-gas-TRAWS-toh-mee) creation of an opening between the bile vessel (ducts) and the stomach

cholangiogram (koh-LAN-jee-oh-gram) record of the bile vessels (ducts)

cholangiography (koh-LAN-jee-AW-grah-fee) procedure for mapping the bile vessels (ducts)

cholangioma (koh-lan-jee-OH-mah) tumor of the bile vessels (ducts)

cholangiopancreatography (koh-LAN-jee-oh-PAN-kree-ah-TAW-grah-fee) procedure for mapping the bile vessels (ducts) and pancreas

cholangitis (KOH-lan-JAI-tis) inflammation of the bile vessels (ducts)

cholecystalgia (KOH-lay-sis-TAL-jah) pain in the gallbladder

cholecystectomy (KOH-lay-sis-TEK-toh-me) surgical removal of the bile (gall) bladder

cholecystitis (KOH-lay-sis-TAI-tis) inflammation of the bile (gall) bladder

cholecystogram (KOH-lay-SIS-toh-gram) record of the bile (gall) bladder

choledochocele (koh-lay-DOH-koh-seel) hernia of the (common) bile duct

choledocholithectomy (KOH-leh-DOH-koh-lih-THEK-toh-mee) surgical removal of a stone from the (common) bile duct

choledocholithiasis (koh-lay-DOH-koh-lith-AI-ah-sis) presence of a stone in the (common) bile duct

choledochotomy (KOH-leh-doh-KAW-toh-mee) incision into the (common) bile duct

cholelith (KOH-lay-lith) gallstone; literally, a stone in the bile

cholelithiasis (KOH-lay-lih-THAI-ah-sis) presence of a gallstone

cholelithotomy (KOH-lay-lih-THAW-toh-mee) incision to remove bile (gall) stones

cholelithotripsy (KOH-lay-lih-THOH-trip-see) crushing of bile (gall) stones

cholemesis (koh-LEM-eh-sis) vomiting bile

chondrectomy (kawn-DREK-toh-mee) removal of cartilage

chondroma (kawn-DROH-mah) a tumor-like growth of cartilage tissue

chondromalacia (KAWN-droh-mah-LAY-shah) abnormal softening of the cartilage

chondro-osteodystrophy (KAWN-droh-AW-stee-oh-DIH-stroh-fee) poor development of bones and cartilage

chondroplasty (KAWN-droh-PLAS-tee) reconstruction of cartilage

chorioamnionitis (KOR-ee-oh-AM-nee-oh-NAI-tis) inflammation of the chorion and amnion

chorioangioma (KOR-ee-oh-AN-jee-OH-mah) blood vessel tumor of the chorion

choriocarcinoma (KOR-ee-oh-KAR-sih-NOH-mah) cancerous tumor of the chorion

chorionitis (KOR-ee-aw-NAI-tis) inflammation of the chorion

chronic obstructive pulmonary disease (COPD) (KRON-ik ob-STRUKT-iv pul-mon-AIR-ee diz-EEZ) a lung disease caused by the continual blockage of lung passages

chylothorax (kai-low-THOR-aks) chyle in the chest

cicatrix (plural cicatrices) (SIK-ah-triks) from Latin, for *scar;* a scar

circulation (SIR-kyoo-LAY-shun) moving of blood from the heart through the vessels and back to the heart

circumcision (SIR-kum-SIH-zhun) surgical removal of the foreskin of the penis

cirrhosis (sir-OH-sis) liver disease named for the change of color in the liver

clonus (CLAH-nis) muscle spasm or twitching

closed reduction (klohzd ree-DUK-shun) returning bones to their proper position without the use of surgery

coagulopathy (coh-AG-yoo-LAW-pah-thee) any disease that deals with problems in blood coagulation

cochlear implant (KOH-klee-ar IM-plant) electronic device that stimulates the cochlea; it can give the sense of sound to those who are profoundly deaf

cochleitis (KOH-klee-AI-tis) inflammation of the cochlea

colectomy (koh-LEK-toh-mee) surgical removal of the colon

colitis (coh-LAI-tis) inflammation of the colon

colonoscopy (COH-lon-AW-skoh-pee) procedure for looking at the colon

colorectal carcinoma (COH-loh-REK-tal KAR-sih-NOH-mah) cancerous tumor of the colon or rectum

colostomy (koh-LAW-stoh-mee) creation of an opening in the colon

colovaginal fistula (COH-loh-VAJ-in-al FIS-tyoo-la) abnormal opening between the colon and vagina

colpitis (kol-PAI-tis) inflammation of the vagina

colpocystitis (KOL-poh-sis-TAI-tis) inflammation of the vagina and urinary bladder

colpopexy (KOL-poh-PEK-see) surgical fixation of the vagina

colpoplasty (KOL-poh-PLAS-tee) surgical reconstruction of the vagina

colpoptosis (KOL-pawp-TOH-sis) downward placement of the vagina

colposcope (KOL-poh-SKOHP) instrument used to examine the vagina

colposcopy (kol-PAW-skoh-pee) procedure for examining the vagina

colpostenosis (KOL-poh-steh-NOH-sis) narrowing in the vaginal opening

comedo (koh-MEE-doh) from Latin, for *to eat up;* a hair follicle plugged with sebum (blackhead, whitehead)

computed axial tomography (CAT or CT) (kom-PYOO-ted AK-see-al taw-MAW-grah-fee) imaging procedure using a computer to produce cross sections along an axis

computed tomography (kom-PYOO-ted tom-O-grah-fee) an imaging procedure using a computer to "cut" or view "slices" of a patient's organs

conductive hearing loss (con-DUK-tiv) sound does not get to the middle/inner ear (due to blockages)

congenital adrenal hyperplasia (kon-JEN-ih-tal ad-REE-nal HAI-per-PLAY-zhah) genetic disease in which the adrenal gland is overdeveloped, resulting in a deficiency of certain hormones and an overproduction of others

congenital anomaly (con-JIN-ih-tal ah-NAW-moh-lee) irregular condition that is present at the time of birth

congenital heart defect (con-JEN-ih-tal HART DEE-fekt) flaw in the structure of the heart, present at birth

congestive cardiomyopathy (con-JES-tiv KAR-dee-oh-mai-AW-pah-thee) heart cavity is unable to pump all the blood out of it (congestive) and becomes stretched (dilated), which causes weak/slow pumping of blood

congestive heart failure (con-JES-tiv HART FAYL-yir) heart failure characterized by the heart cavity being unable to pump all the blood out of it (congestive)

conjunctivitis (con-JUNK-tih-VAI-tis) inflammation of the conjunctiva (also known as pink eye)

constipation (KAWN-stih-PAY-shun) difficulty passing feces

continuous subcutaneous insulin infusion (kun-TIN-yoo-us SUB-koo-TAY-nee-us IN-suh-lin in-FYOO-zhun) continuous injection of insulin into the blood from a pump inserted under the skin

contraction (con-TRAK-shun) shortening or tightening of a muscle (during labor, uterine muscles contract)

corneal abrasion (KOR-nee-al a-BRAY-zhun) scratch on the cornea

corneal transplant (KOR-nee-al TRANZ-plant) replacement of damaged cornea with donated tissue

corneal xerosis (KOR-nee-al ZER-oh-sis) dryness of the cornea

coronary arterectomy (KOR-ah-NAR-ee AR-ter-EK-toh-mee) surgical removal of a coronary artery

coronary artery bypass graft (CABG) (KOR-ah-NAR-ee AR-ter-ee BAI-pas GRAFT) borrowed piece of blood vessel used to bypass a blocked artery in the heart

coronary artery bypass surgery (KOR-ah-NAR-ee AR-ter-ee BAI-pas SIR-jir-ee) surgery to bypass a blocked artery in the heart

coronary circulation (KOR-ah-NAR-ee SIR-kyoo-LAY-shun) circulation of blood from the heart to the heart muscle

coronary thrombosis (KOR-ah-NAR-ee throm-BOH-sis) obstruction of a coronary artery by a clot

corticotropin (KOR-tih-koh-TROH-pin) shorter name for adrenocorticotropic hormone

costalgia (kaws-TAL-jah) rib pain

costectomy (kaws-TEK-toh-mee) removal of a rib

costochondritis (KAW-stoh-kawn-DRAI-tis) inflammation of the cartilage of the rib

cranial hematoma (KRAY-nee-al HEE-mah-TOH-mah) a hematoma beneath the skull

craniectomy (KRAY-nee-EK-toh-mee) removal of a portion of the skull (bone is not replaced)

craniomalacia (KRAY-nee-oh-mah-LAY-shah) abnormal softening of the skull

craniosclerosis (KRAY-nee-oh-skleh-ROH-sis) abnormal hardening of the skull

craniostenosis (KRAY-nee-oh-steh-NOH-sis) abnormal narrowing of the skull

craniosynostosis (KRAY-nee-oh-SIN-aw-STOH-sis) the premature fusing of the skull bones

craniotomy (KRAY-nee-AW-toh-mee) removal of a portion of the skull (bone is later replaced)

crepitation (kreh-pih-TAY-shun) from Latin, for *rattle* or *creaking;* a crackling sound heard in joints

crust (krust) dried substance (i.e., blood, pus) on the skin

cryosurgery (KRAI-oh-SIR-juh-ree) destruction of tissue through freezing

cryptorchidism (krip-TOR-kih-DIZ-um) hidden testicle

culture & sensitivity (KUL-chur and sin-sih-TIH-vih-tee) growing microorganisms in isolation in order to determine which drugs it might respond to

cyanidrosis (sai-yan-ih-DROH-sis) blue sweat

cyanosis (SAI-ah-NOH-sis) a bluish appearance to the skin; a sign that the tissue isn't receiving enough oxygen

cyclokeratitis (SAI-cloh-keh-rah-TAI-tis) inflammation of the ciliary body and cornea

cycloplegia (SAI-kloh-PLEE-jah) paralysis of the ciliary body

cycloplegic (SAI-kloh-PLEE-jik) drug that paralyzes the ciliary body

cyclotomy (sai-KLAW-toh-mee) incision into the ciliary body

cystalgia (sis-TAL-jah) pain in the bladder

cystectomy (sis-TEK-toh-mee) surgical removal of the bladder

cystitis (sis-TAI-tis) inflammation of the bladder

cystocele (SIS-toh-seel) hernia of the bladder

cystodynia (SIS-toh-DAI-nee-ah) pain in the bladder

cystogram (SIS-toh-gram) image of the bladder

cystography (sis-TAW-grah-fee) process for recording/imaging the bladder

cystolith (SIS-toh-lith) stone in the bladder

cystolithectomy (sis-toh-lih-THEK-toh-mee) surgical removal of a stone in the bladder

cystoma (sis-TOH-mah) tumor of the bladder

cystoplegia (SIS-toh-PLEE-jah) bladder paralysis

cystoptosis (sis-TOP-toh-sis) downward displacement of the bladder

cystorrhexis (SIS-toh-REK-sis) rupture of the bladder

cystoscopy (sis-TAWS-koh-pee) process for examining the bladder

cystospasm (SIS-toh-SPAZ-um) involuntary contraction of the bladder

cystostomy (sis-TAW-stoh-mee) creation of an opening in the bladder

cystoureteritis (SIS-toh-yoo-REE-ter-AI-tis) inflammation of the bladder and urethra

cystourethrocele (SIS-toh-yoo-REE-throh-seel) hernia of the bladder and urethra

cytapheresis (SAI-tah-fer-EE-sis) apheresis to remove cellular material

D

dacryoadenalgia (DAK-ree-oh-AD-en-AL-jah) pain in the tear gland

dacryoadenectomy (DAK-ree-oh-AD-en-EK-toh-mee) removal of the tear gland

dacryoadenitis (DAK-ree-oh-AD-en-AI-tis) inflammation of the tear gland

dacryocystalgia (DAK-ree-oh-sis-TAL-jah) pain in the tear sac

dacryocystectomy (DAK-ree-oh-sis-TEK-toh-mee) removal of the tear sac

dacryocystitis (DA-kree-oh-sis-TAI-tis) inflammation of the tear sac

dacryocystorhinostomy (DAK-ree-oh-SIS-toh-rai-NAWS-toh-mee) creation of an opening between the tear sac and the nose

dacryocystotomy (DAK-ree-oh-sis-TAWT-oh-mee) incision into the tear sac

dacryohemorrhea (DAK-ree-oh-HIM-oh-REE-ah) discharge of blood in the tears

dacryolith (DAK-ree-oh-lith) hard formation (stone) in the tear system

dacryolithiasis (DAK-ree-oh-lih-THAI-ah-sis) presence of hard formations (stones) in the tear system

dacryopyorrhea (DAK-ree-oh-pai-REE-ah) discharge of pus in tears

dacryorrhea (DAK-ree-oh-REE-ah) excessive tearing

dacryostenosis (DAK-ree-oh-steh-NOH-sis) narrowing of the tear duct

dactylitis (DAK-tih-LAI-tis) finger inflammation

decubitus ulcer (deh-KYOO-bih-tus UL-sir) bed sore

deep vein thrombosis (DEEP VAYN throm-BOH-sis) the formation of a blood clot deep in the body, most commonly in the leg

delirium (deh-LEER-ee-um) brief loss of mental function

dementia (da-MEN-chah) loss/decline in mental function

dentalgia (den-TAL-jah) tooth pain

dentist (DEN-tist) specialist in teeth

dentistry (DEN-tis-tree) branch of medicine dealing with teeth

dentifrice (DEN-ti-fris) toothpaste

depigmentation (DE-pig-men-TAY-shun) loss of skin pigmentation

dermabrasion (der-mah-BRAY-zhun) rubbing or scraping away the outer surface of skin

dermatitis (der-mah-TAI-tis) inflammation of the skin

dermatoconiosis (der-ma-toh-COH-nee-oh-sis) a skin condition caused by dirt

dermatofibroma (der-MA-toh-fai-BROH-mah) a fibrous skin tumor

dermatolysis (der-mah-TAW-lis-is) loss of skin

dermatomycosis (der-mah-toh-mai-KOH-sis) a fungal skin condition

dermatoscope (dir-MA-toh-SKOHP) instrument used to look at the skin

dermatosis (der-mah-TOH-sis) skin condition

dermoid cyst (DER-moyd SIST) ovarian cyst containing skin and sometimes hair, teeth, bone, or cartilage

dermopathy (der-MAW-pa-thee) skin disease

dermoscopy (der-MAW-skoh-pee) procedure for looking at the skin

diabetes mellitus (DAI-ah-BEE-teez MEH-lih-tis) metabolic disease characterized by excessive urination and hyperglycemia

diabetic ketoacidosis (DAI-ah-BEH-tik KEE-toh-ASS-ih-DOH-sis) acidity of the blood caused by the presence of ketone bodies produced when the body is unable to burn sugar; thus, it must burn fat for energy

diaphoresis (DAI-ah-for-EE-sis) profuse sweating

diaphragmatocele (dai-a-frag-MAT-o-seel) hernia of the diaphragm

diarrhea (DAI-ah-REE-ah) passing of fluid or unformed feces

diastolic pressure (DAI-ah-STAW-lik PRESH-ir) pressure exerted on blood vessels when the heart is relaxed

digital rectal exam (DIJ-ih-tal REK-tal ek-ZAM) examination of the prostate using a finger inserted into the rectum

dilated cardiomyopathy (DAI-lay-ted KAR-dee-oh-mai-AW-pah-thee) see *congestive cardiomyopathy*

diplopia (dih-PLOH-pee-ah) double vision

dipsogenic (DIP-soh-JIN-ik) creating thirst

diuresis (DAI-yur-EE-sis) excessive urination

diuretic (DAI-yur-IT-ik) agent that causes urination

duodenectomy (doo-AW-den-EK-toh-mee) surgical removal of the duodenum

duodenitis (doo-AH-den-AI-tis) inflammation of the duodenum

duritis (dur-AI-tis) inflammation of the dura

dysentery (DIS-en-TER-ee) another name for diarrhea

dysesthesia (DIS-es-THEE-zhah) bad feeling

dyskinesia (dis-kih-NEE-zhah) inability to control movement

dyslexia (dis-LEK-see-ah) difficulty reading

dysmenorrhea (DIS-men-oh-REE-ah) painful menstruation

dysmetabolic syndrome (DIS-meh-tah-BAW-lik SIN-drohm) combination of medical disorders associated with faulty metabolism

dyspareunia (dis-pah-ROO-nee-ah) painful sexual intercourse

dyspepsia (dis-PEP-see-ah) bad digestion

dysphasia (dis-FAY-zhah) difficulty speaking

dysphonia (dis-FON-ia) "bad voice condition"; hoarseness

dysphoria (dis-FOR-ee-ah) a negative emotional state

dysplastic nevus (dis-PLAS-tic NEE-vus) a mole with bad changes/formations (often precancerous)

dyspnea (disp-NEE-ah) difficulty breathing

dysrhythmia (dis-RITH-mee-ah) irregular heartbeat

dystaxia (dis-TAK-see-ah) poor coordination

dystocia (dis-TOH-shee-ah) difficult labor

dystonia (dis-TOH-nee-ah) poor muscle tone

dysuria (dis-YUR-ee-ah) painful urination

E

ear instillation (ee-ir in-stil-AY-shun) ear drops

ear lavage (ee-ir lah-VAJ) rinsing/washing the external ear canal (usually to remove ear wax); from Latin, for *to wash, bathe*

ecchymosis (eh-kih-MOH-sis) from Greek, for *to pour out;* a larger bruise

echocardiogram (EK-oh-KAR-dee-oh-GRAM) image of the heart produced using sound waves; it is the same procedure as an ultrasound performed on pregnant women, but done on the heart

echocardiography (EK-oh-KAR-dee-AW-grah-fee) use of sound waves to produce an image of the heart

echoencephalography (EH-koh-in-SEH-fah-LAW-grah-fee) procedure used to examine the brain using sound waves

eclampsia (eh-KLAMP-see-ah) severe, life-threatening complication of pregnancy characterized by seizures

ectopic pregnancy (ek-TOP-ik PREG-nan-see) implantation of a fertilized egg in a place other than the uterus

ectropion (ek-TROH-pee-on) outward turning of the eyelid, away from the eye

eczema (EK-zeh-mah) from Greek, for *to boil over;* a red, itchy rash that may weep or ooze, then become crusted and scaly

efferent nerve (EH-fir-ent nirv) a nerve that carries impulses away from the central nervous system

effusion (ee-FYOO-zhun) fluid build-up

ejaculation (ee-JAK-yoo-LAY-shun) emission of semen from the urethra

electrocardiogram (eh-LEK-troh-KAR-dee-oh-GRAM) record of the electrical currents of the heart

electrocardiography (eh-LEK-troh-KAR-dee-AW-grah-fee) procedure for recording the electrical currents of the heart

electrocauterization (e-LEK-troh-KAW-ter-ai-ZAY-shun) using electricity to destroy tissue by burning it

electrodesiccation (e-LEK-troh-deh-sih-KAY-shun) using electricity to destroy tissue by drying it

electroencephalography (EEG) (eh-LEK-troh-in-SEH-fah-LAW-grah-fee) procedure used to examine the electrical activity of the brain

electromyogram (eh-lek-troh-MAI-o-gram) record of the electrical activity of a muscle

electromyography (eh-LEK-troh-mai-AW-grah-fee) procedure for measuring the electrical activity of a muscle

elliptocyte (ee-LIP-toh-SAIT) oval-shaped red blood cell

elliptocytosis (ee-LIP-toh-SAI-toh-sis) condition characterized by an increase in the number of oval-shaped red blood cells

embolectomy (EM-boh-LEK-toh-mee) surgical removal of an embolus

embolism (EM-boh-LIZ-um) blockage in a blood vessel caused by an embolus

embolus (EM-boh-lus) mass of matter present in the blood

emphysema (em-fi-ZEE-ma) a disease that causes the alveoli to lose their elasticity; patients can inhale but have difficulty exhaling

empyema (em-pie-EE-mah) pus inside (the chest)

encephalalgia (in-SE-ful-AL-jah) brain pain

encephalitis (in-SEF-ah-LAI-tis) inflammation of the brain

encephalmyeloneuropathy (in-SEF-ah-loh-MAI-el-oh-nir-AW-pah-thee) disease of the brain, spinal cord, and nerves

encephalocele (en-SEF-ah-loh-SEEL) hernia of the brain (normally through a defect in the skull)

encephalography (en-SEH-fah-LOH-grah-fee) procedure for studying the brain

encephalomyelitis (in-SEF-ah-loh-MAI-el-AI-tis) inflammation of the brain and spinal cord

encephalopathy (in-SEF-ah-LAW-pah-thee) disease of the brain

encephalopyosis (in-SEF-ah-loh-pai-OH-sis) a pus-filled abscess in the brain

endarterectomy (END-ar-ter-EK-toh-me) surgical removal of the inside of an artery

endocarditis (EN-doh-kar-DAI-tis) inflammation of the tissue lining the inside of the heart

endocardium (EN-doh-KAR-dee-um) tissue lining the inside of the heart

endocervicitis (EN-doh-SER-vih-SAI-tis) inflammation of the inside of the cervix

endocrine (EN-doh-krin) secrete internally (i.e., into the bloodstream)

endocrinologist (EN-doh-krih-NAW-loh-jist) specialist in internal secretions

endometriosis (EN-doh-MEE-tree-OH-sis) condition in which endometrium cells appear and grow outside the uterus

endometritis (EN-doh-meh-TRAI-tis) inflammation of the endometrium

endometrium (EN-doh-MEE-tree-um) inner layer of uterine tissue

endophthalmitis (EN-dof-thal-MAI-tis) inflammation of the inside of the eye (often a complication from intra-ocular surgery)

endoscope (EN-doh-SKOHP) instrument used to look inside

endoscopic retrograde cholangiopancreatography (EN-doh-SKAW-pik REH-troh-GRAYD KOHL-AN-jee-oh-PAN-kree-ah-TAW-grah-fee) procedure used to examine the bile ducts and pancreas in which an endoscope is passed backward from the digestive tract into the bile duct

endoscope (EN-doh-SKOHP) instrument to look inside

endoscopy (en-DAW-skoh-pee) procedure of looking inside

endotracheal intubation (en-doh-TRAY-kee-al in-too-BAY-shun) insertion of a tube inside the trachea

endovascular neurosurgery (EN-doh-VAS-kyoo-lar NIR-oh-SIR-jir-ee) surgery on the nervous system performed by entering the body through blood vessels

enterectomy (en-ter-EK-toh-mee) surgical removal of the intestines

enterocele (EN-ter-oh-seel) hernia of the intestines

enterodynia (EN-ter-oh-DAI-nee-ah) pain in the intestines

enteropathy (EN-ter-AW-pah-thee) disease of the intestines

enterorrhaphy (en-ter-OR-ah-fee) suture of the intestines

enterotomy (en-ter-AW-toh-mee) incision into the intestines

entropion (en-TROH-pee-on) inward turning of the eyelid, toward the eye

enucleation (eh-NOO-clee-AY-shun) removal of an eye

enuresis (EN-yur-EE-sis) involuntary urination

epicardium (EH-pee-KAR-dee-um) tissue lining the outside of the heart

epidermal (eh-pi-DER-mal) pertaining to the skin

epidermal tumor (eh-pi-DER-mal TOO-mur) tumor on the skin

epididymectomy (EP-ih-DID-ih-MEK-toh-mee) surgical removal of the epididymis

epididymitis (EP-ih-DID-ih-MAI-tis) inflammation of the epididymis

epididymo-orchitis (EP-ih-DID-ih-moh-or-KAI-tis) inflammation of the testicles and epididymis

epididymotomy (EP-ih-DID-ih-MAW-toh-mee) incision into the epididymis

epidural anesthetic (eh-pih-DIR-al an-es-THET-ik) anesthetic applied in the dural region of the spinal cord

epidural hematoma (EH-pi-DIR-al HEE-mah-TOH-mah) a hematoma located on top of the dura

epigastric (eh-pee-GAS-trik) upper center portion of the abdomen

epilepsy (eh-pih-LEP-see) a disease marked by seizures

epinephrine (EH-pee-NEF-rin) hormone secreted by the adrenal gland (from Greek; see also *adrenaline*)

episiorrhaphy (eh-PEE-zee-OR-ah-fee) suture of the vulva

episiostenosis (eh-PEE-zee-oh-stih-NOH-sis) narrowing of the vulvar opening

episiotomy (eh-PEE-zee-AW-toh-mee) incision into the vulva

epistaxis (ep-ee-STAKS-is) nosebleed

erosion (ee-ROH-zhun) loss of skin

erythema (eh-rih-THEE-ma) from Greek, for *redness;* redness

erythrocyanosis (eh-RITH-roh-SAI-an-OH-sis) a red and/or blue discoloration of the skin

erythrocyte (eh-RIH-throh-SAIT) red blood cell

erythrocytosis (eh-RIH-throh-sai-TOH-sis) abnormal increase in the number of red blood cells

erythroderma (eh-RIH-throh-DER-ma) red skin

esophagalgia (eh-SAWF-ah-GAL-jah) pain in the esophagus

esophageal carcinoma (eh-SAWF-ah-JEE-al KAR-sih-NOH-mah) cancerous tumor of the esophagus

esophagectomy (eh-SAW-fah-JEK-toh-mee) surgical removal of the esophagus

esophagitis (eh-SAWF-ah-JAI-tis) inflammation of the esophagus

esophagogastroduodenoscopy (eh-SAW-fah-goh-GAS-stroh-DOO-aw-den-AW-skoh-pee) procedure for looking inside the esophagus, stomach, and duodenum

esophagogastroplasty (eh-SAW-fah-goh-GAS-troh-PLAS-tee) surgical reconstruction of the esophagus and stomach

esophagoscopy (eh-SAW-fah-GAW-skoh-pee) procedure for looking inside the esophagus

esotropia (AY-soh-TROH-pee-ah) inward turning of the eye, toward the nose

euglycemia (YOO-glai-SEE-mee-ah) good blood sugar

eupepsia (yoo-PEP-see-ah) good digestion

euphoria (yoo-FOR-ee-ah) a positive emotional state

eupnea (YOOP-nee-yah) good/normal breathing

euthyroid (YOO-thai-royd) a normal functioning thyroid

eutocia (yoo-TOH-shee-ah) normal labor

excisional biopsy (ek-SIH-zhun-al BAI-op-see) removal of an entire lesion for examination (to cut it out)

excoriation (eks-kor-ee-A-shun) a scratch

exocrine (EKS-oh-krin) secrete externally through ducts to the surface of an organ (i.e., sweat glands and salivary glands)

exophthalmos (EKS-of-THAL-mohs) protrusion of the eye out of the eye socket

exophthalmus (EKS-of-THAL-mus) protrusion of the eye out of the eye socket

exostosis (ek-saw-STOH-sis) an abnormal growth of bone out of another bone

exotropia (EK-soh-TROH-pee-ah) outward turning of the eye, away from the nose

expectorant (eks-PEK-tor-ant) a drug that encourages explusion of material from the lungs

expectoration (eks-pec-tor-A-shun) coughing or spitting material out of the lungs

external fixation (EKS-tir-nal fik-SAY-shun) a fixation of a fractured bone from the outside (i.e., using a cast or splint)

extracorporeal shock wave lithotripsy (ESWL) (EKS-trah-cor-POR-ee-al shok wayv LIH-thoh-TRIP-see) breakdown of kidney stones using sound waves generated outside the body

F

fasciectomy (FA-shee-EK-toh-mee) removal of fascia

fasciitis (FA-shee-AI-tis) inflammation of the fascia

fasciodesis (FA-shoh-DEE-sis) binding of fascia

fascioplasty (FA-shoh-PLAS-tee) reconstruction of fascia

fasciorrhaphy (fah-SHOR-ah-fee) suturing of fascia

fasciotomy (FA-shee-AW-toh-mee) incision into fascia

fecal occult blood test (FOBT) (FEE-kal ah-KULT blud test) test of feces to discover blood not visibly apparent

fetometry (fee-TAW-meh-tree) procedure for measuring the fetus

fissure (FIH-zhur) from Latin, for a *split* or *divide;* a crack in the skin

fistula (FIS-tyoo-la) any abnormal passageway in the body that shouldn't be there

flatus (FLAH-tus) medical term for passing gas

fracture (FRAK-shur) from Latin, for *break;* a bone break

fulguration (FUL-gur-AY-shun) use of electric current to destroy tissue

G

galactorrhea (gah-LAK-toh-REE-ah) discharge of milk

gangliitis (GAN-glee-AI-tis) inflammation of the ganglion

ganglioma (GAN-glee-OH-mah) ganglion tumor

gastralgia (gas-TRAL-jah) stomach pain

gastrectomy (gas-TREK-toh-mee) surgical removal of the stomach

gastritis (gas-TRAI-tis) inflammation of the stomach

gastroduodenostomy (GAS-troh-doo-AH-den-AW-stoh-mee) creation of an opening between the stomach and the duodenum

gastrodynia (GAS-troh-DAI-nee-ah) stomach pain

gastroenteritis (GAS-troh-EN-ter-AI-tis) inflammation of the stomach and intestines

gastroenterocolitis (GAS-troh-EN-ter-oh-coh-LAI-tis) inflammation of the stomach, intestine, and colon

gastroenterologist (GAS-troh-EN-ter-AW-loh-jist) specialist in the stomach and intestines

gastroenterology (GAS-troh-EN-ter-AW-loh-jee) study of the stomach and intestines

gastroenterostomy (GAS-troh-EN-ter-AW-stoh-mee) creation of an opening between the stomach and the intestines

gastroesophageal reflux disease (GERD) (GAS-troh-eh-SOF-ah-JEE-al REE-fluks dih-ZEEZ) disease in which acid comes up from the stomach and damages the esophagus

gastrojejunostomy (GAS-troh-JEH-joo-NAW-stoh-mee) creation of an opening between the stomach and the jejunum

gastromalacia (GAS-troh-mah-LAY-shah) softening of the stomach

gastroparesis (GAS-troh-par-EE-sis) partial paralysis of the stomach

gastropexy (GAS-troh-PEK-see) surgical fixation of the stomach

gastroplasty (GAS-troh-PLAS-tee) surgical reconstruction of the stomach

gastroscope (GAS-troh-SKOHP) instrument for looking at the stomach

gastroscopy (gas-TRAW-skoh-pee) procedure for looking at the stomach

general anesthetic (JIH-nir-al an-es-THET-ik) anesthetic that causes complete loss of consciousness

genu valgum (JEH-noo VAL-gum) bow-legged

genu varum (JEH-noo VAH-rum) knock-kneed

gingival hyperplasia (JIN-jih-val HAI-per-PLAY-zhah) overformation of gum tissue

gingivalgia (JIN-jih-VAL-jah) gum pain

gingivectomy (JIN-jiv-EK-toh-mee) surgical removal of gum tissue

gingivitis (JIN-jih-VAI-tis) inflammation of the gums

gingivoglossitis (JIN-jih-voh-glaw-SAI-tis) inflammation of the gums and tongue

gingivoplasty (JIN-jiv-oh-PLAS-tee) surgical reconstruction of gum tissue

gingivostomatitis (JIN-jih-voh-STOH-mah-TAI-tis) inflammation of the mouth and gums

glomerulonephritis (gloh-MER-yoo-loh-neh-FRAI-tis) inflammation of the kidneys involving primarily the glomeruli

glomerulopathy (gloh-MER-yoo-LAW-pah-thee) disease of the kidney involving primarily the glomeruli

glomerulosclerosis (gloh-MER-yoo-loh-skleh-ROH-sis) hardening of the glomeruli

glossopathy (glaws-AW-pah-thee) disease of the tongue

glossoplasty (GLAWS-oh-PLAS-tee) surgical reconstruction of the tongue

glossoplegia (GLAW-soh-PLEE-jah) paralysis of the tongue

glossorrhaphy (glaws-OR-ah-fee) suture of the tongue

glossotomy (glaws-AW-toh-mee) incision into the tongue

glossotrichia (GLAWS-oh-TRIK-ee-ah) overdevelopment of bumps on the tongue, making the tongue appear to be hairy

glucagon (GLOO-kah-gawn) hormone secreted by the pancreas that stimulates the liver to increase blood sugar levels

glucocorticoid (GLOO-koh-KOR-tih-koyd) a hormone produced by the adrenal cortex with a role in carbohydrate metabolism

gluconeogenesis (GLOO-koh-NEE-oh-JIN-eh-sis) the formation of glucose from noncarbohydrate sources

glucosuria (GLOO-koh-SOO-ree-ah) sugar in the urine

glycemic index (glai-SEE-mik IN-deks) ranking of food based on the way it affects sugar levels in the blood

glycolysis (glai-KAW-lih-sis) breakdown of sugar

glycopenia (GLAI-koh-PEE-nee-ah) deficiency of sugar

glycosuria (GLAI-koh-shur-EE-ah) sugar in the urine

goiter (GOY-ter) swollen thyroid gland

gonadogenesis (goh-NAD-oh-JIN-eh-sis) creation/development of gonads

gonadotropin (goh-NAD-oh-TROH-pin) hormone that stimulates the gonads

gonads (GOH-nadz) the pair of organs used for sexual reproduction; testicles in males and ovaries in females

gonorrhea (GAW-noh-REE-ah) discharge from the gonads

graphospasm (gra-foh-SPAZ-um) writer's cramp

gravida (GRAH-vid-ah) another term for pregnant

gynecologist (GAI-neh-KAW-loh-jist) specialist in medical issues specific to women

gynecology (GAI-neh-KAW-loh-jee) study of medical issues specific to women

gynecomastia (GAI-neh-koh-MAS-tee-ah) development of breast tissue in males

H

hemarthrosis (hee-mar-THROH-sis) blood in a joint

hematemesis (HEM-at-EM-eh-sis) vomiting blood

hemathidrosis (heh-mat-ih-DROH-sis) sweating blood

hematocrit (hee-MAT-oh-krit) test to judge or separate the blood; used to determine the ratio of red blood cells to total blood volume

hematology (HEE-mah-TAW-loh-jee) study of the blood

hematoma (HEE-mah-TOH-mah) mass of blood within an organ, cavity, or tissue

hematopoiesis (heh-MAH-toh-poh-EE-sis) formation of blood cells

hematosalpinx (heh-MAT-oh-SAL-pinks) blockage in a fallopian tube caused by blood

hematuria (HEE-mah-TUR-ee-ah) bloody urination

hemianopsia (HEH-mee-an-OP-see-ah) blindness in half the visual field

hemicolectomy (HEH-mee-koh-LEK-toh-mee) surgical removal of half (a portion) of the colon

heminephrectomy (HEH-mee-neh-FREK-toh-mee) surgical removal of half a kidney

heminephroureterectomy (HEH-mee-NEH-froh-yoo-REE-ter-EK-toh-mee) surgical removal of half a kidney and a ureter

hemiparesis (HEH-mee-puh-REE-sis) partial paralysis on half of the body

hemiplegia (HEH-mee-PLEE-jah) paralysis on half the body

hemodialysis (HEE-moh-dai-AL-ah-sis) procedure for removing waste from the bloodstream

hemoglobin (HEE-moh-GLOH-bin) iron-containing pigment in red blood cells that carries oxygen to the cells

hemoglobinopathy (HEE-maw-GLOH-bin-AW-pah-thee) disease of the hemoglobin

hemolysis (hee-MAW-lih-sis) breakdown of blood cells

hemolytic anemia (HEE-moh-LIH-tik ah-NEE-mee-ah) anemia caused by the destruction of red blood cells

hemophilia (HEE-moh-FEE-lee-ah) condition in which the blood doesn't clot, thus causing excessive bleeding

hemoptysis (heem-op-TIS-is) coughing up blood

hemorrhage (HEM-oh-RIJ) excessive blood loss

hemorrhagic stroke (HEM-oh-RA-jik STROHK) a stroke where blood loss is caused by the rupture of a blood vessel

hemorrhoid (HEM-oh-ROID) inflammation of the veins surrounding the anus

hemorrhoidectomy (HEM-oh-roi-DEK-toh-mee) surgical removal of hemorrhoids

hemostatic (HEE-moh-STAT-ik) drug that stops the flow of blood

hemothorax (heem-o-THOR-aks) blood in the chest

hepatectomy (HEP-ah-TEK-toh-me) surgical removal of the liver

hepaticogastrostomy (heh-PAT-ih-koh-gas-TRAW-stoh-me) creation of an opening between the liver and the stomach

hepaticotomy (heh-PAT-ih-KAW-toh-me) incision into the liver

hepatitis (HEH-pah-TAI-tis) inflammation of the liver

hepatocarcinoma (heh-PAT-oh-KAR-sih-NOH-mah) cancerous tumor of the liver

hepatoma (HEH-pah-TOH-mah) tumor of the liver

hepatomalacia (heh-PAT-oh-mah-LAY-shah) softening of the liver

hepatomegaly (heh-PAT-oh-MEG-ah-lee) enlargement of the liver

hepatopexy (heh-PAT-oh-PEK-see) surgical fixation of the liver

hepatoptosis (heh-PAT-op-TOH-sis) downward displacement of the liver

hepatosclerosis (heh-PAT-oh-skleh-ROH-sis) hardening of the liver

hepatosplenitis (hih-PAT-oh-SPLEEN-ai-tis) inflammation of the liver and spleen

hepatosplenomegaly (heh-PAT-oh-SPLEE-noh-MEH-gah-lee) enlargement of the liver and spleen

hernia (HER-nee-ah) rupture or protrusion of an organ through the wall that normally contains it

herniorrhaphy (her-nee-OR-ah-fee) suture of a hernia

heterograft (HEH-ter-oh-GRAFT) skin transplant taken from a species other than the patient's

hidradenitis (hih-dra-deh-NAI-tis) inflammation of the sweat glands

hidradenoma (hih-drad-eh-NOH-mah) tumor of the sweat gland

hidropoiesis (hih-droh-poh-EE-sis) the formation of sweat

hirsutism (HIR-soo-tizm) excessive growth of facial and body hair in women

homograft (HOH-moh-GRAFT) skin transplant taken from another member of the patient's species

hydrarthrosis (hai-drar-THROH-sis) water (fluid) in a joint

hydrocele (HAI-droh-SEEL) fluid-filled mass in a testicle

hydrocelectomy (HAI-droh-seel-EK-toh-mee) surgical removal of a hydrocele

hydrocephaly (HAI-droh-SEH-fah-lee) abnormal accumulation of spinal fluid in the brain

hydronephrosis (HAI-droh-neh-FROH-sis) kidney condition caused by the obstruction of urine flow

hydrophobia (HAI-druh-FOH-bee-ah) fear of water

hydrosalpinx (HAI-droh-SAL-pinks) blockage in a fallopian tube caused by water (or any clear fluid)

hyperacusis (HAI-per-ah-KOO-sis) excessively sensitive hearing

hyperbilirubinemia (HAI-per-BIH-lee-ROO-bin-EE-mee-ah) excessive bilirubin in the blood

hypercalcemia (HAI-per-kal-SEE-mee-ah) excessive calcium in the blood

hypercapnia (hai-per-CAP-nee-yah) condition of having excessive carbon dioxide in the blood

hypercarbia (hai-per-CAR-bee-yah) excessive carbon dioxide

hypercholesterolemia (HAI-per-koh-LES-ter-aw-LEE-mee-ah) excessive cholesterol in the blood

hypercoagulability (HAI-per-koh-AG-yoo-lah-BIL-ih-tee) increased ability of the blood to coagulate

hyperemesis (HAI-per-EM-eh-sis) excessive vomiting

hyperemesis gravidarum (HAI-per-eh-MEE-sis GRAV-ih-DAR-um) excessive pregnancy-related vomiting; an extreme form of the more common morning sickness

hyperesthesia (HAI-per-es-THEE-zhah) increased sensation

hyperglycemia (HAI-per-glai-SEE-mee-ah) high blood sugar

hypergonadism (HAI-per-GOH-nad-izm) excessive secretion of the sex glands

hyperhidrosis (hai-per-hih-DROH-sis) excessive sweating

hyperkalemia (HAI-per-kah-LEE-mee-ah) excessive potassium in the blood

hyperkeratosis (hai-per-ker-ah-TOH-sis) excessive growth of horny skin

hyperkinesia (hai-per-kih-NEE-zhah) increase in muscle movement or activity

hyperlipidemia (HAI-per-lih-pih-DEE-mee-ah) excessive fat in the blood

hypermastia (HAI-per-MAS-tee-ah) excessively large breasts (can also refer to an abnormal number of breasts)

hypermelanosis (hai-per-mel-an-OH-sis) excessive melanin in the skin

hypernatremia (HAI-per-nah-TREE-mee-ah) excessive salt in the blood

hypernephroma (HAI-per-neh-FROH-mah) cancer of the kidneys; also called *renal cell carcinoma*

hyperopia (HAI-per-OH-pee-ah) farsightedness

hyperparathyroidism (HAI-per-PAR-ah-THAI-roid-IZM) overproduction by the parathyroid glands

hyperphosphatemia (HAI-per-FAWS-fay-TEE-mee-ah) excessive phosphate in the blood

hyperpigmentation (hai-per-pig-men-TAY-shun) excessive pigment in the skin

hyperpituitarism (HAI-per-pih-TOO-ih-tar-IZM) overfunctioning of the pituitary gland

hyperpnea (hai-perp-NEE-ah) heavy breathing

hypersplenism (HAI-per-SPLEE-nizm) increased spleen activity

hypertension (HAI-per-TEN-shun) high blood pressure

hyperthyroidism (HAI-per-THAI-roid-IZM) overproduction by the thyroid

hypertonia (hai-per-TOH-nee-yah) increased muscle tone or tightness

hypertrophic cardiomyopathy (HAI-per-TROH-fik KAR-dee-oh-mai-AW-pah-thee) heart muscle becomes enlarged and blocks blood flow

hypertrophic spondylitis (HAI-per-TROH-fik spon-dih-LAI-tis) overdevelopment of the vertebrae causing inflammation

hypertrophy (hai-PER-troh-fee) overdevelopment of muscle tissue

hyperventilation (hai-per-ven-ti-LAY-shun) overbreathing; condition of having too much air flowing into and out of the lungs; leads to hypocapnia

hypervolemia (HAI-per-voh-LEE-mee-ah) increased blood volume

hypnotic (hip-NAWT-ik) a drug that aids sleep

hypoacusis (HAI-poh-ah-KOO-sis) excessively insensitive hearing

hypocapnia (hai-po-CAP-nee-yah) insufficient carbon dioxide

hypocarbia (hai-po-CAR-bee-yah) insufficient carbon dioxide

hypochondriac (hai-poh-KON-dree-ak) upper side portions of the abdomen

hypodermia (hai-poh-DER-mia) pertaining to beneath the skin

hypogastric (hai-poh-GAS-trik) lower center portion of the abdomen

hypoglycemia (HAI-poh-glai-SEE-mee-ah) low blood sugar

hypoglycemic (HAI-poh-glai-SEE-mik) pertaining to low blood sugar

hypogonadism (HAI-poh-GOH-nad-izm) undersecretion of the sex glands

hypohidrosis (hai-poh-hih-DROH-sis) diminished sweating

hypokinesia (hai-poh-kih-NEE-zhah) decrease in muscle movement or activity

hypomagnesemia (HAI-poh-MAG-nee-SEE-mee-ah) deficient magnesium in the blood

hypomania (HAI-poh-MAY-nee-ah) a mental state just below mania

hypomastia (HAI-poh-MAS-tee-ah) abnormally small breasts

hypomelanosis (hai-poh-mel-an-OH-sis) diminished melanin in the skin

hyponatremia (HAI-poh-nah-TREE-mee-ah) low sodium in the blood

hypoparathyroidism (HAI-poh-PAR-ah-THAI-roid-IZM) underproduction by the parathyroid

hypoperfusion (HAI-poh-per-FYOO-zhun) inadequate flow of blood

hypophysectomy (hai-POF-is-EK-toh-mee) removal of the pituitary gland

hypophysitis (hai-PAWF-ih-SAI-tis) inflammation of the pituitary gland

hypopigmentation (hai-poh-pig-men-TAY-shun) diminished pigment in the skin

hypopituitarism (HAI-poh-pih-TOO-ih-tar-IZM) condition caused by the undersecretion of the pituitary gland

hypopnea (hai-POP-nee-ah) shallow breathing

hypospadias (HAI-poh-SPAY-dee-as) birth defect in which the opening of the urethra is on the underside, instead of the end, of the penis

hypotension (HAI-poh-TEN-shun) low blood pressure

hypothyroidism (HAI-poh-THAI-roid-IZM) underproduction by the thyroid

hypotonia (hai-poh-TOH-nee-yah) decrease in muscle tone or tightness

hypoventilation (hai-po-ven-ti-LAY-shun) underbreathing; condition of having too little air flowing into and out of the lungs; leads to hypercapnia

hypovolemia (HAI-poh-voh-LEE-mee-ah) decreased blood volume

hypoxemia (hai-poks-EEM-ee-yah) insufficient oxygen in the blood

hypoxia (hai-POKS-ee-yah) insufficient oxygen

hysteralgia (HIS-ter-AL-jah) pain in the uterus

hysterectomy (HIS-ter-EK-toh-mee) surgical removal of the uterus

hysterocele (HIS-ter-oh-SEEL) hernia of the uterus

hysterodynia (HIS-ter-oh-DAI-nee-ah) pain in the uterus

hysterography (HIS-ter-AW-grah-fee) procedure for imaging the uterus

hysteropexy (HIS-ter-oh-PEK-see) surgical fixation of the uterus

hysteroptosis (HIS-ter-awp-TOH-sis) downward displacement of the uterus into the vagina

hysterorrhexis (HIS-ter-oh-REK-sis) rupture of the uterus

hysterosalpingectomy (HIS-ter-oh-SAL-pin-JEK-toh-mee) surgical removal of the uterus and fallopian tube

hysterosalpingogram (HIS-ter-oh-sal-PIN-goh-gram) record of the uterus and fallopian tubes

hysteroscope (HIS-ter-oh-SKOHP) instrument for examining the uterus

hysteroscopy (HIS-ter-AW-skoh-pee) procedure for examining the uterus

hysterotomy (HIS-ter-AW-toh-mee) incision into the uterus

I

ichthyosis (ik-thee-OH-sis) a condition in which the skin is dry and scaly resembling fish scales

icterus (IK-ter-us) see *jaundice*

idiopathic (IH-dee-oh-PAH-thik) having no known cause or origin

ileitis (IH-lee-AI-tis) inflammation of the ileum

ileocolitis (IH-lee-oh-koh-LAI-tis) inflammation of the ileum and colon

ileocolostomy (IH-lee-oh-koh-LAW-stoh-mee) creation of an opening between the ileum and colon

ileorrhaphy (IH-lee-OR-ah-fee) suture of the ileum

ileostomy (IH-lee-AW-stoh-mee) creation of an opening in the ileum

ileotomy (IH-lee-AW-toh-mee) incision into the ileum

immunocompromised (ih-MYOO-noh-COM-proh-MAIZD) having an immune system incapable of responding normally and completely to a pathogen or disease

immunodeficiency (ih-MYOO-noh-deh-FIH-shin-see) immune system with decreased or compromised response to disease-causing organisms

immunoglobulin (im-MYOO-noh-GLAW-byoo-lin) protein that provides protection (immunity) against disease

immunologist (IM-myoo-NAW-loh-jist) specialist in the immune system

immunology (IM-myoo-NAW-loh-jee) study of the immune system

immunosuppression (ih-MYOO-noh-suh-PREH-shun) reduction in the activity of the body's immune system

impetigo (im-peh-TAI-goh) from Latin, for *to attack;* a highly contagious bacterial infection of the skin

in vitro fertilization (in VEE-troh FER-tih-lih-ZAY-shun) fertilization of an egg done in a test tube

incision and drainage (I&D) (in-SIH-zhun and DRAY-nij) to cut into a wound to allow trapped infected liquid to drain

incisional biopsy (in-SIH-zhun-al BAI-op-see) removal of a portion of a lesion for examination (to cut into)

incontinence (in-CON-tih-nentz) inability to control urination

induced abortion (in-DOOST ah-BOR-shun) the intentional termination of pregnancy

inferior vena cava (in-FEER-ee-or VEE-nah CAY-vah) portion of the vena cava that gathers blood from the lower portion of the body

inguinal (IN-gwin-al) lower side portions of the abdomen

insomnia (in-SOM-nee-ah) inability to sleep

insulin (IN-suh-lin) hormone secreted by the pancreas that controls the metabolism and uptake of sugar and fats

insulinoma (IN-suh-lin-OH-mah) tumor that secretes insulin (found in the insulin-producing cells in the pancreas)

interictal (IN-ter-IK-tal) time between seizures

internal fixation (IN-tir-nal fik-SAY-shun) the fixation of a fractured bone from the inside (i.e., using screws, pins, plates, etc.)

intracerebral hematoma (IN-trah-seh-REE-bral HEE-mah-TOH-mah) a hematoma located inside the brain

intracerebral hemorrhage (IN-trah-seh-REE-bral HIH-moh-rih) excessive bleeding inside the brain

intracorporeal lithotripsy (IN-trah-cor-POR-ee-al LIH-thoh-TRIP-see) breakdown of kidney stones using a device placed inside the body

intradermal (in-tra-DER-mal) pertaining to inside the skin

intraocular lens implant (IN-trah-AW-kyoo-lar lenz IM-plant) insertion of a new lens inside the eye

intrapartum (IN-trah-PAR-tum) time during birth

intravitreal antibiotic (IN-trah-VEE-tree-nus AN-tai-bai-AW-tiks) antibiotic administered directly into the vitreous gel liquid

iridalgia (IH-rid-AL-jah) pain in the iris

iridectomy (EAR-id-EK-toh-mee) removal of the iris

iridemia (EAR-ih-DEE-mee-ah) bleeding from the iris

iridocyclectomy (EAR-ih-doh-sai-KLEK-toh-mee) removal of the iris and ciliary body

iridocyclitis (EAR-ih-doh-sai-KLAI-tis) inflammation of the iris and ciliary body

iridokeratitis (EAR-ih-doh-keh-rah-TAI-tis) inflammation of the iris and cornea

iridokinesis (IR-ih-doh-kin-EE-sis) movement of the iris

iridopathy (EAR-ih-DOP-ah-thee) disease of the iris

iridotomy (EAR-id-AW-toh-mee) incision into the iris

iritis (ai-RAI-tis) inflammation of the iris

iron deficiency anemia (AI-ern deh-FIH-shin-see ah-NEE-mee-ah) anemia caused by inadequate iron intake

ischemia (ih-SKEE-mee-ah) blockage of blood flow to an organ

ischemic stroke (ih-SKEE-mik STROHK) a stroke where blood loss is caused by a blockage

J

jaundice (JAWN-dis) yellowing of skin, tissue, and fluids caused by increased levels of bilirubin in the blood

jejunitis (JE-joo-NAI-tis) inflammation of the jejunum

jejunoileitis (je-JOO-noh-IH-lee-AI-tis) inflammation of the jejunum and ileum

jejunorrhaphy (JE-joo-NOR-ah-fee) suture of the jejunum

jejunostomy (JE-joo-NAW-stoh-mee) creation of an opening in the jejunum

jejunotomy (JE-joo-NAW-toh-mee) incision into the jejunum

K

keloid (KEE-loid) overgrowth of scar tissue

keratalgia (KEH-rah-TAL-jah) pain in the cornea

keratitis (KEH-rah-TAI-tis) inflammation of the cornea

keratogenic (keh-RA-toh-jen-ik) causing horny tissue development

keratomalacia (ker-AH-toh-mah-LAY-shah) abnormal softening of the cornea

keratopathy (KEH-rah-TOP-ah-thee) disease of the cornea

keratoplasty (ker-A-toh-PLAS-tee) surgical reconstruction of the cornea

keratosis (keh-rah-TOH-sis) horny tissue condition

keratotomy (KER-ah-TAW-toh-mee) incision into the cornea

ketogenesis (KEE-toh-JIN-eh-sis) creation of ketone bodies

ketogenic diet (KEE-toh-JIN-ik DAI-et) diet that aids in the production of ketones in the body

ketolysis (kee-TAW-lih-sis) breakdown of ketones

ketonuria (kee-toh-NUR-ee-ah) presence of ketones in the urine

ketosis (kee-TOH-sis) condition characterized by elevated levels of ketone bodies in the blood

kidney dialysis (KID-nee dai-AL-ah-sis) procedure for removing waste from the blood (a shorter name for hemodialysis)

kleptomania (KLEP-toh-MAY-nee-ah) desire to steal

kyphosis (kai-FOH-sis) humped back—abnormal forward curvature of the upper spine

L

labyrinthectomy (LAB-uh-rinth-EK-toh-mee) removal of the labyrinth

labyrinthitis (LAB-uh-rinth-AI-tis) inflammation of the labyrinth

labyrinthotomy (LAB-uh-rinth-AW-toh-mee) incision into the labyrinth

lacrimation (LAH-krih-MAY-shun) the formation of tears (i.e., crying)

lactation (lak-TAY-shun) production of milk

lactogenic (LAK-toh-JIN-ik) causing the formation of milk

lactorrhea (LAK-toh-REE-ah) discharge of milk

laparocele (LAP-ar-oh-seel) abdominal hernia

laparoenterostomy (LAP-ar-oh-EN-ter-AW-stoh-mee) creation of an opening between the abdomen and the intestines

laparonephrectomy (LAP-ah-roh-neh-FREK-toh-mee) surgical removal of a kidney through the abdomen

laparoscope (LAP-ar-oh-skohp) instrument for looking inside the abdomen

laparoscopic adrenalectomy (LAP-rah-SKAW-pik ad-REE-nal-EK-toh-mee) removal of an adrenal gland by means of a laparascope

laparoscopic surgery (LAP-rah-SKAW-pik SIR-jir-ee) use of a laparoscope to perform minimally invasive surgery

laparoscopy (LAP-ar-AW-skoh-pee) procedure for looking inside the abdomen

laparosplenectomy (LAP-ah-roh-splee-NEK-toh-mee) surgical removal of the spleen through the abdomen

laparotomy (LAP-ar-AW-toh-mee) incision into the abdomen

laryngectomy (la-rin-JEK-toe-mee) removal of the larynx

laryngitis (la-rin-JAI-tis) inflammation of the larynx

laryngoplasty (la-rin-GO-plas-tee) reconstruction of the larynx

laryngotracheobronchitis (la-rin-go-tray-key-o-bron-KAI-tis) inflammation of the larynx, trachea, and bronchi

leukemia (loo-KEE-mee-ah) cancer of the blood or bone marrow characterized by the abnormal increase in white blood cells

leukocyte (LOO-koh-sait) white blood cell

leukocytosis (LOO-koh-sai-TOH-sis) increase in the number of white blood cells

leukoderma (loo-koh-DER-mah) white skin

leukopenia (LOO-koh-PEE-nee-ah) deficiency in white blood cells

leukorrhea (LOO-koh-REE-ah) white vaginal discharge

lipectomy (lih-PEK-toh-mee) removal of fatty tissue

liposuction (LAI-poh-SUK-shun) removal of fatty tissue using a vacuum

lithectomy (lih-THEK-toh-mee) surgical removal of a stone in the bladder

lithocystotomy (LIH-thoh-SIS-TAW-toh-mee) incision into the bladder to remove a stone

lithonephritis (LIH-thoh-neh-FRAI-tis) inflammation of the kidneys caused by stones

lithonephrotomy (LIH-thoh-neh-FRAW-toh-mee) incision into a kidney to remove a stone

lithotripsy (LIH-thoh-TRIP-see) breakdown of a stone

lobectomy (loh-BEK-toh-mee) removal of a lobe

lobotomy (loh-BAW-toh-mee) incision into a lobe

local anesthetic (LOH-kal an-es-THET-ik) any anesthetic that does not affect consciousness

lordosis (lor-DOH-sis) swayback—abnormal forward curvature of the lower spine

lumbar (LUM-bar) middle side portions of the abdomen

lumbar puncture (LP) (LUM-bar PUNK-chir) inserting a needle into the lumbar region of the spine in order to collect spinal fluid

lymphadenectomy (lim-FAD-eh-NEK-toh-mee) surgical removal of a lymph gland (node)

lymphadenitis (LIM-fad-eh-NAI-tis) inflammation of a lymph gland (node)

lymphadenopathy (lim-FAD-eh-NAW-pah-thee) any disease of a lymph gland (node); used to refer to noticeably swollen lymph nodes, especially in the neck

lymphadenotomy (lim-FAD-eh-NAW-toh-mee) incision into a lymph gland (node)

lymphangiectasia (lim-FAN-jee-ek-TAY-zhah) dilation of a lymph vessel, normally noticed by swelling in the extremities

lymphangiogram (lim-FAN-jee-oh-GRAM) record of the study of lymph vessels

lymphangiography (lim-FAN-jee-AW-grah-fee) procedure to study the lymph vessels

lymphangitis (LIM-fan-JAI-tis) inflammation of the lymph vessels

lymphedema (LIMF-ah-DEE-mah) swelling caused by abnormal accumulation of lymph

lymphocyte (LIM-foh-SAIT) lymph cell

lymphoma (lim-FOH-mah) tumor originating in lymphocytes

lymphopenia (LIM-foh-PEE-nee-ah) abnormal deficiency in lymph

M

macerate (MAS-ir-ayt) from Latin, for *to make soft;* to soften the skin

macrocephaly (MA-kroh-SEH-fah-lee) abnormally large head

macrocytosis (MAH-kroh-sai-TOH-sis) condition characterized by large red blood cells

macromastia (MAK-roh-MAS-tee-ah) abnormally large breasts

macrosomia (MAK-roh-SOH-mee-ah) baby with a large body

macrotia (mah-KROH-shee-ah) abnormally large ears

macule (MA-kyool) from Latin, for *spot* or *stain;* small, flat, discolored area (freckle)

magnetic resonance angiography (MRA) (mag-NET-ik REH-zawn-ants AN-gee-AW-grah-fee) procedure used to examine blood vessels

malignant cutaneous neoplasm (mah-LIG-nant kuh-TAY-nee-us NEE-oh-plaz-um) a harmful new formation of the skin tissue (i.e., skin cancer)

malignant melanoma (ma-LIG-nant meh-lah-NOH-mah) a harmful tumor of melanin cell

mammogram (MAM-oh-GRAM) record of a breast exam

mammoplasty (MAM-oh-PLAS-tee) surgical reconstruction of a breast

manic depression (bipolar) (MAN-ik de-PREH-shun) a psychiatric disorder characterized by alternating bouts of excitement and depression

mastalgia (mas-TAL-jah) breast pain

mastectomy (mas-TEK-toh-mee) surgical removal of a breast

mastitis (mas-TAI-tis) inflammation of the breast

mastoidalgia (MAS-toid-AL-jah) pain in the mastoid

mastoidectomy (MAS-toy-DEK-toh-mee) removal of the mastoid

mastoiditis (MAS-toy-DAI-tis) inflammation of the mastoid

mastoidocentesis (mas-TOY-doh-sin-TEE-sis) puncture of the mastoid

mastopexy (MAS-toh-PEK-see) surgical fixation of a breast

mastoptosis (MAS-top-TOH-sis) downward displacement (drooping) of the breast

meatal stenosis (mee-AY-tal steh-NOH-sis) narrowing of the opening of the urethra

meatoplasty (mee-AT-toh-PLAS-tee) surgical reconstruction of the opening of the urethra

meatorrhaphy (MEE-ah-TOR-ah-fee) suture of the opening of the urethra

meatoscope (mee-AT-oh-SKOHP) instrument for examining the opening of the urethra

meatoscopy (MEE-ah-TAW-skoh-pee) process for examining the opening of the urethra

meatotomy (MEE-ah-TAW-toh-mee) incision into the opening of the urethra

menarche (MEN-ar-kee) beginning or first menstruation

meningioma (meh-NIN-jee-OH-mah) tumor of the meninges

meningitis (MEH-nin-JAI-tus) inflammation of the meninges

meningocele (meh-NIN-goh-seel) a hernia of the meninges

meningoencephalitis (meh-NIN-goh-in-SEF-ah-LAI-tis) inflammation of the meninges and brain

meningopathy (MEH-nin-GAW-pah-thee) disease of the meninges

menopause (MEN-oh-pawz) cessation of menstruation

menorrhagia (MEN-oh-RAY-jah) excessive menstrual flow

menorrhalgia (MEN-oh-RAL-jah) painful menstruation

metabolism (meh-TAB-oh-LIZM) breakdown of matter into energy

metacarpectomy (MEH-tah-kar-PEK-toh-mee) removal of a bone of the hand

metatarsalgia (meh-tah-tar-SAL-jah) pain in the bones of the foot

metrocolpocele (MEH-troh-KOL-poh-seel) hernia of the uterus and prolapse into the vagina

metromenorrhagia (MEH-troh-MEN-oh-RAY-jah) excessive menstrual bleeding at irregular intervals

metrophlebitis (MEH-troh-fleh-BAI-tis) inflammation of the blood vessels of the uterus

metrorrhagia (MEH-troh-RAY-jah) menstrual bleeding at irregular times

microcephalus (MAI-kroh-SEF-ah-lus) baby with a small head

microcephaly (MAI-kroh-SEH-fah-lee) abnormally small head

microcytosis (MAI-kroh-sai-TOH-sis) condition characterized by small red blood cells

micromastia (MAI-kroh-MAS-tee-ah) abnormally small breasts

microtia (mai-KROH-shee-ah) abnormally small ears

miosis (mai-OH-sis) abnormal contraction of the pupil (from Greek, for *to lessen*)

miotic (mai-AW-tik) drug that causes the abnormal contraction of the pupil

mononucleosis (MAW-noh-NOO-klee-OH-sis) condition characterized by an abnormally large number of mononuclear leukocytes

monoparesis (MAW-noh-puh-REE-sis) partial paralysis of one limb

monoplegia (MAW-noh-PLEE-jah) paralysis of one limb

mucolytic (myoo-koh-LIT-ik) a drug that aids in the breakdown of mucus

murmur (MIR-mir) abnormal heart sound

muscular dystrophy (MUS-kyoo-lar DIS-troh-fee) disorder characterized by poor muscle development

myalgia (mai-AL-jah) muscle pain

myasthenia (mai-as-THEH-nee-ah) muscle weakness

mycodermatitis (mai-koh-der-mah-TAI-tis) inflammation of the skin caused by fungus

mycosis (mai-KOH-sis) fungus condition

mydriasis (mi-DRAI-ah-sis) abnormal dilation of the pupil

mydriatic (MID-ree-AT-ik) drug that causes the abnormal dilation of the pupil

myectomy (mai-EK-toh-mee) removal of muscle

myelitis (MAI-el-AI-tis) inflammation of the spinal cord

myelocele (MAI-el-oh-SEEL) a hernia of the spinal cord

myelodysplasia (MAI-el-oh-dis-PLAY-zhah) disease characterized by poor production of blood cells by the bone marrow

myelogram (MAI-el-oh-gram) image of the spinal cord, usually done using x-ray

myeloma (MAI-eh-LOH-mah) cancerous tumor of the bone marrow

myelomalacia (MAI-el-oh-mah-LAY-shah) abnormal softening of the spinal cord

myelomeningocele (MAI-el-oh-meh-NIN-goh-seel) a hernia of the spinal cord and meninges

myelopathy (MAI-el-AW-pah-thee) disease of the spinal cord

myelopoiesis (MAI-eh-loh-poh-EE-sis) formation of bone marrow

myocardial infarction (MAI-oh-KAR-dee-al in-FARK-shun) death of heart muscle tissue

myocardial ischemia (MAI-oh-KAR-dee-al ih-SKEE-mee-ah) blockage of blood to the heart muscle

myocarditis (MAI-oh-kar-DAI-tis) inflammation of the heart muscle

myocardium (MAI-oh-KAR-dee-um) heart muscle tissue

myocele (MAI-oh-seel) hernia of muscle tissue

myoclonus (mai-AWK-loh-nus) violent muscle contraction

myodesis (MAI-oh-DEE-sis) binding of muscle

myodynia (mai-oh-DAI-nee-ah) muscle pain

myofasciitis (MAI-oh-FA-shee-AI-tis) inflammation of the muscle and fascia

myography (mai-AW-grah-fee) procedure for studying muscles

myolysis (mai-AW-lih-sis) loss of muscle tissue

myoma (mai-OH-mah) a muscle tumor

myomalacia (mai-oh-mah-LAY-shah) softening of a muscle

myomectomy (MAI-oh-MEK-toh-mee) surgical removal of a tumor in the muscle (usually refers to the muscle of the uterine wall)

myometritis (MAI-oh-meh-TRAI-tis) inflammation of the myometrium

myometrium (MAI-oh-MEE-tree-um) the middle layer of uterine muscle tissue

myopathy (mai-AW-pah-thee) muscle disease

myopia (mai-OH-pee-ah) nearsightedness

myoplasty (MAI-oh-PLAS-tee) muscle reconstruction

myorrhaphy (mai-OR-ah-fee) muscle suture

myosarcoma (MAI-oh-sar-KOH-mah) a cancerous muscle tumor

myosclerosis (mai-oh-skleh-ROH-sis) hardening of a muscle

myositis (MAI-oh-SAI-tis) muscle inflammation

myospasm (MAI-oh-spaz-um) involuntary muscle contraction

myotasis (mai-AW-tah-sis) stretching of a muscle

myotomy (mai-AW-toh-mee) incision into muscle

myotonia (mai-oh-TOH-nee-ah) muscle tone

myringectomy (MIR-in-JEK-toh-mee) removal of the eardrum

myringitis (MIR-in-JAI-tis) inflammation of the eardrum

myringodermatitis (mir-IN-goh-DER-mah-TAI-tis) inflammation of the eardrum and surrounding skin

myringomycosis (mir-IN-goh-mai-KOH-sis) fungal condition of the eardrum

myringoplasty (mir-IN-goh-PLAS-tee) surgical reconstruction of the eardrum

myringotomy (mir-in-GAW-toh-mee) incision into the eardrum

myxedema (MIX-eh-DEE-mah) swelling of the skin caused by deposits under the skin

N

narcolepsy (NAR-coh-LEP-see) a disease characterized by sudden, uncontrolled sleepiness

nasogastric tube (NAY-soh-GAS-trik TOOB) tube inserted through the nose into the stomach

nasolacrimal (NAY-zoh-LAH-krih-mal) pertaining to the nose and tear system

nasopharyngoscope (nay-zoh-fa-RIN-go-skope) an instrument to look at the nose and throat

natal (NAY-tal) pertaining to birth

nebulizer (neh-byoo-LAI-zir) a machine that administers respiratory medication by creating a "cloud" or mist that is inhaled by the patient

necrosis (neh-KROH-sis) tissue death

necrotizing fasciitis (NEH-kroh-TAI-zing FA-shee-AI-tis) inflammation of the fascia causing the death of tissue

neonatal (NEE-oh-NAY-tal) pertaining to new birth (normally the first 28 days after birth)

neonatologist (NEE-oh-nay-TAW-loh-jist) specialist in the neonatal period

neonatology (NEE-oh-nay-TAW-loh-jee) study of the neonatal period

nephralgia (neh-FRAL-jah) pain in the kidney

nephrectomy (neh-FREK-toh-mee) surgical removal of a kidney

nephritis (neh-FRAI-tis) inflammation of the kidney

nephrocele (NEH-froh-seel) hernia of a kidney

nephrocystanastomosis (NEH-froh-SIST-ah-NAS-tah-MOH-sis) opening of a passageway between kidney and bladder

nephrogram (NEF-roh-gram) image of a kidney

nephrography (neh-FRAW-grah-fee) procedure for imaging a kidney

nephrohypertrophy (NEH-froh-hai-PER-troh-fee) overdevelopment of the kidney

nephrolithiasis (NEH-froh-lih-THAI-ah-sis) the presence of stones in the kidney

nephrolithotomy (NEH-froh-lih-THAW-toh-mee) incision into a kidney to remove a stone

nephrologist (neh-FRAW-loh-jist) specialist in the kidneys

nephrology (neh-FRAW-loh-jee) study of the kidneys

nephroma (neh-FROH-mah) kidney tumor

nephromalacia (NEH-froh-mah-LAY-shah) abnormal softening of a kidney

nephromegaly (NEH-froh-MEG-ah-lee) abnormal enlargement of a kidney

nephropathy (neh-FRAW-pah-thee) any kidney disease

nephropexy (NEH-froh-PEK-see) surgical fixation of a kidney

nephroptosis (nef-rop-TOH-sis) downward displacement of a kidney

nephrorrhaphy (neh-FROR-ah-fee) suture of a kidney

nephrosclerosis (NEH-froh-skleh-ROH-sis) abnormal hardening of a kidney

nephroscopy (ne-FRAW-skoh-pee) procedure for examining a kidney

nephrosis (neh-FROH-sis) kidney condition

nephrosonography (NEF-roh-soh-NAW-grah-fee) procedure for imaging a kidney using sound waves

nephrosplenopexy (NEF-roh-SPLEE-noh-PEK-see) surgical fixation of the spleen and a kidney

nephrostomy (neh-FRAW-stoh-mee) creation of an opening in a kidney

nephrotomy (neh-FRAW-toh-mee) incision into a kidney to remove a stone

nephrotoxin (NEH-froh-TOK-sin) an agent poisonous to the kidney

nephroureterectomy (NEH-froh-yoo-REE-ter-EK-toh-mee) surgical removal of a kidney and ureter

neuralgia (nur-AL-jah) nerve pain

neurasthenia (NIR-as-THEN-ee-ah) nerve weakness

neurectomy (nir-EK-toh-mee) removal of a nerve

neuritis (nir-AI-tis) nerve inflammation

neuroarthropathy (NIR-oh-ar-THRAW-pah-thee) disease of the joint associated with nerves

neurodynia (NUR-oh-DAI-nee-ah) nerve pain

neuroencephalomyelopathy (NIR-oh-in-SEF-ah-loh-MAI-el-AW-pah-thee) disease of the nerves, brain, and spinal cord

neurogenic (NIR-oh-JIN-ik) originating from/created by nerves

neuroglycopenia (NIR-oh-GLAI-koh-PEE-nee-ah) deficiency of sugar that interferes with normal brain activity

neurolysis (nir-AW-lih-sis) destruction of nerve tissue

neuroma (nir-OH-mah) a nerve tumor

neuropathy (nir-AW-pah-thee) disease of the nervous system

neuropharmacology (nir-oh-FAR-mah-KAW-loh-jee) the study of the effects of drugs on the nervous system

neuroplasty (NIR-oh-PLAS-tee) reconstruction of a nerve

neurorrhaphy (nir-OR-ah-fee) suturing of a nerve (often the severed ends of a nerve)

neurosclerosis (NIR-oh-skleh-ROH-sis) hardening of nerves

neurosis (neh-ROH-sis) a nerve condition

neurotomy (nir-AW-toh-mee) incision into a nerve

neutropenia (NOO-troh-PEE-nee-ah) deficiency in neutrophil

nevus (NEE-vus) from Latin, for *birthmark* or *mole;* a mole

nocturia (nok-TUR-ee-ah) nighttime urination

nocturnal enuresis (nok-TIR-nal EN-yur-EE-sis) nighttime involuntary urination

nodule (NAWD-jyool) a solid mass that extends deeper into the skin

normocyte (NOR-moh-sait) normal-sized red blood cell

normotension (NOR-moh-TEN-shun) normal blood pressure

nystagmus (nih-STAG-mus) involuntary back-and-forth movement of the eyes (from Greek, for *to nod*)

O

obstetrician (OB-steh-TRIH-shun) specialist in pregnancy, labor, and delivery of newborns

obstetrics (ob-STEH-triks) branch of medicine dealing with pregnancy, labor, and delivery of newborns

obstructive lung disorder (ob-STRUKT-iv) a lung disorder caused by a blockage

occlusion (oh-KLOO-zhun) closing or blockage of a passage

oculomycosis (AW-kyoo-loh-mai-KOH-sis) a fungal eye condition

oculopathy (AW-kyoo-LAW-pah-thee) disease of the eye

oculoplasty (AW-kyoo-loh-PLAS-tee) surgical reconstruction of the eye

odontalgia (OH-dawn-TAL-jah) tooth pain

odontectomy (oh-dawn-TEK-toh-mee) surgical removal of a tooth

odontoclasis (OH-dawn-TAWK-lah-sis) breaking of a tooth

odontodynia (oh-DAWN-toh-DAI-nee-ah) tooth pain

oligocythemia (AW-lih-goh-sih-THEE-mee-ah) deficiency in the number of red blood cells

oligohydramnios (AW-lih-goh-hai-DRAM-nee-ohs) not enough amniotic fluid

oligomenorrhea (AW-lih-goh-MEN-oh-REE-ah) infrequent or light menstrual periods

oligospermia (AW-lih-goh-SPER-mee-ah) condition characterized by low sperm production

oliguria (aw-lih-GYIR-ee-ah) low urine output

onychectomy (aw-nik-EK-toh-mee) removal of a nail

onychia (oh-NIK-ee-ah) a nail condition

onychocryptosis (AW-nih-koh-krip-TOH-sis) an ingrown nail

onychodystrophy (AW-ni-koh-DIS-troh-fee) poor nourishment (and development) of the nail

onycholysis (AW-nih-KAWL-is-is) the loss of a nail

onychomalacia (AW-nih-koh-mah-LAY-shah) abnormal softening of a nail

onychomycosis (AW-nih-koh-mai-KOH-sis) a fungal condition of the nail

onychopathy (aw-nik-AW-pah-thee) nail disease

onychophagia (aw-nih-koh-FAY-jah) eating (biting) the nail

onychotomy (aw-ni-KAW-toh-mee) incision into a nail

oophorectomy (OH-aw-for-EK-toh-mee) surgical removal of an ovary

oophoritis (OH-aw-for-AI-tis) inflammation of an ovary

oophorocystectomy (oh-AW-for-oh-sis-TEK-toh-mee) surgical removal of an ovarian cyst

oophorocystosis (OH-aw-FOR-oh-SIS-toh-sis) ovarian cysts

oophoroma (OH-aw-for-OH-mah) ovarian tumor

oophorotomy (oh-AW-for-AW-toh-mee) incision into an ovary

open reduction (OH-pen ree-DUK-shun) returning bones to their proper position through the use of surgery

ophthalmalgia (OFF-thal-MAL-jah) eye pain

ophthalmatrophy (AWF-thal-MAW-troh-fee) atrophy (wasting away) of the eye

ophthalmectomy (AWF-thal-MEK-toh-mee) removal of the eye

ophthalmic (awf-THAL-mik) pertaining to the eye

ophthalmitis (AWF-thal-MAI-tis) inflammation of the eye

ophthalmologist (AWF-thal-MAW-loh-jist) eye specialist

ophthalmomycosis (awf-THAL-moh-mai-KOH-sis) fungal eye condition

ophthalmomyitis (awf-THAL-moh-mai-AI-tis) inflammation of the eye muscles

ophthalmopathy (AWF-thal-MOH-pah-thee) eye disease

ophthalmoplegia (off-THAL-moh-PLEE-jah) eye paralysis

ophthalmoscope (awf-THAL-mah-SKOHP) instrument for looking at the eye

optic (AWP-tik) pertaining to the eye

optic neuritis (OP-tik nir-AI-tis) inflammation of the optic nerve

optokinetic (AWP-toh-kih-NEH-tik) pertaining to eye movement

optometrist (awp-TAW-meh-trist) specialist in measuring the eye

optomyometer (AWP-toh-MAI-oh-MEE-tir) device used to determine the strength of eye muscles

orchialgia (OR-kee-AL-jah) testicle pain

orchichorhea (OR-kee-kor-EE-ah) involuntary jerking movement of the testicles

orchidectomy (OR-kid-EK-toh-mee) surgical removal of a testicle

orchiditis (OR-kih-DAI-tis) inflammation of the testicles and epididymis

orchidopexy (OR-kid-oh-PEK-see) surgical fixation of a testicle

orchidoptosis (OR-kih-dop-TOH-sis) downward displacement of a testicle

orchidotomy (OR-kid-AW-toh-mee) incision into a testicle

orchiectomy (OR-kee-EK-toh-mee) surgical removal of a testicle

orchiepididymitis (OR-kee-EP-ih-DID-ih-MAI-tis) inflammation of the testicles and epididymis

orchiodynia (OR-kee-oh-DAI-nee-ah) testicle pain

orchiopathy (OR-kee-AW-pah-thee) disease of the testicles

orchiopexy (OR-kee-oh-PEK-see) surgical fixation of a testicle

orchioplasty (OR-kee-oh-PLAS-tee) surgical reconstruction of a testicle

orchitis (or-KAI-tis) inflammation of the testicles and epididymis

orthodontics (or-thoh-DAWN-tiks) branch of medicine dealing with the straightening of teeth

orthodontist (or-thoh-DAWN-tist) specialist in straightening teeth

orthopnea (or-thop-NEE-ah) able to breathe only in an upright position

orthotics (or-THAW-tiks) a device that aids in the straightening or stabilizing of a part of the body

ostalgia (aws-TAL-jah) bone pain

ostealgia (aws-tee-AL-jah) bone pain

ostectomy (aws-TEK-toh-mee) removal of a bone

osteectomy (aws-tee-EK-toh-mee) removal of a bone

osteitis (AW-stee-AI-tis) bone inflammation

osteoacusis (AW-stee-oh-ah-KOO-sis) hearing through bone

osteoarthritis (AW-stee-oh-ar-THRAI-tis) inflammation of the joints, specifically those that bear weight

osteocarcinoma (AW-stee-oh-KAR-sih-NOH-mah) bone cancer tumor

osteochondritis (AW-stee-oh-kon-DRAI-tis) inflammation of bone and cartilage

osteochondroma (AW-stee-oh-kon-DROH-mah) a tumor made up of bone and cartilage

osteodynia (aws-tee-oh-DAI-nee-ah) bone pain

osteodystrophy (aw-stee-oh-DIH-stroh-fee) poor bone development

osteogenesis imperfecta (AW-stee-oh-JIN-eh-sis IM-per-FEK-tah) a disease in which the bones do not develop correctly; also known as brittle bone disease

osteolysis (aw-stee-AW-lih-sis) bone loss

osteomalacia (AW-stee-oh-mah-LAY-shah) softening of the bone

osteometry (aw-stee-AW-meh-tree) procedure for measuring bone

osteomyelitis (AW-stee-oh-MAI-eh-LAI-tis) inflammation of the bone and bone marrow

osteonecrosis (aw-stee-oh-nih-KROH-sis) death of bone

osteopathy (AW-stee-AW-pah-thee) bone disease

osteopenia (AW-stee-oh-PEE-nee-yah) reduction in bone volume

osteoplasty (AWS-tee-oh-PLAS-tee) reconstruction of a bone

osteoporosis (AW-stee-oh-por-OH-sis) loss of bone density

osteosarcoma (AW-stee-oh-sar-KOH-mah) cancerous tumor arising out of bone cells

osteosclerosis (aw-stee-oh-skleh-ROH-sis) abnormal hardening of bone

osteotomy (AWS-tee-AW-toh-mee) incision into a bone

otalgia (oh-TAL-jah) ear pain

otitis externa (oh-TAI-tis eks-TERN-nah) inflammation of the outer ear

otitis media (oh-TAI-tis MEH-dee-ah) inflammation of the middle ear

otodynia (OH-toh-DAI-nee-ah) ear pain

otolaryngologist (OH-toh-LAH-rin-GAW-loh-jist) specialist in the ear and throat

otomycosis (oh-toh-mai-KOH-sis) a fungal ear condition

otoneurologist (OH-toh-nih-RAW-loh-jist) specialist in the nerve connections between the ear and brain

otoplasty (OH-toh-PLAS-tee) surgical reconstruction of the ear

otopyorrhea (OH-toh-PAI-oh-REE-ah) discharge of pus from the ears

otorhinolaryngologist (OH-toh-RAI-noh-LAH-rin-GAW-loh-jist) specialist in the ear, nose, and throat

otorrhea (OH-toh-REE-ah) discharge from the ear

otosclerosis (oh-toh-skleh-ROH-sis) hearing loss caused by the hardening of the bones of the middle ear

otoscope (OH-toh-SKOHP) instrument for looking in the ear

otoscopy (oh-TAW-skoh-pee) procedure for looking in the ear

otosteal (oh-TAWS-tee-all) pertaining to the bones of the ear

ototoxic (OH-toh-TOK-sik) drug that is damaging to the ear/hearing

ovaralgia (OH-var-AL-jah) pain in the ovaries

ovarialgia (oh-VAR-ee-AL-jah) pain in the ovaries

ovarian cystectomy (oh-VAR-ee-an sis-TEK-toh-mee) surgical removal of an ovarian cyst

ovariocentesis (oh-VAR-ee-oh-sin-TEE-sis) surgical puncture of an ovary

ovariocyesis (oh-VAR-ee-oh-sai-EE-sis) ectopic pregnancy in an ovary

ovariorrhexis (oh-VAR-ee-oh-REK-sis) rupture of an ovary

ovariostomy (oh-VAR-ee-AW-stoh-me) creation of an opening into an ovary

ovaritis (OH-var-AI-tis) inflammation of an ovary

oximetry (ok-SIM-ah-tree) a procedure to measure oxygen levels

oxytocin (OK-see-TOH-sin) agent that stimulates uterine contractions and accelerates labor

P

pachyderma (pa-kih-DER-mah) tough skin

palatoplasy (pal-e-toe-PLAS-tee) reconstruction of the palate

palpitation (PAL-pih-TAY-shun) rapid or irregular beating of the heart

pancreatalgia (PAN-kree-ah-TAL-jah) pain in the pancreas

pancreatectomy (PAN-kree-ah-TEK-toh-mee) surgical removal of the pancreas

pancreatic pseudocyst (PAN-kree-at-ik SOO-doh-sist) abnormally expanded area in the pancreas resembling a cyst

pancreatitis (PAN-kree-ah-TAI-tis) inflammation of the pancreas

pancreatoduodenectomy (PAN-kree-at-oh-DOO-aw-den-EK-toh-mee) surgical removal of the pancreas and duodenum

pancreatography (PAN-kree-ah-TAW-graw-FEE) procedure for mapping the pancreas

pancreatolith (PAN-kree-AT-oh-lith) stone in the pancreas

pancreatolithectomy (PAN-kree-ah-toh-lith-EK-toh-mee) removal of a stone in the pancreas

pancreatolithiasis (PAN-kree-at-oh-lih-THAI-ah-sis) presence of a stone in the pancreas

pancytopenia (PAN-SAI-toh-PEE-nee-ah) deficiency in all cellular components of the blood

panhypopituitarism (PAN-HAI-poh-pih-TOO-ih-tar-IZM) defective or absent function of the entire pituitary gland

pansinusitis (pan-sai-nus-AI-tis) inflammation of all sinuses

Pap (Papanicolaou) smear (PAP SMEER) test used to detect cancer cells, most commonly in the cervix

papilledema (PAH-pil-ah-DEE-mah) swelling of the optic nerve where it enters the retina

papule (PA-pyool) from Latin, for *pimple;* a small, solid mass

paralysis (puh-RAH-lu-sis) complete loss of sensation and motor function

parathyroidectomy (PAR-ah-THAI-roid EK-toh-mee) removal of the parathyroid

parathyroidoma (PAR-ah-THAI-roid-OH-mah) tumor of the parathyroid

paresis (puh-REE-sis) partial paralysis characterized by varying degrees of sensation and motor function

paresthesia (PAR-es-THEE-zhah) abnormal sensation (usually numbness or tingling in the skin)

paronychia (par-aw-NIH-kee-ah) a condition of the tissue around a nail

patch (pach) large, flat discolored area

pectoralgia (PEK-tor-AL-jah) chest pain

pectoriloquy (pek-tor-IH-low-kwee) speaking from the chest; used as a means of finding masses in the lung

pectus carinatum (PEK-tus car-ee-NAH-tum) a chest that protrudes like the keel of a ship

pectus excavatum (PEK-tus eks-cuh-VAH-tum) a chest that is hollowed out

pelvic sonograph (PEL-vik SAW-noh-GRAF) instrument for imaging the pelvis using sound waves

pelvicephalometry (PEL-vih-SEF-eh-LAW-meh-tree) procedure for measuring the head size of the baby and the pelvis size of the mother

pelvimetry (pel-VIM-eh-tree) procedure for measuring the pelvis

percussion (per-KUH-shun) the body surface; in this context, to cause vibrations that can help locate fluid build-up in the chest

percutaneous (per-kyoo-TAY-nee-us) pertaining to through the skin

percutaneous coronary intervention (PER-kyoo-TAY-nee-us KOR-ah-NAR-ee IN-ter-VEN-shun) alternative treatment for the coronary artery that passes instruments up a patient's blood vessels into the heart

perfusion (per-FYOO-zhun) circulation of blood through tissue

pericardial effusion (PER-ee-KAR-dee-al ee-FYOO-zhun) fluid pouring out into the tissue around the heart

pericardiocentesis (PER-ee-KAR-dee-oh-sin-TEE-sis) puncture of the tissue around the heart

pericardiotomy (PER-ee-KAR-dee-AW-toh-mee) incision into the tissue around the heart

pericarditis (PER-ee-kar-DAI-tis) inflammation of the tissue around the heart

pericardium (PER-ee- KAR-dee-um) tissue around the heart

perimetritis (PEH-ree-meh-TRAI-tis) inflammation of the perimetrium

perimetrium (PER-ee-MEE-tree-um) tissue on the outside of the uterus, the outer layer of the uterus

perinatal (PEH-ree-NAY-tal) time around birth (normally ranging from 28 weeks of pregnancy to 28 days after pregnancy)

perinatologist (PEH-ree-nay-TAW-loh-jist) specialist in the perinatal period

perinatology (PER-ee-nay-TAW-loh-jee) branch of medicine dealing with the perinatal period

perineocele (PER-ih-NEE-oh-seel) hernia in the perineum region

perineoplasty (PER-ih-NEE-oh-PLAS-tee) surgical reconstruction of the perineum

perineorrhaphy (PER-ih-nee-OR-ah-fee) suture of the perineum

perineotomy (PER-ih-nee-AW-toh-mee) incision into the perineum

periodontitis (PER-ee-OH-don-TAI-tis) inflammation of the region around the teeth

peritoneoscopy (PER-ih-TOH-nee-AW-skoh-pee) procedure for looking at the peritoneum

peritonitis (PER-ih-toh-NAI-tis) inflammation of the peritoneum

petechia (puh-TEE-kee-yah) small bruise

phacoemulsification (FAY-koh-ee-MUL-sih-fih-KAY-shun) fragmentation of an existing lens in order to remove and replace it

phacomalacia (FAH-koh-mah-LAY-shah) abnormal softening of the lens

phacosclerosis (FAH-koh-skleh-ROH-sis) abnormal hardening of the lens

phacoscope (FAY-koh-SKOHP) instrument for looking at the lens

phagocytosis (FAG-oh-sai-TOH-sis) process in which phagocytes (a type of white blood cell) destroy (or eat) foreign microorganisms or cell debris

phakitis (fah-KAI-tis) inflammation of the lens

phimosis (fih-MOH-sis) contraction of the foreskin of the penis, preventing it from being retracted

phlebalgia (fleh-BAL-jah) pain in a vein

phlebarteriectasia (FLEB-ar-TER-ee-ek-TAY-zhah) dilation of blood vessels

phlebectomy (fleb-EK-toh-mee) surgical removal of a vein

phlebitis (fleh-BAI-tis) inflammation of the veins

phlebologist (fleb-AW-loh-jist) specialist in veins

phlebology (fleb-AW-loh-jee) study of veins

phlebophlebostomy (FLEB-oh-fleb-AW-stoh-mee) procedure to create an opening between two veins

phlebosclerosis (FLEB-oh-skleh-ROH-sis) hardening of a vein

phlebostenosis (FLEB-oh-sten-OH-sis) narrowing of the veins

phlebotomist (fleh-BAW-toh-mist) specialist in drawing blood

phlebotomy (fleh-BAW-toh-mee) incision into a vein (another name for drawing blood)

photophobia (FOH-toh-FOH-bee-ah) excessive sensitivity to light

phrenoplegia (fre-no-PLEE-jah) paralysis of the diaphragm

phrenoptosis (fre-nop-TOE-sis) drooping of the diaphragm

phrenospasm (fre-no-SPAZ-um) involuntary contraction of the diaphragm

pituitary adenoma (pih-TOO-ih-TEH-ree AD-en-OH-mah) tumor on the pituitary gland

pituitary dwarfism (pih-TOO-ih-TER-ee DWAR-fizm) abnormally short height caused by undersecretions of growth hormone from the pituitary gland

pituitary gigantism (pih-TOO-ih-TER-ee jai-GAN-tizm) abnormally tall height caused by oversecretion of growth hormone from the pituitary gland

pituitary infarction (pih-TOO-ih-TEH-ree in-FARK-shun) death of the pituitary gland

placenta previa (plah-SIN-tah PREE-vee-ah) condition in which the placenta is attached to the uterus near the cervix

plaque (PLAK) a solid mass on the surface of the skin

plasmapheresis (PLAZ-mah-fer-EE-sis) apheresis to remove plasma

plateletpheresis (PLAYT-let-fer-EE-sis) apheresis to remove platelets (for the purpose of donating them to patients in need of platelets)

pleural effusion (PLUR-al ef-YOO-zhun) fluid pouring out into the pleura

pleuralgia (plur-AL-jah) pain in the pleura

pleurisy (PLUR-ih-see) inflammation of the pleura; another word for pleuritis

pleuritis (plur-AI-tis) inflammation of the pleura

pleurodynia (plur-oh-DAI-nee-ah) pain in the pleura

pleuropexy (ploo-rah-PEK-see) reattachment of the pleura

pneumatic otoscopy (new-MA-tik oh-TAW-skoh-pee) procedure for looking in the ear using air

pneumatocele (new-MAT-o-seel) hernia of the lung

pneumoconiosis (new-moh-con-i-O-sis) a lung condition caused by dust

pneumohemothorax (new-moh-hee-moh-THOR-aks) air and blood in the chest

pneumonectomy (new-mon-EK-toe-mee) removal of a lung

pneumonia (new-MOH-nee-yah) a lung condition

pneumonitis (new-moh-NAI-tis) inflammation of the lung

pneumothorax (new-moh-THOR-aks) air in the chest

poikilocytosis (POI-kih-loh-sai-TOH-sis) condition characterized by red blood cells in a variety of shapes

poliomyelitis (POH-lee-oh-MAI-el-AI-tis) inflammation of the gray matter of the spinal cord

polyadenopathy (PAW-lee-AD-en-AW-pah-thee) disease involving many glands

polycystic kidney disease (PAW-lee-SIS-tik KID-nee dih-ZEEZ) disease characterized by the formation of many fluid-filled cysts in the kidneys

polycythemia (PAW-lee-sih-THEE-mee-ah) excess of red blood cells

polydactyly (paw-lee-DAK-tih-lee) having more than the normal number of fingers (or toes)

polydipsia (PAW-lee-DIP-see-ah) excessive thirst

polyhydramnios (PAW-lee-hai-DRAM-nee-ohs) excessive amniotic fluid

polymenorrhea (PAW-lee-MEN-oh-REE-ah) menstrual periods occurring with greater than normal frequency

polymyositis (PAW-lee-MAI-oh-SAI-tis) inflammation of multiple muscles

polyneuritis (PAW-lee-nir-AI-tis) inflammation of multiple nerves

polyneuropathy (PAW-lee-nir-AW-pah-thee) disease affecting multiple nerves

polyphagia (PAW-lee-FAY-jah) excessive eating

polysomnography (paw-lee-som-NAH-gra-fee) recording multiple aspects of sleep

polyuria (PAW-lee-YOO-ree-ah) excessive urination

positron emission tomography (PET) scan (PAWZ-ih-trawn ee-MISH-un taw-MAW-gra-fee) an imaging procedure that uses radiation (positrons) to produce cross-sections of the brain

postictal (post-IK-tal) time after a seizure

postnatal (post-NAY-tal) pertaining to after birth

postpartum (post-PAR-tum) pertaining to after birth

postpartum alopecia (post-PAR-tum al-oh-PEE-shah) baldness experienced by women after a pregnancy

preeclampsia (PREE-eh-KLAMP-see-ah) condition characterized by high blood pressure and high levels of protein in the urine

preictal (pree-IK-tal) time before a seizure

prenatal (pree-NAY-tal) pertaining to before birth

presbycusis (PREZ-bih-KOO-sis) loss of hearing in old age

presbyopia (PREZ-bee-OH-pee-ah) decreased vision caused by old age

priapism (PREE-ap-izm) persistent and painful erection

proctitis (prok-TAI-tis) inflammation of the anus and rectum

proctologist (prok-TAW-loh-jist) specialist in the anus, rectum, and colon

proctology (prok-TAW-loh-jee) branch of medicine dealing with the anus, rectum, and colon

proctoplasty (PROK-toh-PLAS-tee) surgical reconstruction of the anus and rectum

proctoptosis (prok-TOP-toh-sis) downward displacement of the rectum and anus

proctoscope (PROK-toh-skohp) instrument for looking at the anus and rectum

proctoscopy (prok-TAW-skoh-pee) procedure for looking at the anus and rectum

prosopagnosia (PRAW-soh-pag-NOH-zhah) inability to recognize faces

prostatectomy (PROS-tat-TEK-toh-mee) surgical removal of the prostate

prostatitis (PROS-tah-TAI-tis) inflammation of the prostate

prostatocystitis (PROS-ta-toh-sis-TAI-tis) inflammation of the prostate and bladder

prostatolith (pros-TAT-oh-lith) a stone in the prostate

prostatolithotomy (PROS-TAT-oh-lih-THAW-toh-mee) incision into a prostate to remove a stone

prostatomegaly (PROS-ta-toh-MEH-gah-lee) abnormal enlargement of the prostate

prostatorrhea (PROS-ta-toh-REE-ah) discharge from the prostate

prostatovesiculectomy (pros-TAT-oh-veh-SIK-yoo-LEK-toh-mee) surgical removal of the prostate and seminal vesicles

prostatovesiculitis (PROS-ta-toh-veh-SIK-yoo-LAI-tis) inflammation of the prostate and seminal vesicles

prosthesis (pros-THEE-sis) a device that is added to a body to replace a missing part or lost function

pruritus (prur-AI-tis) from Latin, for *burning nettle;* swollen, raised, itchy areas of the skin

pseudocyesis (SOO-doh-sai-EE-sis) false pregnancy

pseudoesthesia (SOO-des-THEE-zhah) false sensation

psychiatrist (sai-KAI-ah-trist) doctor who specializes in treatment of the mind

psychiatry (sai-KAI-ah-tree) branch of medicine that focuses on the treatment of the mind

psychogenic (SAI-koh-JIN-ik) originating in/created by the mind

psychologist (sai-KAW-loh-jist) doctor who specializes in the study of the mind

psychology (sai-KAW-loh-jee) branch of medicine that focuses on the study of the mind

psychopathy (sai-KAW-pah-thee) a mental illness

psychopharmacology (SAI-koh-FAR-mah-KAW-loh-jee) the study of the effects of drugs on mental processes

psychosis (sai-KOH-sis) a mind condition (involves some sort of break with reality interfering with rational thought or daily functioning)

psychosomatic (SAI-koh-soh-MA-tik) pertaining to the relationship between the body and the mind

psychotropic (SAI-koh-TROH-pik) drugs that are able to turn the mind

pterygium (ter-IH-jee-um) winglike growth of conjunctival tissue extending to the cornea (from Greek, for *wing*)

pulmonary angiography (pul-mon-AIR-ee an-jee-O-grah-fee) an imaging procedure for recording pulmonary blood vessel activity

pulmonary circulation (PUL-mon-AIR-ee SIR-kyoo-LAY-shun) circulation of blood from the heart to the lungs

pulmonary edema (pul-mon-AIR-ee ah-DEE-ma) swelling in the lungs

pulmonary embolism (pul-mon-AIR-ee em-bol-IZ-um) blockage in the pulmonary blood supply

pulmonary function testing (pul-mon-AIR-ee funk-shun TES-ting) a group of tests used to evaluate the condition of the lungs

pulmonary neoplasm (pul-mon-AIR-ee nee-oh-PLAZ-sum) new growth (tumor) in the lung

pustule (PUS-tyool) from Latin, for *little blister;* a pus-filled blister

pyarthrosis (pai-ar-THROH-sis) pus in a joint

pyelitis (PAI-el-AI-tis) inflammation of the renal pelvis

pyelocystitis (PAI-el-oh-sis-TAI-tis) inflammation of the renal pelvis and bladder

pyelocystostomosis (PAI-el-oh-SIS-toh-staw-MOH-sis) creation of an opening between the renal pelvis and bladder

pyelogram (PAI-el-oh-GRAM) image of the renal pelvis

pyelolithotomy (PAI-el-oh-lih-THAW-toh-mee) incision into a renal pelvis to remove a stone

pyelonephritis (PAI-el-oh-neh-FRAI-tis) inflammation of the kidney and renal pelvis

pyelopathy (PAI-el-AW-pah-thee) disease of the renal pelvis

pyeloplasty (PAI-el-oh-PLAS-tee) surgical reconstruction of a renal pelvis

pyelostomy (PAI-el-AW-stoh-mee) creation of an opening in a renal pelvis

pyelotomy (PAI-el-AW-toh-mee) incision into a renal pelvis

pyeloureterectasia (PAI-el-oh-yoo-REE-ter-ek-TAY-zhah) dilation of the renal pelvis and ureter

pyloric stenosis (PAI-lor-ik steh-NOH-sis) narrowing of the sphincter at the base of the stomach

pyonephritis (PAI-oh-neh-FRAI-tis) inflammation of the kidney caused by pus

pyonephrolithiasis (PAI-oh-NEH-froh-lih-THAI-ah-sis) the presence of pus and stones in the kidney

pyopyeloectasis (PAI-oh-PAI-el-oh-EK-tah-sis) pus in a dilated renal pelvis

pyosalpinx (PAI-oh-SAL-pinks) blockage in a fallopian tube caused by pus

pyothorax (pai-oh-THOR-aks) pus in the chest

pyromania (PAI-roh-MAY-nee-ah) desire to set fires

pyuria (pai-YUR-ee-ah) pus in the urine

R

rectalgia (rek-TAL-jah) rectum pain

rectitis (rek-TAI-tis) inflammation of the rectum

rectocele (REK-toh-seel) hernia or protrusion of the rectum into the vagina

rectopexy (REK-toh-PEK-see) surgical fixation of the rectum

regional anesthetic (REE-jih-nal an-es-THET-ik) anesthetic that is injected into a nerve causing loss of sensation over a particular area

renal angiogram (REE-nal AN-jee-oh-GRAM) image of a kidney blood vessel

renal angiography (REE-nal AN-jee-AW-grah-fee) process of imaging a kidney blood vessel

renal angioplasty (REE-nal AN-jee-oh-PLAS-tee) surgical reconstruction of a kidney blood vessel

renal arteriogram (REE-nal ar-TER-ee-oh-GRAM) image of a kidney artery

renal cell carcinoma (REE-nal SELL KAR-sih-NOH-mah) cancer of the kidneys; also known as *hypernephroma*

renal failure (REE-nal FAY-el-yur) kidney failure

renal ischemia (REE-nal ih-SKEE-mee-ah) deficiency of blood in a kidney

reperfusion injury (REE-pir-FYOO-zhun IN-jir-ee) injury to tissue that occurs after blood flow is restored

resectoscope (rih-SEK-toh-SKOHP) instrument for examining and cutting (usually the prostate)

restrictive cardiomyopathy (ree-STRIK-tiv KAR-dee-oh-mai-AW-pah-thee) heart muscle hardens, restricting the expansion of the heart and thus limiting the amount of blood it can pump to the rest of the body

restrictive lung disorder (re-STRIKT-iv) a lung disorder caused by the limiting of air into the lungs

reticulocyte (reh-TIK-yoo-loh-SAIT) immature red blood cell

retinal (REH-tih-nal) pertaining to the retina

retinitis (REH-tih-NAI-tis) inflammation of the retina

retinopathy (REH-tih-NOP-ah-thee) disease of the retina

retinopexy (reh-TIH-noh-PEK-see) surgical fixation (reattachment) of a retina

retinoscope (RET-in-aw-SKOP) instrument for looking at the retina

retinoscopy (RET-in-AWS-koh-pee) procedure for looking at the retina

retinosis (REH-tih-NOH-sis) retinal condition

retinotomy (REH-tih-NAW-toh-mee) incision into the retina

retrograde pyelogram (REH-troh-grayd PAI-el-oh-GRAM) image of the renal pelvis produced by injecting a contrast dye from the bladder to the kidney

rheumatoid arthritis (ROO-mah-toyd ar-THRAI-tis) inflammation of the joint; called rheumatoid because its symptoms resemble those of rheumatic fever

rhinitis (rai-NAI-tis) inflammation of the nasal passages

rhinorrhagia (rai-no-RAY-jah) excessive blood flow from the nose (another term for nosebleed)

rhinorrhea (rai-no-REE-yah) runny nose

rhinosalpingitis (RAI-noh-SAL-pin-JAI-tis) inflammation of the nose and eustachian tubes

rhytidoplasty (rih-tih-doh-PLAS-tee) reconstruction of wrinkled skin

S

salpingectomy (SAL-pin-JEK-toh-mee) surgical removal of a fallopian tube

salpingitis (SAL-pin-JAI-tis) inflammation of a fallopian tube

salpingocyesis (sal-PING-goh-sai-EE-sis) ectopic pregnancy in a fallopian tube

salpingo-oophorectomy (sal-PING-goh-OH-aw-for-EK-toh-mee) surgical removal of a fallopian tube and ovary

salpingocele (sal-PING-goh-seel) hernia of a fallopian tube

salpingo-oophoritis (sal-PING-goh-OH-aw-for-AI-tis) inflammation of a fallopian tube and ovary

salpingopexy (sal-PING-goh-PEK-see) surgical fixation of a fallopian tube

salpingopharyngeal (sal-PING-goh-fah-RIN-jee-al) pertaining to the eustachian tubes and the throat

salpingoscope (sal-PING-goh-skohp) instrument for looking at the eustachian tubes

scale (SKAYL) skin flaking off

schizophrenia (SKIT-zoh-FREH-nee-ah) a mental illness characterized by delusions, hallucinations, and disordered speech

sclerectasia (SKLER-ek-TAY-zhah) overexpansion of the sclera

sclerodermatitis (skleh-roh-der-mah-TAI-tis) inflammation of the skin accompanied by thickening and hardening

scleroiritis (SKLER-oh-ai-RAI-tis) inflammation of the sclera and iris

sclerokeratitis (SKLER-oh-KEH-rah-TAI-tis) inflammation of the sclera and cornea

sclerokeratoiritis (SKLER-oh-KEH-ra-toh-ai-RAI-tis) inflammation of the sclera, cornea, and iris

scleromalacia (SKLEH-roh-mah-LAY-shah) abnormal softening of the sclera

scleronychia (skleh-raw-NIH-kee-ah) thickening and hardening of the nails

sclerosing cholangitis (skleh-ROH-sing KOH-lan-JAI-tis) inflammation and hardening of the bile vessels (ducts)

sclerotomy (skler-AW-toh-mee) incision into the sclera

scoliosis (SKOH-lee-OH-sis) crooked back, or abnormal lateral curvature of the spine

scotoma (skaw-TOH-mah) dark spot in the visual field

scotopia (skaw-TOH-pee-ah) the adjustment of the eye to seeing in darkness

seborrheic dermatitis (se-boh-RAY-ik der-mah-TAI-tis) inflammation of the skin caused by the discharge of oil (sebum)

seminoma (SEM-oh-NOH-mah) type of testicular cancer arising from sperm-forming tissue

sensorineural hearing loss (SEN-sor-ee-NIR-al) sound is not transmitted from the inner ear to the brain (due to problems with the sense organs or nerves)

septic arthritis (SEP-tik ar-THRAI-tis) inflammation of the joint caused by infection

septicemia (SEP-tih-SEE-mee-ah) presence of disease-causing microorganisms in the blood

septoplasty (sep-toe-PLAS-tee) reconstruction of a septum

sialagogic (sai-AL-ah-GAW-jik) agent that causes salivation

sialoadenectomy (sai-AL-oh-AD-en-EK-toh-mee) surgical removal of a salivary gland

sialoadenitis (sai-AL-oh-AD-en-AI-tis) inflammation of the salivary glands

sialoadenosis (sai-AL-oh-AD-en-OH-sis) condition of the salivary glands

sialoangiectasis (SAI-ah-loh-AN-jee-EK-tah-sis) overexpansion of the salivary vessels

sialolith (sai-AL-oh-lith) stone in the saliva

sialolithiasis (sai-AL-oh-lih-THAI-ah-sis) presence of salivary stones

sialolithotomy (sai-AL-oh-lih-THAW-toh-mee) incision to removal salivary stones

sialorrhea (SAI-ah-loh-REE-ah) excessive salivation

sialostenosis (SAI-ah-loh-steh-NOH-sis) narrowing of the salivary glands

sigmoidoscope (sig-MOY-doh-skohp) instrument for looking at the sigmoid colon

sigmoidoscopy (sig-moy-DAW-skoh-pee) procedure for looking at the sigmoid colon

sinusitis (sai-nus-AI-tis) inflammation of the sinus

sleep apnea (sleep AP-nee-ah) a condition where the patient ceases to breathe while asleep

somnambulism (sawm-NAM-byoo-liz-um) sleep walking

sonography (saw-NAW-grah-fee) use of sound waves to produce diagnostic images; also called an ultrasound

sonohysterography (SOH-noh-HIS-ter-AW-grah-fee) procedure using sound waves to examine the uterus

speculum (SPEH-kyoo-lum) device for examining a body cavity, most commonly the vagina

spermatocele (sper-MAT-oh-SEEL) hernia or distention of the epididymis caused by sperm cells

spermatogenesis (sper-MAT-oh-JIN-eh-sis) creation of sperm

spermatolysis (SPER-mah-TAW-lih-sis) destruction of sperm cells

spermicide (SPER-mih-sahyd) agent that kills sperm

spermolytic (SPER-moh-LIH-tik) agent that kills sperm

spherocyte (SFEE-roh-SAIT) red blood cell that assumes a spherical shape

spherocytosis (SFEER-oh-sai-TOH-sis) condition in which red blood cells assume a spherical shape

sphygmomanometer (SFIG-moh-mah-NAW-meh-ter) fancy name for the device used to measure blood pressure

spider angioma see *telangiectasia*

spinal stenosis (SPAI-nal stih-NOH-sis) abnormal narrowing of the spine

spirometry (speer-O-me-tree) a procedure to measure breathing

splenalgia (splee-NAL-jah) pain in the spleen

splenectomy (spleh-NEK-toh-mee) surgical removal of the spleen

splenectopy (splee-NEK-toh-pee) displacement of the spleen, sometimes called floating spleen

splenitis (splee-NAI-tis) inflammation of the spleen

splenodynia (SPLEE-noh-DAI-nee-ah) pain in the spleen

splenolysis (splee-NAW-lih-sis) breakdown (destruction) of spleen tissue

splenomalacia (SPLEE-noh-mah-LAY-shah) softening of the spleen

splenomegaly (SPLEE-noh-MEH-gah-lee) enlargement of the spleen

splenopathy (splee-NAW-pah-thee) any disease of the spleen

splenoptosis (SPLEE-nawp-TOH-sis) downward displacement (drooping) of the spleen

splenorrhexis (SPLEE-noh-REK-sis) rupture of the spleen

spondylitis (spawn-dih-LAI-tis) inflammation of the vertebra

spondyloarthropathy (SPAWN-dih-loh-ar-THRAW-pah-thee) joint disease of the vertebrae

spondylodynia (spawn-dih-loh-DAI-nee-ah) vertebra pain

spondylolisthesis (SPAWN-dih-loh-lis-THEE-sis) the slipping or dislocation of a vertebra

spondylolysis (SPAWN-dih-LO-li-sis) loss of vertebra structure

spondylomalacia (spawn-dih-loh-mah-LAY-shah) softening of the vertebra

spondylosis (SPAWN-dih-LOH-sis) vertebra condition

spondylosyndesis (SPAWN-dih-loh-sin-DEE-sis) fusing together of multiple vertebrae

spontaneous abortion (spawn-TAY-nee-is ah-BOR-shun) the naturally occurring termination of pregnancy; also known as a miscarriage.

sputum (SPYOO-tum) mucus discharged from the lungs by coughing

squamous cell carcinoma (SKWAY-mus sell kar-sih-NO-mah) cancerous tumor of squamous skin cells

steatitis (stay-ah-TAI-tis) inflammation of fat tissue

steatoma (STAY-ah-TOH-ma) a fatty tumor

steatorrhea (STAY-at-oh-REE-ah) excessive fat discharged in the feces

sternotomy (stir-NAW-toh-mee) incision into the sternum

stomatitis (STOH-mah-TAI-tis) inflammation of the mouth

stomatodynia (stoh-MAT-oh-DAI-nee-ah) mouth pain

stomatogastric (stoh-MAT-oh-GAS-trik) pertaining to the mouth and stomach

stomatomycosis (stoh-MAT-oh-mai-KOH-sis) fungus condition of the mouth

stomatoplasty (stoh-MAT-oh-PLAS-tee) surgical reconstruction of the mouth

stomatosis (STOH-mah-TOH-sis) mouth condition

strabismus (struh-BIZ-mus) condition where the eyes deviate when looking at the same object (from Latin, for *to squint*)

stress electrocardiogram (stres eh-LEK-troh-KAR-dee-oh-GRAM) image of the heart produced using sound waves while the patient experiences increases of exercise stress

stress urinary incontinence (SUI) (stress YUR-ih-NAR-ee in-CON-tih-nentz) loss of bladder control caused by the application of external pressure

stroke (STROHK) loss of brain function caused by interruption of blood flow/supply to the brain

subcutaneous (sub-kyoo-TAY-nee-us) pertaining to beneath the skin

subdural hematoma (sub-DIR-al HEE-mah-TOH-mah) a hematoma located beneath the dura

subluxation (sub-luk-SAY-shun) partial dislocation of a joint

superior vena cava (soo-PEER-ee-or VEE-nah CAY-vah) portion of the vena cava that gathers blood from the upper portion of the body (head and arms)

syncope (SIN-koh-pee) fainting; losing consciousness due to temporary loss of blood flow to the brain

syndactyly (sin-DAK-tih-lee) fusion (sometimes called webbing) of fingers or toes

synesthesia (SIN-es-THEE-zhah) condition where one sensation is experienced as another

systemic circulation (sih-STEM-ik SIR-kyoo-LAY-shun) circulation of blood from the heart to the rest of the body

systolic pressure (sih-STAW-lik PRESH-ir) pressure exerted on blood vessels when the heart is contracting

T

tachycardia (TAK-ih-KAR-dee-ah) rapid heartbeat

tachypnea (ta-KIP-nee-yah) rapid breathing

tardive dyskinesia (TAR-div DIS-kin-EE-zhah) condition characterized by the loss of muscle control

tarsectomy (tar-SEK-toh-mee) removal of all or a portion of the ankle

tarsoclasia (TAR-soh-KLAY-zhah) the surgical fracture of the ankle (i.e., to treat clubfoot)

tarsoptosis (tar-sawp-TOH-sis) flat feet

telangiectasia (tel-an-jee-ek-TAY-zhuh) the overexpansion of the blood vessel, sometimes called a spider angioma because of how it looks on the skin

tenalgia (ten-AL-jah) tendon pain

tendectomy (ten-DEK-toh-mee) removal of a tendon

tendonitis (TEN-dah-NAI-tis) tendon inflammation

tendoplasty (TEN-doh-PLAS-tee) reconstruction of a tendon

tenodesis (TEN-oh-DEE-sis) binding of a tendon

tenolysis (ten-AW-lih-sis) freeing/loosening a tendon

tenonectomy (TEN-oh-NEK-toh-mee) removal of a tendon

tenoplasty (TEN-oh-PLAS-tee) reconstruction of a tendon

tenorrhaphy (ten-OR-ah-fee) suture of a tendon

tenotomy (ten-AW-toh-mee) incision into a tendon

teratogenic (TER-ah-toh-JIN-ik) causing the formation of birth defects

teratology (TER-ah-TAW-loh-jee) branch of medicine dealing with the study of birth defects and their causes

teratoma (TER-ah-TOH-mah) see *dermoid cyst*

testicular carcinoma (tes-TIK-yoo-lar KAR-sih-NOH-mah) testicular cancer

testitis (tes-TAI-tis) inflammation of the testicles and epididymis

thelarche (thee-LAR-kay) beginning of breast development

thoracalgia (thor-a-KAL-jah) chest pain

thoracentesis (thor-a-sin-TEE-sis) puncture of the chest

thoracocentesis (thor-a-koh-sin-TEE-sis) puncture of the chest

thoracoplasty (thor-a-koh-PLAS-tee) reconstruction of the chest

thoracoscopy (thor-a-KOS-koh-pee) examination of the chest

thoracostomy (thor-a-KOS-toe-mee) creation of an opening in the chest

thoracotomy (thor-a-KAH-toe-mee) incision into the chest

thrombocyte (THROM-boh-sait) cell that helps blood clot (also known as a platelet)

thrombocytopenia (THROM-boh-SAI-toh-PEE-nee-ah) deficiency in the number of platelets (clot cells)

thrombocytosis (THROM-boh-sai-TOH-sis) increase in the number of platelets (clot cells)

thromboembolism (THROM-boh-EM-boh-LIZ-um) blockage of a vessel (embolism) caused by a clot that has broken off from where it formed

thrombogenic (THROM-boh-JIN-ik) capable of producing a blood clot

thrombolytic (THROM-boh-LIH-tik) drug that breaks down blood clots

thrombophlebitis (THROM-boh-fleh-BAI-tis) inflammation of a vein caused by a clot

thrombosis (throm-BOH-sis) formation of a blood clot

thrombus (THROM-bus) blood clot

thymectomy (thai-MEK-toh-mee) surgical removal of the thymus

thymic hyperplasia (THAI-mik HAI-per-PLAY-zhah) overdevelopment of the thymus

thymoma (thai-MOH-mah) tumor of the thymus

thymopathy (thai-MAW-pah-thee) disease of the thymus

thyrocele (THAI-roh-seel) see *goiter*

thyroid function tests (THAI-roid FUNK-shun TESTS) tests performed to evaluate the function of the thyroid

thyroidectomy (THAI-roid-EK-toh-mee) removal of the thyroid

thyroiditis (THAI-roid-AI-tis) inflammation of the thyroid

thyroidotomy (THAI-roid-AW-toh-mee) incision into the thyroid

thyroidotoxin (thai-ROI-doh-TOK-sin) substance poisonous to the thyroid gland

thyromegaly (THAI-roh-MEH-gah-lee) enlargement of the thyroid

thyroparathyroidectomy (THAI-roh-PAR-ah-THAI-roid-EK-toh-me) removal of the thyroid and parathyroid glands

thyroptosis (THAI-rop-TOH-sis) downward displacement (drooping) of the thyroid

thyrotoxicosis (THAI-roh-TOKS-ih-KOH-sis) condition caused by the exposure of body tissue to excessive levels of thyroid hormone (an extreme version of this is known as "thyroid storm")

thyrotropin (THAI-roh-TROH-pin) hormone that stimulates the thyroid

tibialgia (tih-bee-AL-ja) tibia (shin) pain

tinnitus (tih-NAI-tis) ringing in the ears (from Latin, for *to ring* or *jingle*)

tocodynagraph (TOH-koh-DAI-nah-GRAF) instrument for recording the strength of labor contractions

tocography (toh-KAW-grah-fee) procedure for recording the strength of labor contractions

tocolytic (TOH-koh-LIH-tik) agent that stops or delays premature labor and contractions

tonic (TAW-nik) pertaining to muscle tone (normally weak or unresponsive)

tonic-clonic seizure (TAW-nik CLAH-nik SEE-zhir) a seizure characterized by both a tonic and a clonic phase

tonometer (TOH-naw-MEE-tir) instrument for measuring tension or pressure in the eye (intraocular pressure)

tonsillectomy (TON-sil-EK-toh-mee) surgical removal of a tonsil

tonsillitis (TON-sil-AI-tis) inflammation of a tonsil

topical anesthetic (TAW-pih-kal an-es-THET-ik) local anesthesia applied to the surface of the area to be anesthetized

tracheitis (tray-kee-AI-tis) inflammation of the trachea

tracheomalacia (tray-kee-oh-ma-LAY-shah) softening of the trachea

tracheostenosis (tray-kee-oh-sten-OH-sis) narrowing of the trachea

tracheostomy (tray-kee-AH-stoh-mee) creation of an opening in the trachea

tracheotomy (tray-kee-AH-toe-mee) incision into the trachea

transcranial Doppler sonography (tranz-KRAY-nee-al DAW-plir saw-NAW-gra-fee) an imaging technique that produces an image of the brain using sound waves sent through the skull

transdermal (trans-DER-mal) pertaining to through the skin

transesophageal electrocardiogram (TRANZ-eh-SOF-ah-JEE-al EK-oh-KAR-dee-oh-GRAM) record of the heart using sound waves performed by inserting the sonograph into the esophagus

transfusion (tranz-FYOO-zhun) infusion into a patient of blood from another source

transient ischemic attack (TIA) (TRAN-zee-ent ih-SKEE-mik ah-TAK) a mini-stroke caused by the blockage of a blood vessel that resolves (goes away) within 24 hours

transrectal ultrasonography (TRANZ-REK-tal UL-trah-soh-NAW-grah-fee) procedure involving a probe inserted into the rectum using high-frequency sound waves to scan through the rectum to nearby tissue (most commonly, the prostate)

transurethral resection of the prostate (TURP) (TRANS-yoo-REE-thral ree-SEK-shun of the PROS-tayt) procedure of removing all or part of the prostate by the insertion of a resectoscope into the urethra

transvaginal sonography (TRANZ-VAJ-ih-nal soh-NAW-grah-fee) imaging procedure using sound waves emitted from device inserted in the vagina

trichiasis (trih-KAI-ah-sis) condition caused by eyelashes growing backward and coming in contact with the eye

trichomycosis (trik-koh-mai-KOH-sis) a fungal condition of the hair

tumor (TOO-mur) a larger solid mass

tympanic perforation (tim-PAN-ik per-fer-AY-shun) tear or hole in the eardrum

tympanocentesis (tim-PAN-oh-sin-TEE-sis) puncture of the eardrum

tympanolabyrinthopexy (tim-PAN-oh-lab-uh-rinth-oh-PEK-see) surgical fixation of the eardrum to the labyrinth

tympanometry (tim-pan-AW-meh-tree) procedure for measuring the eardrum

tympanoplasty (tim-PAN-oh-PLAS-tee) surgical reconstruction of the eardrum

tympanosclerosis (tim-PAN-oh-skleh-ROH-sis) hardening of the eardrum

tympanostomy (TIM-pan-AW-stoh-mee) creation of an opening in the eardrum

U

ulcer (UL-sir) from Latin, for *sore;* a sore

ultrasonography (UL-trah-soh-NAW-grah-fee) imaging procedure using high-frequency sound waves

umbilical (um-BIL-ih-kal) middle center portion of the abdomen

uremia (yoo-REE-mee-ah) presence of urinary waste in the blood

ureteralgia (yur-EE-ter-AL-jah) pain in the ureter

ureteritis (yoo-REE-ter-AI-tis) inflammation of a ureter

ureterocele (yoo-REE-ter-oh-SEEL) hernia of the ureter

ureteroileostomy (yoo-REE-ter-oh-IL-ee-AW-stoh-mee) creation of an opening between a ureter and the ileum, a portion of the small intestine

ureterolithiasis (yoo-REE-ter-oh-lih-THAI-ah-sis) presence of stones in a ureter

ureteronephrectomy (yoo-REE-ter-oh-neh-FREK-toh-mee) surgical removal of a kidney and ureter

ureteroplasty (yoo-REE-ter-oh-PLAS-tee) surgical reconstruction of a ureter

ureteropyelitis (yoo-REE-ter-oh-PAI-el-AI-tis) inflammation of a ureter and renal pelvis

ureteropyelonephritis (yoo-REE-ter-oh-PAI-el-oh-neh-FRAI-tis) inflammation of a kidney, renal pelvis, and ureter

ureterorrhaphy (yoo-REE-ter-OR-ah-fee) suture of the ureter

ureteroscopy (yoo-REE-ter-AW-skoh-pee) process of examining a ureter

ureterostenosis (yoo-REE-ter-oh-steh-NOH-sis) narrowing of a ureter

urethrectomy (yoo-ree-THREK-toh-mee) surgical removal of the urethra

urethritis (yoo-ree-THRAI-tis) inflammation of the urethra

urethrocele (yoo-REE-throh-seel) hernia or prolapse of the urethra into the vagina

urethrocystitis (yoo-REE-throh-sis-TAI-tis) inflammation of the urethra and bladder

urethrodynia (yoo-REE-throh-DAI-nee-ah) pain in the urethra

urethrogram (yoo-REE-throh-GRAM) image of the urethra

urethropexy (yoo-REE-throh-PEK-see) surgical fixation of the urethra

urethroplasty (yoo-REE-throh-PLAS-tee) surgical reconstruction of the urethra

urethrorrhea (yoo-REE-throh-REE-ah) discharge from the urethra

urethroscope (yoo-REE-throh-SKOHP) instrument for examining the urethra

urethroscopy (yoo-ree-THRAW-skoh-pee) process of examining the urethra

urethrospasm (yoo-REE-throh-SPAZ-um) involuntary contraction of the urethra

urethrostenosis (yoo-REE-throh-steh-NOH-sis) narrowing of the urethra

urethrotomy (yoo-ree-THRAW-toh-mee) incision into the urethra

urinalysis (YUR-ih-NAL-ih-sis) analysis of the urine

urinary catheterization (YUR-ih-NAR-ee KATH-eh-ter-ih-ZAY-shun) insertion of a catheter into the bladder to drain urine

urinary tract infection (UTI) (YUR-ih-NAR-ee trakt in-FEK-shun) infection of the urinary tract

urocyanosis (YUR-oh-SAI-ah-NOH-sis) blue urine

urodynia (YUR-oh-DAI-nee-ah) painful urination

urologist (yur-AW-loh-jist) specialist in the urinary tract

urology (yur-AW-loh-jee) study of the urinary tract

uropathy (yur-AW-pah-thee) disease of the urinary tract

uropoesis (YUR-oh-poh-EE-sis) formation of urine

urostomy (yur-AW-stoh-mee) creation of an opening in the urinary tract, normally to divert urine flow away from a diseased bladder

uroxanthin (YUR-oh-ZAN-thin) substance in urine that makes it yellow

uterine prolapse (YOO-ter-in PROH-laps) downward displacement of the uterus into the vagina

V

vaginitis (VAJ-ih-NAI-tis) inflammation of the vagina

vaginodynia (VAJ-ih-noh-DAI-nee-ah) vaginal pain

vaginomycosis (VAJ-ih-noh-MAI-koh-sis) fungal condition of the vagina

vaginoperineoplasty (VAJ-ih-noh-PER-ih-NEE-oh-PLAS-tee) suture of the vagina and perineum

vaginoperineorrhaphy (VAJ-ih-noh-PER-ih-nee-OR-ah-fee) suture of the vagina and perineum

vaginoperineotomy (VAJ-ih-noh-PER-ih-nee-AW-toh-mee) incision into the vagina and perineum

vaginoplasty (vah-JI-noh-PLAS-tee) surgical reconstruction of the vagina

vaginoscope (VAJ-ih-noh-SKOHP) instrument used to examine the vagina

vaginosis (VAJ-ih-NOH-sis) condition of the vagina

valvectomy (val-VEK-toh-mee) surgical removal of a heart valve

valvotomy (val-VAW-toh-mee) incision into a heart valve

valvulitis (VAL-vyoo-LAI-tis) inflammation of a heart valve

valvuloplasty (VAL-vyoo-loh-PLAS-tee) surgical reconstruction of a heart valve

varicocele (VAR-ih-koh-SEEL) overexpansion of the blood vessels of the testicles, leading to a soft tumor

varicose veins (VAR-ih-kohs VAYNS) enlarged, dilated vein toward the surface of the skin

varicotomy (VAR-ih-KAW-toh-mee) surgical removal of a varicose vein

vas deferens (VAS DEH-frenz) vessel carrying sperm from the testicles

vascular endoscopy (VAS-kyoo-lar en-DAW-skoh-pee) procedure to look inside a blood vessel

vascular lesion (VAS-kyoo-lar LEE-zhun) wounds related to blood vessels

vasculitis (VAS-kyoo-LAI-tis) inflammation of blood vessels

vasectomy (vah-SEK-toh-mee) surgical removal of the vas deferens

vasoconstrictor (VAS-oh-kin-STRIK-tor) drug that constricts or narrows the diameter of a blood vessel

vasodilator (VAS-oh-DAI-lay-tor) drug that causes the relaxation or expansion of a blood vessel

vasopressor (VAS-oh-PRES-or) drug that constricts or narrows the diameter of a blood vessel

vasospasm (VAS-oh-SPAZ-um) involuntary contraction of a blood vessel

vasovasostomy (VAS-oh-vah-SAW-stoh-mee) creation of an opening between two vessels; technical term for a vasectomy reversal

vena cava (VEE-nah CAY-vah) large-diameter vein that gathers blood from the body and returns it to the heart

venectomy (vee-NEK-toh-mee) surgical removal of a vein

venogram (VEE-noh-gram) record of a vein

venosclerosis (VEE-noh-skleh-ROH-sis) hardening of a vein

venospasm (VEE-noh-SPAZ-um) involuntary contraction of a vein

venostasis (VEE-noh-STA-sis) trapping of blood in an extremity due to compression

ventilation–perfusion scan (ven-ti-LAY-shun–per-FYOO-shun skan) a scan that tests whether a problem in the lungs is caused by airflow (ventilation) or blood flow (perfusion)

ventricular septal defect (VSD) (ven-TRIK-yoo-lar SEP-tal DEE-fekt) defectflaw in the septum that divides the two ventricles of the heart

ventriculotomy (ven-TRIK-yoo-LAW-toh-mee) incision into a ventricle

vertigo (VER-tih-goh) sensation of moving through space (while stationary); from Latin, for *to whirl around*

verucca (vah-ROO-kah) from Latin, for *wart;* a wart

vesicle (VEH-sih-kul) from Latin, for *little bladder;* a small blister

vesicocele (VES-ih-koh-SEEL) hernia of the bladder

vesicostomy (VEH-sih-KAW-stoh-mee) creation of an opening in the bladder

vesicotomy (VEH-sih-KAW-toh-mee) incision into the bladder

vesicoureteral reflux (VUR) (VES-ih-koh-yoo-REE-ter-al REE-fluks) abnormal flow of urine from the bladder back into the ureters

vesicovaginal fistula (VES-ih-koh-VAJ-ih-nal FIS-tyoo-lah) abnormal opening between the urinary bladder and the vagina

vesiculectomy (veh-SIK-yoo-LEK-toh-mee) surgical removal of the seminal vesicles

vestibular neuritis (ves-TIH-byoo-lar nir-AI-tis) inflammation of the vestibular nerve

vestibulitis (ves-TIH-byoo-LAI-tis) inflammation of the vestibule

vestibulotomy (ves-TIH-byoo-LAW-toh-mee) incision into the vestibule

vitiligo (vih-tih-LAI-goh) see *patch*

vitrectomy (vih-TREK-toh-mee) the removal of the vitreous liquid from the eye

voiding (VOI-ding) another term for urination

voiding cystourethrogram (VOI-ding SIS-toh-yoo-REE-throh-GRAM) imaging procedure of the bladder and urethra produced during urination

vulvitis (vul-VAI-tis) inflammation of the vulva

vulvodynia (VUL-voh-DAI-nee-ah) pain in the vulva

vulvovaginitis (VUL-voh-VAJ-ih-NAI-tis) inflammation of the vulva and vagina

X

xanthoderma (zan-thoh-DER-mah) yellow skin

xanthoma (zan-THOH-mah) a yellow tumor

xanthosis (zan-THOH-sis) yellowing of the skin

xenograft (ZEE-noh-graft) see *heterograft*

xeroderma (zeh-roh-DER-mah) dry skin

xerophthalmia (ZER-off-THAL-mee-ah) dry eyes

xerosis (ze-ROH-sis) condition of dryness

PHOTO CREDITS

PREFACE

p. iv(top): © AbleStock.com/360/GettyImages; iv(bottom): © JGI/Daniel Grill/Blend Images/Getty Images RF; p. v: © Larry Williams/Blend Images/Corbis RF; p. vi(top): © Adrian Green/Photographer's Choice/Getty Images; p. vii(top): © Fotosearch/Getty Images RF; vii(bottom): © Steve Gschmeissner/Science Source; p. viii(top): © Eye of Science/Science Source; vii(bottom): © Mike Kemp/Getty Images RF; p. ix(top): © Photodisc/B2M Productions/Getty Images RF; p. ix(bottom): © Stockbyte/Visage/Getty Images RF; p. x(top): © Asia selects/Getty Images RF; p. x(bottom): © Larry Williams/Comet/Corbis; xv(Subjective): © Feliz Aggelos/Photodisc/Getty Images RF; p. xv(Objective): © OJO Images/Getty Images RF; p. xv(Assessment): © Image Source/Getty Images RF; p. xv(Plan): © Zephyr/Science Source; p. xv(heath record): © CNRI/Science Source.

ABOUT THE AUTHORS

Steve L Jones, PhD

p. xii(top left and bottom) © Tamber Jones; (top right): © Mike Tims, HBU University Photographer

Andrew Cavanagh, MD

p. xii(top left) © Shelly Basaldu/Austin Regional Clinic; (top right and bottom) © Andy Cavanagh

A Note from the Authors On Why They Wrote This Book

p. xiii: Photo courtesy of the authors

CHAPTER 1

Opener(left): © AbleStock.com/360/Getty Images; Opener(right): © Adie Bush/Cultura/Getty Images RF; p. 2(left): © Jupiterimages/Comstock Images/Getty Images RF; p. 2(right): © Brooklyn Production/Corbis RF; p. 3: © Getty Images/OJO Images RF; p. 5: © Digital Vision/Punchstock RF; p. 7: © S. Olsson/PhotoAlto RF; p. 13(angi/o): © BioPhoto Assoc./Science Source; p. 14: © Comstock Images RF; p. 14: © Scott Camazine/Science Source; p. 16(pediatrics): © Jose Luis Pelaez Inc/Blend Images LLC RF; p. 16(psychologist): © Don Hammond/Design Pics RF; p. 16(leukemia): © Science Photo Library RF/Getty Images RF; p. 17(melanoma): Public Domain National Cancer Institute (NCI); p. 17(cardiogram): © Stockbyte/PunchStock RF; p. 19: © Bob Coyle/McGraw-Hill Education; p. 20: © Jupiterimages/Imagesource RF; p. 21: © Goodshoot/Punchstock RF.

CHAPTER 2

Opener(top): © JGI/Daniel Grill/Blend Images/Getty Images RF; Opener(bottom): © Creatas/PunchStock RF; p. 54: © Ocean/Corbis RF; p. 57: © F. Schussler/PhotoLink/Getty Images RF; p. 74(Dr. appoint): © Terry Vine/Blend Images LLC RF; p. 74(files): © Antenna/fstop/Getty Images RF; p. 74(feet): © Royalty Free/Digital Stock/Corbis RF; p. 74(Doctor): © Tim Pannell/Corbis RF; p. 77: © EyeWire/Getty Images RF; p. 79: © Getty Images/OJO Images RF; p. 82: © Creatas/PunchStock RF; p. 88: © Joe DeGrandis/McGraw-Hill Education RF; p. 91: © Dynamic Graphics/Jupiter Images RF; p. 93: © M. Constantini/PhotoAlto RF; p. 98: © Thinkstock/Jupiterimages RF.

CHAPTER 3

Opener(right): © Larry Williams/Blend Images/Corbis RF; p. 121: © Eye of Science/Science Source; p. 122(bottom): Joe DeGrandis/McGraw-Hill Education; p. 123(top): © Scott Kleinman/The Image Bank/Getty Images; p. 123(middle): © SPL/Custom Medical Stock Photo, Inc.; p. 124(top): © Joe DeGrandis/McGraw-Hill Education; p. 124(bottom): © George Clerk/Vetta/Getty Images RF; p. 124: Siede Preis/Photodisc/Getty Images; p. 125(rhino): © Valerie Shaff/Stone/Getty Images; p. 125(elephant): © Dave King/Dorling Kindersley/Getty Images; p. 125(thick): © Ryan McVay/Photodisc/Getty Images RF; p. 125(dry): © Akira Kaede/Photodisc/Getty Images RF; p. 125(wrinkle): © Ingram Publishing RF; p. 126(middle): © Ingram Publishing RF; p. 126(bottom): Centers for Disease Control and Prevention/Public Health Image Library; p. 127(top): © ImageSource/Digital Vision/Getty Images RF; p. 127(middle): © James Stevenson/SPL/Science Source; p. 127(bottom left SEM): © Dennis Strete/McGraw-Hill Education; p. 127(bottom right SEM): © Dennis Strete/McGraw-Hill Education; p. 127(bottom left): Digital Vision/Getty Images; p. 127(bottom right): Caia Image/Glow Images; p. 131: Digital Vision/Getty Images; p. 133(top): © ImageSource/Digital Vision/Getty Images RF; p. 133(middle): © James Darell/Digital Vision/Getty Images RF; p. 137(left): Centers for Disease Control and Prevention/Public Health Image Library; p. 137(right): © Ingram Publishing RF; p. 138(freckle): © Digital Vision/Getty Images RF; p. 138(papule): © McGraw-Hill Education; p. 138(pustule): © McGraw-Hill Education; p. 138(abscess): Centers for Disease Control and Prevention; p. 139(upper): Centers for Disease Control and Prevention/Public Health Image Library; p. 140(top): © James Darell/Digital Vision/Getty Images RF; p. 142(top): © McGraw-Hill Education; p. 147(basal cell): © Dr. P. Marazzi/Science Source; p. 147(squamous cell): © Biophoto Assoc./Science Source; p. 147(malignant): © James Stevenson/Science Source; p. 147(decubitus ulcer): © Medical-on-line/Alamy; p. 148(top): © Medical-on-line/Alamy; p. 148(bottom): © Dr. P. Marazzi/SPL/Photo Researchers, Inc.; p. 149(top): © James Stevenson/Science Source; p. 149(middle): © Biophoto Assoc./Science Source; p. 149(bottom): Centers for Disease Control and Prevention; p. 157(top): © Christopher Kerrigan/McGraw-Hill Education; p. 157(bottom): © Christopher Kerrigan/McGraw-Hill Education; p. 162: © St Bartholomew's Hospital, London/Science Source; p. 165: © Pam Ostrow/Blend Images LLC/Dream Pictures RF.

CHAPTER 4

Opener: © Adrian Green/Photographer's Choice/Getty Images; p. 180(bottom): © Kallista Images/Getty Images; p. 184(top): © Mike Powell/The Image Bank/Getty Images; p. 187(top): © Tetra Images/Corbis; p. 187(bottom): © JW Ramsay/McGraw-Hill Education; p.191: © Feliz Aggelos/Photodisc/Getty Images RF; p. 193: © Fancy Photography/Veer RF; p. 197(top): © OJO Images/Getty Images RF; p. 205(top): © Image Source/Getty Images RF; p. 207(bottom): © Image Source/Getty Images RF; p. 209: © Realistic Reflections RF; p. 214(top): © Zephyr/Science Source; p. 214(bottom): © Mehau Kulyk/Science Source; p. 215(top): © Burazin/Photographer's Choice/Getty Images RF; p. 215(bottom): © Comstock/Alamy RF; p. 216(middle): © Michael Matisse/Getty Images RF;

p. 224(RICE): © Rick Brandy/McGraw-Hill Education; p. 227: © CNRI/Science Source; p. 232: © Brand X Pictures/PunchStock RF.

CHAPTER 5

Page 245(top): © Photo and Dissection by Christine Eckel/ McGraw-Hill Education; p. 246(top): © Ned Frisk/Blend Images/Getty Images RF; p. 249: © Serge Krouglikoff/The Image Bank/Getty Images; p. 250(bottom): © Jupiter Images Corporation RF; p. 263: Photomondo/Digital Vision/Getty Images; p. 264(top): © Bob Coyle/McGraw-Hill Education; p. 264(bottom): © Living Art Enterprises/Photo Researchers/ Getty Images; p. 265(hematoma): © Medical Body Scans/ Photo Researchers/Getty Images; p. 267(top): © Fuse/Getty Images RF; p. 267(bottom): © Andrea Marini/Digital Vision/ Getty Images RF; p. 276(hydrocephaly): © Medical Body Scans/ Photo Researchers/Getty Images; p. 276(encephalopyosis): © McGraw-Hill Education; p. 276(hemorrhage): © McGraw-Hill Education; p. 287(top): © Image Source/Image Source/Getty Images RF; p. 287(bottom): © fstop123/E+/Getty Images RF; p. 288(top): © McGraw-Hill Education; p. 294: © Tetra Images/ Getty Images RF; p. 296: © Juanmonino/Vetta/Getty Images RF.

CHAPTER 6

Opener: © Fotosearch/Getty Images RF; p. 311(middle left): © Frank P. Wartenberg/Picture Press/Getty Images; p. 313(left top): © Ralph C. Eagle/MD/Science Source; p. 313(left bottom): © Science Photo Library RF/Getty Images RF; p. 314(otoscope): © Photodisc Collection/Getty Images RF; p. 314(woman): © Hill Street Studios/Photolibrary/Getty Images; p. 314(ear): © Joe DeGrandis/
McGraw-Hill Education; p. 314(microphone): © Stockbyte/ Punchstock RF; p. 316(upper right): © Digital Vision/SuperStock RF; p. 316(lower right): © Siede Preis/Getty Images RF; p. 324(middle): © Dr. P. Marazzi/Science Source; p. 325(scotoma): © Design Pics/Ben Welsh RF; p. 326(bottom): © Peter Dazeley/ Photographer's Choice/Getty Images; p. 330(top): © Fuse/ Getty Images RF; p. 330(bottom): © Jose Luis Pelaez Inc./ Blend Images/Getty Images RF; p. 331: © Keith Brofsky/ Getty Images RF; p. 332(top): © Sean Justice/Corbis RF; p. 333(papilledema): © Biophoto Associates/Science Source; p. 334(bottom): © Creatas/PunchStock RF; p. 343(bottom): Centers for Disease Control and Prevention; p.344(cataract): © Paul Whitten/Science Source; p. 344(corneal abrasion): © Dr. P. Marazzi/Science Source; p. 345: © Sue Ford/Science Source; p. 346(top): © BSIP/Science Source; p. 352(top): © Penny Tweedie/The Image Bank/Getty Images; p. 355: © Jupiter Images Corporation RF; p. 364: © Jupiter Images Corporation/Stockbyte/Getty Images RF; p. 367: © Jean-Luc Kokel/Science Source; p. 369: © JLP/Jose L. Pelaez/Corbis.

CHAPTER 7

Opener: © Steve Gschmeissner/Science Source; p. 385(top): © PhotoAlto sas/Alamy RF; p. 387(top): © I. Rozenbaum & F. Cirou/PhotoAlto RF; p. 390(bottom): © C.Sherburne/Photolink/Getty Images RF; p. 395(top): Dr. M. A. Ansary/Science Source; p. 397(bottom): © Dr. M. A. Ansary/Science Source; p. 402: © Purestock/SuperStock RF; p. 411(top): © ER Productions Ltd/Blend Images LLC RF; p. 411(bottom): © McGraw-Hill Education; p. 412(top): © SPL/Science Source; p. 412(bottom): © McGraw-Hill Education; p. 413(top): © McGraw-Hill Education; p. 419(top): © M. Constantini/PhotoAlto RF; p. 420(insulin infusion): © Realistic Reflections RF; p. 429: © Creatas/PunchStock RF; p. 432: © Image Source/Getty Images RF.

CHAPTER 8

Opener: © Eye of Science/Science Source; p. 442(top): © Ed Reschke; p. 443(top): © Science Photo Library RF/Getty Images RF; p. 443(bottom): © SCIEPRO/Getty Images; p. 444(top): © Purestock/Getty Images RF; p. 444(bottom): © Stockbyte/ PunchStock RF; p. 446(tonsils): © lynx/iconotec.com/Glow Images RF; p. 453: © Meckes/Ottawa/Science Source; p. 454(middle): Dr. P. Marazzi/Science Source; p. 454(bottom): © McGraw-Hill Education; p. 457(left): © ERproductions Ltd/Blend Images LLC RF; p. 457(right): © Ed Reschke; p. 458(bottom): © MedicalRF. com/Getty Images RF; p. 460(thrombosis): © Steve Gschmeissner/ Science Source; p. 460(hepatosplenomegaly): © Dr. M. A. Ansary/ Science Source; p. 461(top): © Bollershot Photo/Science Source; p. 463(top): © liquidlibrary/PictureQuest RF; p. 463(bottom): © Creatas/PunchStock RF; p. 470: © Pixtal/AGE Fotostock; p. 471(middle): © Science Source; p. 472(bottom): © Ed Reschke; p. 473(bottom): Centers for Disease Control and Prevention; p. 474: Centers for Disease Control and Prevention; p. 480(top): © Science Photo Library/Getty Images; p. 481(top): © Cristina Pedrazzini/ Science Source; p. 481(bottom): © PhotoLink/Getty Images; p. 485(top): Science Photo Library RF/Getty Images; p. 485(bottom): Ingram Publishing; p. 488: db2stock/Getty Images; p. 490: Rubberball/Nicole Hill/Getty Images; p. 492: PhotoAlto Agency RF Collection/Laurence Mouton/Getty Images.

CHAPTER 9

Page 505(top): © McGraw-Hill Education; p. 507: © Storman/Getty Images RF; p. 509(top): © Ed Reschke; p. 509(bottom): © liquid library/PictureQuest RF; p. 513: © Adam Gault/SPL/Science Photo Library/Getty Images RF; p. 518: © Custom Medical Stock Photo/Alamy RF; p. 519(top right): © Comstock Images/ PictureQuest; p. 525(echocardiogram): © Steve Allen/Brand X Pictures/Getty Images RF; p. 525(electrocardiogram): © Brand X Pictures/Getty Images RF; p. 525(stress electrocardiogram): © MBI/Alamy RF; p. 527: © Keith Brofsky/Getty Images RF; p. 535: © UygarGeographic/Vetta/Getty Images RF; p. 538(bottom): © Simon Fraser/RNC, Newcastle upon type/Science Source; p. 544: © aaM Photography, ltd./Vetta/Getty Images RF; p. 545(top): © Science Photo Library RF/Getty Images RF; p. 545(bottom): © Stockbyte Platinum/Alamy RF; p. 556: © Punchstock/ Image Source RF; p. 559: © Hillstreet Studios/Blend Images LLC RF; p. 562: © Jose Luis Pelaez Inc/Blend Images LLC RF.

CHAPTER 10:

Opener(right): © Photodisc/B2M Productions/Getty Images RF; Opener(left): © Dorling Kindersley/Dave King/Getty Images; p. 584: © istock/360/Alex Raths/Getty Images RF; p. 590(top): © Tetra Images/Alamy RF; p. 597(top): Centers for Disease Control and Prevention; p. 597(bottom): Centers for Disease Control and Prevention; p. 598(top): © Royalty-Free/Corbis RF; p. 598(middle): © McGraw-Hill Education; p. 599: © BSP/Science Source; p. 603: © MedicalRF.com/Getty Images RF; p. 604(middle): © ERproductions Ltd/Blend Images LLC RF; p. 604(middle): © Photo Disc/Medicine Today/Getty Images RF; p. 604(bottom): © Stockbyte/Punchstock RF; p. 609(bottom): © Getty Images/ Brand X RF; p. 612: © PhotoAlto Agency RF Collections/Frederic Cirou/Getty Images RF; p. 616: © Fuse/Getty Images RF.

CHAPTER 11:

Opener(left): © Stockbyte/Visage/Getty Images RF; p. 627(bottom left): © Omikron/Science Source; p. 627(bottom right): © Christopher Robbins/Stockbyte/Getty Images RF; p. 630(top):

© Blend Images/Jose Luis Pelaez Inc/Getty Images RF; p. 631(top): © Jose Luis Pelaez Inc/Men's Health/Blend Images RF; p. 640: © Stockbyte/Punchstock RF; p. 641(top): © Karin Dreyer/Dentist Appointment/Blend Images LLD RF; p. 643(top): Centers for Disease Control and Prevention; p. 648: © Ian Hooton/Science Photo Library/Getty Images RF; p. 649(top): CDC/Minnesota Department of Health R.N. Barr Library, Librarians Melissa Rethlefsen and Marie Jones; p. 652(top): © Royalty-Free/Corbis RF; p. 653(top): © Karin Dreyer/Dentist Appointment/Blend Images LLC RF; p. 653(middle): © Stockbyte/Getty Images RF; p. 653(bottom): © Keith Brofsky/Photodisc/Getty Images RF; p. 661: © David M. Martin, M.D./Science Source; p. 665(middle): © Photo Researchers/Biophoto Associates/Getty Images; p. 671(top): © 3D4Medical/Science Source; p. 671(middle): © Jill Braaten/McGraw-Hill Education; p. 671(bottom): © Pat Watson/ McGraw-Hill Education; p. 675(top): © Stockbyte/ PunchStock RF; p. 685: © Purestock/Getty Images RF; p. 688: © Design Pics/Kristy-Anne Glubish RF; p. 691: © PhotoAlto Agency RF Collections PhotoAlto/M. Constantini/Getty Images RF.

CHAPTER 12:

Opener: © Asia selects/Getty Images RF; p. 708(top): © Medical RF.com/Getty Images RF; p. 710(middle): © Steve Cole/Photodisc/ Getty Images RF; p. 710(bottom): © Biophoto Associates/ Science Source; p. 716(bottom left): © Enigma/Alamy RF; p. 720: © Dr. P. Marazzi/Science Source; p. 727(bottom): © Getty Images/ Brand X Pictures RF; p. 728: © Science Photo Library - Miriam Maslo RF; p. 731: © James Cavallini/Science Source; p. 732: © C. Sherburne/PhotoLInk/Getty Images RF; p. 733(top): © Rick Brady/McGraw-Hill Education; p. 743(top): © McGraw-Hill Education; p. 744(bottom): © McGraw-Hill Education; p. 745(bottom): © McGraw-Hill Education; p. 746(middle): © McGraw-Hill Education; p. 747: © McGraw-Hill Education; p. 748(bottom): © McGraw-Hill Education; p. 756: Medicimage/ Science Source; p. 758(dialysis): © Science Photo Library/Getty Images RF; p. 769(middle): © C. Sherburne/PhotoLInk/Getty Images RF; p. 772: © Digital Vision/Getty Images RF; p. 775: © Glow Images RF; p. 778: © Pixtal/AGE Fotostock RF.

CHAPTER 13:

Opener: © Larry Williams/Comet/Corbis; p. 800(right): © Bananastock/PictureQuest RF; p. 806(right): © Brand X Pictures/ PunchStock RF; p. 812: © PunchStock/BananaStock RF; p. 813(top): © Dr. P. Marazzi/Science Source; p. 819(top): © Adam Gault/SPL/Getty Images RF; p. 819(bottom): Rhoda Baer/ National Cancer Institute (NCI); p. 822(mammogram): Rhoda Baer/ National Cancer Institute (NCI); p. 822(sonohysterography): © BananaStock/PunchStock RF; p. 822(gynecologist): © Photodisc/ Getty Images RF; p. 823(top): © McGraw-Hill Education; p. 826: © Flying Colours Ltd/Digital Vision/Getty Images RF; p. 834: © UHB Trust/The Image Bank/Getty Images; p. 835(top): © UHB Trust/The Image Bank/Getty Images; p. 835(bottom): © McGraw-Hill Education; p. 846: © Biophoto Assoc./Science Source; p. 847(top): © Science Photo Library RF/Getty Images RF; p. 848(top): © Biophoto Associates/Science Source; p. 850(bottom): © Science Photo Library RF/Getty Images RF; p. 855(middle): © Antonia Reeve/Science Source; p. 855(bottom): © ERproductions Ltd/Getty Images RF; p. 858: © PunchStock/ Getty Images RF; p. 862: © Larry Williams/Comet/Corbis RF; p. 865: © Troy Aossey/The Image Bank/Getty Images.

index

A

B

C

D

E

F

G

H

I

J

K

L

M

N

O

P

Q

R

S

T

U

V

W

X

Y

Z